TO Dr Richard Longley —

I have enjoyed interacting with you
and our mutual patients,
and hope this book is of some
value in your practice.

Very best regards

Leslie J De Groot MD

THE
THYROID
AND ITS DISEASES

SIXTH EDITION

THE THYROID AND ITS DISEASES

SIXTH EDITION

Leslie J. De Groot, M.D.

Professor of Medicine
Thyroid Study Unit
Endocrine Section, Department of Medicine
The University of Chicago Pritzker School of Medicine
Chicago, Illinois

P. Reed Larsen, M.D., F.A.C.P.

Professor of Medicine
Harvard Medical School
Chief, Thyroid Division
Brigham and Women's Hospital
Boston, Massachusetts

Georg Hennemann, M.D., Dr., F.R.C.P, F.R.C.P. (Edin)

Professor of Medicine
Rotterdam Academic Hospital
Erasmus University
Rotterdam, The Netherlands

with a contribution by Edwin L. Kaplan, M.D., Professor of Surgery,
The University of Chicago Pritzker School of Medicine,
Chicago, Illinois

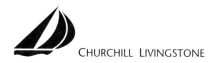

CHURCHILL LIVINGSTONE

New York, Edinburgh, London, Madrid, Melbourne, San Francisco, Tokyo

Library of Congress Cataloging-in-Publication Data

DeGroot, Leslie J.
        The thyroid and its diseases / Leslie J. DeGroot, P. Reed Larsen,
    Georg Hennemann ; with a contribution by Edwin L. Kaplan.—6th ed.
            p. cm.
    Rev. ed. of : The thyroid and its diseases / Leslie J. DeGroot . . .
    [et al.]. 5th ed. c1984
        Includes bibliographical references and index.
        ISBN 0–443–08895–0
        1. Thyroid gland—Diseases. 2. Goiter I. Larsen, P. Reed.
    II. Hennemann, Georg. III. Title.
        [DNLM: 1. Thyroid Diseases. 2. Thyroid Gland—physiology. WK
    200 D321t 1996]
    RC655. T4825 1996
    616.4′4—dc20
    DNLM/DLC
    for Library of Congress   95–36116
                                                          CIP

Sixth Edition© Churchill Livingstone Inc. 1996
Fifth Edition© Churchill Livingstone Inc. 1984

Distributed in the United Kingdom by Churchill Livingstone, Robert Stevenson House, 1–3 Baxter's Place, Leith Walk, Edinburgh EH1 3AF, and by associated companies, branches, and representatives throughout the world.

Accurate indications, adverse reactions, and dosage schedules for drugs are provided in this book, but it is possible that they may change. The reader is urged to review the package information data of the manufacturers of the medications mentioned.

The Publishers have made every effort to trace the copyright holders for borrowed material. If they have inadvertently overlooked any, they will be pleased to make the necessary arrangements at the first opportunity.

Assistant Editor: *Ann Ruzycka*
Production Editor: *Gerald Feldman*
Production Supervisor: *Laura Mosberg Cohen*
Cover Design: *Paul Moran*

Printed in the United States of America

Preface

The organization and practice of medical care are undergoing convulsive changes in the United States and throughout the world. More and more physicians practice in groups and often are now effectively employees of large organizations. Standards of care, protocols for diagnosis and treatment, and limitations on testing and consultations are much on the scene. The scope and importance of the primary care physician is growing, and specialized practice is under pressure.

But at the same time, while patients may be comfortable with a wide variety of care givers when well, they typically want the assistance of a physician highly versed in their illness when seriously ill. To compound the problem, the knowledge-base required for excellent medical practice expands almost explosively, and advances in medical science allow miraculous results from some new treatment almost daily.

Fortunately, however, dedicated and capable young people are still attracted to medicine. It is not yet possible for a computer to replace the human mind. How is the wealth of information needed by the general physician, internist, or specialist to be gained? How is the old material to be related to the just-reported new ideas? Can each family physician review the original data on a problem and independently evaluate the best course of action? Does the required information come from undergraduate course work, teaching during residency, handouts from a pharmaceutical-house detail man, the stacks of read (and unread) journals, or postgraduate refresher courses? Perhaps it will eventually come from the fluttering computer screen.

But as of 1995 and 1996, an effective and still important source of training is a medical text. This text is the sixth revision of a book dedicated to helping physicians provide excellent care and to understanding the pathophysiology and pathomolecular biology that they encounter. The authors now bring with this a tradition extending back over 60 years of presenting all of clinical thyroidology in a readable and cohesive manner. In part this is because of an average of 35 years in the practice of thyroidology among the authors.

More than a decade has passed since the last edition, and there clearly have been substantial advances in the field of clinical thyroidology as well as a logarithmic increase in our knowledge regarding the molecular biology of thyroid hormone action. To substantiate progress in this field, we need only mention the introduction of fine-needle aspiration of thyroid nodules, the use of immunometric TSH assays, the cloning of thyroid hormone receptors, the molecular explanation of thyroid hormone resistance, and the cloning of the activating and inactivating thyroid hormone deiodinases. Since the authors of this textbook are intricately involved in many of these advances, in addition to being thyroid practitioners, we are much aware of the changes that have occurred in our field. One of the reasons for the long delay between editions is that the field of thyroidology has been moving at such a break-neck pace that it is difficult to budget the time to totally rewrite five or six individual chapters on different aspects of thyroid disease, and total rewriting has been the order of the day. It is in fact a labor of love, since the goal of this text is to provide a readable, uniform, and practical guide to the thyroid clinician.

We also have done our best to digest the mountain of clinical and basic research available and present a complete background on the development of the thyroid gland, how the thyroid "system" is regulated, the molecular biology of hormone formation and action, the basic causes of disease, and the process of testing used to sort out the clinical problems.

For this edition we are pleased to welcome our new collaborator, Professor Georg Hennemann, of Rotterdam, a long-time leader in thyroidology in Europe, who brings new perspectives and fresh approaches, and somewhat different experience to this effort, which had previously emanated only from the United States. However, the world of thyroidology is now one, and Professor Hennemann's insights, especially on iodine deficiency and multinodular goiter, conditions more common in Europe, are welcome additions.

Our book is meant to be readable, integrated, and complete in both clinical medicine and basic science. We believe it will be useful reading for students, house staff, fellows, practitioners, and specialists.

A special problem exists with references. Should we throw out the old—but original—observations when information is reformulated 20 years later? In peril of seeming dated, we have kept many of the original citations. We have added, of course, every new concept that we know of, and have tried to add citations of important new studies as they appeared, up to almost the last days before publication.

The authors wish to express their gratitude to the many colleagues who have continued our education during the past decade, the fellows who have carried out the hard work in our laboratories, and to our secretaries.

We especially acknowledge the patience and forbearance (most of the time) of our wives, Helen, Jane, and Atie, to whom we dedicate this book.

Leslie J. De Groot, M.D.
P. Reed Larsen, M.D.
Georg Hennemann, M.D.

Contents

Abbreviations

ADCC	Antibody-dependent cell mediated cytotoxicity	MCHA	Microsomal antibody hemagglutination assay
ADP	Adenosine diphosphate	MHC	Major histocompatibility complex
AMLR	Autologous-mixed lymphocyte reaction	MIF	Migration inhibitory factor
APC	Antigen-presenting cell	MIT	Monoiodotyronsine
ATP	Adenosine triphosphate	MLR	Mixed lymphocyte reaction
ATPase	Adenosine triphosphatase	NAD^+	Nicotine adenine dinucleotide (oxidized)
BEI	Butanol-extractable iodine		
BMR	Basal metabolic rate	NADH	Nicotine adenine dinucleotide (reduced)
cAMP	Cyclic adenosine monophosphate		
CPBA	Competitive protein-binding assay	$NADP^+$	Nicotine adenine dinucleotide phosphate (oxidized)
DF	Dialyzable fraction		
$D-T_3$	D-Triiodothyronine	NADPH	Nicotine adenine dinucleotide phosphate (reduced)
$D-T_4$	D-Thyroxine		
DIT	Diiodotyrosine	PBI	Protein-bound iodine
FSH	Follicle-stimulating hormone	PBMC	Peripheral blood mononuclear cells
FT_3	Free triiodothyronine	PRL	Prolactin
FT_4	Free thyroxine	RA	Retinoic acid
$\%FT_4$	Percent free thyroxine	RAI	Radioactive iodine
FT_3I	Free triiodothyronine index	RAIU	Radioactive iodide uptake
FT_4I	Free thyroxine index	RAR	Retinoic acid receptor
GH	Growth hormone	RFLP	Restriction fragment length poly-morphism
GnRH	Gonadotropin releasing hormone		
hCG	Human chorionic gonadotropin	RIA	Radioimmunoassay
hGH	Human growth hormone	RT_3U	Resin T_3 uptake
HSPs	Heat shock proteins	RT_3	Reverse triiodothyronine
I^-	Iodide	RXR	Retinoid-x-receptor
I_2	Iodine	T_3	Triiodothyronine
IFN-α	Interferon-alpha	T_4	Thyroxine
IL	Interleukin	TBG	Thyroxine-binding globulin
LATS	Long-acting thyroid stimulator	TBIAb	Thyrotropin-binding inhibiting antibody
LATS-P	Long-acting thyroid stimulator protector	TBII	Thyroid-binding inhibitory immunoglobulin
LH	Luteinizing hormone		
LMI	Leukocyte migration inhibition	TBP	Thyroxine-binding protein

TBPA	Thyroxine-binding prealbumin	TPO	Thyroid peroxidase
TCR	T cell antigen receptor	TR-α	Thyroid hormone receptor-alpha
TCR-α	T cell antigen receptor-alpha	TR-β	Thyroid hormone receptor-beta
TDI	Thyrotropin-displacing immuno-globulins	TRE	Thyroid hormone response element
		TRH	Thyrotropin-releasing hormone
Tetrac	Tetraiodothyroacetic acid	Triac	Triiodothyroacetic acid
TG	Thyroglobulin	TSAb	Thyroid-stimulating- antibodies
TGA	Thyroglobulin antibody hemagglu-tination assay	TSBAb	Thyrotropin stimulation blocking antibody
TGI	Thyroid growth-stimulating immunoglobulin	TSH	Thyroid-stimulating hormone
		TSI	Thyroid-stimulating immunoglobulin
THBR	Thyroid hormone binding ratio	TT_3	Total T_3
TNF	Tumor necrosis factor	TT_4	Total T_4
TNF-α	Tumor necrosis factor-alpha	TTR	Transthyretin (formerly termed TBPA)

The Phylogeny, Ontogeny, Anatomy, and Metabolic Regulation of the Thyroid

1

PHYLOGENY

The primary event in the phylogeny of the thyroid was the development of the ability to collect iodide ions and to bind them to protein. These activities have been observed widely among plants and invertebrates. Drechsel[1] recognized in 1896 that sponges and corals contain large quantities of iodine as iodotyrosines, and iodohistidine and bromotyrosine have also been detected. Monoiodotyrosine (MIT) and diiodotyrosine (DIT) have been found in starfish, mollusks, annelids, crustaceans, and insects.[2–4] Thyroxine (T_4) and triiodothyronine (T_3) have also been reported occasionally in these animals, but whether iodothyronines exist in phyla below the chordates is uncertain.[5]

Tong and Chaikoff[6] found a marine alga that concentrates iodide and binds it to tyrosine, forming MIT and DIT. Inhibition of this reaction by catalase indicated that a peroxidase is involved in the oxidation of the trapped iodide, as in the human thyroid. LeLoup[7] has found that a similar oxidative process is involved in active transport of iodide into the gills of the eel. The oxidized iodine is subsequently reduced to iodide and then passively diffused to blood.

Iodinated compounds in the lower forms are usually associated with a horny exoskeleton. It has been suggested that these iodinated substances may be byproducts of the process of "quinone tanning." The formation of benzoquinone cross-linkages in the molecular structure of scleroproteins is probably responsible for hardening of the cuticle, and in the presence of inorganic iodide, benzoquinones can bring about the iodination of proteins in vitro.[8]

1

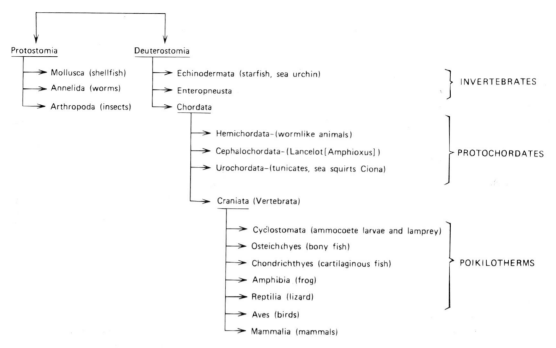

Fig. 1-1. Phylogeny of the development of the thyroid gland.

Thus, the iodination of tyrosine may be mediated quite accidentally by quinones involved in the general tanning reaction of the exoskeleton. After observing the urochordate *Ciona,* however, Roche and co-workers[9] reached an opposite conclusion: they found that the T_4 and $3,5,3'$-T_3 are present in free form, not as part of the polysaccharide exoskeleton. Their results indicated that the thyroid hormone precursors are formed by mechanisms similar to those operating in the vertebrate thyroid. The scleroprotein exoskeleton of the urochordate adult is rich in iodide and contains DIT as well as T_4.[10,11] The cuticular iodoproteins are possibly ingested by the organisms and carried into the gastrointestinal tract, where they may be digested, and the iodoamino acids may be liberated. Gorbman[12] has hypothesized that the protochordates became accustomed to a supply of iodotyrosines and iodothyronines derived from ingesting particles broken off from their scleroprotein covering, and eventually developed a requirement for the iodinated amino acids.

The first evidence of an organ related to the vertebrate thyroid is found in the protochordates, forms intermediate between vertebrates and invertebrates (Fig. 1-1). Three subphyla, the Hemichordata, Urochordata, and Cephalochordata, constitute this group. In the Urochordata and Cephalochordata, an organ known as the *endostyle* lies on the floor of the pharynx and connects with it by a duct. Currently, the significant evolutionary event is believed to have been the development of iodination centers. In the urochordate *Ciona* these centers are at the tip of the endostyle.[13] *Amphioxus,* a member of the Cephalochordata, also has an endostyle, and Barrington[11] has shown that an iodinated glycoprotein is formed in the iodination centers near the tip of the endostyle, probably on the surface of the cell. The endostyle secretes a mucus that passes down the duct into the pharynx and is moved from there into the alimentary canal, presumably carrying iodinated protein along with it. T_4 and T_3 have been reported in this species by Covelli et al.[14] and Tong et al.[15] Dunn, however, found no [125]I T_4 or T_3 in *Ciona* but did provide evidence of T_4 by radioimmunoassay (RIA).[16] Fujita and Sawano[17] found peroxidase activity in the endostyle of *Ciona* using cytochemistry at the electron microscopic level.

It has usually been surmised that these iodoamino acids are produced in the endostyle, but this conclusion is contested by Salvatore.[5] He notes that only a minuscule amount of the total iodine of the animal is present in the endostyle. Further study is needed

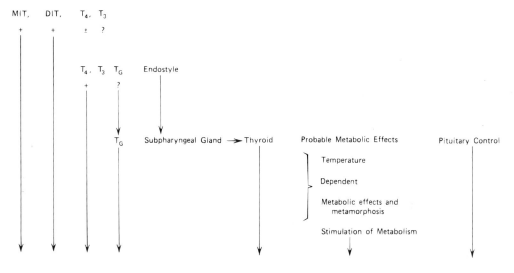

Fig. 1-1. (Continued).

to define the exact relation of this organ to the chordate thyroid. Another organ, the branchial sac (pharynx) of the tunicates, is an alternative candidate for the thyroidal ancestral tree. This organ iodinates proteins of large size (10 and 16 S), forming MIT, DIT, and possibly T_4. The protein has a subunit structure resembling that of thyroglobulin (TG).[18]

Two important conclusions can be drawn from studies on the protochordates. First, in these animals a possible thyroid anlage is present, but it has not yet developed as a discrete unit separate from the pharynx. Second, while no clear role for thyroid hormones has been established, such a role may exist since T_4 has been shown to accelerate metamorphic events in the jellyfish.[19]

The most primitive vertebrate in which a thyroid anlage can be identified with certainty is the ammocoete, the larva of the lamprey, a cyclostome. An open tubular structure in the hypopharynx collects iodide and binds it to a protein, apparently related to TG, forming T_4 and T_3.[20,21] Although this is often referred to as an endostyle, it is not certain that it is homologous to the endostyle of more primitive forms. The term *subpharyngeal gland* has been suggested for this structure.[5] A protease appears in the gland before the ammocoete begins metamorphosis. This protease (presumably) can break down the iodinated protein in the secretion and release of the thyroid hormones. Thus, the evolutionary development of a protease may have allowed the thyroid anlage to become separate from the pharynx, since it could

then release T_4 from its iodoprotein independently of the enzymes of the lower gastrointestinal tract.[22] Thyroid hormone has been found in these larvae, and a T_4-binding protein has been demonstrated as well.[23]

During metamorphosis of the ammocoete into the adult lamprey, the endostyle loses its connection with the pharynx and becomes a thyroid composed of scattered follicles. Plasma concentrations of thyroid hormones are highest in the larvae, prior to formation of a true thyroid, and decrease after metamorphosis.[24] These follicles are not encapsulated, but they have the typical biosynthetic functions associated with hormone formation in adult vertebrates. In the lamprey, the biosynthesis of Tg in larval forms has the same characteristics as that formed in thyroid follicles of the adult form. 3–8 S fractions and a 12 S monomer are suggested to be the precursors of the 18–19 S protein. Total 1 percent in Tg is very low (0.002 percent) and about 5 percent is present in the form of T_3 and T_4.[25] Curiously, the thyroid appears to play no role in the metamorphosis of the ammocoete, although the gland itself undergoes a remarkable change.

The striking relationship of the thyroid to the gastrointestinal tract is apparent in all phylogenetic studies. Dunn[26] has actually found ciliated thyroid cells in the mouse and shark, a reminder of the gland's origin from endoderm. In mammals the gastric mucosa and the salivary glands retain a functional relationship with the thyroid in that they too can concentrate iodide,[27] and the salivary gland contains a peroxidase.

Thus, a thyroid capable of forming iodotyrosines and iodothyronines is present in all extant vertebrates. Its level of function varies widely from species to species and season to season. With the exceptions noted below, thyroid activity in the poikilotherms is very low. Seasonal changes in thyroid activity have been found in both warm- and cold-blooded animals.

Certain morphologic changes occur after the biochemical evolution of the thyroid has ceased. In the adult lamprey and in bony fish, the gland is not encapsulated. The follicles may be widely scattered, either singly or in small clusters, especially along the course of the ventral aorta and in the kidneys.[28] In cartilaginous fish, the thyroid is encapsulated. In the higher vertebrate forms, the thyroid is a one- or two-lobed encapsulated structure.

Function of the Thyroid in Lower Forms

A functioning thyroid is evident in forms as primitive as the lamprey, and thyroid hormone affects protein and lipid metabolism in these forms as in higher vertebrates.[29] Rapid developmental changes analogous to amphibian metamorphosis occur in all vertebrate classes, and thyroid hormones appear to be involved in these events.[30] Radioactive iodine (RAI) ablation of the thyroid in immature trout produces reduced growth, increased pigmentation, a smaller head, poor sex organ development, anemia, and impaired coordination. The condition has been compared to cretinism.[31] In the salmon, the changes that occur before migration from fresh water to salt water (smoltification) coincide with an increased concentration of serum T_4.[32-34] After smoltification, the serum T_4 concentrations fall. Many of the changes occurring during smoltification are analogous to metamorphosis in amphibia. Evidence has also been obtained that the T_4 surge in the salmon is linked to the lunar cycle, although how such a stimulus is internalized is unknown.[35] Thyroid ^{131}I uptake and serum T_4 was measured in *Ambystoma gracile* before, during, and after metamorphosis. Thyroid activity preceded metamorphosis, was highest during metamorphosis, and declined thereafter.[36]

A notable effect of thyroid hormone is the induction of metamorphosis in certain amphibia, first reported by Gundernatsch in 1912.[37] Metamorphosis occurs only when the organism has reached a certain predetermined state of development.[38] T_4 is apparently involved in the metamorphosis of most amphibians. No comparable physiologic event occurs in reptiles, birds, or mammals.

Problems have arisen in relating the phenomenon of metamorphosis to thyroid hormones. In its natural state, the axolotl does not undergo metamorphosis, but large amounts of T_4 can induce it to do so. During laboratory induced (21°C, constant light) metamorphosis, thyroid activation induced by pituitary thyroid-stimulating hormone (TSH) occurs rapidly and is greatest at the onset of metamorphic climax.[39] Certain neoteinic animals, such as *Necturus*, do not undergo limited metamorphosis. Although these animals have a thyroid, it makes little T_4.[12] The limited developmental change they undergo may nevertheless be related to thyroid hormone.

Initially, it was believed that thyroid hormone had little or no stimulatory effect on the oxidative metabolism of cold-blooded species. Now it is known that the effect of the thyroid on metabolic activity in cold-blooded species is strongly dependent on environmental temperature. For example, T_4 causes stimulation of metabolism in lizards at 32°C, but not at low temperatures.[40] The thyroid gland is also more active at higher temperatures (23° to 32°C) than at lower temperatures (10° to 15°C) in snakes, fish, amphibians, turtles, and lizards.[41]

The thyroid physiology of metamorphosis in the bullfrog, *Rana catesbeiana*, has been studied in some detail. Regard et al.[42] found a gradual rise in plasma T_3 and T_4 levels during prometamorphosis in the tadpole that peaked at metamorphic climax (stage XXIII). A 15-fold increase in T_3 and a 10-fold increase in T_4 over basal levels were observed. Two days after metamorphic climax, the levels had fallen to about 20 percent of the peak values, and serum T_4 and T_3 concentrations in the adult bullfrog were low. Thyrotropin-releasing hormone (TRH) is probably not involved in this increase in T_4 and T_3 levels since it fails to stimulate TSH release in tadpoles, lungfish, or axolotl.[43] Thyroid hormone is required for maturation of the median eminence. Thus, Etkin[44] suggests that a "spiraling" feedback mechanism may occur in amphibians. Some hypothalamic-pituitary stimulation leads to increased thyroid hormone synthesis, which further matures the median eminence of the hypothalamus, leading to more TSH secretion, more thyroid hormone, and so on.

Another pituitary hormone, prolactin, may play a role in amphibian metamorphosis, as it has been shown to inhibit T_4-induced axolotl tail fin resorption.[45] Furthermore, organ culture of the *Xenopus* tadpole showed that T_3-induced budding of the hindlimb was inhibited by prolactin.[46] Prolactin inhibits activation of several hydrolytic enzymes seen during metamorphosis in regressing tissue. The prolactin effect can be antagonized by oxytocin. T_4 injected into the hypothalamus of neotenic *Ambystoma tigrinum* induces metamorphosis, possibly by overcoming a prolactin-induced block in the hypothalamus.[47]

Other changes related to thyroid function also occur in the tadpole. Galton[48] recently found that in the tadpole *R. catesbeiana*, peripheral conversion of T_4 and T_3 can take place in the premetamorphic stage. In tadpoles exposed to concentrations of T_4 and T_3 yielding normal plasma hormone values, iopanoic acid, an inhibitor of the deiodinases catalyzing T_4 to T_3 conversion (5'D) and that deiodinating T_3 to 3,3′diiodothyronine (5D) (see Ch. 3), inhibited the physiologic effectiveness of T_4 and enhanced that of T_3. These findings strongly support the hypothesis that this conversion process, leading to production and maintenance of an increased T_3 level, plays an important role in the physiologic action of T_4 in this species. Both deiodinases are present in skin at all stages of development and in the gut and tail during metamorphic climax. In all these tissues enzyme activity increases substantially in thyroid hormone induced climax or during spontaneous metamorphosis. The outer ring (5′) deiodinase has the characteristics of a type II deiodinase (see Ch. 3). Type III (5) deiodinase is highest during premetamorphosis and declines to undetectable concentrations during spontaneous or thyroid hormone induced metamorphic climax.[49] Several groups of investigators have indentified limited capacity, high affinity thyroid hormone receptors in nuclei of *R. catesbeiana* tail fins and livers.[50–54] The sites in tail fin nuclei increase in number as metamorphosis progresses.[50] The results of studies during metamorphic climax suggest that the increases in endogenous T_3 and T_4 occurring at that time saturate a significant fraction of these receptors.[55] Occupancy of the receptors is likely to be critical in inducing metamorphosis in this species.

Receptors for T_3, similar to those found in amphibians, have been demonstrated in hepatic nuclei of lamprey and salmon,[30] and the receptors are similar to those described in mammals (see Ch. 2). The first evidence for c-erbA gene products to be involved in thyroid hormone action in amphibians was provided by Baker and Tata.[56] An α and two β types of thyroid hormone receptors have been detected in *Xenopus laevis*. In contrast to the mammalian genome, there is evidence that there are two α and two β thyroid hormone receptor genes in this species.[57] The DNA and thyroid hormone-binding regions of these receptors are highly conserved with respect to the mammalian and avian counterparts. The α forms predominate at all stages of development while the β forms are clearly detectable only during climax.[56,57] In *R. catesbeiana* a full-length c-erbA cDNA has been cloned.[58] This report shows that tadpole red blood cells express an α but not a β, c-erbA gene. During spontaneous or T_3-induced metamorphosis a 4 to 5-fold increase in red blood cell thyroid hormone receptor α density occurs. This increase could be specifically inhibited by glucocorticoids. Since more *Rana catesbeiana* red blood cells contain glucocosteroid receptors, this suggests a modulating function of glucocosteroids on thyroid hormone receptor expression in these cells during metamorphosis.[58a] In the *Xenopus*, thyroid hormone receptor α mRNA increases during premetamorphosis, reaches a maximum during prometamorphosis, and then falls through climax to the low level seen in the adult. In contrast thyroid hormone receptor β mRNA is barely detectable during premetamorphosis, but the level rises and falls in parallel with the plasma thyroid hormone concentration, peaking at climax. The amount of thyroid hormone receptor α and β mRNAs can be increased rapidly, 3 to 5-and 20 to 50-fold respectively, within 24 hours after exposing young tadpoles to exogenous T_3.[59] This upregulation of the mRNA level is under transcriptional control and inhibited by protein synthesis inhibitors.[59–61] Further studies to explore the autoinduction of the β gene showed that T_3-activated thyroid hormone receptor α and β can regulate its expression.[61a] (For a detailed review of molecular biology in amphibian metamorphosis, see ref. 62.) The homolog of the mamalian cytosolic thyroid hormone binding protein has recently been cloned in the *Xenopus*. The expression of this protein was inversely correlated with tissue-specific transformation during metamorphosis. Thus, a high level of its mRNA was present in the tail during prematamorphosis but was dramatically repressed with the onset of metamorphosis. These and other findings suggest that the cytosolic thyroid hormone binding protein could function to modulate the metamorphic process by regulating the level of intracellular thyroid hormones.[62a]

Hypothalamic and Pituitary Control

There is little evidence for hypothalamic-pituitary control of thyroid function in the cyclostomes or chondrichthyes, but it is present in teleost fish, amphibians, and higher forms. The hypophysis alone can apparently sustain some thyroid function, but hypothalamic control is required for amphibian larvae to pass through a metamorphic climax.[63–65] Although TRH is widely distributed among the vertebrates and protochordates, it seems to control TSH secretion only in mammals and birds.[66] This finding has led to the speculation that TRH is an ancient molecule that has only recently been coopted in association with the development of endothermy.[67]

T_4 directly inhibits pituitary TSH release in goldfish, just as it does in mammals. In addition, thyroid activity is suppressed by a hypothalamic inhibiting factor which prevents pituitary TSH release. Autotransplantation of the pituitary, by removing it from hypothalamic inhibition, is followed by augmented thyroid activity. Production of this factor is increased by T_4 feedback.[68]

A glycoprotein in the mammalian pituitary that is separate from TSH strongly stimulates fish thyroid activity. This was called *heterothyrotropic factor (HTF)* by Fontaine, who first detected it.[69] This factor is now known to be follicle-stimulating hormone (FSH) and luteinizing hormone (LH), the mammalian gonadotropins. The structure of the α subunit of these hormones is identical to the α subunit of TSH, indicating a phylogenetic relationship.

ONTOGENY

The main anlage of the thyroid gland develops as a median endodermal downgrowth from the tongue. It can be seen in the human embryo before the end of the third week. It is located near the primordium of the heart, and as the heart is pulled caudad, the thyroid anlage follows. At about 30 days it has developed into a hollow bilobed structure, and by 40 days the original hollow stalk connecting it to the pharyn-geal floor atrophies and then breaks. Shortly thereafter the lateral extensions of the median anlage make contact with the ultimobranchial bodies developing from the fourth pharyngeal pouches, the so-called lateral anlage of the thyroid. The ultimo-branchial cells are the origin of calcitonin secreting C cells in the thyroid gland and probably contribute to the formation of follicular cells as well.[70] By the eighth week the cells have a tubular arrangement, and cell clusters are apparent. Two weeks later, when the embryo is approximately 80 mm long, follicles are present. Shortly after this time the follicles contain colloid, and the thyroid accumulates and binds iodide by the eleventh or twelfth week (Fig. 1-2). Secondary follicles arise by budding from the primary follicles; they increase in number until the embryo reaches a length of about 160 mm. After this time the follicles increase in size, but the number remains the same. Under intense stimulation, the adult thyroid can form new follicles.

Fujita and Machino[71] have studied the origins of the follicular lumen in the chick embryo. They found that colloid droplets, 1 to 5 μm in diameter and enclosed by a limiting membrane, first appear within the cytoplasm of parenchymal cells. As the droplets enlarge, they approach the cell membrane and come in contact with the droplets of an adjoining cell. The limiting cell membrane disappears, and the droplets fuse. By an extension of this process to cells close to the original droplet, an acinar structure containing colloid and enclosed by a ring of parenchymal cells is formed.

GROSS ANATOMY

Physical Appearance and Anatomic Location

The Germans call the thyroid the "shield gland" (*Schilddrüse*), and the English name, derived from the Greek, means the same thing. Such a term, however, gives an erroneous impression of its shape: the gland as seen from the front is more nearly the shape of a butterfly. (It is interesting to note, however, that the Minoans used a shield which had a shape similar to that of the mammalian thyroid gland.)

The thyroid wraps itself about and becomes firmly fixed by fibrous tissue to the anterior and lateral

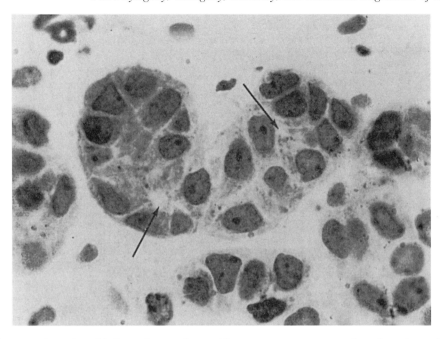

Fig. 1-2. Photograph of thyroid tissue from a fetus with a 50 mm crown-rump length, estimated gestational age 64 days. The arrows indicate two intracellular canaliculi. During incubation of the tissue in organ culture in vitro, there was no uptake or fixation of iodide. The figure shows the earliest stage of formation of colloid spaces. The tissue was fixed in ozmium, embedded in Epon epoxy resin, and sectioned at 1μm thickness ($\times 2,400$). (From Shephard,[213] with permission.)

parts of the larynx and trachea. Anteriorly, its surface is convex; posteriorly, it is concave. The isthmus lies across the trachea anteriorly just below the level of the cricoid cartilage. The lateral lobes extend along either side of the larynx as roughly conical projections reaching the level of the middle of the thyroid cartilage. Their upper extremities are known as the *upper poles* of the gland. Similarly, the lower extremities of the lateral lobes are spoken of as the *lower poles*, although they make no such prominent projections as do the upper (Fig. 1-3).

The weight of the thyroid of the normal nongoitrous adult is 15 to 20 g. The width and length of the isthmus average 20 mm, and its thickness is 2 to 6 mm. The lateral lobes from superior to inferior poles usually measure 4 cm. Their breadth is 15 to 20 mm, and their thickness is 20 to 39 mm.

The thyroid is enveloped by a thin, fibrous, non-stripping capsule that sends septa into the gland substance to produce an irregular, incomplete lobulation. No true lobulation or lobation exists. In fact, the gland is a uniform agglomeration of follicles throughout, packed like berries into a bag; it has no true subdivisions. The lateral lobes lie in a bed between the trachea and the larynx medially and between the carotid sheath and the sternomastoid muscles laterally. The deep cervical fascia, dividing into an anterior and a posterior plane, lines this bed and makes a loosely applied false or surgical capsule for the lateral portions of the gland. In front are the thin, ribbon-like infrahyoid muscles. The thyroid is molded to fit the space available between the neighboring structures perfectly, and is superficially placed. It can usually be outlined by careful palpation in normal humans, unless the neck is thick and short or the sternomastoid muscles are heavily developed.

The shape and attachments of the organ are important in examination and diagnosis. The relation of the thyroid gland to the parathyroids (usually situated on the posterior surface of the gland's lateral lobes within the surgical capsule) and to the recurrent laryngeal nerves, which run in the cleft between the trachea and esophagus just medial to the lateral lobes, are most important to the surgeon. The relationship to the trachea is important from the standpoint of pressure symptoms.

The pyramidal lobe is a narrow projection of thy-

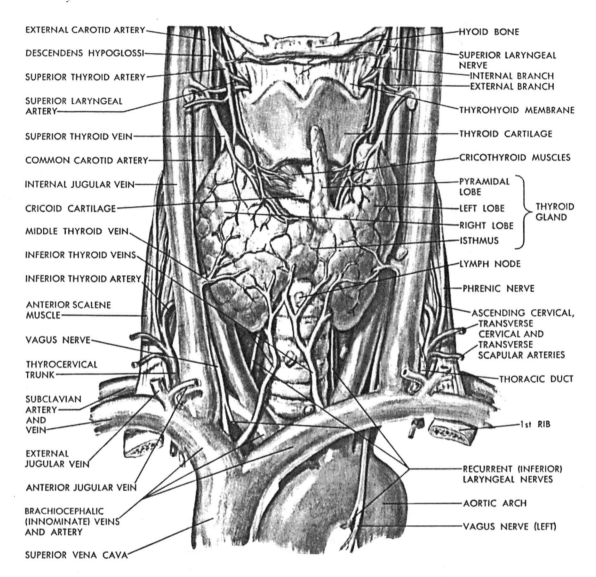

Fig. 1-3. Gross anatomy of the thyroid and its surroundings. (From Netter,[214] with permission.)

roid tissue extending upward from the isthmus and lying on the surface of the thyroid cartilage, to the right or left of the prominence of that structure. It is a vestige of the embryonic thyroglossal tract. The pyramidal lobe is important in its relation to developmental anomalies and also in its propensity to undergo hypertrophy when the rest of the thyroid has been removed. Any pathologic process that is diffuse, for example, Graves' disease or Hashimoto's thyroiditis, may involve the pyramidal lobe. It is therefore an item of some importance diagnostically and in thyroid surgery. Pyramidal lobes are found in about 80 percent of patients.

Blood Supply

The thyroid gland has an abundant blood supply. It has been estimated that the normal flow rate is about 5 ml/g of thyroid tissue each minute. The blood volume of normal humans is about 5 L. This mass moves through the lungs about once a minute, through the kidneys once in 5 minutes, and through the thyroid approximately once an hour. In disease the flow through the gland may be increased up to 100-fold.

This abundant blood supply is provided from the four major thyroid arteries. The superior pair arise from the external carotid and descend several centimeters through the neck to reach the upper poles of the thyroid, where they break into a number of branches and enter the gland. The inferior pair spring from the thyrocervical trunk of the subclavian arteries and enter the lower poles from behind. Frequently, a fifth artery, the thyreoidea ima, from the arch of the aorta, enters the thyroid in the midline. There are free anastomoses among all of these vessels. In addition, a large number of smaller arteriolar vessels derived from collaterals of the esophagus and larynx supply the posterior aspect of the thyroid. The branching of the large arteries takes place on the surface of the gland, where they form a network. Only after much branching are small arteries sent deep into the gland. These penetrating vessels arborize among the follicles, finally sending a follicular artery to each follicle. This, in turn, breaks up into the rich capillary network surrounding the follicle.

The veins emerge from the interior of the gland and form a plexus of vessels under the capsule. These drain into the internal jugular, the brachiocephalic, and occasionally the anterior jugular veins.

Lymphatics

A rich plexus of lymph vessels is in close proximity to the individual follicles, but appears to have no role in thyroid function. The major normal, if not only, secretory pathway is through the venous drainage of the thyroid rather than through the lymphatics. The anatomy of the thyroid lymphatics is considered in Chapter 21.

Innervation

The gland receives fibers from both sympathetic and parasympathetic divisions of the autonomic nervous system. The sympathetic fibers are derived from the cervical ganglia and enter the gland along the blood vessels. The parasympathetic fibers are derived from the vagus and reach the gland by branches of the laryngeal nerves. Both myelinated and nonmyelinated fibers are found in the thyroid, and occasionally in the ganglion cells as well. The nerve supply does not appear to be simply a secretory system. The major neurogenic modifications of thyroid physiology involve blood flow and are reviewed in Chapter 4.

The Follicle: The Secretory Unit

The adult thyroid is composed of follicles, or acini. These have lost all luminal connection with other parts of the body and may be considered, from both the structural and functional points of view, as the primary, or secretory, units of the organ. The cells of the follicles are the makers of hormone; the lumina are the storage depots. In the normal adult gland, the follicles are roughly spherical and vary considerably in size, with an average diameter of 300

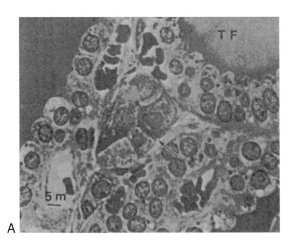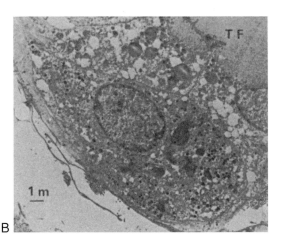

Fig. 1-4. **(A)** Light microscopy of a parafollicular cluster *(arrow)* in relationship to thyroid follicle (TF) (×900). **(B)** Parafollicular cell in characteristic position between follicular cells and follicular basement membrane, not abutting on colloid (TF) (×4,200). Tissue was obtained from normal thyroid tissue of a 26-year-old woman with a solitary thyroid adenomatous nodule. Specimens were fixed in glutaraldehyde and embedded in Araldite-502. (From Teitelbaum et al,[215] with permission.)

μm. The walls consist of a continuous epithelium one cell deep, forming the parenchyma of the thyroid. The epithelium of the normal gland is usually described as cuboidal, the cell height being approximately 15 μm. In the resting gland the cells may become flatter. Under TSH stimulation such as that which occurs with iodide deficiency, the height increases, and the term *columnar* is applied. The height of the epithelium is inversely proportional to the diameter of the lumen of the follicle.

In addition to the acinar cells, there are individual cells or small groups of cells that do not extend to the follicular lumen and which may appear as clusters between follicles (Fig. 1-4). These *light cells*, or C cells, are a distinct category probably derived from the neural crest by the ultimobranchial body, as shown by studies of quail chicks by Le Douarin and Le Lifèvre.[72] The C cells secrete calcitonin (or thyrocalcitonin) in response to an increase in serum calcium.[73] This hormone is important in the regulation of bone resorption and to a lesser extent influences the concentration of serum calcium. Calcitonin acts primarily by suppressing resorption of calcium from bone through an adenylate cyclase-cyclic adenosine monophosphate (cAMP) system. C cells also contain somatostatin, calcitonin gene-related peptide, gastrin-releasing peptide, katacalcin, and helodermin that have either stimulatory or inhibitory activity on thyroid hormone secretion (see the section "Other Regulatory Factors"). The C cells are also the origin of the "medullary" thyroid cancers described in Chapter 18.

Within the follicle and filling its lumen is the homogeneous colloid. This is a mixture of proteins, principally thyroglobulin, but there are other lightweight iodoproteins and albumin as well.

THE FINE STRUCTURE OF THE THYROID CELLS

In the light microscope, the acinar surface of thyroid parenchymal cells appears to be smooth, but the electron microscope shows it to be covered with tiny villi and some pseudopods. The base of the cell abuts a capillary and is separated from it by a two-layer basement membrane visible under the electron microscope. In the usual hematoxylin and eosin stain, the cell cytoplasm is neutrophilic, and colloid droplets may be present. The nucleus is at the base of the cell.

The colloid is variable in tinctorial response but tends to be strongly eosinophilic in resting follicles and pale-staining or even slightly basophilic when the gland is stimulated. In hyperactive follicles the margin of the colloid is scalloped by *resorption vacuoles.* These vacuoles may represent some local variation in the composition of colloid attributable to the hyperactive acinar cells.

The villi are extensions of cytoplasm serving to increase cell secretory surface. Pseudopods extend out into the colloid and surround and ingest it by pinocytosis. Over the course of several hours, the ingested droplets move toward the base of the cell.[74] These droplets of resorbed colloid are then prepared for secretion as hormone by the gland.

The resolving power of the electron microscope has been turned upon the thyroid acinar cell by several investigators, among them Wissig,[75] Dempsey and Peterson,[76] Ekholm and Sjöstrand,[77,78] and Herman.[79] Wissig's and Ekholm's findings are presented here in detail and are typical of the cytologic picture of most species. The entire follicular cell is covered by an uninterrupted plasma membrane (Figs. 1-5 and 1-6). The apical surface of the cell is dome-shaped and is provided with numerous microvilli that are approximately 0.35 μm tall and 0.07 μm broad. This membrane is composed of two dark layers separated by a single pale layer and is 70 Å thick. Terminal bars join opposing cells at the apical margin, and desmosomes often occur on contacting cell surfaces. Vesicular structures, approximately 60 μm broad, appear in the microvilli and contain material that has the same density as colloid. Beneath the apical border there is a band of cytoplasm that is approximately 0.5 μm wide and devoid of organelles, although microtubular and microfilamentous structures are seen in this area.

Beneath this band, a few apical vesicles of 400 to 15,000 Å are seen, and beneath this area and extending to the base of the cell are the channels of the endoplasmic reticulum, also known as *ergoplasmic vesicles.* These vesicles, or channels, are limited by a single membrane (the *α cytomembrane*) approximately 60 to 70 Å thick, and their outer surface is studded with fine granules approximately 130 to 150 Å in diameter. These granules contain ribonucleoprotein and are the ribosomes active in protein synthesis. In some areas the membrane covering the cytomembrane is devoid of ribonucleoprotein particles, and in between the vesicles the ribonucleoprot-

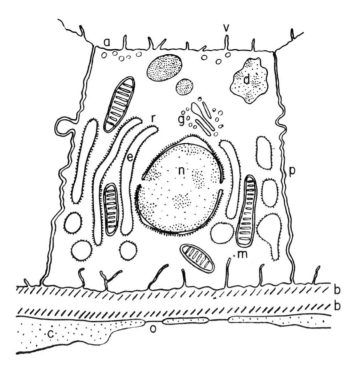

Fig. 1-5. A thyroid follicular cell, including: (a) apical vessel of cell; (e) endoplasmic reticulum; (d) colloid droplets; (v) microvilli; (r) ribosomes on endoplasmic reticulum; (g) Golgi apparatus; (m) mitochondrion; (p) plasma membrane; (c) capillary cells; (n) nucleus; (b) basement membrane; (o) open "pore" endothelial cells. (From Ekholm and Sjöstrand,[77] with permission.)

ein granules may be seen to lie free. The endoplasmic vesicles are very pleiomorphic.

Small vesicles are seen near the apical surface, 50 μm to several microns in diameter, and closed by a single-layer membrane 50 Å in thickness. These droplets appear especially in the apex of the cell and are thought to be secretion droplets. The material within them is frequently quite dense. Large vesicles of up to 1 μm frequently appear in stimulated thyroids. These are called *colloid droplets* because the material within the vesicles is homogeneous and has the density of colloid. Although visible with electron microscopy, these droplets are not visible with light-onicroscopy. The colloid droplets studied by light microscopy may be large resorbed droplets or the fusion of several separate droplets.

The Golgi apparatus is located near the nucleus and consists of small vacuoles and vesicles 400 to 800 Å in diameter. No nucleoprotein granules are found on the surface of these vesicles. The content of the Golgi vesicles has a density similar to that of secretion droplets.

Numerous rod shaped or irregular *mitochondria* are present. Their average diameter is 0.2 μm. They are bordered by a triple layered membrane 160 Å in width consisting of two opaque layers and a less opaque interposed layer. The inner opaque layer is thrown up into folds, or cristae, which run irregularly, along either the long or the short axis of the mitochondrion. The mitochondria contain large quantities of lipoprotein.

The *nucleus* is enclosed within a double-walled envelope whose layers are separated by a less dense area approximately 200 Å thick. The outer nuclear membrane is continuous with the membranes forming the endoplasmic reticulum. The nuclear envelope has characteristic pores 400 Å in diameter.

The abutting plasma membranes of adjacent cells parallel one another and are about 70 Å thick. They are separated by a space 150 Å wide, which contains a material of the same density as the basement membrane. The membrane at the base of the cell is covered on the outer surface by a basement membrane approximately 400 Å in width. A thin layer of fibers

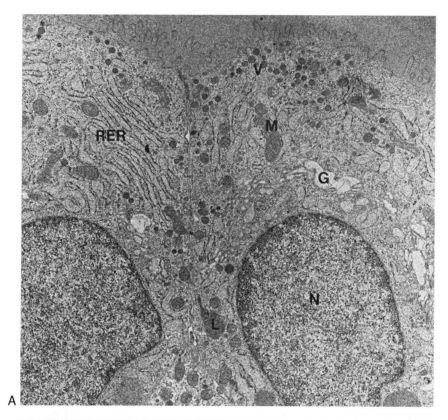

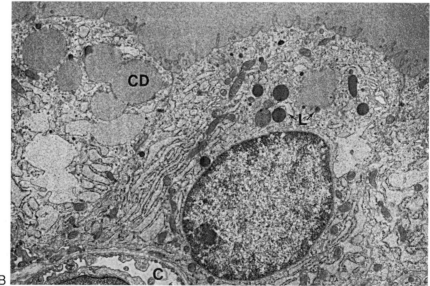

about 400 Å in diameter may occur at the outer surface of the basement membrane. The basement membrane of the follicular cell is separated by a clear area from the basement membrane of the opposing capillary endothelium. At frequent intervals, the wall of the endothelial cell is interrupted by a pore approximately 450 Å in diameter. Here the lumen of the capillary appears to be in direct contact with the basement membrane of the endothelial cell. The thyroid follicle cells are separated by two layers of basement membrane from the capillaries, but the pores in the endothelial lining of the capillaries allow plasma to come in direct contact with basement membrane. This arrangement appears to allow free diffusion of materials into and out of the acinar cell.

The *ribonucleoprotein granules* are involved in the synthesis of protein. They contain measured ribonucleic acids (mRNAs) encoding thyroid cell proteins. Activated amino acids, in combination with specific carrier-transfer RNA, reach the ribosome and are fitted into the RNA template in proper order to form the sequence of residues comprising a protein. The endoplasmic reticulum contains the newly formed protein. This protein should be largely thyroglobulin on its way into the colloid. The function of the Golgi apparatus is the posttranslational folding and glycosylation of the thyroid cell proteins.[80]

METABOLISM OF THE THYROID CELL

The metabolism of the thyroid as related to hormone synthesis and secretion is discussed in Chapter 2. In this section, a review of some general aspects of metabolism of the thyroid acinar cell is provided. The metabolism of the thyroid has been studied by all the usual techniques—in vivo, in situ, or in vitro perfusion, in slices, cells, homogenates, or subcellular fractions. Numerous species, including humans, have been investigated, often with obvious and consistent species-related differences. Conditions of tissue preparation and assays have varied widely. Much of the work has been directed toward elucidating the mechanism of TSH stimulation of the thyroid, seeking the primary site (or sites) of action.

Energy Metabolism

In the human thyroid cell, energy necessary for activities like synthesis of nucleotides, proteins, nuclear acids, and lipids, and transport functions, phagocytosis, lysosome movement, etc. is produced mainly by mitochondrial oxidative phosphorylation (about 85 percent) and to a minor extent by cytosolic aerobic glycolysis.[81] In many respects energy metabolism in the human thyroid cell resembles that in the dog thyroid. The values of oxygen uptake, glucose uptake, and lactate formation are significantly less in the human thyroid cell, however, probably because of a lower cell-colloid ratio in man. Adenosine triphosphate (ATP) concentration in the thyroid cell is around 1 mM and about 90 percent of ribonucleotides are in the form of triphosphates.[82] Free fatty acids are probably the main source of energy in thyroid cells since respiration is maintained for long periods in vitro in the absence of exogenous substrate. Because almost no glycogen is present in these conditions, free fatty acids are probably the endogenous substrates. Glycolytic ATP, however, may be the preferred source of energy for endocytosis of colloid, since inhibition of glycolysis greatly inhibits colloid endocytosis and addition of glucose counteracts this effect.[83] In general, reduced nicotine adenine dinucleotide (NADH) is mainly used in cells for generation of ATP whereas reduced nicotine adenine dinucleotide phosphate (NADPH) serves as an electron donor in reductive biosynthesis. As the

Fig. 1-6. Electron micrographs of rat thyroid. **(A)** Appearance after inactivation of the gland by two daily doses of T_4. The micrograph shows two cell nuclei (N), well developed rough-surfaced endoplasmic reticulum (RER), Golgi apparatus (G), mitochondria (M), lyosomes (L), and numerous dense, apical (exocytocic) vesicles (V). Because of the T_4-induced TSH suppression, no colloid droplets are present (no hormone release); TG synthesis, however, is still active, as indicated by the dense apical vesicle. **(B)** Appearance 20 minutes after intravenous administration of TSH (100 mU) to a rat treated with T_4 for 2 days. The most characteristic features of these cells are the large number of colloid droplets (CD) and the almost complete disappearance of dense apical vesicles; TSH has induced an emptying of these vesicles into the follicle lumen. Other oganelles are similar to those in Figure 1-2. Note the close relation between colloid droplets and lysosomes (L). Part of a capillary (C) is seen at the base of the follicle cells. (Courtesy of Prof. Ragnar Ekholm, Goteborg, Sweden.)

oxidized NADP ($NADP^+$) to oxidized nicotine adenine dinucleotide (NAD^+) ratio is lower in the thyroid mitochondria than in liver mitochondria but does not differ from the ratio in bovine heart and kidney mitochondria, it appears that the primary role of these nucleotides involves energy metabolism.

Mitochondrial inhibitors abolish the stimulatory effect of TSH on thyroid cell respiration.[82] Cyclic AMP does not influence mitochondrial respiration directly. It is therefore assumed that the stimulatory effect of TSH on respiration is secondary to its enhancing effect on energy (i.e., ATP) consuming cellular processes.

Carbohydrate Metabolism

The main route of energy delivery for metabolic processes in the thyroid cell are free fatty acids. Glucose metabolism, however, is important to the thyroid for several reasons. About 70 percent of the glucose taken up by dog or human thyroid slices is transformed to lactate, and a further 5 percent is catabolized through the Embden-Meyerhof pathway and the Krebs cycle.[82] Another 6 percent of glucose

carbon is incorporated into protein and less than 1 percent into lipids and glycogen. The remaining part (about 10 percent) is oxidized through the hexose monophosphate pathway (HMP). Most of the enzymes participating in the Embden-Meyerhof pathway, HMP, and the Krebs cycle have been demonstrated in the human thyroid.[84,85] Since hexokinase instead of glucokinase is present in the thyroid, the rate of phosphorylation of glucose is probably independent of its concentration because of the low Km of hexokinase for glucose.

Glucose metabolism serves several purposes. The incorporation of glucose carbon into proteins is related to the function of the thyroid cell in protein synthesis (i.e., synthesis of thyrogobulin which contains 10 percent carbohydrate). The metabolism of glucose along the HMP is related to the generation of NADPH and pentoses in this pathway. The production of pentoses is obviously necessary for generation of nucleotides. NADPH production is necessary for several reasons (Fig. 1-7). It is needed for generation of H_2O_2 for oxidation and organification of iodide. NADPH may also be an important cofactor in thyroid hormone deiodination. This process is a reductive reaction in which reduced glutathione may

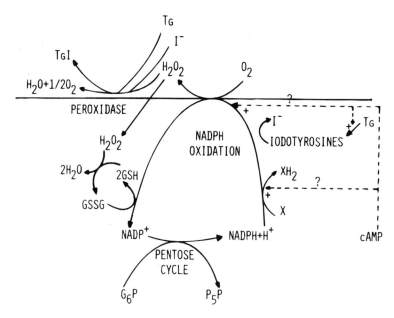

Fig. 1-7. Postulated NADP oxidation-reduction cycle in thyroid. Four mechanisms of NADPH oxidation are outlined: the reduction of any intermediate X by an NADPH-linked dehydrogenase, the deiodination of iodotyrosines released by thyroglobulinolysis, the generation of H_2O_2, and the reduction of H_2O_2 through GSH peroxidase. TG, uniodinated thyroglobulin; TGi, iodinated thyroglobulin; ----- + →, activation. (From Dumont and Vassart,[82] with permission.)

play a regulatory role. NADPH may be important in the reduction of glutathione after it has been oxidized during the deiodination reaction.[86]

TSH enhances carbohydrate metabolism in the dog thyroid.[82] During the stimulation there is a selective increase in the activity of the HMP, while incorporation of glucose into proteins and lipids decreases.[87] The activity of TSH in this sense is probably mediated by cAMP, since this nucleotide can reproduce the TSH effects on glucose uptake, catabolism, incorporation in protein and lipids, and on the HMP pathway. TSH also causes an increase in NADPH and $NADP^+$ concentration through increased NAD^+ kinase activity.[88]

Increased metabolic activity by TSH mainly reflects increased consumption by NADPH dependent processes stimulated by cAMP. For instance, the activity of the HMP pathway is predominantly dependent on the availability of the substrate $NADP^+$ generated during oxidation of NADPH.[82] The variation in activity of the HMP pathway found in various species[89] may reflect the specificity of H_2O_2 generating systems for NADPH versus NADH as coenzyme.[82]

Mitochondrial Respiration

The mitochondrion has appropriately been termed the "powerhouse" of the cell. It provides about 85 percent of generated ATP in the thyroid cell, with only 20 percent coming from glycolysis. The thyroids of different animal species contain mitochondria with similar morphology, having electron transport chain, Krebs cycle enzymes, coupled oxidative phosphorylation, and good respiratory control.[89] The activity of mitochondria is controlled by adenosine diphosphate (ADP) levels.[90] Also respiration linked Ca^{2+} accumulation plays a general and fundamental role in vertebrate cell physiology.[91] Free fatty acids are the preferred substrate of oxidation in the unstimulated thyroid, presumably through mitochondrial pathways.[92] In thyroids of patients with Graves' disease, it was found that mitochondria showed oxidation of tricarboxylic acid cycle intermediates and also of beta-hydroxybutyrate and caproate, which has not been observed in mitochondria of normal human or rat thyroids.[93] Mitochondria of human thyroids show an enzyme pattern characterized by relatively high activities of glucose-6-phosphate dehydrogenase and acid phosphatase and by low activities of the enzymes of the Embden-

Mayerhof pathway, the tricarboxylic acid cycle, and of amino acid metabolism. The findings suggest a favored catabolism of glucose by the HMG pathway.[94] In thyroids of patients operated on for hyperthyroid Graves' disease, all enzyme activities studied were increased.[94] TSH increases oxygen consumption in thyroid slices by 20 to 30 percent within a few minutes, employing a mechanism independent of exogenous substrates. The increased respiration is oligomycin and antimycin sensitive. Thus, respiration is of largely mitochondrial origin and probably represents the effect of TSH in increasing metabolic activities and consequently ATP consumption (see the section "Energy Metabolism"). TSH does not stimulate mitochondrial respiration directly.[95] TSH augments oxidation of pyruvate and acetate by thyroid slices. Compounds such as perchlorate, methimazole, iodide, thiocyanate, and T_4 have no significant direct action on thyroid mitochondria.[96] In isolated thyroid mitochondria, protein synthesis is dependent on intact electron transport and oxidative phosphorylation. It is inhibited by chloramphenicol but not by cycloheximide.[97]

Electron Transport and Oxidative Phosphorylation

The thyroid cell, like other cells, is provided with an electron transport system for shuttling electrons from energy supplying substrates to oxygen. Electrons continually pass from substrate to pyridine nucleotides, then to reductases, and through coenzyme Q and the cytochromes to oxygen, the final acceptor. The activity of these enzymes and their distribution in calf, rat, and human thyroid tissue have been studied in the laboratory of one of the authors.[98–100] In calf thyroid mitochondria, 0.008 μEq NADH and 0.006 μEq NADPH were oxidized per milligram of protein each minute (or 0.07 and 0.04 μEq/g wet tissue/min). Cytochrome oxidase activity was roughly equal to that in muscle, liver, and kidney. Suzuki and Nagashima,[101] in similar investigations, found a greater ratio of flavin to cytochrome oxidase activity than would be expected in the respiratory chain. This suggested the presence of flavin in other enzyme systems that might be involved in H_2O_2 generation and accordingly related to iodination reactions.

The data suggest that the thyroid has a normal electron transport system, but one that is less active than that in the liver. As measured in a test system, probably limited by loss of soluble cytochrome c, NADH oxidase is much more active than NADPH oxidase. The considerable glucose-6-phosphate dehydrogenase and isocitric dehydrogenase activities, in conjunction with low NADPH oxidase and NADPH-cytochrome c reductase activity, ought to keep NADPH in the reduced state, and this has indeed been observed.[102] There is also little, if any, transhydrogenase activity. This situation would also tend to maintain the high ratio of NADPH to NADP, which appears to be necessary for intrathyroidal synthetic mechanisms. β-Hydroxybutyrate and glutamate do not seem to be important oxidative substrates in the thyroid, since their dehydrogenases were not detected. Isocitric dehydrogenase and glucose 6-phosphate dehydrogenase, both NADPH generating enzymes, were found mainly in the soluble fraction of thyroid homogenates, their normal location. More recently unique electron transport, regulated by Ca^{2+} and ATP, that produce H_2O_2, has been described in the apical membrane of porcine thyroid cells.[103] The location of this system suggests its involvement in thyroid hormone synthesis.

RNA and DNA Metabolism

Chronic TSH stimulation produces cell hypertrophy, but the major increase in gland RNA can be ascribed to formation of new cells in a hyperplastic response.[104] Since RNA and DNA synthesis are required for cell growth and division, it is not surprising that TSH stimulation causes rapid and continued increases in synthetic activities. When given in vivo, TSH stimulates uptake and incorporation of RNA precursors within 1 hour and net RNA increases in about 12 hours.[105] TSH also stimulates incorporation of precursors into mRNA thyroid slice by increasing polymerase[106] activity. It is certain that TSH stimulates cell uptake and synthesis of purine and pyrimidine precursors.[107,108] TSH stimulation of purine and pyrimidine synthesis involves, in part, provision of the required ribose.[109] Synthesis of both messenger RNA (mRNA) and ribosomal RNA (rRNA) is stimulated by TSH,[110] but there is no evidence that some species of RNA are selectively formed under the influence of TSH.[107] Increased ratios of mRNA/DNA and transfer RNA/DNA ratios have been described in toxic adenomas and anaplastic carcinomas of human thyroids.[111] RNA degrada-

tion is not known to be influenced by TSH. TSH has been reported to stimulate thyroid nuclear RNA polymerase directly in vitro. Dibutyryl (DB) cAMP stimulates RNA synthesis in vivo, and in slices it activates nuclear RNA polymerase.[112] Thus, cAMP is a "second messenger" in these activities. Data obtained in an immortalized rat thyroid cell line (FRTL$_5$ cells) are consistent with this view.[113]

Formation of polyamines is closely linked to synthesis of new RNA during cell growth, although the mechanism is not known. TSH and cAMP stimulate ornithine decarboxylase, the rate-limiting enzyme in polyamine synthesis.[114]

Protein Metabolism

Thyroid tissue is composed of cells and storage protein, and the kinetic behavior of each compartment varies enormously with the conditions. Thus, in the colloid especially, protein storage and degradation go on concurrently, and the content at any time reflects a balance between these activities.

TSH induces uptake of amino acids by isolated thyroid cells,[115] and stimulates protein synthesis within 30 minutes to 4 hours.[115,116] Because of effects on thyroglobulin (TG) degradation, and dilution of amino acid precursor pools, stimulation of synthesis is more difficult to demonstrate in whole tissues.[107] Yet if thyroid slices are incubated in a high concentration of leucine to obliterate any separate effect of TSH on the cell uptake of amino acid, a clear stimulation of protein synthesis by TSH can be demonstrated in vitro,[117] and also in isolated thyroid cells.[118] Within 12 to 24 hours of chronic TSH stimulation in vivo, net protein content may be decreased by active TG hydrolysis, but protein content is later increased.[119] This response remains nearly linear over four to five weeks as thyroid size in animals quintuples.[104] The response is primarily due to production of new cells, since DNA and protein change in parallel.

Huge polysomes ($\pm$ 40 ribosomal units) connected by mRNA have been demonstrated in the thyroid[120] and were shown to incorporate precursors into TG-related peptides[121] (Fig. 1-8). TSH also shifts thyroid monosomes to polysomes, and this is stimulated by cAMP. This action suggests a direct effect on translation.[122] Phosphorylation of ribosomal proteins by phosphokinase and cAMP may alter their reactivity.[123]

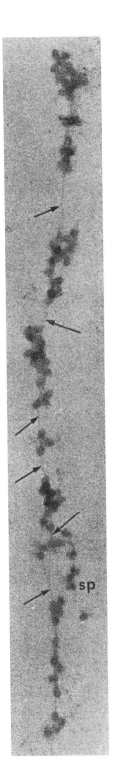

Fig. 1-8. Electron microscopic photograph of an enormous polysome containing 60 or 70 monosomes, the presumed source of TG synthesis. The arrows point to a thread possibly representing mRNA holding the polysome together. (From Keyham et al,[120] with permission.)

cAMP aggregates thyroid ribosomes into polysomes and mimics the action of TSH on protein synthesis in thyroid cells. Since this action is not sensitive to inhibition by actinomycin A, new synthesis of mRNA evidently is not required. cAMP mediates its effect through the activation of aminoacids and the binding of activated aminoacyl-RNA to ribosomes.[124] Chronic cAMP administration can cause gross enlargement of the thyroid.[125]

TG synthesis is discussed in Chapter 2.

Lipid Metabolism

Free fatty acids are the main fuel of the thyroid cell and they may be completely oxidized.[126–128] Sufficient endogenous substrate is present to sustain respiration for several hours during in vitro incubation of thyroid slices.[128] Studies on localization of lipids in human thyroids have shown that small amounts are present only in goiters from thyrotoxic patients, but that appreciable amounts are present in the normal human thyroid (i.e., phospholipids, cholesterol, and gangliosides: 5.2, 4.3 and 0.12 mmol/kg fresh tissue). C cells contain abundant phospholipids.[129–131] The human thyroid contains phospholipids in the following proportion: phosphathidylcholine (41.8 percent), phosphathidylethanolamine (26.9 percent), phosphathidylserine (10.4 percent), phosphathidylinositol (4.4 percent), cardiolipin (3.4 percent), and sphyngomyelin (12.4 percent).[132] TSH enhances the incorporation of precursors into most phospholipids. The effect is believed to reflect a direct stimulation of synthesis of phospholipids. Since TSH also stimulates phospholipid degradation, however, increased phospholipid synthesis under the influence of TSH could also correspond in part to this accelerated turnover.[82]

TSH also stimulates lipogenesis from glucose and incorporation of inositol into phosphoinositide in a glucose free system. TSH specifically enhances synthesis of phosphatidic acid from glycerophosphate after in vivo administration.[133] Since this response is accompanied by colloid droplet formation, which possibly requires formation of membranes, it has been suggested that phospholipid synthesis is secondary to droplet formation.[134] Yet DB cAMP and prostaglandins can, in some species, stimulate droplet formation without altering phospholipid synthesis.[135] In other species, cAMP and DB cAMP stimulate phospholipid formation, but the response does not precisely parallel that of TSH. Thus, cAMP may not be an intermediate in the action of TSH in these reactions.[136]

Mucopolysaccharide or Glucosaminoglycan Metabolism

Bollet et al.[137] found that administration of TSH for 3 to 13 days doubled the glucosaminoglycan (GAG) content of the dog thyroid. Little correlation could be found between thyroid disease state and GAG content in humans.[138] Normal values of 135 μg/100 mg were found, and measurements ranged from 76 in Hashimoto's thyroiditis to 228 in certain instances of "chronic thyroiditis." (These values were determined by the carbazole method; similar values were found by the orcinol method.) It has been shown in the porcine gland that about 90 percent of GAG exists as heparin or heparan sulfate and the remainder as chondroitin sulfate or dermatan sulfate.[139]

Sialic acid (N-acetylneuraminic acid) of the rat thyroid is both in the cells (20 percent) and in the TG (80 percent). thyrotropin injection and thiouracil feeding cause a decrease in total sialic acid and an increase in free sialic acid.[140] Synthesis of the glycoprotein TG is discussed in Chapter 2.

Electrolyte Transport and Metabolism

The mean resting transmembrane potential as studied in rat, rabbit, and guinea pig thyroid cells varies between -60 and -70 mV. The magnitude of the membrane potential was found to be dependent mainly upon the gradient for K^+ across the membrane.[141] A high intracellular K^+ and low Na^+ concentration is maintained by ouabain sensitive Na^+-K^+ ATPase. This ATPase varies in activity in direct relation to chronic TSH stimulation, probably representing cell hypertrophy and hyperplasia.[142] There is no evidence for direct action of TSH on this enzyme.[143] Acute stimulation of thyroid cells induces a depolarization of the cell, which is accompanied by a decrease in membrane resistance.[144,145] The depolarization may correspond to increased permeability to predominantly extracellular cations, such as Na^+ or anions, such as Cl^-, or to a decreased permeability to predominantly intracellular cations, such as K^+. Administration of TSH or veratridine, a sodium channel agonist, depolarized cultured thyroid cells and increased the secretion of radioiodine

from the organically bound pool. Depolarization of the cells by increasing the potassium concentration in the medium failed to promote secretion of radioactive iodine indicating that the sodium influx, rather than the depolarization itself, mediated the response.[146]

PHYSIOLOGICAL CONTROL OF THYROID GLAND FUNCTION

Many substances interact with the thyroid follicular cell to modulate its metabolic activity. The most studied and major control factor of thyroid gland activity is TSH. Other compounds, such as iodide, neurotransmitters, prostaglandins, and growth factors, may also play a regulatory role (Fig. 1-9).

Thyrotropin

TSH is a glycoprotein, consisting of two subunits, an α and a β chain (see Ch. 4). TSH action requires binding to a TSH-specific membrane receptor which activates adenylate cyclase through a G-protein coupled system.

A recent report indicates that the β-unit of human TSH is necessary for recognizing the TSH receptor in FRTL-5 cells while the α-subunit is required for signal transduction.[147] The thyrotropin receptor (TSH-R) is a simple polypeptide chain glycoprotein containing 744 amino acids in the mature protein (after deletion of the 20-amino acid signal peptide) of the human, dog, and rat, and has a calculated molecular weight of approximately 84,500 Dalton (Fig. 1-10). To this weight should be added an unknown molecular mass of carbohydrate chains, the exact weight depending on which of the 6 potential glycosylation sites are in fact glycosylated. The predicted size of the TSH holo receptor is closer to approximately 100,000 Dalton.[148] The former model of TSH-R consisting of an 80,000 Dalton heterodimer of 50,000 Dalton and 30,000 Dalton subunits linked by disulphide bonds is incorrect.[148] The molecule spans across the plasma membrane having a particularly long extracellular domain of 398 amino acids, a seven loop transmembrane domain of 366 amino acids, and a short intracellular tail of 80 amino acids. Intramolecular disulfide bonds are likely to be present between the clusters of highly conserved cysteine residues located at the amino-

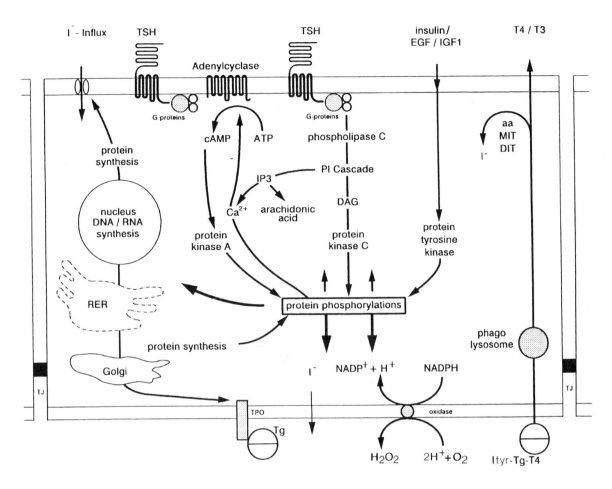

Fig. 1-9. Mechanism of action of thyrotropin, insulin, epidermal growth factor, and insulin-like growth factor-I on the thyroid follicular cell. (Courtesy of Dr. M. den Hartog, Amsterdam, The Netherlands.)

and carboxyl-termini of the extracellular domain.[148,149] Two forms of TSH-R have been reported to exist in thyroid tissue, one with low affinity and one with high affinity.[150] The high affinity site was regarded as physiologically important. There has been controversy about the importance of the low affinity TSH binding site, and recent experiments with a recombinant TSH-R indicated that the low affinity binding site is an artifact.[148]

TSH binds to the extracellular domain of the human TSH-R with a Kd of $\approx 3 \times 10^{-10}$M. Results from experiments using site-directed mutagenesis suggest that a segment between amino acids 32 to 50 is important in either TSH binding or is related to maintaining the correct conformation of the molecule. Furthermore Lys_{201}-Lys_{211} were found to be important in TSH binding.[148] Using synthetic peptides overlapping the complete extracellular sequence of TSH-R, binding inhibition studies revealed that regions 16 to 35, 106 to 125, 226 to 245 and 256 to 275 (the most important) interacted with TSH.[151] On the other hand, based on the ability of these peptides to reverse blocking activity of polyclonal antibodies raised against the extracellular domain of TSH-R for binding of TSH, regions 292 to 311, 367 to 386 and 397 to 415 were identified as important for TSH binding.[152] Others, using the green monkey kidney fibroblast derived from Cos-7 cells transfected with the wild type and with mutant rat TSH-Rs, report that high affinity TSH binding occurs at residues 30 to 37 and 42 to 45 and also at residue 385 and residues 259 to 306. Evidence is

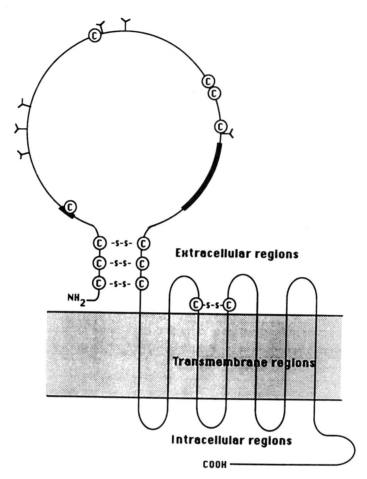

Fig. 1-10. Proposed model of the human TSH-R. Disulfide bonds are shown between highly conserved cysteine residues (C) at the amino- and carboxyl termini of the extracellular region. The black segments represent the regions unique to the TSH-R between amino acid residues 38 to 45 and 317 to 366. The Y symbols depict potential N-linked glycosyliation sites. (From Nagayama and Rapoport,[148] with permission.)

provided that the first two regions are important for TSH binding rather than for increasing cyclic AMP levels. Special attention has recently been directed at residue cysteine-301. A single point mutation at this locus resulted in increased TSH binding but conservation of exerted bioactivity. It is suggested that cysteine-301 is involved in disulfide formation and is important in tertiary structure and that its mutation results in conformational changes of the receptor without loss of functional capacity.[152a] Recently, monoclonal antibodies have been developed against the entire span of the extracellular domain of the human TSH receptor. These antibodies react to discrete conformational and linear epitopes and should enable detailed function-structure studies of the

TSH receptor.[153] For binding of thyroid stimulating antibodies, residue 40 and residues 30 to 33, 34 to 37, 42 to 45, 52 to 56 and 58 to 61 appeared to be important, whereas thyroid stimulating blocking antibodies interact at residue 385 or at residues 295 to 306 and 387 to 395 of the extracellular domain of the TSH receptor.[149,154] From all these studies it is apparent that there are many discrete regions in the extracellular domain of the human TSH-R that bind TSH or TSH-R autoantibodies.

The transmembrane region of the TSH-R consists of about 346 aminoacids with 7 transmembrane segments, 3 extracellular loops, and 3 cytoplasmic loops. The carboxyl-terminal cytoplasmic tail consists of aminoacids all located intracellularly (see Fig.

2-14). There is a high degree of homology between the human, dog, and rat TSH-Rs. Homology with the receptors for LH/CG and FSH is lower.[148] The cytoplasmic part of the TSH receptor is important in coupling to G proteins. Information is rapidly accumulating regarding important domains in the cytoplasmic portion of the TSH-R for activation of phosphatidylinositol bisphosphate (PIP_2) and cAMP signals. Thus, the amino-terminal half of the cytoplasmic tail is essential for full expression of function (i.e., activation of both messenger systems).[155] The first and third cytoplasmic loop are important in PIP_2 signaling but not in cAMP activation,[156,157] while the second loop is important for both pathways.[157]

Binding of TSH to TSH-R leads to activation of adenylate cyclase by interaction with the regulatory (guanine nucleotide binding) G or N protein. Cyclic AMP in its turn activates cAMP dependent protein kinase to transfer the terminal high-energy phosphate of ATP to various acceptors, such as enzymes, ribosomal proteins, histones, chromatin associated proteins, and possibly tubulin. cAMP dependent protein kinases are activated in a dose dependent way.[158,159] Despite all the evidence for the role of cAMP protein kinase dependent mediation of the intracellular effects of TSH, the specific protein substrates for this phosphorylation are not known. Most but not all actions attributed to TSH are promoted by this pathway.[160,161] Exposure of thyroid cells to TSH for 30 min to 4 h leads to a subsequent refractoriness to TSH action over a period of about 20 h,[162] as measured by the subsequent ability of TSH to stimulate cAMP formation, glucose oxidation, or iodide uptake.[163] (This action is, however, not apparent in vivo in man.) Desensitization by TSH may be caused either by decrease in availability of TSH receptors or alteration of coupling between these receptors and the catalytic unit of adenylate cyclase. ADP-ribosylation has been proposed as a possible mechanism for inactivation of the regulatory protein.[164] Later studies, however, could not support this hypothesis since no changes occur with regard to the regulatory protein during desensitization.[165]

The mechanism of desensitization is still a matter of debate. When chinese hamster ovary (CHO) cells are stably transfected with the human TSH-R (hTSH-R), no desensitization was found upon stimulation to TSH by some groups,[166,167] but others[168] did find desensitization to receptor or postreceptor stimulation. Desensitization was also reported to occur in a mouse nonthyroidal cell line (NIH 3T3) stably transfected with hTSH-R, and this was attributed to internalization of TSH receptors.[167] When using a human embryonal kidney cell line (293 cells) stably transfected with hTSH-R or the LH/CG receptor, desensitization occurred when cells were stimulated with their respective hormones. Down-regulation of receptors however was not found.[169] More studies are necessary to understand the process of desensitization by TSH.

The effects caused by TSH encompass many aspects of cell metabolism. Within minutes, TSH causes accumulation of sodium. The TSH stimulated cell develops a swollen apical border, and its intracellular volume increases. Pseudopods appear in 4 to 5 minutes, and colloid droplets increase in number. Colloid is transported more rapidly into the cell, and secretion of T_3, T_4, and iodide is increased. Concurrently, there is stimulation of RNA, protein, and phospholipid synthesis, and oxidation of glucose by the Embden-Meyerhof and HMP pathways. Transport of iodide into the cell increases slowly and probably requires synthesis of new transport proteins. Oxidation and binding of iodide and iodotyrosyl coupling (i.e., hormonogenesis) are increased rapidly, perhaps by increased generation of H_2O_2. All of these responses occur following in vivo stimulation of the thyroid by TSH, and almost every effect has been duplicated in vitro. With a few exceptions cAMP or its more active dibutyryl derivative can reproduce each response both in vivo and in vitro. The actions of TSH on hormonogenesis are especially relevant. Initially, TSH causes an efflux of iodide from the thyroid. Clearance of iodide into the gland gradually increases as the activity of the transport system increases. In the highly stimulated gland, iodide clearance can be nearly 100-fold of normal. Blood flow is remarkably increased to support this clearance. Over subsequent days, TSH causes some induction of the iodide oxidizing enzymes and some increases in enzymes through cell hypertrophy. With continued TSH stimulation there is cell proliferation, and the total iodide binding activity of the thyroid grows in proportion to cell numbers. Stimulation of colloid resorption, proteolysis, and hormone secretion occurs early and becomes so intense that all colloid may disappear. TG synthesis is also greatly enhanced.

Recent investigations were conducted to see if

TSH is also active through receptor mediated cleavage of phosphatidylinositol (Pl). In this other (cAMP independent) second messenger system,[170] binding of the hormone to membrane receptors activates phospholipase C. This substance hydrolyzes phosphatidylinositol biphosphate (PIP_2) to inositol 1,4,5-triphosphate (IP_3) and 1,2-diacyl glycerol (DAG), and these two compounds act as second messengers. IP3 increases free calcium concentration in the cytosol by its release from intracellular stores, such as those in endoplasmatic reticulum and mitochondria. The elevated level of free calcium in the cytosol triggers a great variety of processes: glycogen breakdown, exocytosis, enzyme activation, etc. A well known effect of elevated free calcium is its interaction with calmodulin through which it activates many enzymes and other proteins.[171] DAG activates the enzyme protein kinase C (PKC). The inactive enzyme is located mainly in the cytosol, whereas the active form is membrane bound. Protein kinase C contains a catalytic domain and a regulatory domain. In the absence of activating cofactors (Ca^{2+}, phospholipid, DAG/phorbol ester), the regulatory domain inhibits the kinase activity of the catalytic domain. DAG binding to PKC decreases the inhibitory activity of the regulatory domain resulting in increased affinity of PKC for Ca^{2+}, thereby rendering it active at the physiological levels of this ion. PKC phosphorylates serine and threonine residues in many target proteins. The important general effects of PKC in controlling cell division and proliferation are revealed after its activation by phorbol esters. Such stimulation causes growth of thyroid cells of different species, but inhibits differentiated thyroid function.[172,173–175]

The physiologic significance of the phosphatidylinositol system in the thyrocyte is unknown. Some reports cast doubt upon the significance of this system in cultured thyroid cells of different species.[176–178] There is an increasing concensus, however, that at least in vitro the PIP2 pathway is activated by TSH. PIP2 hydrolysis and increased intracellular free calcium have been found in TSH stimulated FRTL-5 cells.[179–181b] TSH and IGF-I have been reported to synergistically stimulate DAG formation in these cells.[182] Activation of the phosphatidyl pathway by TSH has been found in normal human thyroid cells but not in the dog thyroid.[183–184b] Activation is also seen when human thyrocytes are incubated with ATP, TRH, or bradyki-

nine.[185] Recently it was shown that the PIP2 pathway stimulated iodide organification through its positive effect on H_2O_2 generation in human thyroid slices.[186]

Other Regulatory Factors

Iodine has an autoregulatory function in thyroid cells, especially under conditions of absent or constant TSH stimulation. Iodide in concentrations between 0.01 to 1.0 mM produces a dose dependent inhibition on thyroid cell growth at multiple loci related to both the cAMP dependent and cAMP independent pathways.[187] Inhibitory action of iodide on TSH mediated cAMP formation can be counteracted by agents like methimazole, which prevent iodide organification, indicating that an "oxidized iodine intermediate" may be involved in this response.[188] The effects of iodide on thyroid hormone synthesis are further discussed in Chapter 5.

Insulin-like growth factor-I (IGF-I) acts synergistically with TSH to stimulate adenylate cyclase. A synergistic action between IGF-I and TSH was found in DNA synthesis and thus cell growth.[189] IGF-I stimulates the growth of rat thyroid cells in culture and synergizes the stimulation of DNA synthesis induced by TSH and Graves' IgG.[190] It was later found that at least part of the synergism was due to TSH dependent production of an unidentified amplification factor or factors released from the thyrocytes during incubation.[191] No effect of IGF was found on iodide uptake of FRTL-5 cells.[192] When incubated with sheep thyroid cells, IGFs induced the production of IGF binding proteins (IGFBPs). IGFs exist primarily bound to cell surface receptors or complexed to IGFBPs. The distinct regulation of these IGFBPs by their ligands suggest that these binding proteins may have a biological role in modulating thyroid physiology.[193]

Epidermal growth factor (EGF) receptors have been identified on human thyroid membrane preparations[194] and EGF stimulates the proliferation of thyrocytes from sheep,[195] dogs,[196] pigs,[197] and calves.[198] Using porcine thyroid follicles in collagen gel, it was shown that when EGF was added without TSH, a sequence of events including cell multiplication, migration of thyrocytes, and formation of new follicles could be induced. From these experiments it was suggested that EGF might be involved in the generation of new follicles in the intact gland.[199] Experiments with cultures of human thyroid cells showed that EGF stimulates cAMP production and inhibited TG release during the first 3 days of culture, but stimulated TG release after 12 days of culture.[200] Although EGF stimulates growth of thyroid cells, it has shown to have a marked inhibitory effect on cell differentiation and a small mitogenic effect on human thyrocytes.[201–203] It has been suggested that EGF may play a role in the pathogenesis of human thyroid carcinoma as an increased number of high affinity EGF receptors is found in malignant thyroid growth.[194] When mice were treated with T_4, an increased level of thyroidal EGF mRNA was found, explaining higher levels of immunoreactive EGF in the thyroid. Since EGF inhibits thyroid function, this pathway may act as an autocrine-paracrine regulator. EGF administered in vivo to sheep decreases circulating plasma thyroid hormone levels, supposedly by blocking thyroid hormone secretion. Furthermore, EGF was found to accelerate the peripheral T_4 and T_3 metabolism.[204]

Endothelial cell growth factor, fibroblast growth factor, platelet derived growth factor, and bombesin have been shown to stimulate thymidine incorporation in FRTL-5 cells and they potentiate similar effects of TSH, but at the same time inhibit TSH stimulation of thyrocyte function.[192] Acetylcholine, norepinephrine, prostaglandins F, and TRH have been shown to increase iodide organification and inhibit the action of TSH on thyroid hormone release. These effects are independent of the cAMP pathway. Somatostatin injected into the thyroid artery during surgery in man has been shown to inhibit TSH stimulated thyroid hormone secretion.[205] Other C cell peptides such as calcitonin, calcitonin gene-related peptide, and katacalcin seem to be involved in the inhibition of thyroid hormone secretion, while both gastrin-releasing peptide and helodermin stimulate thyroid hormone secretion.[206,207]

Atrial natriuretic hormone and cytokines (such as tumor necrosis factor-α, interferon-γ, and interleukin-I) seem to inhibit thyroid function.[207,208]

Sympathic nerves enter the thyroid, and receptors for catecholamines appear to exist on the thyroid cell surface. β-Adrenergic agonists stimulate thyroid hormone secretion in animals[208] probably by stimulation of cAMP formation, while the neuropeptide Y potentiates the inhibitory action of noradrenaline on TSH-induced thyroid hormone secretion. Thyroidal nerve fibres have been shown to contain many polypeptides, such as VIP, peptide histidine, isoleucine, neuropeptide Y, substance P, calcitonin gene-related peptide, galanin, and cholecystokinine.[207] Neuropeptide Y has a role in regulation blood flow in the rat.[209] Studies so far have failed to establish any convincing effect of substance P, galanine, and cholecystokinine on basal or TSH stimulated thyroid hormone secretion. Specific receptors for endothelin-1 (ET-1), a vasoactive peptide, have been identified on human thyrocytes in culture. ET-1 exhibits an inhibitory action on TG release by a cAMP-independent pathway. It may also be involved in early goitrogenesis.[210]

Retinoids, vitamin A and its analogues, may modulate differentiation and proliferation of a variety of cells. Recently their effects have been investigated in porcine thyroid cell in culture showing that these compounds inhibit TSH stimulated iodine metabolism by reducing cAMP accumulation and steps subsequent to cAMP production.[211] Hydrocortisone in physiologic concentrations stimulates TSH induced iodide uptake in porcine cells in culture by using a glucocorticoid receptor and by affecting cAMP pathways.[212]

SUMMARY

The thyroid gland is a structure derived from the primitive pharynx, specialized for the production, storage, and release of the thyroid hormones. The precursors of the thyroid hormones and the hormones themselves are found without known function in certain invertebrate species. Beginning with the protochordates, a specialized structure is developed that is concerned with the production of thyroid hormones although, curiously enough, thyroid hormone has no known stimulatory effect on these forms. In all vertebrates, a thyroid is found that secretes thyroid hormone. This hormone produces clear-cut metabolic effects in poikilotherms, although its actual importance for their normal metabolism is not clear. It is responsible for the metamorphosis of most vertebrate larval forms. In birds and mammals, thyroid hormone regulates the metabolic rate.

The thyroid gland of mammals begins as an evagination from the floor of the embryonic pharynx. It descends into the neck, is separated from the gut, is joined by small contributions from the pharyngeal pouches, and develops into the discrete anatomic unit of the adult thyroid gland typified by colloid filled follicles.

The thyroid has an abundant blood supply. The nerve supply seems to be primarily from the autonomic system and has, as its prime function, the regulation of blood flow. There is accumulating evidence for control of secretion by autonomic fibers and catecholamines. The lymphatics of the gland connect with the other lymphatics of the neck and the mediastinum. Although hormone is normally secreted predominantly into the venous effluent of the gland, some release of hormone and iodoproteins into the lymph also occurs.

The functional unit of the thyroid is the follicle, a spheroidal structure lined by parenchymal epithelium, enclosing a gelatinous material known as *colloid*. Colloid is composed primarily of a specific iodinated protein, TG. The appearance of the follicle in the light microscope and its fine structure as disclosed by the electron microscope have been described. In addition to parenchymal cells, the thyroid also contains a specific variety of cells that do not touch the follicular lumen. These cells, known as C cells, secrete calcitonin.

The thyroid carries out a specific biochemical process in the formation and secretion of thyroid hormone. It also has the general intermediary metabolic activities of all tissues. The primary source of cell ATP is mitochondrial oxidative phosphorylation. The cells contain the usual complement of electron transport activities and enzymes of the glycolytic and Krebs cycles. The cell is involved in the synthesis of a predominant protein, TG, and enormous polysomes have been located in the cells that are the site of TG synthesis.

The principal physiologic control of thyroid function is mediated through TSH impinging upon the cell. TSH activates cell membrane adenylate cyclase, through its interaction with the TSH receptor located on the plasma membrane. The mature glycosylated receptor has a molecular weight of approximately 100,000 D. Specific sites on the extracellular domain of the TSH receptor have been identified as critical for TSH binding and signaling. Interaction of TSH with its receptor increases intracellular cAMP by transduction coupled to a Gs α protein, induces increases in oxidation of glucose, synthesis of protein, formation of RNA, uptake of I, and formation and secretion of thyroid hormone. cAMP is presumed to act as an intracellular "second messenger" in most, if not virtually all, of these activities. It has recently been found that TSH may also act via the phosphatidylinositol pathway. The physiologic significance of this pathway, however, has not yet been established.

There are a number of other regulatory factors that may influence thyroid function and growth. Apart from the well known effects of iodine in this respect, neuropeptides belonging to the adrenergic-, cholinergic-, and peptidergic nervous system may be stimulatory or inhibitory. Peptides derived from the C cells, atrial natriuretic factor, growth factors, and cytokines may also be relevant to thyroid function and growth in physiologic and pathologic conditions.

REFERENCES

1. Drechsel HFE: Beiträge zur Chemie einiger Seethiere. II. Über das Achsenskelett der *Gorgonia cavolini*. Z Biol 33:85, 1986

2. Roche J: Biochimie comparée des scléroprotéines iodées des Anthozoaires et des Spongiaires. Experientia 8:45, 1952

3. Berg O, Gorbman A, Kobayashi H: The thyroid hormones in invertebrates and lower vertebrates. p. 302. In Gorbman A (ed): Comparative Endocrinology. John Wiley & Sons, New York, 1959

4. Tong W, Chaikoff IL: [131]I utilization by the aquarium snail and the cockroach. Biochim Biophys Acta 48:347, 1961

5. Salvatore G: Thyroid hormone biosynthesis in Agnatha and Protochordata. Gen Comp Endocrinol, suppl. 2:535, 1969.

6. Tong W, Chaikoff IL: Metabolism of ^{131}I by the marine alga, *Nereocystis leutkana*. J Biol Chem 215:473, 1955

7. Leloup J: Iodoperoxydase branchiale et Absorption des iodures chez l'Anguille. Mecanisme thyroidien de controle. Gen Comp Endocrinol 9:514, 1967

8. Tong W, Chaikoff IL: Activation of iodine utilization in thyroid-gland homogenates by cytochrome C and quinones. Biochim Biophys Acta 37:189, 1960

9. Roche J, Salvatore G, Rametta G: Sur la présence et la biosynthèse d'hormones thyroidiennes chez un Tunicier, *Ciona intestinalis* L. Biochim Biophys Acta 63:154, 1962

10. Cameron AT: The distribution of iodine in plant and animal tissues. J Biol Chem 18:335, 1914

11. Barrington EJW: Some endocrinological aspects of the protochordata. p. 250. In Gorbman A (ed): Com-

parative Endocinology. John Wiley & Sons, New York, 1959

12. Gorbman A: Some aspects of the comparative biochemistry of iodine utilization and the evolution of thyroidal function. Physiol Rev 35:336, 1955

13. Barrington EJW: The distribution and significance of organically bound iodine in the ascidian, *Ciona intestinalis* L. J Marine Biol Assoc UK 36:1, 1957

14. Covelli I, Salvatore G, Sena L, Roche J: Sur la formation d'hormones thyroidiennes et de leurs precurseurs par *Branchiostoma lanceolatum Pallas (Amphioxus)*. Compt Rend Soc Biol 154:1165, 1960

15. Tong W, Kerkof P, Chaikoff IL: Identification of labeled thyroxine and triiodothyronine in *Amphioxus* treated with ^{131}I. Biochim Biophys Acta 56:326, 1962

16. Dunn AD: Studies on iodoproteins and thyroid hormones in ascidians. Gen Comp Endocrinol 40:473, 1980

17. Fujita H, Sawano F: Fine structural localization of endogenous peroxidase in the endostyle of ascidians, *Ciona intestinalis*: a part of phylogenetic studies of the thyroid gland. Arch Histol Jpn 42:319, 1979

18. Suzuki S, Kondo Y: Demonstration of thyroglobulinlike iodinated proteins in the branchial sac of tunicates. Gen Comp Endocrinol 17:402, 1971

19. Spangenberg DB: Thyroxine in early strombilation in *Aurelia aurita*. Amer Zool 14:825, 1974

20. Suzuki S, Kondo Y: Thyroidal morphogenesis and biosynthesis of thyroglobulin before and after metamorphosis in the lamprey, *Lampetra reissneri*. Gen Comp Endocrinol 21:451, 1973

21. Salvatore G, Covelli I, Sena L, Roche J: Fonction thyroïdienne et métabolisme de l'iode chez la larve d'un Cyclostome *(Petromyzon planieri* BI). Compt Rend Soc Biol 153:1686, 1959

22. Gorbman A: Problems in the comparative morphology and physiology of the vertebrate thyroid gland. p. 266. In Gorbman A (ed): Comparative Endocrinology. John Wiley & Sons, New York, 1959

23. Salvatore G, Macchia V, Vecchio G, Roche J: Sur le transport de la thyroxine par les protéines du sérum de l'Ammocoette de *Petromyzon planeri* BI. Compt Rend Soc Biol 153:1693, 1959

24. Wright G, Yonsum JH: Serum thyroxine concentrations in larval and metamorphosing anadromous sea lampreys, *Petromyzon morinus*. J Exp. Zool 2002:27, 1977

25. Monaco F, Andreoli M, La Posta et al: Biosynthesis of thyroglobulin in the endostyle of larva (ammocoetes) of a fresh water lamprey, *Lampetra planeri* B1. C-R-Soc-Biol (Paris) 171:308, 1977

26. Dunn TB: Ciliated cells of the thyroid of the mouse. JNCI 4:555, 1944

27. Brown-Grant K: Extrathyroidal iodide concentrating mechanisms. Physiol Rev 41:189, 1961

28. Baker-Cohen KF: Renal and other heterotopic thyroid tissue in fishes. p. 283. In Gorbman A (ed): Comparative Endocrinology. John Wiley & Sons, New York, 1959

29. Plisetskaya EM, Woo NYS, Murat JC: Thyroid hormones in cyclostomes and fish and their role in regulation of intermediary metabolism. Comp Biochem Physiol 74:179, 1983

30. Dickhoff WW, Darling DS: Evolution of thyroid function and its control in lower vertebrates. Amer Zool 23:697, 1983

31. Matty AJ: Thyroidectomy and its effect upon oxygen consumption of a teleost fish, *Pseudoscarus guacamia*. J Endocrinol 15:1, 1957

32. Leloup J, Fontaine M: Iodine metabolism in lower vertebrates. Ann NY Acad Sci 86:316, 1960

33. Dickhoff WW, Folmar LC, Gorbman A: Changes in plasma thyroxine during smoltification of coho salmon, *Oncorhynchus kisutch*. Gen Comp Endocriol 36:229, 1978

34. Nishikawa K, Hirashima T, Suzuki S, Suzuki M: Changes in circulating L-thyroxine and L-triiodothyronine of the masu salmon, *Oncorhynchus masou*, accompanying the smoltification, measured by radioimmunoassay. Endocrinol Jpn 26:731, 1979

35. Grau EG, Dickhoff WW, Nishioka RS et al: Lunar phasing of the thyroxine surge preparatory to seaward migration of salmonid fish. Science 211:607, 1981

36. Eagleson GW, McKeown BA: Changes in thyroid activity of *Ambystoma gracile* (Baird) during different larval, transforming, and postmetamorphic phases. Can J Zool 56:1377, 1978

37. Gudernatsch JF: Feeding experiments on tadpoles: the influence of specific organs given as food on growth and differentiation. Arch Enwicklungsmech Organ 35:457, 1912

38. Kollros JJ: Thyroid gland function in developing cold-blooded vertebrates. p. 340. In Gorbman A (ed): Comparative Endocrinology. John Wiley & Sons, New York, 1959

39. Norman MF, Carr JA, Norris DO: Adenohypophysial-thyroid activity of the tiger salamander, *Ambystoma trigrinum*, as a function of metamorphosis and captivity. J Exp Zool 242:55, 1987

40. Maker MJ: Metabolic responses of isolated tissues to thyroxine administered in vivo. Endocrinology 74:994, 1964

41. Turner JE, Tipton SR: Environmental temperature and thyroid function in the green water snake, *Natrix cyclopion*. Gen Comp Endocrinol 18:195, 1972

42. Regard E, Taurog A, Nakashima T: Plasma thyroxine and triiodothyronine levels in spontaneously metamorphosing *Rana catesbeiana* tadpoles and in adult *anuran amphibia*. Endocrinology 102:674, 1978

43. Jacobs GF, Michielsen RP, Kuhn ER: Thyroxine and triiodothyronine in plasma and thyroids of the neotenic and metamorphosed axolotl, *Ambystoma mexicanum:* influence of TRH injections. Gen Comp Endocrinol 70:145, 1988

44. Etkin W: Hypothalamic sensitivity of thyroid feedback in the tadpole. Neuroendocrinology 1:293, 1965

45. Platt JE, Brown GB, Erwin SA, McKinley KT: Antagonistic effects of prolactin and oxytocin on tail fin regression and acid phosphatase activity in metamorphosing *Ambystoma tigrinum.* Gen Comp Endocrinol 61:376, 1986

46. Tata JR, Kawahara A, Baker BS: Prolactin inhibits both thyroid hormone-induced morphogenesis and cell death in cultured amphibian larval tissues. Dev Biol 146:72, 1991

47. Norris DO, Gem WA: Thyroxine induced activation of hypothalamic-hypophysial axis in neotenic salamander larvae. Science 194:525, 1976

48. Galton VA: The role of 3,5,3′-triiodothyronine in the physiological action of thyroxine in the premetamorphic tadpole. Endocrinology 124:2427, 1989

49. Galton VA: The role of thyroid hormone in amphibian metamorphosis. TEM 3:96, 1992

50. Yoshizato K, Frieden E: Increase in binding capacity for triiodothyronine in tadpole tail nuclei during metamorphosis. Nature 254:705, 1975

51. Yoshizato K, Kistler A, Frieden E: Binding of thyroid hormones by nuclei of cells from bullfrog tadpole tail fins. Endocrinology 97:1030, 1975

52. Kistler A, Yoshizato K, Frieden E: Binding of thyroxine and triiodothyronine by nuclei of isolated tadpole liver cells. Endocrinology 97:1036, 1975

53. Galton VA: Thyroxine and 3,5,3′-triiodothyronine bind to the same putative receptor in hepatic nuclei of *Rana catesbeiana* tadpoles. Endocrinology 118:114, 1986

54. Galton VA: Binding of thyroid hormones in vivo by hepatic nuclei of *Rana catesbeiana* tadpoles at different stages of metamorphosis. Endocrinology 107:1910, 1980

55. Darling DS, Dickhoff WW, Gorbman A: Comparison of thyroid hormone binding to hepatic nuclei of a rat and a teleost *(Oncorhynch Kisutch).* Endocrinology 111:1936, 1982

56. Baker BS, Tata JR: Accumulation of proto-oncogene c-erb-A related transcripts during *Xenopus* development: association with early acquisition of response of thyroid hormone and estrogen. EMBO J 9:879, 1990

57. Yaoita Y, Shi Y-B, Brown DD: *Xenopus levis* α and β thyroid hormone receptor. Proc Natl Acad Sci USA 87:7090, 1990

58. Schneider MJ, Davey JC, Galton VA: *Rana catesbeiana* tadpole red blood cells express an α, but not a β, c-erbA gene. Endocrinology 133:2488, 1993

58a. Schneider MJ, Galton VA: Effect of glucocorticoids on thyroid hormone action in cultured red blood cells from *Rana catesbeiana* tadpoles. Endocrinology 136:1435, 1995

59. Tata JR: Gene expression during metamorphosis: an ideal model for post-embryonic development. BioEssays 15:239, 1993

60. Kanamori A, Brown DD: The regulation of thyroid hormone receptor β genes by thyroid hormone in *Xenopus levis.* J Biol Chem 267:739, 1992

61. Machuca I, Tata JR: Autoinduction of thyroid hormone receptor during metamorphosis is reproduced in *Xenopus* XTC-2 cells. Mol Cel Endocrinol 87:105, 1992

61a. Muchuca I, Esslemont G, Fairclough L, Tata JR: Analysis of structure and expression of the *Xenopus* thyroid hormone receptor-β gene to explain its autoinduction. Mol Endocrinol 9:96, 1995

62. Shi Y-B: Molecular biology of amphibian metamorphosis. Trends Endocrinol Metab 5:4, 1994

62a. Shi Y-B, Liang VCT, Cheng S-Y: Tissue-dependent developmental expression of a cytosolic thyroid hormone protein gene in *Xenopus:* its role in the regulation of amphibian metamorphosis. FEBS Letters 355:61, 1994

63. Etkin W: Metamorphosis-activating system of the frog. Science 139:810, 1963

64. Dent JN: Maintenance of thyroid function in newts with transplanted pituitary glands Gen Comp Endocrinol 6:401, 1966

65. Voitkevich AA: Neurosecretory control of the amphibian metamorphosis. Gen Comp Endocrinol, suppl. 1:133, 1962

66. Jackson IMD: Evolutionary significance of the phylogenetic distribution of the mammalian hypothalamic releasing hormones. Fed Proc 40:2545, 1981

67. Sawin CT, Bacharach P, Lance V: Thyrotropin-releasing hormone and thyrotropin in the control of thyroid function in the turtle, *Chrysemys picta.* Gen Comp Endocrinol 45:7, 1981

68. Peter RE: Feedback effects of thyroxine in goldfish *Carassius auratus* with an autotransplanted pituitary. Neuroendocrinol 17:273, 1972

69. Fontaine YA: Studies on the heterothyrotropic activity of preparations of mammalian gonadotropins of teleost fish. Gen Comp Endocrinol, suppl. 2:417, 1969

70. Soyama F: Development and differentiation of lateral thyroid. Endocrinol Jpn 20:565, 1973

71. Fujita H, Machino M: On the follicle formation of the thyroid gland in the chick embryo. Exp Cell Res 25:204, 1961

72. LeDouarin N, LeLièvre CH: Démonstration de l'origine neurale des cellules à calcitonine du corps ultimobranchial chez l'embryon de poulet. CR Acad Sci D270:2857, 1970

73. Wolfe HJ, Voelkel EF, Tashjian Jr AH: Distribution of calcitonin-containing cells in the normal adult human thyroid gland: a correlation of morphology with peptide content. J Clin Endocrinol Metab 38: 688, 1974

74. Nadler NJ, Sarkar SK, Leblond CP: Origin of intracellular colloid droplets in the rat thyroid. Endocrinology 71:120, 1962

75. Wissig SL: The anatomy of secretion in the follicular cells of the thyroid gland: the fine structure of the gland in the normal rat. J Biophys Biochem Cytol 7:419, 1960

76. Dempsey EW, Peterson RR: Electron microscopic observations on the thyroid glands of normal, hypophysectomized, cold-exposed, and thiouracil-treated rats. Endocrinology 56:46, 1955

77. Ekholm R, Sjöstrand FS: The ultrastructural organization of the mouse thyroid gland. J Ultrastruct Res 1:178, 1957

78. Ekholm R: Thyroid gland. p. 221. In Kurtz SM (ed): Electron Microscopic Anatomy. Academic Press, San Diego, 1964

79. Herman L: An electron microscope study of the salamander thyroid during hormonal stimulation. J Biophys Biochem Cytol 7:143, 1960

80. Chabaud O, Bouchilloux S, Ronin C, Ferrand M: Localization in a Golgi-rich thyroid fraction of sialyl-, glalactosyl-, and N-acetylglucosaminyltransferases. Biochimie 56:119, 1974

81. Otten J, Dumont JE: Glucose metabolism in normal human thyroid tissue in vitro. Eur J Clin Invest 2: 213, 1972

82. Dumont JE, Vassart G: Thyroid gland metabolism and the action of TSH. p. 311. In DeGroot LJ (ed): Endocrinology 1. Grune & Stratton, Orlando, 1979

83. Dumont JE, Willems C, van Sande J, Nève P: Regulation of the release of thyroid hormones: role of cyclic AMP. Ann NY Acad Sci 185:291, 1971

84. Dumont JE: Carbohydrate metabolism in the thyroid gland. J Clin Endocrinol Metab 20:1246, 1960

85. Rheinwein D, Engelhardt A: Enzymmuster der Menschlichen Schilddrüse I. Normale Schilddrüse. Klin Wochenschr 42:731, 1964

86. Leonard JL, Visser TJ: Biochemistry of deiodination. p. 189. In Hennemann G (ed): Thyroid Hormone Metabolism. Marcel Dekker, New York, 1986

87. Dumont JE, Tondeur-Montenez T: Action de l'hormone thyréotrope sur le métabolisme énergetique du tissue thyroidien. III. Evalution au moyen du ^{14}C glucose des voies du métabolisme du glucose, dans le tissue thyrodien de chien. Biochim Biophys Acta 3:258, 1965

88. Field JB, Epstein SM, Reemer AK, Boyle C: Pyridine nucleotides in the thyroid. Biochim Biophys Acta 121:241, 1964

89. Dumont JE, Vassart G, DeGroot LJ et al: Thyroid mitochondrial respiration. Endocrinology 79:28, 1966

90. Dumont JE: Carbohydrate metabolism in the thyroid gland. J Clin Endocrinol Metab 20:1246, 1960

91. Carafoly EN, Lehninger AL: A survey of the interaction of calcium ions with mitochondria from different tissues and species. Biochem J 122:681, 1971

92. Freinkel N: Action of pituitary thyrotropin on the inorganic phosphorus of thyroid tissue in vitro. Nature 198:889, 1963

93. Inatsuki B, Hiraga M, Anan FK: Studies on the biochemical properties of human thyroid gland mitochondria. J Biochem 74:837, 1973

94. Rheinwein D, Engelhardt A: Enzymmuster der menschlichen Schilddrüse II. Euthyreote und hyperthyreote Strumen. Klin Wochenschr 42:736, 1964

95. Schell E, Dumont JE: Mechanism of action of thyrotropin. In biochemical actions of hormones. p. I:415. Academic Press, San Diego, 1970

96. Lamy FM, Rodesch FR, Dumont JE: Action of thyrotropin on thyroid energetic metabolism. Exp Cell Res 46:518, 1967

97. Mockel J, Dumont JE: Protein synthesis in isolated thyroid mitochondria. Endocrinology 91:817, 1972

98. DeGroot LJ, Dunn AD: Electron-transport enzymes of calf thyroid. Biochim Biophys Acta 92:205, 1964

99. DeGroot LJ, Davis AM: Studies on the biosynthesis of iodotyrosines: the relationship of peroxidase, catalase, and cytochrome oxidase. Endocrinology 70: 505, 1962

100. DeGroot LJ, Dunn AD: Electron transport enzyme activities of human thyroid glands. J Lab Clin Med 71:984, 1968

101. Suzuki M, Nagashima M: Studies on the mechanism of iodination by the thyroid gland. 3. concentration of catalase, flavine, and cytochrome C oxidase in the pig thyroid gland and other tissues. Gunma J Med Sci 10:168, 1961

102. Pastan I, Herring B, Field JB: Changes in diphosphopyridine nucleotide and triphosphopyridine nucleotide levels produced by thyroid-stimulating hormone in thyroid slices in vitro. J Biol Chem 236: PC25, 1961

103. Nakumara Y, Ogihara S, Ohtaki S: Activation by ATP of calcium-dependent NADPH-oxidase generating hydrogen peroxide in thyroid plasma membranes. J Biochem 102:1121, 1987

104. Yamamoto K, DeGroot LJ: Peroxidase and NADPH-

cytochrome c reductase activity during thyroid hyperplasia and involution. Endocrinology 95:606, 1974

105. Ochi Y, DeGroot LJ: Stimulation of RNA and phospholipid synthesis by long-acting thyroid stimulator and by thyroid stimulating hormone. Biochim Biophys Acta 170:198, 1968

106. Kleiman D, Pisarev MA, Spaulding SW: Early effect of thyrotropin on ribonucleic acid transcription in the thyroid. Endocrinology 104:693, 1979

107. Lamy F, Willems C, Lecocq R et al: Stimulation by thyrotropin in vitro of uridine incorporation into the RNA of thyroid slices. Horm Metab Res 3:414, 1971

108. Lindsay RH, Cash AG, Hill JB: TSH stimulation of orotic acid conversion to pyrimidine nucleotides and RNA in bovine thyroid. Endocrinology 84:534, 1969

109. Hall R, Tubman J: The mechanism of action of thyroid stimulation hormone on nucleotide biosynthesis in the thyroid. p. 564. In: Current Topics in Thyroid Research. Academic Press, San Diego, 1965

110. Cartouzou G, Attali JC, Lissitzky S: Acides ribonucleiques messagers de la glande thyroide. 1. RNA a marquage rapide des noyaux et des polysomes. Eur J Biochem 4:41, 1968

111. Besson JE, Briere J, Radisson J et al: Ribosomal and transfer RNA contents of the normal and pathologic human thyroid gland. Biomedicine 27:193, 1977

112. Adiga PR, Murthy PVN, McKenzie JM: Stimulation by thyrotropin, LATS, and dibutyryl 3',5'-AMP of protein and RNA synthesis and RNA polymerase activities in porcine thyroid in vitro. Biochemistry 10:702, 1971

113. Jin S, Harnicek FJ, Neylan D et al: Evidence that adenosine 3',5'-monophosphate mediates stimulation of thyroid growth in FRTL$_5$ cells. Endocrinology 119:802, 1986

114. Sheinman SJ, Burrow GN: In vitro stimulation of thyroid ornithine decarboxylase activity and polyamines by thyrotropin. Endocrinology 101:1088, 1977

115. Tong W: TSH stimulation of ^{14}C-amino acid incorporation into protein by isolated bovine thyroid cells. Endocrinology 80:1101, 1967

116. Wagar G, Ekholm R, Bjorkman U: Action of thyrotropin (TSH) on thyroid protein synthesis in vivo and in vitro. Acta Endocrinol 72:453, 1973

117. Lecocq RE, Dumont JE: Stimulation by thyrotropin of amino acid incorporation into proteins in dog thyroid slices in vitro. Biochim Biophys Acta 281:434, 1972

118. Tong W, Sherwin JR: Stimulatory actions of thyrotropin and dibutyryl cyclic AMP on transcription and translation in the regulation of thyroidal protein synthesis. Biochim Biophys Acta 425:502, 1976

119. Creek RO: Effect of thyrotropin on the weight, protein, ribonucleic acid, and radioactive phosphorus of chick thyroids. Endocrinology 76:1124, 1965

120. Keyham E, Claude A, Lecocq RE, Dumont JE: An electron microscopic study of ribosomes and polysomes isolated from sheep thyroid gland. J Microsc 10:269, 1971

121. Kondo Y, DeNayer P, Salabe G et al: Function of isolated bovine thyroid polyribosomes. Endocrinology 83:1123, 1968

122. Lecocq RE, Dumont JE: In vivo and in vitro effects of thyrotropin on ribosomal pattern of dog thyroid. Biochim Biophys Acta 299:304, 1973

123. Pavlovic-Hournac M, Delbauffe D, Virion A, Nunez J: Protein phosphokinases of bound and free thyroid polyribosomes. FEBS Lett 33:65, 1973

124. Wagar G: Action of cyclic adenosine 3',5' monophosphate on 1-^{14}C-leucine incorporation in a system of rough microsomes from bovine thyroid gland. Acta Endocrinol 81:96, 1976

125. Pisarev MA, DeGroot LJ, Wilber JF: Cyclic-AMP production of goiter. Endocrinology 87:339, 1970

126. Freinkel N: Aspects of the endocrine regulation of lipid metabolism. p. 455. In Dawson MC, Rhodes DN (eds): Metabolism and Physiological Significance of Lipids. John Wiley & Sons, New York, 1965

127. Shah SN, Lossow WJ, Trujillo JL, Chaikoff IC: Metabolic characteristics of preparations of isolated sheep thyroid gland cells. II Fatty acid oxidation. Endocrinology 77:103, 1965

128. Freinkel N: Further observations concerning the action of pituitary thyrotropin on the intermediary metabolism of sheep thyroid tissue in vitro. Endocrinology 66:851, 1960

129. Kasabian SS, Pisarev VB: Histochemical characteristics of lipids in different forms of goiter. Arch Pathol 38:27, 1976

130. Svennerholm L: Gangliosides of human thyroid gland. Biochim Biophys Acta 835:231, 1985

131. Shetalova MV, Isaev El, Mansurov BM: Thyroid tissue phospholipids in different forms of pathology. Probl Endocrinol (Mosk) 28:28, 1982

132. Levis GM, Carli JN, Malamos B: The phospholipids of the thyroid gland. Clin Chim Acta 41:335, 1972

133. Schneider PS: Thyroidal synthesis of phosphatidic acid. Endocrinology 82:969, 1968

134. Scott TW, Good BF, Ferguson KA: Comparative effects of LATS and pituitary thyrotropin on the intermediate metabolism of thyroid tissue in vitro. Endocrinology 79:949, 1966

135. Burke G: On the role of adenyl cyclase activation and endocytosis in thyroid slice metabolism. Endocrinology 86:353, 1970

136. Jacquemin C, Haye B: Action de la TSH sur le meta-

bolisme des phospholipids thyroidiens in vitro. Bull Soc Chim Biol 52:153, 1970

137. Bollet AJ, Beierwaltes WH, Knopf RF et al: Extraocular muscle, skeletal muscle, and thyroid gland mucopolysaccharide response to thyroid-stimulating hormone. J Lab Clin Med 58:884, 1961

138. Bollet AJ, Beierwaltes WH: Acid mucopolysaccharide in the thyroid gland. J Clin Endocrinol Metab 19:257, 1959

139. Shishiba Y, Yanagishita M: Presence of heparan sulfate protcoglycan in thyroid tissue. Endocrinol Jpn 30:637, 1983

140. Wollman SH, Warren L: Effects of thyrotropin and thiouracil on the sialic acid concentration in the thyroid gland. Biochim Biophys Acta 47:251, 1961

141. Green ST, Peterson OH: Thyroid follicular cells: the resting membrane potential and the communication network. Pflugers Arch 391:119, 1981

142. Brunberg JA, Halmi NS: The role of ouabain-sensitive adenosine triphosphatase in the stimulating effect of thyrotropin on the iodide pump of the rat thyroid. Endocrinology 79:801, 1966

143. Stanbury JB: Thyrotropin stimulation of respiration and glucose-1-C oxidation by thyroid slices, as influenced by ouabain and sodium ion. Naunyn-Schmiedebergs Arch Exp Pathol Pharmakol 248:279, 1964

144. Williams JA: Effects of TSH on thyroid membrane properties. Endocrinology 86:1154, 1970

145. Konno N, McKenzie JM: In vitro influence of thyrotropin or long-acting thyroid stimulation on mouse thyroid membrane potential. Metabolism 19:724, 1970

146. Manly SW, Huchsham GJ, Bourkey R: Role of sodium influx in thyrotropin action: effects of the sodium channel agonist veratridine and thyrotropin on radioiodine turnover and membrane potential in cultured porcine thyroid cells. J Endocrinol 110:459, 1986

147. Endo Y, Tetsumoto T, Nagasaki H et al: The distinct roles of α- and β-subunits of human thyrotropin in the receptor-binding and postreceptor events. Endocrinology 127:149, 1990

148. Nagayama Y, Rapoport B: The thyrotropin receptor 25 years after its discovery: new insight after its molecular cloning. Mol Endocrinol 6:145, 1992

149. Kosugi S, Ban T, Akamizu T, Kohn LD: Identification of separate determinants on the thyrotropin recepter reactive with Graves' thyroid-stimulating antibodies and with thyroid stimulating blocking antibodies in idiopathic myxedema: these determinants have no homologous sequence on gonadotropin receptors. Mol Endocrinol 6:168, 1992

150. Goldfine ID, Amir SM, Ingbar SH, Tucker G: The interreaction of radioiodinated thyrotropin with plasma membrane. Biochim Biophys Acta 148:45, 1976

151. Morris JC, Bergert ER, McCormick DJ: Structure-function studies of the human thyrotrophin receptor. J Biol Chem 268:10900, 1993

152. Dallas JS, Desai RK, Cunningham SJ et al: Thyrotropin (TSH) interacts with multiple discrete regions of the TSH receptor: polyclonal rabbit antibodies to one or more of these regions can inhibit TSH binding and function. Endocrinology 134:1437, 1994

152a. Akaminu T, Inoue D, Kosugi S, Kohn LD, Mori T: Further studies of amino acids (206-304) in thyrotropin (TSH)-luteotropin/chorionic gonadotropin (LH/CG) receptor chimeras: cysteine-301 is important in TSH binding and receptor tertiary structure. Thyroid 4:43, 1994

153. Seetharamaiah GS, Wagle NM, Morris JC, Prabhakar BS: Generation and characterization of monoclonal antibodies can bind to discrete conformational or linear epitopes and block TSH binding. Endocrinology 136:2817, 1995

154. Kosugi S, Ban T, Akamizu T et al: Use of thyrotropin receptor (TSHR) mutants to detect stimulating TSHR antibodies in hypothyroid patients with idiopathic myxedema who have blocking TSHR antibodies. J Clin Endocrinol Metab 77:19, 1993

155. Kosugi S, Mori T: The amino-terminal half of the cytoplasmic tail of the thyrotropin receptor is essential for full activities of receptor function. Bioch Bioph Res Comm 200:401, 1994

156. Kosugi S, Mori T: The first cytoplasmic loop of the thyrotropin receptor is important for phosphoinositide signaling but not for agonist-induced adenylate cyclase activation. FEBS Letters 341:162, 1994

157. Kosugi S, Kohn LD, Akamizu T, Mori T: The middle portion in the second cytoplasmic loop of the thyrotropin receptor plays a crucial role in adenylate cyclase activation. Mol Endocrinology 8:498, 1994

158. Spaulding SN, Burrow GN: TSH regulation of cAMP-dependcnt protein kinase activity in the thyroid. Biochem Biophys Res Commun 59:386, 1974

159. Torhu-Delbauffe D, Ohayon R, Pavlovic-Hournac M: Protein kinase patterns in hyperplastic rat thyroids and in human nontoxic nodular goiter. Mol Cell Endocrinol 33:265, 1983

160. Lamy F, Roger P, Contour S et al: Control of thyroid cell proliferation: the example of the dog thyrocyte. Horm Cell Reg 153:168, 1987

161. Dumont JE, Boeynaems JM, de Coster C et al: Biochemical mechanisms in the control of thyroid function and growth. Adv Cyclic Nucleotide Res 9:723, 1978

162. Schumann SJ, Zor U, Chaoth R, Field JB: Exposure of thyroid slices to thyroid stimulating hormone in-

duces refractoriness of the cAMP system to subsequent hormone stimulation. J Clin Invest 57:1132, 1976

163. Field JB, Dekker A, Titus G et al: In vitro and in vivo refractoriness to thyrotropin stimulation of iodine organification and thyroid hormone secretion. J Clin Invest 64:265, 1979

164. Filetti S, Rapoport B: Hormonal stimulation of eukaryotic cell ADP ribosylation: effect of thyrotropin on thyroid cells. J Clin Invest 68:461, 1981

165. Rapoport B, Filetti S, Seto P: On mechanism of escape from desensitization of the cAMP response to TSH in cultured human thyroid cells. Mol Cell Endocrinol 36:181, 1984

166. Chazenbalk GD, Nagayama Y, Kaufman KD, Rapoport B: The functional expression of recombinant human thyrotropin receptors in non-thyroidal eukareotic cells provides evidence that homologous desensitization to thyrotropin stimulation requires a cell-specific factor. Endocrinology 127:1240, 1990

167. Heldin N-E, Gustavsson B, Hermomsson A, Westermark B: Thyrotropin (TSH)-induced receptor internalization in nonthyroidal cells tranfected with a human TSH-receptor complementary deoxyribonucleic acid. Endocrinology 134:2032, 1994

168. Tezelman S, Shaver JK, Grossman RF et al: Desensitization of adenylate cyclase in Chinese hamster ovary cells transfected with human thyroid stimulating hormone receptor. Endocrinology 134:1561, 1994

169. Nagayama, Chazenbalk GD, Takeshita A et al: Studies on homologous desensitization of the thyrotropin receptor in 293 human embryonal kidney cells. Endocrinology 135:1060, 1994

170. Berridge MJ: Inositol thriphosphate and diacylglycerol as second messengers. Biochem J 220:345, 1984

171. Exton JP, Blackmore PF: Calcium mediated hormonal responses. In DeGroot LJ (ed): Endocrinology. WB Saunders, Philadelphia, 1989

172. Roger PP, Reuse S, Servais P et al: Stimulation of cell proliferation and inhibition of differentiated expression by tumor-promoting phorbol esters in dog thyroid cells in primary culture. Cancer Res 46:898, 1986

173. Lombardi A, Veneziani BM, Tramontano D, Ingbar SH: Independent and interactive effects of tetradecanoylphorbol acetate on growth and differentiated functions of FRTL-5 cells. Endocrinology 123:1544, 1988

174. Bacharach LK, Eggo MC, Mak WW, Burrow GN: Phorbol esters stimulate growth and inhibit differentiation in cultured thyroid cells. Endocrinology 116:1603, 1985

175. Ginsberg J, Matowe W, Murray PG: Enhancement

of thyrotropin-stimulated iodide organification in porcine thyroid cells after protein kinase-C inhibition. Endocrinology 132:1815, 1993

176. Berman MI, Thomas Jr CG, Nyfeh SN: Stimulation of inositol phosphate formation in FRTL-5 rat thyroid cells by catecholamines and its relationship to changes in $^{45}CA^{2+}$ efflux and cAMP accumulation. Mol Cell Endocrinol 54:151, 1987

177. Brenner-Gati L, Trowbridge JM, Mucha CS, Gershengron MC: Thyrotropin-induced elevation of 1,2 diaglycerol and stimulation of growth of FRTL-5 cells are not dependent on inositol lipid hydrolysis. Endocrinology 126:1623, 1990

178. Murakami S, Summer CN, Iida-Klein A et al: Physiologic de novo thyroid hormone formation in primary culture of porcine thyroid follicles: adenosine 3′,5′-monophosphate alone is sufficient for thyroid hormone formation. Endocrinology 126:169, 1990

179. Bone EA, Alling OW, Grollman EF: Norepinephrine and thyroid stimulating hormone induce inositol phosphate accumulation in FRTL-5 cells. Endocrinology 119:2193, 1986

180. Field JB, Ealey PA, Marchall NJ, Cockcroft S: Thyroid stimulating hormone stimulates increase in inositol phosphate as well as cyclic AMP in the FRTL-5 rat thyroid cell line. Biochem J 247:519, 1987

181. Corda D, Marcocci C, Kohn LD et al: Association of the changes in cytosolic CA^{2+} and iodide efflux induced by thyrotropin and by the stimulation of α adrenergic receptors in cultured rat thyroid cells. J Biol Chem 260:9230, 1985

181a. Kumura T, Okajima F, Sho K, Kobayashi I, Kondo Y: Thyrotropin-induced hydrogen peroxide production in FRTL-5 thyroid cells is mediated not by adenosine 3′,5′-monophosphate, but by Ca^{2+} signalling followed by phospholipase—An activation and potentiation by an adenosine derivative. Endocrinology 136:116, 1995

181b. Wang X-D, Kiang JG, Smallridge RC: Identification of protein kinase C and its multiple isoforms in FRTL-5 thyroid cells. Thyroid 5:137, 1995

182. Brenner-Gati L, Berg KA, Gershengorn MC: Thyroid stimulating hormone and insulin-like growth factor-I synergize to elevate 1,2-diaglycerol in rat thyroid cells. J Clin Invest 82:114, 1988

183. Laurent E, Mockel J, van Sande J et al: Dual activation by thyrotropin of the phospholipase C and cAMP cascades in human thyroid. Mol Cell Endocrinol 52:273, 1987

183a. D'Arcangelo D, Siletta MG, DiFracesco AL et al: Physiological concentrations of thyrotropin increase cytosolic calcium levels in primary cultures of human thyroid cells. J Endocrinol Metab 80:1136, 1995

184. Lejuene C, Mockel J, Dumont JE: Relative contribu-

tion of phosphoinositides and phosphatidylcholine hydrolysis to the actions of carbamylcholine, thyrotropin (TSH), and pharbol esters on dog thyroid slices: regulation of cytidine monophosphate-phosphatidic acid accumulation and phospholipase-D activity. I. Actions of carmachylcholine, calcium ionophors, and TSH. Endocrinology 135:2488, 1994

184a. Mockel J, Lejeune C, Dumont JE: Relative contribution of phosphoinositides and phosphatidylcholine hydrolysis to the actions of carbamylcholine, thyrotropin (TSH), and pharbol esters on dog thyroid slices: regulation of cytidine monophosphate-phosphatidic acid accumulation and phospholipase-D activity. II. Actions of pharbol esters. Endocrinology 135:2497, 1994

185. Raspé E, Laurent E, Andry G, Dumont JE: ATP, bradykinine, TRH, and TSH activate the Ca^{2+}-phophatidyl inositol cascade of human thyrocytes in primary culture. Mol Cell Endocrinol 81:175, 1991

186. Corvilain B, Laurent E, Lecomte M et al: Role of the cyclic adenosine 3′,5′-monophosphate and the phosphatidylinositol-Ca^{2+} cascades in mediating the effects of thyrotropin and iodide on hormone synthesis and secretion in human thyroid slices. J Clin Endocrinol Metab 79:152, 1994

187. Tramontano D, Veneziani BM, Lombardi A et al: Iodine inhibits the proliferation of rat thyroid cells in culture. Endocrinology 125:984, 1989

188. Rapoport B, West MN, Ingbar SH: On the mechanisms of inhibition by iodine of the thyroid adenylate cyclase response to thyrotropic hormone. Endocrinology 99:11, 1976

189. Brenner-Gati L, Berg KA, Gershengorn MC: Insulin-like growth factor-I potentiates thyrotropin stimulation of adenylcyclase in FRTL-5 cells. Endocrinology 125:1315, 1989

190. Tramontano D, Cushing GW, Moses AC, Ingbar SH: Insulin-like growth factor-I stimulates the growth of rat thyroid cells in culture and synergyzes the stimulation of DNA synthesis induced by TSH and Graves' IgG. Endocrinology 119:940, 1986

191. Takahashi SI, Conti M, van Wijk JJ: Thyrotropin potentiation of insulin-like growth factor-I dependent deoxyribonucleic acid synthesis in FRTL-5 cells: mediation by an autocrine amplification factor(s). Endocrinology 126:736, 1990

192. Pang X-P, Hershman JM: Differential effects of growth factors on (^{3}H)thymidine incorporation and (^{125}I) iodine uptake in FRTL-5 rat thyroid cells. Proc Soc Expt Biol Med 194:240, 1990

193. Bacharach LK, Eggo MC, Burrow GN et al: Regulation of insulin-like growth factor-binding protein messenger ribonucleic acid levels in sheep thyroid cells. Endocrinology 128:1967, 1991

194. Kamamuri A, Abey Y, Yajima Y et al: Epidermal growth factor receptors in plasma membranes of normal and diseased human thyroid glands. J Clin Endocrinol Metab 68:899, 1989

195. Westmark K, Westmark B: Mitogenic effect of epidermal growth factor on sheep thyroid cells in culture. Exp Cell Res 138:47, 1982

196. Roger PP, Dumont JE: Epidermal growth factor controls the proliferation and the expression of differentiation in canine thyroid cells in primary culture. FEBS Lett 144:209, 1982

197. Westmark K, Karlsson FA, Westmark B: Epidermal growth factor modulates thyroid growth and function in culture. Endocrinology 112:1680, 1983

198. Gerard CM, Roger PP: Control of proliferation and differentation in primary cultures of calf thyroid cells. p. 345. In Medeiros-Neto G, Gaitan E (eds): New Frontiers in Thyrodology. Plenum, New York, 1986

199. Westermark K, Nilsson M, Ebendal T, Westermark B: Thyrocyte migration and histiotypic follicle regeneration are promoted by epidermal growth factor in primary culture of thyroid follicles in collagen gel. Endocrinology 129:2180, 1991

200. Tseng Y-CL, Burman KD, Schaudies RP et al: Effects of epidermal growth factor on thyroglobulin and adenosine 3′,5′-monophosphate production by cultured human thyrocytes. J Clin Endocrinol Metab 69:771, 1989

201. Lamy F, Taton M, Dumont JE, Roger PP: Control of protein synthesis by thyrotropin and epidermal growth factor in human thyrocytes: role of morphological changes. Mol Cell Endocrinol 73:195, 1990

202. Osawa S, Spaulding SW: Epidermal growth factor inhibits radioiodine uptake but stimulates deoxyribonucleic acid synthesis in newborn rat thyroids grown in nude mice. Endocrinology 127:604, 1990

203. Nilsson M, Ericsson LE: Effects of epidermal growth factor on basolateral iodide uptake and apical iodide permeability in filter-cultured thyroid epithelium. Endocrinology 135:1428, 1994

204. Corcoran JM, Waters MJ, Eastman CJ, Jorgensen G: Epidermal growth factor: effect on circulating thyroid hormone levels in sheep. Endocrinology 119:214, 1986

205. Ahrén B, Ericsson M, Hetner P et al: Somatostatin inhibits thyroid hormone secretion induced by exogenous TSH in man. J Clin Endocrinol Metab 47:1156, 1978

206. Ahrén B: Thyroid neuroendocrinology: neuroregulation of thyroid hormone secretion. Endocr Rev 7:149, 1986

207. Ahrén B: Regulatory peptides in the thyroid gland:

a review of their localization and function. Acta Endocrinol 124:225, 1991

208. Asakawa H, Miyagawa J-I, Hanafusa T et al: Interferon-τ reduces actin filaments and inhibits thyroid-stimulating hormone-induced formation of microvilli and pseudopods in mouse monolayer thyrocytes. Endocrinology 127:325, 1990

209. Michalkiewiecz M, Huffman LJ, Dey M, Hedge GA: Endogenous neuropeptide Y regulates thyroid bloodflow. Am J Physiol 264:699, 1993

210. Kennedy RL, Haynes WG, Webb DJ: Endothelins as regulators of growth and function in endocrine tissues. Clin Endocrinol 39:259, 1993

211. Arai M, Tsushima T, Isozaki O et al: Effects of retinoids on iodine metabolism, thyroid peroxidase gene expression, and deoxyribonucleic acid synthesis in porcine thyroid cells in culture. Endocrinology 129:2827, 1991

212. Takiyama Y, Tanaka H, Takiyama Y, Makino I: The effects of hydrocortisone and RU486 (mifepristone) on iodide uptake in porcine thyroid cells in primary culture. Endocrinology 135:1972, 1994

213. Shephard TH: Onset of function in the human fetal thyroid: biochemical and radioantographic studies from organ culture. J Clin Endocrinol Metab 27:945, 1967

214. Netter FH: Endocrine system and selected metabolic diseases. In: The Ciba Collection of Medical Illustrations. Vol. 4. Ciba, 1965

215. Teitelbaum SL, Moore KE, Shieber W: Parafollicular cells in the normal human thyroid. Nature 230:334, 1974

Thyroid Hormone Synthesis and Secretion

2

The hormones found in the thyroid and serum are two physiologically potent amino acids, L-thyroxine (tetraiodo thyronine, T$_4$) and L-triiodothyronine (T$_3$). T$_4$ is metabolically active primarily after its deiodination to T$_3$, but it is probably active itself when bound to receptors. In the following discussion, T$_4$ and T$_3$ are referred to collectively as the *thyroid hormones*. Each occurs naturally as the L isomer, and this isomer is implied unless the D isomer is specified.

Dietary iodide is absorbed through the small intestine and transported in the plasma to the thyroid. Plasma iodide is collected by the thyroid, oxidized, and bound to thyroglobulin (TG), where it is found in monoiodotyrosine (MIT) and diiodotyrosine (DIT) as well as in T$_4$ and T$_3$. After a variable period of storage in colloid, TG is resorbed, the peptide bonds of TG are cleaved, and the iodothyronines are liberated into the plasma. The thyroid hormones are transported in the plasma, attached by noncovalent bonds to proteins, and enter the cells of the body where they exert their characteristic stimulatory effects on cell metabolism through actions on gene transcription (Fig. 2-1).

In this chapter, iodine metabolism will be frequently discussed since it is crucial to thyroid hormone formation. T$_4$ is 65 percent iodine by weight, and T$_3$ is 58 percent. The thyroid hormones and their precursors and metabolites are the only iodine-containing compounds in the body that are known to have physiologic significance (Fig. 2-2).

The term *iodide ion* is used to refer to I$-$. *Iodine* is used generically to refer to the iodine molecule in any inorganic form, and molecular iodine is used to refer specifically to I$_2$. An unidentified hypothetical oxidized form related to hormonogenesis is referred to as an *oxidized iodine intermediate*.

AVAILABILITY AND ABSORPTION OF IODINE

The iodine intake of adult humans varies from less than 10 μg/day in areas of extreme deficiency to as much as a few grams per day for persons receiving medicinal iodine. In the United States the average intake in 1960 was about 100 to 150 μg/day, but it has since risen to an average intake of 200 to 500 μg/day and more from water, food, and medicines (see Ch. 5). The use of iodine as a bread conditioner in the baking industry nearly tripled average iodine

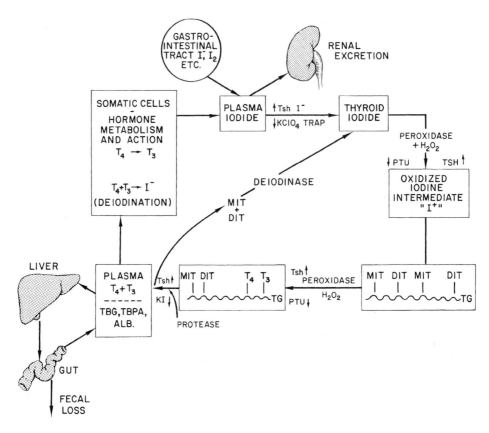

Fig. 2-1. The iodide cycle. Ingested iodide is trapped in the thyroid, oxidized, and bound to tyrosine to form iodotyrosines in TG; coupling of iodotyrosyl residues forms T_4 and T_3. Hormone secreted by the gland is transported in serum. Some T_4 is deiodinated to T_3. The hormone exerts its metabolic effect on the cell and is ultimately deiodinated; the iodide is reused or excreted in the kidney. A second cycle occurs within the thyroid gland, with deiodination of iodotyrosines generating iodide, some of which is reused without leaving the thyroid.

consumption. These additives, however, are now being replaced by other conditioners that do not contain iodine. Conversely, the increasing use of io-dophors as sterilizing agents, as in the milk industry, is adding much iodine to the food chain. Table salt often contains 0.005 to 0.01 percent iodine as a goiter preventive.

In addition to dietary sources, iodine appears in a large number of medical products that may find their way into the patient. It occurs in cough syrups, vitamin preparations, antiseptics, and a variety of substances employed as contrast media in roentgenography. Medicinal sources may provide iodine in amounts much larger than those consumed in an average diet and may cause confusion in the inter-

pretation of laboratory data obtained from patients suspected of having thyroid disease. For example, a patient receiving a saturated solution of potassium iodide as an expectorant could ingest 1 to 3 g of iodine daily. Radiographic contrast material typically contains grams of iodine in covalent linkage, and significant amounts (milligrams) may be liberated in the body. In contrast, some patients on salt restricted or other special diets may actually have low iodine intake.

Dietary iodine is reduced to the oxidation level of iodide before absorption, which occurs throughout the intestine, but principally in the small intestine. Absorption is virtually complete. Iodinated amino acids, including iodotyrosines T_4 and T_3, are trans-

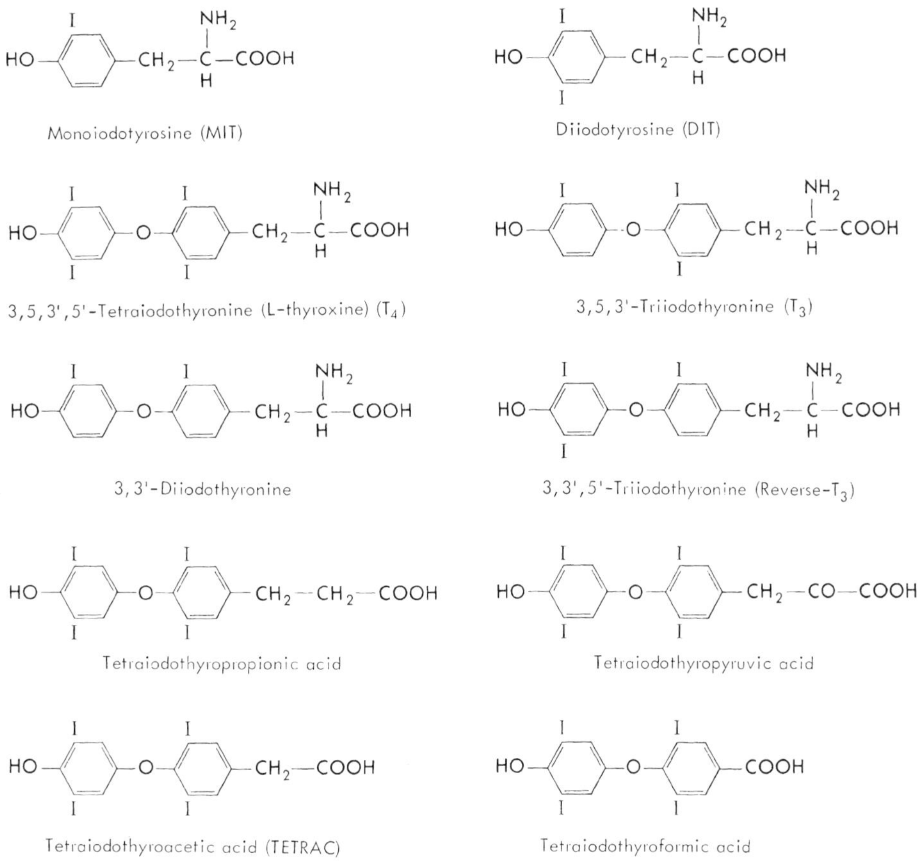

Fig. 2-2. Structural formula of compounds related to T_4.

ported intact across the intestinal wall. Short-chain iodopeptides may also be absorbed without cleavage of peptide bonds.[1] Iodinated dyes used in radiography are absorbed without deiodination, but some deiodination occurs after absorption.

Except in the postabsorptive state, the concentration of inorganic iodide in the plasma is usually less than 1 μg/dl. Absorbed iodide has a volume of distribution numerically equal to about 38 percent of body weight in kilograms.[2] It is largely extracellular, but small amounts are found in red cells, and detectable quantities penetrate the bones.

Iodide is removed from the plasma largely by the kidneys and the thyroid. The renal clearance of iodide is 30 to 50 ml plasma/min[2-4] and is little affected by the iodide load or by excretion of other anions such as chloride. In certain species, such as the rat, iodide clearance is depressed by large chlo-

ride loads. Renal iodide clearance in humans is closely related to glomerular filtration and is less than, but a linear function of, inulin clearance. There is no evidence of tubular secretion or of active transport with a transfer maximum.[5] Reabsorption seems to be partial and passive; it is depressed by an extreme osmotic diuresis. Potassium thiocyanate in humans does not alter renal iodide clearance, nor do thiazide diuretics. Renal clearance of iodide is normal or decreased in hypothyroidism and normal or increased in hyperthyroidism,[2,6] but the changes are indistinct. Iodide is also cleared by the salivary glands and the stomach, but since it is reabsorbed in the small bowel there is no net loss. (This process is evident in whole body isotope scans performed for evaluation of thyroid cancer.) Minute but detectable amounts appear in sweat and in expired air. Large amounts of iodide may appear in the milk of lactating females, mainly during the first 24 hours after ingestion.[7] This iodide would constitute a significant radiation hazard to an infant breast-feeding from a mother receiving ^{131}I for diagnostic tests or treatment.

On iodine diets of about 150 µg/day, the thyroid clears iodide from 10 to 25 ml of serum per minute (average, 17 ml).[2] The total effective clearance rate in humans is thus 45 to 60 ml/min, corresponding to a decrease in plasma iodide of about 12 percent/hr. The thyroidal iodide clearance varies greatly, depending on the average iodide intake and the presence of thyroid pathology. In iodine deficiency it may reach over 100 ml/min. It is reduced to 3 or 4 ml/min after chronic iodine ingestion of 500 to 600 µg/day (Fig. 2-3).

UPTAKE OF IODINE BY THE THYROID

The thyroid cells extract iodide from plasma and concentrate it in the interior of the cell and in the colloid.[8,9] This activity is best described as *iodide transport,* rather than *iodide trapping,* since there is no indication that the iodide is actually held in any complex within the thyroid. The extraction efficiency of the human thyroid is about 0.2—that is, one-fifth of the iodide perfusing the thyroid is removed in each passage through the gland.[10] The concentration of free iodide within the thyroid at any instant is determined by the relationship between the rate of entry of iodide into the thyroid cells and its removal, either through oxidation and

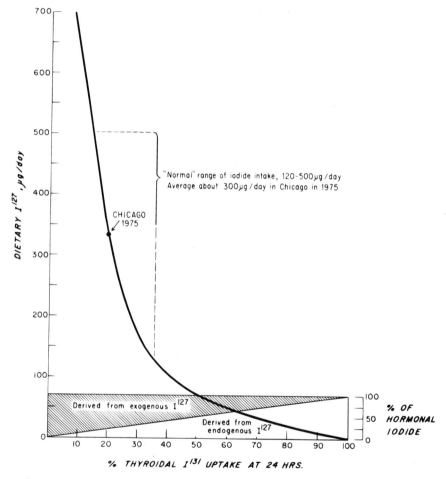

Fig. 2-3. Relationship of RAI intake in diet to the fractional uptake of tracer RAI at 24 hours, the conventional RAIU. With current generous amounts of iodide in the diet, approximately 300 to 500 µg/day, the normal RAIU is 10 to 30 percent.

binding to protein or by passive diffusion back into the blood.

The accumulation of free iodide ions in the thyroid can be readily demonstrated by administration of a drug of the thiocarbamide group, such as propylthiouracil (PTU). These drugs block oxidation and binding of iodide but do not prevent iodide transport. Under these conditions, the normal thyroid maintains a concentration of free iodide 20 of even 50 times higher than that of plasma.[11] This concentration gradient may be several hundred to one in the hyperactive gland of Graves' disease.

Other ions are also concentrated to a variable degree by the thyroid.[12] These ions include bromine (as bromide), astatine (as astatide), and technetium (as pertechnetate, rhenium, and chlorine in the TcO_4, ReO_4, and ClO_4 ions). Fluoride is not concentrated.

Iodide transport is an energy-dependent process requiring O_2 and is inhibited in vitro by CN^- and dinitrophenol. It is inhibited by ouabain, digitoxin, and other cardiac glycosides in vitro, and the inhibition is overcome by potassium.[13] Transport is dependent, therefore, on an adequate potassium level within the thyroid cells and is closely related to membrane ATPase. During gland hyperplasia, iodide transport and cell plasma membrane Na^+-K^+- activated ouabain-sensitive ATPase activity usually vary concordantly.[14] The iodide transporter is currently described as a "Na^+/I^- symporter." Transport of I^- by this membrane protein is driven by an inwardly directed Na^+ gradient produced by the Na^+-/K^+-activated ATPase. The mRNA for the protein has been expressed in frog oocytes,[15] and the cDNA will probably be cloned shortly. There is no evidence that free iodide in the gland exists in any state of oxidation other than iodide ion, or that it is attached to any intracellular receptor. Vilki[16] purified an iodide-complexing lecithin from the thyroid. No direct evidence ties this component to the iodide transport process,[17] but phospholipids are circumstantially related to transport phenomena in several tissues.

Iodide is present both in the thyroid cells and in colloid[8,9]; the cells, however, have a significantly higher concentration.[18] The iodide pump is active at both the base of the cells and the apex. Iodide pumped into the cell diffuses either into colloid or back into interstitial spaces and capillaries.

Iodide that enters the thyroid remains in the free state only briefly before it is further metabolized and bound to tyrosyl residues in protein. A significant proportion of intrathyroidal iodide is free during the first 10 to 20 minutes after administration of a radioactive tracer.[19] With the rapid buildup of protein- bound iodine (PBI) in the colloid, free iodide becomes relatively less significant, and in the steady state it is less than 1 percent of the total gland iodine content. A major fraction of this intrathyroidal free iodide pool is iodide derived from deiodination of MIT and DIT; this iodide is reorganified or leaked from the gland. Data from several laboratories[20,21] suggest that the iodide derived from active transport is somehow functionally separated from that which is generated by deiodination in the gland. The free iodide of the gland becomes organically bound at a rate between 50 and 100 percent of the pool each minute.[11,22] The transport and not the binding process is probably the metabolic control point for hormonogenesis. The proportion of an iodide load bound on any given day seems to vary little whether the gland is presented with one-tenth or five times the normal daily intake. Thus, the iodide-binding process seems to have great ability to accept an excessive load. Iodide transport is most likely governed by thyroid-stimulating hormone (TSH) in order to provide the required average daily thyroidal uptake of iodide; thus, transport activity ultimately controls hormonogenesis.

Iodide transport activity is increased by chronic TSH stimulation and depressed by TSH suppression. The initial response to increased TSH, surprisingly, is depression of the thyroid/serum iodide concentration gradient,[23] followed in a few hours by enhanced iodide transport due to synthesis of new proteins involved in the transport process. Presumably the TSH response involves cyclic adenosine monophosphate (cAMP), since cAMP can induce I^- transport in thyroid cells in vitro.[24]

IODIDE TRANSPORT IN OTHER ORGANS

The salivary glands and the gastric mucosa (both derived, as is the thyroid, from the primitive alimentary tract) also transport iodide and establish a concentration gradient between secretion and plasma that often exceeds 20:1.[25,26] The nature of the transport process may be similar since the three pumps are inhibited, as is the thyroid, by thiocyanate, perchlorate, and cardiac glycosides. Unlike the thyroid, the salivary and gastric glands do not respond to thyrotropic hormone. The choroid plexus also transports iodide, and iodide is freely transported across the placenta and into breast milk.

BIOSYNTHESIS OF T_4 AND T_3

Iodide concentrated by the thyroid cell is rapidly oxidized and bound to tyrosyl residues in TG. The iodotyrosines are coupled more slowly to form T_4 and T_3 (Fig. 2-4). The process requires the presence of iodide, a peroxidase, a supply of H_2O_2, and an iodide acceptor protein. These elements must be appropriately organized anatomically within the cell.

Peroxidase

Numerous laboratories have studied and partially purified thyroid peroxidase,[27–34] an enzyme that oxidizes iodide in the presence of H_2O_2, from a wide variety of thyroid tissues. In crude homogenates of thyroid, the enzyme activity is associated with thyroid cell membranes, but can dissociated from other proteins by use of enzymes such as trypsin or by detergents such as deoxycholate or digitonin. These preparations always contained a hemoprotein that had an absorbency peak at 423 mu when in the reduced form.[33,34] Thus, peroxidase is a heme protein with a prosthetic group that is ferriprotoporphyrin IX or a closely related porphyrin.[35,36] Chemical removal of the prosthetic group inactivates the enzyme, and the heme will recombine with the protein into an active protein.[37] The apoprotein from human thyroids is not always fully saturated with its prosthetic group.[38] Congenitally goitrous children have been identified who have poor peroxidase function because the apoprotein has weak binding for the heme group.[38]

Studies on thyroid "microsomal antigen" led, in our laboratory, to its identification as a pair of 101 to 107 kd proteins. Antibodies against "microsomal antigen" precipitated thyroid peroxidase (TPO), indicating the identity of the antigen long-studied in autoimmune thyroid disease (AITD), and the enzyme long-studied by biochemists.[39,40] A monoclonal antibody raised to purified "microsomal antigen" was used to clone human TPO. Its sequence has now been reported from three laboratories. Two forms of the molecule are produced by alternative

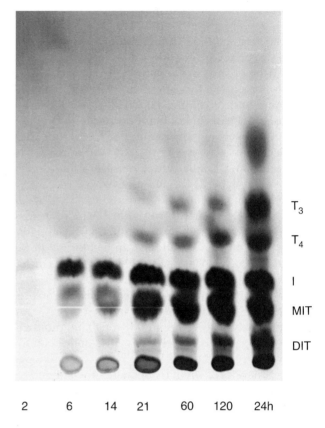

Fig. 2-4. Formation of iodotyrosines and iodothyronines in TG. Rats were pretreated with antithyroid drugs to produce thyroid hyperplasia. Later, ^{131}I was injected, and animals were killed at from two minutes to 24 hours. Thyroids were removed, homogenized, digested with pancreatin, and chromatographed in an ascending system. By 2 minutes MIT and DIT are clearly visible, by 14 minutes traces of T_4 are apparent, and by 21 minutes traces of T_3 are apparent. The material in the iodide spot is largely generated by deiodination of other compounds during enzymatic digestion of the homogenate.

splicing of the mRNA, leaving out one exon in the smaller form.

Kimura et al.[41] cloned two different cDNAs of TPO, one of 3048 and the second of 2877 bp. The large cDNA codes for a protein of 933 aa or 103,026 daltons, and the second has exon 10 coding for 57aa spliced out. Thus it codes for a protein of 96,744 daltons. Both forms are present in normal and abnormal human thyroid tissue. The differences between these MWs and the two forms of the TPO observed in sodium dodecyl sulfate (SDS) gels (107 and

100 kd) results at least in part from carbohydrate groups and iodine added during post-translational processing. There are five characteristic n-glycosylation sites in the TPO molecule,[42] and probably four are occupied by mannose rich oligosaccharides. It should be noted that the exact origin of the 107 and 100 kd forms has not been proven. There is no clear evidence for a different function of the smaller form of TPO, although, lacking one histidine present in the larger form, it may not function enzymatically.[43] Several types of mutations in the TPO gene, causing diminished iodide organification, have been reported (Ch. 2, 16).

TPO shares 46 percent nucleotide and 44 percent aa sequence similarities with human myeloperoxidase, and is clearly from the same gene family. The TPO gene is present on chromosome 2p13, spans over 150 kbp, and has 17 exons.[44,45] It contains domains similar to acetycholinesterase, low density lipoprotein (LDL) receptor, and insulin-like growth factors (IGF) receptor.

TPO mRNA expression is rapidly increased by TSH or cAMP through transcriptional activation.[46] The promoter does not, however, contain a typical cAMP response element. The cDNA has been expressed in several transfection systems which generate authentic TPO, and provide a source of the protein for functional or immunologic studies.[47] Two thyroid specific proteins (TTF-1 and TTF-2) which bind to the promoter of the TPO gene have been cloned,[48] and appear to drive thyroid cell specific expression of this gene. TTF-2 expression is induced by the cAMP cascade, and its binding to the TPO promoter is inhibited by factors which activate the protein kinase C (PKC) pathway.[48]

TPO is synthesized on polysomes, unidirectionally transported into the cell vesicle structures, transported to the Golgi apparatus where it undergoes glycosylation, and is then packaged into exocytotic vesicles along with TG.[49] These vesicles move to and fuse with the apical membrane in a process stimulated by TSH, and TPO is then found in the membrane associated with microvilli.

The apical membrane is internalized by micro- and macropinocytosis, and TPO may be recirculated by this route. TPO is not present in pseudopods or in colloid droplets.

H_2O_2 Supply

By definition, a peroxidase requires H_2O_2 for its oxidative function. In the thyroid this is probably derived from oxidation of pyridine nucleotides. Thyroid cell particles—mixed mitochondria, endoplasmic reticulum, lysozymes, and possibly other structures—oxidize and bind iodide to tyrosine or protein in a catalase-sensitive reaction.[50] The process is stimulated by the addition of nicotine adenine dinucleotide phosphate (NADPH) or nicotine adenine dinucleotide (NADH) and flavin nucleotides.[51–53] The microsomal enzyme NADPH-cytochrome c reductase is possibly responsible for H_2O_2 generation in these particles. Partially purified thyroid peroxidase, NADH-cytochrome c reductase, and a third factor (hematin, cytochrome c, vitamin K_3) have been combined to generate H_2O_2 and oxidize iodide.[54] Antibodies were prepared that combine with and inactivate the reductase, and cause a 50 percent inhibition of iodide binding in thyroid cell particles.[55] This indicates that the NADPH-cytochrome c reductase is one source of H_2O_2 for the peroxidation of iodide. The transfer of reducing equivalents from NADH to NADH-cytochrome B_5 reductase and cytochrome B_5 may be another source of H_2O_2 in the thyroid.[53] Studies by Pommier demonstrate the H_2O_2 is generated by a membrane-associated NADPH-oxidase system,[56] which is Ca^{2+} dependent. Since H_2O_2 generation is largely Ca^{2+} dependent in in vitro systems, this enzyme may be the major source of H_2O_2.

It is possible that NADH is provided by numerous substrate-linked reductions. NADPH might be generated by the HMP oxidation pathway for glucose. The levels of NADH and NADPH are closely linked to glucose oxidation but may be modulated by activity of transhydrogenases, mitochondrial oxidative phosphorylation, and reaction with glutathione[57] or ascorbate.[58] Glutathione reductase and glutathione peroxidase have both been detected in the thyroid. They might divert NADPH or H_2O_2 from use by the peroxidase and could be involved in modulation of iodination in the thyroid. Catalase, which destroys H_2O_2, is present in low concentration in the thyroid and may be an inhibitory factor.[59] Iodide in high concentrations is itself an in vivo inhibitor of iodination through mechanisms that have not been fully defined (see Ch. 5).

TSH actually stimulates NADPH reoxidation in the thyroid, especially by a microsomal respiratory pathway, suggesting a direct linkage to the observed increase in H_2O_2 generation caused by TSH.[60] In vitro studies indicate that TSH can stimulate H_2O_2

generation through both the cAMP cascade and the Ca^{2+} phosphatidylinositol cascade, although the exact linkage is unclear.[61]

Acceptor Molecules

Thyroid peroxidase will iodinate soluble tyrosine and numerous proteins in vitro. In vivo it donates the oxidized iodine intermediate largely to tyrosyl groups in TG (and histidyl residues), but other soluble proteins (e.g., thyroalbumin) and particle-associated insoluble proteins are also iodinated. These proteins are described in detail below.

Certain lipids are also iodinated by the in vitro iodinating systems. Suzuki et al. identified iodinated phosphatidylserine and sphingomyelin; they detected other iodolipids also, but have not yet identified them.[58]

Anatomic Site

Peroxidase has been identified in tissue particles containing mitochondria, lysosomes, and microsomes.[61,62] It is rarely found in significant quantities in the soluble fraction of cell homogenates. Electron microscopic histochemical studies have found the enzyme in the endoplasmic reticulum, Golgi, secretory droplets, and apical cell membranes.[62–63] Exocytotic vesicles contain TG and thyroalbumin, and some have peroxidase in their membranes.[63] The vesicles fuse with the apical membrane and contribute their peroxidase to the membrane; in the process, the proteins are iodinated and transferred to colloid.[64] Peroxidase may be removed from the membrane by "coated pits" into "multivesicular bodies".[64] The cytochrome reductase enzymes are associated with microsomes, i.e., the endoplasmic reticulum. Both exocytosis and H_2O_2 generation are stimulated by TSH.[65] Radioautographic studies show that iodination is occurring at the apical cell border, with the PBI inside the follicle[66–68] (Figs. 2-5 and 2-6). This process probably indicates iodination of protein at the cell border in exocytotic vessels and subsequent transfer into colloid when these vesicles fuse with the apical plasma membrane. Since

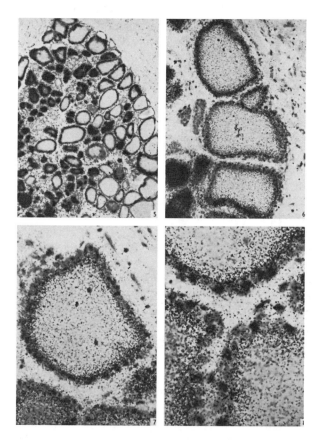

Fig. 2-5. Radioautographs of rat thyroid sections. Animals received iodide shortly before being killed, and radioautographs of thyroid sections were coated with emulsion after being stained by the usual methods. The radioautographs indicated the presence of iodide over the cells, primarily over the colloid, forming a ring reaction at these early intervals.

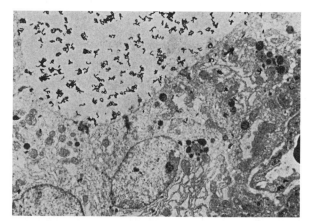

Fig. 2-6. Electron micrograph and radioautograph of a mouse thyroid. The animal received radioactive ^{125}I 25 minutes before death. The radioautograph shows a uniform distribution of grains of ^{125}I over the colloid area and an association of grains with the microvilli ($\times$ 5,700).

isolated cultured thyroid cells can iodinate protein in the incubating medium, it appears that protein outside the cell can also be iodinated.

Mechanism of Tyrosine Iodination

Iodide is oxidized by peroxidase to a reactive intermediate, which then reacts with tyrosine in peptide linkage. Several groups have addressed the exact mechanism of the iodination. Studies by Taurog[68] indicate that I_2 is probably not the reactive iodine intermediate. The reaction may involve single electron oxidations of iodide and peptidyl–tyrosine to free radical states and their subsequent nonenzymatic formation of iodotyrosine.[69] Studies at the University of Chicago suggest that iodide and tyrosine have separate binding sites on the enzyme, are each oxidized by the loss of one electron, and combine to form peptidyl–iodotyrosine, while the reactive intermediates are held on the peroxidase[33,70] (Fig. 2-7). Davidson et al.[71] have found evidence for a reactive oxidized protein-bound intermediate. Ohtaki et al.[34–36] studied rapid spectral absorption

changes in peroxidase reacting with H_2O_2, I^- and tyrosine. Their data indicate that the preferred route is oxidation of enzyme by H_2O_2, followed by a two-electron oxidation of I^- to I^+, which then reacts with tyrosine. Ohtaki and coworkers also provided evidence that TPO catalyzes a two electron oxidation of tyrosine or MIT, and a one-electron oxidation of DIT.[36]

The thiourylene antithyroid drugs propylthiouracil (PTU) and methimazole (MMI) probably inhibit iodination by multiple mechanisms. In low concentration, PTU and MMI compete with tyrosine for activated I^+, and the thiourylenes are metabolized with loss of their –SH group. At high concentrations, TPO is irreversibly inhibited, perhaps by interaction of the antithyroid drug with the heme of TPO.[72] Free DIT is a natural endogenous inhibitor of TPO. As might be expected, iodination of TG is independent of its synthesis. Compounds such as puromycin prevent TG synthesis in vitro but do not impede iodination.

A mechanism of iodide binding involving formation of a reactive sulfenyl–iodide intermediate has

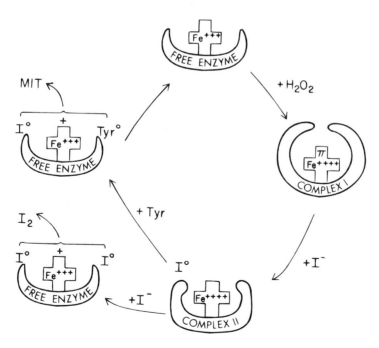

Fig. 2-7. Hypothetical reaction scheme for thyroid peroxidase. In this reaction sequence modeled after that of horseradish peroxidase, H_2O_2 is presumed to oxidize the free enzyme with a loss of two electrons, forming complex I. Iodide is oxidized and binds to the enzyme to form complex II, which may then react either with another iodide molecule or tyrosine. The free radicals of iodide and tyrosine may then unite to form MIT and release the free enzyme.

been proposed. Although sulfenyl iodides may appear in thyroid tissue, their role in thyroid hormone formation is not established.[73] The subunits of TG presumably contain a large number of –SH groups when initially synthesized, but mature iodinated TG has all but two to three such groups oxidized to form –S–S– intrachain bonds. This oxidation goes on pari passu with iodination of TG, and it may be mediated by iodide peroxidase and the oxidized iodine intermediate formed by the peroxidase.

Significant formation of thyroid hormone does not occur outside the thyroid gland.

Regulation of Peroxidation by Iodide

Iodide has an acute inhibitory effect on hormonogenesis and hormone release (Fig. 2-8). This mechanism, known as the "Wolff-Chaikoff block," has resisted final explanation for years.[74,76] A direct inhibition of iodide oxidation by peroxidase, possibly through reduction of the oxidized iodine intermediate by iodide, with formation of I_3, has been proposed by Nunez and coworkers,[76] but direct in vitro inhibition of peroxidase has not been found by others.[70] Possibly I^- somehow reduces H_2O_2 generation, since the Wolff-Chaikoff block can be overcome in vitro by the addition of TSH or an H_2O_2 generating system.[77] Exposure of thyroid tissue to high levels of iodide in vitro causes inhibition of basal adenyl cyclase activity; this may also be related to the block of peroxidase function. The inhibitory action of I^- requires its oxidation to form some intermediate, since methimazole prevents the inhibitory actions of I^-. Various compounds have been proposed, including, recently an iodolactone (an iodinated derivative of arachidonic acid).[78] DIT also regulates thyroid peroxidase in vitro, stimulating T_4 synthesis at low concentrations (0.05 mM) and inhibiting enzyme function at high concentrations (5 mM).[79]

Coupling of Iodotyrosines

Shortly after MIT and DIT are formed, iodinated thyronines appear. The lag period of 14 to 60 minutes[19] presumably is the time necessary for a detectable quantity of labeled iodothyronine to accumulate, rather than the time actually required for the biosynthetic process itself.

The iodothyronine molecule is formed by joining the iodinated hydroxyphenyl group of one iodotyrosine residue to the phenolic hydroxyl of another[80] (Fig. 2-9). This so-called coupling reaction is probably complicated, for it involves a transfer of a large residue between two peptide-linked amino acids. Thyronine itself, the iodine-free backbone of thyroid hormones, is not a constituent of TG, and there is

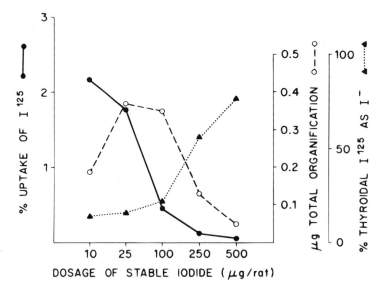

Fig. 2-8. Demonstration of the Wolff-Chaikoff block induced by iodide in the rat. Animals were given increasing doses of stable iodide. Total organification initially increased, but as the dose was increased further, a depression of organification of iodide and an increase in the free iodide present in the thyroid gland occurred.

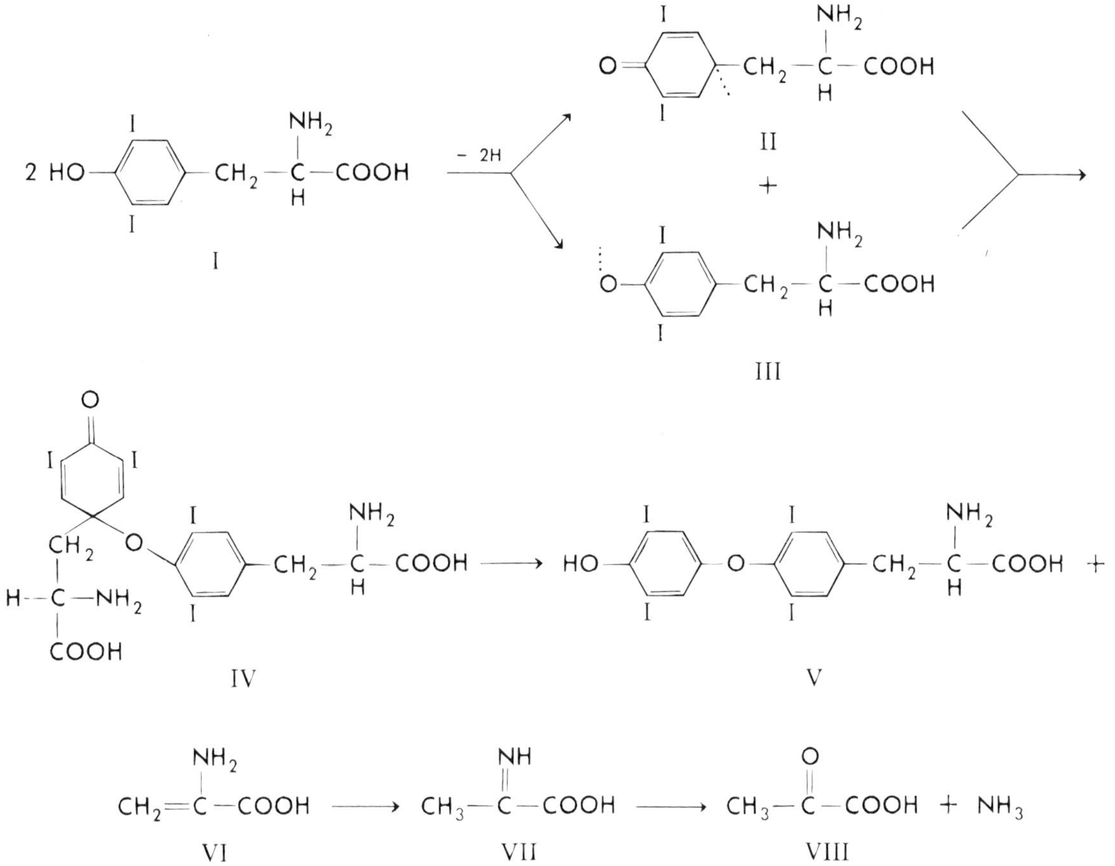

Fig. 2-9. Possible coupling reaction sequence. Oxidation of I (iodotyrosine) may produce II and III, free tyrosyl radicals. These radicals can combine to produce transient product IV, which stabilizes by degrading to V (T_4) and VI (dehydroalanine). The last compound forms compound VII by rearrangement and then, with the addition of water, forms compound VIII (pyruvic acid and ammonia).

no evidence for a synthetic mechanism involving iodination of peptide-bound thyronine. Direct evidence for the postulated sequence comes from observations by Wain.[81] He found that [^{14}C] tyrosine was incorporated into TG, and ultimately the ^{14}C was present in MIT, DIT, and T_4. Gavaret et al.[82] have subsequently observed dehydroalanine in TG after the intramolecular coupling of two iodotyrosyl residues.

Peroxidase mediates coupling.[83,84] Since coupling is an oxidative process, one might expect that some oxidized intermediate (e.g., I$^+$) generated by peroxidase would actually perform the required oxidation, as can I_2. Available data, however, indicate that peroxidase can mediate coupling without involvement of iodine. Further, there is no evidence for a separate coupling enzyme. Given the appropriate steric con-

figuration of the iodothyrosines in the protein, and the presence of peroxidase and an H_2O_2 supply, coupling occurs without other enzyme mediation.

Researchers have suggested that the initial iodination of tyrosyl residues occurs on an immature TG in an uncoiled form, with its tyrosyl groups readily open to the iodinating enzymes. During the next phase of maturation, the molecule may develop a coiled secondary structure as –S–S– bonds and ionic or hydrogen bonds are formed, thereby placing the iodinated tyrosyls in neighboring coils and facilitating the transfer of an iodophenyl group (Fig. 2-10). An alkaline pH or 6 M guanidine, which tend to unfold the TG molecule, hinder T_4 formation during iodination of TG in vitro.[85,86]

The peptide structure of TG imposes important restrictions on the iodination process. Iodination of

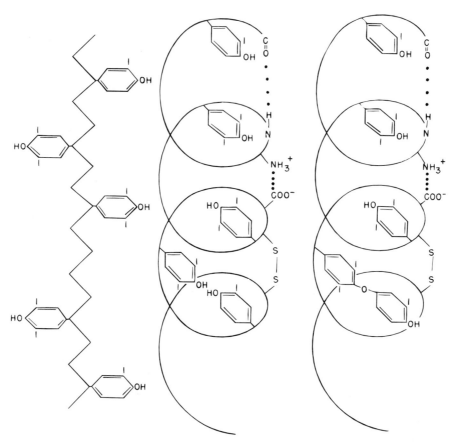

Fig. 2-10. A hypothetical model of the coupling reaction. It is proposed that the immature form of TG is iodinated. During iodination there is formation of disulfide and ionic bonds that mold the molecule into its final tertiary structure, allowing certain iodotyrosyl residues to be appropriately positioned. An oxidative process then forms an intermediate iodophenol free radical, which joins with another iodotyrosine to form T_3 or T_4.

TG follows an ordered sequence such that (in vitro) most molecules are iodinated to the same extent.[87] Formation of T_4 and T_3 involves specific iodotyrosyl donor sites and unique peptide acceptor sequences occurring in TG where coupling takes place.[88–91] Accumulating evidence supports a role for a donor iodotyrosine in the hTG molecule at the following sites: tyrosine 130, tyrosines between aa 2451 and 2597, tyrosine 5 (an important hormonogenic site at which T_4 is formed), sites at Tyr 2553, 2567, and 2746 (possibly specific for T_3),[91] and at Tyr 685 and Tyr 1290.[91] The amino acid sequence in which T_3 is formed may commonly be ser-tyr-ser.[92]

When iodine is added progressively to TG in vitro, first MIT forms, then DIT, and finally T_3 and T_4.[93] Iodine is consumed beyond what is bound to tyrosine

because of oxidation of sulfhydryl groups. Although large amounts of MIT and DIT can be generated in the molecule, formation of T_3 and T_4 is limited. Thus, only certain iodotyrosyl groups are sterically positioned to permit coupling. TG is a good substrate protein for tyrosine iodination and coupling; during in vitro iodination more than 6 percent of added iodine may appear in T_4. TG is not unique in this, however, since other large proteins such as IgM and fibrinogen can also be iodinated and form T_4 almost as readily.

Yip and Klebanoff found that T_4 is formed in vitro when DIT is incubated with L-amino acid oxidase. They suggested that 4-hydroxy diiodophenylpyruvic acid formed by the amino acid oxidase reacted with another molecule of DIT.[94] Enzymes in the thyroid are capable of forming the pyruvate derivative of DIT, and peroxidase could form a reactive hydroperoxide of this compound. In addition diiodophenyl pyruvate hydroperoxide is capable of reacting with DIT to form T_4. Interesting as such possibilities are, there is little evidence that significant amounts of free DIT or MIT occur in the thyroid, or that free iodotyrosines combine with peptidyl–tyrosine in TG.

Kinetics

Radioautographs of thyroid tissue sections demonstrate protein-bound iodine (PBI) 15 to 20 seconds after intravenous administration of radioactive iodine (RAI). In resting glands, bound ^{131}I first appears as a ring at the periphery of the colloid. It then rapidly diffuses through the colloid. In very active glands, the entire colloid is uniformly labeled within 10 to 15 minutes.[66] The speed of mixing is inversely related to the size of the follicle. Within 20 minutes of injection of ^{131}I into rats, 90 to 95 percent of the accumulated iodide in the thyroid is organically bound, and at 24 hours this figure rises to 99 percent.[19]

Most of the accumulated iodide is bound to the soluble protein TG, which is primarily located in the colloid. When the labeled proteins are digested and analyzed by chromatography, labeled iodine is found as MIT and DIT, and after 15 to 60 minutes as T_4 and T_3[19] (Fig. 2-2). Iodine is also bound to intracellular particulate protein. Within the first few minutes of administration of ^{131}I to rats, 10 to 20 percent of the PBI in the thyroid is closely attached to cell particles.

Iodination of TG is progressive, and in the steady state, TG contains 90 to 95 percent of the iodine in the gland. The ratio of MIT to DIT in TG remains quite constant from the earliest minutes of hormonogenesis.[19] Apparently some of the tyrosyl residues are iodinated to the monoiodo-level and others to DIT in a ratio determined by the amount of the oxidized iodine intermediate formed in relation to available tyrosyl receptor groups.[33] In highly stimulated and in iodide-deficient glands, therefore, the ratio of MIT to DIT is greatly increased.

Although formation of MIT in TG occurs within minutes, coupling of iodotyrosyl residues proceeds much more slowly. After an isotope tracer is given in vivo, hours or days may be required before the coupling process achieves a steady-state level of iodothyronine in TG.

When the rat thyroid is in a near equilibrium condition, the DIT fraction comprises about 40 to 45 percent of the iodine, MIT about 20 percent, T_4 about 15 to 25 percent, and T_3 3 to 10 percent.[95] Iodohistidine has been described[96] in TG, as well as minute amounts of 3,3′,5′-triiodothyronine and 3,3′-diiodothyronine. The physiologic significance, if any, of the latter iodinated species is unknown.

Minimal quantities of free (in contrast to peptide-linked) iodinated amino acids are present in the thyroid. Taurog and coworkers[97] found that the specific activity of ^{131}I in free iodinated amino acids is initially less than that in TG, indicating that the free iodinated amino acids are byproducts of TG rather than precursors, and it seems certain that tyrosine is iodinated after its incorporation into this protein. Labeled iodinated amino acids, for instance, are found within TG 15 seconds after injection of iodine[66]; this seems too fast for a de novo synthesis of significant quantities of TG molecules from prelabeled iodotyrosine. Also, thyroidal tRNA does not become "charged" by binding iodotyrosines.[98] In addition, iodination and T_4 synthesis proceed when protein synthesis is abolished by the action of puromycin.

As discussed below, the peptide backbone of TG is made on ribosomes; sugars are then added in the endoplasmic reticulum and the Golgi apparatus. This "noniodinated molecule" is the substrate for iodination. The synthesis and secretion of the protein is a relatively leisurely process requiring hours, in contrast to the rapid process of iodination.[99,100]

TG AND RELATED PROTEINS

Approximately 90 to 95 percent of iodine bound to protein in the gland is in the colloid as part of the TG molecule.[101] From 5 to 10 percent of the iodine is found in the insoluble cell particles, mitochondria, microsomes, and particulate material closely associated with cell nuclei. In addition, other soluble iodinated proteins are found in normal and diseased glands.

TG

The major protein constituent of the thyroid is TG, an enormous (670,000 dalton) glycoprotein that comprises 70 to 80 percent of the protein of the

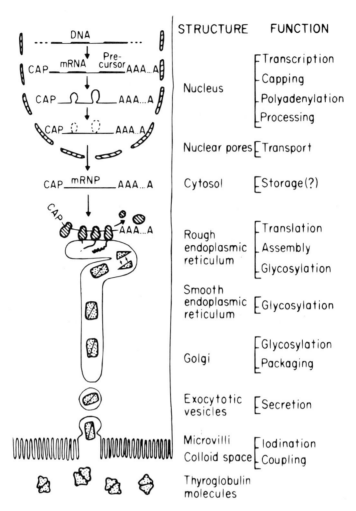

STRUCTURE	FUNCTION
Nucleus	Transcription Capping Polyadenylation Processing
Nuclear pores	Transport
Cytosol	Storage(?)
Rough endoplasmic reticulum	Translation Assembly Glycosylation
Smooth endoplasmic reticulum	Glycosylation
Golgi	Glycosylation Packaging
Exocytotic vesicles	Secretion
Microvilli Colloid space	Iodination Coupling
Thyroglobulin molecules	

Fig. 2-11. The sequence of formation and maturation of the thyroglobulin molecule. The process begins with formation and processing of the mRNA, which is then translated on the rough endoplasmic reticulum. The two subunits are fused, glycosylation follows in the smooth endoplasmic reticulum and in the Golgi, and the molecule is packed into secretory vesicles that approach the microvilli and are iodinated as they are secreted into the colloid space. (From Van Herle et al,[100] with permission.)

gland, coded by a gene on chromosome 8. The protein is formed on large membrane-bound polyribosomes (composed of perhaps 25 to 50 ribosomes)[102] in the endoplasmic reticulum (Fig. 2-11). During in vitro study of TG biosynthesis in thyroid slices, peptides of various sizes appear which are probably fragments or multimers of TG.[103] These are designated according to their sedimentation characteristics as S_{3-8}, S_{12}, S_{17}, S_{19}, and S_{27}.[103] The S_{12} unit represents the 330,000-dalton subunit of TG, and two similar subunits combine to form the noniodinated S_{17} molecule. When 33 S mRNA is translated by in vitro protein-synthesizing systems, the primary product is a 330,000-dalton peptide,[104] encoding in the human a 2748 aa polypeptide with a 19 aa signal peptide. The newly formed TG molecule, comprised of two homo-dimers which may be linked by disulfide bonds, has a sedimentation constant of about 17. This changes to about 19 S on iodination because of conformational shifts induced by iodination and gylcosylation.[105] The protein of the S_{4-5} fraction is probably not in TG monomers, but rather represents other proteins, such as thyroalbumin. The S_{27} fraction represents two closely associated, highly iodinated 19 S molecules.[106] In addition to a polymeric structure, TG may have small peptides associated with it in noncovalent linkage.[107]

cDNAs for both human and animal TGs have been cloned and completely sequenced.[108–109] Although the entire gene has not yet been sequenced, the 5′ flanking DNA comprising the gene promoter has been. Thyroid cell specific proteins such as TTF-1, TFF-2, and Pax-8, bind to specific sequences in the TG promoter to allow its expression in thyroid tissue.[110] Lack of these specific transacting factors in other tissues prevents expression of the gene.

Iodination favors aggregation of TG subunits into the 19 S (or even 27 S) form.[111] A paucity of iodide in the molecule, as in iodide deficiency, produces a TG molecule that is especially easy to dissociate into subunits, probably because fewer disulfide bonds bind the subunits together.[112]

After the peptide is synthesized, carbohydrate chains are added while it is still in the endoplasmic reticulum. It is then transported to the Golgi apparatus, where terminal glycosylation of TG may occur; this glycosylation occurs on subunits of TG before formation of the mature protein. The carbohydrate exists in up to 30 separate units of three different types, composed of aspartic acid-N-acetyl glucosamine, mannose, galactose, fucose, and sialic acid.[100,102,114]

Core carbohydrate units are synthesized as dolichol derivatives, which are transferred en bloc to asparagine, serine, and threonine residues of the TG amino acid skeleton. The carbohydrate units are further processed by deletion and addition of sugars in the endoplasmic reticulum, especially in the Golgi apparatus.[115] After packaging into a secretory droplet in the Golgi apparatus, a terminal sialic acid molecule is added to each of the carbohydrate units. This may be related to the final secretion of the molecule.

The newly formed molecule with its carbohydrate units in place is transported to the colloid and is iodinated in the process.[116] Radioautographic studies confirm this sequence, and show that TG synthesis and transport take several hours.

The Tg molecule contains about 200 cysteine residues, almost all of which exist in the oxidized state as disulfides. This oxidation of free–SH groups to disulfides may occur at an equal rate with the iodination of the molecule, and is believed to relate to the development of the mature molecule's conformation and to the coupling of iodotyrosines. Iodine-poor

TG has a few more free sulfhydryls than normal protein.[117] It is less likely to form 27 S dimers and is more readily degraded by thyroid acid protease than is iodine-rich protein.[118]

TG that has been extensively purified by salt fractionation and gel filtration[119] has been studied after reduction, alkylation, or succinylation, in order to break disulfide bridges bonding subunits together and to permit complete separation of the subunits. The molecule is readily broken into two subunits of about 330,000 daltons, and then into further subunits of ± 160,000 daltons. Smaller subunits of 20,000 to 80,000 daltons may arise from proteolysis of the subunits.[120,121] Formation of these TG fragments is augmented by ongoing iodide peroxidation, suggesting that this peptide bond cleavage may be a normal part of TG iodination.[122]

The amino acid composition of TG in the thyroid is remarkably similar in specimens from different human subjects and even from different species.[108,109,123–125] Each TG molecule contains approximately 140 tyrosyl residues.[126] Only about 40 of the tyrosyl groups are available for iodination, and only 8 to 10 are hormonogenic sites. The average molecule is about 0.5 percent iodine and thus contains an average of 26 iodine atoms per molecule. Normally each molecule carries 2 to 3 T_4 residues, and T_3 is present in some but not all of the TG molecules. The thyroids of rats on diets containing plentiful iodine had molar ratios for the iodine of the iodinated amino acids as follows: DIT = 44; MIT = 28; T_4 = 16; and T_3 = 4. These data indicate there were six DIT residues, seven MIT residues, and one T_4 residue per molecule of TG in the animals, with one T_3 residue in about every third molecule. In the glands of iodine-deficient rats, the iodine molar ratios of the amino acids were: DIT = 24; MIT = 28; T_4 = 12; and T_3 = 6. These data indicate there were four residues of DIT, nine of MIT, one of T_4, and one of T_3 per TG molecule.[19] These data agree with the observations of several investigators that the DIT/MIT ratio and the T_4/T_3 ratio are directly related to the following function:

$$\frac{\text{Oxidized iodine intermediate}}{\text{Available tyrosyl acceptor sites}}$$

This relationship is seen with in vitro systems.[50] In animals given cycloheximide to inhibit TG synthesis, DIT/MIT ratios go up, as does T_4 synthesis.[127] Thus, either an increase in iodide oxidation or a decrease

TABLE 2-1. Iodine and Hormone Content of Thyroid Tissue

Tissue	Total ^{127}I (μg/g)	T_4 (μg/g)	T_3 (μg/g)	T_4I as % of Total I
Normal	630 ± 60	154 ± 3.9	21 ± 3	26 ± 3
Toxic Graves' Gland	450	295	56	42

	$^{127}I\%$	Atoms I / Mole TG	Mole T_4 / Mole TG	Mole T_3 / Mole TG	Mole T_4 / Mole T_3	T_3I as % of Total I	T_4I as % of Total I
Normal	0.42 ± 0.21	22 ± 11	2.5 ± 1.5	0.18 ± 0.1	13 ± 4	2.4 ± 0.05	41 ± 12
Toxic Graves' Gland	0.56 ± 0.12	29 ± 6	3.4 ± 0.6	0.39 ± 0.08	9 ± 2	4.1 ± 0.8	48 ± 10

in TG synthesis favors more formation of DIT and T_4 and less formation of MIT and T_3. The content of T_4 in TG increases, as noted before, in linear relation to ^{127}I content in the range 0.73 to 1.6 percent iodine. Poorly iodinated TG with less than 0.10 percent iodine contains almost no T_4 or T_3.[128] At high levels of iodination, up to six residues of T_4 and two of T_3 may be present in each molecule. Normal human TG has been reported to have a T_4 content of 172 μg/g, a T_3 content of 19 μg/g, and a T_4/T_3 ratio of 13.[129] Larsen[129,130] has reported values for the T4, T3, and iodine content of normal and toxic thyroids (Table 2-1).

The MIT/DIT ratio is also increased in certain pathologic states, including thyrotoxicosis, and in nodules from multinodular goiters.[131] The basis for the alteration is unknown, but it probably represents a limitation in the formation of oxidized iodine among available TG acceptor sites. (This explanation, admittedly, merely restates our ignorance of the process.) In vitro studies of chemical iodination of iodine-poor human TG indicate the same relationships between iodine content and iodoamino acid distribution. With increasing ^{127}I, MIT and DIT, DIT/(MIT + DIT), T_4 and T_3, $T_4/(T_4 + T_3)$, and $(T_4 + T_3)/(MIT + DIT)$ all increase.[128]

The normal human thyroid gland contains enough preformed T_4 to maintain euthyroidism for two months without new synthesis. The TG reserve is thus an excellent buffer against the vicissitudes of dietary iodine intake, both as a store of hormone and as a store of iodine.

T_4 liberated from TG by proteolysis within the gland may be bound by hydrogen bonds to TG. This could serve to protect T_4 from the deiodinase activity of peroxidase present in this tissue or other deiodinases active on iodothyronines.

Thyroalbumin

Soluble iodoproteins distinct from TG may constitute 2 to 13 percent of the iodoprotein in normal human and animal glands and a much higher proportion in abnormal glands.[132–138] One such protein, thyroalbumin, is similar to albumin in its electrophoretic, ultracentrifugal, and solubility characteristics. It contains iodotyrosines and iodothyronines, but their ratios are different from those in TG. Usually there is a high ratio of MIT to DIT and of iodotyrosines to iodothyronines. Earlier studies suggested thyroalbumin was synthesized in the thyroid,[135] and it is certainly iodinated in the gland.[134] Large amounts of an albumin-like protein found in some cystic thyroid lesions suggest that the serum albumin pool readily enters the gland.[101] Recent studies clearly show that "thyralbumin" is serum albumin iodinated in the thyroid.[139] Iodinated albumin has been found in the thyroid glands and sera of patients with Hashimoto's thyroiditis,[136] congenital metabolic defects,[137] thyrotoxicosis,[138] and thyroid carcinoma.[132] This protein may account for some of the 10 to 15 percent of the protein-bound iodine present in normal serum, in a nonbutanol extractable form (in contrast to T_4 and T_3) and thus is described in older literature as "NBEI." Peptides derived from it may appear in the urine. Its half-life in serum is similar to that of serum albumin.

Particulate Iodoproteins

Newly formed TG is associated with thyroid cell membranes and can be dissociated by deoxycholate. These are partially processed molecules[140] with lower carbohydrate and iodine content on their way to colloid. Proteins of smaller size and degradation products of TG are also found in the cell particulate fraction.[141] An iodoprotein attached to cell particles is formed both in vivo and in thyroid tissue slices incubated in vitro.[142] Its turnover rate and resistance to enzymatic hydrolysis indicate that it is distinct from TG. In certain instances of intense thyroid hyperplasia and TG depletion, the particulate protein may be the major fraction of the iodoprotein in the thyroid.[143]

HORMONE STORAGE

Transport of TG from the Cell and Storage in Colloid

The exocytotic vesicles containing TG (and other proteins) are formed in the Golgi apparatus and transported to the cell surface.[144] This process involves folding of the nascent polypeptide in association with molecules such as BiP and chaperonins (which guide the folding), formation of a compact molecule with intrachain disulfide bonds, formation of the dimer, and, through a molecular sorting process, the guiding of the TG molecule to the apical border.[142,143] During this process, the molecule undergoes glycoslyation. The vesicle walls combine with the apical membrane, and the contents are extruded into the colloid space. Microvilli on the apical cell membrane provide increased surface for this secretory activity. Secretory vesicles appear in the villi, which are elongated in active glands. Secretion and iodination are closely coupled, since the exocytotic vesicles carry TPO to the cell membrane where H_2O_2 formation occurs. Secretion of apical vesicles into colloid is regulated by TSH through cAMP and PKA, and in some species by the PKC pathway as well.

Turnover of colloid varies greatly with gland activity. The organic iodide pool, largely in the colloid, turns over at the rate of ± 1 percent per day in normal humans.[2] As the turnover rate increases, less and less colloid is stored, until with extreme hyperplasia none is evident. In such glands, the entire organic iodine content may be renewed each day.[2] In this situation, secretion and reabsorption of colloid are probably still required for hormone formation, although only tiny amounts of colloid are present at any time.

With the obvious exception of iodination, there is no knowledge of the biochemical events occurring in the colloid. Since both iodination of TG and formation of T_4 and T_3 occur in the colloid, there must be either a recirculation of TG through the cell or a reaction of the iodide peroxidase with TG in the colloid. Protease and acid phosphatase may be in the colloid and could induce colloid conditioning before resorption.

HORMONE SECRETION

TG secretion and resorption are functionally linked and proceed in a coordinated fashion. The exocytotic vesicles contribute their membrane to the apical membrane; this membrane is then reinternalized in the resorptive process through formation of colloid droplets.[145] Resorption of TG probably involves an interaction of the protein with membrane receptors. Researchers have identified binding sites for TG on thyroid membranes.[146] Consiglio et al.[147,148] have shown that removal of the terminal sialic acid and galactose from TG carbohydrate units, exposing N-acetylglucosamine residues, augments TG binding and may be involved in uptake of the protein via an N-acetylglucosamine-specific receptor on the cell surface.[148a]

The normal resorptive process includes both macro- and micropinocytosis. Microvilli, or pseudopods, of the cell apical membrane surround a small bit of colloid and pinch it off to form an intracellular colloid droplet[149] (Fig. 2-12). Internalization of colloid by formation of smaller vesicles (micropinocytosis) also occurs, but the role of this pathway is less well established.[144] Increased formation of colloid droplets is one of the earliest effects of TSH stimulation of the gland, occurring within a few minutes. This process may involve microtubules and microfilaments in transporting the droplet.[149,150] It has been estimated[151] that a normal rat thyroid cell forms about one such droplet every 2 to 17 minutes. Once inside the cell, the droplets fuse with an endosome.[152] At this stage, some sorting of thyroglobulin molecules apparently occurs, so that some are recycled back to the colloid space while others are further processed.[153] TG is next passed to a lysosome that has been mobilized from the cell base toward the cell apex, forming a phagosome (Fig. 2-14). The lysosome contains acid proteases, peptidases, and acid phosphatase, probably in an acidic environment.[154–157] Cathepsin D and thiol (cysteine) pro-

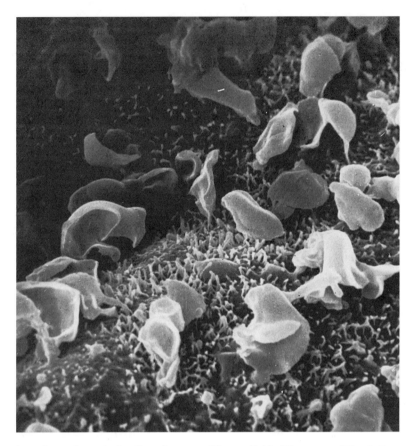

Fig. 2-12. Pseudopods on the apical cell surface engulfing colloid. (Courtesy of Dr. J. Dumont, Boussels.)

teases appear to participate in TG hydrolysis.[158] These proteinases cleave TG to release small peptides containing T_4 and T_3, which are, in turn, later cleaved by exopeptidases to release the hormone.[159]

Glutathione reductase is thought to transfer reducing equivalents to the TG, breaking disulfide linkages and fostering proteolysis. In the phagosome, the TG appears to be completely degraded to its component amino acids, and the released T_4 and T_3 then make their way to the bloodstream. The iodotyrosines are deiodinated by a microsomal flavoprotein deiodinase,[160,161] and the liberated iodide is partially reutilized and partially lost from the cell. This internal iodide cycle is important because three to five times as much iodide is formed inside the gland each day by deiodinase activity as enters the cell from the serum.[2]

The phagosome's fate is to shrink as it digests. It migrates toward the cell base over one to two hours and eventually becomes indistinguishable from a ly-

sosome. Possibly it is recycled. Usually iodine recently bound in the gland is secreted before preexisting material—the "last come, first served" phenomenon. This may occur because newer iodide is near the apical cell surface. In some circumstances, the order of secretion is reversed.[162]

The primary thyroid secretory products are T_4, T_3, and iodide. A small amount of T_4 (about 10 percent is converted by monodeiodination to T_3 in the thyroid by a Type 1 iodothyronine 5′-deiodinase that is inhibited by PTU and is similar to the enzyme present in liver.[163] The extent of deiodination is increased in TSH- or TSAb-stimulated thyroids.[164] T_4 and T_3 thus leave the thyroid in a slightly lower ratio than present in TG, about 10:1 on a weight basis. Average normal secretion in euthyroid humans is 94 to 110 μg T_4 and 10 to 22 μg T_3.[163,164] In peripheral tissues, 30 to 40 percent of T_4 is converted by monodeiodination to T_3, providing about 80 percent of the T_3 available to tissues. Some T_4 is also converted to reverse T_3 (rT3) in the thyroid. Some iodide is secreted by the gland or leaked as a result of inefficiency in reuse of iodide generated through iodotyrosine dehalogenase activity.[2,165,166] This leak is increased as the human gland adapts to high daily iodine intake,[165] possibly in an autoregulatory process, which may serve to prevent excessive TG iodination. Estimates of nonhormonal iodide release vary. Normal glands may release up to 50 μg of iodide each day on an intake of about 100 μg.[2]

A vastly greater iodide leak occurs in diseased glands. Ohtaki et al.[165] found that iodide leak was present in all glands but increased markedly with gland iodine content, presumably reflecting a dependence of iodide leak on iodide intake and found the mean quantity to be about 38 μg when the mean T_4 secretion was 53 μg/day. A small amount of TG is released and can be found in thyroid lymph and in serum.[168] This TG is cleared from the blood with a half-time of about four days. Clearance from the blood is presumed to involve desialation, since removal of asialo-TG is much more rapid than intact TG.[169] TG binds to receptors on thyroid membranes and inhibits binding of TSH to its membrane receptors.[146] TG also inhibits TSH and TSAb stimulation of adenyl cyclase; thus, it may have an inhibitory regulatory feedback effect on thyroid function.[170] Thyroalbumin may be secreted, especially by hyperactive glands. Small amounts of iodotyrosines are normally released, and in very hyperplastic glands, increased iodotyrosines can be detected in blood.[171] The DIT content of normal serum averages 100 ng/100 ml.[172] DIT is increased in thyrotoxicosis and mildly decreased in hypothyroidism, and is present in serum from patients who are fasting. The DIT arises from the thyroid, the diet, and other undisclosed sites.[171]

rT3 is also formed in the thyroid[173] and is secreted in miniscule amounts. Blood levels in normal subjects are about 10 to 30 ng/100 ml. Blood rT3 is largely derived from peripheral conversion of L-T_4 to rT3.[174]

CONTROL OF HORMONE SYNTHESIS

The basic control of iodide organification and hormone synthesis is by the TSH feedback mechanism (see Ch. 4). TSH serves to maintain a sufficiently active iodide transport and iodide peroxidase system to ensure uptake and binding of the required amount of iodide: 70 to 100 μg/day in adult men (Fig. 2-13). Normally the rate of the reaction is set by the iodide transport process, which is directly controlled by TSH levels. Sufficient excess peroxidase and H_2O_2 generating capacity are usually available to bind several times the average daily iodide uptake, should a sudden increase in plasma iodide level occur.[75] TSH stimulation of the thyroid induces increased iodide transport and binding. The acute stimulatory effect of TSH on iodide binding, however, is not due to increased iodide uptake; it may be due to increased provision of H_2O_2. More chronic TSH stimulation leads to increased iodide uptake, H_2O_2 generation, and formation of more peroxidase enzyme. In the human thyroid, TSH appears to exert its positive effects on hormone formation primarily by the phospho-inositide pathway which is activated by high concentrations of TSH.[175]

Regulation of Peroxidation

TSH, acting through its receptors, coupled to Gs proteins, increases cAMP production, which in turn activates protein kinase A. Activation of this pathway leads to cell growth, TPO and TG gene expression, increased I^- transport, increased H_2O_2 generation, and increased hormone secretion.[175,176] Prostaglandins and norepinephrine may have less important effects by the same pathway. Activation of muscarinic receptors in a second signalling pathway leads to hydrolysis of phosphatidylinositol 4,5 phosphate, generation of inositol 1,4,5 phosphate and diacylglycerol, increased intracellular Ca^{2+}, and activation of protein kinase C. This pathway, which can be activated by TSH, may also stimulate iodination, cell growth, and gene expression, but has inhibitory effects on hormone secretion (Fig. 2-14).[176a]

Secretion of thyroid hormone is regulated by TSH through a cAMP-responsive system and also a phosphatidylinositol system (see Ch. 1). Administration of TSH leads to secretion of T_3 within one to two hours, followed by a release of T_4 and TG.

Secretion of hormone in animals can be increased by sympathetic nerve stimulation and directly by α- and β-adrenergic agonists.

Although TSH is the primary determinant of thyroid function, its effect is modulated by a variety of growth factors.[176] The intricacies of these effects remain obscure. EGF stimulates thyroid growth by

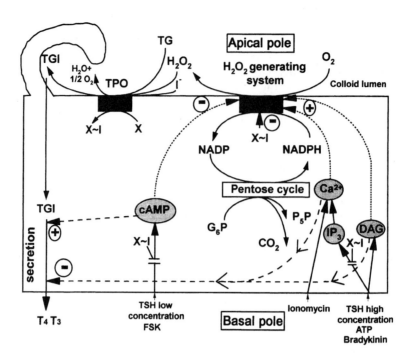

Fig. 2-13. Possible scheme for the control of H_2O_2 generation, iodide organification, hormone secretion, and pentose phosphate pathway activity in human thyroid. cAMP, Second messenger; G_6P, glucose-6-phosphate; P_5P, pentose-5-phosphate; DAG, diacylglycerol; TG, thyroglobulin; X~--, inhibitory action of X~I; + dotted arrow, positive control of H_2O_2 generation; − dotted arrow, negative control of H_2O_2 generation; + dashed arrow, positive control of hormone secretion; − dashed arrow, negative control of hormone secretion. In the human thyroid the TSH-R → cAMP pathway activated at low TSH levels may inhibit iodination, while higher levels of TSH activate the process through the TSH-R → PIP pathway. (From Corvilain et al,[175] with permission.)

binding to a membrane EFG receptor, and coincidentally actually down-regulates hormonogenesis. EGF is secreted by thyroid cells, indicating that growth factors can regulate thyroid cells in an endocrine, paracrine, and autocrine manner.[176] IGF–I and TGF α1, and basic fibroblast growth factor, have similar actions, and IGF-1 is also secreted by thyroid cells.[177] TSH stimulates IGF-1 production by thyroid cells, and TSH + IGF-1 have synergistic effects.[178] Transforming growth factor beta (TGFβ) is also produced in thyroid cells, and appears to function as an autocrine/paracrine inhibitor of thyroid growth by inhibition of TSH, IGF-1, EGF, and TGFα stimulation.[179,180] Like EGF, TGFβ1 inhibits iodide uptake and TPO synthesis, thus having a "dedifferentiating" function.[181] The lymphokines IL-1α, IL-1β, and IFNγ inhibit hormonogenesis during in vitro experiments,[182] and IFNγ inhibits TG synthesis[181] and TPO gene expression.[184–186] IL-1α appears to

induce thyroid nonresponsiveness to TSH.[187] These cytokines may modulate hormonogenesis in patients with autoimmune disease.

SUMMARY

The thyroid hormones, precursors, and degradation products are the only naturally occurring iodine-containing compounds in the body. Hormone biosynthesis is, therefore, intimately related to iodine metabolism. In western nations, iodide intake is plentiful, averaging around 300 μg/day, in contrast to many parts of the world where iodide-deficiency diseases persist.

Dietary iodide is largely absorbed and is cleared by excretion in the urine or by active transport into the thyroid. The accumulated free iodide is rapidly oxidized by thyroid peroxidase and H_2O_2, and

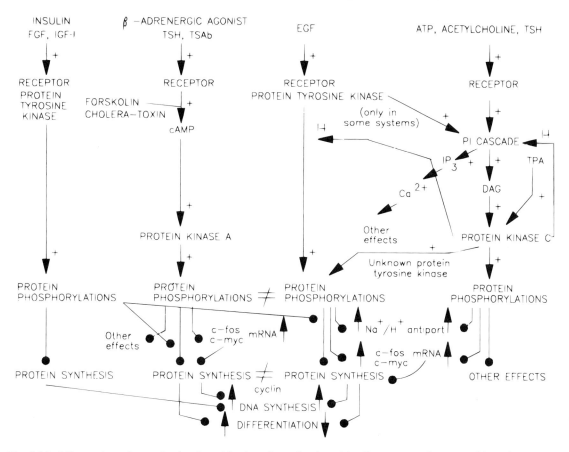

Fig. 2-14. Mitogenic pathways in the thyroids: data from the thyroid cell system are integrated into the present scheme of cell proliferation cascades. DAG, diacylglycerol; EGF, epidermal growth factor; FGF, fibroblast growth factor; IGF, insulin-like growth factor (somatomedin); IP_3, inositol 1,4,5-triphosphate; Pi, phosphatidylinositol; TPA, phorbol ester; TSI, thyroid-stimulating immunoglobulin; ≠, not overlapping patterns; →+, stimulation; ><><, time sequence for which the causal relationships remain to be proved. (From Dumont et al,[177] with permission.)

bound to tyrosine present in the peptide backbone of thyroglobulin. This reaction is believed to occur at the apical cell border so that iodination actually occurs on thyroglobulin present in secretory droplets or present in the colloid space.

The primary substrate for iodination is thyroglobulin, a huge protein of 670,000 kd MW formed from two similar subunits bound together by ionic and disulfide bonds. Thyroglobulin (TG) the protein of which thyroid hormone is formed, is synthesized on the endoplasmic reticulum, glycosylated, and probably phosphorylated as it passes through the Golgi system, and then becomes a substrate for iodination in secretory droplets, where it coexists with TPO in the membrane of the droplets. Thyroid per-

oxidase is a protoporphyrin-IX heme protein that is uniquely expressed in the thyroid. It probably forms iodotyrosines by one electron oxidation of iodide and of tyrosine, and is also responsible for coupling of iodotyrosines within the framework of the thyroglobulin molecule to form the iodothyronines.

Although TG contains approximately 140 tyrosyl residues, only about 40 are available for iodination under most stringent conditions, and fewer—perhaps 8 to 10—are hormonogenic sites. Each molecule, when fully iodinated, normally contains one T_3 molecule and two or three T_4 molecules. Specific tyrosines appear to function as donors for the coupling reaction, and others as the acceptor tyrosine where T_4 and T_3 are formed. Donor tyrosines include those at tyrosine-130 and others in the carboxy terminal portion of the molecule, and important acceptor (hormonogenic) sites exist at tyrosine 5, and possibly at tyrosines 2553, 2567, and 2746. The actual mechanism of the coupling reaction (by thyroid peroxidase, perhaps involving iodine, and augmented by diiodotyrosine) is unknown, but may involve a free radical mechanism involving transfer of an iodophenyl group to the acceptor iodotyrosine molecule.

The iodinated thyroglobulin is stored in colloid for a period ranging from a few hours to 100 days, depending on the activity of the gland, and is then resorbed by macro- and micropinocytosis. The resorption droplets fuse with endosomes. At this stage, some thyroglobulin may be recycled to the colloid space while more is passed to lysosomes in which the molecule is degraded, releasing iodotyrosines and iodothyronines. The iodotyrosines are partially deiodinated, and while much iodide is reused, some is leaked from the thyroid. Some thyroxine is released to the bloodstream, and some is deiodinated to triiodothyronine within the gland.

Hormone synthesis is primarily under the control of thyroid-stimulating hormone (TSH), acting through its receptor and the cyclic-AMP and phosphoinositide pathways. The phosphoinositide pathways appear to be primarily involved in fostering hormone synthesis in the human thyroid, whereas cyclic-AMP may be more involved in regulating secretion. Thyroid growth is regulated by TSH and other growth factors, including insulin, insulin-like growth factors (IGF), and epidermal growth factor (EGF). EGF and similar factors appear to stimulate growth and dedifferentiation, in contrast to the stimulation of differentiated activities of the thyroid by TSH.

REFERENCES

1. Wynn JO: Components of the serum protein-bound iodine following administration of I[131]-labeled hog thyroglobulin. J Clin Endocrinol Metab 21:1572, 1961
2. DeGroot LJ: Kinetic analysis of iodine metabolism. J Clin Endocrinol Metab 26:149, 1966
3. McConahey WM, Keating FR, Power MH: An estimation of the renal and extrarenal clearance of radioiodine in man. J Clin Invest 30:778, 1951
4. Bricker NS, Hlad CJ Jr: Observations on the mechanism of the renal clearance of I[131]. J Clin Invest 34:1057, 1955
5. Perry WF, Hughes JFS: The urinary excretion and thyroid uptake of iodine in renal disease. J Clin Invest 31:457, 1952
6. Berson SA, Yalow RS, Sorrentino J, Roswit B: The determination of thyroidal and renal plasma I[131] clearance rates as a routine diagnostic test of thyroid dysfunction. J Clin Invest 31:141, 1952
7. Weaver JC, Kamm ML, Dobson RL: Excretion of radioiodine in human milk. J Amer Med Assn 173:872, 1960
8. Pitt-Rivers R, Trotter WR: The site of accumulation of iodide in the thyroid of rats treated with thiouracil. Lancet 2:918, 1953
9. Andos G, Wollman SH: Autoradiographic localization of radioiodide in the thyroid gland of the mouse. Am J Physiol 213:198, 1967
10. Pochin EE: Investigation of thyroid function and disease with radioactive iodine. Lancet 2:41, 1950
11. Berson SA, Yalow RS: The iodide trapping and binding functions of the thyroid. J Clin Invest 34:186, 1955
12. Wolff J: Transport of iodide and other anions in the thyroid gland. Physiol Rev 44:45, 1964
13. Wolff J: Thyroidal iodide transport. I. Cardiac glycosides and the role of potassium. Biochim Biophys Acta 38:316, 1960
14. Brunbert JA, Halmi NS: The role of ouabain sensitive adenosine triphosphatase in the stimulating effect of thyrotropin on the iodide pump of the rat thyroid. Endocrinology 79:801, 1966
15. Vilijn F, Carrasco N: Expression of the thyroid sodium/iodide symporter in *Xenopus laevis* oocytes. J Biol Chem 264:11901, 1989
16. Vilki P: An iodide-complexing phospholipid. Arch Biochem Biophys 97:425, 1962
17. Schneider PB, Wolff J: Thyroidal iodide transport. VI. On a possible role for iodide-binding phospholipids. Biochim Biophys Acta 94:114, 1965
18. Chow SY, Yen-Chow YC, Woodbury DM: Compartmentation in the turtle thyroid: water and iodide distribution. Endocrinology 108:2200, 1981
19. DeGroot LJ, Davis AM: The early stage of thyroid hormone formation: studies on rat thyroids in vivo. Endocrinology 69:695, 1961
20. Hildebrandt JD, Scranton JR, Halmi NS: Intrathyroidally generated iodide: its measurement and origins. Endocrinology 105:618, 1979
21. Rosenberg IN, Athans JC, Ahr CS, Behar A: Thyrotropin-induced release of iodide from the thyroid. Endocrinology 69:438, 1961
22. Ingbar SH: Simultaneous measurement of the iodide-concentrating and protein-binding capacities of

the normal and hyperfunctioning human thyroid gland. J Clin Endocrinol Metab 15:238, 1955

23. Halmi NS: Thyroidal iodide transport. Vitam and Horm 19:133, 1961
24. Knopp J, Stolc V, Tong W: Evidence for the induction of iodide transport in bovine thyroid cells treated with thyroid stimulating hormone and dibutyryl cyclic adenosine 3′, 5′-monophosphate. J Biol Chem 245:4403, 1970
25. Brown-Grant K: Extrathyroidal iodide concentrating mechanisms. Physiol Rev 41:189, 1961
26. Alexander WD, Harden RM, Mason DK: Comparison of the concentrating ability of the human salivary gland for bromine, iodine, and technetium. Arch Oral Biol 11:1205, 1966
27. DeGroot LJ, Davis AM: Studies on the biosynthesis of iodotyrosines: a soluble thyroidal iodide-peroxidase tyrosine-iodinase system. Endocrinology 70:492, 1962
28. Nagasaka A, DeGroot LJ, Hati R, Liu C: Studies on the biosynthesis of thyroid hormone: reconstruction of a defined in vitro iodinating system. Endocrinology 88:486, 1971
29. Alexander NM: Purification of bovine thyroid peroxidase. Endocrinology 100:1610, 1977
30. Coval ML, Taurog A: Purification and iodinating activity of hog thyroid peroxidase. J Biol Chem 242:5510, 1967
31. Ljunggren J, Akeson A: Solubilization, isolation, and identification of a peroxidase from the microsomal fraction of beef thyroid. Arch Biochem Biophys 127:346, 1968
32. Rawitch AB, Taurog A, Chernoff SB, Dorris ML: Hog thyroid peroxidase: physical, chemical, and catalytic properties of the highly purified enzyme. Arch Biochem Biophys 194:244, 1979
33. DeGroot LJ, Niepomniszcze H: Biosynthesis of thyroid hormone: basic and clinical aspects. Metabolism 26:665, 1977
34. Ohtaki S, Nakagawa H, Kimura S, Yamazaki I: Analyses of catalytic intermediates of hog thyroid peroxidase during its iodinating reaction. J Biol Chem 256:805, 1981
35. Ohtaki S, Nakagawa H, Nakamura M, Yamazaki I: Reactions of purified hog thyroid peroxidase with H_2O_2, tyrosine, and methylmercaptoimidazone (Goitrogen) in comparison with bovine lactoperoxidase. J Biol Chem 257:761, 1982
36. Ohtaki S, Nakagawa H, Nakamura M, Yamazaki I: One- and two-electron oxidations of tyrosine, monoiodotyrosine, and diiodotyrosine catalyzed by hog thyroid peroxidase. J Biol Chem 257:13398, 1982
37. Krinsky MM, Alexander NM: Thyroid peroxidase: nature of the heme binding to apoperoxidase. J Biol Chem 246:4755, 1971
38. Niepomniszcze H, DeGroot LJ, Hagen GA: Abnormal thyroid peroxidase causing iodide organification defect. J Clin Endocrinol Metab 34:607, 1972
39. Portmann L, Hamada N, Heinrich G, DeGroot LJ: Antithyroid peroxidase antibody in patients with autoimmune thyroid disease: possible identity with antimicrosomal antibody. J Clin Endocrinol Metab 61:1001, 1985
40. Hamada N, Portmann L, DeGroot LJ: Characterization and isolation of thyroid microsomal antigen. J Clin Invest 79:819, 1987
41. Kimura S: Structure and regulation of the human thyroid peroxidase gene. p. 3. In Carayon P, Ruf J (eds): Thyroperoxidase and Thyroid Autoimmunity. John Libbey Eurotext, London, 1990
42. Rawitch AB, Pollock G, Yang SX, Taurog A: The location and nature of the N-linked oligosaccharide units in porcine thyroid peroxidase: studies on the tryptic glycopeptides. p. 69. In Carayon P, Ruf J (eds): Thyroperoxidase and Thyroid Autoimmunity. John Libbey Eurotext, London, 1990
43. Kimura S, Kotani T, McBride OW et al: Human thyroid peroxidase: complete cDNA and protein sequence, chromosome mapping, and identification of two alternately spliced mRNAs. Proc Natl Acad Sci USA 84:5555, 1987
44. de Vijlder JJM, Dinsart C, Libert F et al: Regional localization of the gene for thyroid peroxidase to human chromosome 2pter → p12. Cytogenet Cell Genet 47:170, 1988
45. Barnett PS, Bhatt B, Pagliuca A et al: The thyroid peroxidase gene: accurate localization by non-isotopic in situ hybridization to chromosome 2p13. p. 55. In Carayon P, Ruf J (eds): Thyroperoxidase and Thyroid Autoimmunity. John Libbey Eurotext, London, 1990
46. Abramowicz MJ, Christophe D, Vassart G: Regulation of the TPO gene transcription. p. 11. In Carayon P, Ruf J (eds): Thyroperoxidase and Thyroid Autoimmunity. John Libbey Eurotext, London, 1990
47. Kaufman KD, Filetti S, Seto P, Rapoport B: Expression of recombinant, enzymatically-active, human thyroid peroxidase in eukaryotic cells. p. 17. In Carayon P, Ruf J (eds): Thyroperoxidase and Thyroid Autoimmunity. John Libbey Eurotext, London, 1990
48. Francis-Lang H, Price M, Martin U, Di Lauro R: The thyroid specific nuclear factor, TTF-1, binds to the rat thyroperoxidase promoter. p. 25. In Carayon P, Ruf J (eds): Thyroperoxidase and Thyroid Autoimmunity. John Libbey Eurotext, London, 1990
49. Ericson LE, Johanson V, Molne J et al: Intracellular transport and cell surface expression of thyroperoxidase. p. 107. In Carayon P, Ruf J (eds): Thyroperoxidase and Thyroid Autoimmunity. John Libbey Eurotext, London, 1990

50. DeGroot LJ, Davis AM: Studies on the biosynthesis of iodotyrosines. J Biol Chem 236:2009, 1961

51. Tong W, Taurog A, Chaikoff IL: Activation of the iodinating system in sheep thyroid particulate fractions by flavin cofactors. J Biol Chem 227:773, 1957

52. Suzuki M: Pyridine nucleotide and iodination reaction in the thyroid gland. Gunma Symposia on Endocrinology 3:81, 1966

53. Ohtaki S, Mashimo K, Yamazaki I: Hydrogen peroxide generating system in hog thyroid microsomes. Biochim Biophys Acta 292:825, 1973

54. Hati RN, DeGroot LJ: Studies on the mechanism of iodination supported by thyroidal NADPH-cytochrome c reductase. Acta Endocrinol 74:271, 1973

55. Yamamoto K, DeGroot LJ: Participation of NADPH-cytochrome c reductase in thyroid hormone biosynthesis. Endocrinol 98:1022, 1975

56. Dupuy C, Virion A, Kaniewski J et al: Thyroid NADPH-dependent H_2O_2 generating system: mechanism of H_2O_2 formation and regulation by Ca^{2+}. p. 95. In Carayon P, Ruf J (eds): Thyroperoxidase and Thyroid Autoimmunity. John Libbey Eurotext, London, 1990

57. Bernard B, DeGroot LJ: The role of hydrogen peroxide and glutathione in glucose oxidation by the thyroid. Biochem Biophys Acta 184:48, 1969

58. Suzuki M, Nagashima M, Yamamoto K: Studies on the mechanism of iodination by the thyroid gland: iodide-activating enzyme and an intracellular inhibitor of iodination. Gen Comp Endocrinol 1:103, 1961

59. DeGroot LJ, Davis AM: Studies on the biosynthesis of iodotyrosines: the relationship of peroxidase, catalase, and cytochrome oxidase. Endocrinology 70:505, 1962

60. Perrild H, Loveridge N, Reader SCJ, Robertson WR: Acute stimulation of thyroidal NAD^+ kinase, NADPH reoxidation, and peroxidase activities by physiological concentrations of thyroid stimulating hormone acting in vitro: a quantitative cytochemical study. Endocrinology 123:2499, 1988

61. Bjorkman U, Ekholm R: Hydrogen peroxide generation and its regulation in FRTL-5 and porcine thyroid cells. Endocrinology 130:393, 1992

62. Tice LW, Wollman SH: Ultrastructural localization of peroxidase on pseudopods and other structures of the typical thyroid epithelial cell. Endocrinology 94:1555, 1974

63. Björkman U, Ekholm R, Ericson LE, Ofverholm T: Transport of thyroglobulin and peroxidase in the thyroid follicle cell. Mol Cell Endocrinol 5:3, 1976

64. Björkman U, Ekholm R, Ericson LE: Effects of thyrotropin on thyroglobulin exocytosis and iodination in the rat thyroid gland. Endocrinology 102:460, 1978

65. Björkman U, Ekholm R: Accelerated exocytosis and H_2O_2 generation in isolated thyroid follicles enhance protein iodination. Endocrinology 122:488, 1988

66. Wollman SH, Wodinsky I: Localization of protein-bound I^{131} in the thyroid gland of the mouse. Endocrinology 56:9, 1955

67. Wollman SH, Ekholm R: Site of iodination in hyperplastic thyroid glands deduced from autoradiographs. Endocrinology 108:2082, 1981

68. Taurog A: Thyroid peroxidase-catalyzed iodination of thyroglobulin: inhibition of excess iodide. Arch Biochem Biophys 139:212, 1970

69. Yip CC, Hadley LD: The iodination of tyrosine by myeloperoxidase and beef thyroids: the possible involvement of free radicals. Biochim Biophys Acta 122:406, 1966

70. Yamamoto K, DeGroot LJ: Function of peroxidase and NADPH cytochrome c reductase during the Wolff-Chaikoff effect. Endocrinology 93:822, 1973

71. Davidson B, Neary JT, Strout HV et al: Evidence for a thyroid peroxidase associated "active iodine" species. Biochim Biophys Acta 522:318, 1978

72. Ohtaki S, Nakagawa H, Nakamura M, Yamazaki I: Reactions of purified hog thyroid peroxidase with H_2O_2, tyrosine, and methylmercaptoimidazole (goitrogen) in comparison with bovine lactoperoxidase. J Biol Chem 257:761, 1982

73. Fawcett DM: The formation of sulfenyl iodides as intermediates during the in vitro iodination of tyrosine by calf thyroid homogenates. Can J Biochem 46:1433, 1968

74. Corvilain B, Gerard C, Raspe E et al: Hormonal regulation of iodination. p. 33 In Carayon P, Ruf J (eds): Thyroperoxidase and Thyroid Autoimmunity. John Libbey Eurotext, London, 1990

75. Nagasaka A, Hidaka H: Quantitative modulation of thyroid iodide peroxidase by thyroid stimulating hormone. Biochem Biophys Res Commun 96:1143, 1980

76. Gavaret JM, Pommier J, Deme D et al: In vivo and in vitro regulation by iodide of thyroglobulin iodination and thyroxine synthesis. Horm Metab Res 7:166, 1975

77. Chiraseveenuprapund P, Rosenberg IN: Effects of hydrogen peroxide-generating systems on the Wolff-Chaikoff effect. Endocrinology 109:2095, 1981

78. Dugrillon A, Bechtner G, Uedelhoven WM et al: Evidence that an iodolactone mediates the inhibitory effect of iodide of thyroid cell proliferation but not on adenosine 3',5'-monophosphate formation. Endocrinology 127:337, 1990

79. Deme D, Fimiani E, Pommier J, Nunez J: Free diiodotyrosine effects on protein iodination and thyroid hormone synthesis catalyzed by thyroid peroxidase. Eur J Biochem 51:329, 1975

80. Johnson TB, Tewksbury LB Jr: The oxidation of 3, 5-diiodotyrosine to thyroxine. Proc Natl Acad Sci USA 28:73, 1942

81. Wain WH: The biosynthesis of thyroxine: incorporation of [U-^{14}C] tyrosine into thyroglobulin by mouse thyroid glands in vivo and in vitro. J Endocrinol 56: 173, 1973

82. Gavaret J-M, Cahnmann HJ, Nunez J: Thyroid hormone synthesis in thyroglobulin: the mechanism of the coupling reaction. J Biol Chem 256:9167, 1981

83. Lamas L, Dorris M, Taurog A: Evidence for a catalytic role for thyroid peroxidase in the conversion of diiodotyrosine to thyroxine. Endocrinology 90: 1417, 1972

84. Sugawara M: Coupling of iodotyrosine catalyzed by human thyroid peroxidase in vitro. J Clin Endocrinol Metab 60:1069, 1985

85. Rolland M, Montfort M-F, Lissitzky S: Efficiency of thyroglobulin as a thyroid hormone-forming protein. Biochim Biophys Acta 303:338, 1973

86. Lamas L, Taurog A: The importance of thyroglobulin structure in thyroid peroxidase-catalyzed conversion of diiodotyrosine to thyroxine. Endocrinology 100:1129, 1977

87. Gavaret JC, Deme D, Nunez J: Sequential reactivity of tyrosyl residues of thyroglobulin upon iodination catalyzed by thyroid peroxidase. J Biol Chem 252: 3281, 1977

88. Dunn JT, Dunn AD, Heppner DG Jr, Kim PS: A discrete thyroxine-rich iodopeptide of 20,000 daltons from rabbit thyroglobulin. J Biol Chem 256: 942, 1981

89. Marriq C, Arnaud C, Rolland M, Lissitzky S: An approach to the structure of thyroglobulin. Eur J Biochem 111:33, 1980

90. Dunn JT, Kim PS, Dunn AD: Favored sites for thyroid hormone formation on the peptide chains of human thyroglobulin. J Biol Chem 257:88, 1982

91. Lamas L, Anderson PC, Fox JW, Dunn JT: Consensus sequences for early iodination and hormonogenesis in human thyroglobulin. J Biol Chem 264: 13541, 1989

92. Palumbo G, Gentile F, Condorelli GL, Salvatore G: The earliest site of iodination in thyroglobulin is residue number 5. J Biol Chem 265:1, 1990

93. Edelhoch H: The properties of thyroglobulin. VIII. The iodination of thyroglobulin. J Biol Chem 237: 2778, 1962

94. Yip C, Klebanoff SJ: Synthesis of thyroxine by L-amino acid oxidase. Endocrinology 70:931, 1962

95. Inoue K, Taurog A: Acute and chronic effects of iodide on thyroid radioiodine metabolism in iodine-deficient rats. Endocrinology 83:279, 1968

96. Wolff J, Covelli I: Factors in the iodination of histidine in protein. Europ J Biochem 9:371, 1969

97. Taurog A, Tong W, Chaikoff IL: The monoiodotyrosine content of the thyroid gland. J Biol Chem 184: 83, 1950

98. Alexander NM: Studies on amino acid activating enzymes in thyroid glands. Endocrinology 74:273, 1964

99. Nadler NJ, Leblond CP, Carneiro J: Site of formation of thyroglobulin in mouse thyroid as shown by radioautography with leucine H^3. Proc Soc Exp Biol Med 105:38, 1960

100. Van Herle AJ, Vassart G, Dumont JE: Control of thyroglobulin synthesis and secretion. N Engl J Med 301:239, 1979

101. DeGroot LJ, Carvalho E: Studies on proteins of normal and diseased thyroid glands. J Clin Endocrinol Metab 20:21, 1960

102. Vassart G: Specific synthesis of thyroglobulin on membrane bound thyroid ribosomes. FEBS Lett 22: 53, 1972

103. Chebath J, Chabaud O, Becarevic A et al: Thyroglobulin messenger ribonucleic acid translation in vitro. Eur J Biochem 77:243, 1977

104. Vassart G, Brocas H, Nokin P, Dumont JE: Translation in xenopus oocytes of thyroglobulin mRNA isolated by Poly(U)-sepharose affinity chromatography. Biochim Biophys Acta 324:575, 1973

105. Seed RW, Goldbert IH: Iodination in relation to thyroglobulin maturation and subunit aggregation. Science 149:1380, 1965

106. Salvatore G, Vecchio G, Salvatore M et al: 27S thyroid iodoprotein. J Biol Chem 240:2935, 1965

107. Rolland M, Lissitzky S: Polypeptides non-covalently associated in 19-S thyroglobulin. Biochim Biophys Acta 278:316, 1972

108. Mercken L, Simons M-J, Swillens S et al: Primary structure of bovine thyroglobulin deduced from the sequence of its 8431-base complementary DNA. Nature 316:647, 1985

109. Malthiery Y, Lissitzky S: Primary structure of human thyroglobulin deduced from its 8448-base complementary DNA. Eur J Biochem 165:491, 1987

110. Civitareale D, Lonigro R, Sinclair AJ, Di Lauro R: A thyroid-specific nuclear protein essential for tissue-specific expression of the thyroglobulin promoter. EMBO J 8:2537, 1989

111. Sinadinovic J, Jovanovic M, Kraincanic M, Djurdjevic D: The significance of iodine in the aggregation of subunits into thyroglobulin and in the formation of 27-S iodoprotein. Acta Endocrinol 73:43, 1973

112. Rossi G, Edelhoch II, Tenore A et al: Characterizations and properties of thyroid iodoproteins from severely iodine-deficient rats. Endocrinology 92: 1241, 1973

113. Arima T, Spiro RG: Studies on the carbohydrate

units of thyroglobulin: structure of the mannose-N-acetylglucosamine unit (Unit A) of the human and calf proteins. J Biol Chem 247:1836, 1972

114. Cheftel C, Bouchilloux S, Chabaud O: Glycoprotein biosynthesis in sheep thyroid slices incubated with radioactive glucosamine and leucine. II. A study of microsomal subfractions. Biochim Biophys Acta 170:29, 1968

115. Chabaud O, Bouchilloux S, Ronin C, Ferrand M: Localization in a Golgi-rich thyroid fraction of sialyl-, galactosyl-, and N-acetylglucosaminyltransferases. Biochimie 56:119, 1974

116. Nunez J, Mauchamp J, Macchia V, Roche J: Biosynthese in vitro d'hormones doublement marquees dans des coupes de corps thyroide. II. Biosynthese d'une prethyroglobuline non iodee. Biochim Biophys Acta 107:247, 1965

117. Edelhoch H, Carlomagno MS, Salvatore G: Iodine and the structure of thyroglobulin. Arch Biochem Biophys 134:264, 1969

118. Lamas L, Ingbar SH: The effect of varying iodine content on the susceptibility of thyroglobulin to hydrolysis by thyroid acid protease. Endocrinology 102:188, 1978

119. Salvatore G, Salvatore M, Cahnmann HJ, Robbins J: Separation of thyroidal iodoproteins and purification of thyroglobulin by gel filtration and density gradient centrifugation. J Biol Chem 239:3267, 1964

120. Tarutani O, Ui N: Subunit structure of hog thyroglobulin: dissociation of noniodinated and highly iodinated preparations. Biochim Biophys Acta 181:136, 1969

121. Schneider AB, Edelhoch H: The properties of thyroglobulin. XIX. the equilibrium between guinea pig thyroglobulin and its subunits. J Biol Chem 245:885, 1970

122. Dunn JT, Kim PS, Dunn AD et al: The role of iodination in the formation of hormone-rich peptides from thyroglobulin. J Biol Chem 258:9093, 1983

123. Bismuth J, Rolland M, Lissitzky S: Composition en acides amines de thyroglobulines provenant de sujets euthyroidiens et goitreux. Acta Endocrinol 53:297, 1966

124. Rolland M, Bismuth J, Fondarai J, Lissitzky S: Composition en acides amines de la thyroglobuline de differentes especes animales. Acta Endocrinol 53:286, 1966

125. Dunn JT, Ray SC: Variations of the structure of thyroglobulins from normal and goitrous human thyroids. J Clin Endocrinol Metab 47:861, 1978

126. Robbins J, Rall JE: Proteins associated with the thyroid hormones. Physiol Rev 40:415, 1960

127. Vagenakis AB, Ingbar SH, Braverman LE: The relationship between thyroglobulin synthesis and intra-thyroid iodine metabolism as indicated by the effects of cycloheximide in the rat. Endocrinology 94:1669, 1974

128. Ermans AM, Kinthaert J, Camus M: Defective intra-thyroidal iodine metabolism in nontoxic goiter: inadequate iodination of thyroglobulin. J Clin Endocrinol Metab 28:1307, 1968

129. Larsen PR: Thyroidal triiodothyronine and thyroxine in Graves' disease: correlation with presurgical treatment, thyroid status, and iodine content. J Clin Endocrinol Metab 41:1098, 1975

130. Izumi M, Larsen PR: Triiodothyronine, thyroxine, and iodine in purified thyroglobulin from patients with Graves' disease. J Clin Invest 59:1105, 1977

131. DeCrombrugghe B, Edelhoch H, Beckers C, DeVisscher M: Thyroglobulin from human goiters: effects of iodination on sedimentation and iodoamino acid synthesis. J Biol Chem 242:5681, 1967

132. Robbins J, Wolff J, Rall JE: Iodoproteins in normal and abnormal human thyroid tissue and in normal sheep thyroid. Endocrinology 64:37, 1959

133. Torresani J, Roques M, Peyrot A, Lissitzky S: Mise en evidence, purification, et proprieties d'une iodoalbumine, constituant physiologique de la glande thyroide de rat. Acta Endocrinol 57:153, 1968

134. Jonckheer MH, Karcher DM: Thyroid albumin. I. Isolation and characterization. J Clin Endocrinol Metab 32:7, 1971

135. Otten J, Jonckheer M, Dumont JE: Thyroid albumin. II. In vitro synthesis of a thyroid albumin by normal human thyroid tissue. J Clin Endocrinol Metab 32:18, 1971

136. DeGroot LJ, Hall R, McDermott WV, Davis AM: Hashimoto's thyroiditis: a genetically conditioned disease. N Engl J Med 267:267, 1962

137. DeGroot LJ, Stanbury JB: The syndrome of congenital goiter with butanol-insoluble serum iodine. Am J Med 27:586, 1959

138. Stanbury JB, Janssen MA: Labeled iodoalbumin in the plasma in thyrotoxicosis after I^{125} and I^{131}. J Clin Endocrinol Metab 23:1056, 1963

139. deVijlder VVM, Veenboer GVM, Van Dijk JE: Thyroid albumin originates from blood. Endocrinology 131:578, 1992

140. Kondo Y, Kamiya Y: Purification and some properties of microsome-bound thyroglobulins. Biochim Biophys Acta 427:268, 1976

141. Medeiros-Neto G, Stanbury JB: Particulate iodoproteins in abnormal thyroid glands. J Clin Endocrinol Metab 26:23, 1966

142. Kim PS, Bole D, Arvan P: Transient aggregation of nascent thyroglobulin in the endoplasmic reticulum: relationship to the molecular chaperone, BiP. J Cell Biol 118:541, 1992

143. Kim PS, Kim KR, Arvan P: Disulfide-linked aggregation of thyroglobulin normally occurs during nascent protein folding. Amer J Physiol 265:704, 1993

144. Ericson LE: Ultrastructural aspects on iodination and hormone secretion in the thyroid gland. J Endocrinol Invest 6:311, 1983

145. Engstroöm G, Ericson LE: Effect of graded doses of thyrotropin on exocytosis and early phase of endocytosis in the rat thyroid. Endocrinology 108:399, 1981

146. Hashizume K, Fenzi G, DeGroot LJ: Thyroglobulin inhibition of thyrotropin binding to thyroid plasma membrane. J Clin Endocrinol Metab 46:679, 1978

147. Consiglio E, Salvatore G, Rall JE, Kohn LD: Thyroglobulin interactions with thyroid plasma membranes. J Biol Chem 254:5065, 1979

148. Consiglio E, Shifrin S, Yavin Z et al: Thyroglobulin interactions with thyroid membranes: relationship between receptor recognition of N-acetylglucosamine residues and the iodine content of thyroglobulin preparations. J Biol Chem 256:10592, 1981

148a. Thibault V, Blanck O, Courageot J, et al: The N-acetylglucosamine-specific receptor of the thyroid: purification, further characterization, and expression patterns on normal and pathological glands. Endocrinol 132:468–476, 1993

149. Neve P, Willems C, Dumont JE: Involvement of the microtubule- system in thyroid secretion. Exp Cell Res 63:457, 1970

150. Williams JA, Wolff J: Colchicine-binding protein and the secretion of thyroid hormone. J Cell Biol 54:157, 1972

151. Wollman SH, Loewenstein JE: Rates of colloid droplet and apical vesicle production and membrane turnover during thyroglobulin secretion and resorption. Endocrinology 93:248, 1973

152. Kostrouch Z, Munari-Silem Y, Rajas F et al: Thyroglobulin internalized by thyrocytes passes through early and late endosomes. Endocrinology 129:2202, 1991

153. Kostrouch Z, Bernier-Valentin F, Munari-Silem Y et al: Thyroglobulin molecules internalized by thyrocytes are sorted in early endosomes and partially recycled back to the follicular lumen. Endocrinology 132:2645, 1993

154. Jablonski P, McQuillan MT: The distribution of proteolytic enzymes in the thyroid gland. Biochim Biophys Acta 132:454, 1967

155. Dunn NW, McQuillan MT: Purification and properties of a peptidase from thyroid glands. Biochem Biophys Acta 235:149, 1971

156. Deiss WP, Balasubramaniam K, Peake RL et al: Stimulation of proteolysis in thyroid particles by thyrotropin. Endocrinology 79:19, 1966

157. Peake RL, Cates RJ, Deiss WP Jr: Thyroglobulin degradation: particulate intermediates produced in vivo. Endocrinology 87:494, 1970

158. Yoshinari M, Taurog M: Physiological role of thiol proteases in thyroid hormone secretion. Acta Endocrinol (Copenh) 113:261, 1986

159. Dunn AD, Crutchfield HE, Dunn JT: Proteolytic processing of thyroglobulin by extracts of thyroid lysosomes. Endocrinology 128:3073, 1991

160. Stanbury JB, Morris ML: Deiodination of diiodotyrosine by cell-free systems. J Biol Chem 233:106, 1958

161. Rosenberg IN, Goswami A: Purification and characterization of a flavoprotein from bovine thyroid with iodotyrosine deiodinase activity. J Biol Chem 254:12318, 1979

162. Kobayashi T, Greer MA, Allen CF: Heterogeneity of thyroid iodine turnover: "last come, last served" phenomenon. Endocrinology 94:363, 1974

163. Toyoda N, Nishikawa M, Mori Y et al: Identification of a 27-kilodalton protein with the properties of Type I iodothyronine 5′-deiodinase in human thyroid gland. J Clin Endocrinol Metab 74:533, 1992

164. Toyoda N, Nishikawa M, Mori Y et al: Thyrotropin and triiodothyronine regulate iodothyronine 5′-deiodinase messenger ribonucleic acid levels in FRTL-5 rat thyroid cells. Endocrinology 131:389, 1992

165. Ohtaki S, Moriya S, Suzuki H, Horiuchi Y: Nonhormonal iodine escape from the normal and abnormal thyroid gland. J Clin Endocrinol Metab 27:728, 1967

166. Kubota K, Uchimura H, Mitsuhashi T et al: Effects of intrathyroidal metabolism of thyroxine on thyroid hormone secretion: increased degradation of thyroxine in mouse thyroids stimulated chronically with thyrotrophin. Acta Endocrinol 105:57, 1984

167. Fisher DA, Oddie TH, Thompson CS: Thyroidal thyronine and non-thyronine iodine secretion in euthyroid subjects. J Clin Endocrinol Metab 33:647, 1971

168. Van Herle AJ, Uller RP, Mathews NL, Brown J: Radioimmunoassay for measurement of thyroglobulin in human serum. J Clin Invest 52:1320, 1973

169. Tatumi K, Suzuki Y, Sinohara H: Clearance of circulating desialylated thyroglobulins in the rat. Biochim Biophys Acta 583:504, 1979

170. Bech K, Rasmussen UF, Madsen SN: Influence of thyroglobulin on basal and stimulated human thyroid adenylate cyclase activity. J Clin Endocrinol Metab 53:264, 1981

171. Nelson JC, Weiss RM, Lewis JE et al: A multiple ligand-binding radioimmunoassay of diiodotyrosine. J Clin Invest 53:416, 1974

172. Nelson JC, Weiss RM, Palmer FJ et al: Lewis JF, Wilcox RB: Serum diiodotyrosine. J Clin Endocrinol Metab 41:1118, 1975

173. Chopra IJ: An assessment of daily production and significance of thyroidal secretion of 3,3',5'-triiodothyronine (reverse T3) in man. J Clin Invest 58:32, 1976

174. Laurberg P, Weeke J: Radioimmunological determination of reverse triiodothyronine in unextracted serum and serum dialysates. Scand J Clin Lab Invest 37:735, 1977

175. Corvilain B, Laurent E, Lecomte M et al: Role of cyclic adenosine 3',5'-monophosphate and the phosphatidylinositol-$^{2+}$ cascades in mediating the effects of thyrotropin and iodide on hormone synthesis and secretion in human thyroid slices. J Clin Endocrinol Metab 79:152, 1994

176. Eggo MC, Burrow GN: Integrated regulation of growth and of function. p. 327. In Ekholm R, Kohn LD, Wollman SH (eds): Control of the Thyroid Gland: Regulation of Its Normal Function and Growth. Plenum, New York, 1989

176a. Corvilain B, Laurent E, Lecomte, Vansande J, Dumont J: Role of the cyclic adenosine 3',5'-monophosphate and phosphatidylinositol-Ca $2+$ cascades in mediating the effects of thyrotropin and iodide on hormone synthesis and secretion in human thyroid slices. J Clin Endocrinol Metab 79:152–159, 1994

177. Dumont JE, Maenhaut C, Pirson I et al: Growth factors controlling the thyroid gland. Bailliere's Clin Endocrinol Metab 5:727, 1991

178. Takahashi S-I, Conti M, Van Wyk JJ: Thyrotropin potentiation of insulin-like growth factor-I dependent deoxyribonucleic acid synthesis in FRTL-5 cells: mediation by an autocrine amplification factor(s). Endocrinology 126:736, 1990

179. Grubeck-Leobenstein B, Buchan G, Sadeghi R et al: Transforming growth factor beta regulates thyroid growth: role in the pathogenesis of nontoxic goiter. J Clin Invest 83:764, 1989

180. Colletta G, Cirafici AM, Di Carlo A: Dual effect of transforming growth factor β on rat thyroid cells: inhibition of thyrotropin-induced proliferation and reduction of thyroid-specific differentiation markers. Cancer Res 49:3457, 1989

181. Taton M, Lamy F, Roger PP, Dumont JE: General inhibition by transforming growth factor beta 1 of thyrotropin and cAMP responses in human thyroid cells in primary culture. Molecul Cellul Endocrinol 95:13, 1993

182. Sato K, Sato T, Shizume K et al: Inhibition of ^{125}I organification and thyroid hormone release by interleukin-1, tumor necrosis factor-alpha, and interferon-gamma in human thyrocytes in suspension culture. J Clin Endocrinol Metab 70:1735, 1990

183. Kung AWC, Lau KS: Interferon-gamma inhibits thyrotropin-induced thyroglobulin gene transcription in cultured human thyrocytes. J Clin Endocrinol Metab 70:1512, 1990

184. Yamazaki K, Kanaji Y, Shizume K et al: Reversible inhibition by interferons alpha and beta of ^{125}I incorporation and thyroid hormone release by human thyroid follicles in vitro. J Clin Endocrinol Metab 77:1439, 1993

185. Pang X-P, Hershman JM, Chung M, Pekary AE: Characterization of tumor necrosis factor-α receptors in human and rat thyroid cells and regulation of the receptors by thyrotropin. Endocrinology 125:1783, 1989

186. Ashizawa K, Yamashita S, Nagayama Y et al: Interferon-γ inhibits thyrotropin-induced thyroidal peroxidase gene expression in cultured human thyrocytes. J Clin Endocrinol Metab 69:475, 1989

187. Enomoto T, Sugawa H, Kosugi S et al: Prolonged effects of recombinant human interleukin-1α on mouse thyroid function. Endocrinology 127:2322, 1990

Thyroid Hormone Transport, Cellular Uptake, Metabolism, and Molecular Action

3

This chapter traces the path of the iodothyronines from the thyroid gland to the cell nucleus and reviews the mechanism of their action. Since deiodination of the iodothyronines plays a critical role in activation of thyroxine (T_4), as well as in inactivation of triiodothyronine (T_3), the pathways of iodothyronine deiodination are also reviewed.

Molecular biologic approaches have led to a vast body of published work, filled with new insights, on thyroid hormone-binding proteins, cellular uptake processes, deiodination, and thyroid hormone action. While these studies' insights help explain the physiologic events in this volume, this chapter will focus on their overall biologic implications rather than on the details of their elegant techniques. This information will provide a basis for understanding topics presented in later chapters: the hypothalamic pituitary thyroid axis (Ch. 4), the clinical implications of assays of serum total and free thyroid hormones (Ch. 5 and 6), and thyroid hormone resistance syndromes (Ch. 16).

SERUM THYROID HORMONE-BINDING PROTEINS: TRANSPORT FROM THE SITE OF HORMONE PRODUCTION TO TARGET CELLS

The iodothyronines are virtually insoluble in water, and in all species circulate bound to various plasma proteins. While the type and affinity of binding of these proteins determines the amount of total thyroid hormone in the circulation, it is the minuscule fraction of the total hormone in the unbound form which is maintained constant and correlates most closely with the thyroid state in man and animals. Accordingly, the consensus position is that the thyroid hormone binding proteins, while having an important role in assuring broad and equal distribution of the hydrophobic hormone molecules to the various cells in the body, do not, in and of themselves, have a specific role in thyroid hormone action.[1] For example, transthyretin, (TTR) (formerly termed thyroxine binding prealbumin or TBPA) - the major thyroid hormone-binding protein in mice and as well a prominent T_4 binding protein in humans, can be eliminated from the genome without any effect on thyroid function except to alter total serum hormone levels.[2] This suggests that the role of a specific thyroid hormone binding protein is not essential, or can easily be subsumed by other circulating proteins. The same phenomenon occurs in some humans in whom the major thyroid hormone binding plasma protein, thyroxine-binding globulin (TBG), is not functional. In the present discussion, the three major binding proteins, TBG, TTR, and albumin, will be considered in order of their relative importance as thyroid hormone carrier proteins in humans.

Thyroxine-Binding Globulin

TBG is the major thyroid hormone transport protein in human serum (Table 3-1). This is apparent from Figure 3-1 which shows the distribution of tracer T_4 in human serum after paper electrophoresis. TBG binds approximately 75 percent of the circulating T_4 and a somewhat higher percentage of the circulating T_3. While the electrophoretic mobility of this protein places it in the globulin fraction of the serum proteins, it is not an immunoglobulin, but a globular protein. The term, thyroxine-binding globulin, is a misnomer since it also binds T_3 and reverse T_3, but the name has been retained for consistency. TBG has a molecular mass of approximately 54 kd, about 20 percent of which is carbohydrate. A cDNA for this protein has been isolated, and encodes a 450 amino acid protein with a 20 amino acid signal peptide.[3] The deduced molecular weight is 44 kd. Four glycosylation sites are present. As discussed below, glycosylation of this protein has important effects on

TABLE 3-1. Comparison of Various Properties of the Major Thyroid Hormone-Binding Proteins in Human Plasma

	TBG	TTR	ALB
Mol wt of holoprotein (d)	54,000	54,000 (4 subunits)	66,000
Plasma concentrations (μmol/L)	0.27	4.6	640
T_4 binding capacity as μg T_4/dl	21	350	50,000
Association constants of the major binding site (L/M)			
$\quad T_4$	1×10^{10}	7×10^{7}	7×10^{5}
$\quad T_3$	5×10^{8}	1.4×10^{7}	1×10^{5}
Fraction of sites occupied by T_4 in euthyroid plasma	0.31	0.02	<0.001
Distribution volume (L)	7	5.7	7.8
Turnover rate (%/day)	13	59	5
Dissociation constant (sec^{-1})			
$\quad$For T_4	0.018	0.094	—
$\quad$For T_3	0.16	0.7	—
Distribution of iodothyronines (%/protein)			
$\quad T_4$	68	11	20
$\quad T_3$	80	9	11

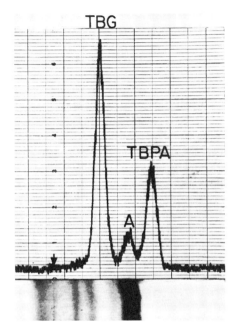

Fig. 3-1. Electrophoretic distribution of T_4-binding proteins. Distribution of tracer [131]I T_4 among the serum proteins is shown, as determined by paper electrophoresis carried out in glycine acetate, pH 8.6. A strip stained for protein is shown in the lower band. The arrow indicates the point of application of protein. TBG, thyroxine-binding globulin; A, albumin; TBPA, thyroxine-binding prealbumin. (From Oppenheimer,[389] with permission.)

its clearance from the plasma and accordingly on its plasma concentration.

Synthesis

Hepatic snythesis and glycosylation of this protein, as well as the various techniques which have been used to study its chemistry in vitro, are shown schematically in Figure 3-2.[4] A major surprise following its molecular cloning was the fact that TBG is a member of the serum protease inhibitor (serpin) superfamily which also includes cortisol-binding globulin.[3] TBG has no anti-protease activity. Cleavage of its active center by elastase has no effect on T_4 binding despite the fact that a major change would be anticipated in its molecular configuration by analogy with alpha 1 antitrypsin or cortisol binding globulin.[4] Thus the "stressed" configuration of the native molecule is not critical to its T_4 binding capacity.

T_4 and T_3 bind to TBG with relatively high affinity, certainly the highest affinity of any of the three human binding proteins.[5–9] The association constant for T_4 is of the order of 10^{10} for the single TBG binding site, and is about 20-fold lower for T_3 (Table 3-1). The TBG concentration in plasma is approximately 270 nmol/L (1.5 mg/dl) and since it can bind one molecule of T_4 or T_3 per mole, the total binding capacity of TBG is slightly less than three times the total T_4 concentration (100 nmol/L) in euthyroid individuals. Thus, about 33 percent of the TBG molecules are occupied by T_4 in the euthyroid individual, and an insignificant number of sites are occupied by T_3. In extreme hyperthyroidism, when serum T_4 concentrations may increase to over 400 nmol/L (30 mg/dl) virtually all of the available binding sites on this protein are occupied. It is the concentration of apo (free) TBG which determines the free fraction of the iodothyronines in human plasma and is the basis for the resin T_3 uptake test and its successors. These tests are still commonly employed estimates of the free fraction of thyroid hormones in clinical practice. The iodothyronines which bind to TBG include reverse T_3, which is bound about 40 percent as tightly as is T_4; d-T_4, with a binding affinity about half that of the L-isomer; tetrac, bound about one quarter as well, and the T_4 and T_3 sulfate conjugates.

The gene coding for TBG is found on the long arm of the human X chromosome.[10] Soon after the identification of TBG, individuals with complete or partial TBG deficiencies were identified.[11,12] Such inherited abnormalities also include families with TBG variants which have reduced T_4 binding affinity, or easily denatured TBG.[13,14] The spectrum of inherited TBG abnormalities has been reviewed in detail.[4,15]

TBG is the only glycosylated protein of the three major human thyroid hormone binding proteins, and the carbohydrate residues of this protein have a major influence on its metabolic clearance.[16] The biological half-life of native TBG is approximately 5 days.[11] If a significant number of the 6 to 10 terminal sialic acid residues are removed, its clearance is markedly accelerated with the half life decreasing to approximately 15 minutes. The variable number of sialic acid residues on the molecule accounts for the micro-heterogeneity of circulating TBG which is found on isoelectric focusing gels.[4] The isoelectric point of most TBG is approximately pH 4 to 5, however, this increases to 6 as the sialic acid residues are removed. This change does not appreciably alter the T_4 binding properties of the molecule, but its heat

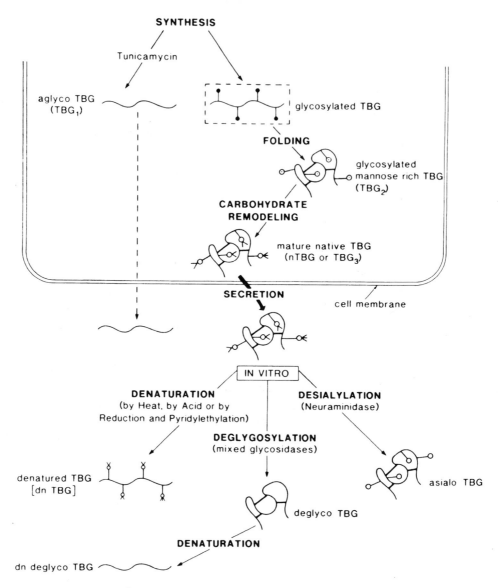

Fig. 3-2. The different forms of TBG and the contribution of oliogosaccharides to TBG secretion and structure. (From Rafetoff,[4] with permission.)

stability is somewhat reduced. The accelerated clearance of asialo-TBG is due to its interaction with the asialo-glycoprotein receptors of the liver. The importance of the liver in the clearance of normal TBG is reflected in the fact that in patients with liver failure, TBG, especially the more highly sialylated molecules with higher isoelectric points, accumulate in the circulation.[17]

The most clinically relevant aspect of TBG physiology occurs in individuals with increases in circulat-

ing estrogen, such as occurs during pregnancy, or in women who are taking oral contraceptives. TBG concentrations are increased two to three fold under these circumstances with maintenance of the normal ratio of occupied to free TBG. Thus the serum T_4 concentrations in pregnancy are generally twice those present in the non-pregnant state. While estrogen increases TBG synthesis in monkey hepatocytes (although not in Hep-G2 cells) its principal effect on TBG is to increase the sialylation of TBG and other glycosylated proteins.[18] This reduces the clearance rate of such proteins, leading to a marked increase in their plasma concentrations.

TBG excess is found rarely on an inherited basis, and this is generally identified only in females since the presence of a single abnormal gene on the X chromosome does not increase TBG.[4,12] The origin of the TBG excess has not been defined, but this presumably occurs due to increases in gene transcription or mRNA stability.[11] The circulating TBG in such patients is normal immunologically, has a normal half life, and a normal distribution on isoelectric focusing gels. This differentiates it from the pattern in patients with estrogen excess, in whom the isoforms with higher isoelectric points are present in greater quantity.[16] TBG deficiency is more common. This deficiency is complete in males and has a prevalence of approximately 1 in 2800. Complete deficiency is less prevalent in females since a homozygous state is required. In females with a single abnormal gene, pregnancy or estrogen causes the expected increase in circulating TBG concentrations.

Aside from the effects of estrogen, hormonal effects on circulating TBG concentrations are modest.

Studies in rhesus monkeys showed that serum TBG changed with thyroid status decreasing in hyperthyroidism and increasing in the hypothyroid state.[19,20] These effects have also been detected in studies using monkey hepatocytes and in Hep G2 cells.[15] The most dramatic effect on circulating TBG levels in humans, aside from that of estrogen, occurs during administration of l asparaginase, an anti-leukemic agent.[21,22] This agent causes an acute inhibition of hepatic TBG synthesis an effect also documented in Hep G2 cells.[23] In vivo this agent must block TBG synthesis nearly completely, since the concentrations of TBG fall with a half life approximately equal to that of the endogenous protein, about 5 days (Fig. 3-3). The remarkable capacity of the human hypothalamic pituitary thyroid axis to deal with an abrupt increase in available T_4 by accelerating T_4 clearance (and presumably decreasing TSH) is seen in the relatively constant value for free T_4 which is maintained during the time when there is an approximately threefold reduction in the concentrations of total T_4 and TBG. The marked increase in the free fraction of T_4 (reflected in the change in the normalized T_3 uptake in Fig. 3-3) demonstrates the dependence of this test on unoccupied

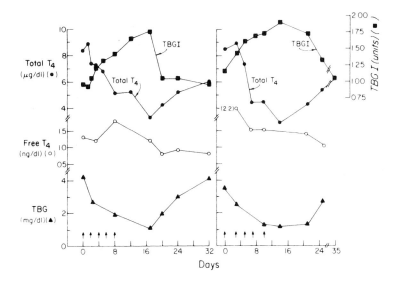

Fig. 3-3. Profile of total thyroxine, thyroxine-binding globulin index, free thyroxine and thyroxine-binding globulin during L-asparaginase treatment of two patients. Arrows indicate the timing of each L-asparaginase dose. Normal values: total T_4, 5 to 10.2 μl/dl; thyroxine-binding globulin index, 0.85 to 1.10; free T_4, 1.92 $\pm$ 0.1 ng per deciliter (mean $\pm$ S.E.); Thyroxine-binding globulin (by radioimmunoassay), 2.1 to 5.2 mg per deciliter. To convert ng/dl of T_4 to nanomoles per liter, multiply by 12.87. (From Garnick and Larsen,[21] with permission.)

TABLE 3-2. Effects of Various Agents or Conditions on Thyroid Hormone-Binding Proteins in Humans

	TBG	TTR	ALB
Estrogen	↑	N	N
Androgen	±↓	N	N
Glucocorticoid	±↓	N	N
L-asparaginase	↓↓	N	±↓
Illness			
Acute	N	↓↓	N
Chronic	↓	↓↓	↓
Liver disease	↑ or ↓	↓↓	↓
AIDS	↑	↓	±↓
Nephrotic syndrome	↓	↓	↓
Opioids	±↑	N	N
5-fluouracil	↑	N	N
Clofibrate	↑	N	N

TBG concentrations which are markedly reduced. Androgens cause slight decreases in TBG, through an unknown mechanism, as do glucocorticoids and anabolic steroids (see Table 3-2). Opioids, heroin, methadone and 5-fluorouracil, promethazine and clofibrate may increase TBG concentrations.[15] Numerous therapeutic agents inhibit the binding of thyroid hormones to TBG, but do not alter its concentration.[24–34] The effects of such agents, which include salicylates and phenytoin, are described in detail in Chapter 5.

Transthyretin

TTR, formerly termed thyroxine-binding prealbumin (TBPA), is a 55 kd protein which consists of four identical subunits, each having a molecular weight of 13.5 kd (see Fig. 3-1). Thus, its molecular weight in the circulation is identical to that of TBG. The term transthyretin (TTR) derives from the fact that this protein, in addition to binding significant quantities of T_4, also is the major transport protein for retinol binding protein, which is in turn the major transport carrier for all *trans* retinoic acid (vitamin A). Its concentration in the serum is 25 μM (about 4.6 mg/dl, about a hundred fold higher than that of TBG, Table 3-1). X-ray crystallographic studies have demonstrated that the tetrameric structure provides two potential binding sites for iodothyronines in a hydrophobic channel.[15] However, the binding of T_4 (or, presumably, T_3) to one of the two

sites in the central core decreases the affinity of the protein for a second iodothyronine. Therefore, it seems likely that only a single binding site is occupied on a given TTR tetramer. While initial studies of this protein some years ago suggested that TTR was not a major carrier for T_3, later results showed that approximately equal quantities of T_3 are transported by this protein and by albumin.[26] The distribution volume of TTR is similar to that of albumin. Its synthetic rate and plasma clearance are much higher than that of TBG, although lower than that of albumin. The half-life of the protein is rapid, about one third of the circulating protein being metabolized per day. Its production and/or disappearance is markedly influenced by the dietary state, accounting for the rapid decrease in the concentration of this protein in humans during starvation or after surgical or medical stress.[35,36] Initial studies suggested that the marked decrease in TTR concentration of about 50 to 60 percent during surgical stress was the cause of the increase in free T_4 which occurs during this period.[35] However, it would appear that the quantity of T_4 made available by such a decrease in TTR concentration could easily be accommodated on TBG and albumin assuming there were no concomitant changes in the levels or binding affinities of these proteins under these circumstances. Because of the relatively large quantities of this protein available, only about 1 to 2 percent of its binding sites are occupied under physiological circumstances, much less than the approximately 33 percent of TBG binding sites similarly occupied at physiological serum T_4 concentrations. Both T_4 and T_3 dissociate rapidly from TTR, these rates being about four times more rapid than that from TBG.[5,6] However, since the quantity of T_4 bound to TBG is seven to eight fold greater, the total T_4 available from the two proteins by dissociation are comparable.[7,8]

Synthesis of TTR occurs primarily in the liver, but has also been identified in both human and rat choroid plexus and in pancreatic islet cells.[37–40] In fact, patients have been identified in whom islet cell tumors were associated with increased T_4 due to increases in serum TTR concentrations.[15,41,42] Synthesis in the choroid plexus accounts for the relatively high concentration of TTR in the cerebrospinal fluid of both humans and rats, where TTR is the major thyroid hormone carrier protein.[37,43] The possibility that TTR in the choroid plexus serves as the transport mechanism for T_4 to enter the central nervous system has been raised by several investigators.[15,37,39,44] Blockade of T_4 binding by administration of a flavonoid compound interferes with labeled T_4 transport to the brain of experimental animals.[45] While the role of TTR in T_4 transport into the brain is under active investigation, the available experimental data do not allow a firm conclusion in this regard. A recent report describes the disruption of the TTR gene in mice using embryonic stem cell gene targeting techniques.[2] Since TTR is the major serum thyroid hormone carrier protein in mice its complete absence will permit definitive studies defining the role of such proteins in thyroid physiology. Based on the results so far available, the animals are phenotypically normal, and plasma levels of total, but not free T_4, are reduced.[2] Serum T_3 concentrations are much less affected, being 65 percent of control. This may be accounted for by a shift in T_3 binding from TTR to circulating albumin and TBG. At the time of this writing, no data are available on T_4 kinetics or the CNS uptake of T_4 in the TTR-deficient animals. Such studies should provide considerable insight into the role of TTR in animals, and by inference, in humans.

Genetic abnormalities which lead to alterations in the affinity of TTR have been described in humans. These abnormalities are discussed in detail in Chapter 16, but include amino acid substitutions which either decrease or increase the affinity of TTR for T_4.[15,42,46-49] In patients in which the TTR variant has an increased affinity of T_4, patients are euthyroid but have an elevated total T_4, and a reduced free fraction, comparable to the situation when TBG concentrations are increased.[46,48] Some TTR variants are associated with decreased affinity for T_4, but, as might be expected from the results in Table 3-1, a reduced TTR affinity does not result in a significant alteration in circulating serum T_4 or T_3 concentrations.[15,42] Alterations in the quantity of TTR, however, can cause discrepant results when free T_4 is estimated using certain T_4 analogues due to binding of the analogue to the abnormal TTR.[49] It is conceivable, since abnormalities causing minor increases or decreases in the affinity of TTR for T_4 do not change serum T_4 concentrations, that genetic abnormalities in this protein may be more common than are currently recognized.

Another aspect of abnormal TTR proteins is their association in four families with the syndrome of familial amyloidotic polyneuropathy (FAP).[15,42,48] In FAP types 1 and 2, TTR shows a reduced affinity for T_4, while in FAP type 4, the affinity of the abnormal TTR for T_4 is increased. The abnormal TTR has been found associated with the amyloid protein which accumulates in the central nervous system and cardiac tissues. A role for the abnormality in T_4 binding in the generation of polyneuropathy has not been established and the two properties may be completely unrelated.

The ratio of binding affinities of T_4, T_3, and other circulating iodothyronines have been evaluated for TTR.[5-9,15] By and large, the affinities for T_3 and reverse T_3 (relative to that for T_4) are similar between TBG and TTR. However, there is a remarkably higher binding affinity of tetrac relative to T_4 for binding to TTR than for that to TBG. Triac is similarly affected indicating that the specificities of the iodothyronine binding site of TTR and TBG depend on the alanine side chain. Crystallographic studies have suggested that this portion of the T_4 molecule is at the open end of the T_4 binding channel of TTR.[50,51] The physiological significance of the higher affinity of TTR for tetrac relative to that of TBG for the same molecule remains to be determined. Other noniodothyronine ligands are also differentially bound, the most notable example being the flavonoid compounds which have a markedly higher binding affinity for TTR than for TBG.[52,53] In terms of a comparison between TTR and other iodothyronine binding proteins, the characteristics of TTR most closely resemble those of the type 1 iodothyronine deiodinase, in which the binding of reverse T_3 or T_4 is quite sensitive to inhibition by the flavonoids.[54] It bears little resemblance to the binding profile for the thyroid hormone nuclear receptors, which have considerably higher binding affinity for T_3 than for T_4. Since TTR is not glycosylated, there is no influence of estrogen administration on the plasma concentration of this protein by post-translational mechanisms.

Albumin

Albumin has one relatively high-affinity binding site for T_4 and five other sites of fifteenfold lower affinity (see Table 3-1). Although the association constants of T_4 for albumin are two orders of magnitude lower than for TTR and four orders of magnitude lower than for TBG, the high concentration of albumin in plasma results in a significant role for this protein in iodothyronine transport in humans. The ratio of the binding affinities of T_3, T_4, and reverse T_3 differ slightly from those of TBG and TTR, with T_3 having a relatively higher binding affinity relative to T_4 than is the case for either TBG or TTR.[7-9,15] This accounts for the higher fraction of T_3 which is albumin, rather than TTR, bound, than might be otherwise expected (see Table 3-1).

The physiologic role of albumin-bound T_4 has been a subject of controversy.[55-62] Some investigators have speculated that this is the source of most of the free hormone which dissociates during passage of plasma through the capillaries, while others have suggested that TBG and TBPA serve this function. A significant issue in this regard is the fact that free fatty acids, which also bind to albumin, can interfere with the binding of T_4 to this protein as well as to the human serum binding proteins in general. Free fatty acids may accumulate in the serum of the starved or ill patient in sufficiently high concentrations that binding of thyroid hormone to the circulating albumin is blocked (see Ch. 6).

From a clinical point-of-view, the most intriguing aspect of albumin iodothyronine binding occurs in the condition known as familial dysalbuminemic hyperthyroxinemia (FDH). In this dominantly-inherited syndrome there is an increase in the amount of a usually minor variant of circulating serum albumin which binds T_4 with increased affinity.[63-68] Thus, such patients present with an elevated serum total T_4. What makes this abnormality more subtle is that, while there is an increase in the affinity of the abnormal albumin for T_4, this is not accompanied by an increase in its T_3-binding affinity. Thus, if patients are screened using an estimate of the free fraction which depends on tracer T_3 (as do many such techniques), the free T_4 fraction is estimated to be normal rather than reduced, as it is shown to be by equilibrium dialysis using tracer T_4. Before the widespread availability and application of immunometric TSH assays to confirm the diagnosis of hyperthyroidism, such patients were often treated with radioiodine or surgery, having been given a diagnosis of biochemical hyperthryoidism. A number of subtypes of FDH have been described, depending on the affinity of albumin for T_4, reverse T_3, and T_3.[15,69,70] This subject is discussed in greater detail in Chapter 6. The variant albumin of FDH also binds with high affinity the T_4 analog used in single-step free T_4 assays. Binding of the tracer analog to the abnormal albumin reduces the binding to the immobilized antibody. Since a similar decrease occurs in sera from patients with a true increase in free T_4 the diagnostic evaluation of such patients may be further confounded.[49]

Lipoproteins

Two lipoproteins, apolipoprotein A1 and apolipoprotein B100, have both been found to bind T_4, and to some extent T_3, with affinities which are similar to those of TTR.[71-73] These proteins are estimated to transport roughly 3 percent of the total T_4 and perhaps as much as 6 percent of the total T_3 in serum. The binding site of apolipoprotein A1 is a region of the molecule that is distinct from that portion which binds to the cellular lipoprotein receptors, and the physiologic role of such binding has not as yet been elucidated.[71] However, given the relatively high concentration of such proteins, the possibility that these may also contribute to the freely dissociable T_4 and T_3 needs to be evaluated further.

The Physiologic Role of the Human Thyroid Hormone Transport Proteins

The recognition almost four decades ago that the thyroid status of individuals remained remarkably constant, despite marked changes in total thyroid hormone due to alterations in thyroid hormone binding proteins, led Robbins and Rall to propose that it is the concentration of free, rather than total, thyroid hormones, that was the best index of thyroid hormone availability.[9,74] The fact that in euthyroid humans, free T_4 and T_3 remain remarkably constant, in spite of marked variations in TBG, TTR, or abnormal albumins, and that the type and affinity of circulating thyroid hormone binding proteins varies markedly between species, both support the concept that hormone availability to cells is determined by the concentration of free hormone. For free hormone concentrations to remain constant requires that the hypothalamic-pituitary axis, the ultimate determinant of thyroid hormone supply, is sensitive to free, not total, thyroid hormone. This axis can respond to both T_4 and serum free T_3 independently, by virtue of the local conversion of T_4 to T_3 within the thyrotroph and central nervous system (see below), adding a further layer of complexity to the system, but it does not alter the underlying principle. The pool of free thyroid hormones is a dynamic one to which significant contributions are made from the thyroid gland, the circulating binding proteins, and the peripheral tissues. Given the rapidity of the association of hormone to both tissues and plasma it is unlikely that a given molecule of T_4, or T_3, remains unbound for more than an instant. On the other hand, when plasma is studied experimentally in the test tube, the contribution of tissue uptake and degradation as well as re-release to the plasma pool are not measured. Thus the system is in equilibrium not with tissues, but with an inert surface. Since the T_4 degradation rate exceeds the available pool of free T_4 many-fold, it is clear that there is normally a rapid net dissociation from the binding proteins into the free form and thence into the cytosol and to sites of T_4 degradation. Net influx into the tissues, however, is not the consequence of a one-time dissociation of thyroid hormones from binding proteins, but the summation of bulk influx and efflux between the tissues and plasma.

Studies of Mendel and Weisinger, and those of Hennemann and colleagues using perfused liver, have clarified the underlying concepts involved in thyroid hormone tissue uptake.[58,61,75–78] The amount of hormone dissociating from the circulating binding proteins per unit time far exceeds the net hormone degraded or excreted by the tissues. The hormone not irreversibly lost during this time is rebound to plasma or cellular proteins. Thus, if we assume that free hormone is a transient state, one may conclude that, while we may not know the instantaneous free hormone concentration in vivo, that concentration is proportional to the free hormone concentration which is measured by equilibrium dialysis in vitro. The rapidity of cellular free hormone uptake was shown in hepatic perfusion studies by Mendel and Cavalieri who found that in the absence of thyroid hormone binding proteins, virtually all labeled T_4 was taken up by the cells in the extreme periphery of the hepatic lobule.[61,62,79,80] These are the first cells which are exposed to the hormone in the protein free bolus. In contrast however, if albumin or TTR was included in the bolus, the distribution of tracer T_4 was equal throughout the lobule. Thus, the role of the binding proteins was to limit the efflux rate of tracer T_4 from capillary insuring that it was not all taken up by the initial layer of cells contacted. This indicates that there is no limitation on the rate of unidirectional T_4 uptake by liver cells at physiological T_4 concentrations. The role of the binding proteins thus appears to be to facilitate even distribution of T_4 and T_3 throughout the organism and not to facilitate uptake.[77]

Whether alterations in the fraction of hormone carried by different proteins, e.g., the effect of increasing TBG in hyperestrogenemic states or decreasing TTR in mice, could change the distribution of hormone among the various tissues within the body is a more complex question. This would depend to a great extent on local factors operating in a given capillary bed, for example, to the transit time of a bolus of plasma through a given capillary bed. For example, it has been proposed that the increase of TBG in pregnancy leads to greater availability of T_4 to the placenta in order to provide a source of iodide to the developing fetus.[81,82] Since there are distinct differences in the half-time of dissociation of T_4 from TBG, TTR, and albumin, it is conceivable that this phenomenon could occur. The longer a bolus of plasma remains in a given location, the greater might be the contribution to tissue T_4 uptake from the T_4-TBG complex.[7,8,58] Under normal circumstances, however, it would appear that it is the T_4 and T_3 bound to albumin which provide the greatest proportion of hormone taken up by the tissues. Yet the specific importance of any particular binding protein is mitigated by the evidence that the sizes of the rapidly exchangeable T_4 pools in liver and kidney in normal and in analbuminemic rats are indistinguishable.[59,77] Furthermore, the 24-hour disposal rate of T_4 is not different from normal in patients with FDH indicating that alterations in serum albumin binding per se do not have a significant influence on the overall rate of T_4 degradation.[67] The fact that in in vitro studies, uptake of labeled thyroid hormones from sera of patients with varying quantities of TBG or of high-affinity albumin was proportional to the free hormone concentration suggests that it is the sum of the association and dissociation constants and the total hormone concentration (not the specific iodothyronine-carrier proteins) which determines tissue T_4 uptake.[83] Thus, while there does not appear to be a specific carrier role for any given protein in determining entry into a given cell, the contributions of hormone from different binding proteins may differ from tissue to tissue, depending on transit time or alterations in any of the binding protein concentration or affinities.[81,82]

From these concepts, it can be concluded that, in equilibrium situations, it is the rate of irreversible thyroid hormone metabolism which influences the net efflux of thyroid hormone from the circulation. Information as to the rate of this efflux is transmitted to the hypothalamic-pituitary axis by the level of free T_4 and T_3. Appropriate adjustments of thyroidal secretion occur consequent to alterations in TSH secretion. This assumes that there is no significant perturbation in the cellular thyroid hormone transport processes. A generalized decrease in cellular uptake, for example, could cause an increase in the free hormone setpoint. Studies which are described in greater detail later in this chapter and in Chapter 4 indicate that the situation in the pituitary and hypothalamus is complicated by the presence of locally produced T_3 which allows this axis to recognize the concentration of serum T_4 indirectly. In states where the uptake and degradation of T_4 are changed by transient alterations in any of the binding proteins, compensatory adjustments occur in TSH production. Thus, the system can remain in equilibrium, despite rapid changes in binding proteins (e.g., Fig. 3-3). However, in states where excess thyroid hormone is supplied, such as in Graves' disease, or states in which thyroid hormone production is reduced, the system fails due to the override of the hypothalamic-pituitary axis on the one hand, or to thyroid gland failure on the other.

Nonetheless, alterations in the concentration of a specific binding protein will influence the fraction of the total T_4 pool which is cleared per unit time. TBG, by virtue of the fact its affinity constant for T_4 is relatively close to the free hormone concentration, may be considered especially important in this circumstance. In the absence of TBG, one might predict that since the amount of T_4 degraded per day is much larger relative to the total T_4 pool than is the case under normal circumstances, minute-to-minute fluctuations in free T_4 concentrations might be greater. If the response time of the hypothalamic axis was slow relative to the rate of fall in free T_4, it could lead to greater TSH release per 24 hours than might occur under normal circumstances. Evidence that this may be the case has been provided in studies showing that serum thyroglobulin concentrations, indirectly reflecting the degree of thyroid stimulation by TSH, are slightly higher in individuals with congenital TBG deficiency than they are in normal subjects.[84]

Taken together, then, it appears that the circulating thyroid hormone binding proteins have a major role in assuring widespread even distribution of these hydrophobic hormones to tissues. The in vivo instantaneous level of free hormone is not known, however, and it is likely to be lower than the free hormone measured in in vitro by equilibrium dialysis. Even so, it is certainly proportional to this. This accounts for the stability of the measured free thyroid hormone concentrations on a minute-to-minute basis in a given individual and between various species regardless of differences in circulating hormone binding proteins.

Theoretically, it would be possible to override this system by administration of an agent which could act like thyroid hormone without producing its metabolic effects. The only substance that may have this effect in humans is phenytoin (diphenylhydantoin). While initially it was though that the depression of the PBI in phenytoin-treated patients was due to competition of the drug with T_4 for TBG-binding, later studies demonstrated that there is about a 20 percent reduction in the concentration of free T_4 in phenytoin-treated patients due to the fact that the fraction of T_4 which is free is not increased.[25,34] This reduction in free T_4 is not associated with a reduction in total T_4 degradation rates, suggesting that tissue uptake of free T_4 was increased in some tissues.[25] Serum TSH is not increased in a phenytoin-treated patients indicating that the hypothalamic-pituitary axis does not interpret the reduced free T_4 as indicative of hypothyroidism.[30,85–87] This indicates that phenytoin resets the hypothalamic-pituitary axis such that it no longer maintains free T_4 concentrations at normal levels. This would occur if phenytoin could act as a thyromimetic agent at the hypothalamic or pituitary level. The mechanism for this effect is not apparent. However, phenytoin treatment also increases the levothyroxine requirements in hypothyroid patients by about 20 percent.[85] It is thought that this occurs due to the induction of T_4 clearance by mechanisms which do not result in the production of T_3. Such effects could reflect increases in the cytochrome p450 enzyme in the liver with a consequent reduction of exogenous exiting T_4 from the liver during its "first pass" through this organ. Treatment with carbimazepine has similar, but more marked effects, in patients with primary hypothyroidism.[88] In patients with intact thyroid glands, T_4 is reduced as in phenytoin-treated patients, but TSH is normal.[86,87,89] It is thus still difficult to reconcile the normal TSH of the phenytoin-treated patient with the reduced free T_4 without postulating a central thyromimetic effect of this drug.

CELLULAR UPTAKE OF THYROID HORMONES

Triiodothyronine

The uptake of T_3 has been evaluated by a number of investigators in many different cells, including rat hepatocytes[90–98] and HEP G2 cells,[99] rat skeletal myoblasts,[100,101] human fibroblasts,[102] erythrocytes,[103] and rat neuroblastoma cells.[104] In addition, studies have been performed in whole rat skeletal muscle,[105,106] brain, liver,[55] and in perfused rat liver.[56,107–111] Saturable sites for T_3 uptake have been identified which have apparent Km values from 60 to 120 nMol for high affinity sites. In most, but not all studies,[97] the uptake of T_3 is inhibited by agents which deplete the cells of ATP (such as KCN), by removal of glucose by ouabain or by removal of extracellular sodium.[91,94] In addition, a monoclonal antibody against a cell membrane protein,[112] or covalent binding of bromoacetyl T_3 to the cell surface[98] inhibits hepatocyte T_3 uptake. The monoclonal antibody bound to a 52 kd protein in the hepatocyte membrane. It should be noted that uptake is not completely blocked by any of the metabolic inhibitors, suggesting that there may be a component of the T_3 uptake process which is energy independent.[94,113] Results of studies in rat hepatocytes have linked the uptake of T_3 with its subsequent sulfation, glucuronidation, and for the sulfate conjugate, with inner ring deiodination.[114,115] T_3-sulfate is a highly effective substrate for inner ring deiodination by the type 1, but not the type 3 deiodinase.[115] These characteristics have allowed the evaluation of the effects of various substances on the cellular uptake of T_3 independent of its deiodination.[76,116] For example, incubation of hepatocytes with ouabain causes an inhibition of inner ring T_3 deiodination without increasing the level of T_3 conjugates (sulfate and glucuronides) in the media indicating it blocks T_3 uptake but not deiodination. On the other hand, PTU causes a marked decrease in deiodination, but this is associated with an increase in the concentration of conjugates in the media indicating PTU does not affect hepatic T_3 uptake. Studies in rat skeletal muscle have furthermore showed that monodansyl ca-

daverine and bacitracin, inhibitors of receptor mediated endocytosis, and metabolic inhibitors, such as oligomyocin, also inhibit T_3 uptake.[100,105] Others have used the rat hepatocyte system to demonstrate inhibition of T_3 uptake by several nonsteroidal anti-inflammatory agents and phenytoin.[96]

All of these results suggest that a stereospecific mechanism for active uptake for T_3 is present in the liver cell. The apparent Km for the uptake process is several orders of magnitude higher than is the level of free hormone in the serum. Thus, cellular transport of T_3 is not saturable under physiologic circumstances. Since it has been difficult to quantitate the concentration gradient across the hepatic cell membrane, it is not certain how much the cellular free T_3 concentration is increased relative to that in the extracellular space by this mechanism although estimates that this ratio is 2 to 3-fold in rat liver have been made using indirect in vivo tracer methods[117] (see below).

Thyroxine

The uptake of T_4 has been studied in many of the same cells.[91,102,118] While again there is some disagreement, the characteristics of T_4 uptake system in rat hepatocytes are similar to those for the T_3 system with high and low affinity systems and apparent Km values several orders of magnitude higher than the free T_4 concentration. By measuring the effects of these agents on deiodination, it was shown that T_4 transport is inhibited by pre-incubation of cells with agents causing ATP depletion, ouabain, bilirubin, non-esterified fatty acids and certain substances accumulating in the sera of patients with renal failure, e.g. 3 α furan fatty acid, 3 carboxy, 4 methyl, 5 propyl 2-furan and indoxyl sulfate.[119] Charcoal treatment of these sera eliminates this inhibition, indicating that the effect is due to the presence of these substances.

Studies of T_4 uptake by rat skeletal muscle suggest that passive entry is the major mechanism for T_4 entry into this tissue.[105] On the other hand, in mouse neuroblastoma cells, evidence for active uptake of 1, but not d, T_4 was apparent, and there was competition for uptake by members of the L system amino acids such as phenylalanine.[118] In human fibroblasts, an active transport system for T_4 has also been identified, with "low" and "high" affinity systems and again the apparent Km for the high affinity system is approximately a hundred fold higher than the free T_4 concentration.[72] Of interest in light of the binding of T_4, but not T_3, to apolipoprotein β in low density lipoproteins, T_4 was also accumulated by such fibroblasts, providing they fully expressed apo B/E receptors.[72] In all of these studies, there was no evidence that any of the circulating binding proteins such as albumin, TTR, or TBG enhanced cellular uptake.

Uptake of Iodothyronines by Intact Organs

There have been many studies of iodothyronine uptake in perfused liver systems. While initial interpretations of these studies were conflicting, the consensus at the present time is that the results are consistent with the predictions from the free T_4 hypothesis discussed earlier. As mentioned, there is virtually complete uptake of tracer T_4 in the periportal cells when rat liver is perfused with protein-free solutions.[61,62] This indicates that there is no restriction of free hormone uptake by cells. In fact, the extraction of free hormone is so complete that were binding proteins not present in the capillary perfusate, distribution of the T_4 (and presumably T_3) would be restricted to hepatic cells first contacted by plasma, assuming that the iodothyronines had not been adsorbed to the endothelial surfaces of the arterial system prior to reaching peripheral tissues. We may reasonably conclude that it is free thyroid hormones which are taken up by cells with no requirement for binding proteins to facilitate that process.[58] Lipoproteins, while potentially increasing T_4 uptake in fibroblasts, are of unknown physiological significance at the present time.[72]

LOCALIZATION OF INTRACELLULAR THYROID HORMONES

The site of thyroid hormone action in regulating metabolic events is the nucleus, where binding of T_3 to a nuclear receptor (TR) initiates a cascade of changes in gene transcription rates (or messenger RNA stability) which eventuate in the phenotypic expression of thyroid hormone effects. The likelihood of active transport of T_3, and probably T_4, across the cell membrane has already been discussed. When thyroid hormone enters the cell, it is rapidly bound to proteins in the cytosol but also rapidly enters the nuclear compartment.[120] Within the

cell, approximately 10 percent of the T_3 is in the nuclear compartment, for all tissues except anterior pituitary.[121] In this tissue, the balance between mechanisms leading to nuclear T_3 accumulation and the concentration and affinity of the cytosolic binding proteins are such that roughly equal fractions of T_3 are found in the nuclear and extranuclear compartments. When cell nuclei are resuspended in physiologic buffers or when TR proteins are expressed in in vitro systems, the affinity constant of the receptors for T_3 is on the order of 10^9 L/M.[122] However, both tracer equilibrium and direct radioimmunoassay studies have demonstrated that in most tissues (e.g., the liver, kidney, and heart) receptors are approximately 50 percent occupied at physiological plasma T_3 concentrations.[121] There are certain exceptions to this rule in that brain and pituitary nuclei have a higher degree of occupancy, on the order of 80 to 90 percent, as a consequence of the T_3 produced locally from cellular T_4 by the type 2 deiodinase.[123] Even considering only those tissues in which virtually all nuclear bound T_3 is derived from plasma, it seems likely either that the free T_3 concentration in the nucleus is much higher than that of plasma or that the functional affinity of the T_3 receptors, must be increased by the nuclear milieu. Otherwise, at the typical ambient plasma T_3 concentrations of approximately 5 to 10 pM, few T_3 receptors would be occupied. One possibility is that a step-up in T_3 concentration of over one hundred-fold occurs at some membrane of the cell to permit this degree of receptor occupancy. This issue has been addressed in some detail and it has been estimated that the free T_3 concentration in the cytoplasm of liver, kidney, and heart ranges from 10 to 15 pM.[124] The estimated free T_3 concentration in rat plasma in the same studies was 9 pM. Thus, by these techniques, the ratio of cytosolic to plasma free T_3 was about 2 to 1. This was confirmed by an independent method using tracer injections. These studies thus suggest that the plasma membrane concentrating mechanism accounts for an approximately twofold increase in free T_3 over that in the plasma. This is still, however, about 30-fold below the concentration required to account for 50 percent occupancy of the nuclear receptors, assuming that the affinity measured in vitro was the same as that in vivo. If so, these results imply that a major concentrative mechanism may operate at the nuclear membrane to enhance T_3 transport into the nucleus.

It is of interest to compare the results of the above

analyses in liver, kidney and heart with those in the brain. As already discussed, tracer kinetic studies had suggested that in this tissue, a substantial amount of tissue T_3 is contributed by T_4 to T_3 conversion in cerebro-cortical tissue.[125,126] These predictions were verified by direct radio immunoassay of brain cytosol.[124] The free cytosolic T_3 concentrations were approximately 40 pM, three to four times that in the liver, kidney and heart. That this increment in T_3 over that present in plasma was derived from local T_4 to T_3 conversion was established by showing that the concentration ratio of isotopic T_3 between cytosol and plasma was 1:1. Thus, these results constitute an independent verification of the significant contribution of locally produced hormone to the nuclear T_3 in the CNS. A similar verification has been performed for pituitary tissue using direct radioimmunoassay of nuclear T_3.[127]

As mentioned, the cytosolic T_3 binding proteins, while having affinities on the order of 10^7 to 10^8 L/M, do not appear to play a significant role in thyroid hormone action. It is of interest that one of these, a 55 kd protein originally identified by its covalent binding of bromoacetyl T_3, is protein disulfide isomerase.[128] This is the same protein to which antibodies were generated when purified liver microsomes were used as an immunogen in attempts to isolate the type 1 deiodinase.[129]

IODOTHYRONINE METABOLISM IN HUMANS

The production rate of T_4 in a 70 kg human is approximately 100 μg (130 nmol) per day deriving entirely from the thyroid gland (see Table 3-3). Tri-

iodothyronine production is approximately 32 μg (50 nmol) per day. There are two sources of T_3. The largest fraction, about 80 percent of the daily production, derives from 5′ monodeiodination of T_4 in peripheral tissues. The remainder is secreted directly by the thyroid gland. A recent study in selenium-deficient rats suggest that in this species as much as 50 percent of daily T_3 production is derived directly from thyroid secretion.[130] Studies showing high levels of expression of type 1 deiodinase in thyroid tissue[131-135] and the earlier demonstration, particularly in the dog thyroid, that PTU reduces the ratio of T_3 to T_4 in thyroid secretion, leads to the conclusion that a significant fraction of the T_3 in thyroid secretion may derive from T_4 to T_3 conversion within that tissue[136,137] However, the ratio of T_4 to T_3 in thyroglobulin from euthyroid humans is approximately 15:1.[138] Thus, hydrolysis of sufficient thyroglobulin to produce 130 nanomoles of T_4 per day would produce about 9 nanomoles of T_3. There is reasonably good agreement that about $\frac{1}{3}$ of the T_4 produced per day in humans is converted to T_3.[139] Since this would yield about 40 nmoles of the estimated total daily production of 50 nmol, there is not a substantial quantity of T_3 left to be accounted for by thyroidal T_4 monodeiodination. In patients with Graves' disease the ratio of T_3 to T_4 in thyroglobulin increases,[138,140] but the type 1 deiodinase activity is markedly stimulated in thyroid and in other tissues.[131,133,135,141,142] In this situation, intrathyroidal T_4 to T_3 conversion may well contribute and perhaps circulating T_4 could be a substrate.[143,144] This may be the explanation for the much greater sensitivity of T_3 production to inhibition by propylthio-

TABLE 3-3. Comparison of Metabolic Parameters of T_4, T_3, and Reverse T_3 (rT_3) in Humans

	T_4	T_3	rT_3
Serum concentrations			
(μg/100 ml)	8	0.14	0.020
(nmol/L)	103	2	0.4
Distribution volume (L)	10	38	90
Metabolic clearance rate (L/day)	1.2	24	110
Disposal or blood production rate			
(μg/day)	101	32	28
(nmol/day)	130	49	43
Fraction from T_4 (%)	—	>80	>95
Fraction excreted undeiodinated in feces (%)	20	?	?
T_4 production unaccounted for as plasma T_3, rT_3, or in feces (%)	11	—	—

uracil in hyperthyroid, compared to euthyroid, humans.[145] Of the remainder of the T_4 produced, approximately 40 percent is deiodinated in the inner ring to form reverse T_3, and a further 20 percent appears in the feces, presumably as the glucuronide conjugate.[25,139] The structures of the parent iodothyronines and the deiodination pathways are illustrated in Figure 3-4. The specific aspects of the metabolic pathways in the deiodination cascade are discussed in greater detail below.

Tracer T_4 disappears from the human circulation in two phases representing distribution into rapidly and slowly equilibrating tissue pools. Disposal of thyroid hormone is assumed to occur, not from the plasma compartment, but from one of the two tissue compartments.[67,75,107,108,139,146,147] This three compartment model of human T_4 metabolism has been employed for many years. The rapid equilibrating tissue pool is assumed to be predominantly liver and kidney. The more slowly equilibrating pool includes skeletal muscle and other tissues which have not been defined. Once equilibration has occurred, the half-life of T_4 disappearance from the circulation is about one week (Table 3-3). Its distribution volume is slightly larger than the albumin space, about 10 liters, and, as indicated, its elimination rate is quite stable, although influenced by thyroid status, nutrition and number of pharmacologic agents (see Ch. 5).

The kinetics of T_3 disappearance in humans are

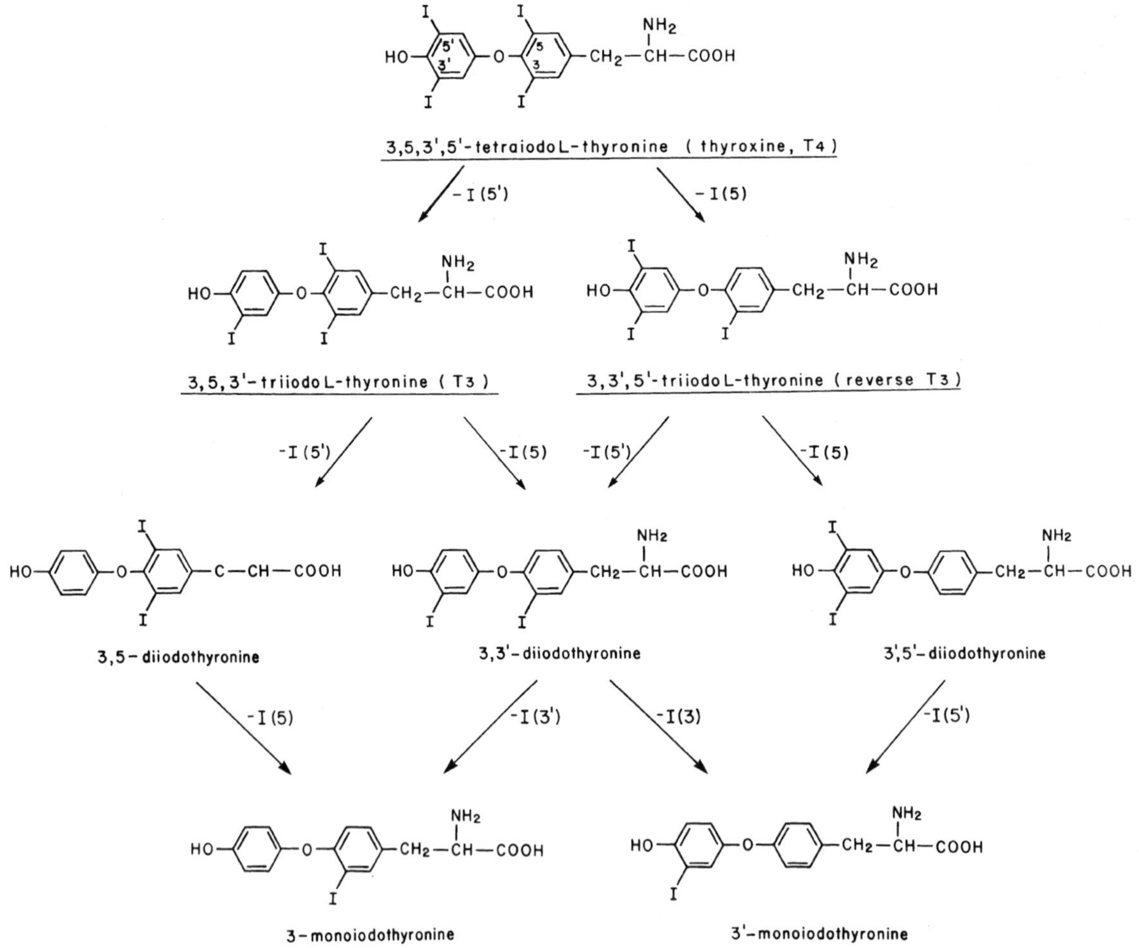

Fig. 3-4. Products produced by the successive monodeiodination of thyroxine in the outer- (5′) and inner (5) rings.

somewhat different.[146,147] The metabolic clearance rate of this hormone is much more rapid (about 24 liters per day) resulting in a half-life of approximately one day for this hormone. T_3 is probably produced both in the rapidly and slowly equilibrating compartments, presumably by the type 1 deiodinase in the kidney, liver (and thyroid?) in the rapid compartment, and by type 2 deiodinase in the slowly equilibrating tissues (see below). The other major circulating iodothyronine is reverse T_3. Its serum concentration is much lower than is that of T_3 (Table 3-3) and its metabolic clearance rate much more rapid. It would appear that roughly equivalent amounts of reverse T_3 and T_3 are produced from T_4 per day.[139] The major pathway for degradation of reverse T_3 in the adult is via 5' deiodination catalyzed by the type 1 iodothyronine deiodinase in liver and kidney. In the fetus, type 1 deiodinase levels are quite low, resulting in relatively high levels of circulating reverse T_3 and low serum T_3 concentrations.[148] Fetal thyroid physiology is discussed further in Chapter 15. Decreases in 5' deiodination are also observed in ill patients or during fasting, with the same results, namely serum T_3 concentration is reduced, but serum reverse T_3 concentration rises.[149] While the effects of illness on thyroid function are examined in greater detail in Chapter 5, this general pattern seems to hold. From a teleological point-of-view, it has been speculated that the fall in serum T_3 concentration in illness and fasting protects against the effects of normal concentrations of T_3 at a time when metabolic processes should be attenuated due to stress. Some evidence has been accumulated to support this concept.[149] It also is possible that the decrease in T_3 supply represents a physiologic disadvantage.[150] It seems likely that the decrease in T_3 production (and reverse T_3 degradation) during fasting or illness is multifactoral and may include reduced hepatic T_4 (and reverse T_3) uptake, reduced hepatic thiol concentration and eventually a decrease in the hepatic content of type 1 deiodinase.[76,123,149]

The other iodothyronines illustrated in Figure 3-4 are of interest as metabolic byproducts and are important primarily in assessing the magnitude of the various pathways for iodothyronine degradation. They have no known physiological role. While the intrinsic half-lives of T_3 and reverse T_3 are shorter than that of T_4, in a hypothyroid patient receiving a stable dose of levothyroxine, the half-life of T_3 and

reverse T_3 in the circulation will parallel that of T_4, since T_4 is the origin of these two iodothyronines. Thus, the only way to reduce T_3 production under these circumstances is to interfere with the action of the 5' deiodinases or to block the uptake of T_4 into deiodinating tissues.

It should also be emphasized that the total body T_4 to T_3 conversion rate estimate of 33 percent in humans is derived from plasma rather than total body T_3 production rates. We recognize that local T_3 production occurs, but it is difficult to quantify this pathway in humans. If there are significant quantities of T_4 converted to T_3 in the central nervous system, and degradation of this T_3 occurred prior to its exit into the plasma, total T_4 to T_3 conversion would be underestimated by sampling only the plasma T_3 pool. While the production of T_3 in such intracellular "hidden" pools does not constitute a major pathway for total body T_4 clearance in quantitative terms, it can be critically important to the cells of tissues such as the brain and pituitary.[126,151,152]

IODOTHYRONINE DEIODINASES

The fact that the major iodothyronine released into the circulation is a prohormone makes the understanding of the deiodination pathways for the iodothyronines essential, not only for evaluating their metabolic degradation, but also for understanding the regulation of thyroid hormone activities. A new phase in the investigation of iodothyronine deiodination began in 1991 with the report of the deduced amino acid sequence of the rat type 1 deiodinase derived from a cDNA isolated by expression cloning.[142] A cDNA encoding the human type 1 deiodinase was isolated soon thereafter and the two were found to be highly homologous.[143] The observation that the active center of this enzyme contained selenocysteine, suspected on the basis of earlier studies of experimental selenium deficiency,[153–157] has allowed many new insights into the regulation of the deiodination process.[54,144,158–161] In addition, identification of some of the special chemical properties of this selenoenzyme, not shared by the types 2 and 3 deiodinases, led to the inference that these deiodinases are unlikely to contain selenocysteine.[162–165] In the case of type 3 deiodinase, this appears to be incorrect in that the type 3 deiodinase of *xenopus laevis*, rat, and human is also a selenoenzyme sharing

TABLE 3-4. Characteristics of Enzymes Converting T$_4$ to T$_3$

Type	1	2
Tissue	Liver (L) Kidney (K) Thyroid (T) Anterior pituitary (AP)	Anterior pituitary (AP) Cerebral cortex (CX) Brown adipose tissue (BAT) Placenta
Substrate	Reverse T$_3$ $\gg$ T$_4$	T$_4$ $\geq$ reverse T$_3$
Active center	Selenocysteine	Cysteine (?)
Molecular weight	28,000	?
Apparent Km for T$_4$	"High" (~3 μM)	"Low" (<5 nM)
Apparent Vmax for T$_4$ (euthyroid rats)	"High" (=30 pmol/min/mg prot)	"Low" (=0.2–1.0 pmol/hr/mg prot)
Inner-ring (5) deiodinase activity	Yes (especially phenolic SO$_4$ conjugates)	No
PTU effect	Inhibit (uncompetitive)	Little or no inhibition
Iopanoic acid	Inhibit (competitive)	Inhibit (competitive)
Gold thioglucose	Competitive (Ki ~ 5–10 nM)	Competitive (Ki ~500 nM)
Hyperthyroidism	↑ (L, T) no effect (K)	↓
Hypothyroidism	↓ (L, K, AP), ↑ T	↑
Neonatal rat	↓ (L); ? (K, T, AP)	↑
Fasting	↓ (L); no effect (K)	↓ or no effect AP; no effect BAT; no effect CX
α_1-adrenergic agents	No effect	In BAT only

significant similarity with the type 1 protein.[166,392,393] In this section, the characteristics of the three deiodinases are reviewed and their role in the regulation of serum and tissue T$_3$ is discussed.

Type 1 Deiodinase

The type 1 deiodinase is often discussed in the context of its role as a 5′ (outer ring) deiodinase converting T$_4$ to T$_3$ (Fig. 3-4 and Table 3-4). This is, however, an oversimplification, since it also catalyzes the inner ring deiodination of T$_4$ to produce reverse T$_3$ and of T$_3$ to produce 3,3′ diiodothyronine (3,3′ T$_2$).[167–169] More notably, when iodothyronines are sulfated at the phenolic hydroxyl, the Vmax/Km ratios for inner ring deiodination of T$_4$-SO$_4$ and T$_3$-SO$_4$ approach that for 5′ deiodination of reverse T$_3$.[115,170] Inner ring deiodination of T$_3$ and T$_3$-SO$_4$ by the rat type 1 deiodinase has recently been confirmed in transient expression assays establishing the unique deiodination potential of this enzyme.[169] A summary of properties and the effects of various pharmacological and physiological conditions on type 1 deiodinase activity are presented in Table 3-4 and a schematic diagram of the deiodination mechanism in Figure 3-5.

At the time that the type 1 deiodinase was cloned, little was known about the regulation of selenocyste-ine insertion in eukaryotic proteins. This presents a problem for the cell since the triplet codon for selenocysteine, UGA, is normally a "stop" codon. It has subsequently been demonstrated that a stem loop sequence in the 3′ untranslated region (3′UT) of the type 1 deiodinase mRNA, termed a SECIS (SElenoCysteine Insertion Sequence) element, is necessary and sufficient for successful translation of this selenoprotein[171–173] (Figure 3-6). This has added yet a further layer of complexity in the study of what initially seemed to be a relatively simple reaction, the removal of an inner or outer ring iodine

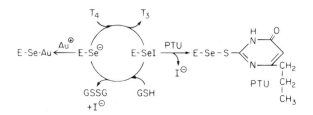

Fig. 3-5. Schematic diagram of the 5′ deiodination of T$_4$ to T$_3$ by the Type I deiodinase. The bisubstrate reaction of the enzyme with T$_4$ and GSH is depicted although the identity of the cytosolic thiol cofactor is still not known. Gold (Au +) and 6 N-propylthiouracil (PTU) are competitive inhibitors of the first and second half-reactions, respectively.

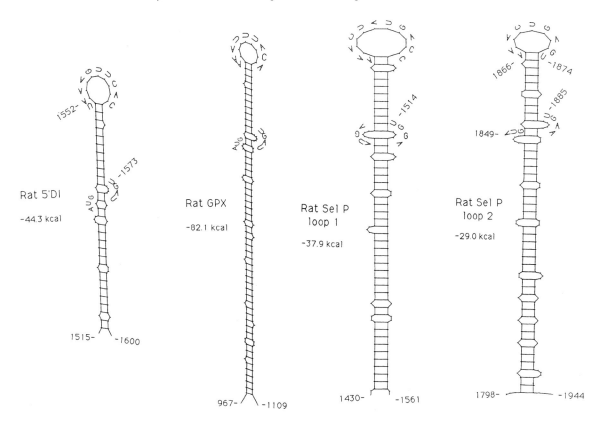

Fig. 3-6. Predicted secondary structures in SECIS elements from rat GPX and rat Sel P stem-loops 1 and 2. Structures were generated using the University of Wisconsin Genetics computer Group Fold program (Zuker and Steigler, 1981). Note the conserved nucleotides in the loops (AAA) and bulges of the stem. (From Berry et al,[172] with permission.)

atom from the iodothyronine nucleus. A similar requirement for sequences in the 3'UT has been found for the *Xenopus laevis* rat and human Type 3 deiodinases.[166,392,393]

Molecular biological techniques have also been used to show that expression type 1 deiodinase mRNA is increased by T_3.[142,174–176] Increases in the type 1 deiodinase mRNA are found in the liver and kidney of T_3 treated rats and mice, after exposure of rat hepatocytes to T_3, or after T_3 treatment of the rat thyroid FRTL 5 cell line.[132] The level of type 1 deiodinase mRNA is reduced in hypothyroid rat liver and kidney, but TSH itself induces an increase in type 1 deiodinase mRNA and enzyme protein in the thyroid cell.[134,135,177] This can explain the comparably altered levels of type 1 enzyme identified in liver of hyper- and hypothyroid rats many years ago.[178] The sera of patients with Graves' disease also increases type 1 deiodinase activity in rat thyroid cells as does T_3 per se.[131] This can explain the elevated type 1 deiodinase activity in Graves' thyroid tissue[131,135,179] which in turn may explain the enhanced susceptibility of T_3 production to inhibition by PTU in patients with Graves' disease.[145] That there may be further regulation of type 1 deiodinase activity by a post translational mechanism has been speculated from the effects of substrates such as reverse T_3 or iopanoic acid to down regulate the level of the enzyme in pituitary cells,[180] a phenomenon first recognized in studies of the type 2 deiodinase in brain and pituitary.[181–183]

Compounds like PTU which block T_3 deiodination while increasing T_3 sulfate conjugates in primary hepatocyte cultures are thought to act by inhibiting deiodination but not the cellular uptake of the iodothyronines since cellular uptake is required for T_3 sulfation.[98] These studies provide persuasive evidence that T_4 uptake into liver and kidney are rate-limiting in T_3 production by the type 1 pathway. It is not known at this time whether sulfation (or glucuronide conjugation) are physiologically-regulated pathways in humans. It would seem likely that sulfation, because it enhances inner ring deiodination, would be a major inactivating pathway for T_4 and T_3 at least in adults.[115]

Lastly, the requirement for a second substrate, a thiol cofactor, in the ping-pong reaction deiodinase mechanism to regenerate the active enzyme is a further step at which deiodination can be regulated in the type 1 pathway (Fig. 3-5). Reduced glutathione or thioredoxin may be this cytosolic co-factor, a decrease in which could explain the rapid inhibition of type 1 iodothyronine deiodination during starvation in humans.[170,184-193] Reduced glutathione production in liver requires NAPDH which in turn is produced primarily by the hexose monophosphate shunt pathway. While this is certainly a likely possibility in the liver, it is not clear what co-factors regulate type 1 deiodination in the thyroid gland. Since the hexose monophosphate shunt pathway is present, the process could be the same. Recent studies have suggested that the rat thyroid, by virtue of its active type 1 deiodinase, could provide substantial quantities of circulating T_3.[130] This could explain why starvation in the rat causes a 50 percent decrease in hepatic type 1 deiodinase activity, but total body T_4 to T_3 conversion is not significantly impaired.[194] While serum T_3 falls in the fasted rat, this reduction can be attributed to the decrease in circulating T_4 due, in turn, to a reduction in TSH release and a change in T_3 distribution space.[194] In addition, type 1 deiodinase mRNA expression in rat kidney is limited to cells in the S-3 segment of the proximal convoluted tubule.[195] These cells are also the site of extensive reduced glutathione production from nonglucose sources. This suggests a potential explanation for persistent T_3 production in the kidney of the fasted rat.[196,197]

In humans, PTU causes a 20 to 30 percent decrease in circulating T_3 when given to hypothyroid individuals receiving replacement levothyroxine.[198,199] On the other hand, acute decreases in serum T_3 of over 50 percent are seen in patients with Graves' disease given propylthyiouracil.[145] This effect is not seen with methimazole, indicating that T_3 production in the hyperthyroid human is considerably more sensitive to PTU than is T_3 production in the euthyroid or hypothyroid human.[200] There are several factors which can explain this

phenomenon. The first is the aforementioned high levels of type 1 deiodinase in the Graves' thyroid. Secondly, hyperthyroidism per se induces type 1 deiodinase in the liver and kidney which would act to increase the proportion of T_3 derived from this pathway (see above). Lastly, the only other pathway for T_3 production from T_4, the Type 2 deiodinase (see below), will be much less important as a potential source of T_3 at elevated serum T_4 concentrations in patients with Graves' disease due to its down regulation as well as its markedly lower Km for T_4 (Table 3-4).

Despite the fact that we have learned a great deal about deiodination by the type 1 pathway, a precise identification of the factor or factors causing the remarkably rapid decreases in serum T_3 and increases in rT_3 during the onset of illness or fasting in humans cannot be defined with certainty. There seems no other mechanism for the dramatic and rapid reduction in T_3 in humans in association with illness or fasting other than by a reduction in T_4 to T_3 conversion. A modest starvation-induced decrease in hepatic type 1 activity alone does not seem sufficient given the lack of a substantial effect of PTU to reduce circulating T_3 in the euthyroid individual. Inhibition of hepatic T_4 uptake, depletion of the hepatic sulfhydryl-containing cytosolic cofactor as well as the decrease in TSH may all contribute to this well recognized but poorly understood phenomenon.

Type 2 Deiodinase

The type 2 iodothyronine deiodinase also converts T_4 to T_3, however, it is not thought to play a major role in the production of plasma T_3 in the adult euthyroid state either in humans or in rats.[123] Rather, its physiology suggests it converts T_4 to T_3 within specific tissues thereby acting to supply T_3 to the nuclei of the cells in which it is expressed (Table 3-4). Type 2 deiodinase does not catalyze inner ring deiodination of the iodothyronines and has a similar low Km for T_4 (about 2 to 3 nM) and reverse T_3 (9 to 10 nM) (Table 3-4). Since catalysis by this enzyme is 3 orders of magnitude less sensitive to PTU than is type 1 deiodination, it may not contain selenocysteine in its active center. However, the fact that the type 3 enzyme also is insensitive and does contain selenocysteine indicates that the possibility is still open. The sensitivity of type 2 deiodinase to competitive inhibition by gold is also consistent with this possibility since the type 3 selenoenzyme is similarly insensitive.[166,392,393]

The important role played by the type 2 deiodinase in T_3 production in brown adipose tissue (BAT) under regulation by the sympathetic nervous system raises the possibility that a similar phenomenon may occur in man.[201] The most comparable human situation to the cold stress used to stimulate type 2 deiodinase in the rodent is that which occurs in the neonate at the time of delivery. The temperature stress at the time of birth would cause comparable stimulation of BAT in the neonate.[202] In the adult human, deposits of BAT are not localized to the interscapular and peri-renal area as they are in the newborn. Studies demonstrating expression of the brown adipocyte specific type 3 adrenergic receptor as well as uncoupling protein mRNA dispersed throughout white adipose tissue raises the possibility that type 2 deiodinase is more widespread and potentially a more important source of T_3 systemically in humans than had been previously appreciated.[203] The activity of the type 2 enzyme is remarkably sensitive to down-regulation by the substrates T_4 or reverse T_3. This was first illustrated by the rapid increase in type 2 enzyme activity found in the brain and pituitary following thyroidectomy, a change which was prevented by maintaining T_4 constant by parenteral injections[181] (Fig. 3-7). The inverse relationship between activity and substrate concentrations has led to the concept that the role of the type 2 enzyme is to facilitate T_3 homeostasis in tissues such as brain, pituitary and brown fat. A decrease in circulating T_4 is associated with an increase in the efficiency of T_4 to T_3 conversion in these tissues due to the increase in type 2 deiodinase.[204,205] Likewise, an increase in serum T_4 (or T_3) leads to a suppression of type 2 deiodinase activity decreasing conversion efficiency in those tissues where this is a rate limiting step in T_3 production.[182,206–208] The increase in type 2 activity, coupled with a reduction in the type 3 deiodinase, can explain the remarkable effectiveness of T_4 as a source of tissue T_3 in the central nervous system of the hypothyroid fetal and newborn rat[204,206,209–211] (Fig. 3-8).

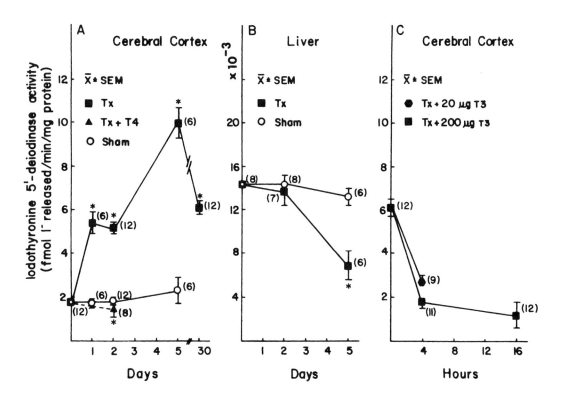

Fig. 3-7. Effects of thyroidectomy or thyroid hormone treatment on cerebral cortex and hepatic iodothyronine 5′-deiodination. Data points are mean ± SEM. (From Leonard et al,[181] with permission.)

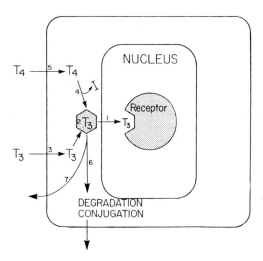

Fig. 3-8. Schematic diagram of the pathways regulating nuclear T_3 in cells such as those in brown adipose tissue, pituitary, or central nervous system in which type 2 deiodinase (step 4) is present. The cystolic T_3 concentration is determined by the rates of reaction indicated by steps 3, 5, 4, 7, and 6. Step 6 is the inner-ring deiodination of T_3 catalyzed by the Type 3 iodothyronine deiodinase. (From Silva and Larsen,[390] with permission.)

There appears to be differential expression and regulation of the type 2 deiodinase in different cells of the anterior pituitary. Enzyme activity has been identified in somatotroph, mammotroph and thyrotroph enriched fractions of dispersed rat anterior pituitary cells.[212,213] However, down regulation of type 2 deiodinase activity by thyroid hormone is limited to the somato- and mammotroph cells.[213] Thus, the increase in type 2 deiodinase activity with hypothyroidism in pituitary is explained primarily by an increase within the somatomammotroph fraction, with no increase in the deiodinase activity in the thyrotrophs. This is critical for the appropriate physiological response of the intact organism to a reduced serum T_4 since an increase in type 2 deiodinase activity in the thyrotroph would mitigate the increase in TSH secretion which is critical to the compensatory response of the pituitary-thyroid axis to impaired thyroid function or iodine deficiency (see Ch. 4).

Type 3 Deiodinase

The third deiodinase is one which catalyzes inner-ring deiodination of T_4 and T_3 thereby inactivating thyroid hormone (Table 3-5). In mammals, the high-

TABLE 3-5. Characteristics of Type 3 (5 or Inner-Ring) Deiodinase

Tissue location	Central nervous system (glial cells), skin, placenta, liver
Substrate preference	T_3 = triac > T_4 (not T_3–SO_4)
Cofactor	Reduced thiols
T_4 Km	~30 nmol
T_3 Km	~3 nmol
Active center	Selenocysteine
PTU	Little or no inhibition
Iopanoic acid	Competitive inhibitor
Gold thioglucose	Poor inhibitor
Hyperthyroidism	Increases activity
Hypothyroidism	Decreases activity
Partial fasting	No change (CNS)

est quantities of this activity have been identified in skin,[214] the placenta[215–219] and the central nervous system[220–222] where it appears to be confined to mature glial cells. However, in *Xenopus laevis* tadpoles, chick embryos, and certain fish, type 3 deiodinase is expressed in liver.[166,223–225] In addition, inner-ring deiodination activity has been demonstrated in the liver in the presence of high concentrations of PTU which indicates that this activity is distinct from that of the inner-ring deiodination catalyzed by the type 1 enzyme.[115] The apparent Km of the type 3 enzyme for either T_3 or T_4 is in the nanomolar range. PTU and gold only weakly inhibit its activity. Interestingly, both triiodopropionic and triiodoacetic (triac) acid are excellent substrates for the enzyme having a Km comparable to that of T_3 but the sulfate conjugates of T_3 and T_4 are poor substrates.[226] This results in an intriguing situation whereby sulfation of T_3 enhances the Vmax/Km ratio for inner-ring deiodination of T_3 by the type 1 enzyme whereas it leads to a marked reduction in the susceptibility to inner-ring deiodination by the type 3 deiodinase.[227,228] As with the types 1 and 2 enzymes, deiodination is facilitated by a thiol co-factor, and the enzyme is found in the microsomal fraction of the cell. Changes in type 3 activity with thyroid status, however, parallel those of the type 1 enzyme. Activity is increased in hyperthyroidism and decreased in the hypothyroid state.[221,229] In fact, one of the major compensatory mechanisms which occurs in the central nervous system of the hypothyroid newborn rat is a decrease in inner-ring deiodinase activity.[206,230] This change, together with the increase in the type 2 deiodinase, results in the marked efficacy of plasma T_4 to maintain a supply of nuclear T_3 to the central nervous system of the iodine deficient or hypothyroid newborn. Since type 3 enzyme also has a selenocysteine active center,[166,392,393] it would be subject to many of the same regulatory pathways for selenoprotein synthesis as the type 1 enzyme.

In terms of human thyroid physiology, the presence of the type 3 deiodinase in placenta presents a critically important barrier to the passage of active iodothyronines from the mother to the fetus[148] (see Ch. 15). The iodothyronines in the amniotic fluid are accessible to this deiodinase which accounts for the extremely high level of reverse T_3 in this compartment. Injection of T_4 into human amniotic fluid causes modest increases in amniotic fluid T_3, presumably from placental type 2 deiodinase, but substantial increments in reverse T_3. In addition, the presence of inner-ring deiodination in the epidermis presents another hurdle to the fetal uptake of active iodothyronine.[214] Nonetheless, it is clear from the studies on congenitally hypothyroid infants that the type 3 deiodinase in the placenta is not absolutely efficient in blocking the access of T_4 to the fetal circulation.[231] The serum T_4 concentrations in the serum of fetuses with complete TPO deficiency are roughly 20 to 50 percent of those in the normal infant despite the absence of T_4 synthesis in the fetal thyroid.

The type 3 deiodinase is presumably the source of much of the circulating reverse T_3 especially when the activity of the type 1 deiodinase is inhibited by PTU or by fasting. Therefore, the fact that serum reverse T_3 rises and serum T_3 falls in the PTU-treated human or rat suggests that the activity of this enzyme is not affected by either perturbation. Likewise, the fetus, which has extremely low type 1 activity, expresses the type 3 enzyme in both skin and in brain. Since T_3 sulfate is not a substrate for the type 3 enzyme,[199,226,232] one would anticipate high levels of T_3 sulfate in the serum of the euthyroid fetus and this has been observed.[228,233,234] Similar increases in circulating T_3 sulfate appear in rats and humans given PTU and during fasting or illness presumably due to the lack of effectivenss of the type 3 deiodinase to metabolize this compound.[234–237]

Integrated Physiologic Role of the Deiodinases

Since the major locus of thyroid hormone action is the cell nucleus and since it is, by and large, T_3 which produces its metabolic effects, the most critical question that must be answered is what are the consequences of the processes discussed above with respect to the quantities of nuclear T_3. As has been emphasized in previous sections, the sources and quantities of T_3 are different among different tissues. A schematic representation of the quantities of T_3, the total nuclear binding capacity for T_3 and the sources of T_3 in some of the major tissues of the rat is shown in Figure 3-9. First, it will be noted that there are considerable differences between tissues in terms of the numbers of T_3 receptor sites available. Brown adipose tissue and anterior pituitary with 6,000 to 8,000 receptor sites per nucleus contain the largest number. The kidney has relatively few, about 1,000, but other tissues such as circulating white cells, fibroblasts, etc. have even fewer. For example, the maximal binding capacity for T_3 in circulating human mononuclear cells is about 200 sites per cell.[238] The spleen and testis also have few specific binding sites for T_3.[121] It should be recalled, however, that when homogenates of heterogeneous tissues such as these are examined, the number of sites in a specific cell type could be much higher than the average depending on the percentage of those receptor positive cells within the tissue. In addition to the variation between tissues in the number of high affinity nuclear T_3 binding sites, there is also a difference between tissues in terms of the fraction of sites occupied and the degree to which intracellular T_3 derived from plasma T_3, termed $T_3(T_3)$, and T_3 produced locally from T_4, termed $T_3(T_4)$, contribute to the occupied receptors. The kidney and liver are typical of most tissues in the body in which virtually all of the T_3 specifically bound to the T_3 receptor is derived directly from plasma. In the cerebral cortex, brown adipose tissue, and anterior pituitary there is a significant contribution to nuclear T_3 from $T_3(T_4)$. This T_3 does not replace that derived from plasma, but is additive such that the degree of saturation of receptors in these tissues is substantially higher than is present in kidney, liver or heart.[123] In the cerebral cortex, for example, virtually all of the available receptors are occupied. The T_3 derived from local T_4 5′ deiodination can, however, be displaced by plasma T_3 by raising its concentration in the plasma. Likewise, should the activity of the type 2 deiodinase be increased, such as occurs in brown fat during cold stress, occupancy by $T_3(T_4)$ will also increase. Under those circumstances, it has been demonstrated that the brown adipocyte nuclear T_3 receptors become

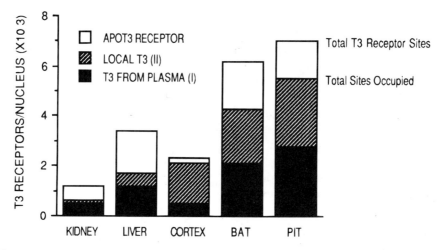

Fig. 3-9. Schematic diagram of the origin of the specifically bound nuclear T_3 in various tissues of the rat. Data are derived from studies in which the sources of specifically bound nuclear T_3 were estimated using double-isotope labeling techniques. In tissues in which the receptor saturation is significantly greater than 50%, the additional T_3 is provided by the type 2 iodothyronine 5′ deiodinase. T_3 in rat plasma is derived largely from the action of the propylthiouracil-sensitive type 1 iodothyronine deiodinase. (From Larsen and Ingbar,[1] with permission.)

saturated.[239] Such a change cannot be effected by increasing the serum T_4 concentration since T_4 per se will down-regulate the type 2 deiodinase. This has been demonstrated in C3H mice which have a genetic deficiency of type 1 deiodinase, and serum T_4 concentrations are approximately twice those of normal controls.[240] Type 2 deiodinase in brain and pituitary of this strain are reduced to about 50 percent and thus the contribution of T_3 produced by type 2 deiodination to the nuclear T_3 pool will remain approximately the same despite a higher T_4 concentration in the tissues. The presence of a type 2 deiodinase, with its potential for increased activity when serum T_4 falls, may be especially important in iodine deficiency. Since the early phases of human hypothyroidism in which serum T_4 is also reduced presents a similar physiology, this condition also benefits from the presence of type 2 deiodinase. However, it seems unlikely that the type 2 deiodinase has evolved for this reason since iodine deficiency is more likely to have provided the potent environmental pressure to maintain the expression of this enzyme.

In considering the physiologic state in humans, it is important to recall that one can theoretically supply T_3 to all nuclei, including those of the brain or anterior pituitary, by administration of T_3. However, to accomplish this on a chronic basis, one would need to maintain a plasma T_3 concentration roughly four times normal to achieve similar degrees of saturation of the cerebro-cortical nuclear receptors as is present due to the combined presence of T_4 and T_3. However, at that elevated plasma T_3 concentration, the quantity of nuclear T_3 in liver, kidney, and heart may be much higher than normal. Thus, because of the intricacies of the mechanisms for T_3 entry into the nucleus, under most circumstances, the T_4 is the most physiologically appropriate mechanism to normalize tissue T_3 concentrations in the brain.

THYROID HORMONE ACTION AT THE MOLECULAR LEVEL

Overview of Thyroid Hormone Action: Nuclear and Non-Nuclear Mediated Effects

The logical conclusion of this chapter is the review of the mechanism of T_3 action in the cell. In this section, the various components of the T_3 receptor-mediated mechanism of thyroid hormone action are discussed. The past decade has witnessed a rapid increase in the application of molecular biological techniques to the study of hormone action leading to revolutionary advances in our understanding of these processes.[241–245] While the details of these pathways are still under intense scrutiny, and, in fact, many critical aspects of the process are still not well understood, the global sequence of events is fairly clear. It is initiated by the binding of T_3 to its receptor. There are two similar nuclear T_3 receptor proteins, the α and β (TRα1 and TRβ1). These proteins have the property of binding T_3 to a high affinity site in the COOH terminal portion of the receptor, which in turn binds to specific DNA sequences present in thyroid hormone responsive genes through a specific protein sequence located near the amino-terminus of the receptor (Fig. 3-10). The specific DNA sequences which allow targeting of thyroid hormone receptors consist of hexamer or octamer nucleotide sequence motifs arranged in specific orientations in thyroid-hormone-responsive genes. These serve as high affinity binding sites for the TRα and/or TRβ. These DNA sequences, termed thyroid hormone response elements or TREs, are usually located in the 5′ flanking or promoter portion of the gene. In addition to specific T_3 binding nuclear receptors, other nuclear proteins, referred to under the general name of thyroid receptor auxiliary proteins (TRAPs), may also be involved in thyroid hormone action by virtue of their capacity to heterodimerize with TRα1 and TRβ1. One group of such proteins are the retinoid-X receptors (RXR) which

have as a ligand a specific metabolic product of retinoic acid, 9 *cis*-retinoic acid. These components are depicted schematically in Figure 3-11 and are discussed in greater detail in subsequent sections. To initiate thyroid hormone effects, T_3 enters the cell, or is generated therein, moves rapidly to the nucleus, interacts with the high affinity site on the TRα or TRβ protein and induces a confirmational change which influences the rate of transcription of the TRE-containing gene. There are two general classes of such genes, those which are positively and those which are negatively regulated by thyroid hormone. A well-studied example of a positively regulated gene is rat growth hormone (rGH). The TSHβ subunit is negatively regulated.

The TR-T_3-TRE responding gene complex satisfies all of the criteria for a thyroid-hormone-regulated process. It includes a mechanism which requires new mRNA synthesis, thus leading to increases or decreases in specific proteins. There is a time requirement for the events to take place which may be as short as minutes or as long as hours depending on the gene involved. It provides a targeting schema for defining genes which are thyroid hormone responsive and those which are not. Through the complexities of the TREs it allows co-stimulation

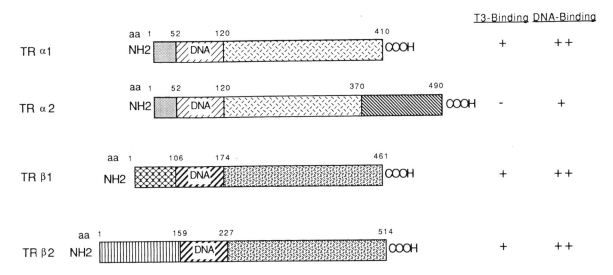

Fig. 3-10. Protein structure of the thyroid hormone receptors and the related α2 protein. The DNA binding portion of the protein is indicated. The portion of the protein carboxy-terminal to this contains the T_3-binding heterodimerization and transactivation domains of the receptors. The role of the amino-terminal sequences is not yet defined. The TRα2 protein is a product of alternate splicing of the TRαmRNA. Because of differences in the extreme carboxy terminal region, it does not bind T_3 nor does it heterodimerize with other nuclear proteins.

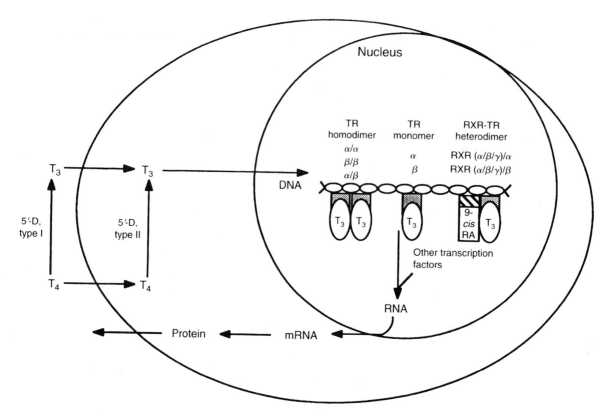

Fig. 3-11. Schematic diagram of the general pathway for thyroid hormone regulated ion of gene expression. The active form of thyroid hormone, triiodothyronine (T_3) is produced by deiodination of thyroxine (T_4) by the enzymes $T_4 5'$-deiodinase (5'-D) Types 1 and 2. T_3 enters the cell or is produced locally and then transported into the nucleus. Transcriptionally active forms of thyroid hormone receptors (TR) include monomers, homodimers, and heterodimers with nuclear protein partners, such as the retinoid-X receptor (RXR). The T_3-receptor complex interacts with specific sequences DNA regulatory regions and modifies gene expression. T_3 causes either increases or decreases in gene expression and may also influence the stability of messenger RNA (mRNA). 9-cis RA denotes 9-cis-retinoic acid, the ligand for RXR. (From Brent,[243] with permission.)

by other ligands in an additive or synergistic fashion. It satisfies the known requirement for high affinity ligands as inducers of thyroid-related effects and provides a mechanism by which a number of different genes can be stimulated in different directions in the same cell. This can explain how the complex T_3 regulated phenotypic events such as metamorphosis occur. The latter process is the most familiar and striking thyroid hormone regulated event in biology.

Before discussing of some of the details of this process, it is important to mention that there are non-nuclear mediated effects of thyroid hormone which have also attracted attention. These include interactions of T_3 with mitochondria,[246] an induc-

tion of calcium ATPase by thyroid hormone in the red cell and other membranes,[247–249] binding of hormone to either plasma membrane or certain cytosolic proteins,[128] and lastly, the regulation of type 2 and, to some extent, type 1 deiodinase activity through substrate induced post-translational down regulation.[181,182,250] This process has been studied in some detail and studies such as those shown in Figure 3-7 indicate that there are rapid changes in type 2 deiodinase which can be demonstrated in physiological systems. In the case of the study illustrated, simply reducing serum T_4 by thyroidectomy in rats leads to a marked increase in type 2 deiodinase activity in the cerebral cortex of the rat, an effect which can be completely prevented by administration of physiological quantities of T_4 following the procedure (Panel A). Shown in Panel B is evidence that thyroidectomy decreases liver Type 1 deiodinase, a change which is first apparent after two days. The elevated Type 2 deiodinase activity of the hypothyroid cerebral cortex is rapidly suppressed by intravenous T_3 (Panel C) although T_4 and reverse T_3 are 10-fold and 5-fold more potent respectively in producing this effect.[182] The down-regulation is not blocked by prior treatment of the animal with agents which block mRNA or protein synthesis. An additional effect of T_4 has been described in cultured glial precursor cells. Polymerization of actin filaments is stimulated by T_4, but not by T_3, again suggesting that this occurs by a non-nuclear mediated process.[251,252] These examples of non-transcriptional changes induced by thyroid hormone serve to remind us that while the nuclear mechanism of thyroid hormone action is certainly the predominant one, an open mind must be maintained to extranuclear events which may have important physiologic implications, even though, at present, they are understood only in phenomenological terms.

In the following section, the various components of the nuclear receptor mediated pathway for thyroid hormone action are reviewed. These will permit the reader to have an appreciation of the current state of our knowledge in this area and provide a background for understanding the molecular basis for thyroid hormone resistance discussed in Chapter 16.

The Nuclear T_3 Receptors

The presence of a nuclear protein which binds T_3 with limited capacity and high affinity was first identified by T_3 tracer studies.[120,253–256] Extraction of these receptors or isolation of nuclei from thyroid hormone responsive cells allowed the determination of the relative binding affinities of different iodothyronines and demonstrated that of the two principal circulating thyroid hormones, T_4 and T_3, T_3 was bound about 10 to 15 times more tightly then was T_4. Since intranuclear T_4 concentrations are somewhat lower than are those of T_3, T_3 occupies virtually all of the nuclear receptors. It was also determined that thyroid hormone responsive tissues such as pituitary and liver have higher binding capacities than do tissues such as the spleen and testis where thyroid hormone effects are difficult to demonstrate. The tissue

with the highest density of receptors is the anterior pituitary (see Fig. 3-9) containing 8,000 to 10,000 receptor molecules per nucleus. Using tracer techniques, it was also recognized that T_3 receptors were found exclusively in the nuclear compartment and could not be identified in the cytosol. This is in contrast to glucocorticoid receptors which are complexed to heat shock proteins in the cytosol until ligand binding occurs.

The concentration of T_3 in the nucleus is such that in most tissues only about half of the available receptors are occupied by ligand at any one time. This situation is dictated by the fact that the hypothalamic-pituitary thyroid axis is set to maintain circulating T_3 and T_4 concentrations at a level which results in this degree of saturation. While one can reason teleologically that a saturation of 50 percent would allow the organism to either decrease or increase thyroid hormone effects by fluctuations in serum T_3 concentrations, the physiologic rationale for this set point is still obscure. For example, there are only rare instances in which a physiological increase in nuclear T_3 occupancy occurs. The best documented example occurs in the brown adipose tissue (BAT) of the rodent exposed to cold stress due to adrenergic activation of type 2 deiodinase. This increase in nuclear T_3 occupancy is required for maximal synthetic rates for the BAT-specific uncoupling protein, a necessary event in the response of the rodent to cold stress.[239] It is difficult to find other examples of such an increase in T_3 occupancy and, in fact, it could be argued that the difference in receptor occupancy for the liver (50 percent) and for the cerebral cortical nuclei (about 90 percent) (Fig. 3-9) reflects the fact that, at least in the adult rat, complete or near complete occupancy of the T_3 receptors in the brain is required for normal cerebro-cortical function. A complete saturation of these receptors on the one hand could explain why there are limited effects of thyroid hormone excess on the central nervous system, and why the effects of hypothyroidism or iodine deficiency during the neonatal period have such dramatic effects on central nervous system development. On the other hand, a reduction in T_3, especially of circulating T_3, does occur in humans under numerous circumstances such as illness or fasting. This would cause nuclear receptor desaturation, particularly in those tissues which contribute in a major way to oxygen consumption and energy utilization in the organism, namely the heart, liver and skeletal muscle. The fact that the T_3 receptors are not completely occupied in the euthyroid state also makes the organism susceptible to the metabolic effects of hyperthyroidism, an event which does not seem to have been anticipated and against which there are few physiologic defenses.

During the search for ligands which could interact with a cDNA sequence encoding a protein highly analogous to the v erb A proto-oncogene, T_3 was found to be the missing ligand.[257,258] The v-erb A proto-oncogene is part of the retrovirus genome which induces erythroblastosis in chickens. Two genes are required for induction of this tumor, the v-erb B oncogene is similar to the EGF receptor and the v-erb A oncogene to the two thyroid hormone receptors. These have been denoted the c-erb Aα and β T_3 receptors because the alpha form initially isolated from a chicken embryo cDNA library[257] had greater similarity to the v-erb A coding sequence than did the human c-erb A β cDNA which was initially cloned from a human placental library.[258] A schematic diagram of the various members of the thyroid receptor family and its subtypes and related proteins are shown in Figure 3-10. The alpha and beta thyroid hormone receptors (TRs) are the products of two different genes. The TRα protein is encoded on chromosome 17 and the human TRβ on chromosome 3. Despite this, there is a high degree of homology between the two.

The major TR proteins, hTRα1 and β1 can be compared in terms of their different functional regions. There is a DNA-binding region in the TRβ1 protein between amino acids 106 and 174 which contains the cysteine coordinated zinc fingers characteristic of the thyroid-steroid receptor gene superfamily. The ligand-binding domain of TRβ is located between residues 239 and 461 and is highly homologous to a similar region in the human TRα. The area of greatest difference between TRα1 and the TRβ1 is in the NH$_2$-terminal region, which is only 52 amino acids in TRα1 protein, but 106 amino acids in TRβ1. This difference has unknown physiological significánce since the entire amino-terminal fragment can be deleted without a detectable change in the functions of the two proteins. It is important to note that the structure-functional aspects of the thyroid hormone receptors resemble those of the other members of this super family, including the retinoic acid, vitamin D, estrogen, androgen, progesterone, glucocorticoid, mineralocorticoid, and a number of other

receptors for which ligands have not yet been identified.[259] In addition to the most prevalent active forms of each receptor, denoted by the subscript 1, there are several gene products which arise due to alternative splicing of the α and β TR mRNAs. For TRα two other variants have been identified. One of these, the TRα2, has alternate exons substituted for the TRα1 final exon beginning at amino acid 370. This protein has interesting properties in that it cannot bind T_3, and yet, amino acids 1–370 are identical to those of the parent hormone.[260-264] Thus, since this protein cannot bind hormone, it is not a receptor per se, and is often termed c-erb A α2 protein. The c-erb A α2 protein can act as an antagonist to the TRα1 and β1 proteins by competing for DNA binding sites.[265,266] Another splicing alternative produces an mRNA termed TRα3 in which again the TRα1 homology ends at amino acid 370, but only the terminal exon contained in TRα2 is present.[260] The significance of this protein is unknown. It presumably could act as an inhibitor in the same way that the TRα2 can, but this has not been documented. No products of alternate splicing of the 3′ region of the mRNA have been identified for TRβ. However, an alternate splicing event produces TRβ2 in which a 159 amino acid terminus is substituted for the 106 amino acid fragment of the TRβ1. While this TRβ isoform was thought initially to be pituitary-specific,[267] it has now been found in several other tissues, particularly in the brain.[268-271]

With the identification of two receptors and a number of different splicing variants, the question immediately was raised as to what physiological role is served by having two such similar receptors, and what role, if any, do the alternately spliced variants play in thyroid physiology? While various studies have elucidated the differential tissue distribution of the TRα and TRβ isoforms,[269,272-274] and documented the effects of the α2 protein to inhibit either TRβ or TRα stimulation of the T_3 response in experimental systems (see above), the ultimate answer to this question is still not known.

One of the initial hypotheses to be tested was whether or not different tissues might express specific receptor subtypes. Many of these studies have employed specific analysis of mRNA expression, but discrepancies between changes in the levels of mRNA and the quantity of T_3 binding proteins during development or under various physiological perturbations led investigators to recognize that more sophisticated analyses of protein expression would be required before significant insights were obtained as to the differential function of these two receptor proteins. However, in terms of general phenomena, in the rat the TRα1 mRNA is present in highest abundance in skeletal and cardiac muscle and brown fat, whereas the TRβ1 mRNA is distributed more generally although it, in turn, is also highly expressed in adult brain, kidney, and liver.[196,275–279] The α2 mRNA is highly expressed in the central nervous system.[260] Despite the absence of mRNAs encoding either TRα1 or TRβ1 in testes, the α2 mRNA is quite high in this tissue.[263] A further level of complexity is found when one examines the response of the mRNA levels to changes in thyroid status. Thyroid hormone excess reduces TRα1 and α2 mRNA in heart, liver and kidney, but there is no change in the T_3-binding capacity.[278] In pituitary tumor cell lines, T_3 decreases the nuclear T_3 binding by about 50 percent.[280] Evaluation of different mRNAs has illustrated that the TRβ2 mRNA is markedly reduced by T_3, but there are no changes in TRβ1 mRNA.[121,278] Also there is a decrease of approximately 50 percent in expression of TRα1 and the α2 protein mRNAs. This further illustrates the complexity of the problem, since it is not possible to determine whether the reduction in the nuclear T_3 binding is due to changes in the level of TRβ2 or TRα1 protein in parallel with their mRNAs. It could also be due to changes in translational efficiency of any one of the three mRNAs together with alterations in the levels of mRNA expression.

In the rat, immunoprecipitation studies suggest that the predominant T_3-binding protein in liver is TRβ1, whereas in brain only 38 percent of T_3 binding protein is immunoprecipitated by a TRβ1 antibody.[281] In heart and kidney the TRα1 and β1 contribute equally to the T_3 receptor population. Several examples of a dissociation between changes in nuclear receptor protein and mRNA have been reported. These include the observation that during fasting in the rat, there is no change in hepatic TRβ1 mRNA, (the major hepatic TR) even though there is a 60 percent fall in total T_3 binding capacity.[282] In addition, there are increases in the immunoprecipitable TRβ1 protein in liver nuclei during maturation in the rat, but no change in the TRβ1 mRNA level.[122,281]

Other potential explanations for the presence of two different T_3 receptor proteins are that they could interact preferentially with different DNA binding sites, that they might bind T_3 or its active derivatives with different affinities, or that different TRs could combine with different auxiliary proteins in the nucleus. Any of these differences would contribute to the differential function of these proteins. It is also possible that the transcriptional stimulation by one TR isoform might be greater than that by the other. In fact, this does appear to be the case, at least in in vitro systems in which the maximal stimulation of transcription by TRα is approximately twice that for TRβ for several thyroid hormone responsive genes.[283,284] Other observations include the fact that TRβ1 binds T_3 with an affinity 6 times higher than that of TRα1, and the affinity of TRβ1 for triac is higher than that for T_3, whereas TRα1 binds T_3 and triac with similar affinities.[285] It has been known for some years that triac is preferentially bound over T_3 in nuclear receptors extracted from various rat tissues, again suggesting that in those tissues at least, the TRβ1 may be expressed to a greater degree. Despite these results it has been difficult to demonstrate the effects of these predicted differences in receptor protein/T_3 binding affinities in dose response relationships in model systems in vitro. In fact, the concentrations of thyroid hormone required for the maximum stimulation of thyroid hormone stimulated transcription in vitro are substantially higher than would be predicted on the basis of the receptor affinity for thyroid hormone.[283,284] The reasons for this are poorly understood, but may have to do with the fact that during expression of the receptors in these experimental systems there may be considerable alteration in the capacity to transport T_3 either into the cells or into the nucleus.

These considerations have special clinical relevance because all of the mutations identified to date which cause the clinical syndrome of thyroid hormone resistance (THR) have been found in the ligand binding domain of the TRβ1 thyroid hormone receptor. Virtually all are inherited as a "dominant negative" phenotype (see Ch. 16). This means that any member of the family in whom one allele of the TRβ1 contains the mutation has phenotypic evidence of resistance despite the fact that three alleles (two TRα genes and one TRβ gene) are entirely normal. Most of the mutations described reduce the T_3 binding affinity of the receptor. The fact that they are limited to the TRβ form strongly suggests that this protein plays a major role in the expression of thyroid hormone effects in humans. The possibility that a comparable mutation in TRα1 would not have deleterious effects on function has been tested and found not to be the case.[284] However, there is evidence that some T_3 receptor binding DNA sequences are more susceptible to inhibition by a mutant TRβ protein than are others.[284,286] The explanation for this phenomenon is under investigation but it may relate to the role of other nuclear proteins which assist the TRs in conferring thyroid hormone effects.

Thyroid Hormone Receptor Auxiliary Proteins (TRAPs)

Thyroid receptor auxiliary proteins were initially recognized as unknown nuclear proteins which enhanced the binding of thyroid hormone receptor to thyroid hormone response elements.[287–291] This function was identified both in assays in which the retardation of migration of TR binding DNA fragments was used as evidence of protein/DNA interactions ("gel-shift assays"), as well by a technique in which biotinylated oligonucleotides were used to complex the TRs which were bound to specific DNA binding sequences from thyroid hormone response genes. While TRs can heterodimerize with retinoic acid receptors,[292] it was recognized that most of the "TRAP" activity in various tissues could be accounted for by the presence of different nuclear DNA binding proteins, the retinoid-X receptors.[293–303] The name retinoid X receptor derives from the fact that these proteins have as their physiological ligand a product of retinoic acid metabolism, 9-*cis* retinoic acid.[293,294,304] While the process of retinoic acid conversion to 9-*cis* retinoic acid can be likened to that of T_4 to T_3 conversion, the important difference is that retinoic acid (RA) and 9-*cis* retinoic acid have distinct nuclear receptors, RAR and RXR. No TRs which bind T_4 with higher affinity than T_3 have been identified. The RXRs, however, like the TRs, do bind the precursor RA but with much lower affinity than they do 9-*cis* retinoic acid. The RXRs have three isoforms (RXRα, β, and γ) encoded by different genes and they are ubiquitously expressed in mammalian tissues. The interaction between the TRs and RXRs (as well as other perhaps as yet unidentified nuclear proteins) is thought to occur between several regions of the TR; a dimerization interface consisting of a series of a heptad repeats in

the ligand binding domain,[292] certain amino acids in the first "zinc finger" domain and residues in the 286–305 portion of TRb.[305–309] On the other hand, homodimerization with another TR occurs between interfaces in the second "zinc finger" of the DNA binding domain as well as certain residues in the 286–305 region.[245,310] Studies using RXR antibodies have demonstrated that these can deplete most, though not all, of the TRAP-like activity in the nuclear extracts of various cells types.[303,311]

The precise physiological role of the RXRs has not as yet been defined. In most experiments, co-expression of RXR proteins causes modest increases in T_3-directed expression of thyroid hormone response element containing reporter genes.[303,312–314] The effect of co-expressing cDNAs encoding these proteins, however, may be underestimated by the fact that endogenous RXR proteins may dampen the effects of the experimentally added RXR proteins. In ES cells which have low expression of RXRs, co-expression of RXRα usually enhances the basal and T_3-induced expression so that with most TREs T_3 induction was not altered.[315] This lack of enhancement of T_3 response is consistent with similar reports in yeast which do not express RXR proteins.[316]

The most striking characteristic of the RXR proteins relates to the contrast between the effects of ligand (T_3) binding on the affinity for DNA of TR-TR homodimers versus RXR TR heterodimers. In gel-shift studies, TR-homodimer binding is disrupted on TREs of the direct or inverted repeat configuration (but not palindromic TREs; see below) such that a single-receptor remains associated with the DNA always on the 3′ half-site.[317–319] With RXR-TR heterodimers, T_3 binding to the TR does not cause a decrease in the affinity for DNA. The complex remains bound to DNA again with the TR persistently present in the 3′ half-site of the direct or inverted repeat.[318,320–322] The mechanism by which T_3-binding alters the confirmation of the TR leading to these differential effects is not understood but it has led to the concept that on genes containing direct-repeat, inverted-repeat or complex configurations of half-sites, such as that of rGH, the RXR-TR-T_3 complex may be the mediator of transcriptional activation.[303,323–325] There are exceptions to this, so that it should be seen primarily as a working hypothesis.[313,326] RXR proteins can homodimerize[322] or heterodimerize with other members of the ligand-activated nuclear receptor superfamily including retinoic acid receptor (RAR), peroxisome proliferator-activated receptor (PPAR), vitamin D receptor (VDR), and others.[293,298,300,327]

Thyroid Hormone Response Elements (TREs)

In order for thyroid hormone to affect the expression of a given gene, there must be a mechanism by which the gene can be recognized. Of the thousands of genes, only a finite number respond either positively or negatively to thyroid hormone. Since T_3 binds with high affinity to nuclear T_3 receptors, and since the presence of these receptors is a prerequisite for a thyroid hormone response, it was logical to infer that specific DNA sequences would be found which bound the receptor. Based on analogies with the glucocorticoid system,[259] it was expected that such TR-binding sequences, termed thyroid hormone response elements (TREs), would be present in duplicate and in a palindromic arrangement, as is the case for glucocorticoid and estrogen response elements. Binding sites for these latter receptors are hexameric sequences. For example, in the case of the estrogen receptor, the nucleotide sequence 5′ AGGTCA 3′ is repeated on the complementary strand of the DNA at a position separated from that on the upper strand by 3 nucleotides. Thus, estrogen and glucocorticoid receptors were presumed to bind to DNA in a homodimeric configuration, one receptor molecule interacting with each of the two hexameric binding sites. Subsequent x-ray crystallographic studies have demonstrated that this is indeed the case with the basic amino acid, cysteine-rich zinc coordination portions of the receptor providing both the critical DNA contacts on the one hand, and the homodimerization interface on the other.[328] It is postulated that the binding of hormone, for example in the case of estrogen receptor, converts the estrogen receptor-DNA complex into a transcriptional enhancer sequence through mechanisms which, while not completely understood, presumably involve interaction with the transcription initiation complex.[259] Thus, such complexes are referred to as "hormone dependent enhancer" sequences since, when occupied by hormone, they affect transcriptional rates as do classical enhancer sequences in other genes. This means that they can be located at various distances from the transcriptional start site and exert positive (or negative) transcriptional effects regardless of their orientation.

It was with this background that the search for response elements in thyroid-hormone-responsive genes was initiated. In the case of thyroid hormone, it was initially necessary to use cells which could respond to T_3, i.e., those which expressed thyroid hormone receptors, since at the time such studies were initiated, the thyroid hormone receptor genes had not yet been cloned.[329] However, soon after such studies were begun, the TRα and β cDNAs were isolated. These could then be introduced into cells along with the artificial promoter-reporters to create an in vitro thyroid hormone responsive system.[330,331] This markedly enhanced the sensitivity and specificity of the paradigm. One of the most intensively studies TREs is that contained in the 5′ flanking region of the rat growth hormone (rGH) gene (Fig. 3-12). Early studies had shown that T_3 increased the transcription of rGH mRNA in normal pituitary tissue in various rat pituitary tumor cell lines.[332,333] The evaluation of the gene demonstrated that the major positive regulatory site for the rGH promoter is located in the 5′ flanking region of the gene between −190 and −160 nucleotides[329,331,333–335] (Figure 3-12). While the hexamer sequence PuGGTCA (Pu = A or G) confers a maximal response, considerable deviation from this idealized sequence is permitted with retention of some function as can be seen when comparing the A, B and C domains of rGH or the TREs in other genes illustrated in Figure 3-13.[336,337] Furthermore, there is new evidence that TR binding may be strongly influenced by the 2 base pairs 5′ to the hexamer and

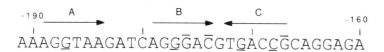

Fig. 3-12. Sequence of the rat growth hormone promoter −190 to −160 with horizontal arrows designating thyroid hormone receptor hexamer-binding half-sites. Horizontal lines indicate G residues protected in a methylation interference-binding assay. (From Brent et al,[241] with permission.)

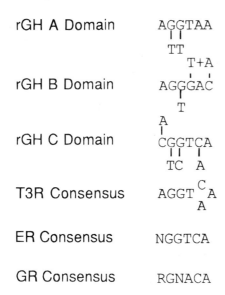

Fig. 3-13. Summary of point mutations in the various domains of the rat growth hormone promoter thyroid hormone receptor-binding site based on a functional analysis in transient transfection assays. Mutations that increased T_3 induction are shown above the sequence, and mutations that decreased response are shown below the sequence. A consensus T_3 receptor (T3R)-binding half-site sequence is shown compared to the consensus-binding half-sites for the estrogen receptor (ER). (From Brent et al,[241] with permission.)

that therefore a complete half-site may, in fact, be an octamer rather than a hexamer.[338–341] The preferred generic octamer for TR binding and function is PyPuPuGGTCA (Py = C or T, Pu = A or G). In some genes a third alternative for the "half-site" orientation is found.[342] This orientation has been termed an inverted palindrome with the receptor orientation arrows pointing in opposite directions. An example is the chicken lysozyme silencer response element (lys sil F-2 element) (Fig. 3-14).

In the early stages of the study of the TRE of the rGH promoter, it was recognized that the nucleotide sequence of the half-site played an important role in determining the potency of the response element. This grew out of studies of the effects of single nucleotide mutations, a summary of which are shown in Figure 3-13.[336] In the A domain, changing either of the two G residues reduces T_3 responsiveness (shown below the sequence). In the B and C domains, the two G residues are also critical. Other mutations which enhance T_3-responsiveness are depicted as altered nucleotides above the sequence.

Thus, in the B domain, changing the third G to T or in the C domain changing the first C to an A also enhances the potency. Changing the fifth C in the C domain to an A reduces the potency and is thus shown below the sequence. These results can be used to determine a consensus half-site, the idealized hexamer PuGGTCA.

These predictions have been tested experimentally using the rGH promoter. If the A domain remains in its wild type sequence, the B domain is mutated to AGGTAA (identical to the A domain) now conforming to a direct repeat with 4-base pair spacer with the B domain, and the C domain is mutated to AGGTCA (on the lower strand) thus forming a palindrome with the B half site, the T_3 response of a heterologous promoter is increased from 3.6-fold to 43-fold.[336] A single G to A mutation in the C domain increases the response 5-fold. Thus it is possible to significantly improve a naturally occurring TRE by making only one or two changes in the 30 bp sequence. The question arises as to why such a potent TRE did not evolve. One possible explanation is revealed in studies showing that with such highly potent artificial TREs, the presence of unoccupied receptor markedly represses transcription, presumably due to its high affinity binding to the TRE.[337,343] This concept is discussed further below under the subject of T_3 responsiveness. Is it also of interest that if one compares the sequences of the human (h) and bovine (b) GH genes in these regions to those of the rGH promoter, there are small but significant differences. In the bGH promoter, even though the A domain is lost, the B/C domain is conserved, and this promoter is T_3-responsive[344] (Fig. 3-14). In the hGH promoter neither the A nor the B domains is conserved explaining why the hGH promoter is not positively responsive to T_3.[267,344,345]

While it is thought that the TRE located between nucleotides -190 and -160 is the major TRE in the rGH gene, other TR binding sites have been identified. These include a single octameric half-site close to the TATA box which imparts a negative T_3 response to this gene.[338] In addition, a positively-responding sequence has been identified in the third intron of the rGH gene.[346] A physiological role for this intronic sequence has yet to be defined (Fig. 3-13).

Studies of the influence of the position of the TRE in the gene on its potency have also been performed using the rGH gene as a model. The TRE can be

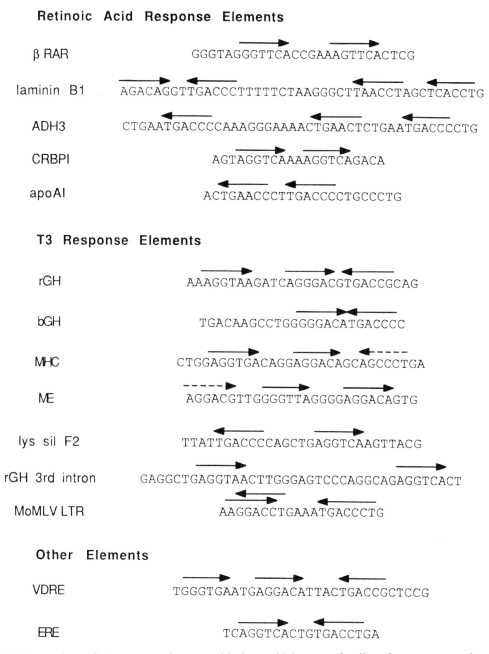

Fig. 3-14. Comparison of T_3 response elements with those which respond to ligand-receptor complexes from other members of the steroid-thyroid hormone nuclear receptor family. Arrows indicate the orientation (5′ to 3′) of the hexamer binding sites in the promoters of the various genes. Also shown are the consensus response elements for vitamin D (VDRE) and estrogen (ERE). (From Williams et al.,[391] with permission.)

inverted or be moved from its normal position to a position 700 nucleotides upstream with only a modest loss in potency. In addition, the element can also be moved to a position only 55 nucleotides upstream of the transcription start site, or to a position just 3′ of the start site and it remains effective in conferring a positive response to T_3 albeit an attenuated one.[347] This subject is discussed further in the context of regulation of TSH expression in Chapter 4. Taken together, these results indicate that the rGH TRE is contained within a 30 nucleotide cassette which can be shifted, inverted, and will still function to confer a positive response to T_3.

Similar mutational analyses have been performed using a number of other thyroid hormone dependent genes (Fig. 3-14). The list is not inclusive, but provides an example of the sequence spectrum of well-documented response elements. In addition, these illustrate the similarity, as well as the degeneracy, in the TRE sequences. For example, while the ABC domain pattern is present in the rat alpha myosin heavy chain, there are differences from the consensus sequence within the 3 half-sites just as in the rGH gene TRE. Such degeneracy is characteristic of TRE half-site sequences which rarely correspond to the generic consensus sequence, PyPuPuG-GTCA.[348]

The consensus hexamer half-site of the TRE is identical to that of the estrogen response element (Fig. 3-14). The hexamer PuGGTCA element is also an effective binding site for the VDR, the RAR, chicken ovalbumin upstream promoter activator (COUP), and the RXRs. How do genes containing such generic half-sites distinguish between these various receptors? This discrimination is in part attributable to the sequence of the individual half-sites, but primarily to the spacing between them and thus their orientation within the α helix. The idealized TRE contains a direct-repeat hexamer separated by four base pairs.[329,349,350] A three-base-pair space between directly repeating hexamers favors vitamin D receptor binding and a five or two base pair spacing, retinoic acid receptor binding (Fig. 3-13). In addition, the RXR nuclear receptors bind to direct repeats separated by a single base pair.[297,299,329,330,349–353] Other orientations of the half-sites are also effective in conferring a T_3 response. These include a palindromic arrangement of the PuGGTCA consensus sequence (as in bGH), with either no or one intervening nucleotide,

though palindromic arrangement with a 3 base pair separation is an estrogen response element (Fig. 3-14).

These examples show the considerable variation and flexibility tolerated in the DNA sequences which confer a T_3 response. Some of these, such as the palindromic arrangement, can also confer a response to retinoic acid.[352] For example, the TREs of the rGH and bGH genes can respond to either ligand.[329,352,354] Part of the explanation for the tolerance of the TRE to so much deviation from the consensus is that the TR is active either as a homodimer, or when complexed to one or another of the other members of the thyroid/retinoic receptor group or, in some cases, even as a monomer. In fact, it is not as yet clear what the T_3-containing active DNA-protein complex within the cell nucleus is. It may differ from cell-to-cell depending on which TR is expressed, its quantity and the nature and number of other nuclear proteins expressed in that tissue. These complexities are discussed further in the following section. In summary, however, it is clear that an identifying tag for a T_3-responsive gene, a sequence which can bind the T_3 receptor, must be present in order for that gene to be regulated by thyroid hormone. In most genes, this tag consists of two closely approximated octamer binding sites which can bind T_3 receptors as well as other nuclear proteins such as retinoic acid or RXR receptors. The position of the TRE in the gene and the nucleotide sequence of the binding site can vary somewhat without loss of the capacity to bind to TRs through a GG di-nucleotide in positions 4 and 5 of the octamer is probably essential. Thus, while we speak of a T_3 response *element* in the singular, this term encompasses a number of variations. The physiologic implications of this degeneracy are still being evaluated. The crystallographic structure of a TRE–TR–RXR complex has been published.[394]

The Mechanism of T_3-Induced Alterations in Gene Transcription

With all that has been learned about the TRE, the ready availability of cloned receptors as well as certain auxiliary proteins, it is perhaps somewhat surprising that we still do not have a precise understanding of why the binding of T_3 to its receptor induces changes in gene transcription. Studies of in vitro transcription systems are only now being reported.[355] As yet, they are more descriptive than mechanistic. There are, however, several general rules that can be cited to help understand the potential explanations for the T_3-directed transcriptional changes. Minimal components for T_3 to stimulate gene transcription include the TR and a suitable TRE in *cis* with a minimal promoter sequence. Apparently even a single high-affinity site can confer T_3 regulation although it is not certain whether such TRS bound to single half-sites are able to cobind RXR.[339-341] For negative regulation, it appears that a single receptor binding site may be functional and T_3-TR binding will decrease transcriptional rates[290,356-360] (see Ch. 4). As mentioned, studies of DNA binding to TREs in vitro suggest the possibility that RXR (or other as yet unidentified nuclear proteins) complex with the TR to induce positive transcriptional effects. T_3 may even alter the level of expression of RXRs[361] further multiplying its effect.

The induction of gene expression by T_3 is initiated by the binding of T_3 (or an analog of T_3 with relatively high affinity) to the T_3 receptor. Such analogs include triac, or even, theoretically, T_4, since this hormone can also bind to the T_3 receptor, although at much lower affinity. However, the effect of T_3 on the TR-DNA complex remains unknown. In transient expression assays already described above, the expression of TRs, together with genes containing TREs with high binding affinity, in the absence of T_3 causes a decrease in the expression of reporter genes controlled by such promoters.[312,337,342,343,353] This can be demonstrated in vitro and is thought to be a consequence of TR interaction with the pre-initiation transcriptional complex.[362] This suppression of TRE-containing promoter gene expression is abrogated by pre-incubation of receptor with triac, but T_3 can not reverse the effect if added in vitro following formation of the pre-initiation complex. This negative effect of unliganded receptor on positively responding thyroid responsive genes has only been demonstrated under artificial circumstances, and it is not yet certain that it is physiologically relevant. However, when one recalls that roughly one-half of the TRs in most cells of a euthyroid vertebrate are not occupied by T_3, it is intriguing to consider the possibility that this may be a mechanism by which a multiplicative effect of thyroid hormone on gene expression could be obtained. It is assumed that interaction of T_3 with TRs induces a conformational change which leads to the exposure of portions of the TR which can then interact with components of

the basal transcription machinery (with or without other proteins) and thereby increase transcription. A termination of the T_3 response would occur through dissociation of T_3 from the receptor (with reversal of the conformational change) or after a dissociation of the T_3-TR-RXR complex from the DNA. Other mechanisms are also possible, such as induction by T_3-TR complexes of local changes in chromatin structure which could enhance the accessibility of transcriptionally active proteins to the promoter of a given gene. An interaction with other as yet unrecognized nuclear proteins with receptor or receptor/RXR protein complexes such as occurs with estrogen receptor is also quite feasible, but such proteins have not yet been identified.[363]

Negative regulation is thought to involve similar mechanisms. The orientation of the TREs, particularly in the TSH beta and alpha subunit genes into a series of direct, or even overlapping repeats with no intervening spacing, suggests there may be special mechanisms involved for negatively regulated genes which do not occur in those positively regulated. Thus it has been shown in model transfections and in vitro using minimal promoters that addition of unliganded TR enhances transcription of negatively regulated genes, and, in turn, the addition of T_3 to such complexes leads to a decrease in transcriptional rates. Other proteins which could be involved in this system have not been defined and it is conceivable that they could be tissue-specific and limited to the cells expressing the negatively regulated genes, such as the thyrotroph. Other possibilities which have been proposed are that T_3-TR complexes could interfere with the binding of a positive regulator of TSHβ gene transcription, such as AP1 (a c-Jun homodimer or c-Jun/c-Fos heterodimer) which is increased in thyrotrophs by TRH or phorbol ester.[357] Such an explanation has been proposed for the negative response which is conferred by the octameric sequence overlying the TATA box of the rGH gene.[338] According to this reasoning T_3-TR complex would interfere with the binding of the TATA-binding protein and associated transcriptional enhancing factors.

The ligand-binding domain of the T_3 receptor contains a 9 heptad "leucine zipper" dimerization interface which forms an amphipathic helix.[292,309] As discussed in greater detail in Chapter 16, mutations in TRβ in families with THR cluster in two areas of the ligand-binding domain on either side of this heterodimerization domain.[309,364.365] While these mutant βTRs bind T_3 with much lower affinity than do wild type receptors, they are thought to compromise the action of the normal alpha and beta TRs by interfering with the accessibility of the latter to the TREs since they do not dissociate from the DNA in the presence of physiologic T_3 concentrations.[366–370]

A further aspect of T_3-regulated gene expression are the effects of T_3 to alter the stability or even editing of the mRNA. Thyroid hormone can alter the half-life of mRNAs encoding growth hormone,[371] malic enzyme,[372–376] apolipoprotein A-I or AII[377] and various enzymes involved in fatty acid synthesis.[377,378] A most striking "post-transcriptional" effect is the editing of the apolipoprotein B mRNA wherein thyroid hormone induces the de-amination of a C to U, resulting in the generation of a stop codon, thus eliminating the synthesis of the full-length protein.[378,379] The specific intermediate steps in these effects of thyroid hormone are not known, but in certain cases appear to require new protein synthesis and are thus, indirectly at least, transcriptional.

Tissue-Specific T_3 Effects

As can be appreciated from the above, there are a number of potential mechanisms by which thyroid hormone could induce tissue specific effects. The mechanism for T_3 entry into the cell, or its production within the cell, could constitute one such mechanism in that this would alter the quantity of T_3 present in the nucleus. Some genes may respond only when all TREs are persistently occupied by T_3-TR complexes. The uncoupling protein gene of brown adipose tissue is an example of one such gene[239,380] and the mitochondrial α glycerophosphate dehydrogenase gene is another.[381] The type of TR expressed in the cell could also influence the degree of thyroid hormone responsiveness, either because there may be an intrinsically higher affinity of T_3 for the TRβform of the receptor or because TRα and β may have differential DNA or TRAP binding affinities. Receptor isoforms could also play a role. Likewise, the non-T_3 binding (c-erb A α 2) protein is especially highly expressed in the brain, pituitary and heart, and could modulate the effects of TRα or β in those tissues.[265,382,383] Furthermore, the nature of the TREs themselves, their binding affinities, the arrangement of the half-sites, and their location within the gene could all affect the magnitude of the response of a specific gene. This has been amply demonstrated in in vitro studies where the activity of these TREs has been compared under identical circumstances.

There is also evidence that some TREs have promoter-specific effects. One of these is the myelin basic protein gene which responds much better to TR beta than to TR alpha.[384] Such TREs may have special affinities or effects on intrinsic homologous promoters which they regulate.[385] Lastly, the types and quantity of auxiliary proteins, such as the DNA-binding RXR family, other as yet uncharacterized DNA binding proteins or even proteins which do not contact DNA, in a given cell type could potentially influence the thyroid hormone response, its magnitude, or even its direction. Phosphorylation of the TRs or RXRs could also influence both the specificity and magnitude of the response by altering binding site specificity of dimerization potential.[386–388] Thus, while we have learned an enormous amount regarding many of the essential components involved in the response to thyroid hormone, much work remains to be done to determine how the relatively simple interaction of T_3 with a high affinity site on the TR has such protean effects on systems ranging from central nervous system organization to metamorphosis.

SUMMARY

Thyroxine is the principal secretory product of the thyroid gland. It is released together with 10-fold lower molar amounts of T_3. T_3 is primarily derived from direct thyroglobulin hydrolysis though in certain situations, such as Graves' disease or iodine-deficiency, there may be an increase in the ratio of T_3 to T_4 in thyroid secretion due to the contribution of intra-thyroidal T_4 5′-deiodination by the type 1 iodothyronine deiodinase. T_4 and T_3 are hydrophobic and circulate almost exclusively in a protein bound form. Only a small fraction of T_4, 0.02 percent, and a somewhat larger fraction of T_3, about 0.3 percent, are free or unbound in the circulation. However, it is the concentrations of these free hormones (about 20 pM for T_4 and 6 pM for T_3) which are maintained constant by the feedback regulatory mechanisms localized in the hypothalamic-pituitary thyrotropic regulatory system. The concentration of thyroid hormone-binding proteins determines the concentration of total hormone in the circulation. Thyroxine-binding globulin (TBG) is the major thyroid hormone-binding protein in human plasma. It is a glycoprotein of approximately 55,000 molecular weight which carries 70 to 80 percent of circulating T_3 and T_4. It is encoded by a gene on the X chromosome and can be totally absent in males with defective genes with no effect on thyroid status. Its clearance is markedly influenced by the number of sialic acid residues on the carbohydrate side chains. These prevent uptake of TBG by the asialo-glycoprotein receptors in the liver and determine its half-life. Either exogenous or endogenous estrogen increases the sialylation of the protein prolonging its half-life and increasing its concentration. Thus, during pregnancy, TBG concentrations are increased two to three fold and somewhat smaller increases occur in patients receiving oral contraceptives or estrogen replacement. The hypothalamic-pituitary axis accommodates to the estrogen-induced increase in circulating TBG by transient increases in T_4 secretion. During the re-equilibration process T_4 and T_3 degradation are also transiently reduced by the slight reduction in free hormone which occurs as the TBG concentration increases. A new steady state ensues with an elevation in total T_4 and T_3 but a normal free hormone concentration.

A second major binding protein for T_4 transport is transthyretin (TTR), a tetrameric protein which also has a molecular weight of approximately 55,000. This protein also transports retinoic acid by virtue of the fact that it binds retinol-binding protein. Transthyretin is markedly reduced during starvation or severe medical illness but this change has little effect on total or free hormone concentrations since the T_4 released binds to TBG and albumin. As with TBG, there are patients with inborn errors of TTR synthesis which cause increases or decreases in TTR concentration. These are quite rare but there is an association of abnormal TTR synthesis with a form of hereditary familial amyloidotic polyneuropathy (FAP). Increases in concentrations of TTR may be recognized by increases in circulating T_4, however, this is associated with a reduction in the free fraction of T_4 but not of T_3, since the latter hormone is relatively weakly bound by this protein. The remainder of thyroid hormones are bound to albumin and lipoproteins. Most albumin molecules have a low affinity for thyroid hormones. The principle point of clinical interest is that in some families a normal variant of albumin which binds T_4 (but not T_3) with increased affinity is over-expressed. This leads to an elevated T_4, but T_3 and serum TSH remain normal. The condition has therefore been termed Familial Dysalbuminemic Hyperthyroxinemia. Such patients can have confusing laboratory results but the normal TSH shows that the patients are euthyroid.

The physiological role of the plasma binding proteins is to ensure even distribution of thyroid hormone throughout the circulation. In their absence, the hydrophobic T_4 or T_3 would be rapidly and nonspecifically bound to the cell surfaces. It is not certain whether a specific binding protein is especially important for delivery of thyroid hormone to any specific tissue. It has been speculated that the increased TBG during pregnancy could serve the role of enhancing thyroid hormone delivery to the placenta to supply substrate for the type 3 deiodinase thus generating iodide for use by the fetus in thyroid hormone synthesis.

Thyroid hormones enter cells by a combination of low affinity, high capacity transport processes and by passive diffusion. The transport process involves interaction of iodothyronines with as yet unidentified carrier molecules or channels and requires ATP. Separate transporters exist for T_3 and T_4. The intracellular distribution of the thyroid hormones is influenced by the concentrations and affinities of the cytosolic binding proteins and the number of thyroid hormone receptors in the nucleus. In most cells, only 10 percent of the T_3 (the active thyroid hormone) is found in the nuclear compartment. The only exception to this is the anterior pituitary, in which approximately 50 percent of the T_3 is in the nucleus. There is the possibility that a transport mechanism also exists at the interface between the cytosol and nuclear compartments in that thyroid hormone receptor saturation in vivo is considerably higher than would be predicted from the concentration of cytosolic and plasma free hormone and the affinity constant of the receptors for T_3.

The metabolic clearance of T_4 and T_3 occurs by successive deiodination of outer and inner rings and glucuronide conjugation in the liver with excretion of T_4 or T_3 into the bile. In humans, about 20 percent of T_4 is excreted into the feces. Three deiodinases have been identified. Type 1 deiodinase is a selenoenzyme which is quite sensitive to inhibition by propylthiouracil or by gold compounds. It is expressed in the liver, kidney, thyroid, and pituitary. It has a relatively high Km for T_4 and catalyzes the outer-ring deiodination of T_4 and reverse T_3 as well as the inner-ring deiodination of T_4, T_3 and their sulfate conjugates. Type 1 deiodinase provides most of the circulating T_3 in animals and humans. Sulfate conjugation of the phenolic hydroxyl of T_4 and T_3 occurs in the liver and leads to hormone inactivation, via loss of an inner-ring iodine atom which is essential for function. Type 1 deiodinase is increased by thyroid hormone and, in the thyroid gland, by increasing intracellular cyclic AMP. It is markedly increased in the hyperthyroid thyroid, liver, and kidney. This may account for the greater sensitivity of T_4 to T_3 conversion to propylthiouracil inhibition in the Graves' disease patient as opposed to that of the euthyroid individual.

Type 2 deiodinase is a low Km, exclusively outer-ring, deiodinase which is relatively insensitive to inhibition by propylthiouracil and gold compounds. It is expressed in the brain, pituitary, brown adipose tissue, and placenta and its physiological role appears to be to provide a supply of interacellular T_3 in those tissues. Over 79 percent of the T_3 in the brain derives from this source. It has been shown that regulation of TSH secretion by circulating T_4 occurs by virtue of the capacity of the thyrotroph to deiodinate T_4 rapidly via the type 2 deiodinase. The activity of this deiodinase is increased in hypothyroidism by a reduction in the degradation rate of the enzyme. Thus, it can serve as a mechanism to enhance the supply of T_3. Type 2 deiodinase is also stimulated by catecholamines in brown adipose tissue. This is an early response of the rodent to cold stress and presumably occurs in the human newborn at the time of parturition. It facilitates mitochondrial uncoupling-protein synthesis and thermogenesis in this organ.

Type 3 deiodinase is an exclusively inner-ring deiodinase expressed in brain, immature skin, liver, and placenta. Its role is to inactivate T_3 by inner-ring deiodination and it does not accept T_3 sulfate as a substrate. It is also a selenoenzyme but is relatively insensitive to inhibition by gold or by propylthiouracil. The synthesis of both type 1 and 3 deiodinase enzymes are complex and require the UGA stop codon mechanism to allow insertion of selenocysteine. Type 3 deiodinase expression is stimulated by thyroid hormone. This has the effect of reducing the rate of T_3 degradation in the hypothyroid state especially in the brain and conversely accelerating it in the hyperthyroid state. Type 3 deiodinase is induced during metamorphosis suggesting that it acts as a homeostatic mechanism during this process. The high levels of type 3 deiodinase in the placenta restrict the access of maternal T_4 and T_3 to the fetus.

The metabolic effects of thyroid hormone are initiated by the binding of T_3 to a nuclear protein termed the thyroid hormone receptor. There are two thyroid hormone receptors in humans, alpha and beta, which have very similar DNA and ligand binding domains but differ in the amino terminal sequence. Separate functions for these two receptors have not been elucidated but the syndrome of resistance to thyroid hormone (RTH) is characterized by mutations in the ligand-binding domain exclusively of the beta receptor. The thyroid hormone responsive genes contain a DNA sequence which serves as a high-affinity binding site for the thyroid hormone receptors probably complexed to other nuclear proteins. These binding sites, which have the optimal consensus octamer sequence PyPuPuGGTCA, are usually arranged as two direct repeats with two nucleotides separating two octamer sequences. This complex is termed a T_3 response element (TRE). When receptors are not occupied by T_3, they are bound to TREs as homodimers and may suppress the transcription of genes stimulated by T_3. When T_3 binds to the receptor, a new complex is formed which for some TREs involves the association of a T_3 receptor with another nuclear protein such as the retinoid-X receptor. It is thought that either the T_3-TR homodimer or RXR-TR heterodimer (or other TR heterodimers) interacts with the transcription-initiation complex to enhance transcription. There are still many unknowns in this process but the TRE and T_3 receptor are essential components. Negative regulation of thyroid-hormone-responsive genes such as that encoding TSH-β occurs by poorly defined mechanisms. For such genes, the unoccupied T_3 receptor may enhance transcription of specific genes perhaps in combination with thyrotroph-specific proteins. Other mechanisms for T_3 effects such as mRNA stabilization or editing or even post-translational modification of proteins also occur but the mechanisms have not been characterized at a molecular level. Nonetheless, the cloning of the thyroid hormone receptors and other nuclear proteins has permitted fundamental insights into the thyroid hormone activation mechanism.

REFERENCES

1. Larsen PR, Ingbar SH: The thyroid. p. 357. In Wilson JE, Foster DW (eds): Williams Textbook of Endocrinology. WB Saunders, Philadelphia, 1992
2. Episkopou V, Maeda S, Nishiguchi S et al: Disruption of the transthyretin gene results in mice with depressed levels of plasma retinol and thyroid hormone. Proc Natl Acad Sci USA 90:2375, 1993
3. Flink IL, Bailey TJ, Gustafson TA et al: Complete amino acid sequence of human thyroxine-binding globulin deduced from cloned DNA: close homology to the serine antiproteases. Proc Natl Acad Sci USA 83:7708, 1986
4. Refetoff S: Inherited thyroxine-binding globulin abnormalities in man. Endocr Rev 10:275, 1989
5. Hiller AP: Human thyroxine-binding globulin and thyroxine-binding pre-albumin dissociation rates. J Physiol 217:625, 1971
6. Hiller AP: The rate of triiodothyronine dissociation from binding sites in human plasma. Acta Endocrinol 80:49, 1975
7. Robbins J, Johnson ML: Theoretical considerations in the transport of the thyroid hormones in blood. p. 1. In Ekins R, Faglia F, Pennisi F, Pinchera A (eds): Free Thyroid Hormones. Excerpta Medica, Amsterdam, 1979
8. Robbins J, Johnson ML: Possible significance of multiple transport proteins for the thyroid hormones. p. 53. In Albertini A, Elkins RP (eds): Free Hormones in Blood. Elsevier, Amsterdam, 1982
9. Robbins J, Rall JE: The iodine-containing hormones. p. 219. In Gray CH, James VHT (eds): Hormones in the Blood. Academic Press, London, 1983
10. Trent JM, Flink IL, Morkin E et al: Localization of the human thyroxine-binding globulin gene to the long arm of the X chromosome (Xq21-22). Am J Hum Gen 41:428, 1987
11. Refetoff S, Fang VS, Marshall JS, Robin NI: Metabolism of thyroxine-binding globulin in man: abnormal rate of synthesis in inherited thyroxine-binding globulin deficiency and excess. J Clin Invest 57:485, 1976
12. Burr WA, Ramsden DB, Hoffenberg R: Hereditary abnormalities of thyroxine-binding globulin concentration: a study of 19 kindreds with inherited increase or decrease of thyroxine-binding globulin. Quart J Med 49:295, 1980
13. Murata Y, Takamatsu J, Refetoff S: Inherited abnormality of thyroxine-binding globulin with no demonstrable thyroxine-binding activity and high

14. serum levels of denatured thyroxine-binding globulin. N Engl J Med 314:694, 1986
14. Refetoff S, Murata Y, Vassart G et al: Radioimmunoassays specific for the tertiary and primary structures of thyroxine-binding globulin (TBG): measurement of denatured TBG in serum. J Clin Endocrinol Metab 59:269, 1984
15. Bartalena L: Recent achievements in studies on thyroid hormone-binding proteins. Endocr Rev 11:47, 1990
16. Ain KB, Refetoff S: Relationship of oligosaccharide modification to the cause of serum thyroxine-binding globulin excess. J Clin Endocrinol Metab 66:1037, 1988
17. Ross DS, Daniels GH, Dienstag JL, Ridgway EC: Elevated thyroxine levels due to increased thyroxine-binding globulin in acute hepatitis. Am J Med 74:564, 1983
18. Ain KB, Mori Y, Refetoff S: Reduced clearance rate of thyroxine-binding globulin (TBG) with increased sialylation: a mechanism for estrogen-induced elevation of serum TBG concentration. J Clin Endocrinol Metab 65:689, 1987
19. Glinoer D, McGuire RA, Dubois A et al: Thyroxine-binding globulin metabolism in rhesus monkeys: effects of hyper- and hypothyroidism. Endocrinology 104:175, 1979
20. McGuire RA, Glinoer D, Albert MA, Robbins J: Comparative effects of thyroxine (T_4) and triiodothyronine on T_4-binding globulin metabolism in rhesus monkeys. Endocrinology 110:1340, 1982
21. Garnick MB, Larsen PR: Acute deficiency of thyroxine-binding globulin during L-asparaginase therapy. N Engl J Med 301:252, 1979
22. Heidemann PH, Stubbe P, Beck W: Transient secondary hypothyroidism and thyroxine-binding globulin deficiency in leukemic children during polychemotherapy: an effect of L-asparaginase. Eur J Pediatr 136:291, 1981
23. Bartalena L, Martino E, Antonelli A et al: Effect of the antileukemic agent L-asparaginase on thyroxine-binding globulin and albumin synthesis in cultured human hepatoma (HEP G2) cells. Endocrinology 119:1185, 1985
24. Austen FK, Rubini ME, Meroney WH, Wolff J: Salicylates and thyroid function. I. Depression of thyroid function. J Clin Invest 37:1131, 1958
25. Larsen PR, Atkinson AJ Jr, Wellman HN, Goldsmith RE: The effect of diphenylhydantoin on thyroxine metabolism in man. J Clin Invest 49:1266, 1970
26. Larsen PR: Salicylate-induced increases in free triiodothyronine in human serum: evidence of inhibition of triiodothyronine binding to thyroxine-binding globulin and thyroxine-binding prealbumin. J Clin Invest 51:1125, 1972

27. Taylor R, Hutton C, Weeke J, Clark F: Fenclofenac-secondary effects upon the pituitary thyroid axis. Clin Endocrinol 19:683, 1983

28. Stockigt JR, Lim C-F, Barlow JW et al: High concentrations of furosemide inhibit serum binding of thyroxine. J Clin Endocrinol Metab 59:62, 1984

29. Wenzel KW: Pharmacological interference with in vitro tests of thyroid function. Metabolism 30:717, 1981

30. Cavalieri RR, Pitt-Rivers R: The effects of drugs on the distribution and metabolism of thyroid hormones. Pharmacol Rev 33:55, 1981

31. McConnel RJ: Abnormal thyroid function test results in patients taking salsalate. JAMA 267:1242, 1992

32. Kurtz AB, Capper SJ, Clifford J et al: The effect of fenclofenac on thyroid function. Clin Endocrinol 15:117, 1981

33. Capper SJ, Humphrey MJ, Kurtz AB: Inhibition of thyroxine binding to serum proteins by fenclofenac and related compounds. Clin Chim Acta 112:77, 1981

34. Chin W, Schussler GC: Decreased serum-free thyroxine concentration in patients treated with diphenylhydantoin. J Clin Endocrinol 28:181, 1968

35. Surks MI, Oppenheimer JH: Postoperative changes in the concentration of thyroxine-binding prealbumin and serum-free thyroxine. J Clin Endocrinol 24:794, 1964

36. Oppenheimer JH, Martinez M, Bernstein G: Determination of the maximal binding capacity and protein concentration of thyroxine-binding prealbumin in human serum. J Lab Clin Med 67:500, 1966

37. Dickson PW, Aldred AR, Marley PD et al: Rat choroid plexus specializes in the synthesis and secretion of transthyretin (prealbumin). J Biol Chem 261:3475, 1985

38. Dickson PW, Howlett GJ, Schreiber G: Rat transthyretin (prealbumin): molecular cloning, nucleotide sequence, and gene expression in liver and brain. J Biol Chem 260:8214, 1985

39. Jacobsson B, Pettersson T, Sandstedt B, Carlstrom A: Prealbumin in the islets of Langerhans. Int Res Commun Syst Med Sci 7:590, 1979

40. Yan C, Costa RH, Darnell JE Jr et al: Distinct positive and negative elements control the limited hepatocyte and choroid plexus expression of transthyretin in transgenic mice. EMBO J 9:869, 1990

41. Rajatanavin R, Leberman C, Lawrence GD et al: Euthyroid hyperthyroxinemia and thyroxine-binding prealbumin excess in islet cell carcinoma. J Clin Endocrinol Metab 61:17, 1985

42. Bartalena L: Thyroid hormone-binding proteins: update 1994. Endocr Rev 3:140, 1994

43. MacDonald PN, Bok D, Ong DE: Localization of cellular retinol-binding protein and retinol-binding protein in cells comprising the blood-brain barrier of rat and human. Proc Natl Acad Sci USA 87:4265, 1990

44. Schreiber G, Aldred AR, Jaworowski A et al: Thyroxine transport from blood to brain via transthyretin synthesis in choroid plexus. Am J Physiol 258:R338, 1990

45. Chanoine JP, Alex S, Fang SL et al: Role of transthyretin in the transport of thyroxine from the blood to the choroid plexus, the cerebrospinal fluid, and the brain. Endocrinology 130:933, 1992

46. Curtis AJ, Scrimshaw BJ, Topliss DJ et al: Thyroxine binding by human transthyretin variants: mutations at position 119, but not positions 54, increase thyroxine-binding affinity. J Clin Endocrinol Metab 78:459, 1994

47. Alves IL, Divino CM, Schussler GC et al: Thyroxine binding in a TTR met 119 kindred. J Clin Endocrinol Metab 77:484, 1993

48. Rosen HN, Moses AC, Murrell JR et al: Thyroxine interactions with transthyretin: a comparison of 10 different naturally occurring human transthyretin variants. J Clin Endocrinol Metab 77:370, 1993

49. Skiest D, Braverman LE, Emerson CH: Concentration of free thyroxine in serum of a patient with euthyroid hyperthyroxinemia secondary to increased thyroxin-binding prealbumin: results by various methods compared. Clin Chem 32:687, 1986

50. Blake CCF, Geisow MJ, Swan IDA: Structure of human plasma prealbumin at 2.5 Å resolution: a preliminary report on the polypeptide chain conformation quaternary structure and thyroxine binding. J Mol Biol 88:1, 1974

51. Blake CCF, Geisow MJ, Oatley SJ et al: Structure of prealbumin: secondary, tertiary, and quaternary interactions determined by Fourier refinement at 1.8 Å. J Mol Biol 121:339, 1978

52. Köhrle J, Fang SL, Yang Y et al: Rapid effects of the flavonoid EMD 21388 on serum thyroid hormone binding and thyrotopin regulation in the rat. Endocrinology 125:532, 1989

53. Lueprasitsakul W, Alex S, Fang SL et al: Flavonoid administration immediately displaces thyroxine (T_4) from serum transthyretin, increases serum-free T_4, and decreases thyrotropin in the rat. Endocrinology 126:2890, 1990

54. Köhrle J: Thyroid hormone deiodination in target tissues—a regulatory role for the trace element selenium? Exp Clin Endocrinol 102:63, 1994

55. Pardridge WM: Carrier-mediated transport of thyroid hormones through the rat blood-brain barrier: primary role of the albumin-bound hormone. Endocrinology 105:605, 1979

56. Pardridge WM: Transport of protein-bound hormones into tissues in vivo. Endocr Rev 2:103, 1981

57. Pardridge WM: Transport of protein-bound thyroid and steroid hormones into tissues in vivo: a new hypothesis on the role of hormone-binding plasma proteins. p. 45. In Albertini A, Elkins RP (eds): Free Hormones in Blood. Elsevier Biomedical, Amsterdam, 1982

58. Mendel CM: The free-hormone hypothesis: a physiologically based mathematical model. Endocr Rev 10:232, 1989

59. Mendel CM, Cavalieri RR, Gavin LA et al: Thyroxine transport and distribution in nagase analbuminemic rats. J Clin Invest 83:143, 1989

60. Mendel CM, Frost PH, Cavalieri RR: Effect of free fatty acids on the concentration of free thyroxine in human serum: the role of albumin. J Clin Endocrinol Metab 63:1394, 1986

61. Mendel CM, Weisiger RA, Cavalieri RR: Uptake of 3,5,3′-triiodothyronine by the perfused rat liver: return to the free hormone hypothesis. Endocrinology 123:1817, 1988

62. Mendel CM, Weisiger RA, Jones AL, Cavalieri RR: Thyroid hormone-binding proteins in plasma facilitate uniform distribution of thyroxine within tissues: a perfused rat liver study. Endocrinology 120:1742, 1987

63. Hennemann G, Krenning EP, Otten M et al: Raised total thyroxine and free thyroxine index but normal free thyroxine. Lancet 1:639, 1979

64. Doctor R, Bos G, Krenning EP et al: Inherited thyroxine excess: a serum abnormality due to an increased affinity for modified albumin. Clin Endocrinol 15:363, 1981

65. Ruiz M, Rajatanavin R, Young RA et al: Familial dysalbuminemic hyperthyroxinemia: a syndrome that can be confused with thyrotoxicosis. N Engl J Med 306:635, 1981

66. Barlow JW, Csicsmann JM, White EL et al: Familial euthyroid thyroxine excess: characterization of abnormal intermediate affinity thyroxine binding to albumin. J Clin Endocrinol Metab 55:244, 1982

67. Mendel CM, Cavalieri RR: Thyroxine distribution and metabolism in familial dysalbuminemic hyperthyroxinemia. J Clin Endocrinol Metab 59:499, 1984

68. Stockigt JR, Dyer SA, Mohr VS et al: Specific methods to identify plasma binding abnormalities in euthyroid hyperthyroxinemia. J Clin Endocrinol Metab 62:230, 1986

69. Montoro M, Collea JV, Frasier SD, Mestman JH: Successful outcome of pregnancy in women with hypothyroidism. Ann Intern Med 94:31, 1981

70. Yabu Y, Amir SM, Ruiz M et al: Heterogeneity of thyroxine binding by serum albumins in normal subjects and patients with familial albuminemic hyperthyroxinemia. J Clin Endocrinol Metab 60:451, 1985

71. Benvenga S: The 27-kilodalton thyroxine (T$_4$)-binding protein is human apolipoprotein A-I: identification of a 68-kilodalton high-density lipoprotein that binds T$_4$. Endocrinology 124:1265, 1989

72. Benvenga S, Robbins J: Enhancement of thyroxine entry into low-density lipoprotein (LDL) receptor-competent fibroblasts by LDL: an additional mode of entry of thyroxine into cells. Endocrinology 126:933, 1990

73. Benvenga S, Cahnmann HJ, Gregg RE, Robbins J: Characterization of the binding of thyroxine to high-density lipoproteins and apolipoproteins A–I. J Clin Endocrinol Metab 68:1067, 1989

74. Robbins J, Rall JE: The interaction of thyroid hormones and protein in biological fluids. Recent Prog Horm Res 13:161, 1957

75. Hennemann G, Docter R: Plasma transport proteins and their role in tissue delivery of thyroid hormone. p. 221. In Greer MA (ed): The Thyroid Gland. Raven Press, New York, 1990

76. Docter R, Krenning EP: Role of cellular transport systems in the regulation of thyroid hormone bioactivity. p. 233. In Greer MA (ed): The Thyroid Gland. Raven Press, New York, 1990

77. Mendel CM, Weisiger RA: Thyroxine uptake by perfused rat liver: no evidence for facilitation by five different thyroxine-binding proteins. J Clin Invest 86:1840, 1990

78. Mendel CM: Thre free hormone hypothesis: distinction from the free hormone transport hypothesis. J Androl 13:107, 1992

79. Weisiger RA: Dissociation from albumin: a potentially rate-limiting step in the clearance of substances by the liver. Proc Natl Acad Sci USA 82:1563, 1985

80. Weisiger RA, Mendel CM, Cavalieri RR: The hepatic sinusoid is not well-stirred: estimation of the degree of axial mixing by analysis of lobular concentration gradients formed during uptake of thyroxine by the perfused rat liver. J Pharm Sci 75:233, 1986

81. Sinha AK, Pickard MR, Ekins RP: Maternal hypothyroxinemia and brain development: I. A hypothetical control system governing fetal exposure to maternal thyroid hormones. Acta Med Austriaca 1:40, 1992

82. Ekins R, Edwards P, Newman B: The role of binding-proteins in hormone delivery. Appendix, p. 3. In Albertini A, Ekins RP (eds): Free Hormones in Blood. Elsevier Biomedical, Amsterdam, 1982

83. Sarne DH, Refetoff S: Normal cellular uptake of thyroxine from serum of patients with familial dysalbuminemic hyperthyroxemia or elevated thyroxine-binding globulin. J Clin Endocrinol Metab 67:1166, 1988

84. Sarne D, Barokas K, Scherberg NH, Refetoff S: Elevated serum thyroglobulin level in congenital thyroxine-binding globulin deficiency. J Clin Endocrinol Metab 57:665, 1983

85. Faber J, Lumholtz IB, Kirkegaard C et al: The effects of phenytoin on the extrathyroidal turnover of thyroxine, 3,5,3′-triiodothyronine, 3,3′,5′-triiodothyronine, and 3′,5′-diiodothyronine in man. J Clin Endocrinol Metab 61:1093, 1985

86. Liewendahl K, Tikanoja S, Helenius T, Majuri H: Free thyroxin and free triiodothyronine as measured by equilibrium dialysis and analog radioimmunoassay in serum of patients taking phenytoin and carbamazepine. Clin Chem 31:1993, 1985

87. Smith PJ, Surks MI: Multiple effects of 5,5′-diphenylhydantoin on the thyroid hormone system. Endocr Rev 5:514, 1984

88. DeLuca F, Arrigo T, Pandullo E et al: Changes in thyroid function tests induced by 2-month carbamazepine treatment in L-thyroxine-substituted hypothyroid children. Eur J Pediatr 145:77, 1986

89. Isojarvi JI, Pakarinen AJ, Myllyla VV: Thyroid function with antiepileptic drugs. Epilepsia 33:142, 1992

90. Govind SR, Rao ML, Thilmann A, Quednau HD: Study of fluxes at low concentrations of L-triiodothyronine with rat liver cells and their plasma-membrane vesicles: evidence for the accumulation of the hormone against a gradient. Biochem J 198:457, 1966

91. Krenning EP, Docter R, Bernard HF et al: Decreased transport of thyroxine (T$_4$), 3,3′,5-triiodothyronine (T$_3$) and 3,3′,5′-triiodothyronine (rT$_3$) into rat hepatocytes in primary culture due to a decrease of cellular ATP content and various drugs. FEBS Lett 140:229, 1982

92. Krenning EP, Docter R, Bernard HF et al: Active transport of triiodothyronine (T$_3$) into isolated rat liver cells. FEBS Lett 91:113, 1978

93. Eckel J, Rao GS, Rao ML, Breuer H: Uptake of L-triiodothyronine by isolated rat liver cells: a process partially inhibited by metabolic inhibitors: attempts to distinguish between uptake and binding to intracellular proteins. Biochem J 182:473, 1979

94. Krenning E, Docter R, Bernard B et al: Regulation of the active transport of 3,3′,5-triiodothyronine (T$_3$) into primary cultured rat hepatocytes by ATP. FEBS Lett 119:279, 1978

95. Krenning E, Docter R, Bernard B et al: Characteristics of active transport of thyroid hormone into rat hepatocytes. Biochim Biophys Acta 676:314, 1981

96. Topliss DJ, Kolliniatis E, Barlow JW et al: Uptake of 3,5,3′-triiodothyronine by cultured rat hepatoma cells is inhibitable by nonbile acid cholephils, diphenylhydantoin, and nonsteroidal antiinflammatory drugs. Endocrinology 124:980, 1989

97. Blondeau J-P, Osty J, Francon J: Characterization of the thyroid hormone transport system of isolated hepatocytes. J Biol Chem 263:2685, 1988

98. Docter R, Krenning EP, Bernard HF et al: Inhibition of uptake of thyroid hormone into rat hepatocytes by preincubation with N-bromoacetyl-3,3′,5-triiodothyronine. Endocrinology 123:1520, 1988

99. Movius EG, Phyillaier MM, Robbins J: Phloretin inhibits cellular uptake and nuclear receptor binding of triiodothyronine in human hep G2 hepatocarcinoma cells. Endocrinology 124:1988, 1989

100. Pontecorvi A, Lakshmanan M, Robbins J: Intracellular transport of 3,5,3′-triiodo-L-thyronine in rat skeletal myoblasts. Endocrinology 121:2145, 1987

101. Pontecorvi A, Lakshmanan M, Robbins J: Different intracellular and intranuclear transport of triiodothyronine enantiomers in rat skeletal myoblasts. Endocrinology 123:2922, 1988

102. Docter R, Krenning EP, Bernard HF, Henneman G: Active transport of iodothyronines into human cultured fibroblasts. J Clin Endocrinol Metab 65:624, 1987

103. Osty J, Jego L, Francon J, Blondeau J-P: Characterization of triiodothyronine transport and accumulation in rat erythrocytes. Endocrinology 123:2303, 1988

104. Gonçalves E, Lakshmanan M, Robbins J: Triiodothyronine transport into differentiated and undifferentiated mouse neuroblastoma cells (NB41A3). Endocrinology 124:293, 1989

105. Centanni M, Robbins J: Role of sodium in thyroid hormone uptake by rat skeletal muscle. J Clin Invest 80:1068, 1987

106. Pontecorvi A, Robbins J: Energy-dependent uptake of 3,5,3′-triiodo-L-thyronine in rat skeletal muscle. Endocrinology 119:2755, 1986

107. van der Heijden JTM, Krenning EP, van Toor H et al: Three-compartmental analysis of effects of D-propranolol on thyroid hormone kinetics. Am J Physiol 255:E80, 1988

108. van der Heyden JTM, Docter R, van Toor H et al: Effects of caloric deprivation on thyroid hormone tissue uptake and generation of low-T$_3$ syndrome. Am J Physiol 251:E156, 1986

109. Docter R, De Jong M, van der Hoek HJ et al: Development and use of a mathematical two-pool model of distribution and metabolism of 3,3′,5-triiodothyronine in a recirculating rat liver perfusion system: albumin does not play a role in cellular transport. Endocrinology 126:451, 1990

110. Pardridge WM: Plasma protein-mediated transport of steroid and thyroid hormones. Am J Physiol 252:E158, 1987

111. Pardridge WM, Landaw EM: Steady state model of

3,5,3′-triiodothyronine transport in liver predicts high cellular exchangeable hormone concentration relative to in vitro free hormone concentration. Endocrinology 120:1059, 1987

112. Mol JA, Krenning EP, Docter R et al: Inhibition of iodothyronine transport into rat liver cells by a monoclonal antibody. Endocrinology, suppl. 115: T17, 1984

113. Krenning EP, Docter R, Bernard B et al: Characteristics of active transport of thyroid hormone into rat hepatocytes. Biochim Biophys Acta 676:314, 1981

114. Otten MH, Mol JA, Visser TJ: Sulfation preceding deiodination of iodothyronines in rat hepatocytes. Science 221:81, 1983

115. Visser TJ: Importance of deiodination and conjugation in the hepatic metabolism of thyroid hormone. p. 255. In Greer MA (ed): The Thyroid Gland. Raven Press, New York, 1990

116. Henneman G, Krenning EP, Polhuys M et al: Carrier-mediated transport of thyroid hormone into rat hepatocytes is rate-limiting in total cellular uptake and metabolism. Endocrinology 119:1870, 1986

117. Rivkees SA, Bode HH, Crawford JD: Long-term growth in juvenile acquired hypothyroidism. N Engl J Med 318:599, 1988

118. Lakshmanan M, Gonçalves E, Lessly G et al: The transport of thyroxine into mouse neuroblastoma cells, NB41A3: the effect of L-system amino acids. Endocrinology 126:3245, 1990

119. Lim C-F, Bernard BF, De Jong M et al: A furan fatty acid and indoxyl sulfate are the putative inhibitors of thyroxine hepatocyte transport in uremia. J Clin Endocrinol Metab 76:318, 1993

120. Oppenheimer JH, Schwartz HL, Koerner D, Surks MI: Limited binding capacity sites for L-triiodothyronine in rat liver: nuclear-cytoplasmic interrelation, bind constants, and cross-reactivity with L-thyroxine. J Clin Invest 53:768, 1974

121. Oppenheimer JH, Schwartz HL, Surks MI: Tissue differences in the concentration of triiodothyronine nuclear binding sites in the rat: liver, kidney, pituitary, heart, brain, spleen, and testis. Endocrinology 95:897, 1974

122. Schwartz HL, Strait KA, Ling NC, Oppenheimer JH: Quantitation of rat-tissue thyroid hormone binding receptor isoforms by immunoprecipitation of nuclear triiodothyronine binding capacity. J Biol Chem 267:11794, 1992

123. Larsen PR, Silva JE, Kaplan MM: Relationships between circulating and intracellular thyroid hormones: physiologic and clinical implications. Endocr Rev 2:87, 1981

124. Oppenheimer JH, Schwartz HL: Stereospecific transport to triiodothyronine from plasma to cytosol and from cytosol to nucleus in rat liver, kidney, brain, and heart. J Clin Invest 75:147, 1985

125. Crantz FR, Larsen PR: Rapid thyroxine 3,5,3′-triiodothyronine conversion and nuclear 3,5,3′-triiodothyronine binding in rat cerebral cortex and cerebellum. J Clin Invest 65:935, 1980

126. Crantz FR, Silva JE, Larsen PR: Analysis of the sources and quantity of 3,5,3′-triiodothyronine specifically bound to nuclear receptors in rat cerebral cortex and cerebellum. Endocrinology 110:367, 1982

127. Larsen PR, Bavli SZ, Castonguay M, Jove R: Direct radioimmunoassay of nuclear 3,5,3′-triiodothyronine in rat anterior pituitary. J Clin Invest 65:675, 1980

128. Obata T, Kitagawa S, Gong QH et al: Thyroid hormone down-regulates p55, a thyroid hormone-binding protein that is homologous to protein disulfide isomerase and the beta subunit of prolyl-4-hydroxylase. J Biol Chem 263:782, 1988

129. Boado RJ, Campbell DA, Chopra IJ: Nucleotide sequence of rat liver iodothyronine 5′-monodeiodinase (5′ MD): its identity with the protein disulfide isomerase. Biochem Biophys Res Comm 155:1297, 1988

130. Chanoine JP, Braverman LE, Farwell AP et al: The thyroid gland is a major source of circulating T_3 in the rat. J Clin Invest 91:2709, 1993

131. Toyoda N, Nishikawa M, Horimoto M et al: Graves' immunoglobulin G stimulates iodothyronine 5′-deiodinating activity in FRTL-5 rat thyroid cells. J Clin Endocrinol Metab 70:1506, 1990

132. Toyoda N, Nishikawa M, Horimoto M et al: Synergistic effect of thyroid hormone and thyrotropin on iodothyronine 5′-deiodinase in FRTL-5 rat thyroid cells. Endocrinology 127:1199, 1990

133. Sugawara M, Lau R, Wasser HL et al: Thyroid T_4 5′-deiodinase activity in normal and abnormal human thyroid glands. Metabolism 33:332, 1984

134. Erickson VJ, Cavalieri RR, Rosenberg LL: Thyroxine-5′-deiodinase of rat thyroid, but not that of liver, is dependent on thyrotropin. Endocrinology 111: 434, 1982

135. Ishii H, Inada M, Tanaka K et al: Triiodothyronine generation from thyroxine in human thyroid: enhanced conversion in Graves' thyroid tissue. J Clin Endocrinol Metab 52:1211, 1981

136. Laurberg P, Boye N: Outer- and inner ring monodeiodination of thyroxine by dog thyroid and liver: a comparative study using a particulate cell fraction. Endocrinology 110:2124, 1982

137. Laurberg P, Boye N: Propylthiouracil, ipodate, dexamethasone, and periods of fasting induce different variations in serum rT_3 in dogs. Metabolism 33:323, 1984

138. Izumi M, Larsen PR: Triiodothyronine, thyroxine, and iodine in purified thyroglobulin from patients with Graves' disease. J Clin Invest 59:1105, 1977

139. Engler D, Burger AG: The deiodination of the iodothyronines and of their derivatives in man. Endocr Rev 5:151, 1984

140. Larsen PR: Thyroidal triiodothyronine and thyroxine in Graves' disease correlation with presurgical treatment, thyroid status, and iodine content. J Clin Endocrinol Metab 41:1098, 1975

141. Kaplan MM: Changes in the particulate subcellular component of hepatic thyroxine-5'-monodeioinase in hyperthyroid and hypothyroid rats. Endocrinology 105:548, 1979

142. Berry MJ, Banu L, Larsen PR: Type I iodothyronine deiodinase is a selenocysteine-containing enzyme. Nature 349:438, 1991

143. Mandel SJ, Berry MJ, Kieffer JD et al: Cloning and in vitro expression of the human selenoprotein, type I iodothyronine deiodinase. J Clin Endocrinol Metab 75:1133, 1992

144. Berry MJ, Larsen PR: The role of selenium in thyroid hormone action. Endocr Rev 13:207, 1992

145. Abuid J, Larsen PR: Triiodothyronine and thyroxine in hyperthyroidism. J Clin Invest 54:201, 1974

146. Cavlieri RR, Steinberg M, Searle GL: The distribution kinetics of triiodothyronine: studies of euthyroid subjects with decreased plasma thyroxine-binding globulin and patients with Graves' disease. J Clin Invest 49:1041, 1970

147. Nicoloff JT, Low JC, Dussault JH, Fisher DA: Simultaneous measurement of thyroxine and triiodothyronine peripheral turnover kinetics in man. J Clin Invest 51:473, 1972

148. Burrow GN, Fisher DA, Larsen PR: Mechanisms of disease: maternal and fetal thyroid function. N Engl J Med 331:1072, 1994

149. Wartofsky L, Burman KD: Alterations in thyroid function in patients with systemic illness: the "euthyroid sick syndrome." Endocr Rev 3:164, 1982

150. Wartofsky L: The low T_3 or "sick euthyroid syndrome": update 1994. Endocr Rev 3:248, 1994

151. van Doorn JD, van der Heide D, Roelfsema F: Sources and quantity of 3,5,3'-triiodothyronine in several tissues of the rat. J Clin Invest 72:1778, 1983

152. Silva JE, Leonard JL, Crantz FR, Larsen PR: Evidence for two tissue specific pathways for in vivo thyroxine 5' deiodination in the rat. J Clin Invest 69:1176, 1982

153. Beckett GJ, Beddows SE, Morrice PC et al: Inhibition of hepatic deiodination of thyroxine is caused by selenium deficiency in rats. Biochem J 248:443, 1987

154. Beckett GJ, MacDougal DA, Nicol F, Arthur JR: Inhibition of type I and II iodothyronine deiodinase activity in rat liver, kidney, and brain produced by selenium deficiency. Biochem J 259:887, 1989

155. Arthur JR, Nicol F, Beckett GJ: Hepatic iodothyronine 5'-deiodinase: the role of selenium. Biochem J 272:537, 1990

156. Arthur JR, Nicol F, Rae PWH, Beckett GJ: Effects of selenium deficiency on the thyroid gland and on plasma and pituitary thyrotropin and growth hormone concentrations in the rat. Clin Chem Enzymol Commun 3:209, 1990

157. Behne D, Kyriakopoulos A, Meinhold H, Kohrle J: Identification of type I iodothyronine 5'-deiodinase as a selenoenzyme. Biochem Biophys Res Comm 173:1143, 1990

158. Contempre B, Dumont JE, Bebe N et al: Effect of selenium supplementation in hypothyroid subjects of an iodine and selenium deficient area: the possible danger of indiscriminate supplementation of iodine-deficient subjects with selenium. J Clin Endocrinol Metab 73:213, 1991

159. Vanderpas JB, Contempre B, Duale NL et al: Iodine and selenium deficiency associated with cretinism in northern Zaire. Amer J Clin Nutr 52:1087, 1990

160. Meinhold H, Campos-Barre A, Behne D: Effects of selenium and iodine deficiency on iodothyronine deiodinases in brain, thyroid, and peripheral tissue. Acta Med Austriaca 19:8, 1992

161. Berry MJ, Larsen PR: Selenocysteine and the structure, function, and regulation of iodothyronine deiodination: update 1994. Endocr Rev 3:265, 1994

162. Berry MJ, Kieffer JD, Harney JW, Larsen PR: Selenocysteine confers the biochemical properties of the type I iodothyronine deiodinase. J Biol Chem 266:14155, 1991

163. Berry MJ, Kieffer JD, Larsen PR: Evidence that cysteine, not selenocysteine, is in the catalytic site of type II iodothyronine deiodinase. Endocrinology 129:550, 1991

164. Berry MJ, Maia AL, Kieffer JD et al: Substitution of cysteine for selenocysteine in type I iodothyronine deiodinase reduces the catalytic efficiency of the protein but enhances its translation. Endocrinology 131:1848, 1992

165. Safran M, Farwell AP, Leonard JL: Evidence that type II 5'-deiodinase is not a selenoprotein. J Biol Chem 266:13477, 1991

166. St. Germain DL, Schwartzman RA, Croteau W et al: A thyroid hormone-regulated gene in *Xenopus laevis* encodes a type III iodothyronine 5-deiodinase. Proc Natl Acad Sci USA 91:7767, 1994

167. Chopra IJ, Chua Teco GN: Characteristics of inner ring (3 and 5) monodeiodination of 3, 5-diiodothyronine in rat liver: evidence suggesting marked similarities of inner- and outer ring deiodinases for iodothyronines. Endocrinology 110:89, 1982

168. Fekkes D, Hennemann G, Visser TJ: Evidence for a single enzyme in rat liver catlysing the deiodination of the tyrosyl and the phenolic ring of iodothyronines. Biochem J 201:673, 1982

169. Moreno M, Berry MJ, Horst C et al: Activation and inactivation of thyroid hormone by type I iodothyronine deiodinase. FEBS lett 344:143, 1994

170. Balsam A, Ingbar SH: The influence of fasting, diabetes, and several pharmacological agents of the pathways of thyroxine metabolism in rat liver. J Clin Invest 62:415, 1978

171. Berry MJ, Banu L, Chen Y et al: Recognition of UGA as a selenocysteine codon in type I deiodinase requires sequences in the 3' untranslated region. Nature 353:273, 1991

172. Berry MJ, Banu L, Harney JW, Larsen PR: Functional characterization of the eukaryotic SECIS elements which direct selenocysteine insertion at UGA codons. EMBO J 12:3315, 1993

173. Berry MJ, Harney JW, Ohama T, Hatfield DL: Selenocysteine insertion or termination: factors affecting UGA codon fate and complementary anticodon-codon mutations. Nucl Acids Res 22:3753, 1994

174. Berry MJ, Kates AL, Larsen PR: Thyroid hormone regulates type I deiodinase messenger RNA in rat liver. Mol Endocrinol 4:743, 1990

175. Menjo M, Murata Y, Fujii T et al: Effects of thyroid and glucocorticoid hormones on the level of messenger ribonucleic acid for iodothyronine type I 5'-deiodinase in rat primary hepatocyte cultures grown as spheroids. Endocrinology 133:2984, 1993

176. O'Mara BA, Dittrich W, Lauterio TJ, St. Germain DL: Pretranslational regulation of type I 5'-deiodinase by thyroid hormones and in fasted and diabetic rats. Endocrinology 133:1715, 1993

177. Borges M, Ingbar SH, Silva JE: Iodothyronine deiodinase activities in FRTL5 cells: predominance of type I 5'-deiodinase. Endocrinology 126:3059, 1990

178. Kaplan MM, Utiger RD: Iodothyronine metabolism in liver and kidney homogenates from hypothyroid and hyperthyroid rats. Endocrinology 103:156, 1978

179. Ishii H, Inada M, Tanaka K et al: Induction of outer- and inner ring monodeiodinases in human thyroid gland by thyrotropin. J Clin Endocrinol Metab 57:500, 1983

180. St. Germain DL, Croteau W: Ligand-induced inactivation of type I iodothyronine 5'-deiodinase: protection by propylthiouracil in vivo and reversibility in vitro. Endocrinology 125:2735, 1989

181. Leonard JL, Kaplan MM, Visser TJ et al: Cerebral cortex responds rapidly to thyroid hormones. Science 214:571, 1981

182. Leonard JL, Silva JE, Kaplan MM et al: Acute post-transcriptional regulation of cerebrocortical and pituitary iodothyroinine 5'-deiodinase by thyroid hormone. Endocrinology 114:998, 1984

183. St. Germain D: The effects and interactions of substrates, inhibitors, and the cellular thiol-disulfide balance on the regulation of type II iodothyronine 5'-deiodinase. Endocrinology 122:1860, 1988

184. Portnay GI, O'Brien JT, Bush J et al: The effect of starvation on the concentration and binding of thyroxine and triiodothyronine in serum and on the response to TRH. J Clin Endocrinol Metab 39:191, 1974

185. Chopra IJ, Solomon DH, Chopra U et al: Pathways of metabolism of thyroid hormones. Recent Prog Horm Res 34:521, 1978

186. Chopra IJ, Smith SR: Circulating thyroid hormones and thyrotropin in adult patients with protein-calorie malnutrition. J Clin Endocrinol Metab 40:221, 1975

187. Spaulding SW, Chopra IJ, Sherwin RS, Lyall SS: Effects of caloric restriction and dietary composition on serum T_3 and rT_3 in man. J Clin Endocrinol Metab 42:197, 1976

188. Visser TJ, van der Does-Tobe I, Docter R, Hennemann G: Subcellular localization of a rat liver enzyme-converting thyroxine into triiodothyronine and possible involvement of essential thiol groups. Biochem J 157:479, 1976

189. Chopra IJ: Sulfhydryl groups and the monodeiodination of thyroxine to triiodothyronine. Science 199:904, 1978

190. Leonard JL, Rosenberg IN: Thyroxine 5'-deiodinase activity of rat kidney: observations on activation by thiols and inhibition by propylthiouracil. Endocrinology 103:2137, 1978

191. Balsam A, Ingbar SH: Observations on the factors that control the generation of triiodothyronine from thyroxine in rat liver and the nature of the effect induced by fasting. J Clin Invest 63:1145, 1979

192. Harris ARC, Fang SL, Hinerfeld L et al: The role of sulfhydryl groups on the impaired hepatic 3',3,5-triiodothyronine generation from thyroxine in the hypothyroid, starved, fetal, and neonatal rodent. J Clin Invest 63:516, 1979

193. Gavin LA, McMahon FA, Moeller M: Dietary modification of thyroxine deiodination in rat liver is not mediated by hepatic sulfhydryls. J Clin Invest 65:943, 1980

194. Kinlaw WB, Schwartz HL, Oppenheimer JH: Decreased serum triiodothyronine in starving rats is due primarily to diminished thyroidal secretion of thyroxine. J Clin Invest 75:1238, 1985

195. Lee WS, Berry MJ, Hediger MA, Larsen PR: The type I iodothyronine 5'-deiodinase mRNA is localized to the S3 segment of the rat kidney proximal tubule. Endocrinology 132:2136, 1993

196. Kaplan MM, Tatro JB, Breibart R, Larsen PR: Comparison of thyroxine and 3,3′,5′-triiodothyronine metabolism in rat kidney and liver homogenates. Metabolism 28:1139, 1979

197. Ferguson DC, Hoenig H, Jennings AS: Triiodothyronine production by the perfused rat kidney is reduced by diabetes mellitus but not by fasting. Endocrinology 117:64, 1984

198. Geffner DL, Azukizawa M, Hershman JM: Propylthiouracil blocks extrathyroidal conversion of thyroxine to triiodothyronine and augments thyrotropin secretion in man. J Clin Invest 55:224, 1975

199. Saberi M, Sterling FH, Utiger RD: Reduction in extrathyroidal triiodothyronine production by propylthiouracil in man. J Clin Invest 55:218, 1975

200. LoPresti JS, Eigen A, Kaptein E et al: Alteration in 3,3′,5′-triiodothyronine metabolism in response to propylthiouracil, dexamethasone, and thyroxine administration in man. J Clin Invest 84:1650, 1989

201. Silva JE, Larsen PR: Adrenergic activation of triiodothyronine production in brown adipose tissue. Nature 305:712, 1983

202. Houstek J, Vizek K, Stanislav P et al: Type II iodothyronine 5′-deiodinase and uncoupling protein in brown adipose tissue of human newborns. J Clin Endocrinol Metab 77:382, 1993

203. Krief S, Lonnqvist F, Raimbault S et al: Tissue distribution of β3-adrenergic receptor mRNA in man. J Clin Invest 91:344, 1993

204. Silva JE, Larsen PR: Comparison of iodothyronine 5′-deiodinase and other thyroid-hormone-dependent enzyme activities in the cerebral cortex and hypothyroid neonatal rat. J Clin Invest 70:1110, 1982

205. Silva JE, Gordon MB, Crantz FR et al: Qualitative and quantitative differences in the pathways of extrathyroidal triiodothyronine generation between euthyroid and hypothyroid rats. J Clin Invest 73:898, 1984

206. Silva JE, Leonard JL: Regulation of rat cerebrocortical and adenohypophyseal type II 5′-deiodinase by thyroxine, triiodothyronine, and reverse triiodothyronine. Endocrinology 116:1627, 1985

207. Obregon MJ, Larsen PR, Silva JE: The role of 3,3′,5′-triiodothyronine in the regulation of type II iodothyronine 5′-deiodinase in the rat cerebral cortex. Endocrinology 119:2186, 1986

208. Kaiser CA, Goumaz MO, Burger AG: In vivo inhibition of the 5′-deiodinase type II in brain cortex and pituitary by reverse triiodothyronine. Endocrinology 119:762, 1986

209. Silva JE, Matthews PS: Production rates and turnover of triiodothyronine in rat developing cerebral cortex and cerebellum. J Clin Invest 74:1035, 1984

210. Morreale de Escobar G, Calvo R, Obregon MJ, Escobar del Rey F: Contribution of maternal thyroxine to fetal thyroxine pools in normal rats near term. Endocrinology 126:2765, 1990

211. Morreale de Escobar G, Obregon MJ, Ruiz de Ona C, Escobar del Rey F: Transfer of thyroxine from the mother to the rat fetus near term: effects on brain 3,5,3′-triiodothyronine deficiency. Endocrinology 122:1521, 1988

212. Koenig RJ, Watson AY: Enrichment of rat anterior pituitary cell types by metrizamide density gradient centrifugation. Endocrinology 115:314, 1984

213. Koenig RJ, Leonard JL, Senator D et al: Regulation of thyroxine 5′-deiodinase activity by T3 in cultured rat anterior pituitary cells. Endocrinology 115:324, 1984

214. Huang TS, Chopra IJ, Beredo A et al: Skin is an active site for the inner ring monodeiodination of thyroxine to 3,3′,5′-triiodothyronine. Endocrinology 117:2106, 1985

215. Roti E, Fang SL, Green K et al: Human placenta is an active site of thyroxine and 3,3′,5-triiodothyronine tyrosyl ring deiodination. J Clin Endocrinol Metab 53:498, 1981

216. Castro MI, Braverman LE, Alex S et al: Inner-ring deiodination of 3,5,3′-triiodothyronine in the in situ perfused guinea pig placenta. J Clin Invest 76:1921, 1985

217. Emerson CH, Bambini G, Alex S et al: The effect of thyroid dysfunction and fasting on placenta inner-ring deiodinase activity in the rat. Endocrinology 122:809, 1988

218. Meinhold H, Campos-Barros A, Walzog B et al: Effects of selenium and iodine deficiency on type I, type II, and type III iodothyronine deiodinases and circulating thyroid hormones in the rat. Exp Clin Endocrinol 101:87, 1993

219. Obregon MJ, Mallol J, Pastor RM et al: L-thyroxine and 3,5,3′-triiodothyronine in rat embryos before onset of fetal thyroid function. Endocrinology 114:305, 1984

220. Kaplan MM, Visser TJ, Yaskoski KA, Leonard JL: Characteristics of iodothyronine tyrosyl-ring deiodination by rat cerebral cortical microsomes. Endocrinology 112:35, 1983

221. Kaplan MM, Yaskoski KA: Phenolic and tyrosyl-ring deiodination of iodothyronines in rat brain homogenates. J Clin Invest 66:551, 1980

222. Kaplan MM, Yakoski KA: Maturational patterns of iodothyronine phenolic and tyrosyl-ring deiodinase activities in rat cerebrum, cerebellum, and hypothalamus. J Clin Invest 67:1204, 1980

223. Galton VA, Hiebert A: Hepatic iodothyronine 5-deiodinase activity in *Rana catesbeiana* tadpoles at differ-

ent stages in the life cycle. Endocrinology 121:42, 1987

224. Darras VM, Berghman LR, Vanderpooten A, Kuhn ER: Growth hormone acutely regulates type III deiodinase in chicken liver. FEBS lett 310:5, 1992

225. Mol K, Kaptein E, Darras VM et al: Different thyroid hormone-deiodinating enzymes in tilapia (*Oreochromis niloticus*) liver and kidney. FEBS Lett 321:140, 1993

226. Santini F, Chopra IJ, Hurd RE et al: A study of the characteristics of the rat placental iodothyronine 5-monodeiodinase: evidence that is distinct from the rat hepatic iodothyronine 5′-monodeiodinase. Endocrinology 130:2325, 1992

227. Polk DH, Reviczky A, Wu SY et al: Metabolism of sulfoconjugated thyroid hormone derivatives in developing sheep. Amer Journal Physiol 266:E892, 1994

228. Chopra IJ, Wu SY, Chua Teco GN, Santini F: A radioimmunoassay for measurement of 3,5,3′-triiodothyronine sulfate; studies in thyroidal and non-thyroidal disease, pregnancy, and neonatal life. J Clin Endocrinol Metab 75:189, 1992

229. McCann UD, Shaw EA, Kaplan MM: Iodothyronine deiodination reaction types in several rat tissues: effects of age, thyroid status, and glucocorticoid treatment. Endocrinology 114:1513, 1984

230. Silva JE, Matthews PS: Production rates and turnover of triiodothyronine in rat developing cerebral cortex and cerebellum: responses to hypothyroidism. J Clin Invest 74:1035, 1984

231. Vulsma T, Gons MH, DeVijlder JMM: Maternal fetal transfer of thyroxine in congenital hypothyroidism due to a total organification defect of thyroid dysgenesis. N Engl J Med 321:13, 1989

232. Santini F, Chopra IJ, Wu SY et al: Metabolism of 3,5,3′-triiodothyronine sulfate by tissues of the fetal rat: a consideration of the role of desulfation of 3,5,3′-triiodothyronine sulfate as a source of T_3. Pediatr Rev 31:541, 1992

233. Santini F, Cortelazzi D, Baggiani AM et al: A study of the serum 3,5,3′-triiodothyronine sulfate concentration in normal and hypothyroid fetuses at various gestational stages. J Clin Endocrinol Metab 76:1583, 1993

234. Wu S-Y, Huang W-S, Polk D et al: The development of a radioimmunoassay for reverse triiodothyronine sulfate in human serum and amniotic fluid. J Clin Endocrinol Metab 76:1625, 1993

235. Rooda SJE, Kaptein E, Rutgers M, Visser TJ: Increased plasma 3,5,3′-triiodothyronine sulfate in rats with inhibited type I iodothyronine dediodinase activity, as measured by radioimmunoassay. Endocrinology 124:740, 1989

236. Rooda SJE, Kaptein E, Visser TJ: Serum triiodothyronine sulfate in man measured by radioimmunoassay. J Clin Endocrinol Metab 69:552, 1989

237. LoPresti JS, Mizuno L, Nimalysuria A et al: Characteristics of 3,5,3′-triiodothyronine sulfate metabolism in euthyroid man. J Clin Endocrinol Metab 73:703, 1991

238. Buergi U, Larsen PR: Nuclear triiodothyronine binding in mononuclear leukocytes in normal subjects and obese patients before and after fasting. J Clin Endocrinol Metab 54:1199, 1982

239. Bianco AC, Silva JE: Nuclear 3,5,3′-triiodothyronine (T_3) in brown adipose tissue: receptor occupancy and sources of T_3 as determined by in vivo techniques. Endocrinology 120:55, 1987

240. Berry MJ, Grieco D, Taylor BA et al: Physiological and genetic analyses of inbred mouse strains with a type I iodothyronine 5′ deiodinase deficiency. J Clin Invest 92:1517, 1993

241. Brent GA, Moore DD, Larsen PR: Thyroid hormone regulation of gene expression. Annu Rev Physiol 53:17, 1991

242. Glass CK, Holloway JM: Regulation of gene expression by the thyroid hormone receptor. Biochim Biophys Acta 1032:157, 1990

243. Brent GA: The molecular basis of thyroid hormone action. N Engl J Med 331:847, 1994

244. Lazar MA: Thyroid hormone receptors: multiple forms, multiple possibilities. Endocr Rev 14:184, 1993

245. Glass CK: Differential recognition of target genes by nuclear receptor monomers, dimers, and heterodimers. Endocr Rev 15:391, 1994

246. Sterling K, Campbell GA, Brenner MA: Purification of the mitochondrial triiodothyronine (T_3) receptor from rat liver. Acta Endocrinol (Copenh) 105:391, 1984

247. Davis FB, Cody V, Davis PJ et al: Stimulation by thyroid-hormone analogues of red blood cell Ca^{2+}-ATPase activity in vitro: correlations between hormone structure and biologic activity in a human cell system. J Biol Chem 258:12373, 1983

248. Dube MP, Davis FB, Davis PJ et al: Effects of hyperthyroidism and hypothyroidism on human red blood cell Ca^{2+}-ATPase activity. J Clin Endocrinol Metab 62:253, 1986

249. Warnick PR, Davis PJ, Davis FB et al: Rabbit skeletal muscle sarcoplasmic reticulum $Ca(^{2+})$-ATPase activity: stimulation in vitro by thyroid-hormone analogues and bipyridines. Biochim Biophys Acta 1153:184, 1993

250. St. Germain DL: Regulatory effect of lithium on thyroxine metabolism in murine neural and anterior pituitary tissue. Endocrinology 120:1430, 1987

251. Farwell AP, Lynch RM, Okulicz WC et al: The actin cytoskeleton mediates the hormonally regulated translocation of type II iodothyronine 5′-deiodinase in astrocytes. J Biol Chem 265:18546, 1990

252. Farwell AP, DiBenedetto DJ, Leonard JL: Thyroxine targets different pathways of internalization of type II iodothyronine 5′-deiodinase in astrocytes. J Biol Chem 268:5055, 1993

253. Samuels HH, Tsai JS: Thyroid hormone action in cell culture: demonstration of nuclear receptors in intact cells and isolated nuclei. Proc Natl Acad Sci USA 70:3488, 1973

254. Schadlow A, Surks M, Schwartz H, Oppenheimer J: Specific triiodothyronine binding sites in the anterior pituitary of the rat. Science 176:1252, 1972

255. Oppenheimer JH, Koerner D, Schwartz HL, Surks MI: Specific nuclear triiodothyronine binding sites in rat liver and kidney. J Clin Endocrinol Metab 35:330, 1972

256. Surks MI, Koerner DH, Oppenheimer JH: In vitro binding of L-triiodothyronine to receptors in rat liver nuclei: kinetics of binding extraction properties and lack of requirement for cytosol proteins. J Clin Invest 55:50, 1975

257. Sap J, Munoz A, Damm K et al: The c-erb-A protein is a high-affinity receptor for thyroid hormone. Nature 324:635, 1986

258. Weinberger C, Thompson CC, Ong ES et al: The c-erb-A gene encodes a thyroid hormone receptor. Nature 324:641, 1986

259. Evans RM: The steroid and thyroid hormone receptor superfamily. Science 240:889, 1988

260. Mitsuhashi T, Nikodem VM: Regulation of expression of the alternative mRNAs of the rat α-thyroid hormone receptor gene. J Biol Chem 264:8900, 1989

261. Obata T, Kitagawa S, Gong QH et al: Thyroid hormone down-regulates p55, a thyroid hormone-binding protein that is homologous to protein disulfide isomerase and the beta-subunit of prolyl-4-hydroxylase. J Biol Chem 263:782, 1988

262. Nakai AS, Seino A, Sakurai A et al: Characterization of a thyroid hormone-receptor expressed human kidney and other tissues. Proc Natl Acad Sci USA 85:2781, 1988

263. Benbrook D, Phahl M: A novel thyroid hormone receptor encoded by a cDNA clone from a human testis library. Science 238:788, 1987

264. Lazar MA, Hodin RA, Darling DS, Chin WW: Identification of a rat c-*erb* A α-related protein which binds deoxyribonucleic acid but does not bind thyroid hormone. Mol Endocrinol 2:893, 1988

265. Koenig RJ, Lazar MA, Hodin RA et al: Inhibition of thyroid hormone action by a nonhormone-binding c-erbA protein generated by alternative mRNA splicing. Nature 337:659, 1989

266. Katz D, Lazar MA: Dominant negative activity of an endogenous thyroid hormone receptor variant (α2) is due to competition for binding sites on target genes. J Biol Chem 268:20904, 1993

267. Isaacs RE, Findell PR, Mellon P et al: Hormonal regulation of expression of the endogenous and transfected human growth hormone gene. Mol Endocrinol 1:569, 1987

268. Cook CB, Kakucska I, Lechan RM, Koenig RJ: Expression of thyroid hormone receptor β2 in rat hypothalamus. Endocrinology 130:1077, 1992

269. Bradley DJ, Towle HC, Young WS III: Spatial and temporal expression of α- and β thyroid hormone receptor mRNAs, including the β subtype, in the developing mammalian nervous system. J Neurosci 12:2288, 1992

270. Lechan RM, Qi Y, Berrodin TJ et al: Immunocytochemical delineation of thyroid hormone receptor beta 2-like immunoreactivity in the rat central nervous system. Endocrinology 132:2461, 1993

271. Schwartz HL, Lazar MA, Oppenheimer JH: Widespread distribution of immunoreactive thyroid hormone beta 2 receptor (TR beta 2) in the nuclei of extrapituitary rat tissues. J Biol Chem 269:24777, 1994

272. Macchia E, Nakai A, Janiga A et al: Characterization of site-specific polyclonal antibodies to c-erbA peptides recognizing human thyroid hormone receptors α1, α2, and β and native 3, 5, 3′-triiodothyronine receptor, and study of tissue distribution of the antigen. Endocrinology 126:3232, 1990

273. Sjösberg M, Vennström B, Forrest D: Thyroid hormone receptors in chick retinal development: differential expression of mRNAs for α and N-terminal variant β receptors. Development 114:39, 1992

274. Wills KN, Zhang X, Pfahl M: Coordinate expression of functionally distinct thyroid hormone receptor alpha isoforms during neonatal brain development. Mol Endocrinol 5:1109, 1991

275. Izumo S, Mahdavi V: Thyroid hormone receptor α isoforms generated by alternative splicing differentially activates myosin HC gene transcription. Nature 334:539, 1988

276. Murray MB, Zilz ND, McCreary NL et al: Isolation and characterization of rat cDNA clones for two distinct thyroid hormone receptors. J Biol Chem 263:12770, 1988

277. Mahdavi V, Chambers AP, Nadal-Ginard B: Cardiac α- and β- myosin heavy chain genes are organized in tandem. Proc Natl Acad Sci USA 81:2626, 1984

278. Hodin RA, Lazar MA, Chin WW: Differential and tissue-specific regulation of the multiple rat c-erbA

messenger RNA species by thyroid hormone. J Clin Invest 85:101, 1990

279. Forrest D, Sjöberg M, Vennström B: Contrasting developmental and tissue-specific expression of α and β thyroid hormone receptor genes. EMBO 9:1519, 1990

280. Samuels HH, Stanley F, Shapiro LE: Dose-dependent depletion of nuclear receptors by L-triiodothyronine: evidence for a role of induction of growth hormone synthesis in cultured GH1 cells. Proc Natl Acad Sci USA 73:3877, 1976

281. Strait KA, Schwartz HL, Perez-Castillo A, Oppenheimer JH: Relationship of c-erbA mRNA content in tissue triiodothyronine nuclear-binding capacity and function in developing and adult rats. J Biol Chem 265:10514, 1990

282. Lane JT, Gadbole M, Strait KA et al: Prolonged fasting reduces rat hepatic β1 thyroid hormone receptor protein without changing the level of its messenger ribonucleic acid. Endocrinology 129:2881, 1991

283. Thompson CC, Evans RM: *Trans*-activation by thyroid hormone receptors: functional parallels with steroid hormone receptors. Proc Natl Acad Sci USA 86:3494, 1989

284. Zavacki AM, Harney JW, Brent GA, Larsen PR: Dominant negative inhibition by mutant thyroid hormone receptors is thyroid hormone response element and receptor isoform specific. Mol Endocrinol 7:1319, 1993

285. Schueler PA, Schwartz HL, Strait KA et al: Binding of 3,5,3'-triiodothyronine (T_3) and its analogs to the in vitro translational products of c-erbA protooncogenes: differences in the affinity of the α- and β-forms for the acetic acid analog and failure of the human testis and kidney α2 products to bind T_3. Mol Endocrinol 234:227, 1990

286. Meier CA, Parkinson C, Chen A et al: Interaction of human β1 thyroid hormone receptor and its mutants with DNA and retinoid X receptor β: T_3 response element-dependent dominant negative potency. J Clin Invest 92:1986, 1993

287. Murray MB, Towle HC: Identification of nuclear factors that enhance binding of the thyroid hormone receptor to a thyroid hormone response element. Mol Endocrinol 2:1434, 1989

288. O'Donnell AL, Koenig RJ: Mutational analysis identifies a new functional domain of the thyroid hormone receptor. Mol Endocrinol 4:715, 1990

289. O'Donnell AL, Rosen ED, Darling DS, Koenig RJ: Thyroid hormone receptor mutations that interfere with transcriptional activation also interfere with receptor interaction with a nuclear protein. Mol Endocrinol 5:94, 1991

290. Burnside J, Darling DS, Carr FE, Chin WW: Thyroid hormone regulation of the rat glycoprotein hormone α-subunit gene promoter activity. J Biol Chem 264:6886, 1989

291. Darling DS, Beebe JS, Burnside J et al: 3,5,3'-triiodothyronine (T_3) receptor-auxiliary protein (TRAP) binds DNA and forms heterodimers with the T_3 receptor. Mol Endocrinol 5:73, 1991

292. Forman BM, Samuels HH: Interactions among a subfamily of nuclear hormone receptors: the regulatory zipper model. Mol Endocrinol 4:1293, 1990

293. Bugge TH, Pohl J, Lonnoy O, Stunnenberg HG: RXRα, a promiscuous partner of retinoic acid and thyroid hormone receptors. EMBO J 11:1409, 1992

294. Mangelsdorf DJ, Ong ES, Dyck JA, Evans RM: Nuclear receptor that identifies a novel retinoic acid response pathway. Nature 345:224, 1990

295. Yu VC, Delsert C, Anderson B et al: RXRβ: a coregulator that enhances binding of retinoic acid, thyroid hormone, and vitamin D receptors to their cognate response elements. Cell 67:1251, 1991

296. Leid M, Kastner P, Lyons R et al: Purification, cloning, and RXR identification of the HeLa cell factor which RAR or TR heterodimerizes to bind target sequences efficiently. Cell 68:377, 1992

297. Glass CK, Devary OV, Rosenfeld MG: Multiple cell type-specific proteins differentially regulate target sequence recognition by the alpha retinoic acid receptor. Cell 63:729, 1990

298. Kliewer SA, Umesono K, Manglesdorf DJ, Evans RM: Retinoid X receptor interacts with nuclear receptors in retinoic acid, thyroid hormone, and vitamin D3 signaling. Nature 355:446, 1992

299. Zhang X-K, Hoffman B, Tran PB-V et al: Retinoid X receptor is an auxiliary protein for thyroid hormone and retinoic acid receptor. Nature 355:441, 1992

300. Hermann T, Hoffmann B, Zhang X et al: Heterodimeric receptor complexes determine 3,5,3'-triiodothyronine and retinoid signaling specificities. Mol Endocrinol 6:1153, 1992

301. Marks SM, Hallenbeck PL, Nagata T et al: H-2RIIBP (RXRβ) heterodimerization provides a mechanism for combinatorial diversity in the regulation of retinoic acid and thyroid hormone responsive genes. EMBO J 11:1419, 1992

302. Marks SM, Levi B-Z, Segars JH et al: H-2RIIBP expressed from a baculovirus vector binds to multiple hormone response elements. Mol Endocrinol 6:219, 1992

303. Hsu J-H, Zavacki AM, Harney JW, Brent GA: Retinoid-X receptor (RXR) differentially augments thyroid hormone response in cell lines as a function of the response element and endogenous RXR content. Endocrinology 136:421, 1995

304. Heyman RA, Mangelsdorf DJ, Dyck JA et al: 9-cis

retinoic acid is a high-affinity ligand for the retinoid X receptor. Cell 68:397, 1992

305. Kurokawa R, Yu V, Naar A et al: Differential orientation of the DNA-binding domain and carboxy-terminal dimerization interface determines binding site selection by nuclear receptor heterodimers, abstracted. Genes Dev 7:1423, 1993

306. Mader S, Chen J-Y, Chen Z et al: The patterns of binding of RAR, RXR, and TR homo- and heterodimers to direct repeats are dictated by the binding specificities of the DNA binding domains. EMBO J 12:5029, 1993

307. Zechel C, Shen X-Q, Chambon P, Gronemeyer H: Dimerizaton interfaces formed between the DNA binding domains determine the cooperative binding of RXR/RAR and RXR/TR heterodimers to DR5 and DR4 elements. EMBO J 13:1414, 1994

308. Perlmann T, Rangarajan PN, Umesono K, Evans RM: Determinants for selective RAR and TR recognition of direct repeat HREs. Genes Dev 7:1411, 1993

309. Au-Fleigner M, Helmer E, Casanova J et al: The conserved ninth C-terminal heptad in thyroid hormone and retinoic acid receptors mediates diverse responses by affecting heterodimer but not homodimer formation. Mol Cell Biol 13:5725, 1993

310. Lee JW, Gulick T, Moore DD: Thyroid hormone receptor dimerization function maps to a conserved subregion of the ligand binding domain. Mol Endocrinol 6:1867, 1992

311. Sugawara A, Yen PM, Darling DS, Chin WW: Characterization and tissue expression of multiple triiodothyronine receptor-auxillary proteins and their relationship to the retinoid-X receptors. Endocrinology 133:965, 1993

312. Graupner G, Wills KN, Tzukerman M et al: Dual regulatory role for thyroid-hormone receptors allows control of retinoic-acid receptor activity. Nature 340:653, 1989

313. Simonides WS, van Hardeveld C, Larsen PR: Identification of sequences in the promoter of the fast isoform of sarcoplasmic reticulum Ca-ATPase (SERCA1) required for transcriptional activation by thyroid hormone, abstracted. Thyroid 2:S102, 1992

314. Rosen ED, O'Donnell AL, Koenig RJ: Ligand-dependent synergy of thyroid hormone and retinoid X receptors. J Biol Chem 267:22010, 1992

315. Hsu J-H, Zavacki AM, Harney JW, Brent GA: Retinoid-X receptor (RXR) differentially augments thyroid hormone response in cell lines as a function of the response element and endogenous RXR content. Endocrinology 136:7227, 1995

316. Hall BL, Smit-McBride Z, Privalsky ML: Reconstitution of retinoid-X receptor function and combinational regulation of other nuclear hormone receptors in the yeast *Saccharomyces cerevisiae*. Proc Natl Acad Sci USA 90:6929, 1993

317. Ribeiro RCJ, Kushner PJ, Apriletti JW et al: Thyroid hormone alters in vitro DNA binding of monomers and dimers of thyroid hormone receptors. Mol Endocrinol 6:1142, 1992

318. Andersson ML, Nordstrom K, Demczuck S et al: Thyroid hormone alters the DNA binding properties of chicken thyroid hormone receptors α and β. Nucl Acids Res 20:4803, 1992

319. Miyamoto T, Suzuki S, DeGroot LJ: High-affinity and specificity of dimeric binding of thyroid hormone receptors to DNA and their ligand-dependent dissociation. Mol Endocrinol 7:224, 1993

320. Hartong R, Wang N, Kurokawa R et al: Delineation of three different thyroid hormone-response elements in promoter of rat sarcoplasmic reticulum Ca^{2+}ATPase gene. J Biol Chem 269:13021, 1994

321. Ikeda M, Rhee M, Chin WW: Thyroid hormone receptor monomer, homodimer, and heterodimer (with retinoid-X receptor) contact different nucleotide sequences in thyroid hormone response elements. Endocrinology 135:1628, 1995

322. Zechel C, Shen X-Q, Chen J-Y et al: The dimerization interfaces formed between the DNA binding domains of RXR, RAR and TR determine the binding specificity and polarity of the full-length receptors to direct repeats. EMBO J 13:1425, 1994

323. Force WR, Tillman JB, Sprung CN, Spindler SR: Homodimer and heterodimer DNA binding and transcriptional responsiveness to triiodothyronine (T_3) and 9-cis-retinoic acid are determined by the number and order of high-affinity half-sites in a T_3 response element. J Biol Chem 269:8863, 1994

324. Beebe JS, Darling DS, Chin WW: 3,5,3'-triiodothyronine receptor auxiliary protein (TRAP) enhances receptor binding by interactions within the thyroid hormone response element. Mol Endocrinol 5:85, 1991

325. Sugawara A, Yen PM, Chin WW: 9-cis retinoic acid regulation of rat growth hormone gene expression: potential role of multiple nuclear hormone receptors. Endocrinology 135:1956, 1994

326. Hallenbeck PL, Phyillaier M, Nikodem VM: Divergent effects of 9-cis-retinoic acid receptor on positive and negative thyroid hormone receptor-dependent gene expression. J Biol Chem 268:3825, 1993

327. Castelein H, Gulick T, Declercq PE et al: The peroxisome proliferator activated receptor regulates malic enzyme gene expression. J Biol Chem 269:26754, 1994

328. Freedman LP: Anatomy of the steroid receptor zinc finger region. Endocr Rev 129:145, 1992

329. Koenig RJ, Brent GA, Warne RL et al: Thyroid hormone receptor binds specifically to a site in the rat growth promoter required for response to thyroid hormone. Proc Natl Acad Sci USA 84:5670, 1987

330. Glass CK, Holloway JM, Devary OV, Rosenfeld MG: The thyroid hormone receptor binds with opposite transcriptional effects to a common sequence motif in thyroid hormone and estrogen response elements. Cell 54:313, 1988

331. Koenig RJ, Warne RL, Brent GA et al: Isolation of a cDNA clone encoding a biologically active thyroid hormone receptor. Proc Natl Acad Sci USA 85:5031, 1988

332. Samuels HH, Stanley F, Casanova J: Relationship of receptor affinity to the modulation of thyroid hormone synthesis by L-triiodothyronine and iodothyronine analogs in cultured GH_1 cells. J Clin Invest 63:1229, 1979

333. Samuels HH, Forman BM, Horowitz ZD, Ye Z-S: Regulation of gene expression by thyroid hormone. J Clin Invest 81:957, 1988

334. Larsen PR, Harney JW, Moore DD: Sequences required for cell-type specific thyroid hormone regulation of the rat growth hormone promoter activity. J Biol Chem 261:14373, 1986

335. Glass CK, Franco R, Weinberger C et al: A c-erb-A binding site in the rat growth hormone gene mediates *trans*-activation by thyroid hormone. Nature 329:738, 1987

336. Brent GA, Harney JW, Chen Y et al: Mutations of the rat growth hormone promoter which increase and decrease response to thyroid hormone define a consensus thyroid hormone response element. Mol Endocrinol 3:1996, 1989

337. Brent GA, Larsen PR, Harney JW et al: Functional characterization of the rat growth hormone promoter elements required for induction by thyroid hormone with and without a co-transfected β type thyroid hormone receptor. J Biol Chem 264:178, 1989

338. Kim H-S, Crone DE, Sprung CN et al: Positive and negative thyroid hormone response elements are composed of strong and weak half-sites 10 nucleotides in length. Mol Endocrinol 6:1489, 1992

339. Katz RW, Koenig RJ: Nonbiased identification of DNA sequences that bind thyroid hormone receptor α1 with high affinity. J Biol Chem 268:19392, 1993

340. Katz RW, Koenig RJ: Specificity and mechanism of thyroid hormone induction from an octomer response element. J Biol Chem 269:18915, 1994

341. Schrader M, Becker-Andre M, Carlberg C: Thyroid hormone receptor functions as monomeric ligand-induced transcription factor on octameric half-sites. J Biol Chem 269:6444, 1994

342. Baniahmad A, Köhne AC, Renkawitz R: A transferable silencing domain is present in the thyroid hormone receptor, in the v-erbA oncogene product, and in the retinoic acid receptor. EMBO J 11:1015, 1992

343. Brent GA, Dunn MK, Harney JW et al: Thyroid hormone aproreceptor represses T_3-inducible promoters and blocks activity of the retonoic acid receptor. N Biologist 1:329, 1989

344. Brent GA, Harney JW, Moore DD, Larsen PR: Multi-hormonal regulation of the human, rat, and bovine growth hormone promoters: differential effects of 3′,5′-cyclic adenosine monophosphate, thyroid hormone, and glucocorticoids. Mol Endocrinol 2:792, 1988

345. Cattini PA, Anderson TR, Baxter JD et al: The human growth hormone gene is negatively regulated by triiodothyronine when transfected into rat pituitary tumor cells. J Biol Chem 261:13367, 1986

346. Sap J, de Magistris L, Stunnenberg H, Vennström B: A major thyroid hormone response element in the third intron of the rat growth hormone gene. EMBO 9:887, 1990

347. Brent GA, Williams GR, Harney JW et al: Effects of varying the position of thyroid hormone response elements within the rat growth hormone promoter: implications for positive and negative regulation by 3,5,3′-triiodothyronine. Mol Endocrinol 5:542, 1991

348. Williams GR, Brent GA: Thyroid hormone response elements. p. 217. In Weintraub B (ed): Molecular Endocrinology Basic Concepts and Clinical Correlations. Raven Press, New York, 1994

349. Koenig RJ, Brent GA, Larsen PR, Moore DD: Direct repeats. Nature 345:584, 1990

350. Umesono K, Murakami KK, Thompson CC, Evans RM: Direct repeats as selective response elements for the thyroid hormone, retinoic acid, and vitamin D3 receptors. Cell 65:1255, 1991

351. Zhang X, Lehmann J, Hoffmann B et al: Homodimer formation of retinoid-X receptor induced by 9-cis retinoic acid. Nature 358:587, 1992

352. Umesono K, Giguere V, Glass CK et al: Retinoic acid and thyroid hormone induce gene expression through a common responsive element. Nature 336:262, 1988

353. Glass CK, Lipkin SM, Devary OV, Rosenfeld MG: Positive and negative regulation of gene transcription by a retinoic acid-thyroid hormone receptor heterodimer. Cell 59:697, 1989

354. Bedo G, Santisteban P, Aranda A: Retinoic acid regulates growth hormone gene expression. Nature 339:231, 1989

355. Suen C-S, Yen PM, Chin WW: In vitro transcriptional studies of the roles of the thyroid hormone (T_3) response elements and minimal promoters in T_3-stim-

ulated gene transcription. J Biol Chem 269:1314, 1994

356. Wondisford FE, Farr EA, Radovick S: Thyroid hormone inhibition of human thyrotropin β-subunit gene expression is mediated by a *Cis*-acting element located in the first exon. J Biol Chem 264:14601, 1989

357. Wondisford FE, Steinfelder H, Nations M, Radovick S: AP-1 antagonizes thyroid hormone receptor action on the thyrotropin β-subunit gene. J Biol Chem 268:2749, 1993

358. Carr FE, Burnside J, Chin WW: Thyroid hormones regulate rat thyrotropin β gene promoter activity expressed in GH₃ cells. Mol Endocrinol 3:709, 1989

359. Carr FE, Wong NCW: Characteristics of a negative thyroid hormone response element. J Biol Chem 269:4175, 1994

360. Chatterjee VKK, Lee JK, Rentoumis A, Jameson JL: Negative regulation of the thyroid-stimulating hormone α gene by thyroid hormone: receptor interaction adjacent to the TATA box. Proc Natl Acad Sci USA 86:9114, 1989

361. Mano H, Mori R, Ozawa T et al: Positive and negative regulation of retinoid-x receptor gene expression by thyroid hormone in the rat. J Biol Chem 269:1591, 1994

362. Fondell JD, Roy AL, Roeder RG: Unliganded thyroid hormone receptor inhibits formation of a functional preinitiation complex: implications for active repression. Genes Dev 7:1400, 1993

363. Halachmi S, Marden E, Martin G et al: Estrogen receptor-associated proteins: possible mediators of hormone-induced transcription. Science 264:1455, 1994

364. Refetoff S, Weiss RE, Usala SJ: The syndromes of resistance to thyroid hormone. Endocr Rev 14:348, 1993

365. Refetoff S, Weiss RE, Wing JR et al: Resistance to thyroid hormone in subjects from two unrelated families is associated with a point mutation in the thyroid hormone receptor β gene resulting in the replacement of the normal proline 453 with serine. Thyroid 4:249, 1994

366. Yen PM, Sugawara A, Refetoff SR, Chin WW: New insights on the mechanism(s) of the dominant negative effect of mutant thyroid hormone receptor in generalized resistance to thyroid hormone. J Clin Invest 90:1825, 1992

367. Jameson JL: Thyroid hormone resistance: pathophysiology at the molecular level (editorial). J Clin Endocrinol Metab 74:708, 1992

368. Jameson JL: Mechanisms by which thyroid hormone receptor mutations cause clinical syndromes of resistance to thyroid hormone. Thyroid 4:485, 1994

369. Nagaya T, Madison LD, Jameson JL: Thyroid hormone receptor mutants that cause resistance to thyroid hormone: evidence for receptor competition for DNA sequences in target genes. J Biol Chem 267:13014, 1992

370. Nagaya T, Jameson JL: Thyroid hormone receptor dimerization is required for dominant negative inhibition by mutations that cause thyroid hormone resistance. J Biol Chem 268:15766, 1993

371. Murphy F, Pardy K, Seah V, Carter D: Post-transcriptional regulation of rat growth hormone gene expression: increased message stability and nuclear polyadenylation accompany thyroid hormone depletion. Mol Cell Biol 12:2624, 1992

372. Dozin B, Magnuson MA, Nikodem VM: Tissue-specific regulation of malic enzyme mRNAs by triiodothyronine. Biochemistry 24:5581, 1985

373. Dozin B, Magnuson MA, Nikodem VM: Thyroid hormone regulation of malic enzyme synthesis: dual tissue-specific control. J Biol Chem 261:10290, 1986

374. Song M-KH, Dozin B, Grieco D et al: Transcriptional activation and stabilization of malic enzyme mRNA precursor by thyroid hormone. J Biol Chem 263:17970, 1988

375. Back DW, Wilson SB, Morris SM Jr, Goodridge AG: Hormonal regulation of lipogenic enzymes in chick embryo hepatocytes in culture: thyroid hormone and glucagon regulate malic enzyme mRNA level at post-transcriptional steps. J Biol Chem 261:12555, 1986

376. Salati LM, Ma XJ, McCormick CC et al: Triiodothyronine stimulates and cyclic-AMP inhibits transcription of the gene for malic enzyme in chick embryo hepatocytes in culture. J Biol Chem 266:4010, 1991

377. Stobl W, Chan L, Patsch W: Differential regulation of hepatic apolipoprotein A-I and A-II gene expression by thyroid hormone in rat liver. Atherosclerosis 97:161, 1992

378. Bostrom K, Garcia Z, Poksay Z: Apolipoprotein B mRNA editing: direct determination of the edited base and occurrence in the nonapolipoprotein B-producing cell lines. J Biol Chem 265:22446, 1990

379. Driscoll DM, Casanova E: Characterization of the apolipoprotein B mRNA editing activity in enterocyte extracts. J Biol Chem 265:21401, 1990

380. Bianco AC, Kieffer JD, Silva JE: Adenosine 3′,5′-monophosphate and thyroid hormone control of uncoupling protein messenger ribonucleic acid in freshly dispersed brown adipocytes. Endocrinology 130:2625, 1992

381. Oppenheimer JH, Schwartz HL, Mariash CN et al: Advances in our understanding of thyroid hormone action at the cellular level. Endocr Rev 8:288, 1987

382. Katz D, Lazar MA: Dominant negative activity of an endogenous thyroid hormone receptor variant (α2)

is due to competition for binding sites on target genes. J Biol Chem 268:20904, 1993

383. Katz D, Berrodin TJ, Lazar MA: The unique C-termini of the thryoid hormone receptor variant, c-erb A α2, and thyroid hormone receptor α1 mediate different DNA-binding and heterodimerization properties. Mol Endocrinol 6:805, 1992

384. Farsetti A, Desvergne B, Hallenbeck P et al: Characterization of myelin basic protein thyroid hormone response element and its function in the context of native and heterologous promoters. J Biol Chem 267:15784, 1992

385. Strait KA, Zou L, Oppenheimer JH: β1 isoform-specific regulation of a triiodothyronine-induced gene during cerebellar development. Mol Endocrinol 6:1874, 1992

386. Lin K-H, Ashizawa K, Cheng S-Y: Phosphorylation stimulates the transcriptional activity of the human β thyroid hormone nuclear receptor. Biochemistry 89:7737, 1992

387. Sugawara A, Yen PM, Apriletti JW et al: Phosphorylation selectively increases triiodothyronine receptor homodimer binding to DNA. J Biol Chem 269:433, 1994

388. Bhat MK, Ashizawa K, Cheng S-Y: Phosphorylation enhances the target gene sequence-dependent dimerization of thyroid hormone receptor with retinoid-X receptor. Biochemistry 91:7927, 1994

389. Oppenheimer, JH: N Engl J Med 289:1153, 1968

390. Silva JE, Larsen PR: Regulation of thyroid hormone expression at the pre-receptor and receptor levels. In Hennemann G (ed) Thyroid Hormone Metabolism. Marcel Dekker, New York, 1986

391. Williams GR, Harney JW, Moore DD et al: Differential capacity of wild type promoter elements for binding and trans-activation by retinoic acid and thyroid hormone receptors. Mol Endocrinol 6:1527, 1992

392. Croteau W, Whittemore SL, Schneider MJ, St. Germain DL: Cloning and expression of a cDNA for a mammalian Type III iodothyronine deiodinase. J Biol Chem 270:16569, 1995

393. Salvatore D, Low SC, Berry MJ et al: Type 3 iodothyronine deiodinase: cloning; in vitro expression; functional analysis of the placental selenoenzyme. J Clin Invest 95:1995

394. Rastinejad F, Perlmann T, Evans RM, Sigler PB: Structural determinants of nuclear receptor assembly of DNA direct repeats. Nature 375:203, 1995

Normal Physiology of the Hypothalamic-Pituitary-Thyroidal System and Its Relation to the Neural System and Other Endocrine Glands

4

The activity of the thyroid gland is predominantly regulated by the concentration of the pituitary glycoprotein hormone, thyroid-stimulating hormone (TSH). In the absence of pituitary or thyrotroph function, hypothyroidism ensues. Thus, regulation of thyroid function in normal individuals is to a large extent determined by the factors which regulate the synthesis and secretion of TSH. Those factors, reviewed in this chapter, consist principally of thyrotropin-releasing hormone (TRH) and the feedback effects of circulating thyroid hormones at the hypothalamic and pituitary levels. The consequence of the dynamic interplay of these two dominant influences on TSH secretion—the positive effect of TRH on the one hand and the negative effects of thyroid hormones on the other—result in a remarkably stable concentration of TSH in the circulation and consequently little alteration in the level of circulating

113

thyroid hormones from day to day and year to year. This regulation is so carefully maintained that an abnormal serum TSH in most patients indicates the presence of a disorder of thyroid gland function. The utility of TSH measurements has been recognized and its use has remarkably increased in recent years due to the development of immunometric methodologies for the accurate quantitation of this protein in serum. Thus, an understanding of the regulatory influences on TSH secretion underlies both normal thyroid physiology and the pathophysiology of thyroid diseases.

This chapter is organized into two sections. The first portion reviews basic studies of TSH synthesis, post-translational modification, and release. The second deals with physiologic studies in humans which serve as the background to the diagnostic use of TSH measurements and reviews the results of TSH assays in a pathophysiologic context.

THE REGULATION OF THYROID-STIMULATING HORMONE SYNTHESIS AND SECRETION: MOLECULAR BIOLOGY AND BIOCHEMISTRY

The Thyroid-Stimulating Hormone Molecule

Thyroid-stimulating hormone (TSH) is a heterodimer consisting of α and β subunits tightly, but noncovalently, bound.[1] While the molecular weight of the deduced amino acid sequence of mature α plus TSH β subunits is approximately 38,000 d, additional carbohydrate (15 percent by weight) results in a significantly higher molecular weight estimate based on sizing by polyacrylamide gel electrophoresis. The α subunit is common to TSH, follicle stimulating hormone (FSH), luteinizing hormone (LH), and chorionic gonadotropin (CG). The β subunit confers specificity to the molecule since it interacts with the thyroid cell TSH receptor and is rate-limiting in the formation of the mature heterodimeric protein. The human α subunit gene is located on chromosome 6 and the TSH β gene on human chromosome 1.[2] The organization of the TSH β gene is somewhat variable between the mouse, rat, and human.[1,3] Much more work has focused the murine TSH β gene due to the availability of the mouse thyrotropic tumor line TtT 97.[4-7]

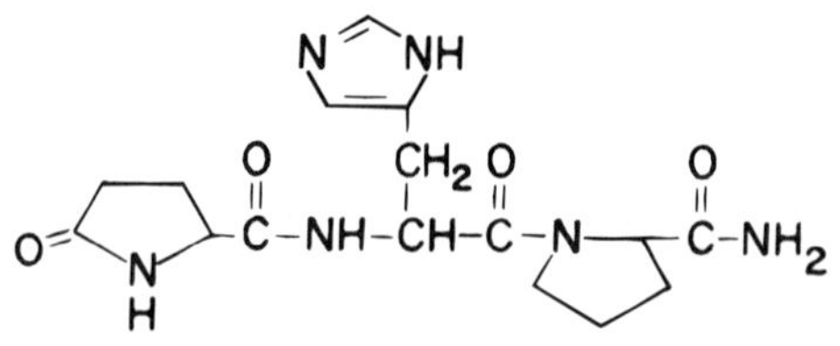

(Pyro)Glu-His-Pro(NH$_2$)

Fig. 4-1. Structure of TRH.

The formation of mature TSH involves several post-translational steps including the excision of signal peptides from both subunits and cotranslational glycosylation with high mannose oligosaccharides.[8] As the glycoproteins are successively transferred from the rough endoplasmic reticulum to the golgi apparatus, the trimming of mannose and further addition of fucose, galactose, and sialic acid occurs.[9] The primary intracellular role of these glycosylation events may be to allow proper folding of the α and TSH β subunits permitting their heterodimerization and also preventing intracellular degradation.[9,10]

To attain normal bioactivity, TSH must be properly glycosylated, a process which requires the interaction of the neuropeptide thyrotropin releasing hormone (TRH), with its receptor on the thyrotroph[11-15] (Fig. 4-1). The requirement for TRH in this process is illustrated by the fact that in patients with central hypothyroidism due to hypothalamic-pituitary dysfunction, normal or even slightly elevated levels of radioimmunoassayable, but biologically subpotent TSH, are found in the circulation in the presence of a reduced free T_4.[14,16,17] Chronic TRH administration to such patients normalizes the glycosylation process, enhancing both its TSH-receptor binding affinity as well as its capacity to activate adenyl cyclase. This, in turn, can normalize thyroid function in such patients.[18] Glycosylation of the molecule can also influence the rapidity of clearance of TSH from the circulation.

Specific amino acids in the βTSH subunit are critical for the dimerization of this protein with the α subunit. The peptide sequence CAGYC (cysteine-alanine-glycine-tyrosine-cysteine) is highly conserved in TSH β, LH β, CG β, and FSH β.[19] In several families with an autosomal recessive form of hypothyroidism due to TSH deficiency, a mutation has been identified which changes the glycine residue in the CAGYC sequence to arginine.[19,20] If a combina-

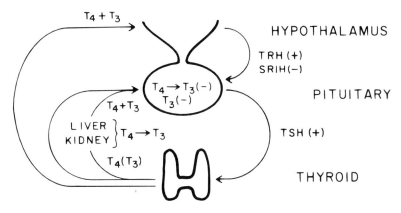

Fig. 4-2. Basic elements in the regulation of thyroid function. TRH is a necessary tonic stimulus to TSH synthesis and release. TRH synthesis is regulated directly by thyroid hormones. T_4 is the predominant secretory product of the thyroid gland, with peripheral deiodination of T_4 to T_3 in the liver and kidney supplying roughly 80 percent of the circulating T_3. Both circulating T_3 and T_4 directly inhibit TSH synthesis and release independently; T_4 via its rapid conversion to T_3. SRIH = somatostatin.

tion of α and the mutant TSH β subunit mRNAs are injected into *Xenopus* oocytes, no intact TSH heterodimer is formed, unlike what occurs when a similar experiment is performed with a normal TSH β mRNA. This illustrates an important role of the CAGYC peptide in influencing the tertiary structure of the TSH β subunit thereby facilitating the heterodimerization process.

Thyroid Hormone Regulation of TSH Synthesis and Secretion

Thyroid hormone is the major regulator of TSH production[21] (Fig. 4-2). T_3 acts by binding to the thyrotroph nuclear T_3 receptor, and T_4 acts by its intra-pituitary or intra-hypothalamic conversion to T_3. Both regulate the synthesis and release of TSH at the pituitary level as well as indirectly affecting TSH synthesis by their effects on the synthesis of TRH and other neuropeptides.

Thyroid Hormone Effects on TSH Synthesis

Thyroid hormone regulation of TSH β subunit transcription is complex and, at least in the rat and mouse, involves control of gene transcription at both start sites of the gene[3,22–28] (Fig. 4-3). Studies of the human, rat, and mouse TSH β genes have demonstrated that they contain DNA hexamer half sites with strong similarity to the T_3 response elements

(TREs) found in genes which are positively regulated by thyroid hormone[29–32] (see Ch. 3). The sequences in the TSH β gene are diagrammed in Figure 4-3 and their similarity to the typical hexamer binding sites in positively regulated genes and in the rat α subunit gene is seen by comparison to the TRE sequences from positively regulated genes[33] (Fig. 3-15). The molecular biology of negative regulation by thyroid hormone is still poorly understood. Nonetheless, these conserved TRE-like sequences presumably are the site on the TSH gene to which the T_3 receptor binds. The subsequent binding of T_3 to similar receptor-DNA complexes suppresses transcription of both α and TSH β subunit genes.[3,24,34,35] The negative transcription conferred by these TRE sequences is retained even if they are transferred to a different gene or placed in a different position within a heterologous gene.[33,36–38] This suggests that the negative transcriptional response to thyroid hormone is intrinsic to this TRE structure.

Hypothyroidism in the rat increases TSH production 15- to 20-fold over that in the euthyroid state. This change can be attributed to several factors. First, the stimulatory effects of TRH discussed below are unopposed by the negative effects of T_3. Secondly, in addition to an increase in the transcription rate per cell, there is a 3- to 4-fold increase in the absolute number of thyrotrophs in the hypothyroid pituitary.[39] Thus, the roughly 20-fold increase in TSH production is due both to an increased number of cells

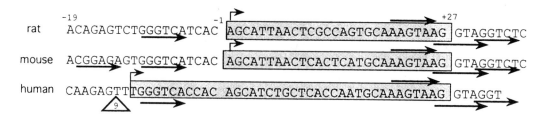

Fig. 4-3. DNA sequences of the putative nTREs in the rat, mouse, and human TSH β subunit gene promoters. A comparison of the proximal promoter regions of the rat, mouse, and human TSH β subunit genes is shown. The straight arrows denote TRE consensus half-sites identified by functional and TR binding assays. The first exons (relative to the downstream promoter for the rat and mouse genes) are shaded, and the bent arrows denote the sites of transcription initiation. Note a nine-nucleotide deletion in the human gene relative to the rodent genes indicated by the triangle just 5′ of the transcriptional start site. (From Chin et al,[3] with permission.)

and to a 3- to 5-fold increase in TSH secretion per cell. Electron microscopic studies have shown near total depletion of secretory granules in the thyrotrophs of hypothyroid animals, a change that is reversed soon after administration of thyroid hormone.[40]

Thyroid Hormone Effects on Release of TSH

The acute administration of T_3 to the hypothyroid rat causes a rapid and marked decrease in the level of serum TSH[21,41–44] (Fig. 4-4). This decrease occurs prior to the decrease in pituitary α and TSH β mRNAs.[45–48] During the period that circulating TSH is falling, pituitary TSH content remains unchanged or increases slightly.[49] The suppression of TSH release is rapid, beginning within 15 minutes of intravenous T_3 injection, but is preceded by the appearance of T_3 in pituitary nuclei.[42] In the experimental setting in the rat, as the bolus of injected T_3 is cleared and the plasma T_3 level falls, nuclear T_3 decreases followed shortly by a rapid increase in plasma TSH. Both the chronological and quantitative relationships between receptor bound T_3 and TSH release are preserved over this time.[42]

The mechanism for this effect of T_3 is unknown. Suppression of basal TSH release is difficult to study in vitro. Accordingly, the T_3 induced blockade of TRH-induced TSH release has been used as a model for this event. This T_3 effect is inhibited by blockers of either protein or mRNA synthesis.[50,51] The effect is not specific for TRH since T_3 will also block calcium ionophore, phorbol ester, or potassium-induced TSH release.[52,53] Furthermore, T_3 will also block the TRH-induced increase in intracellular cal-

cium which precedes TSH release.[54] Thus, T_3 inhibits TSH secretion regardless of what agent is used to initiate that process.

T_4 can cause an equally rapid suppression of TSH via its intrapituitary conversion to T_3[42,55] (Fig. 4-2). This T_4 to T_3 conversion process is catalyzed by the type 2 deiodinase (see Ch. 3). An effect of T_4 per se can be demonstrated if its conversion to T_3 is blocked by a general deiodinase inhibitor such as iopanoic acid.[56,57] In this case, the T_4 in the cell rises to concentrations sufficient to occupy a significant number of receptor sites even though its intrinsic binding affinity for the receptor is only 1/10 that of T_3. A similar effect can be achieved by rapid displacement of T_4 from its binding proteins by flavonoids.[58] It seems likely, however, that under physiologic circumstances the feedback effects of T_4 on TSH secretion and synthesis can be accounted for by its intracellular conversion to T_3.

Based on the analyses of the sources of nuclear T_3 in the rat pituitary (Fig. 3-11, Ch. 3), one would predict that approximately half of the feedback suppression of TSH release in the euthyroid state can be attributed to the T_3 derived directly from plasma; the remainder accounted for by the nuclear receptor bound T_3 derived from intrapituitary T_4 to T_3 conversion.[59–61] Various physiologic studies in both rats and humans confirm this concept in that a decrease in either T_4 or T_3 leads to an increase in TSH.[62–68] The effect of T_4 is best illustrated in the iodine deficient rat model (Fig. 4-5). In this paradigm, rats are placed on a low iodine diet and serum T_3, T_4, and TSH quantitated at frequent times thereafter.[69–71] Despite the fact that serum T_3 concentra-

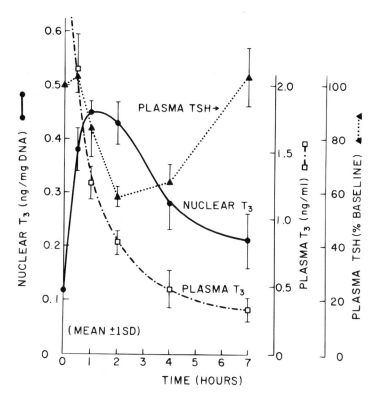

Fig. 4-4. Time course of specific pituitary nuclear T_3 binding and changes in plasma TSH in hypothyroid rats after a single intravenous injection of 70 ng T_3 per 100 g of body weight. Since the maximal capacity of thyroid hormone binding in pituitary nuclear proteins is about 1 ng T_3/mg DNA, the peak nuclear T_3 content of 0.44 ng T_3/mg corresponds to 44 percent saturation. The plasma level falls to about 55 percent of its initial basal level by 90 minutes after T_3 injection, demonstrating that there is both a chronologic and a quantitative correlation between nuclear T_3 receptor saturation and suppression of TSH release. (From Silva and Larsen,[42] with permission.)

tions remain constant, there is a marked increase in TSH as the serum T_4 falls. In humans, iodine deficiency produces similar effects.[72,73] The most familiar example of the independent role of circulating T_4 in suppression of TSH is found in patients in the early phases of primary hypothyroidism in whom serum T_4 is slightly reduced, serum T_3 is normal or even high normal range, but serum TSH is elevated[74,75] (Table 4-1).

The Role of Thyrotropin-Releasing Hormone in TSH Secretion

Thyrotropin-releasing hormone (TRH) is critical for the synthesis and secretion of TSH either in the presence or absence of thyroid hormones. Destruction of the parvocellular region of the rat hypothalamus, which synthesizes the TRH relevant for TSH

regulation, causes hypothyroidism.[41,76] Hypothalamic TRH synthesis is in turn regulated by thyroid hormones and thus TRH synthesis and release is an integral part of the feedback loop regulating thyroid status (see Fig. 4-2). TRH also interacts with thyroid hormone at the thyrotroph raising the set-point for thyroid hormone inhibition of TSH release.[41] The data supporting these general concepts are reviewed in subsequent sections.

Control of Thyrotroph-Specific TRH Synthesis

TRH is synthesized as a large pre-pro-TRH protein in several tissues.[77-83] In addition to the hypothalamus, it has been identified in the brain, β cells of the pancreas, the C cells of the thyroid gland, the myocardium, reproductive organs including the prostrate and testis, and in the spinal cord. This dis-

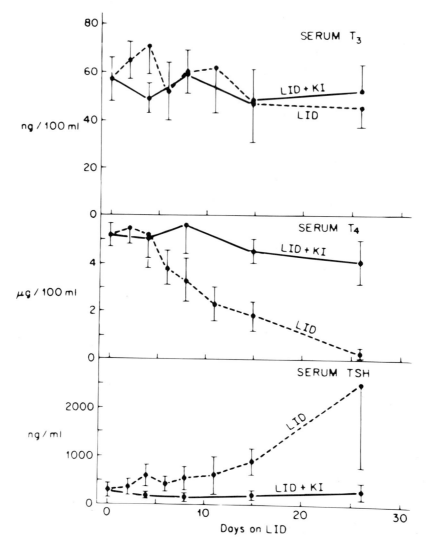

Fig. 4-5. Serum T_3, T_4, and TSH concentrations (mean ± SD) in rats receiving a low iodine diet (LID), with or without potassium iodide (KI) supplementation in the drinking water. (From Riesco et al,[71] with permission.)

TABLE 4-1. Serum Concentration of Thyroid Hormones and TSH in Patients with Primary Hypothyroidism of Increasing Severity

Group[a]	T_4 (µg/dl)	T_3 (ng/dl)	TSH (µU/ml) Basal	After 200 µg TRH
Control	7.1 ± 0.9	115 ± 31	1.3 ± 0.5	11 ± 4.6
1	6–9	119 ± 40	5.3 ± 2.3	39 ± 15
2	4–6	103 ± 20	13 ± 10	92 ± 50
3	2–4	101 ± 35	63 ± 56	196 ± 120
4	<2	43 ± 28	149 ± 144	343 ± 326

Results are mean ± SD.
[a] Patients were categorized according to the severity of thyroid disease based on serum T_4 concentrations.
(Adapted from Bigos et al,[75] with permission.)

cussion focuses on the regulation of TRH synthesis in the parvocellular region of the paraventricular nuclei (PVN) since the TRH produced therein is that regulating TSH secretion. The human pre-pro-TRH molecule contains 5 progenitor sequences for TRH.[77–79,84,85] These five peptides consist of a gln-his-pro-gly peptide preceded and followed by lys-arg or arg-arg dipeptides. The basic dipeptides are the cleavage sites for release of the tetra-peptide progenitor sequence. The glycine residue is the source of the terminal amide for the proline residue of TRH (Fig. 4-1). In addition to the pro-TRH peptides which are released from the pre-pro TRH molecule, intervening non-TRH peptides which have potential physiological function are co-released.[86] The 5′ flanking sequence of the TRH gene has potential glucocorticoid and cyclic AMP response elements (GRE and CRE).[84] There are also at least two potential negative TREs located in this portion of the gene which offer regulatory sites for thyroid hormone control of TRH gene transcription. TRH is released from axon terminals close to the hypothalamic-pituitary portal plexus which travel through the median eminence.[76] The TRH-producing neuron bodies are densely innervated by both catecholamine and neuropeptide Y containing axons which may also regulate the synthesis of the pre-pro-TRH molecule. Somatostatin containing axons also contribute to the negative regulation of TRH synthesis.[87]

Substantial advances in recent years have increased our understanding of the role of thyroid hormones in the regulation of TRH synthesis.[86,88–92] Direct regulation by thyroid hormone of pre-pro-TRH mRNA concentrations in the PVN has been demonstrated using in situ hybridization.[88,89,91] Increases in TRH mRNA levels occur during primary or secondary hypothyroidism and decreases in TRH mRNA result from implantation of a small crystal of T_3 adjacent to the PVN confirming earlier studies in primates.[89,93] The physiological source of the T_3 causing down-regulation of TRH mRNA in the hypothalamus is the subject of ongoing investigations. Somewhat surprisingly, the PVN do not contain the type 2 5′ iodothyronine deiodinase which is thought to be the source of at least 80 percent of the intracellular T_3 in the central nervous system[43,94] (see Ch. 3). However, studies with T_3 containing mini-pumps implanted into thyroidectomized rats indicate that, for normalization of circulating TSH and hypothalamic pre-pro-TRH mRNA, T_3 concentrations about

twice normal have to be maintained in rat plasma.[90] These results are in agreement with earlier studies on the T_3 requirements for normalization of TSH in thyroidectomized rats.[65,66] Thus, for both systems (TRH and TSH), feedback regulation requires a source of T_3 in addition to that provided by the ambient levels of this hormone. While this T_3 seems likely to be produced locally from T_4, the anatomic location of such a process has not been identified. It is possible that T_4 to T_3 conversion occurs elsewhere in the CNS and the T_3 is transported in synaptosomes to the PVN.[95]

TRH Interaction with Pituitary Thyrotrophs and with Thyroid Hormone

TRH binds to a specific receptor in the plasma membrane of the thyrotroph to induce the release of TSH and to stimulate TSH synthesis. The TRH receptor has only recently been cloned and has been identified as a G-protein-coupled receptor with seven highly conserved transmembrane domains[96,97] TRH-receptor mRNA is increased by glucocorticoids and decreased by thyroid hormone as well as by TRH itself.[98,99] The second messengers for induction of the thyrotroph response to TRH are calcium and cyclic GMP.[100–102] TRH causes an acute increase in intracellular calcium in the thyrotrophs via release from internal stores secondary to increases in inositol triphosphate, due to hydrolysis of phosphatidyl inositol in the cell membrane.[100,103,104] G protein activation of phospholipase C is responsible for this hydrolysis. While extracellular calcium is required for TRH stimulation of prolactin synthesis and release from the mammotrophs, intracellular calcium stores appear to be adequate for its effects in the thyrotroph.[105–107] In transfection systems in which the TSHβ gene promoter has been linked to a reporter gene, both phorbol esters and the calcium ionophore, ionomycin, stimulate TSH gene transcription confirming that TRH can act through these second messengers.[108,109]

Thyroid hormone inhibits the effects of TRH on TSH release by a mechanism which requires protein synthesis (see above). Both the effects of phorbol ester, a protein kinase C activator, and calcium ionophore are blocked by pre-incubation of pituitary cells with thyroid hormones. As mentioned, this effect of thyroid hormone requires time and protein synthesis but is otherwise poorly characterized.[50–53]

TABLE 4-2. Predominant Effects of Various Agents on TSH Secretion

Stimulatory	Inhibitory
Thyrotropin-releasing hormone (TRH)	Thyroid hormones and analogs
Prostaglandins (?)	Dopamine
α-Adrenergic agonists (? via TRH)	Somatostatin
	Gastrin
	Cholecystokinin
	Serotonin
	Glucocorticoids
	Interleukin 1β and 6
	Tumor-necrosis factor α

Presumably the same mechanisms are involved in thyroid hormone regulation of basal TSH secretion.

Thyroid hormone thus regulates TSH secretion by multiple pathways. These are schematically illustrated in Figure 4-2 and consist of inhibition of the synthesis of TRH receptor in thyrotroph TSHβmRNA as well as of the release of performed, intact TSH. Which specific mechanism is operational in a given physiological situation may depend on the level of circulating thyroid hormones and the duration of the thyroid hormone excess or deficiency. Together, the intricate relationships between thyroid hormone and TSH secretion account for the exquisite sensitivity of measurements of the circulating TSH concentration as a generally reliable indicator of thyroid status.

Other Influences on TSH Secretion

A number of other hormones, neuropeptides, and physiologic circumstances influence TSH release from the thyrotroph (Table 4-2). Somatostatin blocks TSH secretion acutely, although long-term treatment with somatostatin analog does not cause hypothyroidism in man.[87,110–114] Somatostatin receptors cause activation of Gi proteins which in turn inhibit adenylate cyclase. Dopamine, acting through the DA_2 class of dopamine receptors, also inhibits TSH synthesis and release, again through a decrease in adenylate cyclase.[115–119] While central stimulation of α-adrenergic pathways increases TSH release, presumably through increased TRH, in vitro, α1 adrenergic agonists also enhance TSH release by mechanisms which are independent of those activated by TRH.[120,121] It is thought that this mechanism is also linked to adenylate cyclase activation

since agents increasing intracellular cyclic AMP in thyrotrophs can increase TSH release.[105,122] Thus an intricate set of relationships within the central nervous system controls the TRH-producing neurons in the medial basal hypothalamus. Alterations in any of these mechanisms can influence TRH and consequently TSH release. The relative importance of these neural pathways in human physiology is unknown.

Cytokines have recently been demonstrated to have important effects on TRH or TSH release. Both IL-1β and tumor necrosis factor α (cachectin) inhibit TSH release.[123–126] At the same time, IL-1β stimulates the release of corticotropin-releasing hormone. Interleukin-1β is produced in rat thyrotrophs and is markedly increased by administration of bacterial lipopolysaccharide.[127] It could thus reduce TSH secretion by either autocrine or paracrine mechanisms. Interleukin 6 is produced by the folliculo-stellate cells of the anterior pituitary and thus may also regulate TSH release in a paracrine fashion.[128]

PHYSIOLOGIC REGULATION OF TSH SECRETION IN HUMANS

A number of experimental paradigms have been used to mimic clinical situations that affect the hypothalamic-pituitary-thyroid axis in man. However, with the exception of the studies of thyroid status and iodine deficiency, such perturbations have limited application to humans due to differences in the more subtle aspects of TSH regulation between species. For example, starvation is a severe stress and markedly reduces TSH secretion in rats, but not in humans. Cold stress increases TSH release in the adult rat but not in the adult human. Thus, it is more relevant to evaluate the consequences of various pathophysiologic influences on TSH concentrations in humans rather than to extrapolate from results in experimental animals. This approach has the disadvantage that, in many cases, the precise mechanism responsible for the alteration in TSH secretion cannot be identified. This deficit is offset by the enhanced relevance of the human studies for understanding clinical pathophysiology.

Normal Physiology

The concentration of TSH can now be measured with exquisite sensitivity using immunometric techniques (see below). In euthyroid humans, this concentration is 0.4 to 5.0 mU/L. This normal range is to some extent method-dependent in that the various assays use reference preparations of slightly varying biologic potency. There is no crystalline human TSH preparation, so it is not possible to provide a precise molar equivalent for TSH concentrations.

Free α subunit is also detectable in serum with a normal range of 1 to 5 μg/L, but free TSH β is not detectable.[129,130] Both the intact TSH molecule and the α subunit increase in response to TRH. The α-subunit is also increased in post-menopausal women; thus the level of gonadal steroid production needs to be taken into account in evaluating α subunit concentrations in women. In most patients with hyperthyroidism due to TSH-producing thyrotroph tumors, there is an elevation in the ratio of α subunit to total TSH.[10,110,111,129–136] In the presence of normal gonadotropin this ratio is calculated by assuming a molecular weight for TSH of 28,000 and for α subunit of 13,600 dalton. The approximate specific activity of TSH is 0.2 mU/μg. To calculate the molar ratio of α subunit to TSH, the concentration of α subunit (in μg/L) is divided by the TSH concentration (in mU/L) and this result multiplied by 10. The normal ratio is less than 1.0 and it is usually elevated in patients with TSH-producing pituitary tumor but is normal in patients with thyroid hormone resistance unless they are post menopausal.

The volume of distribution of TSH in humans is slightly larger than the plasma volume, the half-life is about one hour, and the daily TSH turnover between 40 and 150 mU/day.[137,138] Patients with primary hypothyroidism have serum TSH concentrations greater than five and up to several hundred mU/L.[75] In patients with hyperthyroidism due to Graves' disease or autonomous thyroid nodules, TSH is suppressed with levels which are inversely proportional to the severity and duration of the hyperthyroidism, to as low as 0.004 mU/L.[139–141]

TSH secretion in humans is pulsatile.[142–145] The pulse frequency is slightly less than two hours and the amplitude approximately 0.6 mU/L. The frequency and amplitude of pulsations increases during the evening reaching a peak at sleep onset, thus accounting for the circadian variation in basal serum TSH levels.[146–148] The maximal serum TSH is reached between 2100 and 0200 hours and the difference between the afternoon nadir and peak TSH concentrations is 1 to 3 mU/L. Sleep prevents the further rise in TSH as reflected in the presence of further increases in TSH to 5 to 10 mU/ml during sleep deprivation.[149,150] There is little, if any, significant seasonal change in basal TSH nor are there any gender-related differences in either the amplitude or frequency of the TSH pulses.[145]

Age does not have a major effect on serum TSH with the exception of the extremes. There is a marked increase in serum TSH in neonates which peaks within the first few hours of delivery returning towards normal over the next few days (see Ch. 15). It is thought to be a consequence of the marked reduction in environmental temperature at birth. Serum TSH concentrations in apparently euthyroid patients over the age of 70 may be somewhat reduced although usually this is a pathologic finding indicating either exogenous or endogenous thyrotoxicosis.[151]

TSH in Pathophysiologic States

Nutrition

In the rat, starvation causes a marked decrease in serum TSH and thyroid hormones. While there is an impairment of T_4 to T_3 conversion in the rat liver due to a decrease in both thiol co-factor and later in the type 1 deiodinase,[152–155] the decrease in serum T_3 in the fasted rat is primarily due to the decrease in T_4 secretion consequent to TSH deficiency.[156,157] In humans, starvation and moderate to severe illness are also associated with a decrease in serum TSH.[158–164] In the acutely-fasted man, serum TSH falls only slightly and TRH infusion will normalize TSH early in fasting.[165,166] This suggests that the thyrotroph remains responsive during short-term fasting and that the decrease in TSH is likely due to changes due to decreased TRH release. There is evidence to support this in animal studies.[167] Fasting-induced changes in dopaminergic tone do not seem to be sufficient to explain the TSH changes.[119,162] A further contributing cause of the decreased TSH release in fasting may be an abrupt increase in the free fraction of T_4 due to the inhibition of hormone binding by free fatty acids.[168] This would cause an increase in pituitary T_4 and, hence, in pituitary nuclear T_3. Fasting causes a decrease in the amplitude of TSH pulses, not in their frequency.[169]

Illness

The changes in circulating TSH which occur during fasting are more exaggerated during illness. In moderately ill patients, serum TSH may be slightly reduced but the serum free T_4 does not fall and is often mildly increased.[168,170-173] However, if the illness is severe and/or prolonged, serum TSH will decrease and both serum T_4 (and of course T_3) decrease during the course of the illness (see Ch. 5). This may be due to decreased nocturnal TSH secretion.[174-176] Since such changes are short-lived, they do not usually cause symptomatic hypothyroidism. They are often associated with an impaired TSH release after TRH.[162,177] However, the illness-induced reductions in serum T_4 and T_3 will often be followed by a rebound increase in serum TSH as the patient improves. This may lead to a transient serum TSH elevation in association with the still subnormal levels of circulating thyroid hormones and thus be mistaken for primary hypothyroidism.[178] On occasion, transient TSH elevation occurs while the patient is still ill. The pathophysiology of this apparent thyroid gland resistance to TSH is not understood.[179] The transient nature of these changes is reflected in normalization of the pituitary-thyroid axis after complete recovery.

Neuropsychiatric Disorders

Certain neuropsychiatric disorders may also be associated with alterations in TSH secretion. In patients with anorexia nervosa or depressive illness, serum TSH may be reduced or TRH-induced TSH release blunted.[180-186] Such patients often have decreases in the evening enhancement of TSH secretion.[147] The etiology of these changes is not known though it has been speculated that they are a consequence of TRH deficiency.[187] However, the opposite proposition—namely, that excessive TRH secretion is associated with some forms of depression—has also been raised.[182,188,189] The latter is supported by observations that TRH concentrations in cerebrospinal fluid of some depressed patients are elevated.[190,191] There may be a parallel in such patients between increases in TRH and those of ACTH secretion.[181,192] In agreement with this are the increased serum T_4 and TSH levels sometimes found at the time of admission to psychiatric units.[184,193-195]

The suppression of the hypothalamic-pituitary thyroid axis in illness and starvation raises the possibility that interleukin-1 (IL-1) tumor necrosis factor (TNF) α and/or IL-6 inhibition of TRH and/or TSH secretion could play causative roles.[126] Interleukin-1a may also inhibit these processes indirectly by inducing IL-6 secretion by the pituitary cells and both of these cytokines can inhibit pro-TRH, and TSHβmRNA synthesis in rats.[128]

Effects of Hormones and Neuropeptides

Dopamine and Dopamine Agonists

Dopamine and dopamine agonists inhibit TSH release by mechanisms discussed earlier.[115] Dopamine infusion can overcome the effects of thyroid hormone deficiency in the severely ill patient, suppressing the normally elevated TSH of the patient with primary hypothyroidism nearly into the normal range.[117,196] Dopamine causes a reduction of the amplitude of TSH pulsatile release, but not in its frequency.[128,174] However, chronic administration of dopamine agonists, for example in the treatment of prolactinoma, does not lead to central hypothyroidism despite the fact that there is marked decrease in the size of the pituitary tumor and inhibition of prolactin secretion.

Glucocorticoids

The acute administration of pharmacological quantities of glucocorticoids will transiently suppress TSH.[197,200] TSH secretion recovers and T_4 production rates are generally not impaired. In Cushings' syndrome, TSH may be normal or suppressed and, in general, there is a decrease in serum T_3 concentrations relative to those of T_4.[198] High levels of glucocorticoid inhibit basal TSH secretion slightly and may influence the circadian variation in serum TSH.[144] Perhaps as a reflection of this, a modest serum TSH elevation may be present in patients with Addison's disease.[201-203] TSH normalizes with glucocorticoid therapy alone if primary hypothyroidism is not also present.

Gonadal Steroids

Aside from the well described effects of estrogen on the concentration of thyroxine binding globulin (TBG), estrogen and testosterone have only minor influences on thyroid economy (see Ch. 5 and 14). TSH release after TRH is enhanced by estradiol treatment perhaps because estrogens increase TRH receptor number.[204,205] Treatment with the testosterone analog, fluoxymesterone, causes a significant decrease in the TSH response to TRH in hypogonadal men.[206] This may be due to an increase in T_4 to T_3 conversion by androgen.[207] This and the small estrogen effect may account for the lower TSH response to TRH in men than in women although there is no difference in basal TSH levels between the sexes. This is one of the few instances where there is not a close correlation between basal TSH levels and the response to TRH (see below).

Growth Hormone

The possibility that hypothyroidism could be induced by growth hormone (GH) replacement in GH-deficient children was raised in early studies.[208,209] However, these patients received human pituitary GH which in some cases was contaminated with TSH, perhaps inducing TSH antibodies. More recent studies employing recombinant GH have shown no significant changes in TSH concentrations during therapy of adults with GH deficiency.[210] Growth hormone did cause an increase in serum free T_3, a decrease in free T_4, and an increase in the T_3 to T_4 ratio in both T_4-treated and T_4 untreated patients. This suggests that the GH-induced increase in IGF1 stimulates T_4 to T_3 conversion.

Combined deficiencies of GH, prolactin and TSH occur as a congenital abnormality in the rare families with mutations in Pit-1 protein or GHRH receptor.[211-213] In such patients, there is a common cause for the decreased secretion of TSH and GH but the one is not related to the other.

Catecholamines

Acute infusions of α- or β-adrenergic blocking agents or agonists for short periods of time do not affect basal TSH. Furthermore, there is no effect of chronic propranolol administration on TSH secretion even though there may be modest inhibition of peripheral T_4 to T_3 conversion if amounts in excess of 160 mg/day are given.[214]

The Response of TSH to TRH in Humans and the Role of Immunometric TSH Assays

In the last decade, the application of TSH measurements to the evaluation of patients with thyroid disease has undergone a revolutionary change. This is due to the widespread application of the immunometric TSH assay. This assay uses monoclonal antibodies which bind one epitope of TSH and do not interfere with the binding of a second monoclonal or polyclonal antibody to a second epitope. The principle of the test is that TSH serves as the link between an immobilized antibody binding TSH at one epitope and a labeled (radioactive, chemiluminescent or other tag) monoclonal directed against a second portion of the molecule. This approach has improved both sensitivity and specificity by several orders of magnitude. Technical modifications have led to successive "generations" of TSH assays with progressively greater sensitivities.[140,215,216] The first generation TSH assay is considered to be the standard radioimmunoassay which generally has minimal detection limits of 1 to 2 mU/L. The "second" generation (first generation immunometric) assay improved the sensitivity to 0.1 to 0.2 mU/L and the "third" reduced the sensitivity to approximately 0.005 mU/L. Third generation assays are currently being introduced into many clinical laboratories. From a technical point-of-view, the American Thyroid Association recommendations are that third generation assays should be able to quantitative TSH in the 0.010 to 0.020 mU/L range on an interassay basis with a coefficient of variation of 20 percent or less.[217] The most recent development is an assay with a minimal usable sensitivity of 0.0004 mU/L. Such assays are currently available only in specialized laboratories. It would appear that the third generation assays will provide sufficient sensitivity for even the most rigorous clinical applications. As assay sensitivity has improved, the normal range has not changed, remaining between approximately 0.5 and 5.0 mU/L in most laboratories. However, the TSH concentrations in the sera of patients with severe thyrotoxicosis secondary to Graves' disease have been lower with each successive improvement in the TSH assays using a fourth generation assay, the serum TSH is less than 0.004 mU/L in patients with severe hyperthyroidism.[141] While the potential for such high sensitivity is inherent to the technology the clinician should always ascertain that the performance in his/her clinical laboratory meets the appropriate sensitivity criteria before assuming that an assay stipulated to be "second" or "third" generation is achieving that sensitivity on site.[216]

The primary consequence of the availability of the sensitive TSH assays is to allow the substitution of a

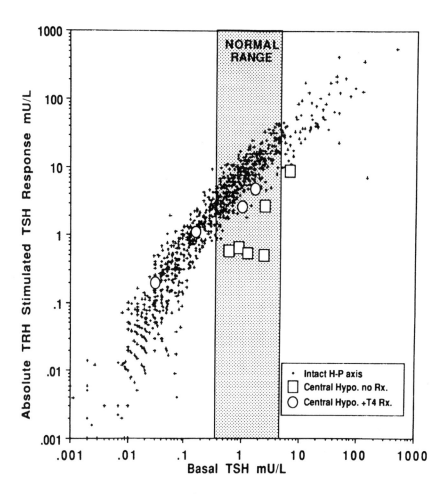

Fig. 4-6. Relationship between basal and absolute (TRH stimulated-basal TSH) TRH-stimulated TSH response in 1,061 ambulatory patients with an intact hypothalamic-pituitary (H-P) axis compared with that in untreated and T$_4$-treated patients with central hypothyroidism. (From Spencer et al,[141] with permission.)

basal TSH measurement for the TRH test in patients suspected of thyrotoxicosis.[139–141,218–220] Nonetheless, it is appropriate to review the results of TRH tests from the point-of-view of understanding thyroid pathophysiology, particularly in patients with hyperthyroidism or autonomous thyroid function. There is a tight correlation between the basal TSH and the magnitude of the TRH-induced peak TSH. (Fig. 4-6) Using a normal basal TSH range of 0.5 to 5 mU/L, the TRH response 15 to 20 minutes after 500 μg TRH (intravenously) ranges between 2 and 30 mU/L. The lower responses are found in patients with lower (but still normal) basal TSH levels.[141] These results are quite consistent with older studies using radioimmunoassays.[221] When the TSH re-

sponse to TRH of all patients (hypo-, hyper- and euthyroid) is analyzed in terms of a "fold" response, the highest response (approximately 20-fold) occurs at a basal TSH of 0.5 mU/L and falls to less than 5 at either markedly subnormal or markedly elevated basal serum TSH concentrations[141] (Fig. 4-7). Thus a low response can have two explanations. The low response in patients with hyperthyroidism and a reduced basal TSH is due to refractoriness to TRH or depletion of pituitary TSH as a consequence of chronic thyroid hormone excess. In patients with primary hypothyroidism, the low fold-response reflects only the lack of sufficient pituitary TSH to achieve the necessary increment over the elevated basal TSH.

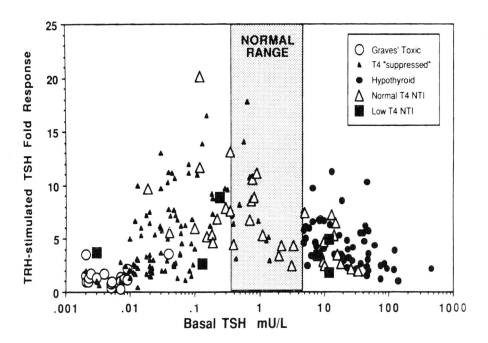

Fig. 4-7. Relationship between basal TSH and fold response in ambulatory patients with varying thyroid conditions versus sick hospitalized patients with NTI and either normal or low T$_4$ levels. (From Spencer et al,[141] with permission.)

Perhaps of most interest pathophysiologically is the response to TRH in patients with non-thyroidal illness and either normal or low free T$_4$ indices (Fig. 4-7). Results from these patients fit within the normal distribution in terms of the relationship between basal TSH (whether suppressed or elevated) and the fold-response to TRH. Thus the information provided by a TRH infusion test adds little to that obtained from an accurate basal TSH measurement.[222] With respect to the evaluation of sick patients, while basal TSH values are on average higher than in patients with thyrotoxicosis, there is still some overlap between these groups.[141,170,223] This indicates that even with second or third generation TSH assays, it may not be possible to establish that thyrotoxicosis is present based on a serum TSH measurement in a population which includes severely ill patients.

An abnormal relationship between the basal TSH and the TRH-response is found in patients with central hypothyroidism. Here the fold TSH response to TRH is lower than normal.[16,141,224] Again, however, TRH testing does not add substantially to the evaluation of such patients in that the diagnosis of central hypothyroidism is established by finding a normal or slightly elevated basal TSH in the presence of a significantly reduced free T$_4$ concentration. While statistically lower and sometimes delayed increments in TSH release after TRH infusion are found in patients with pituitary as opposed to hypothalamic hypothyroidism, the overlap in the TSH increments found in patients with these two conditions is sufficiently large that other diagnostic technologies, such as MRI, must be used to provide definitive localization of the lesion in patients with central hypothyroidism.[16,17,224]

One may conclude from these results that the TRH test is primarily of historical and physiological interest and for use by clinicians who do not have access to sensitive TSH assays. Provocative testing with TRH may still be useful in the follow-up of patient's with Cushings' disease, acromegaly, or in the post-operative evaluation of patients with TSH-producing pituitary tumors.

CLINICAL APPLICATION OF TSH MEASUREMENTS AND SUMMARY

Table 4-3 lists conditions in which basal TSH values may be altered as practical examples of the pathophysiology of the hypothalamic-pituitary thyroid

TABLE 4-3. Conditions Which May Be Associated with Abnormal Serum TSH Concentrations

	Expected TSH (μU/ml)	Thyroid Status	Free T$_4$ Index
TSH reduced			
1. Hyperthyroidism	<0.1	↑	↑, T$_3$↑
2. "Euthyroid" Graves' disease	0.2–0.5	N(↑)	N(T$_3$↑)
3. Autonomous nodules	0.2–0.5	N(↑)	N(T$_3$↑)
4. Excess thyroid hormone treatment	0.1–0.5	N, ↑	N, ↑
5. Thyroiditis	0.1–0.5	N, ↑	N, ↑
6. Illness with or without dopamine	0.1–5.0	N	↑, N, ↓
7. First trimester pregnancy	0.2–0.5	N(↑)	N(↑)
8. Hyperemesis gravidarum	0.2–0.5	N(↑)	↑(N)
9. Hydatidiform mole	0.1–0.4	↑	↑
10. Acute psychosis or depression (rare)	0.4–10	N	N(↑)
11. Elderly (small fraction)	0.2–0.5	N	N
12. Glucocortoids (inconsistent)	0.1–0.5	N	N
13. Congenital TSH deficiency			
a.) PIT1 + 1 Deficiency	0	↓	↓
b.) CAGYC mutant	0	↓	↓
TSH elevated			
1. Primary hypothyroidism	6–500	↓	↓
2. Recovery from severe illness	5–30	N	N, ↓
3. Iodine deficiency	6–150	N, ↓	↓
4. Thyroid hormone resistance	1–15	↑	↑
5. Thyrotroph tumor	3–15	↑	↑
6. Hypothalamic-pituitary dysfunction	1–20	↓	↓
7. Psychiatric illness (especially bipolar disorder)	0.4–10	N	N
8. Test artifact (endogenous anti-mouse γ globulin antibodies)	19–500	N	N
9. Addison's disease	5–30	N	N

axis. This subject is also discussed in Chapter 6 from the standpoint of clinical diagnosis. This section also serves as a summary of the clinically relevant points in this chapter.

Clinical Situations Associated with Subnormal TSH Values

The most common cause of a reduced TSH in a non-hospitalized patient is thyroid hormone excess. This may be due to endogenous hyperthyroidism or excess exogenous thyroid hormone. The degree of suppression of basal TSH is in proportion to the degree and duration of the excess thyroid hormone. The reduced TSH is the pathophysiological manifestation of the activation of the negative feedback loop.

While a low TSH in the presence of elevated thyroid hormones is logical, it results from multiple causes. Prolonged excessive thyroid hormone causes physiological "atrophy" of the thyroid stimulatory limb of the hypothalamic-pituitary thyroid axis. Thus, TRH synthesis is reduced, TRH mRNA in the PVN is absent, TRH receptors in the thyrotroph may

be reduced; and the concentration of TSH β and α subunits and both mRNAs in the thyrotroph are virtually undetectable. Therefore, it is not surprising that several months are usually required for the re-establishment of TSH secretion after the relief of thyrotoxicosis. This is especially well seen in patients with Graves' disease after surgery or radioactive iodine, in whom TSH remains suppressed despite a rapid return to a euthyroid or even hypothyroid functional status.[225,226] Since TRH infusion will not increase TSH release in this situation, it is clear that the thyrotroph is transiently dysfunctional.[227] A similar phenomenon occurs after excess thyroid hormone treatment is terminated, and after the transient hyperthyroidism associated with thyroiditis, though the period of suppression is shorter under the latter circumstances.[228] This cause of reduced circulating thyroid hormones and reduced or normal TSH should be distinguishable from central hypothyroidism by the history.

Severe illness is a common cause of TSH suppression although it is not often confused with thyrotoxicosis. Quantitation of thyroid hormones will generally resolve the issue.[168] Patients receiving high-dose glucocorticoids acutely may also have suppressed TSH values although chronic glucocorticoid therapy does not cause sufficient TSH suppression to produce hypothalamic-pituitary hypothyroidism (see above).

Exogenous dopamine suppresses TSH release. Infusion of 5 to 7.5 μg/kg/min to normal volunteers causes an approximately 50 percent reduction in the concentrations of TSH and consequent small decreases in serum T_4 and T_3 concentrations.[196] In critically ill patients, this effect of dopamine can be superimposed on the suppressive effects of acute illness on thyroid function, reducing T_4 production to even lower levels. Dopamine is sufficiently potent to suppress TSH to normal levels in sick patients with primary hypothyroidism.[196] This needs to be kept in mind when evaluating severely ill patients for this condition. Dopamine antagonists such as metoclopramide or domperidone cause a small increase in TSH in humans. However, somewhat surprisingly, patients receiving the dopamine agonist, bromergocryptine, do not become hypothyroid. Although dopa causes a statistically significant reduction in the TSH response to TRH, patients receiving this drug also remain euthyroid.

The capacity of hCG to function as a thyroid stimulator is discussed in Chapter 14. This may be manifested in patients with normal pregnancy as a slightly subnormal TSH during the first trimester (0.2 to 0.4 mU/L) or by frank, though mild, hyperthyroidism in patients with choriocarcinoma or molar pregnancy.[229]

Patients with acute psychosis or depression and those with agitated psychoses may have high thyroid hormone levels and suppressed or elevated TSH values. The etiology of the alterations in TSH are not known. Those receiving lithium for bipolar illness may also have elevated TSH values due to impairment of thyroid hormone release. Patients with underlying autoimmune thyroid disease or multi-nodular goiter are especially susceptible.[230] A small fraction of elderly patients, particularly males, have subnormal TSH levels with normal serum thyroid hormone concentrations. It is likely that this reflects mild thyrotoxicosis if it is found to be reduced on repeated determinations.

Causes of an Elevated TSH

Primary hypothyroidism is the most common cause of an elevated serum TSH. The serum free T_4 is low normal or reduced in such patients but the serum free T_3 values remain normal until the level of thyroid function has markedly deteriorated.[75] Another common cause of an elevated TSH in an iodine-sufficient environment is the transient elevation which occurs during the recovery phase after a severe illness.[178,179] In such patients a "reawakening" of the hypothalamic-pituitary thyroid axis occurs pari passu with the improvement in their clinical state. In general, such patients do not have underlying thyroid dysfunction. Iodine deficiency is not a cause of elevated TSH in Central and North America but may be in certain areas of Western Europe, South America, Africa, and Asia.

The remainder of the conditions associated with an elevated TSH are extremely rare. In a patient who has an elevated free T_4 index, the presence of TSH at normal or increased levels should lead to a search for either resistance to thyroid hormone or a thyrotroph tumor. Hypothalamic-pituitary dysfunction may be associated with normal or even modest increases in TSH are explained by the lack of normal TSH glycosylation in the TRH-deficient patient. The diagnosis is generally made by finding a serum free T_4 index which is reduced to a greater extent than expected from the coincident serum TSH. Psychiatric illness may be associated with either elevated or suppressed TSH, but the abnormal values are not usually in the range normally associated with symptomatic thyroid dysfunction. The effect of glucocorticoids to suppress TSH secretion has already been mentioned. This is of relevance in patients with Addison's disease in whom TSH may be slightly elevated in the absence of primary thyroid disease.

Lastly, while most of the artifacts have been eliminated from the immunometric TSH assays, there remains the theoretical possibility of an elevated value due to the presence of endogenous antimouse gamma globulin antibodies.[231] These antibodies, like TSH, can complex the two TSH antibodies resulting in artificially elevated serum TSH assay results in euthyroid patients. Such artifacts can usually be identified by finding non-linear results upon assay of serial dilutions of the suspect serum with that from patients with a suppressed TSH.

REFERENCES

1. Shupnik MA, Ridgway EC, Chin WW: Molecular biology of thyrotropin. Endocr Rev 10:459, 1989
2. Naylor SL, Chin WW, Goodman HM et al: Chromo-

some assignment of genes encoding the alpha and beta subunits of glycoprotein hormones in man and mouse. Somatic Cell Mol Genet 9:757, 1983

3. Chin WW, Carr FE, Burnside J, Darling DS: Thyroid hormone regulation of thyrotropin gene expression. Recent Prog Horm Res 48:393, 1993

4. Cacicedo L, Pohl SL, Reichlin S: Effects of thyroid hormones and thyrotropin-releasing hormone on thyrotropin biosynthesis by mouse pituitary tumor cells in vitro. Endocrinology 108:1012, 1981

5. Gershengorn MC: Regulation of thyrotropin production by mouse pituitary thyrotropic tumor cells in vitro by physiologic levels of thyroid hormones. Endocrinology 102:1128, 1978

6. Alexander LM, Gordon DF, Wood WM et al: Identification of thyrotroph-specific factors and *cis*-acting sequences of the murine thyrotropin β subunit gene. Mol Endocrinol 3:1037, 1989

7. Berry MJ, Banu L, Chen Y et al: Recognition of UGA as a selenocysteine codon in type I deiodinase requires sequences in the 3' untranslated region. Nature 353:273, 1991

8. Magner JA: Thyroid-stimulating hormone: biosynthesis, cell biology, and bioactivity. Endocr Rev 11:354, 1990

9. Weintraub BD, Strannard BS, Magner JA et al: Glycosylation and posttranslation processing of thyroid-stimulating hormone: clinical implications. Recent Prog Horm Res 41:577, 1985

10. Weintraub BD, Stannard BS, Linnekin D, Marshall M: Relationship of glycosylation to de novo thyroid-stimulating hormone biosynthesis and secretion by mouse pituitary tumor cells. J Biol Chem 255:5715, 1980

11. Amir SM, Kubota K, Tramontano D et al: The carbohydrate moiety of bovine thyrotropin is essential for full bioactivity but not for receptor recognition. Endocrinology 120:345, 1987

12. Amir S, Menezes-Ferreira MM, Shimohigashi Y et al: Activities of deglycosylated thyrotropin at the thyroid membrane receptor-adenylate cyclase system. J Endocrinol Invest 8:537, 1986

13. Gesundheit N, Fink DL, Silverman LA, Weintraub BD: Effect of thyrotropin-releasing hormone on the carbohydrate structure of secreted mouse thyrotropin: analysis by lectin affinity chromatography. J Biol Chem 262:5197, 1987

14. Taylor R, Weintraub BD: Altered thyrotropin (TSH) carbohydrate structures in hypothalamic hypothyroidism created by paraventricular nuclear lesions are corrected by in vivo TSH-releasing hormone administration. Endocrinology 125:2198, 1989

15. Menezes-Ferreira MM, Petrick PA, Weintraub BD: Regulation of thyrotropin (TSH) bioactivity by TSH-releasing hormone and thyroid hormone. Endocrinology 118:2125, 1986

16. Faglia G, Bitensky L, Pinchera A et al: Thyrotropin secretion in patients with central hypothyroidism: evidence for reduced biologic activity of immunoreactive thyrotropin. J Clin Endocrinol Metab 48:989, 1979

17. Petersen VB, McGregor AM, Belchetz PE et al: The secretion of thyrotrophin with impaired biologic activity in patients with hypothalamic-pituitary disease. Clin Endocrinol 8:397, 1978

18. Beck-Peccoz P, Amir S, Menezes-Ferreira MM et al: Decreased receptor binding of biologically inactive thyrotropin in central hypothyroidism: effect of treatment with thyrotropin-releasing hormone. N Engl J Med 312:1085, 1985

19. Hayashizaki Y, Hiraoka Y, Endo Y, Matsubara K: Thyroid-stimulating hormone (TSH) deficiency caused by a single base substitution in the CAGYC region of the β-subunit. EMBO J 8:2291, 1989

20. Hayashizaki Y, Hiraoka Y, Tatsumi K: Deoxyribonucleic acid analyses of five families with familial inherited thyroid-stimulating hormone deficiency. J Clin Endocrinol Metab 71:792, 1990

21. Reichlin S, Utiger RD: Regulation of the pituitary-thyroid axis in man: relationship of TSH concentration to concentration of free and total thyroxine in plasma. J Clin Endocrinol Metab 27:251, 1967

22. Shupnik MA, Ridgway EC: Thyroid hormone control of thyrotropin gene expression in rat anterior pituitary cells. Endocrinology 121:619, 1987

23. Kourides IA, Gurr JA, Wolf O: The regulation and organization of thyroid-stimulating hormone genes. Recent Prog Horm Res 40:79, 1984

24. Carr FE, Burnside J, Chin WW: Thyroid hormones regulate rat thyrotropin β gene promoter activity expressed in GH$_3$ cells. Mol Endocrinol 3:709, 1989

25. Carr FE, Ridgway EC, Chin WW: Rapid simultaneous measurement of rat α and thyrotropin (TSH) β-subunit messenger ribonucleic acids (mRNAs) by solution hybridization: regulation of TSH subunit mRNAs by thyroid hormones. Endocrinology 117:1272, 1985

26. Gurr JA, Januszeski MM, Tidikis IM et al: Thyroid hormone regulates expression of the thyrotropin β subunit gene from both transcription start sites in the mouse and rat. Mol Cell Endocrinol 71:185, 1990

27. Gurr JA, Kourides IA: Regulation of thyrotropin biosynthesis: discordant effect of thyroid hormone on α and β subunit mRNA levels. J Biol Chem 258:10208, 1983

28. Chatterjee VKK, Lee JK, Rentoumis A, Jameson JL: Negative regulation of the thyroid-stimulating hormone α gene by thyroid hormone: receptor interac-

tion adjacent to the TATA box. Proc Natl Acad Sci USA 86:9114, 1989

29. Wondisford FE, Farr EA, Radovick S: Thyroid hormone inhibition of human thyrotropin β-subunit gene expression is mediated by a *cis*-acting element located in the first exon. J Biol Chem 264:14601, 1989

30. Wondisford FE, Radovick S, Moates JM et al: Isolation and characterization of the human thyrotropin β subunit gene: differences in gene structure and promoter function from murine species. J Biol Chem 263:12538, 1988

31. Bodenner DL, Mroczynski MA, Weintraub BD et al: A detailed functional and structural analysis of a major thyroid hormone inhibitory element in the human thyrotropin β subunit gene. J Biol Chem 266: 21666, 1991

32. Darling DS, Burnside J, Chin WW: Binding of thyroid hormone receptors to the rat thyrotropin β gene. Mol Endocrinol 3:1359, 1989

33. Brent GA, Williams GR, Harney JW et al: Effects of varying the position of thyroid hormone response elements within the rat growth hormone promoter: implications for positive and negative regulation by 3,5,3'-triiodothyronine. Mol Endocrinol 5:542, 1991

34. Burnside J, Darling DS, Carr FE, Chin WW: Thyroid hormone regulation of the rat glycoprotein hormone α subunit gene promoter activity. J Biol Chem 264: 6886, 1989

35. Shupnik MA, Ardisson LJ, Meskell MJ et al: Triiodothyronine (T_3) regulation of thyrotropin subunit gene transcription is proportional to T_3 nuclear receptor occupancy. Endocrinology 118:367, 1986

36. Zenke M, Munoz A, Sap J et al: v-erbA oncogene activation entails the loss of hormone-dependent regulator activity of c-erbA. Cell 61:1035, 1990

37. Morita S, Fernandez-Mejia C, Melmed S: Retinoic acid selectively stimulates growth hormone secretion and messenger ribonucleic acid levels in rat pituitary cells. Endocrinology 124:2052, 1989

38. Wondisford FE, Steinfelder H, Nations M, Radovick S: AP-1 antagonizes thyroid hormone receptor action on the thyrotropin β-subunit gene. J Biol Chem 268:2749, 1993

39. Koenig RJ, Watson AY: Enrichment of rat anterior pituitary cell types by metrizamide density-gradient centrifugation. Endocrinology 115:314, 1984

40. Farquhar MG, Rinehart JF: Cytologic alterations in the anterior pituitary gland following thyroidectomy: an electron microscope study. Endocrinology 55:857, 1954

41. Martin JB, Boshans R, Reichlin S: Feedback regulation of TSH secretion in rats with hypothalamic lesions. Endocrinology 87:1032, 1970

42. Silva JE, Larsen PR: Pituitary nuclear 3,5,3'-triiodothyronine and thyrotropin secretion: an explanation for the effect of thyroxine. Science 198:617, 1977

43. Larsen PR, Silva JE, Kaplan MM: Relationships between circulating and intracellular thyroid hormones: physiologic and clinical implications. Endocr Rev 2:87, 1981

44. Spira O, Birkenfeld A, Avni A, et al: TSH synthesis and release in the thyroidectomized rat: effect of T_3. Acta Endocrinol 92:502, 1979

45. Franklyn JA, Wood DF, Balfour NJ, Sheppard MC: Effect of triiodothyronine on thyrotropin β- and α messenger RNAs in the pituitary of the euthyroid rat. Mol Cell Endocrinol 60:1, 1988

46. Franklyn JA, Wood DF, Balfour NJ et al: Effect of hypothyroidism and thyroid hormone replacement in vivo on pituitary cytoplasmic concentrations of thyrotropin β- and α subunit mRNAs. Endocrinology 120:2279, 1987

47. Shupnik MA, Chin WW, Habener JF, Ridgway EC: Transcriptional regulation of the thyrotropin subunit genes by thyroid hormone. J Biol Chem 260: 2900, 1985

48. Chin WW, Shupnik MA, Ross DS et al: Regulation of the α- and thyrotropin β subunit messenger ribonucleic acids by thyroid hormones. Endocrinology 116:873, 1985

49. Silva JE, Larsen PR: Peripheral metabolism of homologous thyrotropin in euthyroid and hypothyroid rats: acute effects of thyrotropin-releasing hormone, triiodothyronine, and thyroxine. Endocrinology 102:1783, 1978

50. Vale W, Burgus R, Guillemin R: On the mechanism of action of TRF: effects of cycloheximide and actinomycin on the release of TSH stimulated in vitro by TRF and its inhibition by thyroxine. Neuroendocrinology 3:34, 1968

51. Bowers CY, Lee KL, Schally AV: A study on the interaction of the thyrotropin-releasing factor and L-triiodothyronine: effects of puromycin and cycloheximide. Endocrinology 82:75, 1968

52. Gard TG, Bernstein B, Larsen PR: Studies on the mechanism of 3,5,3'-triiodothyronine-induced suppression of secretagogue-induced thyrotropin release in vitro. Endocrinology 1:44, 1981

53. Koenig RJ, Senator D, Larsen PR: Phorbol esters as probes of the regulation of thyrotropin secretion. Biochem Biophys Res Comm 125:353, 1984

54. Schrey MP, Larsen PR: Evidence for a possible role of Ca^{2+} in the 3,3,3'-triiodothyronine inhibition of thyrotropin-releasing hormone-induced secretion of thyrotropin by rat anterior pituitary in vitro. Endocrinology 108:1690, 1981

55. Silva JE, Larsen PR: Contributions of plasma triiodo-

thyronine and local thyroxine monodeiodination to triiodothyronine to nuclear triiodothyronine receptor saturation in pituitary, liver, and kidney of hypothyroid rats: further evidence relating saturation of pituitary nuclear triiodothyronine receptors and the acute inhibition of thyroid-stimulating hormone release. J Clin Invest 61:1247, 1978

56. Larsen PR, Dick TE, Markovitz MM et al: Inhibition of intrapituitary thyroxine to 3,5,3'-triiodothyronine conversion prevents the acute suppression of thyrotropin release by thyroxine in hypothyroid rats. J Clin Invest 64:117, 1979

57. Obregon MJ, Pascual A, Mallol J et al: Evidence against a major role of L-thyroxine at the pituitary level: studies in rats treated with iopanoic acid (Telepaque). Endocrinology 106:1827, 1980

58. Lueprasitsakul W, Alex S, Fang SL et al: Flavonoid administration immediately displaces thyroxine (T₄) from serum transthyretin, increases serum-free T₄, and decreases thyrotropin in the rat. Endocrinology 126:2890, 1990

59. Silva JE, Dick TE, Larsen PR: Contribution of local tissue thyroxine monodeiodination to the nuclear 3,5,3'-triiodothyronine in pituitary, liver, and kidney of euthyroid rats. Endocrinology 103:1196, 1978

60. Larsen PR: Thyroid-pituitary interactions: feedback regulation of thyrotropin secretion by thyroid hormones. N Engl J Med 306:23, 1982

61. Larsen PR, Bavli SZ, Castonguay M, Jove R: Direct radioimmunoassay of nuclear 3,5,3'-triiodothyronine in rat anterior pituitary. J Clin Invest 65:675, 1980

62. Saberi M, Utiger RD: Augmentation of thyrotropin responses to thyrotropin-releasing hormone following small decreases in serum thyroid-hormone concentrations. J Clin Endocrinol Metab 40:435, 1975

63. Geffner DL, Azukizawa M, Hershman JM: Propylthiouracil blocks extrathyroidal conversion of thyroxine to triiodothyronine and augments thyrotropin secretion in man. J Clin Invest 55:224, 1975

64. Larsen PR, Frumess RD: Comparison of the biologic effects of thyroxine and triiodothyronine in the rat. Endocrinology 100:980, 1977

65. Connors JM, Hedge GA: Feedback effectiveness of periodic versus constant triiodothyronine replacement. Endocrinology 106:911, 1980

66. Connors JM, Hedge GA: Feedback regulation of thyrotropin by thyroxine under physiological conditions. Am J Physiol 240:E308, 1981

67. Suzuki H, Kadena N, Takeuchi K, Nakagawa S: Effects of three-day oral cholecystography on serum iodothyronines and TSH concentrations: comparison of the effects among some cholecystographic agents and the effects of iopanoic acid on the pituitary-thyroid axis. Acta Endocrinol 92:477, 1979

68. Suzuki H, Noguchi K, Nakahata M et al: Effect of iopanic acid on the pituitary-thyroid axis: time sequence of changes in serum iodothyronines, thyrotropin, and prolactin concentrations and responses to thyroid hormones. J Clin Endocrinol Metab 53:779, 1981

69. Abrams GM, Larsen PR: Triiodothyronine and thyroxine in the serum and thyroid glands of iodine-deficient rats. J Clin Invest 52:2522, 1973

70. Fukuda H, Yasuda N, Greer MA et al: Changes in plasma thyroxine, triiodothyronine, and TSH during adaptation to iodine deficiency in the rat. Endocrinology 97:307, 1975

71. Riesco G, Taurog A, Larsen PR, Krulich L: Acute and chronic responses to iodine deficiency in rats. Endocrinology 100:303, 1977

72. Patel YC, Pharoah POD, Hornabrook RW, Hetzel BS: Serum triiodothyronine, thyroxine, and thyroid-stimulating hormone in endemic goiter: a comparison of goitrous and nongoitrous subjects in New Guinea. J Clin Endocrinol Metab 37:783, 1973

73. Chopra IJ, Hershman JM, Hornabrook RW: Serum thyroid hormone and thyrotropin levels in subjects from endemic goiter regions of New Guinea. J Clin Endocrinol Metab 40:326, 1975

74. Wennlund A: Variation in serum levels of T₃, T₄, FT₄, and TSH during thyroxine replacement therapy. Acta Endocrinol 113:47, 1986

75. Bigos ST, Ridgway EC, Kourides IA, Maloof F: Spectrum of pituitary alterations with mild and severe thyroid impairment. J Clin Endocrinol Metab 46:317, 1978

76. Jackson I: Thyrotropin-releasing hormone. N Engl J Med 306:145, 1982

77. Richter K, Kawashima E, Egger R, Kreil G: Biosynthesis of thyrotropin-releasing hormone in the skin of *Xenopus laevis*: partial sequence of the precursor deduced from cloned cDNA. EMBO J 3:617, 1984

78. Lechan RM, Wu P, Jackson IMD et al: Thyrotropin-releasing hormone precursor: characterization in rat brain. Science 231:159, 1986

79. Yamada M, Wondisford FE, Radovick S et al: Assignment of human preprothyrotropin-releasing hormone (TRH) gene to chromosome 3. Som Cell Mol Gen 17:97, 1991

80. Engler D, Scanlon M, Jackson IMD: Thyrotropin-releasing hormone in the systemic circulation of the neonatal rat is derived from the pancreas and other extraneural tissues. J Clin Invest 67:800, 1981

81. Leduque P, Wolf B, Aratan-Spire S et al: Immunocyto-chemical localization of thyrotropin-releasing hormone (TRH) in the β-cells of adult hypothyroid pancreas. Reg Peptides 10:281, 1985

82. Gkonos PJ, Tavianini MA, Liu CC, Roos BA: Thyro-

tropin-releasing hormone gene expression in normal thyroid parafollicular cells. Mol Endocrinol 3: 2101, 1989

83. Jeffcoate SL, White N, Hokfelt T et al: Localization of thyrotropin-releasing hormone in the spinal cord of the rat by immunohistochemistry and radioimmunoassay. J Endocrinol 69:9P, 1976

84. Lee SL, Stewart K, Goodman RH: Structure of the gene encoding rat thyrotropin-releasing hormone. J Biol Chem 263:16604, 1988

85. Yamada M, Radovick S, Wondisford FE et al: Cloning and structure of human genomic DNA and hypothalamic cDNA encoding human preprothyrotropin-releasing hormone. Mol Endocrinol 4:551, 1990

86. Bulant M, Roussel JP, Astier H et al: Processing of thyrotropin-releasing hormone prohormone (pro-TRH) generates a biologically active peptide, pre-pro-TRH-(160-169), which regulates TRH-induced thyrotropin secretion. Proc Natl Acad Sci USA 87: 4439, 1990

87. Arimura A, Schally AV: Increase in basal and thyrotropin-releasing hormone-stimulated secretion of thyrotropin by passive immunization with antiserum to somatostatin. Endocrinology 98:1069, 1976

88. Segerson TP, Kauer J, Wolfe H et al: Thyroid hormone regulates TRH biosynthesis in the paraventricular nucleus of the rat hypothalamus. Science 238: 78, 1987

89. Dyess EM, Segerson TP, Liposits Z et al: Triiodothyronine exerts direct cell-specific regulation of thyrotropin-releasing hormone gene expression in the hypothalamic paraventricular nucleus. Endocrinology 123:2291, 1988

90. Kakucska I, Rand W, Lechan RM: Thyrotropin-releasing hormone (TRH) gene expression in the hypothalamic paraventricular nucleus is dependent upon feedback regulation by both triiodothyronine and thyroxine. Endocrinology 130:2845, 1992

91. Koller KJ, Wolff RS, Warden MK, Zoeller RT: Thyroid hormones regulate levels of thyrotropin-releasing hormone mRNA in the paraventricular nucleus. Proc Natl Acad Sci USA 84:7329, 1987

92. Strait KA, Zou L, Oppenheimer JH: $\beta 1$ isoform-specific regulation of a triiodothyronine-induced gene during cerebellar development. Mol Endocrinol 6: 1874, 1992

93. Belchetz PE, Gredley G, Bird D, Himsworth RL: Regulation of thyrotropin secretion by negative feedback of triiodothyronine on the hypothalamus. J Endocrinol 76:439, 1978

94. Riskind PN, Kolodny JM, Larsen PR: The regional hypothalamic distribution of type II 5′-monodeiodinase in euthyroid and hypothyroid rats. Brain Res 420:194, 1987

95. Dratman MB, Crutchfield FL: Synaptosomal [^{125}I]triiodothyronine after intravenous [^{125}]thyroxine. Am J Physiol 235:E638, 1978

96. Straub RE, Frech GC, Joho RH, Gershengorn MC: Expression cloning of a cDNA encoding the mouse pituitary thyrotropin-releasing hormone receptor. Proc Natl Acad Sci USA 87:9514, 1990

97. Zhao D, Yang J, Jones KE et al: Molecular cloning of a complementary deoxyribonucleic acid encoding the thyrotropin-releasing hormone receptor and regulation of its messenger ribonucleic acid in rat GH cells. Endocrinology 130:3529, 1992

98. Gershengorn MC: Biohormonal regulation of the thyrotropin-releasing hormone receptor in mouse pituitary thyrotropic tumor cells in culture. J Clin Invest 62:937, 1978

99. Fujimoto J, Gershengorn MC: Evidence for dual regulation by protein kinases A and C of thyrotropin-releasing hormone receptor mRNA in GH$_3$ cells. Endocrinology 129:3430, 1991

100. Brenner-Gati L, Gershengorn MC: Effects of thyrotropin-releasing hormone on phosphoinositides and cytoplasmic free calcium in thyrotropic pituitary cells. Endocrinology 118:163, 1986

101. Oron Y, Gillo B, Straub RE, Gershengorn MC: Mechanism of membrane electrical response to thyrotropin-releasing hormone in *Xenopus* oocytes injected with GH$_3$ pituitary cell messenger ribonucleic acid. Mol Endocrinol 1:918, 1987

102. Gershengorn MC, Thaw C: TRH stimulates biphasic elevation of cytoplasmic free calcium in GH$_3$ cells: further evidence that TRH mobilizes cellular and extracellular Ca^{2+}. Endocrinology 116:591, 1985

103. Martin TJF: Thyrotropin-releasing hormone rapidly activates the phosphodiester hydrolysis of polyphosphoinositides in GH$_3$ pituitary cells: evidence for the role of a polyphosphoinositide-specific phospholipase C in hormone action. J Biol Chem 258:14816, 1983

104. Recbecchi MJ, Gershengorn MC: Thyroliberin stimulates rapid hydrolysis of phosphatidylinositol 4, 5-bisphosphate by a phosphodiesterase in rat mammotropic pituitary cells. Biochem J 216:287, 1983

105. Gershengorn MC, Rebecchi MJ, Geras E, Areval CO: Thyrotropin-releasing hormone (TRH) action in mouse thyrotropic tumor cells in culture: evidence against a role for adenosine 3′,5′-monophosphate as a mediator of TRH-stimulated thyrotropin release. Endocrinology 256:153, 1980

106. Gershengorn MC: Thyrotropin-releasing hormone action: mechanism of calcium-mediated stimulation of prolactin secretion. Recent Prog Horm Res 116: 591, 1985

107. Geras E, Rebecchi MJ, Gershengorn MC: Evidence

that stimulation of thyrotropin and prolactin secretion by thyrotropin-releasing hormone occur via different calcium-mediated mechanisms: studies with verapamil. Endocrinology 110:901, 1982

108. Carr FE, Shupnik MA, Burnside J, Chin WW: Thyrotropin-releasing hormone stimulates the activity of the rat thyrotropin β subunit gene promoter transfected into pituitary cells. Mol Endocrinol 3:717, 1989

109. Carr FE, Galloway RJ, Reid AH et al: Thyrotropin-releasing hormone regulation of thyrotropin β-subunit gene expression involves intracellular calcium and protein kinase C. Biochemistry 30:3721, 1991

110. Comi RJ, Gesundheit N, Murray L: Response of thyrotropin-secreting pituitary adenomas to a long-acting somatostatin analogue. N Engl J Med 317:12, 1987

111. Beck-Peccoz P, Mariotti S, Guillausseau PJ: Treatment of hyperthyroidism due to inappropriate secretion of thyrotropin with somatostatin analogue SMS 201-995. J Clin Endocrinol Metab 68:208, 1989

112. Berelowitz M, Maeda K, Harris S, Frohman LA: The effect of alterations in the pituitary-thyroid axis on hypothalamic content and in vitro release of somatostatin-like immunoreactivity. Endocrinology 107:24, 1980

113. Weeke J, Hansen AAP, Lundbaek K: Inhibition by somatostatin of basal levels of serum thyrotropin (TSH) in normal men. J Clin Endocrinol Metab 41:168, 1975

114. Weeke J, Christensen SE, Hansen AP et al: Somatostatin and the 24th levels of serum TSH, T_3, T_4, and reverse T_3 in normals, diabetics, and patients treated for myxedema. Acta Endocrinol 94:30, 1980

115. Spaulding SW, Burrow GN, Donabedian R, Van Woert M: L-dopa suppression of thyrotropin-releasing hormone response in man. J Clin Endocrinol Metab 35:182, 1972

116. Besses GS, Burrow GN, Spaulding SW, Donabedian RK: Dopamine infusion acutely inhibits the TSH and prolactin response to TRH. J Clin Endocrinol Metab 41:985, 1975

117. Leebaw WF, Lee LA, Woolf PD: Dopamine affects basal and augumented pituitary hormone secretion. J Clin Endocrinol Metab 47:480, 1978

118. Miyai K, Yamamoto T, Azukizawa M et al: Inhibition of thyrotropin and prolactin secretions in primary hypothyroidism by 2-Br-α-ergocryptine. J Clin Endocrinol Metab 40:334, 1974

119. Pourmand M, Rodriguez-Arnao MD, Weightman DR et al: A novel agent for the investigation of anterior pituitary function and control in man. Clin Endocrinol 12:211, 1980

120. Krulich L, Giachetti A, Marchlewska KOJ: On the role of the central noradrenergic and dopaminergic systems in the regulation of TSH secretion in the rat. Endocrinology 100:496, 1977

121. Krulich L, Mayfield A, Steele MK et al: Differential effects of pharmacological manipulations of central $\alpha 1$- and $\alpha 2$-adrenergic receptors on the secretion of thyrotropin and growth hormone in male rats. Endocrinology 110:796, 1982

122. Dieguez C, Foord SM, Peters JR et al: $\alpha 1$ adrenoreceptors and $\alpha 1$-adrenoreceptor-mediated thyrotropin release in cultures of euthyroid and hypothyroid rat anterior pituitary cells. Endocrinology 117:624, 1985

123. Ozawa M, Sato K, Han DC et al: Effects of tumor necrosis factor-α/cachectin on thyroid hormone metabolism in mice. Endocrinology 123:1461, 1988

124. Pang XP, Hershman JM, Mirell CJ, Pekary AE: Impairment of hypothalamic-pituitary-thyroid function in rats treated with human recombinant tumor necrosis factor-α (cachectin). Endocrinology 125:76, 1989

125. Dubuis JM, Dayer JM, Siegrist-Kaiser CA, Burger AG: Human recombinant interleukin-1β decreases plasma thyroid hormone and thyroid-stimulating hormone levels in rats. Endocrinology 123:2175, 1988

126. Van der Poll T, Romijn JA, Wiersinga WM, Sauerwein HP: Tumor necrosis factor: a putative mediator of the sick euthyroid syndrome in man. J Clin Endocrinol Metab 71:1567, 1990

127. Koenig JI, Snow K, Clark BD et al: Intrinsic pituitary interleukin-1 beta is induced by bacterial lipopolysaccharide. Endocrinology 126:3053, 1990

128. van Haasteren GA, van der Meer MJ, Hermus AR et al: Different effects of continuous infusion of interleukin-1 and interleukin-6 on the hypothalamic-hypophysial-thyroid axis. Endocrinology 135:1336, 1994

129. Kourides IA, Ridgway EC, Weintraub BD et al: Thyrotropin-induced hyperthyroidism: use of alpha and beta subunit levels to identify patients with pituitary tumors. J Clin Endocrinol Metab 45:534, 1977

130. Kuzuya N, Kinji I, Ishibashi M: Endocrine and immunohistochemical studies on thyrotropin (TSH)-secreting pituitary adenomas: responses of TSH, α-subunit, and growth hormone to hypothalamic-releasing hormones and their distribution in adenoma cells. J Clin Endocrinol Metab 71:1103, 1990

131. Gesundheit N, Petrick PA, Nissim M et al: Thyrotropin-secreting pituitary adenomas: clinical and biochemical heterogeneity. Ann Intern Med 11:827, 1989

132. Faglia G, Beck-Peccoz P, Piscitelli G, Medri G: Inappropriate secretion of thyrotropin by the pituitary. Horm Res 26:79, 1987

133. Oppenheim DS, Kana AR, Sangha JS, Klibanski A: Prevalence of α-subunit hypersecretion in patients with pituitary tumors: clinically non-functioning and somatotroph adenomas. J Clin Endocrinol Metab 70:859, 1990

134. Fiskin RA, Walker BA, Buxton PH: A pituitary thyrotropinoma causing thyrotoxicosis and amenorrhoea/galactorrhoea: studies of α subunit in the tumor and in blood. J R Soc Med 82:298, 1989

135. Beck-Peccoz P, Piscitelli G, Amir S: Endocrine, biochemical, and morphological studies of a pituitary adenoma secreting growth hormone, thyrotropin (TSH), and α-subunit: evidence for secretion of TSH with increased bioactivity. J Clin Endocrinol Metab 62:704, 1986

136. Weintraub BD, Gershengorn MC, Kourides IA, Fein H: Inappropriate secretion of thyroid-stimulating hormone. Ann Intern Med 95:339, 1981

137. Ridgway EC, Weintraub BD, Maloof F: Metabolic clearance and production rates of human thyrotropin. J Clin Invest 53:895, 1974

138. Kourides IA, Re RN, Weintraub BD et al: Metabolic clearance and secretion rates of subunits of human thyrotropin. J Clin Invest 59:508, 1977

139. Spencer CA, Lai-Rosenfeld AO, Guttler RB et al: Thyrotropin secretion in thyrotoxic and thyroxine-treated patient: assessment by a sensitive immunoenzymometric assay. J Clin Endocrinol Metab 63:349, 1986

140. Spencer CA, LoPresti JS, Patel A et al: Applications of a new chemiluminometric thyrotropin assay to subnormal measurement. J Clin Endocrinol Metab 70:453, 1990

141. Spencer CA, Schwarzbein D, Guttler RB et al: Thyrotropin (TSH)-releasing hormone stimulation test responses employing third- and fourth generation TSH assays. J Clin Endocrinol Metab 76:494, 1993

142. Greenspan SL, Klibanski A, Schoenfeld D, Ridgway EC: Pulsatile secretion of thyrotropin in man. J Clin Endocrinol Metab 63:661, 1986

143. Brabant G, Ranft U, Ocran K et al: Thyrotropin: an episodically secreted hormone. Acta Endocrinol 112:315, 1986

144. Brabant G, Brabant A, Ranft U: Circadian and pulsatile thyrotropin secretion in euthyroid man under the influence of thyroid hormone and glucocorticoid administration. J Clin Endocrinol Metab 65:83, 1987

145. Brabant G, Frank K, Ranft U: Physiological regulation of circadian and pulsatile thyrotropin secretion in normal man and woman. J Clin Endocrinol Metab 70:403, 1990

146. Weeke J: Circadian variation of the serum thyrotropin level in normal subjects. Scand J Clin Lab Invest 32:337, 1973

147. Bartalena L, Placidi GF, Martino E et al: Nocturnal serum thyrotropin (TSH) surge and the TSH response to TSH-releasing hormone: dissociated behavior in untreated depression. J Clin Endocrinol Metab 71:650, 1990

148. Rose SR, Nisula BC: Circadian variation of thyrotropin in childhood. J Clin Endocrinol Metab 68:1086, 1989

149. Parker DC, Pekary AD, Hershman JM: Effect of normal and reversed sleep-wake cycles upon nyctohemeral rhythmicity of plasma thyrotropin: evidence suggestive of an inhibitory influence in sleep. J Clin Endocrinol Metab 43:318, 1976

150. Parker DC, Rossman LG, Pekary AE, Hershman JM: Effect of 64-hour sleep deprivation on the circadian waveform of thyrotropin (TSH): further evidence of sleep-related inhibition of TSH release. J Clin Endocrinol Metab 64:157, 1987

151. Sawin CT, Geller A, Wolf PA et al: Low serum thyrotropin concentrations as a risk factor for atrial fibrillation in older persons. N Engl J Med 331:1249, 1994

152. Balsam A, Ingbar SH: The influence of fasting, diabetes, and several pharmacologic agents of the pathways of thyroxine metabolism in rat liver. J Clin Invest 62:415, 1978

153. Balsam A, Ingbar SH: Observations on the factors that control the generation of triiodothyronine from thyroxine in rat liver and the nature of the effect induced by fasting. J Clin Invest 63:1145, 1979

154. Harris ARC, Fang SL, Hinerfeld L et al: The role of sulfhydryl groups on the impaired hepatic 3′,3,5-triiodothyronine generation from thyroxine in the hypothyroid, starved, fetal, and neonatal rodent. J Clin Invest 63:516, 1979

155. Kaplan MM: Subcellular alterations causing reduced hepatic thyroxine 5′-monodeiodinase activity in fasted rats. Endocrinology 104:58, 1979

156. Kaplan MM, Tatro JB, Breibart R, Larsen PR: Comparison of thyroxine and 3,3′,5′-triiodothyronine metabolism in rat kidney and liver homogenates. Metabolism 28:1139, 1979

157. Kinlaw WB, Schwartz HL, Oppenheimer JH: Decreased serum triiodothyronine in starving rats is due primarily to diminished thyroidal secretion of thyroxine. J Clin Invest 75:1238, 1985

158. Portnay GI, O'Brien JT, Bush J et al: The effect of starvation on the concentration and binding of thyroxine and triiodothyronine in serum and on the response to TRH. J Clin Endocrinol Metab 39:191, 1974

159. Chopra IJ, Solomon DH, Chopra U et al: Pathways of metabolism of thyroid hormones. Recent Prog Horm Res 34:521, 1978

160. Chopra IJ, Smith SR: Circulating thyroid hormones and thyrotropin in adult patients with protein-calorie malnutrition. J Clin Endocrinol Metab 40:221, 1975

161. Spaulding SW, Chopra IJ, Sherwin RS, Lyall SS: Effects of caloric restriction and dietary composition on serum T_3 and rT_3 in man. J Clin Endocrinol Metab 42:197, 1976

162. Wartofsky L, Burman KD: Alterations in thyroid function in patients with systemic illness: the "euthyroid sick syndrome." Endocr Rev 3:164, 1982

163. Wehman RE, Gregerman RI, Burns WH et al: Suppression of thyrotropin in the low-thyroxine state of severe nonthyroidal illness. N Engl J Med 312:546, 1985

164. Hugues J, Burger AG, Pekary AE, Hershman JM: Rapid adaptations of serum thyrotropin, triiodothyronine and reverse triiodothyronine levels to short term starvation and refeeding. Acta Endocrinol 105:194, 1984

165. Carlson HE, Drenick EJ, Chopra IJ, Hershman JM: Alterations in basal and TRH-stimulated serum levels in thyrotropin, prolactin, and thyroid hormones in starved obese men. J Clin Endocrinol Metab 45:707, 1977

166. Mortimer CH, Besser GM, Goldie DJ et al: The TSH, FSH, and prolactin responses to continuous infusions of TRH and the effects of oestrogen administration in normal males. Clin Endocrinol 3:97, 1974

167. Blake NG, Eckland DJ, Foster DJ, Lightman SL: Inhibition of hypothalamic thyrotropin-releasing hormone messenger ribonucleic acid during food deprivation. Endocrinology 129:2714, 1991

168. Kaplan MM, Larsen PR, Crantz FR et al: Prevalence of abnormal thyroid function test results in patients with acute medical illnesses. Am J Med 72:9, 1982

169. Romijn JA, Adriaanse R, Brabant G et al: Pulsatile secretion of thyrotropin during fasting: a decrease of thyrotropin pulse amplitude. J Clin Endocrinol Metab 70:1631, 1990

170. Ehrmann DA, Weinberg M, Sarne DH: Limitations to the use of a sensitive assay for serum thyrotropin in the assessment of thyroid status. Arch Intern Med 149:369, 1989

171. Faber J, Kirkegaard C, Rasmussen B et al: Pituitary-thyroid axis in critical illness. J Clin Endocrinol Metab 65:315, 1987

172. Hamblin PS, Dyer SA, Mohr VS et al: Relationship between thyrotropin and thyroxine changes during the recovery from severe hypothyroxinemia of critical illness. J Clin Endocrinol Metab 62:717, 1986

173. Kehlet H, Klauber PV, Weeke J: Thyrotropin, free and total triiodothyronine, and thyroxine in serum during surgery. Clin Endocrinol 10:131, 1979

174. Romijn JA, Wiersinga WM: Decreased nocturnal surge of thyrotropin in non-thyroidal illness. Journal of Clinical Endocrinology and Metabolism 70:35, 1990

175. Bartalena L, Martino E, Brandi LS: Lack of nocturnal serum thyrotropin surge after surgery. J Clin Endocrinol Metab 70:293, 1990

176. Custro N, Scafidi V, Gallo S, Notarbartolo A: Deficient pulsatile thyrotropin secretion in the low thyroid hormone state of severe non-thyroidal illness. Eur J Endocrinol 130:132, 1994

177. Maturlo SJ, Rosenbaum RL, Pan C, Surks MI: Variable thyrotropin response to thyrotropin-releasing hormone after small decreases in plasma free thyroid hormone concentrations in patients with non-thyroidal diseases. J Clin Invest 66:451, 1980

178. Bacci V, Schussler GC, Kaplan TB: The relationship between serum triiodothyronine and thyrotropin during systemic illness. J Clin Endocrinol Metab 54:1229, 1982

179. Brent GA, Hershman JM, Braunstein GD: Patients with severe nonthyroidal illness and serum thyrotropin concentrations in the hypothyroid range. Am J Med 81:463, 1986

180. Loosen PT, Prange AJ: Serum thyrotropin response to thyrotropin-releasing hormone in psychiatric patients. Am J Psychiatry 139:405, 1982

181. Kirkegaard C, Carroll BJ: Dissociation of TSH and adrenocortical disturbances in endogenous depression. Psychiatry Res 3:253, 1980

182. Targum SD, Greenberg RD, Harmon RL: Thyroid hormone and the TRH stimulation test in refractory depression. J Clin Psychiat 45:345, 1984

183. Loosen PT: The TRH-induced response in psychiatric patients: a possible neuroendocrine marker. Psychoneuroendocrinology 10:237, 1985

184. Spratt DI, Pont A, Miller MB et al: Hyperthyroxinemia in patients with acute psychiatric disorders. Am J Med 73:41, 1982

185. Morley JE, Shafer RB: Thyroid function screening in new psychiatric admissions. Arch Intern Med 142:592, 1982

186. Gewirtz GR, Malaspina D, Hatterer JA et al: Occult thyroid dysfunction in patients with refractory depression. Am J Psychiatry 145:1012, 1988

187. Karlberg BE, Kjellman BF, Kagedal B: Treatment of endogenous depression with oral thyrotropin. Acta Psychiatr Scand 58:389, 1978

188. Gold MS, Pottash AL, Extein I et al: The TRH test in the diagnosis of major and minor depression. Psychoneuroendocrinology 6:159, 1981

189. Chopra IJ, Solomon DH, Huang TS: Serum thyrotropin in hospitalized psychiatric patients: evidence for hyperthyrotropinemia as measured by an ultra-

sensitive thyrotropin assay. Metabolism 39:538, 1990

190. Loosen PT: Thyroid function in affective disorders and alcoholism. Endocrinol Metab Clin N Amer 17: 55, 1988

191. Banki CM, Bissette G, Arato M, Nemeroff CB: Elevation of immunoreactive CSF TRH in depressed patients. Am J Psychiatry 142:1526, 1988

192. Gibbons JL, McHugh PR: Plasma cortisol in depressive illness. J Psych Res 1:162, 1962

193. Chopra IJ, Solomon DH, Huang TS: Serum thyrotropin in hospitalized psychiatric patients: evidence for hyperthyrotropinemia as measured by an ultrasensitive thyrotropin assay. Metabolism 39:538, 1990

194. Morley JE, Shafer RB, Elson MK et al: Amphetamine induced hyperthyroxinemia. Ann Intern Med 93: 707, 1980

195. O'Shanick GD, Ellinwood EH Jr: Persistent elevation of thyroid stimulating hormone in women with bipolar affective disorder. Am J Psychiatry 139:513, 1982

196. Kaptein EM, Spencer CA, Kamiel MB, Nicoloff JT: Prolonged dopamine administration and thyroid hormone economy in normal and critically ill subjects. J Clin Endocrinol Metab 51:387, 1980

197. Ree RN, Kourides AA, Ridgway EC et al: The effect of glucocorticoid administration of human pituitary secretion of thyrotropin and prolactin. J Clin Endocrinol Metab 43:338, 1976

198. Duick DS, Wahner HW: Thyroid axis in patients with Cushing's syndrome. Arch Intern Med 139:767, 1979

199. Nicoloff JT, Fisher DA, Appleman MD Jr: The role of glucocorticoids in the regulation of thyroid function in man. J Clin Invest 49:1922, 1970

200. Duick DS, Warren DW, Nicoloff JT et al: Effect of single dose dexamethasone on the concentration of serum triiodothyronine in man. J Clin Endocrinol Metab 39:1151, 1974

201. Gharib HE, Hodgson SF, Gastineau CF et al: Reversible hypothyroidism in Addison's disease. Lancet 734, 1972

202. Farah DA, Boag D, Moran F, McIntosh S: High concentrations of thyroid-stimulating hormone in untreated glucocorticoid deficiency: indications of primary hypothyroidism? Br Med J 172:285, 1982

203. Topliss DJ, White EL, Stockigt JR: Significance of thyrotropin excess in untreated primary adrenal insufficiency. J Clin Endocrinol Metab 50:52, 1980

204. Faglia G, Beck-Peccoz P, Ferrari C et al: Enhanced plasma thyrotropin response to thyrotrophin-releasing hormone following oestradiol administration in man. Clin Endocrinol 2:207, 1974

205. Gershengorn MC, Marcus-Samuels BE, Geras E: Estrogens increase the number of thyrotropin-releasing hormone receptors on mammotropic cells in culture. Endocrinology 105:171, 1979

206. Morley JE, Sawin CT, Carlson HE et al: The relationship of androgen to the thyrotropin and prolactin response to thyrotropin-releasing hormone in hyponadal and normal men. J Clin Endocrinol Metab 52: 173, 1981

207. Arafah BM: Decreased levothyroxine requirement in women with hypothyroidism during androgen therapy for breast cancer. Ann Intern Med 121:247, 1994

208. Lippe BM, Van Herle AJ, LaFranchi SH et al: Reversible hypothyroidism in growth-hormone deficient children treated with growth hormone. J Clin Endocrinol Metab 40:143, 1975

209. Porter BA, Refetoff S, Rosenfeld RL et al: Abnormal thyroxine metabolism in hyposomatotrophic dwarfism and inhibition of responsiveness to TRH during GH therapy. Pediatrics 51:668, 1975

210. Jorgensen JOL, Pedersen SA, Laurberg P et al: Effects of growth-hormone therapy on thyroid function of growth hormone-deficient adults with and without concomitant thyroxine-substituted central hypothyroidism. J Clin Endocrinol Metab 69:1127, 1989

211. Radovick S, Nations M, Du Y et al: A mutation in the POU-homeodomain of Pit-1 responsible for combined pituitary hormone deficiency. Science 257: 1115, 1992

212. Pfaffle RW, DiMattia GE, Parks JS et al: Mutation of the POU-specific domain of Pit-1 and hypopituitarism without pituitary hypoplasia. Science 257:1118, 1992

213. Tatsumi K, Miyai K, Notomi T et al: Cretinism with combined hormone deficiency caused by a mutation in the Pit-1 gene. Nat Genet 1:56, 1992

214. Lotti G, Delitala L, Devilla L et al: Reduction of plasma triiodothyronine (T_3) induced by propranolol. Clin Endocrinol 6:405, 1977

215. Wehmann RE, Rubenstein HA, Pugeat MM, Nisula BC: Extended clinical utility of a sensitive and reliable radioimmunoassay of thyroid-stimulating hormone. South Med J 76:969, 1983

216. Klee GG, Hay ID: Sensitive thyrotropin assays: analytic and clinical performance data. Mayo Clin Proc 63:1123, 1988

217. Hay ID, Bayer MF, Kaplan MM et al: American Thyroid Association assessment of current free thyroid hormone and thyrotropin measurements and guidelines for future clinical assays. Clin Chem 37:2002, 1991

218. Toft AD: Use of sensitive immunoradiometric assay for thyrotropin in clinical practice. Mayo Clin Proc 63:1035, 1988

219. Ross DS, Ardisson LJ, Meskell MJ: Measurement of

thyrotropin in clinical and subclinical hyperthyroidism using a new chemiluminescent assay. J Clin Endocrinol Metab 64:684, 1989

220. Seth J, Kellett HA, Caldwell G et al: A sensitive immunoradiometric assay for serum thyroid-stimulating hormone: a replacement for the thyrotropin-releasing hormone test? Br J Med 289:1334, 1984

221. Sawin CT, Hershman JM, Chopra IJ: The comparative effect of T_4 to T_3 on the TSH response to TRH in young adult men. J Clin Endocrinol Metab 44:273, 1977

222. Borst GC, Osburne RC, O'Brian JT et al: Fasting decreases thyrotropin responsiveness to thyrotropin-releasing hormone: a potential cause of misinterpretation of thyroid function tests in the critically ill. J Clin Endocrinol Metab 57:380, 1983

223. Gow SM, Elder A, Caldwell G: An improved approach to thyroid function testing in patients with non-thyroidal illness. Clin Chim Acta 158:49, 1986

224. Faglia F, Beck-Peccoz P, Ferrari C et al: Plasma thyrotropin response to thyrotropin-releasing hormone in patients with pituitary and hypothalamic disorders. J Clin Endocrinol Metab 37:595, 1973

225. Toft AD, Irvine WJ, Hunter WM et al: Anomalous plasma TSH levels in patients developing hypothyroidism in the early months after ^{131}I therapy for thyrotoxicosis. J Clin Endocrinol Metab 39:607, 1974

226. Toft AD, Irvine WJ, McIntosh D et al: Temporary hypothyroidism after surgical treatment of thyrotoxicosis. Lancet 2:817, 1976

227. Thein-Wai W, Larsen PR: Effects of weekly thyroxine administration on serum thyroxine, and 3,5,3'-triiodothyronine, thyrotropin, and the thyrotropin response to thyrotropin-releasing hormone. J Clin Endocrinol Metab 50:560, 1980

228. Vagenakis AG, Braverman LE, Azizi F: Recovery of pituitary thyrotropic function after withdrawal of prolonged thyroid-suppression therapy. N Engl J Med 293:681, 1975

229. Gow SM, Kellett HA, Seth J et al: Limitations of new thyroid function tests in pregnancy. Clin Chim Acta 152:325, 1985

230. Emerson CH, Dyson WL, Utiger RD: Serum thyrotropin and thyroxine concentration in patients receiving lithium carbonate. J Clin Endocrinol Metab 36:338, 1973

231. Boscato LM, Stuart MC: Heterophilic antibodies: a problem for all immunoassays. Clin Chem 34:27, 1988

Effects of Drugs, Disease, and Other Agents on Thyroid Function; The Nonthyroidal Illness Syndrome

5

The sensitive and tightly regulated feedback control system, the autoregulatory mechanisms of the thyroid gland, and the large intrathyroidal and extrathyroidal storage pools of thyroid hormone seem to be designed to provide a constant supply of the hormone to peripheral tissues in the face of perturbations imposed by the external environment, chemicals, and a variety of diseases processes. This characteristic is in marked contrast to that of certain other endocrine organs, such as the adrenal cortex and medulla, which have a limited hormone storage capacity and are geared to respond acutely to alterations of the environment. Nevertheless, even if the response to such perturbations is of limited amplitude, because of the widespread metabolic role of thyroid hormone and the multiple processes involved in its synthesis, secretion, transport, metabolism, and action, it is inconceivable that the system would remain immutable. In fact, the thyroid is not only subject to changes imposed by a great number of exogenous and endogenous perturbations, but the same agent often evokes alterations in various aspects of thyroid hormone economy. For this reason, it is difficult to classify precisely the external and internal influences according to their mode of action; nor is it possible in a limited review to describe all environmental factors and agents. Instead, they will be covered under three broad categories: changes in the external environment, chemicals and drugs, and nonthyroidal diseases. Each of the more important factors and chemical agents will be considered individually for its effect on various aspects of thyroid economy.

RESPONSES TO ALTERATIONS IN THE EXTERNAL ENVIRONMENT

Environmental Temperature

Changes in environmental temperature cause alterations in TSH secretion and in the serum concentration of thyroid hormones and their metabolism. The changes are probably mediated both through control mechanisms involving the hypothalamus and the pituitary and through peripheral effects on the pathways and rates of thyroid hormone degradation and fecal losses. The in vitro effects of temperature on the firmness of binding of T_4 to its transport serum proteins conceivably also play a role in vivo.[1] The overall effects of environmental temperature have been more obvious and easier to demonstrate in animals than in humans.

Effects of Cold

Dramatic, although transient, increases in serum TSH levels have been observed in infants and young children during surgical hypothermia.[2] Also, a prompt and important secretion of TSH occurs in the newborn, in the first few hours after birth, accompanied by an increase in thyroid hormone secretion and clearance.[3,4] Since this TSH surge is partially prevented by maintaining infants in a warm environment, postnatal cooling appears to be responsible in part for the rise in TSH secretion. On the other hand, exposure of adults to cold or even intensive hypothermia has produced no changes,[5,6] or at best minimal increases[7] in serum TSH. More prolonged exposure to cold results in an increase in serum T_4 and T_3 concentrations.[6] These alterations may be partly the consequence of a direct effect of temperature on the rate and pathways of thyroid hormone metabolism, which have been more thoroughly studied in animals.[8,9] It has been more difficult to show

a clear seasonal variation in serum hormone concentration. However, the variation demonstrated in several studies[10,11] has been, as expected, inversely related to the environmental temperature.

Cold exposure in animals leads to thyroid gland hyperplasia, enhanced hormonal secretion, degradation, and excretion, accompanied by an increased demand for dietary iodine. All of these effects are presumably due to an increased need for thyroid hormone by peripheral tissues. The prompt activation of pituitary TSH secretion after cold exposure of rats[12,13] is possibly due in part to a direct effect on the hypothalamus.[14] Exposure to cold has also resulted in augmented TRH production,[15] increased serum levels of this hypothalamic factor,[16] and blunted responses of TSH to exogenous TRH.[17] These effects have not been reproduced by other laboratories[13,18] although an increase in thyroid hormone secretion has been clearly demonstrated.[6,19,20] In rats, it is associated with augmented rates of T_4 and T_3 deiodination, increased conversion of T_4 to T_3, and enhanced hepatic binding and biliary and fecal clearance of the iodothyronines.[8,9,21,22]

Effects of Heat

In general, an increase in ambient temperature has produced effects opposite to those observed during cold exposure, although the effects of heat have not been extensively investigated. As indicated above, thyroid hormone levels in serum tend to be lower during the summer months. A decrease in the serum T_3 concentration, with reciprocal changes in the levels of rT_3, have been observed in normal subjects acutely exposed to heat and during febrile illnesses.[23,24] In the latter condition, the contribution of the rise in body temperature relative to other effects of systemic illness cannot be dissociated. A decrease in the elevated serum TSH level associated with primary hypothyroidism has been induced by increases in body temperature.[25]

High Altitude and Anoxia

Acute elevations in serum T_4 and T_3 concentrations occur in humans during the early period of exposure to high altitude.[26] Increases in the rate of T_4 degradation and thyroidal RAIU have also been reported.[27,28] Moderate, transient increases in oxygen consumption were found in one study. These responses do not appear to be due to sympathetic activation.[28]

The responses of rats exposed to high altitude or anoxia seem to be quite different. Thyroidal iodinative activity and T_4 formation are diminished.[29–31] The partial reversal of these changes by the administration of TSH led the authors of these studies to conclude that the primary effect is probably diminished TSH secretion.

Alterations in Light

Pinealectomy induces a moderate increase in thyroid weight,[32] and continuous light exposure[33] increases the T_4 secretion rate of rats by about 20 percent. These studies suggest that melatonin has an inhibitory effect on thyroid gland function.[34] Although the retinas of rat pups reared in total darkness are totally devoid of the normal complement of TRH, the content of TRH in the hypothalamus remains unaltered.[35] The diurnal variation in hypothalamic TRH content, reflecting both rhythmic synthesis and secretion, is, however, blunted in the absence of cyclical light changes. The effect of light on the thyroid economy of humans, if any, is unknown.

Nutrition

Since thyroid hormone plays a central role in the regulation of total body metabolism, it is not surprising that various nutritional factors would cause profound alterations in the regulation, supply, and disposal of this thermogenic hormone. Although many substances naturally occurring in the diet affect the thyroid economy, the most striking and important effects are related to alterations in total calorie intake and the supply of iodine. The changes accompanying calorie deprivation seem to be homeostatic in nature and produce alterations in thyroid hormone in an overall direction toward conservation of energy through reduction in catabolic expenditure. The changes observed with a deficiency or excess of iodine supply generally serve to maintain an adequate synthesis and supply of thyroid hormone, principally through modifications in thyroidal iodide accumulation and binding.

Starvation and Fasting

Description of the most important changes in thyroid function during starvation and their underlying mechanisms is the result of work carried out during the previous decade. The most dramatic effect is a decrease in the serum TT_3 within 24 to 48 hours of the initiation of fasting.[36–40] Because changes in the free T_3 fraction are usually small, the absolute concentration of FT_3 is also reduced, clearly into the hypothyroid range. It has now been unequivocally demonstrated that the marked reduction in serum T_3 is caused by a reduction in its generation from T_4 rather than by an acceleration in its metabolic clearance rate.[41,42] It is accompanied by a concomitant and reciprocal change in the concentration of total and free rT_3. The increase in the serum rT_3 concentration tends to begin later and to return to normal at the time serum T_3 is being maintained at a low level with continuous calorie deprivation.[38,39] Little change occurs in the concentrations of TT_4 and FT_4 and the production and metabolic clearance rates of T_4.[38,39,41,42] When small changes have been observed, they were generally in the direction of an increase in the FT_4 concentration. They are attributed to decreased concentration of the carrier proteins in serum, as well as to their diminished association with the hormone caused by the inhibitory effect of free fatty acids (FFA) the level of which increases during fasting.[40,43]

Decreased outer ring monodeiodination (5′-deiodinase activity) would explain both the decreased generation of T_3 from T_4 and the accumulation of rT_3. This hypothesis seems to be fully supported by in vitro studies using liver tissue from fasted fats.[44] It is further supported by the finding of increased generation and serum concentration of $3′,5′-T_2$ and $3′-T_1$ and decreased $3,5-T_2$ and $3,3′-T_2$.[44–47] However, a less important increase in the monodeiodination of the inner ring of T_4 (5-deiodination)[42] explains the temporal dissociation of changes in serum T_3 and rT_3 concentration. An increase in the nondeiodinative pathway of T_4 degradation with the formation of Tetrac has been also reported.[48]

Considerable controversy remains regarding the mechanisms responsible for the observed changes in the rates of the deiodinative pathways of iodothyronines. Decreased generation of nonprotein sulfhydryls (NP-SH) as a cause of the reduction in 5′-deiodinase activity was suggested on the basis of the observed enhancement in enzyme activity by the in vitro addition of dithiothreitol. Reduced glutathione and NADPH had a similar effect.[49] Although Chopra's[50] direct measurements of NP-SH in tissue during fasting seemed to confirm this hypothesis, the

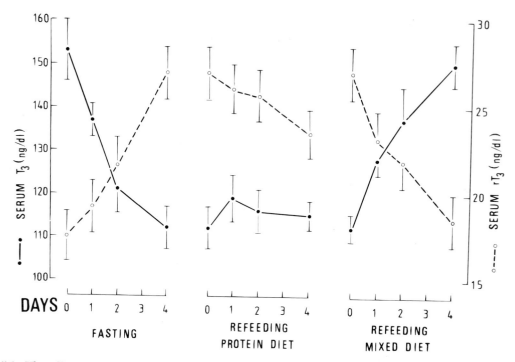

Fig. 5-1. The effect of food deprivation and diet composition on the serum concentration of T_3 and rT_3 in humans. Data represent means ± SEM for six subjects. Fasting produces reciprocal changes in these thyronines that are reversed by refeeding a mixed diet. A protein diet has no effect on the concentration of T_3 but partially restores that of rT_3. (Data from Azizi.[39])

precise mechanism appears to be more complex. Decreased tissue NP-SH content does not always correlate with the inhibition of T_3 generation, which may be restored by glucose refeeding independently of changes in NP-SH content.[50,51]

Composition of the diet rather than reduction in the total calorie intake seems to determine the occurrence of decreased T_3 generation in peripheral tissues during food deprivation. The dietary content of carbohydrate appears to be the key ingredient since as little as 50 g glucose reverses toward normal the fast-induced changes in T_3 and rT_3.[52] Replacement of dietary carbohydrate with fat results in changes typical of starvation.[39,53] Refeeding of protein may partially improve the rate of T_3 generation, possibly by acting as a source of glucose through gluconeogenesis.[54] Yet, dietary glucose is not the sole agent responsible for all changes in iodothyronine metabolism associated with starvation. For example, the increase in serum rT_3 concentration may not be solely dependent on carbohydrate deprivation since a pure protein diet partially restores the level of rT_3 but not that of T_3[39] (Fig. 5-1). The composition of

the antecedent diet also has an effect on the magnitude of the serum T_3 fall during fasting.[39,52] It is possible that the cytoplasmic redox state, measured in terms of the lactate/pyruvate ratio rather than glucose itself, regulates the rate of deiodinative pathways of iodothyronines.[55]

The basal serum TSH level during calorie deprivation is either normal or low and the response to TRH is blunted,[37–39] an unexpected finding in view of the consistent and profound decrease in serum FT_3 levels. Several hypothesis have been proposed to explain this paradox. Because the pituitary is able to continue to respond appropriately during fasting to both suppressive and stimulatory signals,[56] it has been suggested that starvation only "resets" the set point of feedback regulation. A more plausible hypothesis, supported by experimental data,[57,58] does not invoke a change in the set point of the pituitary but rather proposes that the pituitary is regulated by the intracellular concentration of T_3, which may remain unaltered through factors ensuring its continuous local generation during starvation, whereas a decrease is typically found in other tissues. This hypothesis gives credence to the preservation of a closer inverse relationship between serum FT_4 and TSH than between FT_3 and TSH. Hypothalamic TRH content in starved rats appears to be normal,[59] but low values have also been reported under specific conditions.[60] Neonatal starvation in rats leads to diminished TRH and TSH production, with resultant hypothyroidism and growth retardation.[61]

Starvation produces a greater than 50 percent decrease in the maximal binding capacity of T_3 to rat liver nuclear receptors within 48 hours.[62] Although accompanied by a diminution of almost equal magnitude in the nuclear T_3 content, it is unlikely that the observed change represents a down regulation of the receptor by the hormone. Indeed, even the more profound diminution of nuclear T_3 content associated with hypothyroidism does not produce changes in the maximal binding capacity of T_3 in rat liver nuclei. The increase in glucagon concentration also does not appear to be the mediator in starvation-induced changes in nuclear T_3 receptor. The affinity of the rat liver T_3 receptor is not affected by starvation.[62,63] Studies in humans used circulating mononuclear cells and probably due to the limited choice of tissue, results have been either controversial or negative.[64]

Review of the possible mechanisms governing the alterations in thyroid economy during calorie deprivation would be incomplete without mentioning the changes produced in other hormonal systems as well as the general effects on the organism. Among them are the increase in plasma cortisol and suppression of adrenergic stimuli.[65] Both changes are known to induce independently a decrease in the serum T_3 concentration by inhibition of T_4 to T_3 conversion in peripheral tissues (see below). Accordingly, they may be partly responsible for the decrease in T_3 neogenesis during starvation. It is also unclear to what extent thyroid function is modulated by changes in the internal milieu secondary to the many metabolic changes of starvation. In addition to a direct effect of glucose, changes in FFA, ketosis, and the redox state are a few examples of potential factors that could play a role.

Two questions of theoretical and practical importance concern the investigators working in this field. Do the observed changes in thyroid function produce some degree of hypothyroidism, and if so, is this state beneficial to the energy-deprived organism? Although the suppressed serum TSH response

to TRH suggests that the starving organism does not suffer from a significant deprivation in thyroid hormone, other observations indicate the contrary. The decreased pulse rate, systolic time interval, oxygen consumption, and decrease in activity of some liver enzymes are suggestive of hypothyroidism at the level of peripheral tissues.[66] Furthermore, administration of T_3 to restore its serum level to normal during fasting increased the production and excretion of urea and 3-methylhistidine.[56,57] Larger doses of T_3, given during fasting, had even more profound effects. These effects included dramatic increased in the excretion of urea and creatine, and increased plasma levels of ketones and FFA indicating an accelerated protein and fat breakdown.[68] Such evidence leaves little doubt that the decrease in T_3 generation during calorie deprivation has an energy- and nitrogen-sparing effect. It is tempting to speculate that the result is beneficial in the adaptation to malnutrition through reduction in metabolic expenditure.

Fasting is not only a useful model for studying the effects of calorie deprivation on thyroid hormone but is also the prototype of the "low T_3 syndrome."[69] The latter is produced by a number of chemical agents and drugs, and accompanies a variety of nonthyroidal illnesses. It is possible that malnutrition, concomitant in a number of acute and chronic illnesses, is in part responsible for some of the observed changes in thyroid physiology.

Protein-Calorie Malnutrition

As in the case of starvation, protein-calorie malnutrition is associated with a low serum T_3 concentration and increased rT_3 levels, probably due to similar changes in iodothyronine monodeiodination. However, important differences exist between the abnormalities in thyroid function observed in protein-calorie malnutrition and acute calorie deprivation. Most reports indicate important decreases in TBG and TTR concentrations, and there are also indications of hormone binding abnormalities.[70,71] As a consequence, the free concentrations of both T_4 and T_3 are usually normal.[70,72] Recovery is associated with restoration of the level of serum thyroid hormones and binding proteins. Despite an accelerated turnover time, the absolute amount of extrathyroidal T_4 disposed each day is reduced. Refeeding restores the T_4 kinetics to normal.[70] The thyroidal RAIU is reduced due to a defect in the iodine-concentrating mechanism.[73] The most striking difference between starvation and protein-calorie malnutrition is the finding the latter of an exaggerated and sustained TSH response to TRH, with basal TSH levels either elevated or normal.[70,72,74]

The experimental model of protein malnutrition in the rat yielded different results from those observed in humans. Serum T_4 and T_3 levels were found to be both elevated.[75] However, in the lamb, as in humans, chronic malnutrition leads to a lower rate of T_4 utilization.[76]

Overfeeding and Obesity

Overfeeding produces an increase in the serum T_3 concentration as a result of an increased conversion of T_4 to T_3. It is particularly marked when the excess calories are given in the form of carbohydrates.[77] Thus, it appears that the effect of overnutrition on iodothyronine metabolism is the opposite of that of starvation. This finding gives further credence to the speculation that changes in thyroid hormone may serve to modulate the homeostasis of energy expenditure.

Although it has been reported that serum T_3 concentrations correlate with body weight,[78] it appears that this phenomenon reflects instead increases in calorie intake. In fact, the bulk of information indicates that obese subjects have normal thyroid function and hormone metabolism.[79] Furthermore, no abnormalities in the hypothalamic-pituitary-thyroid axis have been demonstrated.

Minerals

Iodine

Of the many minerals that may affect thyroid function, iodine is the most important. It is a prerequisite substrate for thyroid hormone synthesis and also interacts with the function of the thyroid gland at several levels.

Acute administration of increasing doses of iodide enhances total hormone synthesis until a critical level of intrathyroidal iodide is reached. Beyond this level, iodide organification and hormone synthesis are blocked (the acute Wolff-Chaikoff block). Chronic or repeated administration of moderate to large doses of iodine causes a decrease in iodide transport resulting a decrease in its intrathyroidal concentration. The latter relieves the Wolff-Chaikoff

block and is known as the escape or adaptation phenomenon. Although the exact mechanism of the block and escape are unknown, they appear to be autoregulatory in nature since they are independent of pituitary TSH secretion. One mechanism through which iodide acts is via desensitization of the thyroid gland to TSH. This action occurs without a change in TSH receptor number, and may be via an action on adenylyl cyclase.[80] More detailed description is provided in Chapters 2 and 3.

Another effect of large doses of iodine, apparently independent of TSH and hormone synthesis, is the prompt inhibition of hormone release. It has been exploited to achieve rapid amelioration of thyrotoxicosis in Graves' disease and toxic nodular goiters (see Chs. 11 and 17). In normal persons, the inhibitory effect of large doses of iodine on thyroid hormone release produces a transient decrease in the serum concentration of T_4 and T_3. It causes, in turn, a compensatory increase in serum TSH, which stimulates hormone secretion and thus counteracts the effect of iodine.[81,82] The mechanisms of thyroidal autoregulation are believed to serve the purpose of accommodating wide and rapid fluctuations in iodine supply.

The most intriguing effects of iodine are the involution of hyperplasia and the decrease in vascularity that occur when the ion is administered to patients with diffuse toxic goiter. Under different circumstances, iodide may intensify the hyperplasia and produce a goiter (Chs. 9 and 11).

Iodine deficiency used to be the leading cause of goiter and remains so in certain parts of the world. When severe, it can cause hypothyroidism and cretinism, described in detail in Chapter 20. In the United States and the rest of the developed world, untoward effects from excess iodine supplementation or the use of iodine-containing compounds are more common than problems related to iodine deficiency.

Excess iodine can be responsible for the development of goiter, hypothyroidism, and thyrotoxicosis. It should be emphasized, however, that these complications usually arise in persons with underlying defects of thyroid function who are unable to utilize the normal adaptive mechanisms. Iodide-induced goiter (iodide goiter), without or with hypothyroidism (iodide myxedema), is encountered with greater frequency in patients with Hashimoto's thyroiditis or previously treated Graves' disease.[83,84] Other predisposed persons include those who have undergone partial thyroid gland resection, patients with defects of hormonogenesis, and some with cystic fibrosis.[85] Drugs such as phenazone,[86,87] lithium,[88] sulfadiazine,[89] and cycloheximide[90] may act synergistically with iodide to induce goiter and/or hypothyroidism.

More rarely, ingestion of excess iodide may cause thyrotoxicosis (iodide-induced thyrotoxicosis or Jodbasedow). This was observed with the introduction of iodine prophylaxis in areas of endemic iodine deficiency.[91,92] It has also been observed after the administration of iodide in excess to patients with nodular thyroid disease residing in areas of moderate iodine deficiency or even iodine sufficiency.[93,94] Although the exact mechanism of induction of thyrotoxicosis remains obscure, it may be related to the stimulation of increased thyroid hormone synthesis in areas of the gland with autonomous nodular activity.

Ingestion of excess iodide by a gravid woman may cause an iodide goiter in the fetus, and if the gland is large enough it may result in asphyxia during the postnatal period (Ch. 14). Consumption of Kombu, the iodine-rich seaweed, is responsible for the occurrence of endemic goiter in the Japanese island of Hokkaido.[95] It has also been suggested that the the increase in dietary iodine content in the United States during the last three decades is responsible for the higher recurrence rate of thyrotoxicosis in patients previously treated with antithyroid drugs.[96]

Calcium

Calcium is said to be goitrogenic when in the diet in excess. Administration of 2 g calcium per day was associated with decreased iodide clearance by the thyroid.[97] The action is unknown, but it may in some way make overt a borderline dietary iodine deficiency.

Nitrate

Nitrate in the diet (0.3 to 0.9 percent) can interfere with ^{131}I uptake in the thyroid of rats and sheep.[98] This concentration is found in some types of hay and in silages.

Bromine

Bromine is concentrated slightly by the thyroid and interferes with the thyroidal ^{131}I uptake in animals[99] and humans, possibly by competitive inhibition of iodide transport into the gland.

Rubidium

Rubidium is goitrogenic in rats.[100] However, the mechanism of action is unknown.

Fluorine

Fluorine is not concentrated by the thyroid but has a mild antithyroid effect, possibly by inhibiting the iodide transport process.[101] In large amounts, it is goitrogenic in animals. The amounts of fluorine consumed in areas with endemic fluorosis are not sufficient to interfere with thyroid function or to produce goiter.[102,103] However, other data suggest that dietary fluorine may exacerbate an iodine deficiency and thus modulate the distribution of goiter in areas with low iodine intake.[104]

Cobalt

Cobalt inhibits iodide binding by the thyroid.[105] The mechanism is unknown. It is sufficiently active to have been used in the treatment of thyrotoxicosis.[106]

Lithium

Lithium ion is goitrogenic when used in the treatment of manic-depressive psychosis and can induce myxedema.[107] Experimentally, lithium increases thyroid weight and slows thyroid iodine release.[108] When lithium carbonate was given to human subjects in doses of 900 mg four times daily, there was a significant decrease in the rate of release of thyroidal iodine in euthyroid and hyperthyroid subjects.[109] Lithium also decreases the rate of degradation of T_4 in both hyperthyroid and euthyroid subjects.[110] Inhibition of thyroid hormone release may be the dominant effect of the ion. Therefore, the decrease in serum T_3 concentration is greater in hyperthyroid patients, and changes in the rT_3 level, if any, are minimal.[111–113]

A number of mechanisms have been suggested for the effects of lithium. One well-documented phenomenon is a potentiation of an iodide-induced block of binding and hormone release,[88,114] perhaps because lithium is concentrated by the thyroid[115] and increases the intrathyroidal iodide concentration[109,111] (Fig. 5-2). Although it has been shown that lithium inhibits the adenylate cyclase activity in the thyroid gland as well as in other tissues,[116] it also blocks the cAMP-mediated translocation of thyroid hormone. The latter effect, which is probably re-

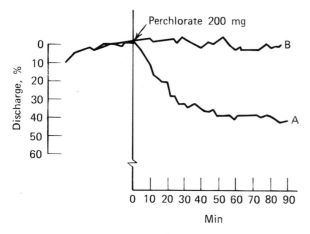

Fig. 5-2. The potassium perchlorate discharge test was carried out in a euthyroid patient during lithium treatment with serum lithium concentrations of 0.8 to 1.3 mEq/liter and during a period without lithium for 10 days. After the administration of radioiodide thyroidal isotope, content was measured for three hours before and 90 minutes after the administration of 200 mg perchlorate. The iodide perchlorate discharge test result was negative in patients not receiving lithium (B) but was strongly positive in patients under lithium (A) treatment. (From Andersen,[114] with permission.)

sponsible for the inhibition of hormone release, appears to be due to the stabilization of thyroid cell microtubules promoted by lithium.[117] The increase in serum TSH concentration and its response to TRH most likely represents an early manifestation of hypothyroidism rather than a direct effect of lithium on the hypothalamic-pituitary axis.[118] The prevalence of goiter has been reported to be as high as 37 percent.[118]

Lithium is reported to produce exophthalmos during chronic therapy; the condition regresses when treatment is stopped. The phenomenon is a protrusion of the globe but does not involve the other changes of infiltrative ophthalmopathy of Graves' disease.[118,119]

Physical and Emotional Stress

Perhaps the most dramatic study of emotional stress is that reported by Kracht,[120] who found that stress provoked thyrotoxicosis in wild rabbits. Although some stress models may prompt secretion of thyroid hormone in animals,[120,121] this effect is unlikely to occur in humans, at least for a sustained

period of time. The stress-induced increase in adrenocortical activity tends not only to suppress TSH release but also to inhibit T_3 neogenesis. A major problem in the analysis of available date is to separate effects due to stress from those caused by the agents used to induce the stress. Many of the changes in thyroid function described in this chapter under headings such as starvation, temperature, and nonthyroidal illness may be due in part to stress.

Surgery

Surgery has been used as a means to study the effect of stress on thyroid physiology in animals.[122] Studies in humans have been prompted by the suspicion that thyroid hormone may mediate the postoperative metabolic changes leading to increased oxygen consumption and protein wastage. Some discrepancies in available data stem from lack of uniformity in the groups of patients studied in terms of preoperative state or disease, type of surgery, types of anesthetic agents and other drugs used, and the postoperative course, including nutrition and the period of recovery.

The most striking change in thyroid function is a decrease in the serum TT_3 and FT_3 concentrations shortly after surgery; rT_3 concentrations are elevated in the postoperative period.[123,124] The combined findings suggest a diversion in the normal deiodinative pathways of T_4. FT_4 levels may also be depressed in the postoperative period, but to a lesser degree.[124] The TTR but not the TBG level is sharply reduced.[125] This clear reduction in the concentration of the active forms of thyroid hormone during the postoperative period is preceded by a small, short-term increase in FT_4 and FT_3 concentrations during surgery.[123,124] The magnitude of the subsequent reduction in T_3 level appears to correlate with the severity of trauma and the morbidity during the postoperative course.[123] The serum TSH concentration also tends to diminish,[124] except during surgery performed in children under the conditions of hypothermia.[2]

Because surgical trauma produces a prompt elevation in plasma cortisol levels and food intake is curtailed during the pre-, intra-, and postoperative periods, the possibility that glucocorticoids and starvation are the principal contributors to the observed changes in thyroid function has been given strong consideration. However, Brandt et al.[126]

showed equally profound diminution in the serum T_3 concentration when surgery was carried out with epidural anesthesia, which abolishes the plasma cortisol surge. Similarly, the almost routine use of glucose infusion should have been able to prevent the changes in serum T_3 and rT_3 levels if starvation played a major role in producing the changes observed during surgery.

Acute Mental Stress

Data on the effect of emotional stress on thyroid function in humans are principally derived from studies in patients with psychiatric disturbances. Thus, even if only patients with acute psychiatric decompensation are considered, the results are colored by the nature of the mental illness, its antecedent history, and the use of drugs. An early suggestion of enhanced hormonal secretion came from the observation of elevated protein-bound iodine (PBI) levels in the serum of psychiatric patients presumably under emotional stress and in medical students in the course of examinations.[127] In more recent studies, elevations of the FT_4 have been consistently found during admission of acute psychiatric patients. The incidence ranged from 7 to 18 percent.[128–130] In one study, an equal number of patients (9 percent) had a low FT_4I.[128] In most instances, values became normal with time and treatment of the psychiatric illness. The TSH response to TRH is blunted or even absent in most psychiatric patients with elevated FT_4I.[130] Significant abnormalities in the serum T_3 concentration are rare.

CHEMICALS AND DRUGS

Goitrogens

A number of compounds have the ability to inhibit thyroid hormone synthesis (Fig. 5-3). Irrespective of their mechanism of action, they are collectively called *goitrogens*, because as a result of a decrease in serum thyroid hormone level, TSH secretion is enhanced, causing goiter formation. Some goitrogens occur naturally in food, and others are in drugs with goitrogenic side effects. The least toxic and those possessing the highest thyroid-inhibiting activity are used in the treatment of hyperthyroidism.

Dietary Goitrogens

The discovery of natural and synthetic substances that impair the synthesis of thyroid hormone are landmarks in the history of pharmacology.[131] These substances are discussed in more detail in Chapter 20. Although iodide deficiency is, without doubt, the major cause of endemic goiter and cretinism throughout the world, dietary goitrogens may play a contributing role in some endemics, and may possibly be the dominant factor in certain areas. The dietary goitrogens fall into several categories, more than one of which may occur in the same food.

Certain foods contain cyanogenic glucosides,[132] compounds that, upon hydrolysis by glucosidase, release free cyanide. These foods include almond seeds and such important dietary items as cassava, sorghum, maize, and millet. Cassava contains enough cyanogenic glucoside to be lethal if large quantities are consumed raw. Ordinarily, the root is extensively soaked, then dried and powdered. Most of the cyanide is lost in this process; that left in the root is liberated after ingestion and converted to SCN-. Chronic poisoning due to cassava is responsible for a tropical neuropathy in Nigeria[133] and Tanzania, and is suspected of being a contributing cause of goiter in Central Africa.[134,135]

Other important classes of antithyroid compounds arise from hydrolysis of the thioglucosides.[132,136,137] These compounds are metabolized in the body to goitrin or thiocyanates and isothiocyanates, and ultimately to other sulfur containing compounds, or are excreted as such. They are important in the goitrogenic activity of seeds of plants of the genus *Brassica* and the *cruciferae, compositae*, and *unbelliferae*. Among the plants containing these compounds are cabbage, kale, brussel sprouts, cauliflower, kohlrabi, turnip, rutabaga, mustard, and horseradish. Cattle may ingest these goitrogens and pass them to humans through milk, as observed in Australia,[138] Finland,[139,140] and England.[141] The isothiocynate, cheiroline, occurs in the leaves of choumoellier and may be related to a focal area of endemic goiter in Australia. The goitrogen is thought to be transmitted from forage to cows, to milk, and finally to children. Although there is considerable circumstantial evidence relating these compounds to endemic goiter, it has been difficult to prove their role with certainty.

Thiocyanate is a well known inhibitor of iodide trapping when in high concentration in blood. The

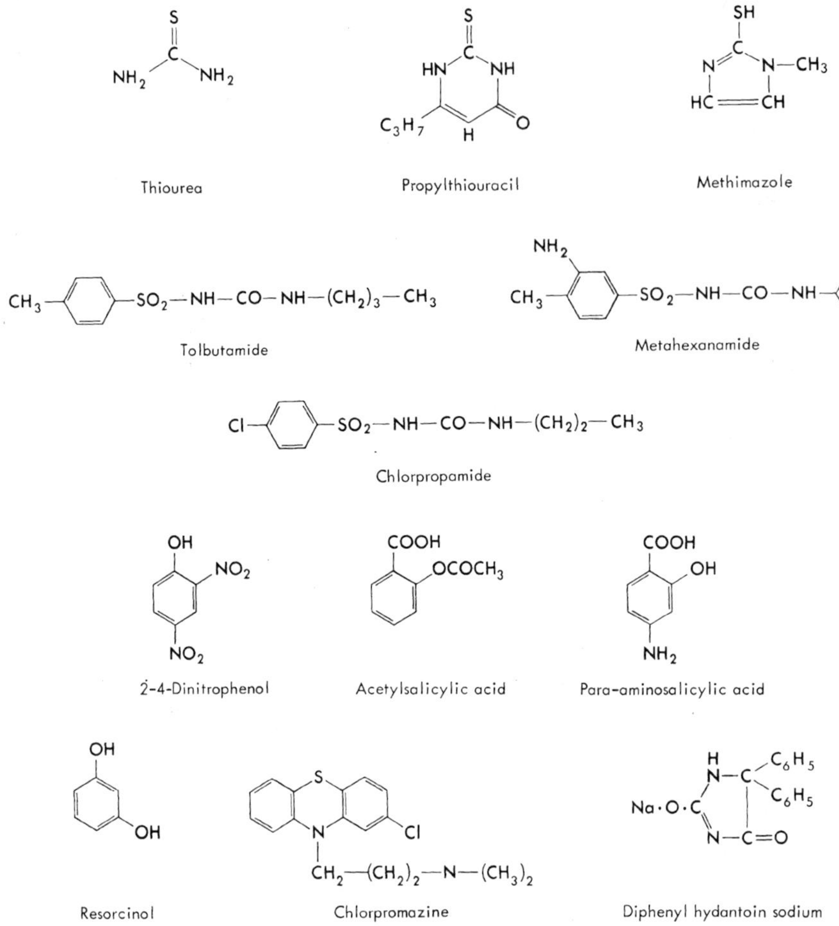

Fig. 5-3. Structural formulas of some drugs that affect the thyroid.

blood levels obtained by ingestion of dietary goitrogens are rarely of this degree. Inhibition of iodide trapping, and thyroid peroxidase activity, and augmentation of urinary iodide loss, as demonstrated by Delange and Ermans and co-workers, all may play a role in the goitrogenic activity.[132,134,135]

Astwood et al. and Greer[142,143] found that turnips contain progoitrin, which is a mustard oil thioglycoside. It undergoes rearrangement by enzymes in human enteric bacteria, or in the turnip, to be converted to goitrin, an active goitrogenic thioglycoside, L-5-vinyl-2-thio-oxazolidone.[144,145] Goitrin inhibits oxidation of iodine and its binding to thyroid protein in the same way as do the thiocarbamides.

Several endemics of goiter have been attributed to dietary goitrogens, usually acting together with iodine deficiency. Goitrin is apparently present in cow's milk in Finland.[146] In the Pedgregoso region of Chile, pine nuts of the tree *Araucaria americana* are made into a flour and consumed in large amounts, and may be related to endemic goiter.[147,148] In the Cauca river valley of Colombia, sulfur-containing compounds found in the water supply, derived from sedimentary rocks containing a large amount of organic matter, are believed to be responsible for endemic goiter.[149] At least, extracts from these waters are goitrogenic in rats.

Other mechanisms may also contribute to dietary goitrogenicity. Thus, diets high in soybean components or other materials increasing fecal bulk may cause excess fecal loss of T_4 and increase the need for this hormone.[150–153] These diets are low in iodine content, and soybean has been thought but not proven to contain a goitrogen.

The goitrogens, by blocking hormone synthesis, deplete the thyroid of iodide; this reduction itself increases the sensitivity of the gland to TSH.[154] This sensitivity, in turn, further promotes goitrogenicity.

Antithyroid Drugs

According to their principal mode of action on thyroidal iodine metabolism, antithyroid drugs are divided into two categories: (1) the monovalent anions, which inhibit iodide transport into the thyroid gland, and (2) a large number of compounds that act through inhibition of thyroidal iodide binding and iodotyrosine coupling. The most important representatives of this latter category of compounds are the group of thionamides. The effect of the drugs in the first category is counteracted by exposure to excess iodine, whereas iodine has no, and at times even potentiates, the action of drugs in the second category. Other drugs inhibit thyroid hormone secretion or act through yet unknown mechanism. A list of these agents is provided in Table 5-1.

Monovalent Anions

Certain monovalent anions (SCN^-, ClO_4^-, NO_3^-) inhibit transport of iodide into the thyroid gland and thereby depress iodide uptake and hormone formation.[164,166] Thiocyanate stimulates efflux of iodide from the thyroid as well,[167] and also inhibits iodide binding and probably coupling.[168,169] A large number of complex anions, such as monofluorosulfonate, difluorophosphate, and fluoroborate,[170] inhibit iodide transport. Of these, fluoroborate,[171] like perchlorate,[172] is concentrated by the thyroid gland. These ions have a molecular volume and charge similar to those of iodide, and may compete with iodide for transport.[170,171] Perchlorate is sufficiently active to be useful clinically.[173] Perchlorate and thiocyanate also displace T_4 from thyroid hormone-binding serum proteins in vivo and in vitro and cause a transient elevation of free T_4.[174]

Thionamides

The thionamide and thiourylene drugs do not prevent transport of iodide into the thyroid gland, but rather impair covalent binding of iodide to TG.[175–177] They are competitive substrates for thyroid iodide peroxidase, preventing the peroxidation of iodide by this enzyme. In small doses, the thiocar-bamides inhibit formation of iodothyronines from iodotyrosyl precursors. When slightly larger amounts are present, iodination of MIT and tyrosine is prevented.[177,178] Minute amounts (10^{-8} M) have, paradoxically, a stimulatory effect on iodination in thyroid slices.[179]

The basic structure necessary for the antithyroid action of these drugs is

where X may be C, N, or O[180,181] (Fig. 5-3). The thiocarbamides are metabolized in the thyroid gland by transsulfuration.[182] The enzyme responsible is also involved in the iodide peroxidase enzyme system.[183] Glands under TSH stimulation metabolize the antithyroid drugs at an accelerated rate, as has been shown for thiourea.[184]

Iodide is released more rapidly from a gland blocked by PTU than from one blocked by perchlorate.[165,185] This action occurs presumably because PTU prevents the utilization of all iodide available to the gland (transported from the blood or formed in the gland by deiodination of iodotyrosines), whereas potassium perchlorate prevents uptake of iodide but does not inhibit reutilization of iodide derived from within the gland. T_4 disappears from the PTU-blocked rat thyroid at a faster rate than do iodotyrosines.[185]

In addition to the effects on the thyroid gland, PTU (and, to a much lesser extent, methimazole) partially inhibits the peripheral deiodination of T_4[186–191] and its hormonal action.[188,192–194] PTU acts directly on body tissues to inhibit the normal formation of T_3 from T_4.[191,195] Coincidentally, fecal excretion of T_4 increases.[186] In order to inhibit goiter induced by antithyroid drugs in rats, one must maintain the T_4 concentration in blood at a higher level that is normal for the species.[188,192] Presumably, inhibition of T_4 monodeiodination by the antithyroid drug leads to a buildup of T_4 in blood and diminishes the availability of T_3 in the tissues.[191] Higher doses of T_4 or higher blood levels may be sufficient to push the reaction toward T_3 and allow formation of quantities sufficient to prevent goiter.

Metabolism of the antithyroid drugs has been observed after administration of ^{35}S-labeled drugs. Me-

TABLE 5-1. Agents Inhibiting Thyroid Hormone Synthesis and Secretion

Substance	Common Use
Block iodide transport into the thyroid gland	
Monovalent anions (SCN^-, ClO_4^-, NO_3^-)[a]	Not in current use; ClO_4^- test agent
Complex anions (monofluorosulfonate, difluorophosphate, fluoroborate)[a]	—
Minerals (bromine, fluorine)	In diet
Lithium[a]	Treatment of manic-depressive psychosis
Ethionamide	Antituberculosis drug
Impair TG iodination and iodotyrosine coupling	
Thionamides and thiourylenes, (PTU, methimazole, carbimazole)[a]	Antithyroid drugs
Sulfonamides (acetazolamide, sulfadiazine sulfisoxazole)[a]	Diuretic, bacteriostatic
Sulfonylureas (carbutamide, tolbutamide, metahexamide, ?chloropropamide)[a]	Hypoglycemic agents
Salicylamides (*p*-aminosalicylic acid, *p*-aminobenzoic acid)[a]	Antituberculosis drugs
Resorcinol[155]	Cutaneous antiseptic
Amphenone[156] and aminoglutethimide[157,158]	Antiadrenal and anticonvulsive agents
Thiocyanate[a]	No current use; in diet
Antipyrine (phenazone)[a]	Antiasthmatic
Aminotriazole[159]	"Cranberry poison"
Amphenidone[160]	Tranquilizer
2,3-Dimercaptopropanol (BAL)[161]	Chelating agent
Ketoconozole	Antifungal agent
Inhibitors of thyroid hormone secretion	
Iodide (in large doses)[a]	Antiseptic, expectorant, and others
Lithium[a]	See above
Mechanism unknown	
p-bromdylamine maleate[162]	Antihistaminic
Phenylbutazone[163]	Antiinflammatory agent
Minerals (calcium, rubidium, cobalt)[a]	—
Interleukin II	Chemotherapeutic agent
γ-Interferon	Activiral and chemotherapeutic agent

[a] References given in the text.

thimazole is rapidly absorbed from the gastrointestinal tract in humans. It reaches a peak plasma level about an hour after administration, and then declines gradually to near zero levels at 24 hours. These drugs are accumulated and degraded in the thyroid, since they are substrates of the peroxidase.[196,197] Carbimazole is accumulated as its metabolic product, methimazole. The concentration ratio between thyroid and plasma for unmetabolized methimazole in rats may approach 25, eight hours after administration of the drug. The metabolic products derived from the drug are excreted in the urine, largely during the first day.

Other Goitrogenic Compounds

A number of other drugs, including the aminoheterocyclic compounds and substituted phenols, act as goitrogens principally by impairing TG iodination (Fig. 5-3). They are in general far less potent in their goitrogenic effect than the thionamides. None are used therapeutically as antithyroid drugs; rather, goitrogenesis is an undesirable side effect of their use. Some the compounds have multiple effects and thus influence thyroid physiology at various levels. These compounds are individually discussed in greater detail. A comprehensive list is provided in Table 5-1.

Sulfonamides

Sulfonamides, particularly those containing an aminobenzene grouping, have antithyroid activity. Acetazoleamide (Diamox), the diuretic agent, has a strong effect on animals and humans.[198,199] Its action, prevention of intrathyroidal iodide binding, is not related to carbonic anhydrase inhibition. Sulfadiazine and sulfisoxazole have a similar action, probably through a synergistic effect on iodide.[89]

Sulfonylureas

Sulfonylureas, derivatives of sulfonamides and used as hypoglycemic-antidiabetic agents, also inhibit the synthesis of thyroid hormone. They include carbutamide, tolbutamide, methahexamide, and possibly chlorpropamide, but not the phenylethyl biguanide (Fig. 5-3). They impair thyroidal RAIU and cause goiter in the rat.[200,201] Carbutamide is much more potent than tolbutamide. Carbutamide, 2 g/day (but not 1 g/day), may reduce the thyroidal RAIU in humans to 20 percent of control values, but the uptake gradually rises as treatment is continued and is normal after 20 weeks. From 1 to 2 g tolbutamide per day does not affect RAIU in humans.[202] Thus, in the usual dose range, tolbutamide will not depress thyroid function.

Chlorpropamide in large doses (3 to 7 g) depresses the RAIU in humans; the common therapeutic doses (up to 1 g daily) usually have no effect on serum T_4.[203] A mild antithyroid action is often reflected in a rise in RAIU, which may be found after the agents are withdrawn.

These drugs inhibit hormone synthesis by inhibition of iodide binding. In most instances, the pituitary compensates for the effect and maintains a euthyroid state by increased synthesis of TSH. Nevertheless, hypothyroidism is said to be more common in diabetic patients on sulfonylureas than in patients treated by other means.[204]

Sulfonylureas also block binding of T_4 to the carrier proteins in serum and thus depress the T_4 concentrations.[205] This effect is most pronounced after intravenous administration.

Effects of Miscellaneous Compounds and Drugs

General Mechanism of Action

A large number of chemical compounds may affect thyroid function and economy. The list has rapidly grown with the introduction of new diagnostic agents, drugs, and food additives. This section is not intended to provide an all-encompassing review. Rather, the more commonly encountered compounds are listed, and those enjoying wider use or having an effect of particular interest in understanding the mechanism of drug interaction are described in greater detail.

Drugs affect the thyroid system at all levels of the hypothalamic-pituitary-thyroid axis as well as the transport, metabolism, and excretion of T_4 and its derivatives. Some hormones and drugs may affect thyroid hormone transport in blood by altering the concentration of the binding proteins in serum. Thyroid hormone transport may also be affected by substances that compete with the binding of thyroid hormone to its carrier proteins (Table 5-2). TBG synthesis is increased by estrogens[222–225] and decreased by androgens and anabolic steroids.[225,226] The most extensively studied compounds that interfere competitively with thyroid hormone binding to the carrier proteins in serum are salicylates, diphenylhydantoin, and heparin.[214,227–233] In general, the effect is a diminution in the serum concentration of total (bound) T_4, and to lesser extent T_3, without a significant effect on the absolute concentration of the metabolically active fractions of FT_4 and FT_3, or usually their free indices (FT_4I and FT_3I). In the steady state, the quantity of thyroid hormone reaching peripheral tissues and the pathways and amount of hormone degradation remain unaltered. However, before this steady state is reached, an acute perturbation in the equilibrium between free and bound hormone brings about transient changes in thyroid hormone secretion and degradation. The hypothalamic-pituitary-thyroid axis participates in the reestablishment of the new steady state. For example, as illustrated in Figure 5-4, an abrupt increase in the concentration of TBG shifts the equilibrium between total and bound hormone, causing a decrease in the concentration of free hormone. The consequences are fourfold. First, there is a shift in the exchangeable hormone from tissues to blood. Second, a decreased hormone content in tissues diminishes its absolute degradation rate. Third, a decline in hormone concentration in tissues activates the hypothalamic-pituitary axis, causing an increase in TSH secretion. Fourth, the latter acts on the thyroid gland to step up its hormonal secretion and reestablish an appropriate thyroid hormone/TBG ratio. Thus, a normal thyroid hormone concentration in serum and tissues and hormonal production and disposal rates are reestablished. TSH concentration returns to normal, and a new steady state is maintained at the expense of an increased intravas-

TABLE 5-2. Compounds that Affect Thyroid Hormone Transport Proteins in Serum

Substance	Common Use
Increase TBG concentration	
Estrogens[a]	Ovulatory suppressants, anticancer agents
Heroin and methadone[206]	Opiates (in addicts)
Clofibrate[207]	Hypolipemic agent
5-Fluorouracil[208]	Anticancer agent
Perphenazine[209]	Tranquilizer
Decrease TBG concentration	
Androgens and anabolic steroids[a]	Virilizing, anticancer, and anabolic agents
Glucocorticoids[a]	Antiinflammatory, immunosuppressive, and anticancer agents; decrease intracranial pressure
L-Asparaginase[210]	Antileukemic agent
Nicotinic acid[211,212]	Hypolipidemic agent
Interfere with thyroid hormone binding to TBG and/or TTR	
Salicylates and salsalate[a]	Antiinflammatory, analgesic, antipyrexic, and antituberculosis agents
Diphenylhydantoin and analogs[a]	Anticonvulsive and antiarrhythmic agents
	Antianxiety agent
Furosemide[213]	Diuretic
Sulfonylureas[a]	Hypoglycemic agents
Heparin[a]	Anticoagulant
Dinitrophenol[a]	Uncouples oxidative phosphorylation
Free fatty acids[214,215]	—
o,p´-DDD[216]	Antiadrenal agent
Phenylbutazone[217]	Antiinflammatory agent
Halofenate[218]	Hypolipemic agent
Fenclofenac[219]	Antirheumatic agent
Orphenadrine[220]	Spasmolytic agent
Monovalent anions (SCN^-, ClO_4^-)[a]	Antithyroid agents
Thyroid hormone analogs, including dextroisomers[221]	Cholesterol reducing

[a] References given in the text.

cular pool and a decreased fractional turnover rate and total distribution space of thyroid hormone.[234,235] The reverse sequence of events accompanies an acute decrease in TBG concentration (Fig. 5-4).

Some of the agents that may alter the extrathyroidal metabolism of thyroid hormone are listed in Table 5-3. Several drugs with wide use in clinical practice inhibit the conversion of T_4 to T_3 in peripheral tissues. Glucocorticoids,[241,242] amiodarone,[243,244] and propranolol[245–247] are a few examples. As expected, their most profound effect on thyroid function is a decrease in the serum concentration of T_3[241,243,245] usually with a concomitant increase in the rT_3 level.[241,243] An increase in the serum T_4 concentration has also been observed on occasion.[243,247] The serum TSH concentration may also occasionally rise,[243] provided the drug does not have a direct inhibitory effect on the hypothalamic-

pituitary axis.[248] In the absence of inherent abnormalities in thyroid hormone secretion or in its regulation, TSH levels should return to normal and hypothyroidism should not ensue from the chronic administration of compounds the only effect of which is to interfere partially with T_4 monodeiodination.

Other mechanisms by which some compounds affect the extrathyroidal metabolism of thyroid hormone are acceleration of the overall rates of deiodinative and nondeiodinative routes of hormone disposal. Examples of drugs acting principally through the former mechanism are diphenylhydantoin and phenobarbital,[249–251] and via the latter the cholesterol lowering resin, colestipal.[239] These drugs should increase the secretion of hormone from the thyroid gland in order to compensate for the enhanced hormonal loss through degradation or fecal excretion. In normal individuals the thyroid

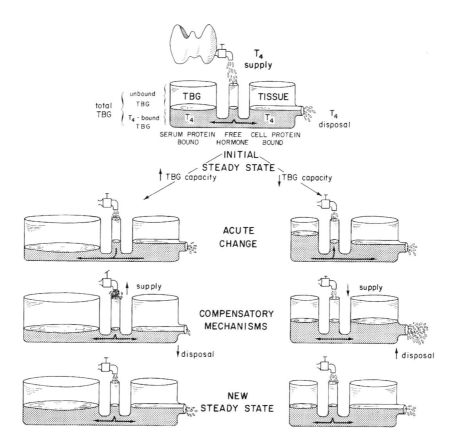

Fig. 5-4. Graphic representation of the sequence of events after an acute change in serum TBG concentration in a subject with normally controlled thyroid hormone secretion and metabolism. The communicating vessel principle is used for analogy. The width of the two large vessels represents available T_4-binding capacity in serum (TBG) and in peripheral cells (TISSUE), which are partially saturated by T_4 (*gray areas*). The fluid represents thyroid hormone (T_4 in this example, although an analogous diagram can be drawn for T_3). The height of fluid in the small central vessels represents free T_4 concentration in equilibrium with bound T_4 in each of the large vessels. FT_4 is proportional to the level of saturation of the binding sites in serum (TBG) and in cells (TISSUE). Thyroidal secretion (supply) of hormone is represented by the input of fluid through the faucet, and hormone metabolism (disposal) by the overspill of the tissue reservoir. For further details see text. (From Refetoff and Nicoloff,[476] with permission.)

hormone concentration in blood should remain unaltered. Furthermore, it has been anticipated, as well as observed, that hypothyroid patients receiving such drugs require higher doses of exogenous hormone to maintain a eumetabolic state (Ch. 9).

Acute increases in serum T_4 and FT_4 concentration after the injection of insulin or during halothane anesthesia have been attributed to an enhanced release of T_4 normally stored in the liver.[252,253]

The last two decades have seen a prodigious growth in the list of substances that act on the hypo-thalamic-pituitary axis (Table 5-4). Although many of these compounds occupy an important place in the modern pharmaceutical armamentarium, only a few have significant effect on thyroid function via this central mechanism. Furthermore, persons without a thyroid abnormality under treatment rarely show clear changes in the basal serum TSH. Rather, the response of TSH to the administration of TRH may be altered, or the high levels of serum TSH in primary hypothydroidism may undergo a further increase or a significant diminution.

TABLE 5-3. Agents that Alter the Extrathyroidal Metabolism of Thyroid Hormone

Substance	Common Use
Inhibit conversion of T_4 to T_3	
PTU[a]	Antithyroid drug
Glucocorticoids (hydrocortisone, prednisone, dexamethasone)[a]	Antiinflammatory and immunosuppressive; decrease intracranial pressure
Decrease intracranial pressure	
Propranolol[a]	β-Adernergic blocker (antiarrhythmic, antihypertensive)
Iodinated contrast agents [ipodate (orgrafin), iopanoic acid (Telepaque)][a]	Radiologic contrast media
Amiodarone[a]	Antianginal and antiarrhythmic agent
Clomipramine[236]	Tricylic antidepressant
Stimulators of hormone degradation or fecal excretion	
Diphenylhydantoin[a]	Anticonvulsive and antiarrhythmic agent
Carbamazepine[237]	Anticonvulsant
Phenobarbital[a]	Hypnotic, tranquilizing, and anticonvulsive agent
Cholestyramine[238] and colestipol[239]	Hypolipemic resins
Soybeans[151,152]	Diet
Rifampin[240]	Antituberculosis drug

[a] References given in the text.

Although the aim of the next three paragraphs is to provide a general impression of the mechanism of action of these compounds, because of some inconsistencies in available information, it is premature to draw definite conclusions. A major problem in interpretation is the variability of experimental designs. These variables include doses, routes of administration, duration and time of treatment, drug combinations, age and sex of subjects, hormonal status at the time of testing, and time of blood sampling. Furthermore, observed responses are biased not only by the technical constraints of serum TSH measurements but also by the method of data analysis. For example, results of TSH responses to TRH have been expressed in terms of changes in the absolute value, increments or decrements from the basal level, and percent of the basal value at either the peak and nadir of the response or the integrated area over the duration of the response.

The most potent suppressors of pituitary TSH secretion are thyroid hormone and its analogs. They act on the pituitary gland by blocking TSH secretion through the mechanisms discussed in Chapter 4. Some of the TSH-inhibiting agents listed in Table 5-4, namely, fenclofenac and salicylates, may act by increasing the free thyroid hormone level due to interference with its binding to serum proteins. Other agents appear to have a direct inhibitory effect on the pituitary and possibly on the hypothalamus. The most notable is dopamine and its agonists. They have been shown to suppress the basal TSH levels in euthyroid persons[286,287] and in patients with primary hypothyroidism.[269,286–288] More uniformly, they suppress the TSH response to the administration of TRH.[270,287,289,290] It is thus not surprising that a great number of dopamine antagonists induce an amplification of TSH secretion.[150–155] Increases in the basal TSH and in its response to TRH have been observed in euthyroid persons,[254,257] as well as in patients with primary hypothyroidism[252–258] who have been given these drugs. A notable exception to this rule, which casts some doubt on the assumed mechanism of action of dopamine antagonists, is pimozide. This neuroleptic dopamine blocker has actually been shown to reduce the elevated serum TSH level in patients with primary hypothyroidism.[291]

Iodine and some iodide-containing organic compounds cause a rapid increase in the basal and TRH-stimulated levels of serum TSH. This effect is undoubtedly due to a decrease in the serum thyroid hormone concentration either by inhibition of hormone synthesis and secretion by the thyroid gland[81,82] or by a selective decrease in the concentration of T_3.[292] The latter effect is mediated through the inhibition of T_3 generation from T_4. A more se-

TABLE 5-4. Agents that May Affect TSH Secretion

Substance	Common Use
Increase serum TSH concentration and/or its response to TRH	
Iodine (iodide and iodine-containing compounds)[a]	Radiologic contrast media, antiseptic expectorants, antiarrhymic and antianginal agents
Lithium[a]	Treatment of bipolar psychoses
Dopamine receptor blockers (metclopramide,[254,255] domperidone[255,256])	Antiemetic
Dopamine-blocking agent (sulpiride[257])	Tranquilizer
Decarboxylase inhibitor (benserazide[258])	—
Dopamine-depleting agent (monoiodotyrosine[255])	—
L-Dopa inhibitors (chloropromazine,[259] biperidine,[260] haloperidol[260])	Neuroleptic drugs
Cimetidine (histamine receptor blocker)[261]	Treatment of peptic ulcers
Clomifene (antiestrogen)[262]	Induction of ovulation
Spironolactone[263]	Antihypertensive agent
Amphetamines[264]	Anticongestants and antiappetite
Decrease serum TSH concentration and/or its response to TRH	
Thyroid hormones (T_4 and T_3)	Replacement therapy, antigoitrogenic and anticancer agents
Thyroid hormone analogs (D-T_4,[265] 3,3′,5-Triac,[266] etiroxate-HCl,[267] 3,5-dimethyl-3-isopropyl-L-thyronine[268])	Cholesterol-lowering and weight reducing agents
Dopaminergic agents (agonists)	
Dopamine[a]	Antihypotensive agent
L-Dopa[a] (dopamine precursor)	Diagnostic and anti-Parkinsonian agent
2-Brom-α-ergocryptine[a]	Antilactation and pituitary tumor suppressive agent
Fusaric acid (inhibitor of dopamine β-hydroxylase[269])	—
Pyridoxine (coenzyme of dopamine synthesis[270])	Vitamin and antiheuropathic agent
Other dopaminergic agents (perbidil,[271] apomorphine,[271] lisuride[272])	Treatment of cerebrovascular diseases and migraine
Dopamine antagonist (pimozide)[a]	Neuroleptic agent
α-Noradrenergic blockers (phentolamine,[273] thioridazine[274])	Neuroleptic agents
Serotonin antagonists (metergoline,[275] cyroheptadine,[276] methysergide[277])	Antimigraine agents and appetite stimulators
Serotonin agonist (5-hydroxytryptophan[278])	—
Glucocoricoids[a]	Antiinflammatory, immunosuppressive, and anticancer agents
	Reduction of intracranial pressure
Acetylsalicylic acid[a]	Antiinflammatory, antipyrexic and analgesic agent
Growth hormone[279b]	Growth-promoting agent
Somatostatin[280,281]	—
Opiates (morphine,[282] leucine-eukephaline,[283] heroin[284])	Analgesic agents
Clofibrate[285]	Hypolipemic agent
Fenclofenac[218]	Antirheumatic agent

[a] References given in the text.
[b] In hyposomatotrophic dwarfs.

lective, tissue-specific inhibition of T_4 to T_3 conversion appears to be responsible for the TSH-stimulating effect of the radiographic contrast agent iopanoic acid. Indeed, a predominant block on the intrapituitary conversion of T_4 to T_3 has been demonstrated.[58] It should be noted that iodine induced thyroid hormone hypersecretion is not due to increased TSH.[94] A decrease in the free thyroid hormone concentration in serum, albeit minimal in magnitude, may also be responsible for the increase in TSH levels observed during treatment with clomifene.[262]

It has been postulated that some agents may act by modifying the effect of TSH on its target tissue. For example, theophylline may potentiate the action of TSH through its inhibitory effect on phosphodiesterase, which may lead to an increase in the intracellular concentration of cAMP.[293] In fact, the presence of the pituitary is required to demonstrate that methylxanthines augment the goitrogenic effect of a low-iodine diet in the rat.[294] One of the postulated effects of diethyl ether anesthesia in the rat is inhibition of the action of TSH on the thyroid gland,[295] although it has also been reported to induce a transient redistribution of T_4 between serum and tissues.[296]

A handful of drugs seem to act by blocking some of the peripheral tissue effects of thyroid hormone. Others appear to mimic one or several manifestations of the thyroid hormone effect on tissues. Guanethidine releases catecholamines from tissues.[297] It has a beneficial effect in thyrotoxicosis, including a decrease in BMR, pulse rate, and tremulousness.[298,299] This agent probably has no direct effect on the thyroid gland, but may depress those manifestations of thyrotoxicosis that are mediated by sympathetic pathways. The sympatholytic agents phentolamine and dibenzyline have been reported both to depress and to stimulate thyroid function in animals. Their action is not clear, and clinically it is not impressive.[300–302] Among a number of α-adrenergic blocking agents tested, only phentolamine showed an inhibitory effect on the TSH response to TRH.[273]

Among the multiple effects the β-adrenergic blocker, propranolol, has on thyroid hormone economy, it appears to reduce the peripheral tissue responses to thyroid hormone (see Chs. 3 and 11). In contrast, dinitrophenol enhances oxygen con-

sumption by a direct effect on tissues and thus mimics one of the actions of thyroid hormone.[303]

Specific Agents

Estrogens

Hyperestrogenism, either endogenous (caused by pregnancy, hydatidiform moles, or estrogen-producing tumors) or exogenous (due to the administration of estrogens), is accompanied by an increase in TBG and a decrease in TTR concentrations in serum.[222–224] Estrogens are the most common cause of TBG elevation, and this effect can be produced even from their topical application. The magnitude of TBG increase is in part dose related and occurs in women as well as in men. Estrogen increases the complexity of oligosaccharide side chains and, as a consequence, the number of sialic acids in the TBG molecule which in turn prolongs its survival in serum.[304] The concentrations of other serum proteins, including several that bind hormones, such as cortisol-binding globulin and sex-hormone binding globulin, are also increased.[305]

The consequences of increased TBG concentration in serum are higher serum levels of T_4, T_3, and rT_3 and, to a lesser extent, other metabolites of T_4 deiodination. The fractional turnover rate of T_4 is depressed principally due to an increase in the intravascular T_4 pool. On the other hand, the FT_4 and FT_3 concentrations and the absolute amount of hormone degraded each day remain normal.[234,235] Transient changes in these parameters during the early changes in TBG concentration can be anticipated as described above.

The effect of estrogen, if any, on the control of TSH secretion is controversial. Contradictory results suggesting a stimulatory[306] and an inhibitory[307,308] effect have been obtained by different investigators. Although women show a greater TSH responsiveness to TRH than men,[308–310] administration of pharmacologic doses of estrogens does not appear to have a significantly enhancing effect.[311,312]

Some of the effects of pregnancy on thyroid function are also mediated by an estrogen-induced increase in the serum TBG concentration. The effects on thyroidal and renal iodide clearance and BMR are mediated by different mechanisms (see Ch. 3).

The effects of estrogens on the rat do not parallel those observed in humans. Estrogens do not induce changes in the concentration of serum T_4-binding proteins in the rat.[22] Thus, investigations carried out in this species are not helpful for interpretating the effects of estrogens observed in humans.

Androgens

Androgens decrease the concentration of TBG in serum and thereby reduce the level of T_4 and T_3.[225,313] The TTR concentration, however, is increased.[225] As with estrogens, the concentration of free hormone remains unaffected, and the degradation rate of T_4 is normal at the expense of an accelerated turnover rate.[225] TSH levels are normal.[307] anabolic steroids with weaker androgenic action have the same effect, although similar changes observed during danazol therapy have been attributed to its androgen-like properties.[226]

Salicylates

Salicylate and its noncalorigenic congeners (Fig. 5-3) compete for thyroid hormone-binding sites on serum TTR and TBG.[227–230] As a result, the serum concentrations of T_4 and T_3 decline and their free fractions increase.[230] The turnover rate of T_4 is accelerated, but degradation rates remain normal.[227,228] Salicylate and its noncalorigenic congeners suppress the thyroidal RAIU but do not retard iodine release from the thyroid gland.[314] Thus, the impaired response of TSH to TRH[315] and the hypermetabolic effect[316] of this drug were attributed to the increase in the FT_4 and FT_3 fractions. If this proposed explanation were correct, hormonal release from the serum-binding proteins should produce only a temporary suppression of the thyroidal RAIU and transient hypermetabolism. In fact, both effects have been observed during chronic administration of salicylates.[227,228] In addition, this mechanism of action does not explain the lack of calorigenic effect of some salicylate congeners despite their ability to also displace thyroid hormone from its serum-binding proteins.

In vitro studies have demonstrated an inhibitory effect of salicylate on the outer ring monodeiodination of both T_4 and rT_3,[317] but lack of typical changes in serum iodothyronine levels suggests that this action is less important in vivo.

Acetylsalicylic acid mimics in several ways the action of thyroid hormone. For example, it lowers the serum cholesterol level,[318] but it does not provide a therapeutic effect in myxedema, or lower TSH levels.[319] Administration of 8 g aspirin daily raises the BMR to normal in myxedema, accelerates the circulation, and increases sweating, but it has no effect on the skin change, the electrocardiogram, or the mental state.[318]

Because of some analogies between the effects of salicylates and nitrophenol, uncoupling of oxidative phosphorylation has been suggested as one of its possible mechanisms of action. If this were the case, direct chemical action does not appear to be involved since analogs of salicylate that do not uncouple oxidative phosphorylation in vitro are active in vivo.[320]

p-Aminosalicylic acid and p-aminobenzoic acid are closely related chemically to salicylate. They inhibit iodide binding in the thyroid gland and are goitrogenic.[321,322] These agents also displace thyroid hormone from its serum protein-binding sites.[323] Abnormalities of thyroid function tests have been also reported in patients treated with salsalate.[324]

Heparin

Patients receiving heparin chronically have increased FT_4 and FT_3.[232,233] Reciprocal changes in serum TSH have been reported.[233] These changes may occur because heparin interacts with the T_4-binding proteins to alter the steric configuration of the binding sites and reduce the affinity of the proteins for T_4 and T_3 or because heparin causes elevation of free fatty acids, which compete for T_4 binding.[210]

Glucocorticoids

Physiologic amounts, as well as pharmacologic doses, of glucocorticoids influence thyroid function. Their effects are variable and multiple, depending on the dose and on the endocrine status of the individual. The type of glucocorticoid and the route of administration may also influence the magnitude of the effect.[325] Known effects include (1) decrease in the serum concentration of TBG and increase in that of TTR;[326,327] (2) inhibition of the outer ring deiodination of T_4 and probably rT_3;[241,242] (3) suppression of TSH secretion;[248,328,329] (4) a possible disease in hepatic binding of T_4; and (5) increase in renal clearance of iodide.[330,331]

The decrease in the serum concentration of TBG caused by the administration of pharmacologic doses, of glucocorticoids results in a decrease in the serum total T_4 concentration and an increase in its free fraction and the rein uptake test result. The absolute concentration of FT_4 and FT_4I remain normal.

The more profound decrease in the concentration of serum T_3 compared to T_4 associated with the administration of pharmacologic doses of glucocorticoids cannot be ascribed to their effect on serum TBG. It is due to the decreased conversion of T_4 to T_3 in peripheral tissues. Thus, glucocorticoids reduce the serum T_3/T_4 ratio and increase that of rT_3/T_4 in hypothyroid patients receiving replacement doses of thyroid hormone.[241] This effect of the steroid is rapid and may be seen within 24 hours.[241,242]

Earlier observations of cortisone-induced depression of uptake and clearance of iodide by the thyroid[330,331] can now be attributed to the effect of this steroid on TSH secretion. Pharmacologic doses of glucocorticoids suppress the basal TSH level in euthyroid subjects and in patients with primary hypothyroidism, and decrease their TSH response to TRH.[248,328,329] The latter effect is less marked in the presence of hypothyroidism.[329] Normal adrenocortical secretion appears to have a suppressive influence on pituitary TSH secretion because patients with primary adrenal insufficiency have a significant elevation of TSH.[332] Tashjian et al.[333] showed that hydrocortisone increased the number of TRH receptors in cultures of rat pituitary tumors. The mechanism of glucocorticoid action on the hypothalamic-pituitary axis is covered in Chapter 4.

No single change in thyroid function can be ascribed to a specific mode of action of glucocorticoids. For example, a diminished thyroidal RAIU may be due to the combined effects of TSH suppression and increased renal clearance of iodide. Similarly, a low serum TT_4 level is the result of suppressed thyroidal secretion due to diminished TSH stimulation as well as the decreased serum level of TBG. One of the common problems in clinical practical is to separate the effect of glucocorticoid action on pituitary function from that of other agents and those caused by acute and chronic illness. This situation arises often since steroids are commonly used in a variety of autoimmune and allergic disorders as well as in the treatment of septic shock. The diagnosis of coexisting true hypothyroidism is difficult, if not impossible. Due to the suppressive effects of glucocorticoids on the hypothalamic-pituitary axis, the low levels of serum T_4 and T_3 may not be accompanied by an increase in the serum TSH concentration, which would otherwise be diagnostic of primary hypothyroidism. In such circumstances, a depressed rather than an elevated serum rT_3 level may be helpful in the detection of coexistent primary thyroid failure.

Pharmacologic doses of glucocorticoids induce a prompt decline in serum T_4 and T_3 concentrations in thyrotoxic patients with Graves' disease.[241] Amelioration of the symptoms and signs in such patients may also be accompanied by a decrease in the elevated thyroidal RAIU and a diminution of the TSH receptor antibody titer.[327,334] This effect of glucocorticoids may be due in part to its immunosuppressive action since it has been shown that administration of dexamethasone to hypothyroid patients with Hashimoto's thyroiditis causes an increase in the serum concentration of both T_4 and T_3.[335]

Iodinated Contrast Agents

The principal effect of some iodine-containing radiologic contrast media is inhibition of T_4 to T_3 conversion. In fact, they may be the most potent of all agents known to interfere with this step of iodothyronine metabolism. A triiodo- and a monoamino-benzene ring with a proprionic acid chain appear to be required because iodinated contrast agents without this chemical structure have little or no effect.[336] Two of these agents, namely, ipodate (Oragrafin) and iopanoic acid (Telepaque), are used for oral cholecystography.

A decrease in the rate of deiodination of the outer ring of thyronines causes a profound decrease in the serum T_3 concentration and an increase in the rT_3 and T_4 levels.[336,337] The serum T_4 concentration may reach values well within the thyrotoxic range.[336] These changes are accompanied by an increase in serum TSH secretion.[292] The latter is particularly notable, if not characteristic of these agents, probably because of their potent inhibitory effect on T_3 generation in pituitary tissue.[58] These agents have been used to study the regulation of thyroid hormone action via the process of iodothyronine deiodination.[58,338] Changes persist for at least two to four weeks after their administration.[336]

Iodocontrast agents also decrease the hepatic uptake of T_4[339] and inhibit T_3 binding to its nuclear receptors.[340] The antithyroidal effect of the iodine present in these agents is believed to be responsible for the falling T_4 level and amelioration of the symptoms and signs of thyrotoxicosis when they are administered to patients with Graves' disease.[340]

Amiodarone

Changes in thyroid function observed during the administration of this drug are similar to those seen with iodine-containing contrast agents. They include a marked decrease in serum T_3, an increase in rT_3, and a more modest elevation in the T_4 concentration.[243,341] Basal and TRH-stimulated TSH levels are increased. The principal mechanism of action is believed to be inhibition of T_3 generation from T_4.

Amiodarone also contains 37 percent iodine, a characteristic shared with the iodine-containing contrast media, but the principal effect on thyroid function appears to be due to its structural resemblance to thyroid hormone rather than to its iodine content. In contrast, the more rare occurrence of amiodarone-induced thyrotoxicosis is caused by the excess iodine released from the drug and is observed more frequently in areas of mild iodine deficiency.[342] The drug is used as an antianginal and antiarrhythmic agent and the bradycardia that almost invariably occurs when the drug is used in high doses, may suggest the presence of hypothyroidism.[342] Measurement of serum TSH, the most useful test in the differential diagnosis of hypothyroidism, may also give misleading results. If hypothyroidism is suspected, it is appropriate to obtain a measurement of the serum rT_3 concentration. A failure to show high serum levels of this thyronine in a patient receiving amiodarone can be considered indicative of hypothyroidism.

Diphenylhydantoin (Dilantin)

Diphenylhydantoin (DPH) (Fig. 5-3) competes with thyroid hormone binding to TBG.[230,231] This effect of DPH and diazepam, a related compound, has been exploited to study the conformational requirements for the interaction of thyroid hormone with its serum carrier protein.[231,343] It appears that the angle formed between the two phenyls and the hydantoin group of DPH is nearly identical to that formed between the two phenyls linked by an ether bond in T_4.[231] Although the affinity of DPH for TBG is far below that of T_4, when used in therapeutic doses the serum concentration achieved is high enough to cause a significant occupancy of the hormone-binding sites on TBG. This effect of DPH is only partly responsible for the decrease in the total concentration of T_4 and T_3 in serum.

DPH accelerates the conjugation and clearance of T_4 and T_3 by the liver and probably enhances the conversion of T_4 to T_3.[249,344] The net result is a decrease in the serum concentration of T_4 and rT_3 and, less consistently, that of T_3[345,346] because the enhanced degradation of T_3 is compensated for by an increase in its generation from T_4. Yet, basal TSH- and TRH-stimulated values are within the normal range[345,346] or slightly elevated.[237,347] Calculated indices of FT_4 are usually reduced, but the FT_4 measured by dialysis is normal.[249,345]

Both DPH and diazepam are commonly used in clinical practice, the former as an anticonvulsive and antiarrhythmic agent and the latter as anxiolytic. Reduced serum levels of thyroid hormone in patients having therapeutic blood levels of DPH should not be viewed as indicative of thyroid dysfunction unless the TSH level is elevated. DPH may significantly increase the required dose of thyroid hormone replacement in athyreotic individuals.[348]

Phenobarbital

Chronic administration of phenobarbital to animals induces increased binding of thyroid hormone to liver microsomes and increased deiodinating activity.[250,251,349] Phenobarbital administration reduces the biologic effectiveness of the hormone by diverting it to microsomal degradative pathways. In humans, phenobarbital augments fecal T_4 clearance by nearly 100 percent,[350] but serum T_4 and FT_4 levels remain near normal because of compensatory increases in T_4 secretion. It is not apparent that barbiturates have an important effect on thyroid mediated metabolic action in normal humans. The augmented hepatic removal of T_4 induced by phenobarbital lower the absolute T_3 disposal by nearly 25 percent, increase T_4 clearance, and lower T_4 and FT_4I in patients with Graves' disease but does not produce a clinical response.[350]

Propranolol

Propranolol, a β-adrenergic blocker, is commonly used as an adjunct in the treatment of thyrotoxicosis Propranolol is also used in its own right in the treatment of cardiac arrhythmias and hypertension. Information regarding its effects on thyroid hormone action, and application in the symptomatic treatment of thyrotoxicosis is found in Chapters 3 and 11, respectively.

Propranolol does not affect the secretion or overall turnover rate of T_4, nor TSH release or its regulatory mechanisms.[351,352] A small to moderate lowering effect on serum T_3 has been reported in euthyroid subjects as well as in patients with hyperthyroidism or with myxedema under L-T_4 replacement therapy.[245,247,353,354] Reciprocal increases in serum rT_3 and 3′,5′,-T_2 levels have also been reported.[354] Such data, combined with the finding by some investigators of minimal increases in serum T_4[247] levels, suggest a mild blocking effect of this drug on the 5′-deiodination of iodothyronines. This effect does not appear to be related to the β-adrenergic-blocking action of propranolol, since other β-blocking agents do not share the deiodinase-blocking property.[355,356]

Clearly, the ameliorating effects of propranolol on the clinical manifestations of thyrotoxicosis are related to its β-adrenergic blocking action, rather than its effect on thyronine metabolism. Reduction of tachycardia, anxiety, and tremor is useful in the management of patients.[357–359] Whether it alters the hypermetabolism of thyrotoxicosis is debatable.

Reserpine

Reserpine formerly had wide use as an antihypertensive agent but has been replaced by more effective agents. Reserpine alters the manifestations of thyrotoxicosis by reducing anxiety, tachycardia, and tremulousness.[360] This effect may arise from depression of autonomic centers or possibly from depletion of catecholamines in the peripheral tissues.[361] Reserpine may depress the formation of iodotyrosines in thyroid tissue in vitro, but this action does not seem to be important clinically. Reserpine does not alter the results of thyroid function tests other than the BMR.[360]

Nitrophenols

2,4-Dinitrophenol (Fig. 5-3) elevates the BMR, lowers the serum concentration T_4, accelerates the peripheral metabolism of T_4, and depresses the thyroidal RAIU and secretion.[277,362,363] The action is probably complex. The drug stimulates the metabolism by uncoupling oxidative phosphorylation in mitochondria.[364] T_4 in vitro also uncouples oxidative phosphorylation. Part of the effect of dinitrophenol

may be to mimic the action of thyroid hormone on hypothalamic or pituitary receptor control centers; this effect would account for the diminished thyroid activity. Dinitrophenol also displaces thyroid hormone from T_4-binding serum proteins.[229] This action could lower the total hormone concentration in serum but should have no persistent effect on thyroid function. Dinitrophenol increases biliary and fecal excretion of T_4, and this action largely accounts for the rapid removal of hormone from the circulation.[365] Deiodination of T_4 is also increased.[366] Both of these effects may be related to displacement of hormone from TTR or to changes in metabolism of hormone in the liver.

2,4-Dinitrophenol does not share some of the most important properties of T_4. It cannot initiate metamorphosis of tadpoles[367] or provide a substitute for hormonal therapy in myxedema.

Dopaminergic Agents

It is now reasonably well established that endogenous brain dopamine plays a physiologic role in the regulation of TSH secretion through its effect on the hypothalamic-hypophyseal axis.[254,368,369] Dopamine exerts a suppressive effect on TSH secretion and can be regarded as antagonistic to the stimulatory action of TRH at the pituitary level.[286,289,369] Much of the information regarding the role of dopamine on the control of TSH secretion in humans has been derived from observations made during the administration of agents with dopamine-agonistic and -antagonistic activity (see Table 5-4 and Ch. 4).

Dopamine infusion is commonly used in the care of acutely ill hypotensive patients. It lowers the basal serum TSH level in both euthyroid and hypothyroid patients and blunts its response to the administration of TRH.[254,286,289,370]

L-dopa, the precursor of dopamine, used in the treatment of Parkinson's disease and as a test agent in the diagnosis of pituitary diseases, also suppresses the basal and the TRH-stimulated serum TSH level in euthyroid subjects as well as in patients with primary hypothyroidism[287,290] (Fig. 5-5).

A similar effect has been observed during the administration of 2-brom-α-ergocryptine (bromocryptine), a dopamine agonist used in the treatment of some pituitary tumors and to suppress lactation during the puerperal period. Although the agent has been shown definitely to diminish the high serum

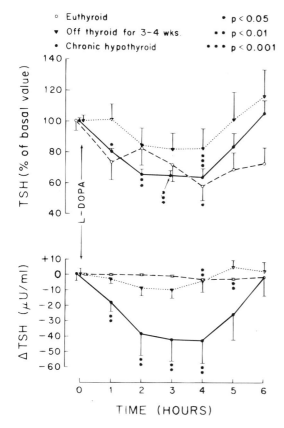

Fig. 5-5. Effect of L-dopa on serum TSH in patients with hypothyroidism of long duration (chronic hypothyroidism), hypothyroidism of short duration (not receiving thyroid hormone for three to four weeks), and in euthyroidism. Mean ± SEM levels for TSH are expressed as a percentage of the mean basal TSH value and as the absolute increments or decrements from the mean basal TSH value. Results were analyzed by the Student t test and the statistical significance is indicated. (From Refetoff et al,[287] with permission.)

TSH levels in patients with primary hypothyroidism,[288] a significant inhibitory effect on TRH-induced TSH secretion has not been clearly demonstrated.[371,372]

The exact mechanism whereby dopaminergic drugs inhibit pituitary TSH secretion remains unknown, although a direct interaction with pituitary receptors has been suggested.[373] Furthermore, although some authors have cautioned that prolonged infusion of dopamine may induce secondary hypothyroidism and thus worsen the prognosis of severely ill patients,[374] there is no evidence that chronic treatment with dopaminergic drugs induces hypothy-

roidism in less critically ill patients.[290] These drugs and the somatostatin analogue, octreotide, have been used with variable success in the treatment of some rare pituitary-induced thyrotoxicoses.[375,376] When measurements of the basal or stimulated serum TSH levels are used in the differential diagnosis of primary and secondary hypothyroidism, the concomitant use of drugs with dopamine-agonistic or -antagonistic activity should be taken into account in the interpretation of results.

NONTHYROIDAL DISEASES

Abnormalities of thyroid function are often detected in patients known to have another disease. Two reasons can be given to explain this occurrence: (1) a direct effect of the nonthyroidal illness mediated through stress, metabolic changes, specific organ involvement or the use of drugs; and (2) a true association between the nonthyroidal illness and primary thyroid disease due to a common etiologic mechanism or a coincidental occurrence for other reasons. This section is devoted to the influence of a variety of nonthyroidal diseases on thyroid economy, the association between primary thyroid diseases and other diseases being covered in greater detail in Chapters 7, 9, and 10. However, it should be emphasized that this distinction can at times be nebulous.

General Aspects

Nonthyroidal illnesses may affect the thyroid economy at all levels, including hormone secretion, transport, and metabolism. The most remarkable and consistent alterations common to most disease processes are those involving thyroid hormone transport and the pathways of its metabolism. Common to most acute and chronic systemic illnesses is a profound diminution in serum T_3 concentration that, on occasion, may fall to levels undetectable by routine clinical assays (less than 20 ng/dl). It is this finding and the apparent lack of symptoms and signs compatible with hypothyroidism that gave rise to the popular terms *low T_3 syndrome* and *euthyroid sick syndrome*. These appellations are rather unfortunate. The former, which describes the observation of decreased serum T_3 concentration, does not take into account the possibility that hormone levels in tissues may not be as profoundly decreased or that the intracellular T_3 concentration could be appropriate for concomitant changes in its tissue receptor density. The term *euthyroid sick* implies that the patient is functionally hormone sufficient. Yet, many patients exhibit various signs suggestive of hyper- or hypometabolism. Whether these metabolic changes are thyroid hormone dependent is debatable, although current beliefs ascribe to alterations of thyroid hormone the function of energy conservation in the face of increased catabolic expenditure imposed by the intercurrent disease process.[69]

The serum T_3 concentration is usually disproportionately low compared to corresponding decreases in the transport proteins and T_4 levels.[354,377–380] In such instances, the absolute level of FT_3 is also diminished. The mechanism responsible for this selective diminution of T_3 in serum has been recently clarified. It is not due to increases in the degradation or disposal rates of T_3 or to a diminution in the fraction contributed by direct thyroidal secretion. Rather, it principally involves the monodeiodinative pathways of hormone degradation by peripheral tissues, with a decrease in the conversion of T_4 to T_3.[378–380] The increase in serum rT_3 concentration, which commonly accompanies low serum T_3 values, is probably due to a delay in its clearance rather than to an enhanced generation from T_4.[354,381,382] This result is in agreement with the finding of diminished 5'-deiodinase activity in animal tissues obtained from experimental disease models.[44,383] The enzyme is responsible not only for the generation of T_3 but also for the further degradation of rT_3. Additional support for this hypothesis is provided by recent observations on the deiodinative degradation of T_3 and rT_3, with the formation of metabolites containing two iodine atoms. More specifically, the rate of generation and the serum concentration of $3,3'$-T_2 are decreased,[246,382] whereas those of $3',5'$-T_2 are maintained.[246] A diagrammatic illustration of the metabolic cascade of T_4 deiodination can be found in Figure 2-20. For the overall description of the normal pathways of sequential deiodination of iodothyronines, see Chapter 3.

As indicated above, a reciprocal increase in serum rT_3 concentration has been observed in almost all clinical circumstances, with significant depression of the T_3 level. A notable exception to this rule is chronic renal failure, where normal rT_3 values have been reported despite a marked depression in the serum T_3 concentration.[246,381,384] Profound and persistent reciprocal changes between serum T_3 and rT_3 concentrations as well as falling T_4 levels have been equated with a worsening prognosis. Notably, delayed recovery from acute febrile illness,[385] progressive liver[386] and kidney[387] failure, the outcome and complications of surgical procedures,[123] the extent of myocardial damage after myocardial infarction,[388] and the degree of metabolic imbalance in diabetic ketoacidosis[389,390] have all been correlated with the magnitude of the changes in circulating levels of these thyronines. Conversely, reversal to normal appears to accompany clinical improvement.

The monodeiodinative degradation is not the only pathway of thyroid hormone metabolism to be perturbed in nonthyroidal illnesses. Indeed, the nondeiodinative pathway of T_4 degradation can be markedly increased. Estimates made in diabetic patients in Pittman's laboratory[380] indicate an increase to 47 percent from the normal 23 percent (Fig. 5-6). This route of hormone disposal includes oxidative deamination and decarboxylation to yield Tetrac and Triac, as well as conjugation and fecal loss.

Hormonal production and secretion by the thyroid gland remain normal or reduced in nonthyroidal illness. This finding may appear surprising considering that one of the main degradative pathways of the principal product of hormonal secretion, T_4, is inhibited. An increase in the rates of alternative pathways of T_4 degradation seems to be responsible for the maintenance of a normal disposal and thus production rate. Kinetic studies indicate a slight increase in the T_4 clearance rate, a diminution in serum T_4 concentration, and the absolute degradation rate of both T_4 and T_3 are typically reduced (Table 5-5).[379,391] In liver cirrhosis, T_4 degradation is also depressed. In turn, the production rate of T_4 is also decreased, thus stabilizing its concentration in serum.[392,393] Increased T_4 production rates have been observed in disorders associated with excessive hormone losses. Significant amounts of protein-bound hormone can be lost in patients suffering from nephrotic syndrome or protein-losing enteropathy.[394,395]

From the foregoing discussion, it is anticipated that under conditions of normal secretion, thyroidal RAIU should also be normal. Unfortunately, this is not always the case in patients with nonthyroidal illness. The RAIU may be increased due to iodine deficiency caused by nutritional factors or delayed renal clearance of the administered isotope in patients with impaired renal function or congestive heart fail-

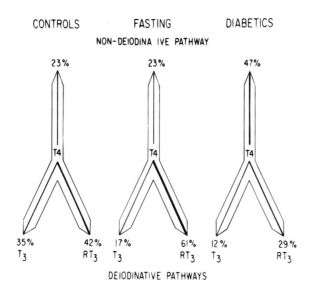

Fig. 5-6. Nondeiodinative and monodeiodinate (conversion to T_3 and rT_3) pathways of T_4 disposal in normal fed subjects, during fasting, and in patients with diabetes mellitus. Data are expressed as the percentage of TT_4 disposed. (Reprinted from *Thyroid Today*,[380] with the permission of Travenol Laboratories, Flint Division, Deerfield, Illinois.)

TABLE 5-5. Thyroid Function and T_4 and T_3 Metabolism in Renal Failure

	Normal Control Subjects	Uremic Patients		
		Before Hemodialysis	After Hemodialysis	After Renal Transplantation
Creatinine (mg/dl)	1.0 ± 0.2	10.0 ± 2.3[a]	12.2 ± 3.5[a]	1.6 ± 0.6
TBG capacity (μg T_4/dl)	18.3 ± 5.4	16.4 ± 3.0	16.5 ± 4.0	22.0 ± 6.4
FT_4I	7.1 ± 1.0	7.0 ± 2.4	6.6 ± 1.5	7.8 ± 1.1
TSH (μU/ml)	2.8 ± 1.2	3.2 ± 1.5	2.7 ± 2.5	3.3 ± 2.1
T_4				
Concentration (μg/dl)	6.6 ± 0.9	4.6 ± 0.9	5.9 ± 1.4	6.9 ± 1.6
Turnover rate (%/day)	10.2 ± 0.9	7.0 ± 1.1[b]	9.6 ± 1.9	9.9 ± 2.3
Metabolic clearance rate (liters/day)	1.2 ± 0.2	1.1 ± 0.1	1.4 ± 0.4	1.2 ± 0.3
Disposal (μg/day)	80 ± 9	59 ± 9	81 ± 26	72 ± 12
T_3				
Concentration (ng/dl)	140 ± 7	68 ± 15[a]	83 ± 17[a]	130 ± 16
Metabolic clearance rate (liters/day)	18.6 ± 3.6	14.6 ± 3.0	12.5 ± 3.1[a]	17.9 ± 2.4
Disposal (μg/day)	25.9 ± 4.0	10.1 ± 3.6[a]	10.1 ± 2.3[a]	23.5 ± 5.3
T_4 and T_3 conversion (%)	37.2 ± 5.8	15.7 ± 3.1	12.8 ± 1.7[a]	34.0 ± 15
Thyroidal T_3 secretion (μg/dl)	1.8 ± 1.2	3.7 ± 2.2	1.7 ± 1.1	3.4 ± 3.3

[a] $P < 0.01$ compared to normal subjects.
[b] $P < 0.05$

ure. Conversely, RAIU may be suppressed by iodide excess often due to the administration of iodine-containing drugs or radiologic contrast media, especially when combined with impaired renal excretion. Certain drugs may also suppress the RAIU through their inhibitory effect on TSH secretion.

Nonthyroidal illness is not associated with thyroid gland enlargement. The rule does not apply to patients with renal failure in whom goiter has been reported to occur in one-third to one-half of cases.[379,396] With this exception, the presence of goiter in a patient with nonthyroidal illness should always raise the suspicion of primary thyroid disease.

Abnormalities in thyroid hormone transport due to nonthyroidal illness take two forms: changes in the concentration of hormone carrier proteins in serum and interference with their association with the hormone. Most profound and prompt is a decrease in serum TTR concentration accompanying virtually all nonthyroidal illnesses and noxious insults.[222,397] This decrease has a questionable effect on the overall transport because of the relatively low affinity of TBTR for the hormone. More important, although of lesser magnitude, are the changes in TBG concentration. They have a greater effect on the total and free concentrations of T_4 because the affinity of TBG for T_4 is approximately one order of magnitude greater than that for T_3. Nonthyroidal illnesses are generally associated with minimal to moderate decreases in TBG-binding capacity.[379,385,397] Exceptions to this rule are acute porphyria, lysinuric protein intolerance hypogammaglobulinemia, and infectious hepatitis, which cause increased TBG levels.[398–401] Although increases or decreases in serum TBG concentration may produce proportional changes in the total concentration of T_4 in serum, they should not change the absolute concentration of FT_4, provided the patient is in a steady state and hormonal production and disposal remain unaltered. This finding has been confirmed in patients with inherited TBG abnormalities by measurement of FT_4 using equilibrium dialysis or by estimation of the FT_4I.[235] In general, FT_4 values in patients with a variety of unrelated nonthyroidal illnesses have been reduced or within normal limits. However, changes in either direction have been observed.[402–405] The prevalence of abnormal FT_4 values varies according to the selection of patients, as well as the technique used for the estimation of the FT_4 concentration, and has been reported

to be as high as 25 percent during the admission of patients for acute medical illnesses.[403,405] There is little agreement concerning the proportion of elevated compared to low values, which in some studies have been equally distributed,[405] whereas other studies showed predominantly high[342] or low[403] values. Such discrepancies are mostly attributed to factors related to the method used for the estimation of FT_4.[402–404] Also, on occasion, FT_4 values may be increased far beyond the expected from the moderate reduction in TBG levels. This result has been attributed to the presence of inhibitors of thyroid hormone binding in the serum of patients with nonthyroidal illness.[406–408] Some of these compounds are allegedly of tissue origin leaking from organs of the diseased patient.[408] Others are normal serum constituents that are present in high concentrations under specific conditions. They include FFA[42,211] and a number of substances that may accumulate in uremic serum.[409]

Serum TSH levels are within the normal limits or reduced in nonthyroidal illness. This general statement is made with the knowledge that exceptions exist. However, taking into account the low serum total and free T_3 levels, as well as on occasion low T_4 levels, clear elevations of TSH values would have been anticipated. More usual is the finding of a normal, blunted, or even suppressed TSH response to the administration of TRH.[379,390,410,411] These findings indicate the possibility of either a limited TSH reserve or a diminished sensitivity of the pituitary to the feedback regulation by thyroid hormone. The latter possibility was raised by the results of Maturlo et al.,[412] who found that a further reduction in FT_4 and FT_3 levels failed to increase the serum TSH levels or augment its response to TRH in one-half of their patients with nonthyroidal illness. Another possibility to be considered is that intrapituitary thyroid hormone concentration and their metabolic pathways are regulated independently of other tissues. Supporting data are limited, although in an experimental uremic rat model pituitary T_3 levels were found to be normal despite a marked reduction in total and nuclear liver T_3 content.[413]

The question of whether euthyroidism, or, more precisely, the thyroid hormone-dependent metabolic state, is preserved in nonthyroidal illness despite the occurrence of profound changes in thyroid function remains unanswered. Hypothyroidism may be suggested on the basis of decreased neogenesis of T_3, a thyronine that mediates most, if not all, of the biologic effects of thyroid hormone. Yet, it may be argued that the tissue concentration of the hormone may be appropriate to saturate the decreased number of tissue receptors. Several studies in animals have clearly demonstrated that a variety of diseases and starvation reduce the total binding capacity of the nuclear T_3 receptors.[62,63,413–416] Because serum TSH levels are clearly elevated in patients with even subclinical hypothyroidism, the failure to observe not only an elevation in the basal TSH value in patients with nonthyroidal illness but also the lack of an augmented TSH response to TRH has been advanced as the ostensible evidence that such patients are indeed euthyroid. This observation is far from constituting proof since it is known that nonthyroidal illness may suppress the secretion of TSH even inpatients with documented primary hypothyroidism.[417] It appears clear that to define the thyroid status of sick patients, one should turn to the assessment of the metabolic state. Unfortunately, direct observations made in patients with nonthyroidal illnesses are complicated by lack of precise methods for dissociating the metabolic effects dependent upon the action of thyroid hormone from those mediated by other factors related to nonthyroidal illness. Work with experimental animal models is plagued by the same inherent difficulties. Some indications suggesting diminished thyroid hormone effect in peripheral tissues have been obtained.[418] Currently, the most popular theory is based on studies carried out during starvation (see the section on starvation and fasting) and on teleologic considerations. It suggests that the diminished provision of biologically active thyroid hormone and the absence of a compensatory stimulation of hormone secretion serve the purpose of energy conservation in the face of increased metabolic demands imposed upon the diseased organism. Thus, at the present time, no answer can be provided to the ultimate question posed by the clinician: Should patients with nonthyroidal illnesses be supplemented with thyroid hormone?

A review of the possible mechanisms responsible for the observed alterations of thyroid function in nonthyroidal illness would be incomplete without mentioning the contribution of extraneous and unrelated factors that may affect the overall picture. There is no question that severe chronic illnesses are usually associated with nutritional deficiencies. A number of elemental compounds have a direct ef-

fect on the thyroid. Furthermore, calorie deprivation, in particular lack of carbohydrates, produces changes in thyroid function quite similar to those observed in nonthyroidal illness. The effects of nonspecific stress also must not be overlooked. These effects have been covered in the preceding sections of this chapter. Patients often receive drugs that affect the hypothalamic-pituitary-thyroid axis as well as hormone metabolism. Those drugs used with greater frequency and most likely to affect the economy of the thyroid are also covered in the preceding sections of this chapter. Their contribution should be taken into account in the assessment of patients. Finally, aging seems to affect most aspects of thyroid function[419,420]; for example, serum T_3 levels decline with age. However, the validity of this observation has been questioned since the prevalence of nonthyroidal illnesses also increases with advancing age.[421,422] The same argument may be applied to those studies that have reported changes with age in the control and secretion of TSH.

The diagnostic implications concerning thyroid function in acute and chronic nonthyroidal illnesses can be summarized as follows. Normal serum T_3 levels do not exclude the possibility of thyrotoxicosis (T_4 toxicosis). Primary hypothyroidism of a mild to moderate degree cannot be ruled out on the basis of normal basal or TRH-stimulated TSH levels. In the absence of gross alterations in TBG concentration, measurement of the serum T_4 level and its free fraction are more useful indices in the diagnosis of concurrent hyper- or hypothyroidism. The distinction between nonthyroidal illness and true hypothyroidism may be aided by the serum rT_3 value. The level of thyroid gland activity cannot be evaluated by the RAIU test in patients who have recently received iodine containing contrast media or drugs, under conditions of iodine deficiency, or in patients with impaired excretory function due to renal failure. The clinician should be familiar with the effects of drugs and other chemical agents that may interfere with individual tests of thyroid function.

The aim of the preceding discussion was to review in its broadest sense the effects of nonthyroidal illness on various aspects of thyroid function. It should, however, be emphasized that each disease process may not only produce different changes within the general framework described above but may also give rise to distinct and unique alterations in a particular aspect of the thyroid system. These changes are presented in the following section.

Specific Illnesses

Liver Disease

Since the liver plays several different and important roles in thyroid economy, liver diseases may not only manifest more severe changes common to other nonthyroidal illnesses but may also show aberrations unique to the involvement of this organ. The alterations in thyroid function are dependent upon the degree of liver cell damage and the type of pathology.

The liver is the site of synthesis of all thyroid hormone-binding proteins and is responsible for removal of the desialylated product of TBG degradation.[423,424] Decreases in serum TBG and TTR concentrations have been observed in hepatic cirrhosis,[392,397] but these changes may be variable. Consequently, serum T_4 concentrations may be normal,[378,410] but more likely slightly decreased.[397] In marked contrast, infectious hepatitis causes an increase in the serum TBG level.[401] For this reason, serum T_4 levels are also elevated, and in contrast to patients with cirrhosis or other nonthyroidal illnesses, the concentration of T_3 is not depressed.[401]

The liver is also an important organ for T_4 degradation and T_3 neogenesis, and is perhaps the organ from which an important proportion of the circulating T_3 is derived. It is thus not surprising that serum T_3 is reduced in proportion to the extent of hepatic damage,[377,378,386,410] and a significant reduction correlates with a poor prognosis.[386,410] The concentration of rT_3 in serum is increased.[377,381] Among a variety of nonthyroidal illnesses studies, hepatic failure is probably unique for the finding of reduced T_4 turnover and production rate.[392,393] Undoubtedly, impairment of the nondeiodinative pathways of T_4 disposal through deamination, decarboxylation, conjugation, and biliary excretion are in part responsible, since reduction in the deiodinative conversion of T_4 to T_3 from a normal of 35.7 percent to 15.6 percent[378] is no greater than that observed in other nonthyroidal illnesses.[379,380]

Another distinction between patients with other nonthyroidal illnesses and those with liver disease is the finding that the latter may have elevated serum TSH levels[378] and no blunting of the TSH responses to TRH.[378,410] The RAIU is frequently elevated in patients with hepatic cirrhosis, but the uptake falls to normal during prolonged hospitalization.[425] This phenomenon may occur because the patients are often placed on diets deficient in iodide, which is repleted by the inpatient treatment.

Hepatic failure produces tremor, weight loss, and weakness, and may be accompanied by tachycardia an, more rarely, proptosis. These findings, combined with the abnormalities in liver function that may accompany thyrotoxicosis (see Ch. 10), can present a diagnostic dilemma. To complicate matters further, there is a propensity for patients with chronic active hepatitis and primary biliary cirrhosis to develop hypothyroidism, which may also give rise to abnormalities in liver function (see Ch. 9). The hypothyroidism is due to the increased prevalence of Hashimoto's thyroiditis in patients with autoimmune liver diseases.[426,427]

Kidney Disease

The alterations in thyroid function observed in patients with renal disease cover a wide and varied spectrum. This fact is probably related to the severity and duration of impaired renal function, as well as to the type of pathology and mode of treatment. Also, because the kidney is the main organ that competes with the thyroid in the clearance of plasma iodide, alterations specifically related to this function, and not usually encountered with other nonthyroidal illnesses, are anticipated.

With severe impairment of renal function, a decrease in serum T_3 concentration, common to other nonthyroidal illnesses, is observed.[377,379,384,411] It is apparently not due to the contribution of the kidney to the overall deiodinative process, since anephric patients do not demonstrate a more profound decrease in their serum T_3 level.[379] Rather, as in other nonthyroidal illnesses, the rate of conversion of T_4 to T_3 is decreased.[379] We found it to be in average 13 percent as compared to 37 percent in normal control persons. Chronic hemodialysis did not product a significant improvement, but successful renal transplantation reversed the process to normal[379] (Table 5-5).

In contrast to other nonthyroidal illnesses, and probably unique to uremia, serum rT_3 levels do not show an increase reciprocal to the diminished T_3

concentration. In general, serum rT_3 levels have been found to be normal.[381,384]

No impairment in the turnover rate of T_4 has been demonstrated,[379] and total serum T_4 values have been normal[428,429] or slightly diminished.[379] Frank decreases in serum T_4 levels[377,411,430] are probably the consequence of a general deterioration in the clinical state.[387] Serum TBG levels are also usually normal[430] or slightly decreased.[379,431] The latter finding concurs with the levels of TT_4.[379] In this context, patients suffering from the nephrotic syndrome form a separate group. TT_4 and TBG concentrations in serum may be low due to urinary losses associated with proteinuria.[432] In fact, as much as one-third to three-fourths of the T_4 normally secreted by the thyroid may be lost through this route.[394,395] These findings do not appear to represent a uniform feature in patients with the syndrome. The correlation between the degree of hypothyroxinemia, proteinuria, and urinary T_4 loss suggests that they are dependent upon the severity of the nephrotic syndrome.[394]

Estimations of the FT_4 levels in patients with renal failure by equilibrium dialysis or indirectly by the FT_4I are either normal[379,411,429,431] or slightly decreased.[387,430] When the values clearly deviate from normal, and especially when they are found to be elevated, the presence of inhibitors or competitors of T_4 binding to serum proteins should be suspected. Heparin, used during hemodialysis as an anticoagulant, may be responsible.[232,233] Furthermore, substances such as phenols, indoles, and urea, which are found in excess in the serum of patients with uremia, have been shown to inhibit T_4 binding to proteins.[409]

With a few exceptions, most data indicate that serum TSH values in uremic patients are within the normal range.[379,387,429,430] The typical TSH response to TRH is blunted (decreased and delayed).[379,411] The delay may be due to decreased urinary clearance of either substances. Thus, it is unlikely that abnormalities in TSH are responsible for the changes in thyroidal RAIU often encountered in patients with impaired renal function. Because of reduced renal clearance, serum iodide may be elevated as much s 10-fold.[433] The rate of thyroidal RAI clearance is secondarily depressed, giving rise to a low RAIU at 2, 4, and 24 hours after the administration of the isotope. Ultimately, due to delayed renal clearance, the RAIU may rise to levels above normal at 36 and 48 hours.[379,433] The absolute

RAIU by the thyroid is increased, and the patients are in positive iodide balance.[433] The results of these kinetic studies of iodine have been confirmed by the finding of increased intrathyroidal iodine content measured directly by fluorescent scanning.[379]

Another unusual finding, not common to other nonthyroidal illnesses, is the presence of goiter in one-third to one-half of patients with chronic renal failure.[379,396] The cause is unknown, but autoimmune disease of the thyroid does not appear to be involved since no thyroid autoantibodies have been detected.[379] Experimental work in the rat implicates the excess iodine and other goitrogens, such as fluoride, which could be absorbed during hemodialysis.[434]

Successful renal transplantation results in normalization of all abnormalities of thyroid function, with the exception of the response to TRH.[379,431] Persistent blunting is probably directly related to the use of glucocorticoids to suppress graft rejection. Chronic hemodialysis produces little or no change.[379,430]

The question of whether the impairment of thyroid function gives rise to hypothyroidism is particularly pertinent in patients with chronic renal failure. The clinical appearance of pallor, puffy face, dry skin, and weakness, with complaints of fatigue and constipation, are suggestive of this diagnosis. In addition, nephrotic patients have edema and hyperlipidemia, uremic children may show growth and bone retardation, and deep tendon reflexes may be sluggish due to neuropathy. Assessment of the metabolic status through a number of nonspecific tests suggested to Spector et al.[429] that uremic patients are euthyroid. Experimental evidence for the presence of hypothyroidism at the peripheral tissue level was found in a uremic rat model.[413,418] The reduction in the serum T_3 level was associated with concomitant decreases in whole liver and nuclear T_3 content and nuclear T_3 receptor-binding capacity, but not in affinity, and the activities of two thyroid hormone-dependent liver enzymes (α-glycerophosphate dehydrogenase and malic dehydrogenase). These changes were similar to those observed in thyroidectomized animals and were restored to normal by T_3 administration (Fig. 5-7). The same animals had normal intrapituitary T_3 content, which explains the failure to observe TSH elevation despite low serum and liver T_3 concentrations. Since these abnormalities were not observed in control animals given the same food, factors other than nutrition must contrib-

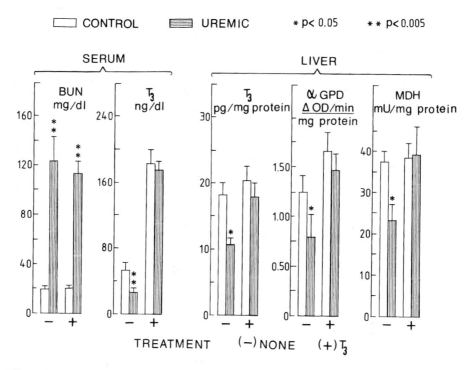

Fig. 5-7. Effect of uremia on T_3 and liver enzymes and the response to T_3 treatment. Six weeks after partial nephrectomy, low serum and liver T_3 concentrations were accompanied by a decrease in the activities of two thyroid hormone-dependent liver enzymes, α-glycerophosphate dehydrogenase (αGPD) and malate dehydrogenase (MDH). T_3 replacement (0.4 μg/100 g body weight/day) for four weeks corrected the T_3 deficiency and low enzyme activities in the liver of the uremic rats without altering the severity of azotemia. Values are expressed in terms of mean ± SEM.

ute to the observed changes in hormone metabolism and its tissue distribution.

Diabetes Mellitus

Although test results of thyroid function in well-controlled diabetics are within the normal range,[380,435] the high prevalence of this illness and the common occurrence of poor control give it an important place among nonthyroidal illnesses likely to cause alterations in thyroid function. When such abnormalities occur in diabetics, they show, in common with other nonthyroidal illnesses, a decreased serum T_3 concentration, with a reciprocal increase in the rT_3 level.[389,436] These changes are secondary to alterations in the relative rates of thyronine metabolism through normal pathways, which can be elicited even in the absence of clear abnormalities in their concentration in serum.[435,437] Detailed studies in Pittman's laboratory have demonstrated a decrease in the rates of T_4 conversion to both T_3 and rT_3, as well as a

decrease in the metabolic clearance rate of both triiodothyronines. This global inhibition of T_4 monodeiodination without a proportional decrease in the overall clearance of T_4 suggested a marked increase in the alternative nondeiodinative pathway of T_4 disposal (Fig. 5-6). This finding contrasts to changes in thyronine metabolism observed during fasting and other nonthyroidal diseases so far studied. In fasting, the nondeiodinative pathway of T_4 degradation remains unaltered, whereas the decrease of T_4 to T_3 conversion is compensated for by an increase in the generation of rT_3.[380]

A large number of studies have documented the expected changes in serum iodothyronine, albeit often of moderate degree. These alterations correlated well with the level of fasting glucose,[435] the magnitude of metabolic imbalance,[389,390] and the degree of hyperglycemia after insulin withdrawal.[438] The opposite correlation between glucose and levels of triiodothyronines in starvation is far from being

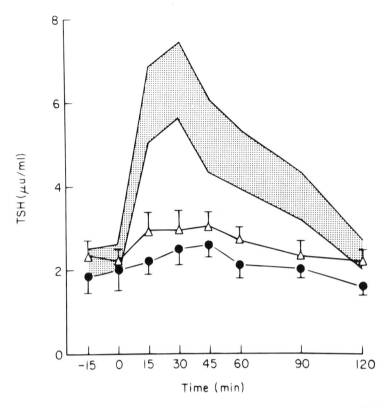

Fig. 5-8. Serum TSH concentrations in response to the intravenous administration of 200 μg TRH during ketoacidosis *(circles)* and five days after full recovery *(triangles)*. Values are expressed in terms of mean $\pm$ SEM, and stippled area represents the responses of normal controls. (From Naeije et al,[390] with permission.)

contradictory to the observations made in diabetics since reduced glucose use is a common feature in both conditions. There is a possibility of an independent effect of insulin, perhaps stress induced, since it lowers the serum T_3 level during hypoglycemia.[439]

In addition to the abnormalities of thyroid hormone metabolism, diabetes mellitus affects the function of the pituitary and thyroid glands. However, evidence for the existence of such defects has been obtained only in patients during ketoacidosis or in experimental animals. The TSH response to TRH is almost completely abolished in ketoacidosis[390] (Fig. 5-8), and the serum TRH concentration but not the hypothalamic content is reduced in the diabetic rat.[440] Administration of exogenous TSH does not correct the impaired hormonal secretion by the thyroid gland of the diabetic mouse.[441]

Most of the abnormalities of thyroid function observed in diabetic men have been confirmed in the rat with streptozotocin induced diabetes mellitus. The decreased concentration of serum T_4 and T_3 can

be corrected with insulin treatment.[442] A decrease in the conversion of T_4 to T_3 similar to that observed during starvation has been shown in vitro using liver slices, but alterations in the sulfhydryl content in tissues could not be demonstrated,[380] suggesting a specific reduction or inhibition of the conversion of rT_3 to $3,3'-T_2$ and of $3',5'-T_2$ to $3'-T_1$.[383] Reduced maximal binding capacity but not affinity of the nuclear T3-binding receptor has been reported in the lung and liver of diabetic rats.[415,416]

Finally, it should be remembered that altered thyroid function in diabetes is likely to be due to primary hypothyroidism because of the association between Hashimoto's thyroiditis and diabetes mellitus. Reported figures for the prevalence of primary hypothyroidism in diabetes range from 4 to 17 percent.[442,444]

Myocardial Infarction

The changes in thyroid function observed in myocardial infarction can be taken as an example of effects of an acute illness combined with stress and accentu-

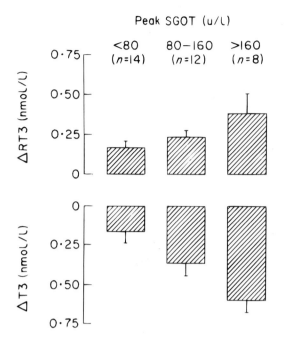

Fig. 5-9. Changes in serum rT_3 and T_3 concentrations after myocardial infarction as a function of the extent of myocardial damage. Maximal increments ($\Delta rT;3$) and decrements (ΔT_3) calculated from the values obtained on the 14th day postinfarction are divided into three groups according to the peak serum glutamic oxaloacetic transaminase (SGOT) levels used as an estimate of the infarct size. Values are means ± SEM. (From Wiersinga et al,[477] with permission.)

ated by caloric restriction and the use of drugs (amiodarone, propranolol, and glucocorticoids). The principal perturbation is an inhibition of the 5'-deiodination of thyronines, which results in a decrease in T_3 and an increase in rT_3 concentrations.[354,445] Further in the deiodinative cascade, a decrease in $3,3'-T_2$ and an increase in the $3',5'-T_2$ levels occur.[354] Changes in serum T_4 concentration are minimal, with values reported as normal,[354,388] slightly decreased,[445] or increased.[446] The last may be due in part to hemoconcentration.[446] The secretion rate of T_4 remains unaltered.[446] Small transient increases in serum TSH concentration have been observed.[388] Although diet and drugs may play a role in the alterations of thyroid function, the acute myocardial insult itself undoubtedly has an effect. In fact, the degree of myocardial injury, as measured by the increases in glutamic-oxaloacetic transminase, correlates with the degree of reciprocal changes in T_3 and rT_3[388] (Fig. 5-9). Also, the magnitude of rT_3 ele-

vation correlated with decreased survival, and a delayed return of the concentration of these triiodothyronines to normal, was associated with a complicated course of the illness.[388,445] More profound changes of thyroid function during the postinfarction period are preceded by higher mean serum cortisol levels.[447]

Infectious and Febrile Illnesses

With minor variations, the general characteristics of the alterations of thyroid function in infectious diseases are similar to those encountered with other nonthyroidal illnesses. Serum T_3 levels are depressed and rT_3 levels increased, probably due to decreased conversion of T_4 to T_3 and clearance of rT_3.[448,449] The levels of serum T_3 and, to a certain extent, those of rT_3 appear to decrease and increase, respectively, with the height of fever in hyperpyrexic patients.[26,385] It is unclear whether body temperature is the principal factor responsible for this relationship, since the clinical severity of the infection also correlates with the height of fever.[385] Furthermore, T_3 levels are as markedly depressed in sepsis associated with hypothermia.[450]

T_4 levels have been found to be normal[24,385] or high,[451] but more commonly reduced.[385,449] More consistent is the finding of increased free fraction and absolute FT_4 concentration,[24,449] probably due to a decrease or interference in binding to TBG.[385,452] The T_4 disappearance rate is accelerated, but secretion is usually decreased.[452,453] Serum TSH values are reduced or normal.[385,451] In one study of hypothermic patients, some with sepsis, TSH elevation during the recovery period was associated with survival, whereas persistent suppression was associated with death.[450]

A major role has been attributed to calorie deprivation in the genesis of alterations in thyroid function.[449] Undoubtedly, stress and the resultant increase in cortisol secretion are also contributing factors.

Malignancies

Abnormalities of thyroid function common to other nonthyroidal illnesses occur with advanced malignant diseases and deterioration in the general state of health. Changes specific to particular types of malignancies have also been found. Hepatocellular carcinomas can give rise to increased TBG levels, probably due to concomitant hepatitis. The high incidence of hypothyroidism in patients with lymphoma or Hodgkin's disease is due to thyroid damage as a result of irradiation, probably potentiated by the iodide contrast medium used in the preradiotherapy staging by lymphangiography.[454,455] Trophoblastic tumors produce thyroid-stimulating substances that may cause hyperthyroidism (see Ch. 13). A high incidence of thyroid function abnormalities has been reported in patients with lung cancer. Most of the abnormalities were typical of nonthyroidal illness and were associated with a bad prognosis. Only 3 patients with definite primary hypothyroidism were reported in a group of 204 patients.[456] The alleged association between hypothyroidism and breast cancer appears to be ill founded.[457]

Tumor-bearing rats have decreased thyroidal activity, decreased hormone binding to serum proteins, and enhanced hormonal degradation and clearance, with a resultant decrease in hormone concentration in serum.[414,458]

Anorexia Nervosa

Changes in thyroid function observed in patients with anorexia nervosa are not dissimilar to those found during calorie deprivation, described earlier in this chapter. Associated symptoms and signs may suggest the presence of hypothyroidism. They are dry, cool skin, low body temperature, constipation and amenorrhea in the presence of a low BMR and serum cholesterol level, and prolonged deep tendon reflex relaxation time.[459,460] The low serum T_3 concentration, high rT_3 concentration, and blunted TSH response to TRH[459-461] have a tendency to improve, if not totally normalize, with weight gain.[460,461]

Psychiatric Illnesses

Abnormalities in thyroid function observed on admission of acute psychiatric patients, and their subsequent changes with treatment, are covered in the section on acute mental stress. In depression, serum T_3 concentrations are either normal[259,462] or depressed,[463] but FT_3 values are not changed.[462] Elevations in the rT_3, $3,3'-T_2$, $3',5'-T_2$, and $3'-T_1$ levels, all products of rT_3 degradation, have been reported.[462,464] the nocturnal rise of TSH and its response to TRH are blunted.[463,465] The latter response has been proposed as a test in the differential

diagnosis of depression since it was not observed in schizophrenia.[466] The test may also be useful in predicting a sustained recovery after electroconvulsive therapy. In addition, TRH may stimulate GH release in depression,[465] and is also observed in other nonendocrine diseases including hepatic and renal failure and anorexia nervosa.[467-469]

Illnesses Associated with Increased Prevalence of Thyroid Disease

In a number of diseases, the greater frequency of abnormalities of thyroid function is attributed to an increased prevalence of primary thyroid diseases rather than to an effect of the nonthyroidal illness on thyroid function. The co-occurrence of several organ-specific autoantibodies in some autoimmune diseases is considered to be evidence for the direct involvement of the thyroid gland. Thus, the high prevalence of hypothyroidism in *pernicious anemia, Sjögren syndrome, lupus erythematosus, rheumatoid arthritis,* and *Addison's disease* appears to be due to thyroid destruction caused by Hashimoto's thyroiditis. The same reasoning has been advanced to explain the presence of primary hypothyroidism in patients with *diabetes mellitus, chronic active hepatitis,* and *primary biliary cirrhosis.* Increased prevalence of Hashimoto's thyroiditis, with or without hypothyroidism, has also been observed in some chromosomal abnormalities such as *Turner, Down,* and *Kleinfelter syndromes.* Graves' thyrotoxicosis, also an autoimmune disease, is more prevalent in patients with *myasthenia gravis* and *idiopathic thrombocytopenic purpura.* The association of thyroid diseases with other autoimmune diseases is discussed in Chapter 7.

An increased incidence of goiter and thyrotoxicosis has been reported in patients with *ulcerative colitis* and *regional enteritis.*[470] Children with *celiac disease* and patients with *cerebrotendinous xanthomatosis (cholestanolosis)*[471] may have a propensity to develop mild hypothyroidism.[472] Tangier disease is associated with both hypo- and hyperthyroidism.

Hereditary cystinosis is frequently complicated by thyroid gland atrophy caused by deposition of cystine crystals in thyroid cells.[473] In addition, Bercu et al.[474] have suggested that some patients with cystinosis have pituitary resistance to thyroid hormone.

Pseudohypoparathyroidism is often associated with hypothyroidism. Multiple endocrine gland hyperactivity in the *McCune Albright Syndrome* and *pseudohypo-*

parathyroidism with and without Albright hereditary osteodystrophy are associated with hyperthyroidism and hypothyroidism, respectively. In both instances, the etiology of the defects is mutations in the G-protein α_s which couples the hormone receptors to adenylyl cyclase.[475] In the McCune Albright syndrome, somatic mutations resulting in the substitution of Arg 201 with His or Cys, decrease GTPase activity which leads to the constitutive activation of the G-protein and TSH independent hyperthyroidism. Different germ line mutations reduce coupling of the G-protein to the receptor, resulting in hypothyroidism.

SUMMARY

This chapter considers the effects of various environmental factors, drugs and chemicals, and nonthyroidal diseases on thyroid function.

In animals, cold exposure causes a prompt increase in TSH secretion, which gives rise to thyroid hormone release and leads to thyroid gland hyperplasia. Part of this effect is due to an apparent increase in the need for thyroid hormone by peripheral tissues and to an excessive rate of hormone degradation and excretion. In humans, hypothermia causes a dramatic TSH secretion in the newborn, but this repose is almost totally lost after the first few years of life. Exposure to heat has an opposite effect, although of lesser magnitude. A small seasonal variation in serum thyroid hormone levels that follow this general pattern has been reported.

Simulated altitude and anoxia depress thyroid hormone formation in rats, but in humans serum T_4 and T_3 concentrations, T_4 degradation, and oxygen consumption are at least temporarily augmented by high altitude.

Starvation has a profound effect on thyroid function, causing a decrease in serum T_3 concentration and a reciprocal increase in rT_3 level. These changes are due to a selective inhibition of the 5'-monodeiodination of iodothyronines by peripheral tissues. Reduction in carbohydrate intake rather than total calorie deprivation appears to be the determinant factor. These alterations in thyroid function are believed to reduce the catabolic activity of the organism and thus to conserve energy in the face of decreased calorie intake. Chronic malnutrition is accompanied by similar changes. Overfeeding has opposite although transient effects.

Physical and emotional stresses can have variable and opposite effects. Increased thyroid hormone secretion and serum levels have been observed in stressed animals and in acute psychiatric patients on admission. The physical stress of surgery causes a prompt decrease in the serum T_3 concentration, probably as a consequence of decreased T_3 neogenesis. This effect of surgery cannot be fully explained on the basis of increased adrenocortical activity or calorie deprivation.

Many minerals alter the synthesis of thyroid hormone, mainly through their interference with iodide concentration and binding by the thyroid gland. The action of iodine is only briefly covered here since it is discussed in Chapters 2 and 13. Calcium, nitrate, bromine, rubidium, and fluorine are allegedly goitrogenic. Lithium carbonate, used in the usual doses for the treatment of affective disorders, can produce goiter in susceptible persons. It inhibits iodide binding and hormonal release from the thyroid gland, probably through a synergistic action with iodide.

Numerous dietary goitrogens, including cyanogenic glucosides, thioglucosides, thiocyanate, and goitrin, are present in a wide variety of foods, and are believed to contribute to the occurrence of endemic goiter in some areas of the world.

Monovalent anions such as thiocyanate and perchlorate inhibit iodide transport into the thyroid and cause goiter.

Thionamide drugs such as PTU and the related compound, methimazole, inhibit thyroid peroxidase and thus prevent thyroid hormone synthesis. In addition, PTU but not methimazole inhibits the conversion of T_4 to T_3 in peripheral tissues.

Under appropriate circumstances, sulfonamides, sulfonylureas, salicylamides, resorsinol, amphenone, aminoglutethamide, antipyrine, aminotriazole, amphenidone, 2,3-dimercaptopropanolol, and phenylbutazone have antithyroid action.

A growing list of drugs and diagnostic agents have been found to affect thyroid economy by modulating the regulation of the hypothalamic-pituitary-thyroid axis, as well as by interfering with thyroid hormone transport, metabolism, excretion, and action. Some drugs, such as salicylates, diphenylhydantoin, and glucocorticoids, act at several levels. Several compounds, most notably estrogens, diphenylhydantoin, diazepam, heparin, halophenate, fenclofenac, and some biologically inactive thyroid hormone analogs compete with binding of thyroid hormone to its carrier proteins in serum. The only consequence of drugs affecting hormone transport is a decrease or increase in the concentration of total but not free hormone in serum.

Glucocorticoids, drugs such as propranolol, and amiodarone and some iodinated contrast media, inhibit the extrathyroidal generation of T_3. The result is a decrease in serum T_3 and an increase in rT_3 concentrations, with a slight increase or no change in T_4 values. Thyroid hormone disposal is accelerated by diphenylhydantoin and phenobarbital, which increase several of the pathways of hormone degradation, and by hypolipemic resins, which increase the fecal loss of hormone. Homeostasis is usually maintained by a compensatory increase in thyroid hormone secretion.

Some drugs act through inhibition or stimulation of TSH secretion. Most notable of the former effect are dopamine agonists such as L-dopa and bromocryptine, as well as some α-adrenergic blockers, glucocorticoids, acetylsalicylic acid, and opiates. A variety of dopamine antagonists as well as cimetidine, clomifene, and spirolactone appear to increase TSH secretion. These compounds seem to interfere with the normal dopaminergic suppression of the hypothalamic-pituitary axis. Observed changes in TSH secretion are not associated with significant metabolic alterations. Some of the drugs have an apparent effect on TSH secretion through changes induced at the levels of the free and active forms of the thyroid hormone. A handful of drugs appear to block or antagonize the action of thyroid hormone on tissues. These drugs include guanethidine, propranolol, and dinitrophenol.

Nonthyroidal illnesses induce important transient or sustained effects on thyroid function. Some of the alterations may be due in part to stress, poor nutrition, and medications, all inevitable companions of patients with severe acute or chronic illnesses. Others are a direct consequence of the systemic illness or specific organ involvement. The typical pattern comprises decreased T_3 and increased rT_3 concentrations in serum and a suppressed TSH response to TRH, with only a minimal downward trend for serum T_4 and TBG concentrations. The magnitude of these changes appears to correlate with the severity of the illness and the extent of tissue insult, and is usually indicative of a poor prognosis. Yet, it has been suggested that these changes in thyroid function serve the purpose of conserving energy by a diminished provision of biologically active thyroid hormone in order to compensate for the increased metabolic demands imposed by the disease. Evidence suggesting euthyroidism despite a profound decrease in serum T_3 concentration, as well as for hypothyroidism, have been advanced. However, no definite conclusions can be drawn concerning the wisdom of thyroid hormone supplementation.

Some diseases do not follow the general pattern of thyroid hormone alterations associated with nonthyroidal illnesses. For example, TBG concentration may be elevated rather than depressed in infectious hepatitis; rT_3 levels are not diminished in chronic renal failure; total and free T_4 and/or T_3 levels may be high during acute psychiatric decompensation; and TSH secretion may be augmented rather than depressed in patients with liver cirrhosis. Thus, caution should be exercised in interpreting laboratory tests of thyroid function and determining the significance of clinical symptoms and signs in patients with nonthyroidal illnesses.

The clinician should be thoroughly familiar with the effects of drugs, nonthyroidal illnesses, and other extraneous factors on thyroid function, and these factors should all be considered in the differential diagnosis of primary thyroid disease.

REFERENCES

1. Bernstein G, Oppenheimer JH: Factors influencing the concentration of free and total thyroxine in patients with nonthyroidal disease. J Clin Endocrinol Metab 26:195, 1966
2. Wilber JF, Baum D: Elevation of plasma TSH during surgical hypothermia. J Clin Endocrinol Metab 31:372, 1970
3. Fisher DA, Odell WD: Acute release of thyrotropin in the newborn. J Clin Invest 48:1670, 1969
4. Fisher DA, Oddie TH: Neonatal thyroidal hyperactivity: Response to cooling. Am J Dis Child 107:574, 1964
5. Hershman JM, Read DG, Bailey AL et al: Effect of cold exposure on serum thyrotropin. J Clin Endocrinol Metab 30:430, 1970
6. Nagata H, Izumiyama T, Kamata K et al: An increase of plasma triiodothyronine concentration in man in a cold environment. J Clin Endocrinol Metab 43:1153, 1976
7. Golstein-Golaire J, Van Haelst L, Bruno OD et al: Acute effects of cold on blood levels of growth hormone, cortisol, and thyrotropin in man. J Appl Physiol 29:622, 1970

8. Balsam A, Sexton FC: Increased metabolism of iodothyronines in the rat after short-term cold adaptation. Endocrinology 97:385, 1975

9. Bernal J, Escobar del Rey F: Effect of the exposure to cold on the extrathyroidal conversion of L-thyroxine to triiodo-L-thyronine, and on intramitochondrial α-glycerophosphate dehydrogenase activity in thyroidectomized rats on L-thyroxine. Acta Endocrinol 78:481, 1975

10. DuRuisseau JP: Seasonal variation of PBI in healthy Montrealers. J Clin Endocrinol Metab 25:1513, 1965

11. Smals AGH, Ross HA, Kloppenborg PWC: Seasonal variation in serum T_3 and T_4 levels in man. J Clin Endocrinol Metab 44:998, 1977

12. Panda JN, Turner CW: Effect of thyroidectomy and low environmental temperature (4.4°C) upon plasma and pituitary thyrotrophin in the rat. Acta Endocrinol 54:485, 1975

13. Emerson CH, Utiger RD: Plasma thyrotropin-releasing hormone concentrations in the rat. J Clin Invest 56:1564, 1975

14. Andersson B: Hypothalamic temperature and thyroid action. p. 50. In Brain-Thyroid Relationships, Aba Foundation Study Group 18, 1964

15. Montoya E, Seibel MJ, Wilber JF: Thyrotropin-releasing hormone secretory physiology: studies by radioimmunoassay and affinity chromatography. Endocrinology 96:1413, 1975

16. Szabo M, Frohman LA: Suppression of cold-stimulated thyrotropin secretion by antiserum to thyrotropin-releasing hormone. Endocrinology 101:1023, 1977

17. Hefco E, Krulich L, Illner P, Larsen PR: Effect of acute exposure to cold on the activity of the hypothalamic-pituitary-thyroid system. Endocrinology 97:1185, 1975

18. Jobin M, Ferland L, Coté J, Labrie F: Effect of exposure to cold on hypothalamic TRH activity and plasma levels of TSH and prolactin in the rat. Neuroendocrinology 18:204, 1975

19. Melander A, Rerup C: Studies on thyroid activity in the mouse. Acta Endocrinol 58:202, 1968

20. Yamada T, Kajihara A, Onaya T et al: Studies on acute stimulatory effect of cold on thyroid activity and its mechanism in the guinea pig. Endocrinology 77:968, 1965

21. Balsam A Leppo, LE: Augmentation of the peripheral metabolism of L-triiodothyronine and L-thyroxine after acclimation to cold: Multifocal stimulation of the binding of iodothyronines by tissues. J Clin Invest 53:980, 1974

22. Galton VA, Nisula BC: Thyroxine metabolism and thyroid function in the cold-adapted rat. Endocrinology 85:79, 1969

23. Epstein Y, Udassin R, Sack J: Serum 3,5,3′-triiodothyronine and 3,3′,5′-triiodothyronine concentrations during acute heat load. J Clin Endocrinol Metab 49:677, 1979

24. Ljunggren JG, Klalner G, Tryselius M: The effect of body temperature on thyroid hormone levels in patients with nonthyroidal illness. Acta Med Scand 202:459, 1977

25. O'Malley BP, Davies TJ, Rosenthal FD: TSH responses to temperature in primary hypothyroidism. Clin Endocrinol 13:87, 1980

26. Rastogi GK, Malhotra MS, Srivastava MC et al: Study of the pituitary-thyroid functions at high altitude in man. J Clin Endocrinol Metab 44:447, 1977

27. Moncloa F, Guerra-Garcia R, Subauste C et al: Endocrine studies at high altitude. I. Thyroid function in sea-level natives exposed for two weeks to an altitude of 4,300 meters. J Clin Endocrinol Metab 26:1237, 1966

28. Surks MI, Beckwitt HJ, Chidsey CA: Changes in plasma thyroxine concentration and metabolism, catecholamine excretion, and basal oxygen consumption in man during acute exposure to high altitude. J Clin Endocrinol Metab 27:789, 1967

29. Mulvey PF, Macaione JMR: Thyroidal dysfunction during simulated altitude conditions. Fed Proc 23:1243, 1969

30. Surks MI: Effect of hypoxia and high altitude on thyroidal iodine metabolism in the rat. Endocrinology 78:307, 1966

31. Surks MI: Effect of thyrotropin on thyroidal iodine metabolism during hypoxia. Am J Physiol 216:436, 1969

32. Pazo JH, Houssay AB, Davison TA, Chait RJ: On the mechanism of the thyroid hypertrophy in pinealectomized rats. Acta Physiol Lat Am 18:332, 1968

33. Singh DV, Turner CW: Effect of light and darkness upon thyroid secretion rate and on the endocrine glands of female rats. Proc Soc Exp Biol Med 131:1296, 1969

34. Singh DV, Narang GD, Turner CW: Effect of melatonin and its withdrawal on thyroid hormone secretion rate of female rats. J Endocrinol 43:489, 1969

35. Martino E, Seo H, Lernmark A, Refetoff S: Ontogenetic pattern of thyrotropin-releasing hormone-like material in rat hypothalamus, pancreas, and retina: selective effect of light deprivation. Proc Natl Acad Sci 77:4345, 1980

36. Portnay GI, O'Brian JT, Bush J et al: The effect of starvation on the concentration and binding of thyroxine and triiodothyronine in serum and on the response to TRH. J Clin Endocrinol Metab 39:191, 1974

37. Merimee TJ, Fineberg ES: Starvation-induced alter-

ations of circulating thyroid hormone concentrations in man. Metabolism 25:79, 1976

38. Carlson HE, Drenick EJ, Chopra IJ, Hershman JM: Alterations in basal and TRH-stimulated serum levels of thyrotropin, prolactin, and thyroid hormones in starved obese men. J Clin Endocrinol Metab 45: 707, 1977

39. Azizi F: Effect of dietary composition on fasting-induced changes in serum thyroid hormones and thyrotropin. Metabolism 27:935, 1978

40. Scriba PC, Bauer M, Emmert D et al: Effects of obesity, total fasting, and realimentation on L-thyroxine (T$_4$), 3,5,3'-L-triiodothyronine (T$_3$), 3,3',5'-L-triiodothyronine (rT$_3$), thyroxine binding globulin (TBG), cortisol, thyrotrophin, cortisol binding gloublin (CBG), transferrin, α_2-haptoglobin, and complement C'3 in serum. 91:629, 1979

41. Vagenakis AG, Portnay GI, O'Brian JT et al: Effect of starvation on the production and metabolism of thyroxine and triiodothyronine in euthyroid obese patients. J Clin Endocrinol Metab 45:1305, 1977

42. Suda AK, Pittman CS, Shimizu T, Chambers JB Jr: The production and metabolism of 3,5,3'-triiodothyronine and 3,3',5'-triiodothyronine in normal and fasting subjects. J Clin Endocrinol Metab 47:1311, 1978

43. Stokholm KH: Decrease in serum free triiodothyronine, thyroxine-binding globulin, and thyroxine-binding prealbumin whilst taking a very low-calorie diet. Int J Obest 4:133, 1980

44. Balsam A, Ingbar SH: The influence of fasting, diabetes, and several pharmacologic agents on the pathways of thyroxine metabolism in rat liver. J Clin Invest 62:415, 1978

45. Chopra IJ, Geola F, Solomon DH, Maciel RMB: 3',5'-diiodothyroxine in health and disease: studies by a radioimmunoassay. J Clin Endocrinol Metab 47: 1198, 1978

46. Chopra IJ: A radioimmunoassay for measurement of 3'-monoiodothyronine. J Clin Endocrinol Metab 51:117, 1980

47. Pangaro L, Burman KD, Wartofsky L et al: Radioimmunoassay for 3,5-diiodothyronine and evidence for dependence on conversion from 3,5,3'-triiodothyronine. J Clin Endocrinol Metab 50:1075, 1980

48. Pittman CS, Shimizu T, Burger A, Chambers JB Jr: The nondeiodinative pathways of thyroxine metabolism: 3,5,3',5'-tetraiodothyroacetic acid turnover in normal and fasting human subjects. J Clin Endocrinol Metab 50:712, 1980

49. Balsam A, Ingbar SH: Observations on the factors that control the generation of triiodothyronine from thyroxine in rat liver and the nature of the defect induced by fasting. J Clin Invest 63:1156, 1979

50. Chopra IJ: Alterations in monodeiodination of iodothyronines in the fasting rat: effects of reduced nonprotein sulfhydryl groups and hypothyroidism. Metabolism 29:161, 1980

51. Gavin LA, McMahon FA, Moeller M: Dietary modification of thyroxine deiodination in rat liver is not mediated by hepatic sulfhydryls. J Clin Invest 65: 943, 1980

52. Burman KD, Dimond RC, Harvey GS et al: Glucose modulation of alterations in serum iodothyronine concentrations induced by fasting. Metabolism 28: 291, 1979

53. Danforth E, Sims EAH, Horton ES, Goldman RF: Correlation of serum triiodothyronine concentrations with dietary composition. Diabetes 24:406, 1975

54. Harris ARC, Fang SL, Vagenakis AG, Braverman LE: Effect of starvation, nutriment replacement, and hypothyroidism on in vitro hepatic T$_4$ to T$_3$ conversion in the rat. Metabolism 27:1680, 1978

55. Burger AG, Berger M, Wimpfheimer K, Danforth E: Interrelationships between energy metabolism and thyroid hormone metabolism during starvation in the rat. Acta Endocrinol 93:322, 1980

56. Gardner DF, Kaplan MM, Stanley CA, Utiger RD: Effect of triiodothyronine replacement on the metabolic and pituitary responses to starvation. N Engl J Med 300:579, 1979

57. Silva JE, Dick TE, Larsen PR: The contribution of local tissue thyroxine monodeiodination to nuclear 3,5,3'-triiodothyronine in pituitary, liver, and kidney of euthyroid rats. Endocrinology 103:1196, 1978

58. Cheron RG, Kaplan MM, Larsen PR: Physiologic and pharmacologic influences on thyroxine to 3,5,3'-triiodothyronine conversion and nuclear 3,5,5'-triiodothyronine binding in rat anterior pituitary. J Clin Invest 64:1402, 1979

59. Harris ARC, Fang SL, Azizi F et al: Effect of starvation on hypothalamic-pituitary-thyroid function in the rat. Metabolism 27:1074, 1978

60. Morley JE, Russell RM, Reed A et al: The interrelationship of thyroid hormones with vitamin A and zinc nutritional status in patients with chronic hepatic and gastrointestinal disorders. Am J Clin Nutr 34:1489, 1981

61. Shambaugh GE III, Wilber JF: The effect of caloric deprivation upon thyroid function in the neonatal rat. Endocrinology 94:1145, 1974

62. DeGroot LJ, Coleoni AH, Rue PA et al: Reduced nuclear triiodothyronine receptors in starvation-induced hypothyroidism. Biochem Biophys Res Commun 79:173, 1977

63. Schussler GC, Orlando J: Fasting decreases triiodothyronine receptor capacity. Science 199:686, 1978

64. Buergi V, Larsen PN: Nuclear triiodothyronine binding in mononuclear leukocytes in normal subjects and obese patients before and after fasting. J Clin Endocrinol Metab 54:1199, 1982

65. Jung RT, Shetty PS, James WPT: Nutritional effects on thyroid and catecholamine metabolism. Clin Sci 58:183, 1980

66. Huang HS, Pittman CS: Effects of thyroid hormone evaluated by cardiac systolic time interval in fasted subjects. J Formosan Med Ass 83:1087, 1994

67. Vignati L, Finley RJ, Haag S, Aoki TT: Protein conservation during prolonged fast: a function of triiodothyronine levels. Trans Assoc Am Physicians 16:169, 1978

68. Carter WJ, Shakir KM, Hodges S et al: Effect of thyroid hormone on metabolic adaptation to fasting. Metabolism 24:1177, 1975

69. Wartofsky L, Burman D: Alterations in thyroid function in patients with systemic illness: the "euthyroid sick syndrome." Endocr Rev 3:164, 1982

70. Ingenbleek Y, Malvaux P: Peripheral turnover of thyroxine and related parameters in infant protein-calorie malnutrition. Am J Clin Nutr 33:609, 1980

71. van der Westhuyzen JM: Plasma-T_3 assay in Kwashiorkor. Lancet 2:965, 1973

72. Chopra IJ, Smith SR: Circulating thyroid hormones and thyrotropin in adult patients with protein-calorie malnutrition. J Clin Endocrinol Metab 40:221, 1975

73. Ingenbleek Y, Beckers C: Thyroidal iodide clearance and radioiodide uptake in protein-calorie malnutrition. Am J Clin Nutr 31:408, 1978

74. Pimstone B, Becker D, Hendricks S: TSH response to synthetic thyrotropin-releasing hormone in human protein-calorie malnutrition. J Clin Endocrinol Metab 36:779, 1973

75. Tulp OL, Krupp PP, Danforth E Jr, Horton ES: Characteristics of thyroid function in experimental protein malnutrition. J Nutr 109:1321, 1979

76. Falconer IR, Marchant B: Thyroxine utilization in lambs in natural and controlled environments. J Endocrinol 46:363, 1970

77. Danforth E Jr, Horton ES, O'Connell M et al: Dietary-induced alterations in thyroid hormone metabolism during overnutrition. J Clin Invest 64:1336, 1979

78. Bray GA, Fisher DA, Chopra IJ: Relation of thyroid hormones to body weight. Lancet 1:1206, 1976

79. Glass AR, Burman KD, Dahms WT, Boehm TM: Endocrine function in human obesity. Metabolism 30:89, 1981

80. Filetti S, Rapoport B: Evidence that organic iodine attenuates the adenosine 3′,5′-monophosphate response to thyrotropin. Endocrinology 113:1608, 1983

81. Vagenakis AG, Downs P, Braverman LE et al: Control of thyroid hormone secretion in normal subjects receiving iodides. J Clin Invest 52:528, 1973

82. Vagenakis AG, Rapoport B, Azizi F et al: Hyper-response to thyrotropin-releasing hormone accompanying small decreases in serum thyroid hormone concentration. J Clin Invest 54:913, 1974

83. Braverman LE, Ingbar SH, Vagenakis AG et al: Enhanced susceptibility to iodide myxedema in patients with Hashimoto's disease. J Clin Endocrinol Metab 32:515, 1971

84. Braverman LE, Woeber KA, Ingbar SH: Induction of myxedema by iodide in patients euthyroid after radioiodine or surgical treatment of diffuse toxic goiter. N Engl J Med 281:816, 1969

85. Azizi F, Bentley D, Vagenakis A et al: Abnormal thyroid function and response to iodides in patients with cystic fibrosis. Trans Assoc Am Physicians 87:111, 1974

86. Begg TB, Hall R: Iodide goiter and hypothyroidism. Q J Med 32:351, 1963

87. Pasternak DP, Socolow EL, Ingbar SH: Synergistic interaction of phenazone and iodide on thyroid hormone biosynthesis in the rat. Endocrinology 84:769, 1969

88. Shopsin B, Shenkman L, Blum M, Hollander CS: Iodine and lithium-induced hypothyroidism: documentation of synergism. Am J Med 55:695, 1973

89. Milne K, Greer MA: Comparison of the effects of propylthiouracil and sulfadiazine on thyroidal biosynthesis and the manner by which they are influenced by supplemental iodide. Endocrinology 71:580, 1962

90. Vagenakis AG, Ingbar SH, Braverman LE: The relationship between thyroglobulin synthesis and intrathyroid iodine metabolism as indicated by the effects of cycloheximde in the rat. Endocrinology 94:1669, 1974

91. Jackson AS: Iodine hyperthyroidism: an analysis of fifty cases. Boston Med Surg J 193:1138, 1925

92. Vidor GI, Stewart JD, Wall JR et al: Pathogenesis of iodide induced thyrotoxicosis: studies in northern Tasmania. J Clin Endocrinol Metab 37:901, 1973

93. Ermans AM, Camus M: Modifications of thyroid function induced by chronic administration of iodide in the presence of "autonomous" thyroid tissue. Acta Endocrinol 70:463, 1972

94. Vagenakis AG, Wang CA, Burger A et al: Iodide-induced thyrotoxicosis in Boston. N Engl J Med 287:523, 1972

95. Suzuki H, Higuchi T, Sawa K et al: "Endemic coast goiter" in Hokkaido, Japan. Acta Endocrinol 50:161, 1965

96. Wartofsky L: Low remission after therapy for Graves'

disease: possible relation of dietary iodine with anti-thyroid therapy results. JAMA 226:1083, 1973

97. Boyle JA, Greig WR, Fulton S, Dalakos TG: Excess dietary calcium and human thyroid function. J Endocrinol 34:532, 1966

98. Bloomfield RA, Welsch CW, Garner GB, Muhrer ME: Effect of dietary nitrate on thyroid function. Science 134:1690, 1961

99. Clode W, Sobral JM, Baptista AM: Bromine interference in iodine metabolism and its goitrogenic action. p. 65. In Pitt-Rivers R (ed): Advances in Thyroid Research. Pergamon Press, New York, 1961

100. Bach I, Braun S, Gati T et al: Effect of rubidium on the thyroid. p. 505. In Pitt-Rivers R (ed): Advances in Thyroid Research. Pergamon Press, New York, 1961

101. Galletti PM, Joyet G: Effect of fluorine on thyroidal iodine metabolism in hyperthyroidism. J Clin Endocrinol Metab 18:1102, 1958

102. Gedalia I, Brand N: The relationship of fluoride and iodine in drinking water in the occurrence of goiter. Arch Int Pharmacodyn Ther 142:312, 1963

103. Siddiqui AH: Incidence of simple goiter in areas of endemic fluorosis. J Endocrinol 20:201, 1960

104. Day TK, Powell-Jackson PR: Fluoride water hardness, and endemic goiter. Lancet 1:1135, 1972

105. Paley KR, Sobel ES, Yalow RS: Effect of oral and intravenous cobaltous chloride on thyroid function. J Clin Endocrinol Metab 18:850, 1958

106. Pimentel-Malaussera E, Roche M, Lavrisse M: Treatment of eight cases of hyperthyroidism with cobaltous chloride. JAMA 167:1719, 1958

107. Pousset GB Jr, Berthezene F, Tourniare J, Devic M: Myxoedeme au lithium. Ann Endocrinol 34:549, 1973

108. Berens SC, Bernstein RS, Robbins J, Wolff J: Antithyroid effects of lithium. J Clin Invest 49:1357, 1970

109. Spaulding SW, Burrow GN, Bermudez F, Himmelhoch JM: The inhibitory effect of lithium on thyroid hormone release in both euthyroid and thyrotoxic patients. J Clin Endocrinol Metab 35:905, 1972

110. Carlson HE, Temple R, Robbins J: Effect of lithium on thyroxine disappearance in man. J Clin Endocrinol Metab 36:1251, 1973

111. Burman KD, Diamond RC, Earll JM et al: Sensitivity to lithium in treated Graves' disease: effects on serum T_4, T_3, and reverse T_3. J Clin Endocrinol Metab 43:606, 1976

112. Blomqvist N, Lindstedt G, Lundberg PA, Walinder J: No inhibition by Li^+ of thyroxine monodeiodination to 3,5,3'-triiodothyronine and 3,3',5'-triiodothyronine (reverse triiodothyronine). Clin Chim Acta 79:457, 1977

113. Linquette M, Lefebre J, Van Parys C, Wemeau JL: Le lithium dans le traitement des thyrotoxicoses. Ann d'Endocrinol 39:15, 1978

114. Andersen BF: Iodide perchlorate discharge test in lithium-treated patients. Acta Endocrinol 73:35, 1973

115. Berens SC, Wolff J, Murphy DL: Lithium concentration by the thyroid. Endocrinology 87:1085, 1970

116. Wolff J, Berens SC, Jones AB: Inhibition of thyrotropin-stimulated adenyl cyclase activity of beef thyroid members by low concentration of lithium ion. Biochem Biophys Res Commun 39:77, 1970

117. Bhattacharya B, Wolff J: Stabilization of microtubules by lithium ion. Biochem Biophys Res Commun 73:383, 1976

118. Lazarus JH, Joh R, Bennie EH et al: Lithium therapy and thyroid function: a long-term study. Psych Med 11:85–92, 1981

119. Segal RL, Rosenblatt S, Eliasoph I: Endocrine exophthalmos during lithium therapy of manic-depressive disease. N Engl J Med 289:136, 1973

120. Kracht J: Fright thyrotoxicosis in the wild rabbit, a model of thyrotrophic alarm reaction. Acta Endocrinol 15:355, 1954

121. Falconer IR, Hetzel BS: Effect of emotional stress and TSH on thyroid vein hormone level in sheep with exteriorized thyroids. Endocrinology 75:42, 1964

122. Haibach H, McKenzie JM: Increased free thyroxine postoperatively in the rat. Endocrinology 81:435, 1967

123. Hagenfeldt I, Melander A, Thorell J et al: Active and inactive thyroid hormone levels in elective and acute surgery. Acta Chir Scand 145:77, 1979

124. Chan V, Wang C, Yeung RTT: Pituitary-thyroid responses to surgical stress. Acta Endocrinol 88:490, 1978

125. Socolow EL, Woeber KA, Purdy RH et al: Preparation of ^{131}I-labeled human serum prealbumin and its metabolism in normal and sick patients. J Clin Invest 44:1600, 1976

126. Brandt MR, Skovsted L, Kehlet H, Hansen JM: Rapid decrease in plasma triiodothyronine during surgery and epidural analgesia independent of afferent neurogenic stimuli and of cortisol. Lancet 2:1333, 1976

127. Tingley JO, Morris AW, Hill SR, Pittman JA: The acute thyroid response to emotional stress. Ala J Med Sci 2:297, 1965

128. Cohen KL, Swigar ME: Thyroid-function screening in psychiatric patients. JAMA 242:254, 1979

129. Levy RP, Jensen JB, Laus VG et al: Serum thyroid hormone abnormalities in psychiatric disease. Metabolism 30:1060, 1981

130. Spratt DI, Pont A, Miller MB et al: Hyperthyroxi-

nemia in patients with acute psychiatric disorders. Am J Med 73:41, 1982

131. Chesney AM, Clawson TA, Webster B: Endemic goiter in rabbits. I. Incidence and characteristics. Johns Hospkins Hosp Bull 43:261, 1928

132. Ermans AM, Delange F, Van Der Velden M, Kinthaert J: Possible role of cyanide and thiocyanate in the etiology of endemic cretinism. p. 455. In Stanbury JB, Kroc RL (eds): Human Development and the Thyroid Gland: Relation to Endemic Cretinism. Plenum Press, New York, 1972

133. Monekasso GL, Wilson J: Plasma thiocyanate and vitamin B_{12} in Nigerian patients with degenerative neurological disease. Lancet 1:1062, 1971

134. Delange F, Ermans AM: Role of a dietary goitrogen in the etiology of endemic goiter on Idjwi Island. Am J Clin Nutr 24:1354, 1971

135. Delange F, Thilly C, Ermans AM: Iodine deficiency, a permissive condition in the development of endemic goiter. J Clin Endocrinol Metab 28:114, 1968

136. Langer P, Greer MA: Antithyroid activity of some naturally occurring isothiocyanates in vitro. Metabolism 17:596, 1968

137. Langer P: Antithyroid action in rats of small doses of some naturally occurring compounds. Endocrinology 79:1117, 1966

138. Clements FW, Wishart JW: A thyroid-blocking agent in the etiology of endemic goiter. Metabolism 5:623, 1956

139. Peltola P: The goitrogenic effect of milk obtained from the region of endemic goiter in Finland. p. 10. In Pitt-Rivers R (ed): Advances in Thyroid Research. Pergamon Press, New York, 1961

140. Peltola P, Krusius FE: Effect of cow's milk from the goiter-endemic district of Finland on thyroid function. Acta Endocrinol 33:603, 1960

141. Kilpatrick R, Broadhead GD, Edmonds CJ et al: Studies on goiter in the Sheffield region. p. 273. In Pitt-Rivers R (ed): Advances in Thyroid Research. Pergamon Press, New York, 1961

142. Astwood EB, Greer MA, Ettlinger MG: L-5-vinyl-2-thiooaxazolidone, an antithyroid compound from yellow turnip and from bassica seeds. J Biol Chem 181:121, 1949

143. Greer MA: The isolation and identification of progoitrin from bassica seed. Arch Biochem Biophys 99:369, 1962

144. Langer P, Michajlovskij N: Studies on the antithyroid activity of naturally occurring L-5-vinyl-2-thiooxazolidone and its urinary metabolite in rats. Acta Endocrinol 62:21, 1969

145. Krusius FE, Peltola P: The goitrogenic effect of naturally occurring L-5-vinyl- and L-5-phenyl-2-thio-oxazolidone in rats. Acta Endocrinol 53:342, 1966

146. Arstila A, Krusius FE, Peltola P: Studies on the transfer of thio-oxazolidone-type goitrogens into cow's milk in goiter-endemic districts of Finland and in experimental conditions. Acta Endocrinol 60:712, 1969

147. Barzelatto J, Beckers C, Stevenson C et al: Endemic goiter in Pedgregoso (Chile). I. Description and function studies. Acta Endocrinol 54:577, 1967

148. Linazasoro JM, Sanchez-Martin JA, Jiminez-Diaz C: Goitrogenic effect of walnuts. Lancet 2:501, 1966

149. Gaitan E, Wahner HW, Correa P et al: Endemic goiter in the Cauca Valley. I. Results and limitations of twelve years of iodine prophylaxis. J Clin Endocrinol Metab 28:1730, 1968

150. McCarrison R: The goitrogenic action of soybean and ground-nut. Indian J Med Res 21:179, 1933

151. Van Wyk JJ, Arnold MB, Wynn J, Pepper F: The effects of a soybean product on thyroid functions in humans. Pediatrics 24:752, 1959

152. Pinchera A, MacGillivray MH, Crawford JD, Freeman AG: Thyroid refractoriness in an athyrotic cretin fed soybean formula. N Engl J Med 273:83, 1965

153. Yamada T: Effect of fecal loss of thyroxine on pituitary-thyroid feedback control in the rat. Endocrinology 82:327, 1968

154. Bray GA: Increased sensitivity of the thyroid in iodine-depleted rats to the goitrogenic effects of thyrotropin. J Clin Invest 47:1640, 1968

155. Bull GM, Fraser R: Myxedema from resorcinol ointment applied to leg ulcers. Lancet 1:851, 1950

156. Selenkow HA, Rivera A, Thorn GW: The effects of amphenone on thyroid function in man. J Clin Endocrinol Metab 17:1131, 1957

157. Pittman JA, Brown RW: Antithyroid and antiadrenocortical activity of aminoglutethimide. J Clin Endocrinol Metab 26:1014, 1966

158. Rallison ML, Kumagai LF, Tyler FH: Goitrous hypothyroidism induced by aminoglutethmide, anticonvulsant drug. J Clin Endocrinol Metab 27:265, 1967

159. Jukes TH, Shaffer CB: Antithyroid effects of aminotriazole. Science 132:296, 1960

160. Pittman JA, Brown RW: Antithyroid action of amphenidone. J Clin Endocrinol Metab 22:100, 1962

161. Current JV, Hales IB, Dobyns BM: The effect of 2,3-dimercaptopropanol (BAL) on thyroid function. J Clin Endocrinol Metab 20:13, 1960

162. Sharpe AR Jr. Inhibition of thyroidal ^{131}I uptake by parabromdylamine maleate. J Clin Endocrinol Metab 21:739, 1961

163. Linsk JA, Paton BC, Persky M et al: Asaacs M, Kupperman HS. The effect of phenylbutazone and a related analogue (G25671) upon thyroid function. J Clin Endocrinol Metab 17:416, 1957

164. Wyngaarden JB, Stanbury JB, Rapp B: The effects

of iodide, perchlorate, thiocyanate, and nitrate administration upon the iodide-concentrating mechanism of the rat thyroid. Endocrinology 52:568, 1953

165. Ermans AM, Goossens F: Influence du perchlorate et du methimazol sur l'excretion urinaire de l'iode chez l'homme. Arch Int Pharmacodyn Ther 132:487, 1961

166. Stewart RDH, Murray IPC: An evaluation of the perchlorate discharge test. J Clin Endocrinol Metab 26:1050, 1966

167. Scranton JR, Nissen WM, Halmi NS: The kinetics of the inhibition of thyroidal iodide accumulation by thiocyanate: a reexamination. Endocrinology 85:603, 1969

168. Frohman LA, Klocke FJ: Recurrent thiocyanate intoxication, with pancytopenia, hypothyroidism, and psychosis. N Engl J Med 268:701, 1963

169. Taurog A, Potter GD, Chaikoff IL: Conversion of inorganic ^{131}I to organic ^{131}I by cell-free preparations of thyroid tissue. J Biol Chem 213:119, 1955

170. Anbar M, Guttman S, Lewitus Z: Effect of monofluorosulphanate, difluorophosphate, and F borate ions on the iodine uptake of the thyroid gland. Nature 183:1517, 1959

171. Anbar M, Guttman S, Lewitus Z: The accumulation of fluoroborate ions in thyroid glands of rats. Endocrinology 66:888, 1960

172. Chow SY, Chang LR, Yen MS: A comparison between the uptakes of radioactive perchlorate and iodide by rat and guinea pig thyroid glands. J Endocrinol 45:1, 1969

173. Crooks J, Wayne EJ: A comparison of potassium perchlorate, methylthiouracil, and carbimazole in the treatment of thyrotoxicosis. Lancet 1:401, 1960

174. Michajlovskij N, Langer P: Increase of serum free thyroxine following the administration of thiocyanate and other anions in vivo and in vitro. Acta Endocrinol 75:707, 1974

175. Rosenberg IN: The antithyroid activity of some compounds that inhibit peroxidase. Science 116:503, 1952

176. DeGroot LJ, Davis AM: Studies on the biosynthesis of iodotyrosines: a soluble thyroidal iodide-peroxidase tyrosine-iodinase system. Endocrinology 70:492, 1962

177. Yamazaki E, Noguchi A, Slingerland DW: Effect of methylthiouracil and iodide on the iodinated constituents of thyroid tissue in Graves' disease. J Clin Endocrinol Metab 20:889, 1960

178. Iino S, Yamada T, Greer MA: Effect of graded doses of propylthiouracil on biosynthesis of thyroid hormones. Endocrinology 68:582, 1961

179. Mulvey PF Jr, Slingerland DW: The in vitro stimulation of thyroidal activity by propylthiouracil. Endocrinology 70:7, 1962

180. Selenkow HA, Collaco FM: Clinical pharmacology of antithyroid compounds. Clin Pharmacol Ther 2:191, 1961

181. Astwood EB: Mechanisms of action of various antithyroid compounds. Ann NY Acad Sci 50:419, 1949

182. Maloff F, Spector L: The desulfuration of thiourea by thyroid cytoplasmic particulate fractions. J Biol Chem 234:949, 1959

183. Maloof F, Soodak M: Cleavage of disulfide bonds in thyroid tissue by thiourea. J Biol Chem 236:1689, 1961

184. Mitchell ML, Sanchez-Martin JA, Harden AB, O'Rourke ME: Failure of thiourea to prevent hormone synthesis by the thyroid gland of man and animals treated with TSH. J Clin Endocrinol Metab 21:157, 1961

185. Mayberry WE, Astwood EB: The effect of propylthiouracil on the intrathyroid metabolism of iodine in rats. J Biol Chem 235:2977, 1960

186. Escobar del Rey F, Morreale de Escobar G: The effect of propylthiouracil, methylthiouracil, and thiouracil on the peripheral metabolism of L-thyroxine in thyroidectomized L-thyroxine maintained rats. Endocrinology 69:456, 1961

187. Van Middlesworth L, Jones SL: Interference with deiodination of some thyroxine analogs in the rat. Endocrinology 69:1085, 1961

188. Escobar del Rey F, Morreale de Escobar G, Garcia-Garcia MD, Mouriz Garcia J: Increased secretion of thyrotrophic hormone in rats with a depressed peripheral deiodination of thyroid hormone and a normal or high plasma PBI. Endocrinology 71:859, 1962

189. Slingerland DW, Burrows BA: Inhibition by propylthiouracil of the peripheral metabolism of radiothyroxine. J Clin Endocrinol Metab 22:511, 1962

190. Furth ED, Rives K, Becker DV: Nonthyroidal action of propylthiouracil in euthyroid, hypothyroid, and hyperthyroid man. J Clin Endocrinol Metab 26:239, 1966

191. Oppenheimer JH, Schwartz HL, Surks MI: Propylthiouracil inhibits the conversion of L-thyroxine to L-triiodothyronine: An explanation of the antithyroxine effect of propylthiouracil and evidence supporting the concept that triiodothyronine is the active hormone. J Clin Invest 51:2493, 1972

192. Stasilli NR, Kroc RL, Edlin R: Selective inhibition of the calorigenic activities of certain thyroxine analogues with chronic thiouracil treatment in rats. Endocrinology 66:872, 1960

193. Bray GA, Hildreth S: Effect of propylthiouracil and methimazole on the oxygen consumption of hypothyroid rats receiving thyroxine or triiodothyronine. Endocrinology 81:1018, 1967

194. Ruegamer WR, Warren JS, Barstow M, Beck W: Effects of thiouracil on rat liver alpha-glycerophosphate dehydrogenase and serum PBI responses to L-thyroxine. Endocrinology 81:277, 1967

195. Chopra IJ, Solomon DH, Chopra U et al: Pathways of metabolism of thyroid hormones. Recent Prog Horm Res 34:521, 1978

196. Pittman JA, Beschi RJ, Smitherman TC: Methimazole: its absorption and excretion in man and tissue distribution in rats. J Clin Endocrinol Metab 33:182, 1971

197. Marchant B, Alexander WD, Lazarus JH et al: The accumulation of ^{35}S antithyroid drugs by the thyroid gland. J Clin Endocrinol Metab 34:847, 1972

198. Krieger DT, Moses A, Ziffer H et al: Effect of acetazoleamide on thyroid metabolism. Am J Physiol 196:291, 1959

199. Gabrilove JL, Alvarez AA, Soffer LJ: Effect of acetazoleamide (Diamox) on thyroid function. J Appl Physiol 13:491, 1958

200. Brown J, Solomon DH: Mechanism of antithyroid effects of a sulfonylurea in the rat. Endocrinology 63:473, 1958

201. Tranquade RE, Solomon DH, Brown J, Greene R: The effect of oral hypoglycemic agents on thyroid function in the rat. Endocrinology 67:293, 1960

202. Nikkilä EA, Jakobson T, Josipii SG, Karlsson K: Thyroid function in diabetic patients under long-term sulfonylurea treatment. Acta Endocrinol 33:623, 1960

203. Skinner NS Jr, Hayes RL, Hill SR Jr: Studies on the use of chlorpropamide in patients with diabetes mellitus. Ann NY Acad Sci 74:830, 1959

204. Hunton RB, Wells MV, Skipper EW: Hypothyroidism in diabetics treated with sulphonylurea. Lancet 2:449, 1965

205. Hershman JM, Konerding K: Effects of sulfonylurea drugs on the thyroid and serum protein binding of thyroxine in the rat. Endocrinology 83:74, 1968

206. Azizi F, Vagenakis AG, Portnay GI et al: Thyroxine transport and metabolism in methadone and heroin addicts. Ann Intern Med 80:194, 1974

207. McKerron CG, Scott RL, Asper SP, Levy RI: Effects of clofibrate (Atromid S) on the thyroxine-binding capacity of thyroxine-binding globulin and free thyroxine. J Clin Endocrinol Metab 29:957, 1969

208. Beex L, Ross A, Smals P, Kloppenborg P: 5-Fluorouracil-induced increase of total thyroxine and triiodothyronine. Cancer Treat Rep 61:1291, 1977

209. Oltman JE, Friedman S: Protein-bound iodine in patients receiving perphenazine. JAMA 185:726, 1963

210. Garnick MB, Larsen PR: Acute deficiency of thyroxine-binding globulin during L-asparaginase therapy. N Engl J Med 301:252, 1979

211. Cashin-Hemphill L, Spencer CA, Nocoloff JT et al: Alterations in serum thyroid hormonal indices with colestipol-niacin therapy. Ann Intern Med 107:324, 1987

212. O'Brien T, Silverberg JD, Nguyen TT: Nicotinic-acid-induced toxicity associated with cytopenia and decreased levels of thyroxine-binding globulin. Mayo Clin Proc 67:465, 1992

213. Stockigt JR, Lim CF, Barlow JW et al: Interaction of furosemide with serum thyroxine-binding sites: In vivo and in vitro studies and comparison with other inhibitors. J Clin Endocrinol Metab 60:1025, 1985

214. Hollander CS, Scott RL, Burgess JA et al: Free fatty acids: a possible regulator of free thyroid hormone levels in man. J Clin Endocrinol Metab 27:1219, 1967

215. Tabachnick M, Hao YL, Korcek L: Effect of oleate, diphenylhydantoin, and heparin on the binding of ^{125}I-thyroxine to purified thyroxine-binding globulin. J Clin Endocrinol Metab 36:392, 1973

216. Marshall JS, Tompkins LS: Effect of o,p'-DDD and similar compounds on thyroxine-binding globulin. J Clin Endocrinol Metab 28:386, 1968

217. Abiodun MO, Bird R, Havard CW, Sood NK: The effects of phenylbutazone on thyroid function. Acta Endocrinol 72:257, 1973

218. Davis PJ, Hsu TH, Bianchine JR, Morgan JP: Effects of a new hypolipidemic agent, MK-185, on serum thyroxine-binding globulin (TBG) and dialysable fraction thyroxine. J Clin Endocrinol Metab 34:200, 1972

219. Taylor R, Clark F, Griffiths ID, Weeke J: Prospective study of effect of fenclofenac on thyroid function tests. Br J Med 281:911, 1980

220. Wiersinga WM, Fabius AJ, Touber JL: Orphenadrine, serum thyroxine, and thyroid function. Acta Endocrinol 86:522, 1977

221. Pages RA, Robbins J, Edelhoch H. Binding of thyroxine and thyroxine analogs to human serum prealbumin. Biochemistry 12:2773, 1973

222. Oppenheimer JH: Role of plasma proteins in the binding, distribution, and metabolism of the thyroid hormones. N Engl J Med 278:1153, 1968

223. Man EB, Reid WA, Hellegers AE, Jones WS: Thyroid function in human pregnancy. III. Serum thyroxine-binding prealbumin (TBPA) and thyroxine-binding globulin (TBG) of pregnant women aged 14 through 43 years. Am J Obstet Gynecol 103:338, 1969

224. Glinoer D, Fernandez-Deville M, Ermans AM: Use of direct thyroxine-binding globulin measurement in the evaluation of thyroid function. J Endocrinol Invest 1:329, 1978

225. Braverman LE, Ingbar SH: Effects of norethandrolone on the transport in serum and peripheral turn-

over of thyroxine. J Clin Endocrinol Metab 27:389, 1967

226. Graham RL, Gambrell RD: Changes in thyroid function tests during danazol therapy. Obstet Gynecol 55:395, 1980

227. Austen FK, Rubini ME, Meroney WH, Wolff J: Salicylates and thyroid function. I. Depression of thyroid function. J Clin Invest 37:1131, 1958

228. Wolff J, Austen FK: Salicylates and thyroid function. II. The effect on the thyroid-pituitary interrelation. J Clin Invest 37:1144, 1958

229. Christensen LK: Thyroxine-releasing effect of salicylate and of 2,4-dinitrophenol. Nature 183:1189, 1959

230. Larsen PR: Salicylate-induced increases in free triiodothyronine in human serum: evidence of inhibition of triiodothyronine binding to thyroxine-binding globulin and thyroxine-binding prealbumin. J Clin Invest 51:1125, 1972

231. Oppenheimer JH, Tavernetti RR: Displacement of thyroxine from human thyroxine-binding globulin by analogs of hydantoin: Steric aspects of the thyroxine-binding site. J Clin Invest 41:2213, 1962

232. Schatz DL, Sheppard RH, Steiner G et al: Influence of heparin on serum free thyroxine. J Clin Endocrinol Metab 29:1015, 1969

233. Hershman JM, Jones CM, Bailey AL: Reciprocal changes in serum thyrotropin and free thyroxine produced by heparin. J Clin Endocrinol Metab 34:574, 1972

234. Dowling JT, Frienkel N, Ingbar SH: The effect of estrogens upon the peripheral metabolism of thyroxine. J Clin Invest 39:1119, 1974

235. Refetoff S, Fang VS, Marshall JS, Robin NI: Metabolism of thyroxine-binding globulin (TBG) in man: abnormal rate of synthesis in inherited TBG deficiency and excess. J Clin Invest 57:485, 1976

236. Schlienger JL, Kapfer MT, Singer L, Stephan F: The action of clomipramine on thyroid function. Horm Metab Res 12:481, 1980

237. Rootwelt K, Ganes T, Johannessen SI: Effect of carbamazepin, phenytoin, and phenobarbitone on serum levels of thyroid hormones and thyrotropin in humans. Scand J Clin Lab Invest 38:731, 1978

238. Northcutt RC, Stiel MN, Nollifield JW, Stant EG Jr.: The influence of cholestyramine on thyroxine absorption. JAMA 208:1857, 1969

239. Witztum JL, Jacobs LS, Schonfeld G: Thyroid hormone and thyrotropin levels in patients placed on colestipol hydrochloride. J Clin Endocrinol Metab 46:838, 1978

240. Isley WL: Effect of rafampin therapy on thyroid function tests in a hypothyroid patient on replacement L-thyroxine. Ann Int Med 107:517, 1987

241. Chopra IJ, Williams DE, Orgiazzi J, Solomon DH: Opposite effects of dexamethasone on serum concentrations of 3,3',5'-triiodothyronine (reverse T_3) and 3,3',5-triiodothyronine (T_3). J Clin Endocrinol Metab 41:911, 1975

242. Duick DS, Warren DW, Nicoloff JT et al: Effect of a single dose of dexamethasone on the concentration of serum triiodothyronine in man. J Clin Endocrinol Metab 39:1151, 1974

243. Burger A, Dinichert D, Nicod P et al: Effects of amiodarone on serum triiodothyronine, reverse triiothyronine, thyroxine, and thyrotropin. J Clin Invest 58:255, 1976

244. Savoie JC, Massin JP, Thomopoulos P, Leger F: Iodine-induced thyrotoxicosis in apparently normal thyroid glands. J Clin Endocrinol Metab 41:685, 1975

245. Lotti G, Delitala G, Devilla L et al: Reduction of plasma triiodothyronine induced by propranolol. Clin Endocrinol 6:405, 1977

246. Faber J, Kirkegaard C, Lumholtz IB et al: Measurements of serum 3',5'-diiodothyronine and 3,3'-diiodothyronine concentrations in normal subjects and in patients with thyroid and nonthyroid disease: studies of 3',5'-diiodothyronine metabolism. J Clin Endocrinol Metab 48:611, 1979

247. Wiersinga WM, Touber JL: The influence of β-adrenoreceptor blocking agents on plasma thyroxine and triiodothyronine. J Clin Endocrinol Metab 45:293, 1977

248. Re RN, Kourides IA, Ridgway EC et al: The effect of glucocorticoid administration on human pituitary secretion of thyrotropin and prolactin. J Clin Endocrinol Metab 43:338, 1976

249. Larsen PR, Atkinson AJ, Wellman HN, Goldsmith RE: The effect of diphenylhydantoin on thyroxine metabolism in man. J Clin Invest 49:1266, 1970

250. Schwartz HL, Kozyreff V, Surks MI, Oppenheimer JH: Increased deiodination of L-thyroxine and L-triiodothyronine by liver microsomes from rats treated with phenobarbital. Nature 221:1262, 1969

251. Schwartz HL, Bernstein G, Oppenheimer JH: Effect of phenobarbital administration on the subcellular distribution of ^{125}I-thyroxine in rat liver: importance of microsomal binding. Endocrinology 84:270, 1969

252. Blum C, Corvette C, Beckers C: Effect of insulin-induced hypoglycemia on thyroid function and thyroxine turnover. Eur J Clin Invest 3:124, 1973

253. Johnstone RE, Kennel EM, Brummond W Jr et al: Effect of halothane anesthesia on muscle, liver, thyroid, and adrenal-function tests in man. Clin Chem 22:217, 1976

254. Scanlon MF, Weightman DR, Shale DJ et al: Dopamine is a physiologic regulator of thyrotropin (TSH) secretion in normal man. Clin Endocrinol 10:7, 1979

255. Scanlon MF, Rodriguez-Arnao MD, Pourmand M et al: Catecholaminergic interactions in the regulation of thyrotropin (TSH) secretion in man. J Endocrinol Invest 3:125, 1980

256. Delitala G, Devilla L, Lotti G: Domperidone, an extracerebral inhibitor of dopamine receptors, stimulates, thyrotropin and prolactin release in man. J Clin Endocrinol Metab 50:1127, 1980

257. Massara F, Camanni F, Belforte L et al: Increased thyrotropin secretion induced by sulpiride in man. Clin Endocrinol 9:419, 1978

258. Delitala G, Devilla L, Lotti G: TSH and prolactin stimulation by the decarboxylase inhibitor benserazide in primary hypothyroidism. Clin Endocrinol 12:313, 1980

259. Kirkegaard C, Bjoerum CN, Cohn D et al: Studies of the influence of biogenic amines and psychoactive drugs on the prognostic value of the TRH stimulation test in endogeneous depression. Psychoneuroendocrinology 2:131, 1977

260. Kirkegaard C, Bjoerum N, Cohn D, Lauridsen UB: TRH stimulation test in manic-depressive illness. Arch Gen Psychiatry 35:1017, 1978

261. Nelis GF, Van DeMeene JG: The effect of oral cimetidine on the basal and stimulated values of prolactin, thyroid stimulating hormone, follicle stimulating hormone, and luteinizing hormone. Postgrad Med J 56:26, 1980

262. Feldt-Rasmussen U, Lange AP, Date J, Kern-Hansen M: Effect of clomifen on thyroid function in normal men. Acta Endocrinol 90:43, 1979

263. Smals AG, Kloppenborg PW, Hoefnagesl WH, Drayer JM: Pituitary-thyroid function in spirolactone-treated hypertensive women. Acta Endocrinol 90:577, 1979

264. Morley JE, Shafer RB, Elson MK et al: Amphetamine-induced hyperthyroxinemia. Ann Int Med 93:707, 1980

265. Gloebel B, Weinheimer B: TRH-test during D-T$_4$ application. Nuc-Compact 8:44, 1977

266. Medeiros-Neto G, Kallas WG, Knobel M et al: Triac (3,5,3'-triiodothyroacetic acid) partially inhibits the thyrotropin response to thyrotropin-releasing hormone in normal and thyroidectomized hypothyroid patients. J Clin Endocrinol Metab 50:223, 1980

267. Emrich D: Untersuchungen zum einfluss von Etiroxat-XCL auf den Jodstoffwechsel beim menschen. Arzneim Forsch 27:422, 1977

268. Tamagna EI, Hershman JM, Jorgensen EC: Thyrotropin suppression by 3,5-dimethyl-3'-isopropyl-L-thyronine in man. J Clin Endocrinol Metab 48:196, 1979

269. Yoshimura M, Hachiya T, Ochi Y et al: Suppression of elevated serum TSH levels in hypothyroidism by fusaric acid. J Clin Endocrinol Metab 45:95, 1977

270. Delitala G, Rovasio P, Lotti G: Suppression of thyrotropin (TSH) and prolactin (PRL) release by pyridoxine in chronic primary hypothyroidism. J Clin Endocrinol Metab 45:1019, 1977

271. Masala A, Delitala G, Devilla L et al: Effect of apomorphine and peribedil on the secretion of thyrotropin and prolactin in patients with primary hypothyroidism. Metabolism 27:1608, 1978

272. Delitala G, Wass JAH, Stubbs WA et al: The effect of lisurgide hydrogen maleate, an ergot derivative, on anterior pituitary hormone secretion in man. Clin Endocrinol 11:1, 1979

273. Nilsson KO, Thorell JI, Hökfelt B: The effect of thyrotrophin-releasing hormone on the release of thyrotrophin and other pituitary hormones in man under basal conditions and following adrenergic blocking agents. Acta Endocrinol 76:2, 1974

274. Lamberg BA, Linnoila M, Fogelholm R et al: The effect of psychotropic drugs on the SH-response to thyroliberin (TRH). Neuroendocrinology 24:90, 1977

275. Delitala G, Rovasio PP, Masala A et al: Metergoline inhibition of thyrotropin and prolactin secretion in primary hypothyroidism. Clin Endocrinol 8:69, 1978

276. Ferrari C, Paracchi A, Rondena M et al: Effect of two serotonin antagonists on prolactin and thyrotropin secretion in man. Clin Endocrinol 5:575, 1976

277. Collu R: The effect of TRH on the release of TSH, PRL, and GH in man under basal conditions and following methysergide. J Endocrinol Invest 2:121, 1978

278. Yoshimura M, Ochi Y, Miyazaki T et al: Effect of intravenous and oral administration of L-DOPA on HGH and TSH release. Endocrinol Jpn 19:543, 1972

279. Porter BA, Refetoff S, Rosenfield RL et al: Abnormal thyroxine metabolism in hyposomatotrophic dwarfism and inhibition of responsiveness to TRH during GH therapy. Pediatrics 51:668, 1973

280. Siler TM, Yen SS, Guillemin R: Inhibition by somatostatin on the release of TSH induced in man by thyrotropin-releasing factor. J Clin Endocrinol Metab 38:742, 1974

281. Weeke J, Hansen AP, Lundbaek K: Inhibition by somatostatin of basal levels of serum thyrotropin (TSH) in normal men. J Clin Endocrinol Metab 41:168, 1975

282. Thomas JA, Shahid-Salles KS, Donovan MP: Effects of narcotics on the reproduction system. Avd Sex Horm Res 3:169, 1977

283. May P, Mittler J, Manougian A, Erte N: TSH release-inhibiting activity of leucine-enkephaline. Horm Metab Res 11:30, 1979

284. Chan V, Wang C, Yeung RT: Effects of heroin addiction on thyrotropin, thyroid hormones, and prolactin secretion in men. Clin Endocrinol 10:557, 1979

285. Kobayashi I, Shimomura Y, Maruta S et al: Clofibrate and a related compound suppress TSH secretion in primary hypothyroidism. Acta Endocrinol 94:53, 1980

286. Delitala G: Dopamine and TSH secretion in man. Lancet 2:760, 1977

287. Refetoff S, Fang VS, Rapoport B, Friesen HG: Interrelationships in the regulation of TSH and prolactin secretion in man: effects of L-dopa, TRH, and thyroid hormone in various combinations. J Clin Endocrinol Metab 38:450, 1974

288. Miyai K, Onishi T, Hosokawa M et al. Inhibition of thyrotropin and prolactin secretions in primary hypothyroidism by 2-Br-α-ergocryptine. J Clin Endocrinol Metab 39:391, 1974

289. Burrow GN, May PB, Spaulding SW, Donabedian RK: TRH and dopamine interactions affecting pituitary hormone secretion. J Clin Endocrinol Metab 45:65, 1977

290. Spaulding SW, Burrow GN, Donabedian RK, Van Woert M: L-dopa suppression of thyrotropin-releasing hormone response in man. J Clin Endocrinol Metab 35:182, 1977

291. Collu R, Jéquier JC, Leboeuf G et al: Endocrine effects of pimozide, a specific dopaminergic blocker. J Clin Endocrinol Metab 41:981, 1975

292. Kleinman RE, Vagenakis AG, Braverman LE: The effect of iopanoic acid on the regulation of thyrotropin secretion in euthyroid subjects. J Clin Endocrinol Metab 51:399, 1980

293. Faglia G, Ambrosi B, Beck-Peccoz P et al: The effect of theophylline on plasma thyrotropin response (HTSH) to thyrotropin releasing factor (TRF) in man. J Clin Endocrinol Metab 34:906, 1972

294. Wolff J, Varrone S: The methyll xanthines—a new class of goitrogens. Endocrinology 85:410, 1969

295. Oyama T, Potsaid MS, Slingerland DW: Effect of diethyl ether anesthesia on thyroid function of rats: pituitary, adrenal, and thyroid relationship. Endocrinology 65:459, 1959

296. Fore W, Kohler P, Wynn J: Rapid redistribution of serum thyroxine during ether anesthesia. J Clin Endocrinol Metab 26:821, 1966

297. Cass R, Kuntzman R, Brodie BB: Norepinephrine depletion as possible mechanism of action of guanethidine (SU 5864), a new hypotensive drug. Proc Soc Exp Biol Med 103:871, 1960

298. Gaffney TE, Braunwald E, Kahler RL: Effects of guanethidien on triiodothyronine-induced hyperthyroidism in man. N Engl J Med 265:16, 1961

299. Lee WY, Bronsky D, Waldstein SS: Studies of thyroid and sympathetic nervous system interrelationships. II. Effect of guanethidine on manifestations of hyperthyroidism. J Clin Endocrinol Metab 22:879, 1962

300. Ramey ER, Bernstein H, Goldstein MS: Effect of sympathetic blocking agents on the increased oxygen consumption following administration of thyroxine. Fed Proc 14:118, 1955

301. Surtskin A, Cordonnier JK, Lang S: Lack of influence of the sympathetic nervous system on the calorigenic response to thyroxine. Am J Physiol 188:503, 1957

302. Schwartz NB, Hammond GE, Gronert GA: Interaction between thyroxine and dibenzyline on metabolic rate. Am J Physiol 191:573, 1957

303. Cutting WC, Rytand DA, Tainter ML: Relationship between blood cholesterol and increased metabolism from dinitrophenol and thyroid. J Clin Invest 13:547, 1934

304. Ain KB, Mori Y, Reetoff S: Reduced clearance of thyroxine-binding globulin (TBG) with increased sialylation: a mechanism for estrogen-induced elevation of serum TBG concentration. J Clin Endocrinol Metab 65:689, 1987

305. Doe RP, Mellinger GT, Swaim WR, Seal JS: Estrogen dosage effects on serum proteins: a longitudinal study. J Clin Endocrinol Metab 27:1081, 1967

306. Ramey JN, Burrow GN, Polackwich RK, Donabedian RK: The effect of oral contraceptive steroids on the response of thyroid-stimulating hormone to thyrotropin-releasing hormone. J Clin Endocrinol Metab 40:712, 1975

307. Gross HA, Appleman MD, Nicoloff JT: Effect of biologically active steroids on thyroid function in man. J Clin Endocrinol Metab 33:242, 1971

308. Lemarchand-Beraud T, Rappoport G, Magrini G et al: Influences of different physiologic conditions on the gonadotropins and thyrotropin responses to LHRH and TRH. Horm Metab Res, suppl. 5:170, 1974

309. Haigler ED Jr, Hershman JM, Pittman JA Jr, Blaugh CM: Direct evaluation of pituitary thyrotropin reserve utilizing thyrotropin releasing hormone. J Clin Endocrinol Metab 33:573, 1971

310. Snyder PJ, Utiger RD: Response to thyrotropin releasing hormone (TRH) in normal man. J Clin Endocrinol Metab 34:380, 1972

311. Carlson HE, Jacobs LS, Daughaday WH: Growth hormone, thyrothyropin, and prolactin responses to thyrotropin-releasing hormone following diethylstilbestrol pretreatment. J Clin Endocrinol Metab 37:488, 1973

312. Rutlin E, Haug E, Torjesen PA: Serum thyrotrophin, prolactin, and growth hormone, response to TRH during estrogen treatment. Acta Endocrinol 84:23, 1977

313. Federman DD, Robbins J, Rall JE: Effects of methyl testosterone on thyroid function, thyroxine metabolism, and thyroxine-binding protein. J Clin Invest 37:1024, 1958

314. Woeber KA, Barakat RM, Ingbar SH: Effects of salicylate and its noncalorigenic congeners on the thyroidal release of ^{131}I in patients with thyrotoxicosis. J Clin Endocrinol Metab 224:1163, 1964

315. Dussault JH, Turcotte R, Guyda H: The effect of acetylsalicylic acid on TSH and PRL secretion after TRH stimulation in the human. J Clin Endocrinol Metab 43:232, 1976

316. Langer P, Földes O, Michajlovskij N et al: Short-term effect of acethylsalicylic acid on pituitary-thyroid axis and plasma cortisol level in healthy human volunteers. Acta Endocrinol 88:698, 1978

317. Chopra IJ, Solomon DH, Chua Teco GN, Nguyen AH: Inhibition of hepatic outer-ring monodeiodination of thyroxine and 3,3′,5′-triiodothyronine by sodium salicylate. Endocrinology 106:1728, 1980

318. Alexander WD, Johnson KWM: A comparison of the effects of acetylsalicylic acid and DL-triiodothyronine in patients with myxoedema. Clin Sci 15:593, 1956

319. Yamamoto T, Woeber KA, Ingbar SH: The influence of salicylate on serum TSH concentration in patients with primary hypothyroidism. J Clin Endocrinol Metab 34:423, 1972

320. Woeber KA, Ingbar SH: The effects of noncalorigenic congeners of salicylate on the peripheral metabolism of thyroxine. J Clin Invest 43:931, 1964

321. Christensen K: The metabolic effect of p-amino salicylic acid. Acta Endocrinol 31:608, 1959

322. MacGregor AG, Somner AR: The antithyroid action of para-amino salicylic acid. Lancet 2:931, 1954

323. Christensen LK: The metabolic effect of salicylate and other hydroxybenzoates. Acta Pharmacol Toxicol 16:129, 1959

324. McConnell RJ: Abnormal thyroid function in patients taking salsalate. JAMA 267:1242, 1992

325. Gamstedt A, Jarnerot A, Kagedal B, Soderholm B: Corticosteroids and thyroid function. Acta Med Scand 205:379, 1979

326. Oppenheimer JH, Werner SC: Effect of prednisone on thyroxine-binding proteins. J Clin Endocrinol Metab 26:715, 1966

327. Werner SC, Platman SR: Remission of hyperthyroidism (Graves' disease) and altered pattern of serum-thyroxine binding induced by prednisone. Lancet 2:751, 1965

328. Otsuki M, Dakoda M, Baba S: Influence of glucocorticoids on TRF-induced TSH response in man. J Clin Endocrinol Metab 36:95, 1973

329. Dussault JH: The effect of dexamethasone on TSH and prolactin secretion after TRH stimulation. Can Med Assoc J 111:1195, 1974

330. Berson SA, Yalow RS: The effect of cortisone on the iodine-accumulating functions of the thyroid gland in euthyroid subjects. J Clin Endocrinol Metab 12:407, 1952

331. Ingbar SH: The effect of cortisone on the thyroidal and renal metabolism of iodine. Endocrinology 53:171, 1953

332. Topliss DJ, White EL, Stockigt JR: Significance of thyrotropin excess in untreated primary adrenal insufficiency. J Clin Endocrinol Metab 50:52, 1980

333. Tashjian AH, Osborne R, Maina D, Knaian A: Hydrocortisone increases the number of receptors for thyrotropin-releasing hormone on pituitary cells in culture. Biochem Biophys Res Commun 79:333, 1977

334. Benoit FL, Greenspan FS: Corticoid therapy for pretibial myxedema: observations on the long-acting thyroid stimulator. Ann Intern Med 66:711, 1967

335. Yamada T, Ikejiri K, Kotani M, Kusakabe T: An increase of plasma triiodothyronine and thyroxine after administration of dexamethasone to hypothyroid patients with Hashimoto's thyroiditis. J Clin Endocrinol Metab 46:784, 1978

336. Burgi H, Wimpfheimer C, Burger A et al: Changes of circulating thyroxine, triiodothyronine, and reverse triiodothyronine after radiographic contrast agents. J Clin Endocrinol Metab 43:1203, 1976

337. Wu SY, Chopra IJ, Solomon DH, Bennett LR: Changes in circulating iodothyronines in euthyroid and hyperthyroid subjects given ipodate (Oragrafin), an agent for oral cholescystography. J Clin Endocrinol Metab 46:691, 1978

338. Larsen PR, Dick TE, Markovitz BP et al: Inhibition of intrapituitary thyroxine to 3,5,3′-triiodothyronine conversion prevents the acute suppression of thyrotropin release by thyroxine in hypothyroid rats. J Clin Invest 64:117, 1979

339. Felicetta JV, Green WL, Nelp WB: Inhibition of hepatic binding of thyroxine by cholecystographic agents. J Clin Invest 65:1032, 1980

340. DeGroot LJ, Rue PA: Roentgenographic contrast agents inhibit triiodothyronine binding to nuclear receptors in vitro. J Clin Endocrinol Metab 49:538, 1979

341. Nademanee K, Piwonka RW, Singh BN, Hershman JM: Amiodarone and thyroid function. Prog Cardiovascul Dis 31:427, 1989

342. Martino E, Safran M, Aghini-Lombardi F et al: Environmental iodine intake and thyroid dysfunction during chronic amiodarone therapy. Ann Intern Med 101:28, 1984

343. Schussler GC: Diazepan competes for thyroxine binding. J Pharmacol Exp Ther 178:204, 1971

344. Molholm Hansen J, Skovsted L, Birk Lauridsen U

et al: The effect of diphenylhydantoin on thyroid function. J Clin Endocrinol Metab 39:785, 1974

345. Heyma P, Larkins RG, Perry-Kenne D et al: Thyroid hormone levels and protein binding in patients on long-term diphenylhydantoin treatment. Clin Endocrinol 6:369, 1977

346. Cavalieri RR, Gavin LA, Wallace A et al: Serum thyroxine, free T_4, triiodothyronine, and reverse-T_3 in diphenylhydantoin treated patients. Metabolism 28:1161, 1979

347. Hansen JM, Skovsted L, Lauridsen UB et al: The effect of diphenylhydantoin on thyroid function. J Clin Endocrinol Metab 39:785, 1974

348. Blackshear JL, Schultz AL, Napier JS, Stuart DD: Thyroxine replacement requirements in hypothyroid patients receiving phenyltoin. Ann Intern Med 99:341, 1983

349. Oppenheimer JH, Shapiro HC, Schwartz HL, Surks MI: Dissociation between thyroxine metabolism and hormonal action in phenobarbital-treated rats. Endocrinology 88:115, 1971

350. Cavalieri RR, Sung LC, Becker CE: Effects of phenobarbital on thyroxine and triiodothyronine kinetics in Graves' disease. J Clin Endocrinol Metab 37:308, 1973

351. Wartofsky L, Dimond RC, Noel GL et al: Failure of propranolol to alter thyroid iodine release, thyroxine turnover, or the TSH and PRL responses to thyrotropin-releasing hormone in patients with thyrotoxicosis. J Clin Endocrinol Metab 41:485, 1975

352. Woolf PD, Lee LA, Schalch DS: Adrenergic manipulation and thyrotropin releasing hormone (TRH)-induced thyrotropin (TSH) release. J Clin Endocrinol Metab 35:616, 1972

353. Faber J, Friis T, Kirkegaard C et al: Serum T_4, T_3, and reverse T_3 during treatment with propranolol in hyperthyroidism, L-T_4-treated myxedema, and normal man. Horm Metab Res 11:34, 1979

354. Faber J, Kirkegaard C, Lumholtz IB et al: Variations in serum T_3, rT_3, 3,3'-diiodothyronine, and 3',5'-diiodothyronine induced by acute myocardial infarction and propranol. Acta Endocrinol 94:341, 1980

355. Murchison LE, How J, Bewsher PD: Comparison of propranolol and metoprolol in the management of hyperthyroidism. Br J Clin Pharmacol 8:581, 1979

356. How ASM, Khir AN, Bewsher PD: The effect of atenolol on serum thyroid hormones in hyperthyroid patients. Clin Endocrinol 13:299, 1980

357. Hadden DR, Bell TK, McDevitt DG et al: Propranolol and the utilization of radioiodine by the human thyroid gland. Acta Endocrinol 61:393, 1969

358. Wilson WR, Theilen ED, Fletcher FW: Propranolol and its effects in thyrotoxicosis on heart at rest or exercise. J Clin Invest 43:1697, 1964

359. Das G, Krieger M: Treatment of thyrotoxic storm with intravenous administration of propranolol. Ann Intern Med 70:985, 1969

360. Canary JJ, Shaaf M, Duffy BJ Jr, Kyle LH: Effects of oral and intramuscular administration of reserpine in thyrotoxicosis. N Engl J Med 257:435, 1957

361. Waud DR, Kattegoda SR, Krayer O: Threshold dose and time course of norepinephrine depletion of mammalian heart by reserpine. J Pharmacol Exp Ther 124:340, 1958

362. Goldberg RC, Wolff J, Greep RO: Studies on the nature of the thyroid-pituitary interrelationship. Endocrinology 60:38, 1957

363. Goldberg RC, Wolff J, Greep RO: The mechanism of depression of plasma protein-bound iodine by 2,4-dinitrophenol. Endocrinology 56:560, 1955

364. Lardy HA, Wellman H: Oxidative phosphorylations: role of inorganic phosphate and acceptor systems in control of metabolic rates. J Biol Chem 195:215, 1952

365. Escobar del Rey F, Morreale de Escobar G: Studies on the peripheral disappearance of thyroid hormone. IV. The effect of 2,4-dinitrophenol on the ^{131}I distribution in thyroidectomized, L-thyroxine maintained rats, 24 hours after the injection of ^{131}I-labeled L-thyroxine. Acta Endocrinol 29:161, 1958

366. Escobar del Rey F, Morreale de Escobar G: Studies on the peripheral disappearance of thyroid hormone. V. The effect of 2,4-dinitrophenol on the variations of the ^{131}I distribution pattern with time, after the injection of ^{131}I-labeled L-thyroxine into thyroidectomized, L-thyroxine maintained rats. Acta Endocrinol 29:176, 1958

367. Cutting CC, Tainter ML: Comparative effects of dinitrophenol and thyroxin on tadpole metamorphosis. Proc Soc Exp Biol Med 31:97, 1933

368. Reichlin S: Regulation of the hypophysiotropin secretion of the brain. Arch Intern Med 135:1350, 1975

369. Morley JE: Neuroendocrine control of thyrotropin secretion. Endocr Rev 2:396, 1981

370. Kaptein EM, Spencer CA, Kamiel MB, Nicoloff JT: Prolonged dopamine administration and thyroid hormone economy in normal and critically ill subjects. J Clin Endocrinol Metab 51:387, 1980

371. Benker G, Zäh W, Hackenberg K et al: Long-term treatment of acromegaly with bromocriptine: postprandial HGH levels and response to TRH and glucose administration. Horm Metab Res 8:291, 1976

372. Köbberling J, Darrach A, Del Pozo E: Chronic dopamine receptor stimulation using bromocriptine: failure to modify thyroid function. Clin Endocrinol 11:367, 1979

373. Foord SM, Peters J, Scanlon MF et al: Dopaminergic

control of TSH secretion in isolated pituitary cells. FEBS Lett 121:257, 1980

374. Heinen E, Herrmann J, Konigshausen T, Kruskemper HL: Secondary hypothyroidism in severe nonthyroidal illness? Horm Metab Res 13:284–288, 1981

375. Weintraub BD, Gershengorn MC, Kourides IA, Fein H: Inappropriate secretion of thyroid stimulating hormone. Ann Intern Med 95:339, 1981

376. Chanson P, Weintraub BD, Harris AG: Octreotide therapy for thyroid hormone-stimulating hormone-secreting pituitary adenomas. Ann Int Med 119:236, 1994

377. Chopra IJ, Chopra U, Smith SR et al: Reciprocal changes in serum concentration of 3,3′,5′-triiodothyronine (reverse T_3) and 3,3′,5-triiodothyronine (T_3) in systemic illnesses. J Clin Endocrinol Metab 41:1043, 1975

378. Nomura S, Pittman CS, Chambers JB Jr et al: Reduced peripheral conversion of thyroxine to triiodothyronine in patients with hepatic cirrhosis. J Clin Invest 56:643, 1975

379. Lim VS, Fang VS, Katz AI, Refetoff S: Thyroid dysfunction in chronic renal failure: a study of the pituitary-thyroid axis and peripheral turnover kinetics of thyroxine and triiodothyronine. J Clin Invest 60:522, 1977

380. Pittman CS: The effects of diabetes mellitus on thyroid physiology. Thyroid Today, 4:4, 1981

381. Chopra IJ: An assessment of daily production and significance of thyroidal secretion of 3,3′,5′-triiodothyronine (reverse T_3) in man. J Clin Invest 58:32, 1976

382. Geola F, Chopra IJ, Geffner DL: Patterns of 3,3′,5′-triiodothyronine monodeiodination in hypothyroidism and nonthyroidal illnesses. J Clin Endocrinol Metab 50:336, 1980

383. Chopra IJ, Wiersinga W, Harrison F: Alterations in hepatic monodeiodination of iodothyronines in the diabetic rat. Life Sci 28:1765, 1981

384. Gomez F, De La Cueva R, Wauters JP, Lemarchand-Beraud T: Endocrine abnormalities in patients undergoing long-term hemodialysis. Am J Med 68:522, 1980

385. Talwar KK, Sawhney RC, Rastogi GK: Serum level of thyrotropin, thyroid hormones and their response to thyrotropin-releasing hormone in infective febrile illnesses. J Clin Endocrinol Metab 44:398, 1977

386. Walfish PG, Orrego H, Israel Y et al: Serum triiodothyronine and other clinical and laboratory induces of alcoholic liver disease. Ann Intern Med 91:13, 1979

387. Kolendorf K, Moller BB, Rogowski P: The influence of chronic renal failure on serum and urinary thyroid hormone levels. Acta Endocrinol 89:80, 1978

388. Wiersinga WM, Lie KI, Touber JL: Thyroid hormones in acute myocardial infarction. Clin Endocrinol 14:367, 1981

389. Saunders J, Hall SEH, Sonksen PH: Thyroid hormones in insulin-requiring diabetes before and after treatment. Diabetelogia 15:29, 1978

390. Naeije R, Golstein J, Clumeck N et al: A low T_3 syndrome in diabetic ketoacidosis. Clin Endocrinol 8:467, 1978

391. Kaptein EM, Grieb DA, Spencer C et al: Thyroxine metabolism in the low thyroxine state of critical nonthyroidal illnesses. J Clin Endocrinol Metab 53:764, 1981

392. McConnon J, Row VV, Volpe R: The influence of liver damage in man on the distribution and disposal rates of thyroxine and triiodothyronine. Clin Endocrinol 34:144, 1972

393. Faber J, Thomsen HF, Lumholtz IB et al: Kinetic studies of thyroxine, 3,5,3′-triiodothyronine, 3,3′,5′-triiodothyronine, 3′,5′-diiodothyronine, 3,3′-diiodothyronine, and 3′-monoiodothyronine in patients with liver cirrhosis. J Clin Endocrinol Metab 53:978, 1981

394. Gavin LA, McMahon FA, Castle JN, Cavalieri RR: Alterations in serum thyroid hormones and thyroxine-binding globulin in patients with nephrosis. J Clin Endocrinol Metab 46:125, 1978

395. Afrasiabi MA, Vaziri ND, Gwinup G et al: Thyroid function studies in the nephrotic syndrome. Ann Intern Med 90:335, 1979

396. Ramirez G, Jubiz W, Gutch CF et al: Thyroid abnormalities in renal failure: a study of 53 patients on chronic hemodialysis. Ann Intern Med 79:500, 1973

397. Inada M, Sterling M: Thyroxine turnover and transport in Laennec's cirrhosis of the liver. J Clin Invest 46:1275, 1967

398. Hollander CS, Scott RL, Tschudy DP et al: Increased protein-bound iodine and thyroxine-binding globulin in acute intermittent porphyria. N Engl J Med 277:995, 1967

399. Lamberg BA, Perheentupa J, Rajantie J et al: Increase in thyroxine-binding globulin (TBG) in lysinuric protein intolerance. Acta Endocrinol 97:67, 1981

400. Lever A, Bird D, Byfield PGH et al: Increased serum concentration of T_4-binding globulin in patients with hypogammaglobulinaemia. Clin Endocrinol 18:195, 1983

401. Gardner DF, Carithers RL, Galen EA, Utiger RD: Thyroid function tests in patients withy acute and resolved hepatitis B infection. Ann Intern Med 96:450, 1982

402. Kaptein EM, Macintyre SS, Weiner JM et al: Free thyroxine estimates in nonthyroidal illness: compari-

son of eight methods. J Clin Endocrinol Metab 52: 1073, 1981

403. Melmed S, Geola FL, Reed AW et al: A comparison of methods for assessing thyroid function in nonthyroidal illness. J Clin Endocrinol Metab 54:300, 1982

404. Kaplan MM, Larsen PR, Crantz FR et al: Prevalence of abnormal thyroid function test results in patients with acute medical illnesses. Am J Med 72:9, 1982

405. Gooch BR, Isley WL, Utiger RD: Abnormalities in thyroid function tests in patients admitted to a medical service. Arch Intern Med 142:1801, 1982

406. Chopra KJ, Chua Teco GN, Nguyen AH, Solomon DH: In search of an inhibitor of thyroid hormone binding to serum proteins in nonthyroid illnesses. J Clin Endocrinol Metab 49:63, 1979

407. Oppenheimer JH, Schwartz HL, Mariash CN, Kaiser FE: Evidence for a factor in the sera of patients with nonthyroidal illness which inhibits iodothyronine binding by solid matrices, serum proteins, and rat hepatocytes. J Clin Endocrinol Metab 54:757, 1982

408. Chopra IJ, Solomon DH, Teco GNC, Eisenberg JB: An inhibitor of the binding of thyroid hormones to serum proteins is present in extrathyroidal tissues. Science 215:407, 1982

409. Spaulding SW, Gregerman RI: Free thyroxine in serum equilibrium dialysis: effects of dilution, specific ions, and inhibitors of binding. J Clin Endocrinol Metab 34:974, 1972

410. Schlienger JL: Thyroid status in fifty patients with alcoholic cirrhosis. Z Gastroenterol 17:452, 1979

411. Gomez-Pan A, Alvarez-Ude F, Yeo PPB et al: Function of the hypothalamo-hypophysial-thyroid axis in chronic renal failure. Clin Endocrinol 11:567, 1979

412. Maturlo SJ, Rosenbaum RL, Pan C, Surks MI: Variable thyrotropin response to thyrotropin-releasing hormone after small decreases in plasma free thyroid hormone concentrations in patient with nonthyroidal disease. J Clin Invest 66:451, 1980

413. Lim VS, Passo C, Murata Y et al: Reduced triiodothyronine content in liver but not pituitary of the uremic rat model: demonstration of changes compatible with thyroid hormone deficiency in liver only. Endocrinology 114:280, 1984

414. Rosenbaum RI, Maturlo SU, Surks MI: Changes in thyroidal economy in rats bearing transplantable Walker 256 carcinomas. Endocrinology 106:1386, 1980

415. Das DK, Ganguly M: Diabetes, hypophysectomy, or thyroidectomy reduces nuclear L-triiodothyronine-binding capacity of rat lung. Endocrinology 109:296, 1981

416. Burman KD, Lukes YD, Latham KR et al: The effect of dexamethasone, diet control, and hyperglycemia on murine hepatic T_3 receptors. Life Sci 28:1701, 1981

417. Hooper MJ: Diminished TSH secretion during acute nonthyroidal illness in untreated primary hypothyroidism. Lancet 1:48, 1979

418. Lim VS, Henriquez C, Seo H et al: Thyroid function in a uremic rat model: evidence suggesting tissue hypothyroidism. J Clin Invest 66:946, 1980

419. Ingbar SH: Effect of aging on thyroid economy in man. J Am Geriatr Soc 24:49, 1976

420. Havard CWH: The thyroid and aging. Clin Endocrinol Metab 10:163, 1981

421. Jefferys PM, Hoffenberg R, Farran HEA et al: Thyroid-function tests in the elderly. Lancet 1:924, 1972

422. Olsen T, Laurberg P, Weeke J: Low serum triiodothyronine and high serum reverse triiodothyronine in old age: an effect of disease not age. J Clin Endocrinol Metab 47:1111, 1978

423. Marshall JS, Pensky J, Green AM: Studies on human thyroxine-binding globulin. IV. The nature of slow thyroxine-binding globulin. J Clin Invest 51:3173, 1972

424. Refetoff S, Fang VS, Marshall JS: Studies on human thyroxine-binding globulin (TBG). IX. Some physical, chemical, and biological properties of radioiodinated TBG and partially desialylated TBG (STBG). J Clin Invest 56:177, 1975

425. Shipley RA, Buchwald E, Chudzik BS: Thyroidal uptake and plasma clearance of ^{131}I and ^{127}I in cirrhosis of the liver. J Clin Endocrinol Metab 17:1229, 1957

426. Schussler GC, Schaffner F, Hurley J, Shapiro J: Thyroid function in primary biliary cirrhosis, abstracted. Clin Res 27:259A, 1979

427. Crowe J, Christensen E, Butler J et al: Primary biliary cirrhosis: the prevalence of hypothyroidism and its relationship to thyroid autoantibodies in sicca syndrome. Gastroenterology 78:1437, 1980

428. Beckers C, van Ypersele de Strihou C, Coche E et al: Iodine metabolism in severe renal insufficiency. J Clin Endocrinol Metab 29:293, 1969

429. Spector DA, Davis PJ, Helderman JH et al: Thyroid function and metabolic state in chronic renal failure. Ann Intern Med 85:724, 1976

430. Hershman JM, Krugman LG, Kopple JD et al: Thyroid function in patients undergoing maintenance hemodialysis: unexplained low serum thyroxine concentration. Metabolism 27:755, 1978

431. Joasoo A, Murray IPC, Parkin J et al: Abnormalities of in vitro thyroid function tests in renal disease. QJ Med 43:245, 1974

432. Robbins J, Rall JE, Peterman ML: Thyroxine binding by serum and urine proteins in nephrosis: qualitative aspects. J Clin Invest 36:1333, 1957

433. Perry WF, Hughes JFS: The urinary excretion and thyroid uptake of iodine in renal disease. J Clin Invest 41:457, 1952

434. Robertson BF, Prestwich S, Ramirez G et al: The role of iodine in the pathogenesis of thyroid enlargement in rats with chronic renal failure. Endocrinology 101: 1272, 1977

435. Pittman CS, Suda AK, Chambergs JB Jr, Ray GY: Impaired 3,5,3'-triiodothyronine (T$_3$) production in diabetic patients. Metabolism 28:333, 1979

436. Fujii S, Akai T, Tanaka S et al: Thyroid hormone abnormalities in patients with diabetes mellitus. J Clin Invest 4:71, 1981

437. Pittman CS, Suda AK, Chambers JB Jr et al: Abnormalities of thyroid hormone turnover in patients with diabetes mellitus before and after insulin therapy. J Clin Endocrinol Metab 48:854, 1979

438. Madsbad S, Laurberg P, Weeke J et al: Very early changes in circulating T$_3$ and rT$_3$ during development of metabolic derangement in diabetic patients. Acta Med Scand 209:385, 1981

439. Tevaawerk GM, Hurst C, Ursik P, Reese L: Effect of insulin-induced hypoglycemia on the serum concentrations of thyroxine, triiodothyronine. CMA Journal 121:1090, 1979

440. Wilber JF, Banerji A, Prasad C, Mori M: Alterations in hypothalamic-pituitary-thyroid regulation produced by diabetes mellitus. Life Sci 28:1757, 1981

441. Bagchi N, Brown TR, Shivers B et al: Decreased thyroidal response to thyrotropin in diabetic mice. Endocrinology 109:1428, 1981

442. Pericas I, Jolin T: The effect of streptozotocin-induced diabetes on the pituitary thyroid axis in goitrogen-treated rats. Acta Endocrinol 86:128, 1977

443. Feely J, Isles TE: Screening for thyroid dysfunction in diabetics. Br Med J 1:1678, 1979

444. Gray RS, Borsey DQ, Seth J et al: Prevalence of subclinical thyroid failure in insulin-dependent diabetes. J Clin Endocrinol Metab 50:1034, 1980

445. Longhini C, Portaluppi F, Candini G et al: Serum levels of 3,5,3'-triiodothyronine, 3,3',5'-triiodothyronine, and thyroxine in acute myocardial infarction. Ric Clin Lab 9:197, 1979

446. Harland WA, Orr JS, Dunnigan MG, Sequeria RFC: Thyroxine secretion rate after myocardial infarction. Br Heart J 34:1072, 1972

447. Kahana L, Keidar S, Sheinfeld M, Palant A: Endogenous cortisol and thyroid hormone levels in patients with acute myocardial infarction. Clin Endocrinol 19:131, 1983

448. Wartofsky L, Burman KD, Dimond RC et al: Studies on the nature of thyroidal suppression during acute falciparum malaria: integrity of pituitary response to TRH and alterations in serum T$_3$ and reverse T$_3$. J Clin Endocrinol Metab 44:85, 1977

449. Richmond DA, Molitch ME, O'Donnell TF: Altered thyroid hormone levels in bacterial sepsis: the role of nutritional adequacy. Metabolism 29:936, 1980

450. Bacci V, Schussler GC, Kaplan TB: The relationship between serum triiodothyronine and thyrotropin during systemic illness. J Clin Endocrinol Metab 54: 1229, 1982

451. Majarajan G, Etta KM, Singh A et al: Thyroxine triiodothyronine, and thyrotropin levels in meningococcal meningitis, typhoid fever, and other febrile conditions. Clin Endocrinol 9:401, 1978

452. Lutz JH, Gregerman RI, Spaulding SW et al: Thyroxine binding proteins, free thyroxine, and thyroxine turnover interrelationships during acute infectious illness in man. J Clin Endocrinol Metab 35:230, 1972

453. Gregerman RI, Solomon N: Acceleration of thyroxine and triiodothyronine turnover during bacterial pulmonary infections and fever: implications for the functional state of the thyroid during stress and senescence. J Clin Endocrinol Metab 27:93, 1967

454. Glatstein E, McHardy-Young S, Brast N et al: Alterations in serum thyrotropin (TSH) and thyroid function following radiotherapy in patients with malignant lymphoma. J Clin Endocrinol Metab 32:833, 1971

455. Kaplan MM, Garnick MB, Gelber R et al: Risk factors in thyroid abnormalities after neck irradiation for childhood cancer. Am J Med 74:272, 1983

456. Ratcliffe JG, Stack BH, Burt RW et al: Thyroid function in lung cancer. Br Med J 1:210, 1978

457. Macfarlane IA, Robinson EL, Bush H et al: Thyroid function in patients with benign and malignant breast disease. Br J Cancer 41:478, 1980

458. Galton VA, Ingbar SH: Effect of a malignant tumor on thyroxine metabolism and thyroid function in the rat. Endocrinology 79:964, 1966

459. Miyai K, Yamamoto T, Azaukizawa M et al: Serum thyroid hormones and thyrotropin in anorexia nervosa. J Clin Endocrinol Metab 46:334, 1975

460. Croxson MS, Ibbertson HK: Low serum triiodothyronine (T$_3$) and hypothyroidism in anorexia nervosa. J Clin Endocrinol Metab 44:167, 1977

461. Leslie RDG, Isaacs AJ, Gomez J et al: Hypothalamo-pituitary-thyroid function in anorexia nervosa: influence of weight gain. Br Med J 2:526, 1978

462. Kirkegaard C, Faber J: Altered serum levels of thyroxine, triiodothyronines, and diiodothyronines in endogenous depression. Acta Endocrinol 96:199, 1981

463. Weeke A, Weeke J: Disturbed circadian variation of serum thyrotropin in patients with endogenous depression. Acta Psychiatr Scand 57:281, 1978

464. Kirkegaard C, Faber J, Cohn D et al: Serum 3'-monoiodothyronine levels in normal subjects and in patients with thyroid and nonthyroid disease. Acta Endocrinol 97:454, 1981

465. Maeda K, Kato Y, Ohgo S et al: Growth hormone

and prolactin release after injection of thyrotropin-releasing hormone in patients with depression. J Clin Endocrinol Metab 40:501, 1975

466. Gold MS, Pottash ALC, Davies RK: Distinguishing unipolar and bipolar depression by thyrotropin release test. Lancet 2:411, 1979

467. Czernichow P, Dauzet MC, Broyer M, Rappaport R: Abnormal TSH, PRL, and GH response to TSH-releasing factor in chronic renal failure. J Clin Endocrinol Metab 43:630, 1976

468. Panerai AE, Salerno F, Manneschi M et al: Growth hormone and prolactin responses to thyrotropin-releasing hormone in patients with severe liver disease. J Clin Endocrinol Metab 45:134, 1977

469. Maeda K, Kato Y, Yamaguchi N et al: Growth hormone release following thyrotrophin-releasing hormone injection into patients with anorexia nervosa. Acta Endocrinol 81:1, 1976

470. Jäernerot G, Khan AKA, Truelove SC: The thyroid in ulcerative colitis and Crohn's disease. II. Thyroid enlargement and hyperthyroidism. Acta Med Scand 197:83, 1975

471. Schreiner A, Hopen G, Skrede S: *Crebroteninous xanthomatosis* (cholestanolosis): investigation of two sisters and their family. Acta Neurol Scand 51:405, 1975

472. Vanderschueren-Lodeweyckx M, Eggermont E, Cornette C et al: Decreased serum thyroid hormone levels and increased TSH response to TRH in infants with celiac disease. Clin Endocrinol 6:361, 1977

473. Chan AM, Lynch MJG, Bailey JD, Fraser D: Hypothyroidism in cystinosis. Am J Med 48:678, 1970

474. Bercu BB, Orloff S, Schulman JD: Pituitary resistance to thyroid hormone in cystinosis. J Clin Endocrinol Metab 51:1262, 1980

475. Weinstein LS, Shenker A: G protein mutations in human disease. Clin Biochem 26:333, 1993

476. Refetoff S, Nicoloff JT. p. 564. In DeGroot L (ed): Endocrinology. WB Saunders, Philadelphia, 1985

477. Wiersinga WM et al. Clin Endocrinol 8:467, 1978

Evaluation of Thyroid Function in Health and in Disease

6

The possibility of thyroid disease is considered when signs or symptoms suggest hyper- or hypothyroidism or some physical abnormality of the thyroid gland. Evaluation of the patient should begin with a thorough history and physical examination and those routine laboratory tests that are relevant to the care of any patient. It should then proceed to tests of thyroid function designed to establish the level of hormonal activity and the nature of the thyroid disorder. Since most thyroid diseases require prolonged periods of treatment, it is crucial to establish a firm diagnosis before embarking on such a program. Further, a number of medications, in particular those used in the treatment of thyroid disease, may alter the results of thyroid function tests undertaken after therapy has begun.

CLINICAL DIAGNOSIS BY HISTORY AND PHYSICAL EXAMINATION

The history should include an evaluation of all systems in which signs of thyroid dysfunction appear. Inquiry should be made about fatigue, anxiety, tremulousness, insomnia, drowsiness, changes in mood, or a tendency to emotional lability. It is important to know whether there has been hair loss or change in hair or skin texture. Increase or decrease of perspiration should be noted. Symptoms of ocular disease may be present. Altered sensitivity to cold or heat is important. The nails may have become brittle or have developed the characteristic changes described by Plummer (see Chapter 10, Fig. 10-7). Shortness of breath or dyspnea on exertion should

189

be evaluated, as well as any history of tachycardia or rhythm irregularity. Change in appetite or bowel habits, weight loss, thirst, and frequency of urination may be important. The menstrual period may be altered. Occasionally symptoms of arthritis or bursitis may occur. Sometimes neuromuscular signs, such as the carpal tunnel syndrome, ataxia, or muscle weakness, are encountered. Neck pain or tenderness, difficulty in swallowing, dysphagia, hoarseness, or a mass may be noted, and a history of recent change in these symptoms may be significant. Any prior history of thyroid disease or previous therapy should be recorded. A history of exposure of the thyroid gland to irradiation is particularly important. The use of iodide, or iodide-containing compounds, antithyroid drugs, estrogen-containing compounds, amiodarone, phenytoin, and aspirin may be relevant. Also, thyroid disease frequently is present in members of the patient's family.

Attention should be paid to a history of those illnesses that are sometimes found in association with thyroid disease, such as symptoms of pituitary adenoma with impingement on the optic nerves or other structures. Adrenal or ovarian failure or other diseases of possible autoimmune origin must also be considered. Similarly, diseases with clinical manifestations that overlap those commonly found in the presence of altered thyroid states should be identified. Furthermore, a variety of nonthyroidal illnesses may be associated with thyroid disease or result in changes of thyroid function (see Chapter 5). It is the responsibility of the clinician to determine the presence or absence of associated thyroid involvement.

The physical examination should provide a general evaluation of the patient and of specific signs of altered metabolism or local pathology related to the thyroid gland. Typical signs are fine or coarse hair, thin hair, thin nails, Plummer's nails, red palms, red and smooth elbows, excessive sweating, thin or thick skin, change in pigmentation, tremor, restlessness, evidence of weight loss, muscle weakness, tachycardia, cardiac arrhythmia, or signs of congestive failure. Enlargement of the lymph nodes and spleen and alterations in distribution of body hair and secondary sex characteristics should be looked for. Deafness or decreased hearing actuity, enlargement of the tongue, serosal effusions, umbilical hernia, and abnormalities of gait and coordination may be seen. Particular attention should be paid to the eyes in terms of protrusion, chemosis, restricted eye motion, double vision, and swelling of the insertion of the lateral rectus muscle.

Much can be learned by simply observing the thyroid gland and the neck. It is possible in thin persons to ascertain the size and shape of the thyroid gland, observe whether it is symmetric and whether it contains visible lumps. One should note the presence of surgical scars, telangiectasis related to irradiation, dilated veins arising from possible thoracic inlet obstruction, or evidence of old infection. Deviation of the trachea is an important sign. Detailed descriptions of symptoms and clinical signs appear in chapters dealing with specific disease processes.

Examination of the Thyroid Gland

Much of the subsequent diagnostic process depends on a careful examination of the thyroid. Internists and surgeons often disagree as to whether the examination should be made with the physician in front of or behind the patient. The approach is perhaps unimportant, so long as the examiner develops a consistent and thorough technique. Our preferred technique is to have the patient sit on the examining table and to examine from the front and then palpate the left side of the gland with the right hand and the right side of the gland with the opposite hand. The examiner reaches across the sternocleidomastoid muscle with the fingers, pulls a flap of skin toward the midline, and then carefully presses beneath the muscle to find the lobes of the thyroid gland.

Except on rare occasions, when the thyroid gland may be tender, manual examination if done carefully is not objectionable to most patients. The gland usually feels like a bilobed structure with a thin isthmus. The isthmus extends across the front of the trachea, just below the last prominent structure below the larynx, this being the cricoid cartilage. The lobes can be felt on each side of the trachea and are approximately the size of half of an adult's index finger. The consistency of a normal gland is that of firm meat. Being fixed to the trachea, the thyroid moves up and down with deglutition, and this convenient maneuver allows assessment of the lower portion of the gland. One can easily estimate the size and shape of the gland in young and thin persons, but it becomes progressively more difficult as people age and become kyphotic, if they have short necks, or if they are obese or have had prior neck surgery. Extension of the neck may make palpation easier or may, by tightening the skin and strap muscles, make it more difficult. At times it is helpful to examine the patient supine with a pillow under the shoulders in order to extend the neck passively. This position may raise a deep-seated thyroid out of the anterior mediastinum. One should note the size, shape, consistency, and fixation of the thyroid, the presence of lobulations or discrete nodules, their number and location, and the presence or absence of an isthmus and pyramidal lobe. If the gland is enlarged, it is important to look for tracheal deviation. Nodules should be characterized as cystic, if possible, by palpation, transillumination, or needle aspiration (described below). Lymph nodes related to inflammation or tumor may appear above the thyroid, near or in the pyramidal lobe (Delphian nodes), above, lateral to, or below the thyroid lobes, or in any of the other areas of the neck, but particularly in the supraclavicular fossae and anterior cervical chain. Occasionally, one can identify other structures such as nodules or cysts in the remnant of the thyroglossal duct or the pharyngeal cleft systems, the digastric muscles, laryngoceles, or esophageal diverticuli. Rarely, a mass in or next to the thyroid will prove at surgery to be a parathyroid adenoma.

In goiters of any significant size, it is useful to palpate for a vascular thrill and to ascultate for a bruit. These sounds are characteristic of hyperplastic thyroid glands and are most frequently observed in Graves' disease. The bruit is typically a low-pitched to-and-fro murmur. It must be differentiated from a cardiac murmur, a bruit in a carotid artery related to atherosclerosis or, most frequently, from a venous hum.

In older patients, a pulsatile, hard innominate or common carotid artery may be found in the thoracic inlet and mistakenly identified as a thyroid mass. Occasionally, a large, soft mass at the thoracic inlet proves to be a lymphatic sac communicating with the thoracic duct. Cystic hygromas may be confusing in this region. More rarely, abundant subcutaneous padding of the anterior neck (fat pad goiter) or pronounced cervical lordosis (Modigliani's syndrome) may be confused with goiter.[1]

Laryngoscopic examination is important in all patients who report hoarseness or any change in voice, especially if operation on the thyroid gland is planned. It is important to repeat the examination after surgery if any alteration in the voice occurs.

EVALUATION BY LABORATORY TESTS

During the past three decades, clinical thyroidology has witnessed the introduction of a plethora of diagnostic procedures. These laboratory procedures provide greater choice, sensitivity, and specificity and have thus enhanced the likelihood of early detection of occult thyroid diseases presenting with only minimal clinical findings or obscured by coincidental nonthyroid diseases. They also assist in the exclusion of thyroid dysfunction when symptoms and signs closely mimic a thyroid ailment. On the other hand, the wide choice of complementary and overlapping tests indicates that each procedure has its limitations and that no single test is always reliable. The trend in clinical medicine to place a greater reliance upon laboratory aids has depreciated the value of the conventional history and physical findings, which are still crucial in the overall management and in the physician-patient relationship. Therefore, tests discussed in this chapter should be regarded as tools to validate a clinical impression. Only under special circumstances may tests alone be used to make a diagnosis or choose a particular mode of therapy.

Two fundamental questions should be considered in the evaluation of thyroid diseases. First, what is the metabolic status of the patient? Is the patient hormonally deficient (hypothyroid), hormonally sufficient (euthyroid), or is there hormonal excess (thyrotoxicosis)? Second, what is the etiology of the disease? The same process may give rise to a hormonal imbalance or cause an abnormality of thyroid gland anatomy in the absence of hormonal perturbation.

Thyroid tests can be classified into broad categories according to the information they provide at the functional, etiologic, or anatomic levels (Table 6-1).

1. Tests that directly assess the level of the gland activity and integrity of hormone biosynthesis. Tests such as thyroidal radioiodide uptake and perchlorate discharge are carried out in vivo.
2. Tests that measure the concentration of thyroid hormones and their transport in blood. They are performed in vitro and are basic for indirect assessment of thyroid hormone–dependent metabolic activity.

TABLE 6-1. Tests of Thyroid Function and Aids in the Diagnosis of Thyroid Diseases

In vivo tests of thyroid gland activity and integrity of hormone synthesis and secretion
    Thyroidal radioiodide uptake (RAIU)
        Early thyroid RAIU and ^{99m}pertechnetate uptake measurements
    Perchlorate discharge test
    Saliva-to-plasma radioiodide ratio

Measurement of hormone concentration and other iodinated compounds and their transport in blood
    Measurement of total thyroid hormone concentration in serum
        Iodometry
        Radioligand and immunometric assays
            TT_4
            TT_3
    Measurement of total and unsaturated thyroid hormone-binding capacity in serum
        In vitro uptake tests
        TBG measurement
    Estimation of free thyroid hormone concentration
        Dialyzable T_4 and T_3 by isotopic equilibrium
        Free T_4 and T_3 index methods
        Estimation of FT_4 and FT_3 by TBG measurement
        Two-step immunoassays
        Analog (one-step) immunoassays
    Measurements of iodine-containing hormone precursors and products of degradation
        3.3′,5′-triiodothyronine of reverse T_3 (rT_3)
        3,5,-diiodothyronine (3,5-T_2)
        3,3′,-diiodothyronine (3,3′-T_2)
        3′,5′,-diiodothyronine (3′,5′,-T_2)
        3′-monoiodothyronine (3′-T_1)
        3-monoiodothyronine (3-T_1)
        Tetra- and triiodothyroacetic acid (TETRAC and TRIAC)
        3,5,3′-T_3 sulfate (T_3S)
        di- and monoiodityrosine (MIT and DIT)
        Thyroglobulin (TG)

Measurement of thyroid hormone and its metabolities in other body fluids and in tissues
    Urine
    Amniotic fluid
    Cerebrospinal fluid (CSF)
    Milk
    Saliva
    Effusions
    Tissues

Tests assessing the effects of thyroid hormone on body tissues
    Basal metabolic rate (BMR)
    Deep tendon reflex relaxation time (photomotogram)

Tests related to cardiovascular function
Miscellaneous biochemical and physiologic changes related to the action of thyroid hormone on peripheral tissues
Measurement of substances absent in normal serum
    Thyroid autoantibodies
    Thyroid-stimulating immunoglobulins (TSI)
        Thyroid stimulation assays
            Standard in vivo mouse bioassay (LATS)
            In vitro bioassays (animal or human tissue and recombinant TSH receptor)
        Thyrotropin-binding assays
        Thyroid growth-promoting assay
    Other substances with thyroid-stimulating activity
    Exophthalmos-producing substance (EPS)
    Tests of cell-mediated immunity (CMI)
Anatomic and tissue diagnoses
    Thyroid scintiscanning
        Radioiodide and ^{99m}pertechnitate scans
        Other isotope scans
        Fluorescent scans
    Ultrasonography
    X-ray and related procedures
        Computed tomography (CT scanning)
        Angiography
        Lymphography
        Thermography
    Magnetic resonance imaging (MRI)
    Biopsy of the thyroid gland
        Core biopsy (open or closed)
        Percutaneous fine-needle aspiration (FNA)
Evaluation of the hypothalamic-pituitary-thyroid axis
    Thyrotropin (TSH)
    Thyrotropin-releasing hormone (TRH) test
    Other tests of TSH reserve
    Thyroid stimulation test
    Thyroid suppression test
Specialized thyroid tests
    Iodotyrosine deiodinase activity
    Tests for defective hormonogenesis
    Iodine kinetic studies
    Absorption of thyroid hormone
    Turnover kinetics of T_4 and T_3
    Metabolic kinetics of thyroid hormones and their metabolites
    Measurement of the production rate and metabolic kinetics of other compounds
    Transfer of thyroid hormone from blood to tissues
Applications of molecular biology in the diagnosis of thyroid diseases

3. Another category of tests attempts to measure more directly the impact of thyroid hormone on peripheral tissues. Unfortunately, tests available to assess this important parameter are nonspecific, since they are often altered by a variety of nonthyroidal processes.

4. The presence of several substances, such as thyroid autoantibodies, usually absent in healthy individuals, are useful in establishing the etiology of some thyroid illnesses.

5. Invasive procedures such as biopsy in histologic examination or enzymatic studies are occasionally required to establish a definite diagnosis. Gross abnormalities of the thyroid gland, detected by palpation, can be assessed by scintiscanning and by ultrasonography.

6. The integrity of the hypothalamic-pituitary-thyroid axis can be evaluated by (a) the response of the pituitary gland to thyroid hormone excess or deficiency; (b) the ability of the thyroid gland to respond to thyrotropin (TSH); and (c) the pituitary responsiveness to thyrotropin-releasing hormone (TRH). These tests are intended to identify the primary organ affected by the disease process that manifests as thyroid dysfunction; in other words, primary (thyroid), secondary (pituitary), or tertiary (hypothalamic) malfunction.

7. Lastly, a number of special tests will be briefly described. Some are invaluable in the elucidation of rare inborn errors of hormone biosynthesis and others are mainly research tools.

Each test has inherent limitations, and no single procedure is diagnostically adequate for the entire spectrum of possible thyroid abnormalities. The choice, execution, application and interpretation of each test requires the understanding of thyroid physiology and biochemistry dealt with in the preceding chapters. Thyroid tests serve not only in the diagnosis and management of thyroid illnesses but also enhance understanding of specific disease pathophysiology.

In Vivo Tests of Thyroid Gland Activity and Integrity of Hormone Synthesis and Secretion

Common to these tests is the administration to the patient of radioisotopes that the body cannot distinguish from naturally occurring, stable iodine isotopes (^{127}I). In contrast to all other tests, these procedures directly evaluate thyroid gland function. Formerly these tests were used to diagnose hypothyroidism and thyrotoxicosis, but this application has been supplanted by measurement of serum TSH and thyroid hormone concentrations in blood. Also, alterations of thyroid gland activity and in handling of iodine are not necessarily coupled to the amount of hormone produced and secreted. The tests are time consuming, relatively expensive, and expose the patient to irradiation that may not always be inconsequential. Nevertheless, they still are important in investigative medicine and in the diagnosis of inborn errors of thyroid hormonogenesis. Administration of isotopes is required for thyroid gland scanning used to demonstrate ectopic thyroid tissue and to establish the etiology of some forms of thyrotoxicosis. Finally, measurement of the thyroidal radioiodide uptake is the only means for estimating the dose of radioiodide to be delivered in the therapy of thyrotoxicosis and thyroid carcinoma.

To understand the physiologic basis of this category of tests, one should remember the following: Iodine is an integral part of the thyroid hormone molecule. Although several other tissues (salivary glands, mammary glands, lacrimal glands, the choroid plexus, and the parietal cells of the stomach) can extract iodide from blood and generate a positive tissue-to-serum iodide gradient, only the thyroid gland stores iodide for an appreciable period of time.[2] Since the kidneys continually filter blood iodide, the final fate of most iodine atoms is to be trapped by the thyroid gland or to be excreted in the urine. When a tracer of iodide is administered to the patient, it rapidly becomes mixed with the stable extrathyroidal iodide pool and its handling is thereafter identical to that of the stable isotope. Thus, the thyroidal content of radioiodine gradually increases and that in the extrathyroidal body pool gradually declines until virtually no free iodide is left. Normally this end point is reached between 24 and 72 hours.

From data of the radioiodide uptake by the thyroid gland and/or urinary excretion and/or stable iodide concentration in plasma and urine, the following pertinent parameters can be derived: (1) the rate of thyroidal iodine uptake (thyroid iodide clearance), (2) the fractional thyroid radioactive iodide uptake (RAIU), (3) the absolute iodide uptake (AIU) by the thyroid gland, and (4) the urinary excretion of radioiodide, or iodide clearance. After the complete

TABLE 6-2. Commonly Used Isotopes for In Vivo Studies and Radiation Dose Delivered

| Nuclide | Principal Photon Energy (keV) | Physical Decay | | Estimated Radiation Dose (m rads/μCi) Administered | | Average Dose Given for Scanning Purposes (μCi) |
		Mode	Half-Life (days)	Thyroid[a]	Total Body	
$^{131}I^-$	364	β (0.606 Mev)	8.1	1,340	0.08	50
$^{125}I^-$	28	Electron capture	60	835	0.06	50
$^{123}I^-$	159	Electron capture	0.55	13	0.03	200
$^{132}I^-$	670	β (2.12 MeV)	0.10	15	0.1	50[b]
$^{99m}TcO_4^-$	141	Isometric transition	0.25	0.2	0.01	2,500

[a] Calculations take into account the rate maximal uptake and residence time of the isotope, as well as gland size. For iodine isotopes, average data for adult euthyroid persons used were T$\frac{1}{2}$ of uptake 5 hours, biologic T$\frac{1}{2}$ 50 days, maximal uptake 20%, and gland size 15 g. (see also refs. [Quimby, 1970[5]; MIRD, 1975[6]; MIRD, 1976[7]]).

[b] Dose used for early thyroidal uptake studies.

removal of administered radioiodide, from the circulation, depletion of the radioisotope from the thyroid gland can be monitored by direct counting over the gland. Reappearance of the radioiodine in the circulation in protein-bound form can be measured and then used to estimate the intrathyroidal turnover of iodine and the secretory activity of the thyroid gland.

The foregoing tests can be combined with the administration of agents known to normally stimulate or to inhibit thyroid gland activity, thus providing information on the control of thyroid gland activity. Administration of radioiodide followed by scanning allows us to examine the anatomy of functional tissue. The latter two applications of in vivo tests utilizing radioiodide will be discussed under their respective headings.

The potential hazard of irradiation resulting from the administered radioisotopes should always be kept in mind. Children are particularly vulnerable, and doses of x-rays as small as 20 rads to the thyroid gland are associated with increased risk of developing thyroid malignancies.[3] However, it must be noted that there is no proven danger from isotopes used to diagnose thyroid diseases. In vivo administration of radioisotopes is absolutely contraindicated during pregnancy and in breast-feeding mothers.[4] Studies should be deferred if pregnancy is suspected.

A number of radioisotopes are now available. Furthermore, provision of more sophisticated and sensitive detection devices has substantially decreased the dose required to complete the studies. Table 6-2[5-7] lists the most commonly used isotopes for in vivo thyroid studies. Isotopes with slower physical decay,

such as $^{125}I^-$ and $^{131}I^-$, are particularly suitable for long-term studies. Isotopes with faster decay, such as $^{123}I^-$ and $^{132}I^-$, usually deliver a lower irradiation dose and are advantageous in short-term and repeated studies. The peak photon energy gamma emission differs among isotopes, allowing the execution of simultaneous studies with two isotopes.

Thyroidal Radioactive Iodide Uptake

Thyroidal radioactive iodide uptake is the most commonly used thyroid test requiring radioisotope administration. It is usually given orally in a capsule or in liquid form, and the quantity accumulated by the thyroid gland at various intervals of time is measured by epithyroid counting using a gamma scintillation counter. Correction for the amount of isotope circulating in the blood of the neck region, by subtracting counts obtained over the thigh, is of particular importance during the early periods following its administration. A dose of the same radioisotope, usually 10 percent, placed in a neck "phantom" is also counted as a "standard." The percentage of thyroidal RAIU is calculated from the counts cumulated per constant time unit.

The percentage of RAIU 24 hours after the administration of radioiodide is most useful, since in most instances the thyroid gland has reached the plateau of isotope accumulation and because it has been shown that the best separation between high, normal, and low uptake occurs at this time. Normal values for 24-hour RAIU in most parts of North America range from 5 to 30 percent. In many other parts

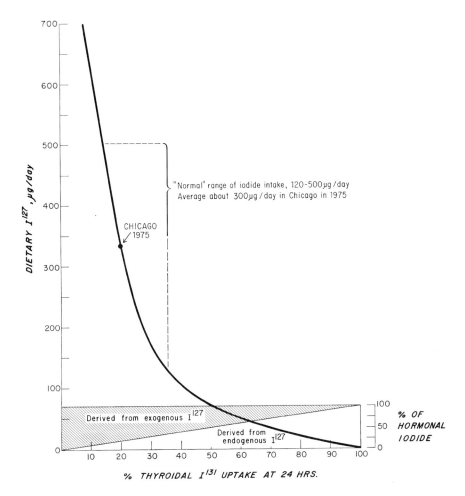

Fig. 6-1. Relation of 24-hour thyroidal radioiodide (^{131}I) uptake (RAIU) to dietary content of stable iodine (^{125}I). The uptake increases with decreasing dietary iodine. With iodine intake below the amount provided from thyroid hormone degradation, the latter contributes a larger proportion of the total iodine taken up by the thyroid. Under current dietary habits in the United States, the average 24-hour thyroidal RAIU is below 20 percent.

of the world, normal values range from 15 to 50 percent. Lower normal values are due to increased dietary iodine intake following the enrichment of foods, particularly mass-produced bread (150 µg of iodine per slice), with this element.[8] Fig. 6-1 shows the inverse relationship between the daily dietary intake of iodine and the RAIU test. The intake of large amounts of iodide (>5 mg/day), mainly from the use of iodine-containing radiologic contrast media, antiseptics, vitamins, and drugs, suppresses the RAIU values to a level hardly detectable using the usual equipment and doses of the isotope. Depending upon the type of iodine preparation and

the period of exposure, depression of RAIU can last for weeks, months, or even years. Most notorious is Lipiodol, formerly used in myelography. Even external application of iodide may suppress thyroidal RAIU. The need to inquire about individual dietary habits and sources of excess iodide intake is obvious.

The test does not measure hormone production and release but merely the avidity of the thyroid gland for iodide and its rate of clearance relative to the kidney. Disease states resulting in excessive production and release of thyroid hormone are most often associated with increased thyroidal RAIU and those causing hormone underproduction with de-

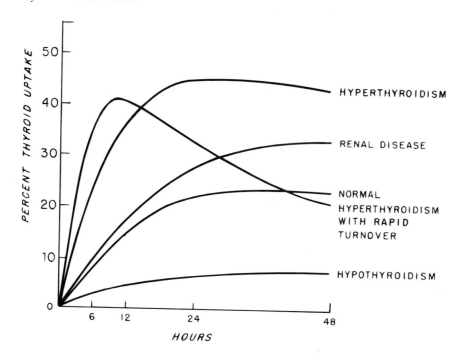

Fig. 6-2. Examples of thyroidal RAIU curves under various pathologic conditions. Note the prolonged uptake in renal disease due to decreased urinary excretion of the isotope, and the early decline in thyroidal radioiodide content in some patients with thyrotoxicosis associated with a small but rapidly turning over intrathyroidal iodine pool.

creased thyroidal RAIU (Fig. 6-2). Important exceptions include high uptake values in some hypothyroid patients and low values in some hyperthyroid patients. Increased thyroidal RAIU with hormonal insufficiency co-occur in the presence of severe iodide deficiency and in the majority of inborn errors of hormonogenesis (see Chapters 16 and 20). In the former, lack of substrate and, in the latter, a specific enzymatic block of hormone synthesis cause hypothyroidism poorly compensated by TSH-induced thyroid gland overactivity. Decreased thyroidal RAIU with hormonal excess is typically encountered in the syndrome of transient thyrotoxicosis (both de Quervain's and painless thyroiditis),[9] ingestion of exogenous hormone (thyrotoxicosis factitia), iodide-induced thyrotoxicosis (jodbasedow disease),[10] and in patients with thyrotoxicosis on moderately high intake of iodide (Table 6-3). High or low thyroidal RAIU as a result of low or high dietary iodine intake, respectively, may not be associated with significant changes in thyroid hormone secretion.

Table 6-3 lists various factors, including diseases,

that affect the value of the 24-hour thyroidal RAIU. Minor changes related to sex and age may be disregarded. Surreptitious spitting and vomiting within hours after administration of the radioisotope could significantly reduce the RAIU.

Several variations of the test have been devised that have particular value under special circumstances. Some of these are briefly described.

Early Thyroid RAIU and Pertechnetate ϱ99m Uptake Measurements

In some patients with severe thyrotoxicosis and low intrathyroidal iodine concentration, the turnover rate of iodine may be accelerated, causing a rapid initial uptake of radioiodide that reaches a plateau before 6 hours and that is followed by a decline through release of the isotope in hormonal or other forms (Fig. 6-2). Although this phenomenon is rare, some laboratories choose to routinely measure early RAIU, usually at 2, 4, or 6 hours. Early measurements require the accurate determination of background activity contributed by the circulating iso-

TABLE 6-3. Diseases and Other Factors Affecting 24-Hour Thyroidal RAIU

Increased RAIU
  Hyperthyroidism (Graves' disease, Plummer's disease, toxic adenoma, trophoblastic disease, pituitary resistance to thyroid hormone, TSH-producing pituitary adenoma)
  Nontoxic goiter (endemic, inherited biosynthetic defects, generalized resistance to thyroid hormone, Hashimoto's thyroiditis)
  Excessive hormonal loss (nephrosis, chronic diarrhea, hypolipidemic resins, diet high in soybean)
  Decreased renal clearance of iodine (renal insufficiency, severe heart failure)
  Recovery of the suppressed thyroid (withdrawal of thyroid hormone and antithyroid drug administration, subacute thyroiditis, iodine-induced myxedema)
  Iodine deficiency (endemic or sporadic dietary deficiency, excessive iodine loss as in pregnancy or in the dehalogenase defect)
  TSH administration
Decreased RAIU
  Hypothyroidism (primary or secondary)
  Defect in iodide concentration (inherited "trapping" defect, early phase of subacute thyroiditis, transient hyperthyroidism)
  Suppressed thyroid gland caused by thyroid hormone (hormone replacement, thyrotoxicosis factitia, struma ovarii)
  Iodine excess (dietary, drugs, and other iodine contaminants)
  Miscellaneous drugs and chemicals

tope. Radioisotopes with a shorter half-life, such as ^{123}I and ^{132}I, are more suitable.

Since thyroidal uptake in the very early period following administration of radioiodide reflects mainly iodide-trapping activity, pertechnetate 99m as the pertechnetate ion ($^{99m}TcO_4^-$) may be used. In euthyroid patients, thyroid trapping is maximal at about 20 minutes and is approximately 1 percent of the administered dose.[11] This test, when coupled with the administration of T_3, can be used to evaluate thyroid gland suppressibility in thyrotoxic patients treated with antithyroid drugs (see below).

Perchlorate Discharge Test

The perchlorate discharge test, used to detect defects in intrathyroidal iodide organification, is based on the following physiologic principle. Iodide is "trapped" by the thyroid gland through an energy-requiring active transport mechanism. Once in the gland, it is rapidly bound to thyroglobulin, and retention no longer requires active transport. Several ions, such as thiocyanate (SCN^-) and perchlorate (ClO_4^-), inhibit active iodide transport and cause the release of the intrathyroidal iodide not bound to thyroid protein. Thus measurement of intrathyroidal radioiodine loss following the administration of an inhibitor of iodide trapping would indicate the presence of an iodide-binding defect.

In the standard test, epithyroid counts are obtained at frequent intervals (every 10 or 15 minutes) following the administration of radioiodide. Two hours later, 1 g of potassium perchlorate ($KClO_4$) is administered orally and repeated epithyroid counts continue to be obtained for an additional 2 hours. In healthy individuals, radioiodide accumulation in the thyroid gland ceases after the administration of the iodide transport inhibitor, but there is little loss of the thyroidal radioactivity accumulated prior to induction of the "trapping" block. A loss of 5 percent or more indicates an organification defect (see Chapter 16).[12] The severity of the defect is proportional to the extent of radioiodide discharged from the gland and is complete when virtually all the activity accumulated by the gland is lost (see Fig. 16-2). The test is positive in the inborn defect of iodide organification, which can be associated with deafness (Pendred's syndrome), during the administration of iodide organification blocking agents, in some cases of Hashimoto's thyroiditis,[13] or following treatment with radioactive iodide.[14]

Several modifications of this test have been devised to increase its sensitivity, thus allowing the detection of minor defects of iodide organification. For example, in the 20-minute perchlorate discharge test, $NaClO_4$ is given intravenously 10 minutes after an intravenous dose of radioiodide while neck radioactivity is recorded continually.[15] In the iodide-perchlorate discharge test, 0.5 mg of stable iodide is given along with the tracer isotope and the test is performed in the manner described for the standard test.[16]

Saliva-to-Plasma Radioiodide Ratio

The saliva-to-plasma radioiodide ratio evaluates the iodide-trapping function, and its principal application is in the diagnosis of congenital defects in this step of iodine metabolism. Like the thyroid gland, some organs, including the salivary glands, concentrate iodide to severalfold the plasma level.[2] Patients unable to concentrate iodide in the thyroid gland also have this defect in other tissues normally possessing this transport process. The test involves administering radioiodide followed 1 hour later by the simultaneous collection of saliva and blood. The saliva-to-plasma ratio (S:P) of isotope in an equal volume of these fluids is normally greater than 10 or 40, depending upon the rate of saliva flow.[17] It is near 1 in patients with congenital trapping defect (see Chapter 16).

Measurement of Hormone Concentration and Other Iodinated Compounds and Their Transport in Blood

Measurements of T_4 and T_3 in serum and the estimation of their free concentration have become the most commonly used tests for evaluating thyroid hormone–dependent metabolic status. This approach has been espoused since the development of simple, sensitive, and specific methods for measuring these iodothyronines and because no specific tests directly measure the metabolic effect of these hormones. Other advantages are the requirement of only a small blood sample and the large number of determinations that can be completed by a laboratory during a regular workday.

The thyroid gland is the principal source of all hormonal iodine-containing compounds or their precursors, and peripheral tissue is the source of the products of degradation. Fig. 6-3 provides their chemical structures and normal concentrations in serum. Note that the concentration of each substance depends not only upon the amount synthesized and secreted but also upon its affinity for carrier serum proteins, distribution in tissues, rate of degradation and, finally, clearance.

The main secretory product of the thyroid gland is T_4, T_3 being next in relative abundance. Both compounds are metabolically active when administered in vivo. They are synthesized and stored in the thyroid gland as a part of a larger molecule, thyroglobulin (TG), which must be degraded to release the two iodothyronines in a ratio favoring T_4 by 10- to 20-fold.[18] Under normal circumstances, only minute amounts of TG escape into the circulation. On a

molar basis, it is the least abundant iodine-containing compound in blood. With the exception of T_4, TG, and small amounts of diiodotyrosine (DIT) and monoiodotyrosine (MIT), all other iodine-containing compounds found in the serum of healthy persons are produced mainly in extrathyroidal tissues by a stepwise process of deiodination of T_4.[19] An alternative pathway of T_4 metabolism that involves deamination and decarboxylation but retention of the iodine residues gives rise to tetraiodothyroacetic acid (TETRAC) and triiodothyroacetic acid (TRIAC).[20,21] Conjugation to form sulfated iodoproteins also occurs.[22] Circulating iodoalbumin is generated by intrathyroidal iodination of serum albumin.[23] Small amounts of iodoproteins may be formed in peripheral tissues[24] or in serum[25,26] by covalent linkage of T_4 and T_3 to soluble proteins. Although the physiologic function of circulating iodine compounds other than T_4 and T_3 remains unknown, measuring changes in their concentration is occasionally of diagnostic value.

Measurement of Total Thyroid Hormone Concentration in Serum Iodometry

Iodine constitutes an integral part of the thyroid hormone molecule. It is thus not surprising that determination of iodine content in serum was the first method suggested almost six decades ago to identify and quantify thyroid hormone.[27]

Measurement of protein-bound iodine (PBI) was the earliest method used routinely to estimate thyroid hormone concentration in serum. The test measures the total quantity of iodine precipitable with the serum proteins,[28] 90 percent of which is T_4. The normal range is 4 to 8 μg I/dl of serum.

Efforts to measure serum thyroid hormone levels with greater specificity and with lesser interference from nonhormonal iodinated compounds led to the development of the butanol-extractable iodine (BEI) and T_4I by column techniques. In the BEI method, sequential extractions with acidified butanol and washes with alkali result in the isolation of iodothyronines. The T_4I by column measures the iodine content in iodothyronines after their isolation from serum by an anion-exchange resin column followed by serial elution with increasing concentrations of acetic acid. All chemical methods for measuring thyroid hormone in serum have been

NAME	Abbreviation	Molecular Weight	FORMULA	NORMAL CONCENTRATION[a] (range)	
				ng / dl	pmol / L
3,5,3',5'-tetraiodothyronine (Thyroxine)	T_4	777	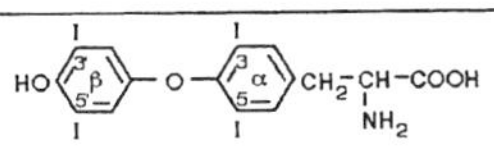	5,000 - 12,000	64,000 - 154,000
3,5,3'-triiodothyronine (Liothyronine)	T_3	651	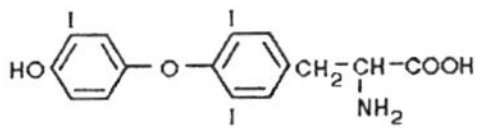	80 - 190[b]	1,200 - 2,900
3,3',5'-triiodothyronine (Reverse T_3)	rT_3	651	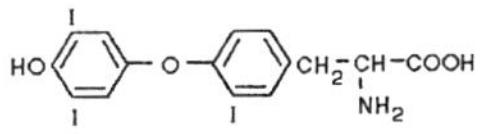	14 - 30	220 - 480
3.5-diiodothyronine	$3,5-T_2$	525	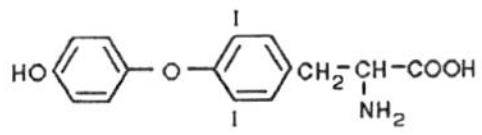	0.20- 0.75[b]	3.8 - 14
3,3'-diiodothyronine	$3,3'-T_2$	525	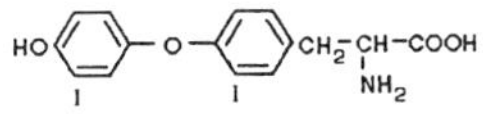	1 - 8[b]	19 - 150
3'5'-diiodothyronine	$3'5'-T_2$	525	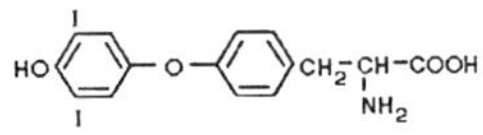	1.5 - 9.0[b]	30 - 170
3'-monoiodothyronine	$3'-T_1$	399	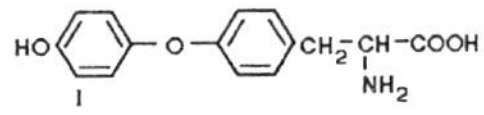	0.6 - 4	15 - 100
3-monoiodothyronine	$3-T_1$	399	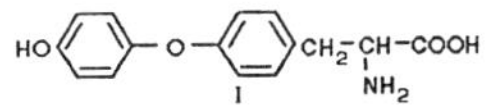	< 0.5 - 7.5	< 13 - 190
3,5,3',5'-tetraiodothyroacetic acid (TETRAC)	T_4A	748	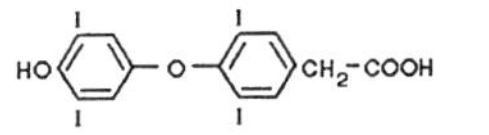	< 8 - 60	< 105 - 800
3,5,3'-triiodothyroacetic acid (TRIAC)	T_3A	622	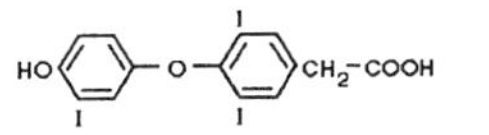	1.6 - 3	26 - 48
3,5-diiodotyrosine	DIT	433	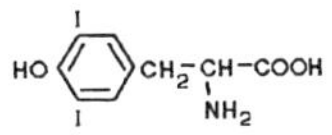	1 - 2	23 - 530
3-monoiodotyrosine	MIT	307	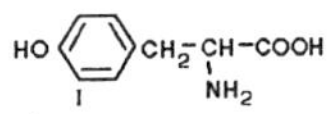	90 - 390[c]	2,900 - 12,700
thyroglobulin	Tg	660,000	glycoprotein made of two identical subunits	< 100 - 2,500	1.5 - 38

Fig. 6-3. Iodine-containing compounds in serum of healthy adults. **(a)** Iodothyronine concentration in the euthyroid population is not normally distributed. Thus, calculation of the normal range on the basis of 95 percent confidence limits for a Gaussain distribution is inaccurate. **(b)** Significant decline with old age. **(c)** Probably an overestimation due to cross-reactivity by related substances.

replaced by the ligand assays, which are devoid of interference by even large quantities of nonhormonal iodine-containing substances.

Iodometry is still used experimentally to measure the iodine content in TG and in special clinical conditions, such as inborn defects of hormonogenesis, when the production and secretion of nonhormonal iodine-containing compounds is suspected. A difference between the PBI and T_4I level greater than 20 percent is found in some patients with inherited or acquired defects of hormonogenesis (see Chapters 8 and 16).

Radioligand Assays

Naturally occurring, iodide-containing compounds in serum can be measured by radioimmunoassays (RIA). The principle of these assays is the competition of the substance (S) being measured with the same isotopically labeled compound (S*) for binding to a specific class of immunoglobulin G (IgG) molecules present in the antiserum (antibody [Ab]). S is the ligand and the Ab is either a polyclonal antiserum to S or a monoclonal IgG. The reaction obeys the law of mass action. Thus, at equilibrium, the amount of S* bound to Ab to form the complex Ab-S* is inversely proportional to the concentration of S and forms the complex Ab-S, provided the amounts of Ab and S* are kept constant.

$$AbS^* + [S] \rightleftharpoons AbS + S^*$$

The radioisotope content in Ab-S* or in the unbound (free) S* is determined after their separation by precipitation of the antibody-ligand complex or adsorption of the free ligand. Some RIAs are carried out with the Ab fixed to a solid support, reacting with S and S* in solution. Increments of known amounts of S are added to a series of reactions to construct a standard curve that describes the curvilinear stoichiometric relationship between Ab-S* and S. It can be converted to a straight line by a number of mathematical transformations, such as the logit-log plot. Blank reactions contain S* but not specific Ab or a large excess of S in a full reaction.[29] The sensitivity of the assay is dependent upon the affinity of the Ab and specific activity of S*. Under optimal conditions, as little as 1 pg of S can be measured.

Production of antisera requires that iodoamino acids be rendered antigenic by conjugation to albumin or to some other large molecule or particle.[30] In the assay, the iodoamino acids need to be liberated from their association with hormone-binding serum proteins, mainly TBG, the affinity constant of which is often equal to that of most antisera. Methods include extraction, competitive displacement of the iodoamino acid being measured, or inactivation of thyroxine-binding globulin (TBG).[31-34] Ideally, binding competitors should displace the iodoamino acid from TBG but interfere little or not at all with the specific immune reaction. This technique allows measurements in samples of whole unprocessed serum. While there is no interference by nonhormonal iodine-containing compounds, some cross-reactivity among related naturally occurring iodoamino acids does exist.[35] Thus, antibodies that possess little or no cross-reactivity should be selected for each assay, particularly when the concentration of the measured substance is lower than that of the cross-reacting congeners. Antisera are rarely able to differentiate the L from the D isomers,[36,37] but this is not crucial in clinical assays. Rarely, some patients develop circulating antibodies against thyronines that interfere with the RIA carried out on unextracted serum samples. Depending on the method used for the separation of bound from free ligand, values obtained may be either spuriously low or high in the presence of such antibodies.[38,39]

A wide choice of commercial kits is available for most RIA procedures, making these assays accessible to all medical centers. RIAs have been adapted for the measurement of T_4 in small samples of dried blood spots on filter paper and are used in screening for neonatal hypothyroidism.[40]

The first method developed to measure an iodoamino acid using the principle described above did not make use of antiserum.[41] The native serum protein TBG was used instead of an antibody to measure T_4 in extracted serum. The method, termed *competitive protein-binding assay (CPBA)*, was gradually supplanted by the RIA.

Other Methods

More recently, assays have been developed that are based on the principle of the radioligand assay but that do not use radioactive material. These assays, which use ligand conjugated to an enzyme, are gradually replacing currently used RIAs. The enzyme-linked ligand competes with the ligand being measured for the same binding sites on the antibody. Quantitation is carried out by spectrophotometry of the color reaction developed after the addition of the enzyme substrate.[42] Both homogeneous (*enzyme-multiplied immunoassay technique [EMIT]*) and heterogeneous (*enzyme-linked immunosorbent assay [ELISA]*) assays for T_4 have been developed.[43-45] In the homogeneous assays, no separation step is required, thus providing easy automation.[43] In one such assay, T_4 is linked to malate dehydrogenase, inhibiting the enzyme activity. The enzyme is activated when the T_4 enzyme conjugate is bound to T_4-specific antibody. Active T_4 conjugates to other enzymes, such as peroxidase[44] and alkaline phosphatase,[45] have also been developed. The assay has been adapted to measure T_4 in dried blood samples used in mass screening programs for neonatal hypothyroidism.[45] Other nonradioisotope immunoassays use *fluorescence excitation* to detect the labeled ligand and *radial diffusion* to separate antibody-bound from free ligand on a solid matrix.

Several techniques distinct from iodometry, radioligand assays, and enzyme-linked immunologic assays, have been devised to measure T_4 and T_3 in serum and in other biologic materials. They include *gas-liquid chromatography*,[46] *neutron activation*,[47] and *double isotope derivative*[48] assays. These methods are likely to remain strictly research tools. A modified version of liquid chromatography can distinguish between D- and L-isomers.[49]

Serum Total Thyroxine

The usual concentration of serum total thyroxine (TT_4) in adults ranges from 5 to 12 μg/dl (64 to 154 nmol/L). When concentrations are below or above this range in the absence of thyroid dysfunction, they are usually the result of an abnormal level of serum TBG. The hyperestrogenic state of pregnancy and administration of estrogen-containing compounds are the most common causes of a significant elevation of serum TT_4 levels in euthyroid persons. Rarely, TBG excess is inherited.[50] Serum TT_4 is virtually undetectable in the fetus until midgestation. Thereafter, it rapidly increases, reaching high-normal adult levels during the last trimester. A further acute but transient rise occurs within hours after delivery.[51] Values remain above the adult range until 6 years of age,[52] but subsequent age-related changes are minimal and not a uniform finding.[53-55] In clinical practice, the same normal range of TT_4 applies to both sexes and all ages above 6 years.

Small seasonal variations and changes related to high altitude, cold, and heat have been described. Rhythmic variations in serum TT_4 concentration are of two types: variations related to postural changes in serum protein concentration[56] and true circadian variation.[31] Postural changes in protein concentration do not alter the free T_4 (FT_4) concentration.

Although levels of serum TT_4 below the normal range are usually associated with hypothyroidism and above this range with thyrotoxicosis, it must be remembered that the TT_4 level may not always correspond to the FT_4 concentration, which represents the metabolically active fraction (see below). The TT_4 concentration in serum may be altered by independent mechanisms: (1) an increase or decrease in the supply of T_4, as seen in most cases of thyrotoxicosis and hypothyroidism, respectively; (2) changes

due solely to alterations in T_4 binding to serum proteins; and (3) compensatory changes in serum TT_4 concentration due to high or low serum levels of T_3. Table 6-4 lists conditions associated with changes in serum TT_4 and their relationship to the metabolic status of the patient.

Serum TT_4 levels are low in conditions associated with decreased TBG concentration, the presence of abnormal TBGs with reduced binding affinity (see Chapter 16), or when the available T_4-binding sites on TBG are partially saturated by competing drugs present in blood in high concentrations (see Table 5-2). Conversely, TT_4 levels are high when the serum TBG concentration is high. The person remains euthyroid provided the feedback regulation of the thyroid gland is intact.

Although changes in transthyretin (TTR) concentration rarely give rise to significant alterations in TT_4 concentration,[57] the presence of a variant serum albumin with high affinity for T_4[58,59] or antibodies against T_4[38,39] produce elevations in the TT_4 concentration, whereas the FT_4 level and and metabolic status remain normal. The variant albumin is inherited as an autosomal dominant trait termed *familial dysalbuminemic hyperthyroxinemia* (*FDH*) (see Chapter 16).

Another possible cause of discrepancy between the observed serum TT_4 concentration and the metabolic status of the patient is divergent changes in the serum TT_3 and TT_4 concentrations with alterations in the serum T_3/T_4 ratio. The most common situation is that of elevated TT_3 concentration. The source of T_3 may be endogenous, as in T_3 thyrotoxicosis, or exogenous, as during ingestion of T_3. In the former situation, contrary to the common variety of thyrotoxicosis, elevation in the serum TT_3 concentration is not accompanied by an increase in the TT_4 level. In fact, the serum TT_4 level is normal and occasionally low.[60] This finding indicates that in T_3 thyrotoxicosis the hormone is predominantly secreted as such rather than arising from the peripheral conversion of T_4 to T_3. Ingestion of pharmacologic doses of T_3 results in thyrotoxicosis associated with severe depression of the serum TT_4 concentration. A moderate hypersecretion of T_3 can be associated with euthyroidism and a low serum TT_4 concentration. This circumstance, occasionally referred to as T_3 *euthyroidism*, may be more prevalent than T_3 thyrotoxicosis. It is believed to constitute a state of compensatory T_3 secretion as a physiologic adaptation

TABLE 6-4. Conditions Associated with Changes in Serum TT$_4$ Concentration and Relation to the Metabolic Status

Metabolic Status	Serum TT$_4$ Concentration		
	High	Low	Normal
Thyrotoxic	Hyperthyroidism (all causes, including Graves' disease, Plummer's disease, toxic thyroid adenoma, early phase of subacute thyroiditis) Thyroid hormone leak (early stage of subacute thyroiditis, transient thyrotoxicosis) Excess of exogenous or ectopic T$_4$ (thyrotoxicosis factitia, struma ovarii) Predominantly pituitary resistance to thyroid hormone	Intake of excessive amounts of T$_3$ (thyrotoxicosis factitia)	Low TBG (congenital or acquired) T$_3$ thyrotoxicosis (untreated or recurrent post therapy); more common in iodine deficient areas Drugs competing with T$_4$-binding to serum proteins (see also entry under euthyroid with low TT$_4$) Hypermetabolism of nonthyroidal origin (Luft's syndrome)

Euthyroid	High TBG (congenital or acquired)
	 T$_4$-binding albuminlike variant
	 Endogenous T$_4$ antibodies
	 Replacement therapy with T$_4$ only
	 Treatment with D-T$_4$
	 Generalized resistance to thyroid hormone
		Low TBG (congenital or acquired)
		 Endogenous T$_4$ antibodies
		
		 Mildly elevated or normal T$_3$
		    T$_3$ replacement therapy
		
		    Iodine deficiency
		    Treated thyrotoxicosis
		    Chronic thyroiditis
		    Congenital goiter
		 Drugs competing with T$_4$-binding to serum proteins
			Normal state

Hypothyroid	Severe generalized resistance to thyroid hormone	Thyroid gland failure
		   Primary (all causes, including gland destruction, severe iodine deficiency, inborn error of hormonogenesis)
		   Secondary (pituitary failure)
		   Tertiary (hypothalamic failure)
			High TBG (congenital or acquired)
			 ?Isolated peripheral tissue resistance to thyroid hormone

of the failing thyroid gland, such as after treatment for thyrotoxicosis, in some cases of chronic thyroiditis, or during iodine deprivation.[61,62] Serum TT$_4$ concentration is also low in healthy persons receiving replacement doses of T$_3$. Conversely, serum TT$_4$ levels are above the upper limit of normal in 15 to 50 percent of patients rendered eumetabolic by administration of T$_4$ alone.[63] Because of the relatively slow rate of metabolism and large extrathyroidal T$_4$ pool, the serum concentration of the hormone varies little with the time of sampling in relation to ingestion of the daily dose.[64]

Two conditions also characteristically occur with a discrepancy between the clinical status and the serum concentration of TT$_4$: (1) the syndrome of resistance to thyroid hormone associated with elevated TT_4 as well as FT_4 and TT_3 levels and usually clinical euthyroidism[65] and (2) the syndrome of hypermetabolism in the absence of thyroid dysfunction described by Luft et al.[66] The latter is a rare mitochondrial defect producing thyroid hormone–independent hypermetabolism.

Serum Total Triiodothyronine

Normal serum TT_3 concentrations in the adult are 80 to 190 ng/dl (1.2 to 2.9 nmol/L). While sex differences are small, differences with age are more dramatic. In contrast to serum TT_4, TT_3 concentration at birth is low, about one-half the normal adult level. It rises within 24 hours to about double the normal adult value followed by a rapid decrease over the subsequent 24 hours to a level in the upper adult range, which persists for the first year of life.[51] A steady decline in the mean TT_3 level has been observed to cover the entire life span, from early childhood to old age.[53-55] It is possible that the change is related to the prevalence of nonthyroidal illness rather than to age alone.[67] Nevertheless, interpretation of borderline values should take into account the patient's age. Although a positive correlation between serum TT_3 level and body weight has been observed, it may be related to overeating.[68] Rapid and profound reductions in serum TT_3 level can be produced within 24 to 48 hours of total calorie or only carbohydrate deprivation.[69-71]

Most conditions causing serum TT_4 levels to increase are associated with high TT_3 concentrations. Thus, serum TT_3 levels are usually elevated in thyrotoxicosis and reduced in hypothyroidism. However, in both conditions the TT_3/TT_4 ratio is elevated relative to normal euthyroid persons. This elevation is due to the disproportionate increase in serum TT_3 concentration in thyrotoxicosis and a lesser diminution in hypothyroidism relative to the TT_4 concentration.[30,36,72] Accordingly, measurement of the serum TT_3 level is a more sensitive test for the diagnosis of hyperthyroidism and that of TT_4 more useful in the diagnosis of hypothyroidism.

There are circumstances in which discrepancies between the serum TT_3 and TT_4 concentrations are disproportionate or in opposite direction (Table 6-

5). It is in such conditions that measurement of T_3 has been most useful. It has helped explain the syndrome of thyrotoxicosis with normal TT_4 and FT_4 levels (T_3 thyrotoxicosis), and in some cases only the free T_3 may be elevated.[60,73] In some patients, treatment of thyrotoxicosis with antithyroid drugs may normalize the serum TT_4 but not TT_3 level, producing a high TT_3/TT_4 ratio. Patients with T_3-predominant Graves' disease and TT_3/TT_4 greater than 20 ng/μg are believed to be less prone to remission.[74] In areas of limited iodine supply[62] and in patients with limited thyroidal ability to process iodide,[61] euthyroidism can be maintained at low serum TT_4 and FT_4 levels by increased direct thyroidal secretion of T_3. Although these changes have a rational physiologic explanation, the significance of discordant serum TT_4 and TT_3 levels under other circumstances is less well understood.

The most common cause of discordant serum concentrations of TT_3 and TT_4 is a selective decrease of serum TT_3 due to decreased conversion of T_4 to T_3 in peripheral tissues. This reduction is an integral part of the pathophysiology of a number of nonthyroidal acute and chronic illnesses and calorie deprivation (see Ch. 5). In these conditions, the serum TT_3 level is often lower than that commonly found in patients with frank primary hypothyroidism, yet these persons do not present clear clinical evidence of hypometabolism. In some individuals, decreased T_4 to T_3 conversion in the pituitary gland[75] or in peripheral tissues[76] is an inherited condition.

A variety of drugs may also produce changes in the serum TT_3 concentration without apparent metabolic consequences (see Chapter 6). Drugs that compete with hormone binding to serum proteins decrease serum TT_3 levels, presumably without affecting the free T_3 concentration (Table 5-5). Some drugs, such as glucocorticoids,[77] depress the serum TT_3 concentration by interfering with the peripheral conversion of T_4 to T_3. Others, such as phenobarbital,[78] depress the serum TT_3 concentration by stimulating the rate of intracellular hormone degradation. The majority have multiple effects. These effects are combinations of those described above, as well as inhibition of the hypothalamic-pituitary axis or thyroidal hormonogenesis.[79]

Changes in serum TBG concentration have an effect on the serum TT_3 concentration similar to that on TT_4 (see Chapter 16). The presence of endoge-

TABLE 6-5. Conditions That May be Associated with Discrepancies Between the Concentration of Serum TT_3 and TT_4

Serum TT_3/TT_4 Ratio	TT_3	TT_4	Metabolic Status		
			Thyrotoxic	Euthyroid	Hypothyroid
↑	↑	N	T_3-thyrotoxicosis (endogenous)	Endemic iodine deficiency (T_3 autoantibodies)[a]	—
↑	N	↓	—	Treated thyrotoxicosis (T_4 autoantibodies)[a]	Endemic cretins (severe iodine deficiency)
↑	↑	↓	Pharmacologic doses of T_3 (exogenous T_3-toxicosis) Partially treated thyrotoxicosis	T_3 replacement (especially 1 to 3 h after ingestion) Endemic iodine deficiency	(T_3 autoantibodies)[a]
↓	↓	N	—	Most conditions associated with reduced conversion of T_4 to T_3 Chronic or severe acute illness[b] Trauma (surgical, burns) Fasting and malnutrition Drugs[c] (T_3 autoantibodies)[a]	—
↓	N	↑	Severe nonthyroidal illness associated with thyrotoxicosis	Neonates (first three weeks of life) T_4 replacement Familial hyperthyroixinemia due to T_4-binding albuminlike variant (T_4 autoantibodies)[a]	—
↓	↓	↑	—	At birth Acute nonthyroidal illness with transient hyperthyroxinemia	(T_4 autoantibodies)[a]

[a] Artifactual values dependent upon the method of hormone determination in serum.

[b] Hepatic and renal failure, diabetic ketoacidosis, myocardial infarction, infectious and febrile illness, malignancies.

[c] Glucocorticoids, iodinated contrast agents, amiodarone, propranolol, propylthiouracil.

nous antibodies to T_3 may result in an elevation of the serum TT_3, but as in the case of high TBG, the concentration of FT_3 is normal and it does not cause hypermetabolism.[38]

Administration of commonly used replacement doses of T_3, usually on the order of 75 μg/day or 1 μg/kg body weight per day,[80] results in serum TT_3 levels in the thyrotoxic range. Furthermore, because of the rapid gastrointestinal absorption and relatively fast degradation rate, the serum level varies considerably according to the time of sampling in relation to hormone ingestion.[64]

Measurement of Total and Unsaturated Thyroid Hormone–Binding Capacity in Serum

Because the concentration of thyroid hormone in serum is dependent on its supply as well as on the abundance of hormone-binding sites on serum proteins, the estimation of the latter facilitates the correct interpretation of values obtained from the measurement of the total hormone concentration. These results may be used to estimate the free hormone concentration, which is important in differentiating changes in serum total hormone concentration due to alterations of binding proteins in euthyroid patients from those due to abnormalities in thyroid gland activity giving rise to hypermetabolism or hypometabolism.

In Vitro Uptake Tests

In vitro uptake tests measure the unoccupied thyroid hormone–binding sites on TBG. They use labeled T_3 or T_4 and some form of synthetic absorbent to measure the proportion of radiolabeled hormone that is not tightly bound to serum proteins. Because ion exchange resins are often used as absorbents, the test became known as the *resin T_3 or T_4 uptake test (T_3U or T_4U)*, describing the technique rather than the entity measured. This name has sometimes led to confusion with the in vivo iodine uptake test. The T_3U test is sometimes referred to as the T_3 *test*. This name is inappropriate and should be reserved to indicate measurement of T_3 concentration.

The test is usually carried out by incubating a sample of the patient's serum with a trace amount of labeled T_3 or T_4. The labeled hormone, not bound to available binding sites on TBG present in the serum sample, is absorbed onto an anion exchange resin and measured as resin-bound radioactivity. Values correlate inversely with the concentration of unsaturated TBG. Various methods use different absorbing materials to remove the hormone not tightly bound to TBG. The original test used red blood cells[81] which were soon replaced by anion exchange resin in the form of beads or sponges[82] and other adsorbing materials. Labeled T_3 is usually used because of its less firm yet preferential binding to TBG. Similar results can be obtained with T_4, after appropriate serum dilution and addition of T_4. The addition of barbital buffer allows selective binding of T_4 to TBG.[83] Irrespective of the materials used, the various assay requirements must be standardized and kept constant. Although the test is not affected by the presence of most nonhormonal iodine–containing compounds, it has been reported that Oragrafin[84] and, to a limited extent heparin,[85] will increase the uptake of tracer by particular absorbents. Depending upon the method, typical normal results for T_3U are 25 to 35 percent or 45 to 55 percent. Thus, it is more valuable to express results of the uptake tests as a ratio of the result obtained in a normal control serum run in the same assay as the test samples. Normal values will then range on either side of 1.0, usually 0.85 to 1.15.

The uptake of the tracer by the absorbent is inversely proportional to the amount of unsaturated binding sites (unoccupied by endogenous thyroid hormone) in serum TBG. Thus, the uptake is increased when the amount of unsaturated TBG is reduced as a result of excess endogenous thyroid hormone or a decrease in the concentration of TBG. In contrast, the uptake is decreased when the amount of unsaturated TBG is increased as a result of a low serum thyroid hormone concentration or an increase in the concentration of TBG. Since the test can be affected by either or both independent variables, serum total thyroid hormone and TBG concentrations, the results cannot be interpreted without knowledge of the hormone concentration. As a rule, parallel increases or decreases in both serum TT_4 concentration and the T_3U test indicate hyperthyroidism and hypothyroidism, respectively, whereas discrepant changes in serum TT_4 and T_3U suggest abnormalities in TBG binding. However, abnormalities in hormone and TBG concentrations may coexist in the same patient. For example, a hypothyroid patient with a low TBG level will typically show a low TT_4 level and normal T_3U result (Fig. 6-4). Because of structural similarities, several nonhormonal compounds compete with thyroid hormone for its binding site on TBG. Some are used as pharmacologic agents and may thus alter the in vitro uptake test as well as the total thyroid hormone concentration in serum. Table 5-2 lists these compounds.

TBG and TTR Measurements

The concentrations of TBG and TTR in serum can be estimated by measurement of their total T_4 binding capacity at saturation[86] or measured directly by immunologic techniques.[87,88] Although the saturation methods provide accurate information on the total binding capacity of individual carrier proteins, they are tedious. They are based on the partition of labeled T_4 among the carrier proteins in serum (TBG, TTR, and albumin) separated by electrophoresis and determined at several increments of added T_4. Values may vary according to the conditions of electrophoresis, in particular the type of buffer and pH. Generally accepted normal values in the adult are 14 to 27 μg T_4/dl serum (180 to 350 nmol/L) for TBG capacity and 220 to 360 μg T_4/dl serum (2.8 to 4.6 μmol/L) for TTR capacity. A simple saturation

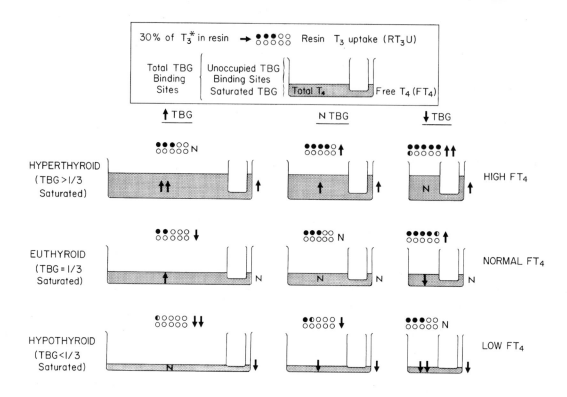

Fig. 6-4. Graphic representation of the relationship between the serum total T_4 concentration, the RT_3U test, and the free T_4 (FT_4) concentration in various metabolic states and in association with changes in TBG. The principle of communicating vessels is used as an illustration. The height of fluid in the small vessel represents the level of FT_4; the total amount of fluid in the large vessel, the total T_4 concentration; and the total volume of the large vessel, the TBG capacity. Dots represent resin beads and black dots, those carrying the radioactive T_3 tracer ($T3^*$). The RT_3U test result (black dots) is inversely proportional to the unoccupied TBG binding sites represented by the unfilled capacity of the large vessel. (From Endocrinology, L.J. DeGroot (ed). 1979, Grune & Straton Inc.)

method, using anion exchange resin rather than electrophoresis, is available for routine use in clinical laboratories.[83]

Immunologic methods for directly measuring proteins are also available. TBG concentration in serum can be determined by RIA,[88] and both TBG and TTR can be measured by Laurell's rocket immunoelectrophoresis,[89,90] by radial immunodiffusion,[91] or by enzyme immunoassay.[87] Another method combines hormone binding to TBG and immunologic techniques.[92] Commercial kits are available for quantifying serum TBG; these employ, with various modifications, the technical principles described above. Some use a competitive partition of the radioiodinated hormone between endogenous TBG and added antiserum against the hormone; others use a

specific TBG antiserum and T_4 or radioiodinated TBG as label. Absolute concentrations in the serum of normal adults vary according to the purity of the standard preparation. The true mean value for TBG is 1.6 mg/dl (260 nmol/L), with a range of 1.1 to 2.2 mg/dl (180 to 350 nmol/L) serum. In adults, the normal range for TTR is 16 to 30 mg/dl (2.7 to 5.0 μmol/L).

The concentrations of TBG and TTR in serum vary with age, sex, pregnancy, and posture. Determining the concentration of these proteins in serum is particularly helpful when evaluating extreme deviations from normal, as in congenital abnormalities of TBG. In most instances, however, the in vitro uptake test, in conjunction with the serum TT_4 level, gives an approximate estimation of the TBG concentration. A numerical value can be derived from the ratio of the T_3U test expressed as a percentage of the normal control and the serum TT_4, known as the *TBG index*.[93]

Estimation of Free Thyroid Hormone Concentration

A minute amount of thyroid hormone circulates in the blood in a free form, not bound to serum proteins. It is in reversible equilibrium with the bound hormone and represents the diffusible fraction of the hormone capable of traversing cellular membranes to exert its effects on body tissues.[94] Although changes in serum hormone–binding proteins affect both the total hormone concentration and the corresponding fraction circulating free, in the euthyroid person the absolute concentration of free hormone remains constant. This finding agrees with the concept of free hormone transfer from blood to tissue. It is thus not surprising that the concentration of free hormone in serum correlates better with the tissue hormone level and its biologic effect.[95] Information concerning this value is probably the most important parameter in the evaluation of thyroid function as it relates to the metabolic status of the patient.

With few exceptions, the free hormone concentration is high in thyrotoxicosis, low in hypothyroidism, and normal in euthyroidism, even in the presence of profound changes in TBG concentration,[96,97] provided the patients is in a steady state (see Fig. 5-4). Notably, FT_4 concentration may be normal or even low in patients with T_3 thyrotoxicosis and in those ingesting pharmacologic doses of T_3. On occasion, the concentration of FT_4 may be outside the normal range in the absence of an apparent abnormality in the thyroid hormone–dependent metabolic status. This is frequently observed in severe nonthyroidal illness during which both high[96–98] and low[99,100] values have been reported. As expected, when a euthyroid state is maintained by the administration of T_3 or by predominant thyroidal secretion of T_3, the FT_4 level is also depressed. More consistently, patients with a variety of nonthyroidal illnesses have low FT_3 levels.[101] This decrease is characteristic of all conditions associated with depressed serum TT_3 concentrations due to a diminished conversion of T_4 to T_3 in peripheral tissues (see Chapter 5). Both FT_4 and FT_3 values may be out of line in patients receiving a variety of drugs (see below). Marked elevations in both FT_4 and FT_3 concentrations in the absence of

hypermetabolism are typical of patients with resistance to thyroid hormone (see Chapter 16).[65] The FT_3 concentration is usually normal or even high in hypothyroid persons living in areas of severe endemic iodine deficiency. Their FT_4 levels are, however, normal or low.[62]

Direct Measurement of Free T_4 and Free T_3

Unfortunately, the precise measurements of absolute FT_4 and FT_3 concentrations are technically difficult and have until recently been limited to research assays. To minimize perturbations of the relationship between the free and bound hormone, these must be separated by ultrafiltration or by dialysis involving minimal dilution and little alteration of the pH or electrolyte composition. The separated free hormone is then measured directly in a radioimmunoassay.[97] These assays are probably the most accurate available, but small, weakly bound, dialyzable substances or drugs may be removed from the binding proteins, and the free hormone concentration measured in their presence may not fully reflect the free concentration in vivo. The broad normal range varies among laboratories and is from 0.8 to 2.7 ng/dl (10 to 35 pmol/L).

Isotopic Equilibrium Dialysis

This method has been the gold standard for the estimation of the FT_4 or FT_3 concentration for almost 30 years. It is based on the determination of proportion of T_4 or T_3 that is unbound, or free, and is thus able to diffuse through a dialysis membrane, i.e., the dialyzable fraction (DF). To carry out the test, a sample of serum is incubated with a tracer amount of labeled T_4 or T_3. The labeled tracer rapidly equilibrates with the respective bound and free endogenous hormones. The sample is then dialyzed against buffer at a constant temperature until the concentration of free hormone on either side of the dialysis membrane has reached equilibrium. The DF is calculated from the proportion of labeled hormone in the dialysate. The contribution from radioiodide present as contaminant in the labeled tracer hormone should be eliminated by careful purification[98] and by various techniques of precipitation of the dialyzed hormone.[96,102] FT_4 and FT_3 levels can be measured simultaneously by addition to the sample of T_4 and T_3 labeled with two different radioiodine isotopes.[103] Ultrafiltration is a modification of the dialysis technique.[98] Results are expressed as the fraction (DFT$_4$ or DFT$_3$) or percent (%FT$_4$ or %FT$_3$) of the respective dialyzed hormones, and the absolute concentrations of FT$_4$ and FT$_3$ are calculated from the product of the total concentration of the hormone in serum and its respective DF. Typical normal values for FT$_4$ in the adult range from 1.0 to 3.0 ng/dl (13 to 39 pmol/L) and, for FT$_3$, from 0.25 to 0.65 ng/dl (3.8 to 10 pmol/L).

Results by these techniques are generally comparable to those determined with the direct, one-step, methods (see below) but are more likely to differ with extremely low or extremely high TBG concentrations or in the presence of circulating inhibitors of protein binding.[104] The measured DF may be altered by the temperature at which the assay is run, the degree of dilution, the time allowed for equilibrium to be reached, and the composition of the diluting fluid.[105] The calculated value is dependent on an accurate measurement of total T$_4$ or T$_3$ and may be incorrect in patients with T$_4$ or T$_3$ autoantibodies.

Index Methods

Because the determination of free hormone by equilibrium dialysis is cumbersome and technically demanding, most clinical laboratories have used a method by which a free T$_4$ index (FT$_4$I) or free T$_3$ index (FT$_3$I) is derived from the product of the TT$_4$ or TT$_3$ (determined by immunoassay) and the value of an in vitro uptake test (see below). While not always in agreement with the values obtained by dialysis, these techniques are rapid and simple. They are more likely to fail at extremely low or extremely high TBG concentrations, in the presence of abnormal binding proteins, in patients with nonthyroidal illness, or in the presence of circulating inhibitors of protein binding.

The theoretical contention that the FT$_4$I is an accurate estimate of the absolute FT$_4$ concentration can be confirmed by the linear correlation between these two parameters. This is true provided results of the in vitro uptake test (T$_3$U or T$_4$U) are expressed as the thyroid hormone binding ratio (THBR), determined by dividing the tracer counts bound to the solid matrix by counts bound to serum proteins.[106] Values are corrected for assay variations using appropriate serum standards and are expressed as the ratio of a normal reference pool.[106,107] The normal range is slightly narrower than the cor-

responding TT$_4$ in healthy euthyroid patients with a normal TBG concentration. It is 6.0 to 10.5 or 77 to 135 when calculated from TT$_4$ values measured by RIA and expressed in μg/dl or nmol/L, respectively. In thyrotoxicosis FT$_4$I is high and in hypothyroidism it is low, irrespective of the TBG concentration. Euthyroid patients with TT$_4$ values outside the normal range as a result of TBG abnormalities have a normal FT$_4$I.[83] Lack of correlation between the FT$_4$I and the metabolic status of the patient has been observed under the same circumstances as those described for similar discrepancies when the FT$_4$ concentration was measured by dialysis.

Methods for estimating the FT$_3$I are also available[103,108] but are rarely used in routine clinical evaluation of thyroid function. Like the FT$_4$I, it correlates well with the absolute FT$_3$ concentration. The test corrects for changes in TT$_3$ concentration resulting from variations in TBG concentration.

Estimation of FT$_4$ and FT$_3$ Based on TBG Measurements

Since most T$_4$ and T$_3$ in serum are bound to TBG, their free concentration can be calculated from their binding affinity constants to TBG and molar concentrations of hormones and TBG.[109,110] A simpler calculation of the T$_4$/TBG and T$_3$/TBG ratios yields values that are similar to but less accurate than the FT$_4$I and FT$_3$I, respectively.[106]

Two-step Immunoassays

In two-step assays, the free hormone is first immunoextracted by a specific bound antibody (first step) that is frequently fixed to the tube (coated tube).[111,112] After washing out serum, labeled tracer is added and allowed to equilibrate between the unoccupied sites on the antibody and those of serum thyroid hormone–binding proteins. The free hormone concentration will be inversely related to the antibody-bound tracer, and values are determined by comparison to a standard curve. Values obtained with this technique are generally comparable to those determined with the direct methods. They are more likely to differ in the presence of circulating inhibitors of protein binding and in sera from patients with nonthyroidal illness.

Analog (One-Step) Immunoassays

In analog assays, a labeled analog of T$_4$ or T$_3$ directly competes with the endogenous free hormone for binding to antibodies.[113] In theory, these analogs are not bound by the thyroid hormone–binding proteins in serum. However, various studies have found significant protein binding to the variant albuminlike protein,[95] to transthyretin, and to iodothyronine autoantibodies.[114] This results in discrepant values to other assays in a number of conditions, including nonthyroidal illness, pregnancy, and in individuals with familial dysalbuminemic hyperthyroxinemia (FDH).[95] While commercial kits have been modified to minimize these problems, their accuracy remains controversial.

In another method the antibody to which the labeled T_4 is attached is contained in nylon microcapsules through which FT_4 from the sample can penetrate, i.e., a form of dialysis. The displacement of the labeled T_4 from the antibody is proportional to the FT_4 concentration in the test sample of serum.[115]

Method Selection for Estimating Free Thyroid Hormone Concentration

None of the available methods for estimating the free hormone concentration in serum provide infallible evaluations of the thyroid hormone–dependent metabolic status. Each test possesses inherent advantages and disadvantages, depending upon specific physiologic and pathologic circumstances. For example, methods based on the measurement of the total thyroid hormone and TBG concentrations cannot be used in patients with absent TBG due to inherited TBG deficiency. Under such circumstances, the concentration of free thyroid hormone depends upon the interaction of the hormone with serum proteins that normally play a negligible role (TTR and albumin). When alterations of thyroid hormone binding do not equally affect T_4 and T_3, discrepant results of FT_4I are obtained when using labeled T_4 or T_3 in the in vitro uptake test. For example, euthyroid patients with the inherited albumin variant (FDH) or having endogenous antibodies with greater affinity for T_4 will have high TT_4 but a normal T_3U test, which will result in an overestimation of the calculated FT_4I. In such instances, calculation of the FT_4I from a T_4U test may provide more accurate results. Conversely, reduced overall binding affinity for T_4 that affects T_3 to a lesser extent will underestimate the FT_4I derived from a T_3U test. Similarly, the T_4U and T_3U for estimating free hormone concentration are satisfactory in the presence of alterations in TBG concentration but not alterations of the affinity of

TBG for the hormone.[116,117] To correct for variations in TBG concentration, a different range of normal values for free hormone indices must be established for each TBG variant with altered affinity for thyroid hormone.

Methods based on equilibrium dialysis are most appropriate when estimating the free thyroid hormone level in patients with all varieties of abnormal binding to serum proteins if the true concentration of total hormone has been accurately determined. Notwithstanding the in vivo experiments of Pardridge et al.,[118] all methods for estimating the FT_4 concentration may give either high or low values in patients with severe nonthyroidal illness who are believed to be euthyroid.[96–100,119,120] This has been attributed, at least in part, to the presence of inhibitors of thyroid hormone binding to serum proteins as well as to the various adsorbents used in the test procedures.[121,122] Some of these inhibitors allegedly leak from the tissues of the diseased patient.[123,124] Such discrepancies are even more pronounced during transient states of hyperthyroxinemia or hypothyroxinemia associated with acute illness, after withdrawal of treatment with thyroid hormone, and in acute changes in TBG concentration (see Chapters 5 and 16).

The contribution of various drugs that interfere with binding of thyroid hormone to serum proteins or with the in vitro tests should also be taken into account when choosing and interpreting tests (see Table 5-2). Although the free thyroid hormone concentration in serum seems to determine the amount of hormone available to body tissues, factors that govern their intracellular binding and metabolism may alter their action. It is for these reasons, as well as because of technical problems, that serum measurements of free hormone in serum occasionally need to be supplemented by tests that measure the tissue effects of thyroid hormone and its pathways of intracellular metabolism. Bioassays that measure the amount of thyroid hormone entering the cell (bioavailable T_4)[125] may find clinical application in the future.

Measurements of Iodine-Containing Hormone Precursors and Products of Degradation

The last two decades have witnessed the development of RIAs for measuring naturally occurring, iodine-containing substances that possess little if any thyromimetric activity. Some of these substances are products of T_4 and T_3 degradation in peripheral tissues. Others are predominantly, if not exclusively, of thyroidal origin. Since they are devoid of significant metabolic activity, measurement of their concentration is of value only in detecting abnormalities in the metabolism of thyroid hormone in peripheral tissues, as well as defects of hormone synthesis and secretion. Such knowledge is often helpful in defining the etiology of some thyroid illnesses or hormonal imbalance. They may be collectively viewed as diagnostic markers.

3,3',5'-Triiodothyronine or Reverse T_3

3,3',5'-Triiodothyronine (rT_3) is principally a product of T_4 degradation in peripheral tissues (see Chapter 3). It is also secreted by the thyroid gland, but the amounts are practically insignificant.[126] Thus, measurement of reverse T_3 (rT_3) concentration in serum reflects both tissue supply and metabolism of T_4 and identifies conditions that favor this particular pathway of T_4 degradation.

When total rT_3 (TrT_3) is measured in unextracted serum, a competitor of rT_3 binding to serum proteins must be added.[127] Several chemically related compounds may cross-react with the antibodies. The strongest cross-reactivity is observed with 3,3'-T_2, but this does not present a serious methodologic problem because of its relatively low levels in human serum. Though cross-reactivity with T_3 and T_4 is lesser, these compounds are more often the cause of rT_3 overestimation due to their relative abundance, particularly in thyrotoxicosis.[128] Free fatty acids interfere with the measurement of rT_3 by RIA.[129]

The normal range in adult serum for TrT_3 is 14 to 30 ng/dl (0.22 to 0.46 nmol/L), although values ranging from 25 to 65 ng/dl have been reported.[101,126,127,130,131] It is elevated in subjects with high TBG and in half of individuals with FDH.[132] Serum TrT_3 levels are normal in hypothyroid patients treated with T_4, indicating that peripheral T_4 metabolism is an important source of circulating rT_3.[126,133] Values are high in thyrotoxicosis and low in untreated hypothyroidism. High values are normally found in cord blood and in newborns.[133,134]

With only a few exceptions, notably uremia, serum TrT_3 concentrations are elevated in all circumstances that cause low serum T_3 levels in the absence of obvious clinical signs of hypothyroidism. These conditions include, in addition to the newborn period, a variety of acute and chronic nonthyroidal illnesses,[131] calorie deprivation, and the influence of a growing list of clinical agents and drugs (see Table 5-3).

Current clinical application of TrT_3 measurement in serum is in the differential diagnosis of conditions associated with alterations in serum T_3 and T_4 concentrations when thyroid gland and metabolic abnormalities are not readily apparent.

The dialyzable fraction of rT_3 in normal adult serum is 0.2 to 0.32 percent, or approximately the same as that of T_3. The corresponding serum FrT_3 concentration is 50 to 100 pg/dl (0.77 to 1.5 pmol/L). In the absence of gross TBG abnormalities, variations in serum FrT_3 concentration closely follow those of TrT_3.[101]

3,5-Diiodothyronine

The normal adult range for total 3,5-diiodothyronine (3,5-T_2) in serum measured by direct RIAs is 0.20 to 0.75 ng/dl (3.8 to 14 pmol/L).[135] The belief that 3,5-T_2 is derived from T_3 is supported by the observations that conditions associated with high and low serum T_3 levels have elevated and reduced serum concentrations of 3,5-T_2, respectively.[136] Thus, high serum 3,5-T_2 levels have been reported in hyperthyroidism and low levels in serum of hypothyroid patients, newborns, during fasting, and in patients with liver cirrhosis.

3,3'-Diiodothyronine

Normal concentrations of 3,3'-diiodothyronine (3,3'-T_2) in adults probably range from 1 to 8 ng/dl (19 to 150 pmol/L).[54,137] Levels are clearly elevated in hyperthyroidism and in the newborn.[131] Values have been found to be normal or depressed in nonthyroidal illnesses,[131,137] in agreement with the demonstration of reduced monodeiodination of rT_3 to 3,3'-T_2.[138] In vivo turnover kinetic studies and measurement of 3,3'-T_2 in serum after the administration of T_3 and rT_3 have clearly shown that 3,3'-T_2 is the principal metabolic product of these two triiodothyronines.

3',5'-Diiodothyronine

Reported concentrations of 3',5'-diiodothyronine (3',5'-T_2) in serum of normal adults have a mean overall range of 1.5 to 9.0 ng/dl (30 to 170 pmol/

L).[54,131,137,139,140] The substances that principally cross-react in the assay are rT_3, $3,3\text{-}LT_2$, and $3\text{-}T_1$. Values are high in hyperthyroidism and in the newborn.[139,140] Being the derivative of rT_3 monodeiodination,[139] $3',5'\text{-}T_2$ levels are elevated in serum during fasting[140,141] and in chronic illnesses[133] in which the level of the rT_3 precursor is also high. Administration of dexamethasone also produces an increase in the serum $3',5'\text{-}T_2$ level.[139]

3´-Monoiodothyronine

The concentration of $3'$-monoiodothyronine ($3'\text{-}T_1$) in serum of normal adults, measured by RIA, has been reported to range from 0.6 to 2.3 ng/dl (15 to 58 pmol/L)[133] and from <0.9 to 6.8 ng/dl (<20 to 170 pmol/L).[131] Its two immediate precursors, $3,3,'$ $3,3'\text{-}T_2$ and $3',5'\text{-}T_2$, are the main cross-reactants in the RIA. Serum levels are very high in hyperthyroidism and low in hypothyroidism. The concentration of $3'\text{-}T_1$ in serum is elevated in all conditions associated with high rT_3 levels, including newborns, nonthyroidal illness, and fasting.[131,134] This finding is not surprising, since the immediate precursor of $3'$-T_1 is $3',5'\text{-}T_2$,[142] a product of rT_3 deiodination, which is also present in serum in high concentration under the same circumstances. The elevated serum levels of $3'\text{-}T_1$ in renal failure are attributed to decreased clearance, since the concentrations of its precursors are not increased.[131]

3-Monoiodothyronine

Experience with the measurement of 3-monoiodothyronine ($3\text{-}T_1$) in serum is limited. Normal values in serum of adult humans using trititium-labeled $3\text{-}T_1$ in a specific RIA ranged from <0.5 to 7.5 ng/dl (<13 to 190 pmol/L).[143] The mean concentration of $3\text{-}T_1$ in serum of thyrotoxic patients and in cord blood was significantly higher. $3\text{-}T_1$ appears to be a product of in vivo deiodination of $3,3'\text{-}T_2$.

Tetraiodothyroacetic Acid and Triiodothyroacetic Acid

The iodoamino acids, tetraiodothyroacetic acid (TETRAC or T_4A) and triiodothyroacetic acid (TRIAC or T_3A), products of deamination and oxidative decarboxylation of T_4 and T_3, respectively, have been detected in serum by direct RIA measurements.[21,76,144] Reported mean concentrations in the serum of healthy adults have been 8.7 ng/dl[144] and 2.6 ng/dl (range, 1.6 to 3.0 ng/dl or 26 to 48 pmol/L)[21] for T_3A and 28 ng/dl (range <8 to 60 mg/dl or <105 to 800 pmol/L)[76] for T_4A. Serum T_4A levels are reduced during fasting and in patients with severe illness,[145] although the percentage of conversion of T_4 to T_4A is increased.[20,146] The concentration of serum T_3A remains unchanged during the administration of replacement doses of T_4 and T_3.[21] It has been suggested that intracellular rerouting of T_3 to T_3A during fasting is responsible for the maintenance of normal serum TSH levels in the presence of low T_3 concentrations.[147]

3,5,3´-T3 Sulfate

A RIA procedure to measure $3,5,3'\text{-}T_3$ sulfate (T3S) in ethanol-extracted serum samples is available.[22] Concentrations in healthy adults range from 4 to 10 ng/dl (50 to 125 pmol/L). Although the principal source of T_3S is T_3, and the former binds to TBG, values are high in newborns and low in pregnancy. This suggests different rates of T_3S generation or metabolism in mother and fetus. T_3S values are high in thyrotoxicosis and in nonthyroidal illness.

Diiodotyrosine and Monoiodotyrosine

Although RIA methods for measuring DIT and MIT have been developed, due to limited experience, their value in clinical practice remains unknown. Early reports gave a normal mean value for DIT in serum of healthy adults of 156 ng/dl (3.6 nmol/L),[148] with progressive decline due to refinement of techniques to values as low as 7 ng/dl with a range of 1 to 23 ng/dl (0.02 to 0.5 nmol/L).[149] Thus, the normal range for MIT of 90 to 390 ng/dl (2.9 to 12.7 nmol/L)[150] is undoubtedly an overestimation. Iodotyrosine that has escaped enzymatic deiodination in the thyroid gland appears to be the principal source of DIT in serum. Iodothyronine degradation in peripheral tissues is probably a minor source of iodotyrosines since administration of large doses of T_4 to healthy subjects produces a decline rather than an increase in the serum DIT level.[149] DIT is metabolized to MIT in peripheral tissues. Serum levels of DIT are low during pregnancy and high in cord blood.

Thyroglobulin

RIA methods are now used routinely for measurement of TG in serum.[151,152] They are specific and, depending upon the sensitivity of the assay, capable of detecting TG in the serum of approximately 90 percent of the euthyroid healthy adults. When antisera are used in high dilutions, there is virtually no cross-reactivity with iodothyronines or iodotyrosines. Results obtained from the analysis of sera containing TG autoantibodies are inaccurate, limiting the applicability of the assay.[152] Thus, interpretation of the test requires prior screening for the presence of such autoantibodies. The presence of thyroid peroxidase antibodies does not interfere with the TG RIA.

TG concentrations in serum of healthy adults range from <1 to 25 ng/ml (<1.5 to 38 pmol/L), with mean levels of 5 to 10 ng/ml.[151,153–155] On a molar basis, these concentrations of TG are minute relative to the circulating iodothyronines; 5,000-fold lower than the corresponding concentration of T_4 in serum. Values tend to be slightly higher in women than in men.[151] In the neonatal period and during the third trimester of pregnancy, mean values are approximately four- and two-fold higher.[154,156] They gradually decline throughout infancy, childhood, and adolescence.[157] The positive correlation between the levels of serum TG and TSH indicates that pituitary TSH regulates the secretion of TG.

Elevated serum TG levels reflect increased secretory activity by stimulation of the thyroid gland or damage to thyroid tissue, whereas values below or at the level of detectability indicate a paucity of thyroid tissue or suppressed activity. TG levels in a variety of conditions affecting the thyroid gland have been reviewed[158] and are listed in Table 6-6.

Interpretation of a serum TG value should consider that TG concentrations may be high under normal physiologic conditions or altered by drugs. Administration of iodine and antithyroid drugs increases the serum TG level, as do states associated with hyperstimulation of the thyroid gland by TSH or other substances with thyroid-stimulating activity. This is due to increased thyroidal release of Tg rather than changes in its clearance.[159] Administration of TRH and TSH also transiently increases the serum level of TG.[160] Trauma to the thyroid gland, as during diagnostic and therapeutic procedures, including percutaneous needle biopsy, surgery, or ^{131}I therapy, can produce a striking, although short-lived, elevation in the TG level in serum.[154,161,162] Pathologic processes with destructive effect on the thyroid gland also produce transient, though more prolonged increases.[163] TG is undetectable in serum

TABLE 6-6. Conditions Associated with Changes in Serum TG Concentration Listed According to Presumed Mechanism

Increased
TSH mediated
Acute and transient (TSH and TRH administration, neonatal period)
Chronic stimulation
Iodine deficiency, endemic goiter, goitrogens
Reduce thyroidal reserve (lingual thyroid)
TSH-producing pituitary adenoma
Generalized resistance to thyroid hormone
TBG deficiency
Non-TSH mediated
Thyroid stimulators
IgG (Graves' disease)
hCG (trophoblastic disease)
Trauma to the thyroid (needle aspiration and surgery of the thyroid gland, ^{131}I therapy)
Destructive thyroid pathology
Subacute thyroiditis
"Painless thyroiditis"
Postpartum thyroiditis
Abnormal release
Thyroid nodules (toxic, nontoxic, multinodular goiter)
Differentiated nonmedullary thyroid carcinoma
Abnormal clearance (renal failure)
Decreased
TSH suppression
Administration of thyroid hormone
Decreased synthesis
Athyreosis (postoperative, congenital)
TG synthesis defect

after total ablation of the thyroid gland, as well as in healthy persons receiving suppressive doses of thyroid hormone.[158] It is thus a useful test in the differential diagnosis of thyrotoxicosis factitia,[164] especially when transient thyrotoxicosis with a low RAIU or suppression of thyroidal RAIU by iodine are alternative possibilities.

The most striking elevations in serum TG concentrations have been observed in patients with metastatic differentiated nonmedullary thyroid carcinoma, even after total surgical and radioiodide ablation of all normal thyroid tissue.[154,165] It usually persists despite full thyroid hormone suppressive therapy, suggesting excessive autonomous release of TG by the neoplastic cells. The determination is thus of particular value in the follow-up and management of metastatic thyroid carcinomas, particularly when they fail to concentrate radioiodide.[153,165] Follow-up of such patients with sequential serum TG determinations facilitates the early detection of tumor recurrence or growth and the assessment of treatment efficacy. Measurement of serum TG is also useful in patients with metastases, particularly to bone, in whom there is no evidence of a primary site and when thyroid malignancy is being considered in the differential diagnosis.[154,165] On the other hand, serum TG levels are of no value in the differential diagnosis of primary thyroid cancer because levels may be within the normal range in the presence of differentiated thyroid cancer and high in a variety of benign thyroid nodules.[153,155,165] Whether early detection of recurrent thyroid cancer after initial ablative therapy could be achieved by serum TG measurement with cessation of hormone replacement therapy is still debatable.[166–168] The problem stems from the fact that TG secretion by the tumor is modulated by TSH and could be suppressed by the administration of thyroid hormone.[166,168]

TG levels are high in the early phase of subacute thyroiditis.[163] Declining serum TG levels during the course of antithyroid drug treatment of patients with Graves' disease may indicate the onset of a remission.[162,169] TG may be undetectable in the serum of neonates with dyshormonogenic goiters due to defects in TG synthesis[170] but very high in some hypothyroid infants with thyromegaly or ectopy.[171] Measurement of serum TG in hypothyroid neonates is useful in differentiating infants with complete thyroid agenesis from those with hypothyroidism due to other causes, and thus in most cases obviates the need for the diagnostic administration of radioiodide.[171,172]

Measurement of Thyroid Hormone and Its Metabolites in Other Body Fluids and in Tissues

Clinical experience with measurement of thyroid hormone and its metabolites in body fluids other than serum and in tissues is limited for several reasons. Analyses carried out in urine and saliva do not appear to give information not obtained from serum analyses. Amniotic fluid, cerebrospinal fluid, and tissues are less readily accessible for sampling. Their likely application in the future will depend on information they could provide beyond that obtained from similar analyses in serum.

Urine

Because thyroid hormone is filtered in the urine predominantly in free form, measurement of the total amount excreted over 24 hours offers an indirect method for estimating the free hormone concentration in serum. The 24-hour excretion of T_4 in healthy adults ranges from 4 to 13 μg and from 1.8 to 3.7 μg, depending upon whether total or only conjugated T_4 is measured. Corresponding normal ranges for T_3 are 2.0 to 4.0 μg and 0.4 to 1.9 μg.[173–175] Striking seasonal variations have been shown for the urinary excretion of both hormones, with a nadir during the hot summer months in the absence of significant changes in serum TT_4 and TT_3. As expected, values are normal in pregnancy and in nonthyroidal illnesses and are high in thyrotoxicosis and low in hypothyroidism.[37,174,175] The test may not be valid in the presence of gross proteinuria and impaired renal function.[176]

Amniotic Fluid

All iodothyronines measured in blood have also been detected in amniotic fluid. Except for T_3, 3,3'-T_2, and 3'-T_2, the concentration at term is lower that in cord serum.[139,140,142,177–179] This fact cannot be fully explained by the low TBG concentration in amniotic fluid. Although the source of iodothyronines in amniotic fluid is unknown, the general pattern more closely resembles that found in the fetal circulation than in the maternal.

The TT_4 concentration in amniotic fluid average 0.5 μg/dl (65 nmol/L), with a range of 0.15 to 1.0 μg/dl, and is thus very low when compared to values in maternal and cord serum.[177–179] The FT_4 concentration is, however, twice as high in amniotic fluid as in serum. The TT_3 concentration is also low relative to maternal serum, being on the average 30 ng/dl (0.46 nmol/L) in both amniotic fluid and cord serum.[179] rT_3, on the other hand, is very high in amniotic fluid, on average 330 ng/dl (5.1 nmol/L) during the first half of gestation, declining precipitously at about the 30th week of gestation to an average of 85 ng/dl (1.3 nmol/L), which is also found at term.[178,179]

Cerebrospinal Fluid

T_4, T_3, and rT_3 concentrations have been measured in human cerebrospinal fluid (CSF).[180–182] The concentrations of both TT_4 and TT_3 are approximately

50-fold lower than those found in serum. However, the concentrations of these iodothyronines in free form are similar to those in serum. In contrast, the level of TrT_3 in CSF is only 2.5-fold lower than that of serum, whereas that of FrT_3 is 25-fold higher. This is probably due to the presence in CSF of a larger proportion of TTR which has high affinity for rT_3.[181] All the thyroid hormone–binding proteins present in serum are also found in CSF, although in lower concentrations.[181] The concentrations of TT_4 and FT_4 are increased in thyrotoxicosis and depressed in hypothyroidism. Severe nonthyroidal illness gives rise to increased TrT_3 and FrT_3 levels.[182]

Milk

TT_4 concentration in human milk is on the order of 0.03 to 0.5 μg/dl.[183] Analytic artifacts were responsible for the much higher values formerly reported.[183,184] TT_3 concentrations range from 10 to 200 ng/dl (015 to 3.1 nmol/L).[184,185] The concentration of TrT_3 ranges from 1 to 30 ng/dl (15 to 460 pmol/L).[184] It is thus unlikely that milk would provide a sufficient quantity of thyroid hormone to alleviate hypothyroidism in the infant.

Saliva

One study suggests that only the free fraction of small nonpeptide hormones that circulate predominantly bound to serum proteins are transferred to saliva and that their measurement in this easily accessible body fluid would provide a simple and direct means to determine their free concentration in blood. This hypothesis was confirmed for steroid hormones[186] not tightly bound to serum proteins. Levels of T_4 in saliva range from 4.2 to 35 ng/dl (54 to 450 pmol/L) and do not correlate with the concentration of free T_4 in serum.[187] This finding is in part due to the transfer of T_4 bound to the small but variable amounts of serum proteins that reach the saliva.

Effusions

TT_4 measured in fluid obtained from serous cavities bears a direct relationship to the protein content and the serum concentration of T_4. Limited experience with TG measurement in pleural effusions from patients with thyroid cancer metastatic to lungs suggests that it may be of diagnostic value.[165]

Tissues

Since the response to thyroid hormone is expressed at the cell level, it is logical to assume that hormone concentration in tissues should correlate best with its action. Methods for extraction, recovery, and measurement of iodothyronines from tissues have been developed, but for obvious reasons data from thyroid hormone measurements in human tissues are limited. Preliminary work has shown that under several circumstances, hormonal levels in tissues such as liver, kidney, and muscle usually correlate with those found in serum.[188]

Measurements of T_3 in cells most accessible for sampling in humans, namely red blood cells, gave values of 20 to 45 ng/dl (0.31 to 0.69 nmol/L) or one-fourth those found in serum.[189] They are higher in thyrotoxicosis and lower in hypothyroidism.

The concentrations of all iodothyronines have been measured in thyroid gland hydrolysates.[18,133,139] In normal glands, the molar ratios relative to the concentration of T_4 are on average as follows: $T_4/T_3 = 10$; $T_4/rT_3 = 80$; $T_4/3,5'-T_2 = 1,400$; T; $i4/3,3'-T_2 = 350$; $T_4/3',5'-T_2 = 1,100$; and $T_4/3'-T_1 = 4,400$. Information concerning the content of iodothyronines in hydrolysates of abnormal thyroid tissue is limited, and the diagnostic value of such measurements has not been established.

Measurement of TG in metastatic tissue obtained by needle biopsy may be of value in the differential diagnosis, especially when the primary site is unknown and the histologic diagnosis is not conclusive.

Tests Assessing the Effects of Thyroid Hormone on Body Tissues

Thyroid hormone regulates a variety of biochemical reactions in virtually all tissues. Thus, ideally, the adequacy of hormonal supply should be assessed by the tissue responses rather than by parameters of thyroid gland activity or serum hormone concentration that are several steps removed from the site of thyroid hormone action. Unfortunately, the tissue responses (metabolic indices) that are easily measured are nonspecific; their alteration by a variety of physiologic and pathologic mechanisms is unrelated to thyroid hormone deprivation or excess. For this reason, these tests have been replaced by direct measurements of thyroid gland activity and hormone concentration in serum that provide greater sensitivity, specificity, and diagnostic accuracy. Yet none of the "specific" tests are true substitutes for tests that measure metabolic and biochemical responses of tissues to thyroid hormone. While mild degrees of thyroid dysfunction may be measured by alterations in the serum concentration of TSH or the TSH response to TRH, it is uncertain whether the pituitary threshold of response to the hormonal supply reflects the status of other tissues. Furthermore, in certain conditions, serum TSH levels may be elevated to maintain a normal hormone supply to peripheral tissue. Similar reasoning, backed by concrete examples, could be used to depreciate the reliance upon tests measuring thyroid hormone concentration in serum. In practice, however, such arguments do not improve the reliability of available tests of hormone action. As a consequence, they are primarily used as confirmatory tests in patients with unusual or uncertain diagnoses.

The following review of biochemical and physiologic changes mediated by thyroid hormone has a dual purpose: (1) to outline some of the changes that may be used as clinical tests in the evaluation of the metabolic status and (2) to point out the changes in various determinations commonly used in the diagnosis of a variety of nonthyroidal illnesses, which may be affected by the concomitant presence of thyroid hormone deficiency or excess.

Basal Metabolic Rate

The basal metabolic rate (BMR) has a long history in the evaluation of thyroid function. It measures oxygen consumption under basal conditions of overnight fast and rest from mental and physical exertion. Since standard equipment for measuring BMR may not be readily available, it can be estimated from the oxygen consumed over a timed interval by analyzing samples of expired air.[190] The test indirectly measures metabolic energy expenditure, or heat production.

Results are expressed as the percentage of deviation from normal after appropriate corrections have been made for age, sex, and body surface area. Low values are suggestive of hypothyroidism, and high values reflect thyrotoxicosis. The various nonthyroidal illnesses and other factors affecting the BMR, including sources of errors, have been reviewed.[191] Although this test is no longer a part of the routine diagnostic armamentarium, it is still useful in research and in the evaluation of patients suspected of having resistance to thyroid hormone.[65]

Deep Tendon Reflex Relaxation Time (Photomotogram)

Delay in the relaxation time of the deep tendon reflexes, visible to the experienced eye, occurs in hypothyroidism. Several instruments have been devised to quantify various phases of the Achilles tendon reflex. Although normal values vary according to the phase of the tendon reflex measured, the apparatus used, and individual laboratory standards, the approximate adult normal range for the half-relaxation time is 230 to 390 msec. Diurnal variation, differences with sex, and changes with age, cold exposure, fever, exercise, obesity, and pregnancy have been reported. However, the main reason for the failure of this test as a diagnostic measure of thyroid dysfunction is the large overlap with values obtained in euthyroid patients and alterations caused by nonthyroidal illnesses.[192] These illnesses include myotonic disorders, pernicious anemia, diabetes mellitus, uremia, neurosyphilis, Parkinson's disease, sarcoidosis, local edema, and disorders of the psyche. Also, hypoglycemia and administration of glucose, epinephrine, reserpine, β-adrenergic blockers, potassium, and large doses of salicylates, amphetamines, glucocorticoids, and estrogens alter the relaxation time.[192] The test is of little value in the diagnosis of thyrotoxicosis and is less reliable in the diagnosis of hypothyroidism in children than in adults. It has no value in cases of mild hypothyroidism.

Tests Related to Cardiovascular Function

Thyroid hormone–induced changes in the cardiovascular system can be measured by noninvasive techniques. One such test measures the time interval between the onset of the electrocardiographic QRS complex (Q) and the arrival of the pulse wave at the brachial artery, detected by the Korotkoff sound (K) at the antecubital fossa. This QK interval can be measured at systolic (QKs) and diastolic (QKd) cuff pressure, the latter being more commonly used.[193] Normal adult values for QKd range from 185 to 235 msec. It is shorter in thyrotoxicosis and prolonged in hypothyroidism, but changes also occur with age and after exercise. Related tests that determine the systolic time interval (STI) measure the pre-ejection

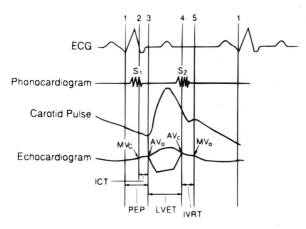

Fig. 6-5. Simultaneous tracings of electrocardiogram (ECG), phonocardiogram, carotid pulse, and echocardiogram. Measurements of the systolic pre-ejection period (PEP), isovolemic contraction time (ICT), left ventricular ejection time (LVET), and isovolumic relaxation time (IVRT) are indicated. (From I Kline, The thyroid, L.E. Braverman & R.D. Utiger (eds). 1991, J.B. Lippincot Co.)

period (PEP), obtained by subtraction of the left ventricular ejection time (LVET) from the total electromechanical systole $(Q - A_2)$.[194] The left ventricular ejection time (LVET), which is also affected by the thyroid status, can be measured by the M mode echocardiogram[195] (Fig. 6-5). The PEP/LVET ratio is most useful in assessing thyroid hormone action in the cardiovascular system.[196] As with other tests of thyroid hormone action, the principal deficiency of these measurements is their alteration in a variety of nonthyroidal illnesses. These conditions include high-output states such as acute febrile illnesses or anemia, pheochromocytoma, aortic valvular stenosis, and ventricular conduction defects. Drugs such as epinephrine and β-adrenergic blocking agents also affect the test results.

Miscellaneous Biochemical and Physiologic Changes Related to the Action of Thyroid Hormone on Peripheral Tissues

Thyroid hormone affects the function of a variety of peripheral tissues. Thus hormone deficiency or excess may alter a number of determinations used to diagnose illnesses unrelated to thyroid hormone dysfunction. Knowledge of determinations that may be affected by thyroid hormone is important in the interpretation of laboratory data (Table 6-7).

Measurement of Substances Absent in Normal Serum

Tests that measure substances present in the circulation only under pathologic circumstances do not establish the level of thyroid gland function, but they are of value in establishing the cause of the hormonal dysfunction or thyroid gland pathology.

Thyroid Autoantibodies

The humoral antibodies most commonly measured in clinical practice are directed against thyroglobulin (TG) or thyroid cell microsomal (MC) proteins. The latter are principally represented by the thyroid peroxidase (TPO).[296–298] More recently, assays have been developed using purified and recombinant TPO.[299] Other circulating immunoglobulins, which are less frequently used as diagnostic markers, are those directed against a colloid antigen, T_4 and T_3. Antibodies against nuclear components are not tissue specific. Immunoglobulins that stimulate the thyroid gland will be discussed in the next section.

A variety of techniques are available for measuring TG and MC antibodies. These procedures include a precipitation reaction, the Ouchterlony diffusion technique, immunoelectro-osmophoresis, cytotoxic assay, competitive binding radioassay, complement fixation reaction,[300] tanned red cell agglutination assay,[301] the Coon's immunofluorescent technique,[302] and enzyme-linked immunosorbent assay.[299,303] Although the competitive binding radioassay[304,305] appears to be the most sensitive of these tests, the new-generation agglutination methods best combine sensitivity and simplicity and have found the widest clinical application. Current commercial kits utilize synthetic beads rather than red cells.

In the assay of TG and MC antibodies by hemagglutination (TgHA and MCHA), particulate material is coated with human TG or solubilized thyroid MC proteins (TPO) and exposed to serial dilutions of the patient's serum. Agglutination of the coated particulates occurs in the presence of antibodies specific to the antigen attached to their surface. To detect false-positive reactions, it is prudent to include a blank for each sample using uncoated particles. Because of the common occurrence of prozone or blocking phenomenon, it is necessary to screen all serum samples through at least six consecutive twofold dilutions.[306] Results are expressed in terms of the high-

TABLE 6-7. Biochemical and Physiologic Changes Related to Thyroid Hormone Deficiency and Excess

Entity Measured	During Hypothyroidism	During Thyrotoxicosis
Metabolism of various substances and drugs		
Fractional turnover rate (antipyrine,[197] dipyrone,[198] PTU, and methimazole,[197] albumin,[199] low-density lipoproteins,[200] cortisol,[201,202] and Fe[203,204])	↓	↑
Serum Amino acids		
Tyrosine (fasting level and after load)[205,206]	↓	↑
Glutamic acid[205]	N	↑
Proteins		
Albumin[207]	↓	↓
Sex hormone–binding globulin[14,208,209]	↓	↑↑
Ferritin[210,211]	↓	↑
Low-density lipoproteins[200]	↓	↑
Fibronectin[212]		↑
Factor VIII–related antigen[212]		↑
Tissue-plasminogen activator[212]		↑
TBG[83]	↑	↓
TBPA[213]	N	↓
Hormones		
Response to glucose[214]	↓	↓
Response to glucagon[215]	↑	↓
Estradiol-17β,[216] testosterone,[14,208,216] and gastrin[217]	↓ or N	↑
Parathyroid hormone concentration[218,219]	↑	↓
Response to PTH administration[219]	↓	↑
Calcitonin[220]	↓	↑
Calcitonin response to Ca^{++} infusion[221]	↓	
Renin activity and aldosterone[222,223]	↓	↑
Catecholamines[224] and noradrenaline[225]	↑	↑
Atrial natriuretic peptide[226,227]	↓	↑
Erythropoietin[201]	N or ↓	↑
LH[216]		N or ↑
Response to GnRH[228]	↑	N
Prolactin and response to stimulation with TRH, arginine, and chlorpromazine[229,230]	↑ or N	↓
Growth hormone		
Response to insulin[231,232]	↓	N or ↓
Response to TRH[233]		No change
Epidermal growth factor[234]	N	↑
Enzymes		
Creatine-phosphokinase,[235,236] lactic dehydrogenase,[236] and glutamic oxaloacetic transminase[236]	↑	↓
Adenylate kinase[237]	N	↑
Dopamine β-hydroxylase[238]	↑	↓
Alkaline phosphatase[219,239]	a	↑
Malic dehydrogenase[240]	↑↑	↑
Angiotensin-converting enzyme,[212,241] alanine aminotransferase,[242] and glutathione S-transferase[242,243]	N	↑
Coenzyme Q$_{10}$[244]		↓

(Continued)

TABLE 6-7 *(Continued)*

Entity Measured	During Hypothyroidism	During Thyrotoxicosis
Others		
1,25,OH-vitamin D_3[245]	↑	N or ↓
Carotene, vitamin A[246]	↑	↓
cAMP,[247] cGMP,[248] and Fe[203,249]	N or ↓	N or ↑
K[250]		↓
Na[251]	↓	
Mg[252]	↑	↓
Ca[219,253]	↓	↑
P[218,219]		↑
Glucose		
Concentration[215,231]	↓	↑
Fractional turnover during IV tolerance test[214]	↓	
Insulin hypoglycemia[231]	prolonged	
Bilirubin[254,255]	↑[b]	↑
Creatinine[256]	N or ↑	↓
Creatine[256]	N or ↑	↑
Cholesterol,[246,257] carotene,[246,257] phospholipids and lethi-cin,[246,257] and triglycerides[257,258]	↑	↓
Lipoprotein[a259]	↑	↓
Apolipoprotein B[259]	↑	↓
Type IV collagen[260]	↓	↑
Type III procollagen[260]	↓	↑
Free fatty acids[261]		↑
Carcinoembryonic antigen[262]	↑	
Osteocalcin[220]	↓	↑
Urine		
cAMP[263]	↓	↑
after epinephrine infusion[264]	No change	↑
cGMP[248]	N or ↓	↑
Mg[252]	↓	↑
Creatinine[256]	N	↓
Creatine[256]	N	↑
Tyrosine[206]	N or ↓	↑
MIT (after) administration of [131]IMIT[265]		↑
Glutamic acid[206]	N	↑↑
Taurine[266]	↓	
Carnitine[267]	↓	↑
Tyramine, tryptamine, and histamine[268]		↑
17-hydroxycorticoids and ketogenic steroids[269]	↓	↑
Pyridinoline (PYD), deoxypyridinoline (DPD)[270]		↑
Hydroxyproline,[271] and hydroxylysyl glycoside[272]		↑
Red blood cells		
Fe[203,249]	↓	↑
Na[273]	N	↑
Zn[274]	N	↓
Hemoglobin[203,249]	↓	↓
Glucose-6-phosphate dehydrogenase activity[275]	N or ↓	↑
Reduced glutathione[276] and carbonic anhydrase[277]	↑	↓
Ca-ATPase activity[278]	↓	↓

(Continued)

TABLE 6-7 *(Continued)*

Entity Measured	During Hypothyroidism	During Thyrotoxicosis
White blood cells		
Alkaline phosphatase[279]	↓	↓
ATP production in mitochondria[280]	?↑	↓
Adipose tissue		
cAMP[247]	N	↓
Lipoprotein lipase[258]		↑
Skeletal muscle		
cAMP[247]	↓	
Sweat glands		↑
Sweat electrolytes[281]	↑	N
Sebium excretion rate[282]	↓	N
Intestinal system and absorption		
Basic electrical rhythm of the duodenum[283]	↓	↑
Riboflavin absorption[284]	↑[a]	↓[a]
Ca absorption[285]		↓
Intestinal transit and fecal fat[286,287]		↑
Pulmonary function and gas exchange		
Dead space,[288] hypoxic ventilatory drive,[289] and arterial PO_2[288]	↓	
Neurologic system and CSF		
Relaxation time of deep tendon reflexes (phomotogram)[290]	↑	↓
CSF proteins[291]	↑	
Cardiovascular and circulatory system		
Timing of the arterial sounds (QKd)[193]	↑	↓
Left ventricular ejection time (LVET), preejection period (PEP) ratio[194]	↓	↓
ECG[292,293]		
Heart rate and QRS voltage	↓	↑
Q-Tc interval		↓
PR interval		↑
T wave	Flat or inverted	Transient abnormalities
Common arrhythmias	Atrioventricular block	Atrial fibrillation
Bones		
Osseous maturation (bone age by x-ray film)[294,295]	Delayed (epiphysial dysgenesis)	Advanced

N = normal; ↑ = increased; ↓ = decreased.
[a] In children.
[b] In neonates.

est serum dilution, or titer, showing persistent agglutination. The presence of immune complexes, particularly in patients with high serum TG levels, may mask the presence of TG antibodies. Assays for the measurement of such TG–anti-TG immune complexes have been developed.[307]

Normally, the test response is negative, but results may be positive in up to 10 percent of the adult population. The frequency of positive test results is higher in women and with advancing age. The presence of thyroid autoantibodies in the apparently healthy population is thought to represent subclinical autoimmune thyroid disease rather than false-positive reactions. TPO antibodies are detectable in approximately 95 percent of patients with Hashimoto's thyroiditis and 85 percent of those with Graves' disease, irrespective of the functional state of the thyroid gland. Similarly, TG antibodies are positive in about 60 and 30 percent of adult patients with Hashimoto's thyroiditis and Graves' disease, respectively.[305,306,308,309] TG antibodies are less frequently detected in children with autoimmune thyroid disease.[310] Although higher titers are more common with Hashimoto's thyroiditis, quantifying the antibody titer carries little diagnostic implication. The tests are of particular value in the evaluation of patients with atypical or selected manifestations of autoimmune thyroid disease (ophthalmopathy and dermopathy). Positive antibody titers are predictive of postpartum thyroiditis.[311] Low antibody titers occur transiently in some patients after an episode of subacute thyroiditis.[312] Patients with multinodular goiter, thyroid adenomas, or secondary hypothyroidism show no increased incidence of thyroid autoantibodies. In some patients with Hashimoto's thyroiditis and undetectable thyroid autoantibodies in their serum, intrathyroidal lymphocytes have been demonstrated to produce TPO antibodies.

Other antibodies directed against thyroid components or other tissues have been described in the serum of some patients with autoimmune thyroid disease. They are less frequently measured, and their diagnostic value in thyroid disease has not been fully evaluated. A small proportion of patients with Hashimoto's thyroiditis and undetectable TG antibodies may have circulating antibodies against a distinct antigen present in the thyroid colloid.[313] Circulating antibodies capable of binding T_4 and T_3 have also been demonstrated in patients with autoimmune thyroid diseases; these antibodies may interfere with the measurement of T_4 and T_3 by RIA techniques.[38,39,314]

Antibodies reacting with nuclear components that are not tissue specific and with cellular components of parietal cells and adrenal, ovarian, and testicular tissues are more commonly encountered in patients with autoimmune thyroid disease.[315] Their presence reflects the frequency of coexistence of several autoimmune disease processes in the same patient (see Chapter 7). Increased incidence of circulating antibodies against *Yersinia enterocolitica* has been observed in patients with a variety of pathologic conditions of the thyroid gland.[316] This is probably due to structural similarity between TSH receptor and a *Y. enterocolitica* protein.

Thyroid-Stimulating Immunoglobulins

Many names have been given to tests that measure abnormal γ-globulins in the serum of some patients with autoimmune thyroid disease, in particular Graves' disease.[317] The interaction of these unfractionated immunoglobulins with thyroid follicular cells usually results in a global stimulation of thyroid gland activity and only rarely causes inhibition. It has been recommended that these assays all be called TSH receptor antibodies (TRAb) with a phrase "measured by . . . . assay" to identify the type of method used for their determination.[106] The tests will be described under three general categories: (1) those measuring the thyroid-stimulating activity using in vivo or in vitro bioassays; (2) tests based on the competition of the abnormal immunoglobulin with binding of TSH to its receptor; and (3) measurement of thyroid growth-promoting activity of immunoglobulins. Tests employ both human and animal tissue material or cell lines.

Thyroid Stimulation Assays

The earliest assays employed various modifications of the McKenzie mouse bioassay.[318,319] The abnormal γ-globulin with TSH-like biologic properties has relatively longer in vivo activity, hence its name, *long-acting thyroid stimulator* (LATS). The assay measures the LATS-induced release of thyroid hormone from the mouse thyroid gland prelabeled with radioiodide. The presence of LATS in serum is pathognomonic of Graves' disease. However, depending upon the assay sensitivity, a variable percent of untreated patients will show a positive LATS response. LATS may be found in the serum of patients with Graves' disease even in the absence of thyrotoxicosis. Although it is more commonly present in patients with ophthalmopathy, especially when accompanied by pretibial myxedema,[320] LATS does not appear to correlate specifically with the presence of thyrotoxicosis, its severity, or course of complications. LATS crosses the placenta and may be found transiently in newborns from mothers possessing the abnormal γ-globulin.[321]

Attempts to improve the ability to detect *thyroid stimulating antibodies (TSAb)* in autoimmune thyroid disease led to the development of several in vitro assays using animal as well as human thyroid tissue. The ability of the patient's serum to stimulate endocytosis in fresh human thyroid tissue is measured by direct count of intracellular colloid droplets formed. Using such a technique, *human thyroid stimulator (HTS)* activity has been demonstrated in serum samples from patients with Graves' disease that were devoid of LATS activity measured by the standard mouse bioassay.[322] TSAb can be detected by measuring the accumulation of cyclic adenosine monophosphate (cAMP) or stimulating adenylate cyclase activity in human thyroid cell cultures and thyroid plasma membranes, respectively.[323] Accumulation of cAMP in the cultured rat thyroid cell line $FRTL_5$ has also been used as an assay for TSAb.[324] Stimulation of release of T_3 from human[325] and porcine[326] thyroid slices is another form of in vitro assay for TSAb. An in vitro bioassay using a cytochemical technique depends upon the ability of thyroid-stimulating material to increase lysosomal membrane permeability to a chromogenic substrate, leucyl-β-naphthylamide, which then reacts with the enzyme naphthylamidase. Quantitation is by scanning and integrated microdensitometry.[327]

The recent cloning of the TSH receptor[328,329] led to the development of an in vitro assay of TSAb using cell lines that express the recombinant TSH receptor.[330,331] This assay, based on the generation of cAMP, is specific for human TSH receptor antibodies that have thyroid-stimulating activity and thus contrasts with assays based on binding to the TSH receptor (see below) that cannot distinguish between antibodies with thyroid-stimulating and TSH-blocking activity. Accordingly, the recombinant human TSH receptor assay measures antibodies relevant to the pathogenesis of autoimmune thyrotoxicosis and is more sensitive than formerly used TSAb assays. For example, 94 percent of serum samples were positive for TSab compared to 74 percent when the same samples were assayed using FRTL-5 cells.[332]

Thyrotropin-Binding Inhibition Assays

The principle of binding-inhibition assays dates to the discovery of another class of abnormal immunoglobulins in patients with Graves' disease—those that prevent human thyroid gland extract from neutralizing the bioactivity of LATS tested in the mouse.[333] This material, known as *LATS protector (LATS-P)*, is species specific, having no biologic effect on the mouse thyroid gland but capable of stimulating the human thyroid.[334] The original assay was cumbersome, which limited its clinical application.

Techniques used currently, which may be collectively termed *radioreceptor assays*, are based on the competition of the abnormal immunoglobulins and TSH for a common receptor-binding site on thyroid cells. The test is akin in principle to the radioligand assays, in which a natural membrane receptor takes

the place of the binding proteins or antibodies. Various sources of TSH receptors are employed, including human thyroid cells,[335] their particulate or solubilized membrane,[336,337] and cell membranes from porcine thyroids[338] or from guinea pig fat cells[339] and, more recently, recombinant human TSH receptor expressed in mammalian cells.[340] Since the assays do not directly measure thyroid-stimulating activity, the abnormal immunoglobulins determined have been given variety of names, such as *thyroid-binding inhibitory immunoglobulins (TBII)* or *antibodies (TBIAb)* and *thyrotropin-displacing immunoglobulins (TDI)*.

Thyroid Growth-Promoting Assays

Assays have also been developed that measure the growth-promoting activity of abnormal immunoglobulins. One such assay is based on the staining by the Feulgen reaction of nuclei from guinea pig thyroid cells in S-phase.[341] Another assay measures the incorporation of tritium-thymidine into DNA in FRTL cells.[342] Whether the *thyroid growth-stimulating immunoglobulins (TGI)* measured by these assays represent a population of immunoglobulins distinct from that with stimulatory functional activity remains a subject of active debate.

Clinical Applications

Measurement of abnormal immunoglobulins that interact with thyroid tissue by any of the methods described above is not indicated as a routine diagnostic test for Graves' disease. It is useful, however, in a few selected clinical conditions: (1) in the differential diagnosis of exophthalmos, particularly unilateral exophthalmos, when the origin of this condition is otherwise not apparent; the presence of TSI would obviate the necessity to undertake more complex diagnostic procedures described elsewhere;[343] (3) in the differential diagnosis of pretibial myxedema or other forms of dermopathy, when the etiology is unclear and it is imperative that the cause of the skin lesion be ascertained; (3) in the differentiation of Graves' disease from toxic nodular goiter, when both are being considered as the possible cause of thyrotoxicosis, when other tests such as thyroid scanning and thyroid autoantibody tests have been inconclusive, and particularly when such a distinction would play a role in determining the course of therapy; (4) when nonautoimmune thyrotoxicosis is suspected in a patient with hyperthyroidism and diffuse or nodular goiter[344,345]; (5) in Graves' disease during pregnancy, when high maternal levels of TSAb are a warning for the possible occurrence of neonatal thyrotoxicosis; (6) in neonatal thyrotoxicosis, where serial TSAb determinations showing gradual decrease may be helpful in distinguishing between intrinsic Graves' disease in the infant and transient thyrotoxicosis resulting from passive transfer of maternal TSAb.[321,346] Some investigators have found the persistence of TSAb's to be predictive of the relapse of Graves' thyrotoxicosis following a course of antithyroid drug therapy.[347]

Other Substances with Thyroid-Stimulating Activity

Some patients with trophoblastic disease develop hyperthyroidism as a result of the production and release of a thyroid stimulator known as *molar* or *trophoblastic thyrotropin* or *big placental TSH*.[348] This material can be detected in the standard mouse bioassay and is distinguished from LATS and TSH by its intermediate length of biologic action. Furthermore, in contrast to LATS, it can be detected in a bioassay that is based on the incorporation of radioactive phosphorus in the thyroid of day-old chicks.[349] It is very likely that the thyroid-stimulating activity in patients with trophoblastic disease is entirely due to the presence of high levels of human chorionic gonadotropin (hCG).[350] Thus the RIA of hCG can be useful in the differential diagnosis of thyroid dysfunction.

Exophthalmos-Producing Substance (EPS)

A variety of tests have been developed for measuring exophthalmogenic activity in serum.[351–354] Although a great uncertainty still exists regarding the pathogenesis of thyroid-associated eye disease, the role of the immune system appears to be central. Exophthalmogenic activity has also been detected in IgG fractions of some patients with Graves' ophthalmopathy. The role of assays to detect specific antibodies is discussed further in Chapter 7.

Tests of Cell-Mediated Immunity

Delayed hypersensitivity reactions to thyroid antigens are present in autoimmune thyroid diseases (see Chapter 7). Cell-mediated immunity (CMI) can be measured in several ways: (1) the migration inhibition test, which measures the inhibition of migration of sensitized leukocytes when exposed to the sensitizing antigen; (2) the lymphotoxic assay, which measures the ability of sensitized lymphocytes to kill target cells when exposed to the antigen; (3) the blastogenesis assay, which scores the formation of blast cells after exposure of lymphocytes to a thyroid antigen; and (4) thymus-dependent (T) lymphocyte subset quantitation utilizing monoclonal antibodies. The tests require fresh leukocytes from the patient, are variable in their response, and are difficult to perform.

Anatomic and Tissue Diagnoses

The purpose of the procedures described in this section is to evaluate the anatomic features of the thyroid gland, localize and determine the nature of abnormal areas, and eventually provide a pathologic or tissue diagnosis. All of these tests are performed in vivo. They cause inconvenience and at times discomfort and thus require the patient's understanding and cooperation.

Thyroid Scintiscanning

Normal and abnormal thyroid tissue can be externally imaged by three scintiscanning methods: (1) with radionuclides that are concentrated by normal thyroid tissues such as iodide isotopes and ^{99m}Tc given as the pertechnetate ion; (2) by administration of radiopharmaceutical agents that are preferentially concentrated by abnormal thyroid tissues; and (3) fluorescent scanning, which uses an external source of americium 241 and does not require administration of radioactive material. Each has specific indications, advantages, and disadvantages.

The physical properties, dosages, and radiation delivered by the most commonly used radioisotopes are listed in Table 6-2. The choice of scanning agents depends on the purpose of the scan, the age of the patient, and the equipment available. Radioiodide scans cannot be performed in patients who have recently ingested iodine-containing compounds. ^{123}I and ^{99m}TcO$_4$$^-$ are the radionuclides of choice because of the low radiation exposure.[355–357] Iodine 131 is still used for detecting functioning metastatic thyroid carcinoma by total body scanning.

A wide variety of imaging instruments is available. Rectilinear scanners have been largely replaced by stationary pinhole collimated Anger-type scanner gamma cameras that view the entire field being scanned. The image is displayed on an oscilloscope, and a Polaroid photograph is obtained for a permanent record. The data can also be stored on magnetic tape. The camera provides better resolution, but greater attention should be given to positioning, since magnification and distortion may cause significant problems.[357] Regardless of the display format, the scan should reproduce as accurately as possible the anatomic configuration of the tissue and the relative concentration of the radioactivity. Oblique and lateral views are helpful for demonstrating "cold" nodules that may be obscured by overlying functioning tissue. If retrosternal goiter is suspected, the proper isotope should be chosen to allow penetration through bony structures.

One of the most critical aspects in the correct interpretation of scans is the provision of anatomic landmarks that allow orientation of position and provide a scale for estimating size. Palpable abnormalities must also be marked in the scanning position. With the gamma camera, landmarks are recorded by obtaining a scan record with small Cobalt 57 marker sources placed over the areas of interest or by markers that obstruct the emission of x-rays.

Radioiodide and Pertechnetate 99m Scans

$^{99m}TcO_4^-$ is concentrated, and all iodide isotopes are concentrated and bound, by thyroid tissue. Depending upon the isotope used, scans are carried out at different times after administration: 20 minutes for $^{99m}TcO_4^-$, 4 or 24 hours for $^{123}I^-$; 24 hours for $^{125}I^-$ and $^{131}I^-$; and 48, 72, and 96 hours when $^{131}I^-$ is used in the search for metastatic thyroid carcinoma. The appearance of the normal thyroid gland on scan may be best described as a narrow-winged butterfly. Each "wing" represents a thyroid lobe, which in the adult measures 5 ± 1 cm in length and 2.3 ± 0.5 cm in width.[358] Common variants include the absence of a connecting isthmus, a large isthmus, asymmetry between the two lobes, and trailing activity extending to the cricoid cartilage (pyramidal lobe). The latter is more commonly found in conditions associated with diffuse thyroid hyperplasia. Occasionally, collection of saliva in the esophagus during $^{99m}TcO_4^-$ scanning may simulate a pyramidal lobe, but this artifact can be eliminated by having the patient drink water.

TABLE 6-8. Indications for Radionuclide Scanning

Detection of anatomic variants and search for ectopic thyroid tissue (thyroid hemiagenesis, lingual thyroid, struma ovarii)
Diagnosis of congenital athyreosis
Determination of the nature of abnormal neck or chest (mediastinal) masses
Evaluation of solitary thyroid nodules (functioning or nonfunctioning)
Evaluation of thyroid remnants after surgery
Detection of functioning thyroid metastases
Evaluation of focal functional thyroid abnormalities (suppressed or nonsuppressible tissue)

Table 6-8 lists the indications for scanning. In clinical practice, scans are most often requested for evaluating the functional activity of solitary nodules. Normally, the isotope is homogeneously distributed throughout both lobes of the thyroid gland. This distribution occurs in the enlarged gland of Graves' disease and may be seen in Hashimoto's thyroiditis. A mottled appearance may be noted in Hashimoto's thyroiditis and can occasionally be seen in Graves' disease, especially after therapy with radioactive iodide. Irregular areas of relatively diminished and occasionally increased uptake are characteristic of large multinodular goiters. The traditional nuclear medicine jargon classifies nodules as *hot, warm,* and *cold,* according to their isotope-concentrating ability relative to the surrounding normal parenchyma (Fig. 6-6). Hot, or hyperfunctioning, nodules are typically benign, although occasionally the presence of malignancy has been reported.[359,360] Cold, or hypofunctioning, nodules may be solid or cystic. Some may prove to be malignant, but most are benign. This differentiation cannot be made by scanning.[77,361] Occasionally, a nodule that is functional on a $^{99m}TcO_4^-$ scan will be found to be cold on an iodine scan; this pattern is found with both benign and malignant nodules. The scan is of particular value in identifying autonomous thyroid nodules, since the remainder of the gland is suppressed. Search for functioning thyroid metastases is best accomplished using 2 to 10 mCi of ^{131}I after ablation of the normal thyroid tissue and cessation of hormone therapy to allow TSH to increase above the upper limit of normal. Administration of bovine TSH is not recommended; however, recombinant human TSH may prove to be useful in allowing scanning without

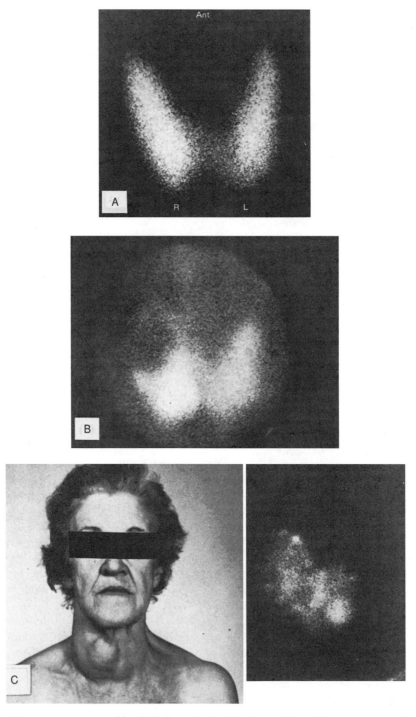

Fig. 6-6. Thyroid scans. **(a)** Normal thyroid imaged with ^{123}I. **(b)** Cold nodule in the right lobe imaged by ^{99m}Tc. **(c)** Elderly woman with obvious multinodular goiter and the corresponding radioiodide scan on right.

requiring cessation of hormone therapy.[362] Uptake is also found outside the thyroid gland in patients with lingual thyroids and in the rare ovarian dermoid tumor containing functioning thyroid tissue.

The scan can be used as an adjunct during TSH stimulation and T_3 suppression tests to localize suppressed normal thyroid tissue or autonomously functioning areas, respectively (see below). Applications other than those listed in Table 6-8 are of doubtful benefit and are rarely justified considering the radiation exposure, expense, and inconvenience. [123]I single photon emission computed tomography (SPECT) may also be useful in evaluating thyroid abnormalities.[363]

Other Isotope Scans

Because most test procedures, short of direct microscopic examination of thyroid tissue, fail to detect thyroid malignancy with any degree of certainty, efforts have been made to find other radioactive materials that would be of diagnostic use. Several such agents that are concentrated by metabolically active tissues, irrespective of their iodide-concentrating ability, have been tried. However, despite claims to the contrary, they have had only limited value or their diagnostic usefulness has not been fully evaluated. These agents include [75]selenium methionine, [125]cerium, [67]gallium citrate, [32]phosphorus, ^{99m}Tc pyrophosphate, and [201]Thallium.[364]

Scanning with ^{131}I-labeled anti-TG to detect occult metastatic thyroid malignancy that fails to concentrate ^{131}I showed promising early results[365]; however, the procedure has not proved clinically useful.

Fluorescent Scans

Fluorescent scans allow thyroid scanning without the administration of radioisotopes. The process involves the focal irradiation of the thyroid gland with a 60-KeV gamma ray derived from a [241]Am source. Its interaction with stable iodine ([127]I) within the gland produces the emission of a characteristic 28.5 KeV K-alpha (fluorescent) x-ray that is picked up by a lithium-drifted silicon detector.[366] The resulting scan shows the distribution of stable iodine within the gland, the content of which can be quantified by the use of appropriate iodide standards. Since the procedure is independent of the iodide-concentrating mechanism of the thyroid gland, fluorescent scanning is not hampered by excess iodide ingestion

or treatment with thyroid hormone, situations under which a radionuclide scan cannot be obtained. Furthermore, because administration of radioisotopes is not required, the scan is safe for children and for women during pregnancy and lactation.

The information derived relates to iodine storage and distribution within the gland, thus differing from that obtained from scans using radionuclides. Nevertheless, nodules that appear to be cold by isotope scanning usually also show decreased [127]I content by fluorescent scanning. The procedure is of particular value in demonstrating suppressed thyroid tissue with potential functioning capability in patients who have been taking replacement thyroid hormone treatment for a prolonged period of time.[367] Despite its apparent usefulness, this technique is not available in most centers.

Ultrasonography

Ultrasonography, or echography, is used to outline the thyroid gland and to characterize lesions differing in density from the surrounding tissue. The technique differentiates interphases of different acoustic densities, using sound frequencies in the megahertz range that are above the audible range. A transducer fitted with a piezoelectric crystal produces and transmits the signal and receives echo reflections. Interfaces of different acoustic densities reflect dense echoes, liquid transmits sound without reflections, and air-filled spaces do not transmit the ultrasound.[368]

In the one-dimensional or A-mode ultrasonogram, the transducer is held in one position for each image. The echoes, a series of spikes recorded on an oscilloscope, are of height proportional to the intensity of the echo and of distance corresponding to the actual space of echo interphases. The two-dimensional, or B-mode, ultrasonogram is performed with scanner that moves the transducer in a horizontal plane across the neck. A composite image of echoes represented by lines and dots in a scale of shades from black to white (gray-scale scan), proportional to the intensity of generated echoes, is assembled electronically. Since air is a poor conductor of ultrasound, contact with the skin is secured using special gels, oil, or water. This contact, as well as holding the transducer perpendicular to the skin, is essential to avoid artifacts.

One of the most useful applications of the ultrasonogram is to differentiate solid from cystic lesions.[368,369] Purely cystic lesions are entirely sonolucent, whereas solid lesions produce multiple echoes due to multiple sonic interphases. Many lesions, called *complex lesions,* are mixed (solid and cystic). Some tumors may have the same acoustic characteristics as the surrounding normal tissue and thus escape echographic detection. While high-resolution ultrasonography can detect thyroid nodules of only a few millimeters,[370] lesions need to be larger than 0.5 cm to allow differentiation between solid and cystic structures. A sonolucent pattern is frequently noted in glands with Hashimoto's thyroiditis, but this has also been described in multinodular glands and in patients with Graves' disease.[368,371,372]

Because sonography localizes the position as well as the depth of lesions, the procedure has been used to guide the needle during aspiration biopsy.[373] In complex lesions, the sonographic guiding ensures sampling from the solid portion of the nodule. With experience and proper calibration, sonography can be used to estimate thyroid gland size.[374,375] Several recent reports have described toxic nodules treated by injecting alcohol under sonographic guidance.[376] Although ultrasonography has found virtually the same applications as scintiscanning, claims that it may differentiate benign from malignant lesions are unfounded. Also, ultrasonography cannot be used to assess substernal goiters because of interference from overlying bone.

The procedure is simple and painless, and at the frequencies of sound used, does not produce tissue damage. Since it does not require the administration of isotopes, it can be safely used in children and during pregnancy. Also, because the procedure is independent of iodine-concentrating mechanisms, it is valuable in the study of suppressed glands.

X-Ray Procedures

A simple x-ray film of the neck and upper mediastinum may provide valuable information regarding the location, size, and effect of goiter on surrounding structures. Roentgenograms may show an asymmetric goiter, an intrathoracic extension of the gland, and displacement or narrowing of the trachea. If there is any suggestion of posterior extension of the mass, it is useful to take films during the swallow of x-ray contrast material. The soft tissue x-ray technique may disclose calcium deposits. Large deposits in

flakes or rings are typical of an old multinodular goiter, whereas foci of finely stippled flecks of calcium are pathognomonic of papillary adenocarcinoma.

Information not related to anatomic abnormalities of the thyroid gland may be obtained from x-ray studies. In children with a history of hypothyroidism, an x-ray film of the hand to determine bone age could aid in estimating the onset and duration of thyroid dysfunction.[294,295] Hypothyroidism leads to retardation in bone age and in infants produces a dense calcification of epiphyseal plates most easily seen at the distal end of the radius. Long-standing myxedema produces pituitary hypertrophy that, especially in children but also in adults, causes enlargement of the sella turcica demonstrable on skull x-ray films.[377]

Computed Tomography and Magnetic Resonance Imaging

Computed tomography provides useful information on the location and architecture of the thyroid gland as well as its relationship to surrounding tissues.[378] The test is, however, too costly relative to other procedures that provide similar information. An important application of CT is the assessment and delineation of obscure mediastinal masses and large substernal goiters.[379] In such instances the substernal location limits the use of ultrasonography and the lack of function, especially during suppressive therapy, limits use of radionuclide scanning. The necessity to infuse iodine-containing contrast agents limits the application of CT in patients being considered for radioiodide therapy.

CT and magnetic resonance imaging (MRI) are clearly indicated in another area of thyroid diseases, namely, in the evaluation of ophthalmopathy.[343] As with CT, MRI is also useful in delineating mediastinal masses.[379]

Other Procedures

Several unrelated methods for the anatomic delineation and characterization of thyroid pathology have been used. Their utility and level of sophistication vary and have limited clinical application. These procedures include (1) angiography with selective injection of radiologic contrast material for delineating tumor masses[380]; (2) lymphography by directly injecting thyroid tissue with contrast material[381] or radionuclide-tagged colloid material[382] that is rapidly transported to local lymph nodes adjacent to hyperplastic glands; and (3) thermography,[383] which differentiates between malignant and benign thyroid lesions, based on the assumption that malignant lesions are more active metabolically and thus increase in infrared energy emission from the overlying dermis. A barium swallow may be useful in evaluating a goiter impinging on the esophagus, while a flow volume loop may be useful in documenting functional impingement on the upper airway.

Biopsy of the Thyroid Gland

Histologic examination of thyroid tissue for diagnostic purposes requires an invasive procedure. The choice of biopsy procedure depends on the intended type of microscopic examination. Core biopsy for histologic examination of tissue while preserving architecture is obtained by closed-needle or open surgical procedure; aspiration biopsy is performed to obtain material for cytologic examination.

Core Biopsy

Closed core biopsy is an office procedure carried out under local anesthesia. A large (about 15-gauge) cutting needle of the Vim-Silverman type is most commonly used.[384] The needle is introduced under local anesthesia through a small skin nick and firm pressure is applied over the puncture site for 5 to 10 minutes after withdrawal of the needle. In experienced hands, complications are rare but may include transient damage to the laryngeal nerve, puncture of the trachea, laryngospasm, jugular vein phlebitis, and bleeding.[385] Because of the fear of disseminating malignant cells, biopsy was restricted for many years to the differential diagnosis of diffuse benign diseases. With improved cytology and biopsy techniques, open biopsy carried out under local or general anesthesia has been virtually abandoned.[385]

Percutaneous Fine-Needle Aspiration

Because of the development of more sophisticated staining techniques for cytologic examination and the realization that fear of tumor dissemination along the needle tract was not well founded,[386,387] percutaneous fine-needle aspiration (FNA) has become increasingly popular.[385,388]

The procedure is exceedingly simple and safe. The patient lies supine, with a small pillow under the shoulders to hyperextend the neck. Local anesthesia is usually not required. The skin is prepared with an antiseptic solution. The lesion, fixed between two gloved fingers, is penetrated with a fine (22- to 27-gauge) needle attached to a syringe. Suction is then applied while the needle is moved within the nodule. A nonsuction technique using capillary action has also been developed. The small amount of aspirated material, usually contained within the needle or its hub, is applied to glass slides and spread. Some slides are air dried and others are fixed before staining. Because biopsy of small nodules may be technically more difficult, the use of ultrasound to guide the needle has been suggested.[373,376] It is important that the slides be properly prepared, stained, and read by a cytologist experienced in interpreting material from thyroid gland aspirates.

The yield of false-positive and false-negative results varies from one center to another, but both occurrences are acceptably low. Various centers have reported that the accuracy of this technique in distinguishing benign from malignant lesions may be as high as 95 percent.[385,388] In one clinic in which the procedure is used routinely, the number of patients operated upon decreased by one-third, whereas the percentage of thyroid carcinomas among the patients who underwent surgery doubled.[389] When results suggest follicular neoplasia, surgery is required, as follicular adenoma cannot be differentiated from follicular cancer by cytology alone. As the sample obtained may not always be representative of the lesion, surgical treatment is indicated for lesions suspected of being malignant on clinical grounds. In such instances, some physicians recommend repeated aspiration biopsies. Other uses of aspiration biopsy include presumed lymphoma or invasive anaplastic carcinoma when biopsy may spare the patient an unnecessary neck exploration. Another application of needle aspiration is to confirm and treat thyroid cysts.

Evaluation of the Hypothalamic-Pituitary-Thyroid Axis

The development of an RIA for the routine measurement of TSH in serum and the availability of synthetic TRH[390,391] have placed increased reliance on tests assessing the hypothalamic-pituitary control of thyroid function. These tests allow the diagnosis of mild and subclinical forms of thyroid dysfunction and provide a means to differentiate between thyroprivic (primary) and trophoprivic, and pituitary (secondary) or hypothalamic (tertiary), thyroid gland failure. Furthermore, as a result of these methodologic advances, classic theories of the feedback mechanisms regulating thyroid gland function have been confirmed.[390–393]

Thyrotropin

Efforts to improve existing assays for measuring TSH have produced over 100 bioassay systems.[394,395] Despite general agreement of results among assays,[395] none were sensitive enough to routinely measure pituitary TSH in serum. The more sensitive bioassays recently developed[322,323,325–327,332–339,341,342,396] are still technically demanding and unsuitable for routine use. The clinical use of these assays is restricted to the measurement of thyroid-stimulating substances of other than pituitary origin (see previous section) and in the characterization of TSH with reduced or increased bioactivity.[397,398]

The routine measurement of TSH in clinical practice initially used RIA techniques. These first-generation assays had a sensitivity level of 1 mU/L, which did not allow the separation of normal from reduced values. A major problem with early TSH RIAs was cross-reactivity with gonadotropins (LH, FSH, and hCG) sharing with TSH a common α subunit.[399] Despite potential errors from immunologic cross-reactivity and the possibility of detecting immunologic material with altered biologic activity,[397,398,400] under the usual circumstances even older RIA methods for measuring pituitary TSH correlated well with values obtained using bioassay techniques.[401] Another uncommon source of error is the presence in the serum sample of heterophilic antibodies induced by vaccination with materials contaminated with animal serum[402] or endogenous TSH antibodies.[403] RIA techniques for measuring TSH in dry blood spots on filter paper are used to screen for neonatal hypothyroidism.[33]

Newer techniques have been developed using multiple antibodies to produce a "sandwich" type assay in which one antibody (usually directed against the α subunit) serves to anchor the TSH molecule and another (usually monoclonal antibodies di-

rected against the β subunit) is either radioiodinated (Immunoradiometric assay, IRMA) or is conjugated with an enzyme (immunoenzymometric [IEMA]) or a chemiluminescent compound (chemiluminescent assay [ICMA]).[112,404] In these assays, the signal should be directly related to the amount of the ligand present rather than being inversely related, as in RIAs measuring the bound tracer.[405] This results in decreased background "noise" and greater sensitivity, decreased interference from related compounds as well as an expanded useful range.[112,404,406] Initial improvements of the TSH assay resulted in assays with a sensitivity limit of 0.1 mU/L, a normal range of approximately 0.5 to 4.5 mU/L, and the ability to distinguish between low and normal TSH values.[112,404,406] Recently, commercial assays have been developed with an even higher sensitivity limit of 0.005 to 0.01 mU/L and a similar normal range but an expanded range between the lower limit of normal and the lower limit of sensitivity.[407,408]

The nomenclature for differentiating these various assays has not been standardized; manufacturers apply various combinations of "high(ly)," "ultra," and "sensitive." It has been recommended that the sensitivity limit be used to define assays, with early radioimmunoassays detecting values ≥ 1 mU/L designated as "first-generation assays," those with a lower sensitivity limit of 0.1 mU/L designated as "second-generation assays," and those with a lower sensitivity limit of 0.01 mU/L designated as "third-generation assays."[112] The determination of the appropriate sensitivity level has also been controversial. Some base it on a coefficient of variation less than 20 percent and others on the lowest level that can be reliably differentiated from the zero TSH standard.[112,406] At a minimum, for a TSH assay to be considered "sensitive," the overlap of TSH values in sera from clinically hyperthyroid and euthyroid individuals should be less than 5 percent and preferably less than 1 percent.[112]

In a number of these third-generation assays, TSH detected in clinically toxic patients and elevated values found in euthyroid subjects were not confirmed when the samples were measured in other assays. In some cases, this has been attributed to the presence of antibodies directed against the animal immunoglobulins used in the assay.[409–411] These act to bind the anchoring and detecting antibodies and lead to an overestimation of TSH. In some cases, this effect may be blocked by the addition of an excess of non-specific immunoglobulin of the same species.[411]

TSH appears abruptly in the pituitary and serum of the fetus at midgestation and can also be detected in amniotic fluid.[51,412,413] The mean TSH level is higher in cord than in maternal blood. A substantial increase, to levels severalfold above the upper range in adults, is observed during the first half-hour of life.[413] Levels decline to near the normal adult range by the third day of life. Minimal changes reported to occur during adult life and in early adolescence[414] have no significant effect on the overall range of normal. In the absence of pregnancy, no significant sex differences have been observed. Although early studies failed to show diurnal TSH variation,[415] significantly higher values have been recorded during the late evening and early night that are partially inhibited by sleep.[416] This diurnal rhythm of TSH is superimposed upon continuous high-frequency, low-amplitude variations. The nocturnal TSH surge persists in patients with mild primary hypothyroidism[417,418] and is abolished in hypothalamic hypothyroidism[417,419] and in some patients during fasting[420] and with nonthyroidal illness.[421,422] It is enhanced by oral contraceptives[423] and is abolished by high levels of glucocorticoids.[424] The presence of seasonal variation has not been a uniform finding, but it is unlikely to affect the clinical interpretation of serum values.[425] Various types of stressful stimuli have no significant effect on the basal serum TSH level, except for a rise during surgical hypothermia in infants but not in adults.[426] Various stimuli, such as administration of insulin, vasopressin, glucagon, bacterial pyrogens, arginine, prostaglandins, and chlorpromazine, which elicit in healthy humans a secretory response of some pituitary hormones, have no effect on serum TSH. However, administration of any of a growing list of drugs has been found to alter the basal concentration of serum TSH and/or its response to exogenous TRH (see Table 5-4).

In the presence of a normally functioning hypothalamic-pituitary system, there is an inverse correlation between the serum concentration of FT_4 and TSH. Changes in the serum concentration of TT_4 as a result of TBG abnormalities or drugs competing with T_4 binding to TBG have no effect on the level of serum TSH. The pituitary is exquisitely sensitive to both minimal decreases and increases in thyroid hormone concentration, with a logarithmic change in TSH levels in response to changes in

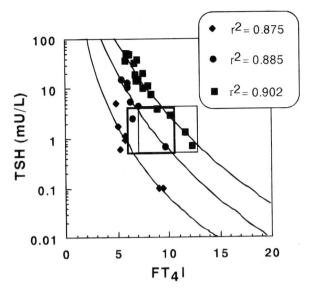

Fig. 6-7. Correlation of the serum TSH concentration and the free thyroxine index (FT_4) in three individuals given increasing doses of L-T_4. Note the logarithmic correlation between TSH and FT_4I and the variable individual requirement of free T_4 to normalize the TSH level. Normal ranges are included in the heavy lined box and those for subjects on L-T_4 replacement in the light lined box. (From D. Sarne and S. Refetoff, Endocrinology, L.J. DeGroot (ed). 1995, Grune & Straton Inc.)

T_4[404,408,427,428] (Fig. 6-7). Thus, serum TSH levels should be elevated in patients with primary hypothyroidism and low or undetectable in thyrotoxicosis. Indeed, in the absence of hypothalamic-pituitary disease, illness, or drugs, TSH is an accurate indicator of thyroid hormone status and the adequacy of thyroid hormone replacement.[404,429]

In patients with primary hypothyroidism from whatever cause, levels may reach 1,000 μU/ml or higher. The magnitude of serum TSH elevation grossly correlates with the severity and in part with the duration of thyroid hormone deficiency.[430,431] TSH concentrations above the upper limit of normal have been observed in the absence of clinical symptoms and signs of hypothyroidism and in the presence of serum T_4 and T_3 levels well within the normal range.[430,432] This condition is most commonly encountered in patients developing hypothyroidism due to Hashimoto's thyroiditis or with limited ability to synthesize thyroid hormone because of prior thyroid surgery, radioiodide treatment, or severe iodine deficiency.[430,432] There is disagreement on whether

TABLE 6-9. Discrepancies Between TSH and Free Thyroid Hormone Levels

Elevated Serum TSH Value Without
Low FT$_4$ or FT$_3$ Values

Subclinical hypothyroidism (inadequate replacement therapy, mild thyroid gland failure)
Recent increase in thyroid hormone dosage
Drugs
Inappropriate TSH secretion syndromes
Laboratory artefact

Subnormal Serum TSH Value Without
Elevated FT$_4$ or FT$_3$ Values

Subclinical hyperthyroidism (excessive replacement therapy, mild thyroid gland hyperfunction, autonomous nodule)
Recent decrease in suppressive thyroid hormone dosage
Recent treatment of thyrotoxicosis (Graves' disease, toxic multinodular goiter, toxic nodule)
Resolution thyrotoxic phase of thyroiditis
Nonthyroidal illness
Drugs
Central hypothyroidism

such patients have subclinical hypothyroidism or a "compensated state" in which euthyroidism is maintained by chronic stimulation of a reduced amount of functioning thyroid tissue through hypersecretion of TSH. Transient hypothyroidism may occur in some infants during the early neonatal period.[434] There are several circumstances in which the usual reverse relationship between the serum level of TSH and T$_4$ is not maintained in patients with proven primary hypothyroidism. Treatment with replacement doses of T$_4$ may normalize or even produce serum levels of thyroid hormone above the normal range before the high TSH levels have reached the normal range.[404,431,435] This is true in patients with severe or long-standing primary hypothyroidism, who may require 3 to 6 months of hormone replacement before TSH levels are fully suppressed. Conversely, serum TSH concentration may remain low or normal for up to 5 weeks after withdrawal of thyroid hormone replacement when serum levels of T$_4$ and T$_3$ have already declined to values well below the lower range of normal.[404,436] The most common example of this discrepancy is in patients maintained on replacement thyroxine. Twenty to forty percent have a T$_4$ or FTI just above the normal range when TSH is "normal"—perhaps because of replacing the thyroid secretion of T$_4$ and T$_3$ with T$_3$ alone. Causes for discrepancies between TSH and free T$_4$ and T$_3$ levels are listed in Table 6-9.

At this time, it is uncertain what TSH level is appropriate for suppressive thyroid hormone therapy. The frequency with which patients have subnormal, but detectable, TSH values depends on both the population studied and the sensitivity of the assay (Fig. 6-8). Using an assay with a sensitivity limit of 0.1 mU/L, 3 to 4 percent of hospitalized patients have been noted to have a subnormal TSH.[432,437] When patients with an undetectable TSH in such an assay were re-evaluated in an assay with a sensitivity limit of 0.005 mU/L, 3 of 77 (4 percent) with thyrotoxicosis and 32 of 37 (86 percent) with nonthyroidal illness or on drugs were found to have a subnormal but detectable TSH level.[407] Thus, the more sensitive the assay, the more likely that patients with clinical thyrotoxicosis will have undetectable serum TSH while those with illness will have a subnormal but detectable level. However, with progressively more sensitive assays, the likelihood of a clinically toxic patient having a detectable TSH will increase, and if patients on suppressive therapy are treated until the TSH is undetectable, the more likely they will have symptoms of thyrotoxicosis.

A persistent absence of a reverse correlation between serum thyroid hormone and TSH concentration has a very different connotation. A low serum level of thyroid hormone without clear elevation of the serum TSH concentration is suggestive of trophoprivic hypothyroidism, especially when associated with obvious clinical stigmata of hypothyroidism.[433] An inherited defect of the TSH receptor has been shown to produce marked persistent hyperthyrotropinemia in the presence of normal thyroid hormone levels.[438] In some cases, a mild elevation of the serum TSH level measured by RIA is probably due to the presence of immunoreactive TSH with reduced biologic activity.[397] Distinction between pituitary and hypothalamic hypothyroidism can be made on the basis of the TSH response to the administration of TRH (see below).

In another group of pathologic conditions, serum TSH levels may not be suppressed despite a clear elevation of serum free thyroid hormone levels. Because such a finding is incompatible with a normal thyroregulatory control mechanism of the pituitary, which is preserved in the more common forms of thyrotoxicosis, it has been termed *inappropriate secretion of TSH*.[439] It implicitly suggests a defective feedback regulation of TSH. When associated with the classic clinical and metabolic changes of thyrotoxico-

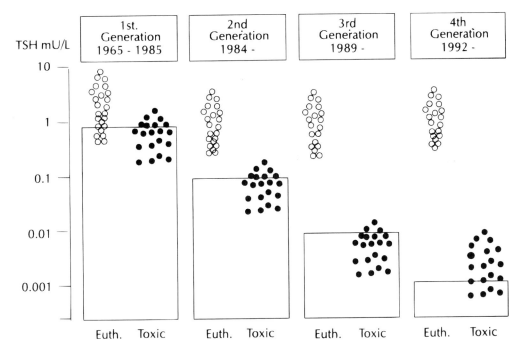

Fig. 6-8. The effect of serum TSH assay sensitivity on the discrimination of euthyroid subject (Euth) from those with thyrotoxicosis (Toxic). (From C. Spencer, Clinical Diagnostics, Eastman Kodak Co., 1992).

sis, it is usually due to TSH-secreting pituitary adenoma or isolated pituitary resistance to the feedback suppression by thyroid hormone.[439] The existence of hypothalamic hyperthyroidism can be questioned.[440] Precise diagnosis requires further studies, including radiologic examination of the pituitary gland and a TRH test. In addition, the presence of high circulating levels of the α subunit of pituitary glycoprotein hormones (α SU), giving rise to a disproportionately high α SU/TSH molar ratio in serum, is characteristic, if not pathognomonic, of TSH-secreting pituitary tumors.[439,441] Normal, and occasionally high, serum TSH levels, associated with a clear elevation in serum FT_4 and FT_3 but no clear clinical evidence of hypothyroidism or symptoms and signs suggestive of both thyroid hormone deficiency and excess, are typical of resistance to thyroid hormone (RTH)[65,442] (see Chapter 16).

Although TSH has been implicated in the pathogenesis of simple, nontoxic goiter, TSH levels are characteristically normal unless hypothyroidism supervenes or iodide deficiency is severe. Elevated TSH levels may occur in the presence of normal thyroid hormone levels and apparent euthyroidism in nonthyroidal diseases[437,443] (see also Chapter 5) and

with primary adrenal failure.[444] A more common occurrence in severe acute and chronic illnesses is a normal or low serum TSH concentration despite low levels of T_3 and even low T_4 levels.[407,429,445] TSH values may be transiently elevated during the recovery phase.[446] Various hypotheses to explain these anomalous findings have been proposed, but a perfectly satisfactory explanation is not at hand.

A specific RIA for the β subunits of human TSH is also available but has not found clinical application.[447]

Thyrotropin-Releasing Hormone

TRH

The hypothalamic tripeptide protirelin (TRH) plays a central role in the regulation of pituitary TSH secretion.[391,392,419] It is thus not surprising that attempts have been made to measure its concentration in a variety of body fluids, with the purpose of deriving information relevant to the function of the thyroid gland in health and in disease. Several methods have been used to quantify TRH,[448–451] but for many reasons, measurement in humans has failed to provide information of diagnostic value. These include high dilution of TRH by the time it reaches the systemic circulation, rapid enzymatic degradation, and ubiquitous tissue distribution.[448,450,451] Mean serum TSH levels of 5 and 6 pg/ml have been reported. It is uncertain whether measurements carried out in urine truly represent TRH.[449]

TRH Test

The TRH test measures increased pituitary TSH in serum in response to the administration of synthetic TRH. The magnitude of the TSH response to TRH is modulated by the thyrotroph response to active thyroid hormone and is thus almost always proportional to the concentration of free thyroid hormone in serum. The response is exquisitely sensitive to minor changes in the level of circulating thyroid hormones, which may not be detected by direct measurement.[427,428] A direct correlation between basal serum TSH values and the maximal response to TRH has been observed even in the absence of thyroid hormone abnormalities, suggesting that there may be a fine modulation of pituitary sensitivity to TRH in the euthyroid state.[452]

TRH normally stimulates pituitary prolactin secretion and, under certain pathologic conditions, the release of GH and ACTH.[391,392] Accordingly, the test has been used to assess a variety of endocrine functions, some unrelated to the thyroid. In clinical practice, the TRH test is used mainly (1) to assess the functional integrity of the pituitary thyrotrophs and thus to aid in differentiating hypothyroidism due to intrinsic pituitary disease from hypothalamic dysfunction, (2) in the diagnosis of mild thyrotoxicosis when results of other tests are equivocal, and (3) in the differential diagnosis of inappropriate TSH secretion, in particular when a TSH-secreting adenoma is suspected.

TRH is effective when given intravenously as a bolus or by infusion,[414,453] intramuscularly,[454] or orally[455] in single or repeated doses. Doses as small as 6 μg can elicit a significant TSH response, and there is a linear correlation between the incremental changes in serum TSH concentrations and the logarithm of the administered TRH dose.[414] The standard test uses a single TRH dose of 400 μg/1.73 m^2 body surface area given by rapid intravenous injection. Serum is collected before and at 15 minutes and then at 30-minute intervals over 120 to 180 minutes, although many clinicians choose to obtain a single

postinjection sample at 15, 20, or 30 minutes. In healthy persons serum TSH increases promptly, with a peak level at 15 to 40 minutes, which is on the average 16 μU/ml, or fivefold the basal level. The decline is more gradual, with a return of serum TSH to the preinjection level by 3 to 4 hours.[414,453] Results can be expressed in terms of the peak level of TSH achieved, the maximal increment above the basal level (ΔTSH), the peak TSH value expressed as a percentage of the basal value, or the integrated area of the TSH response curve. Determination of TSH before and 30 minutes after the injection of TRH provides information concerning the presence or absence of TSH responsiveness but cannot detect delayed or prolonged responses.

The stimulatory effect of TRH is specific for pituitary TSH, its free α and β subunits,[447] and prolactin. Under normal circumstances, no significant changes are observed in the serum levels of other pituitary hormones[456] or potential thyroid stimulators.[457] Responsiveness is present at birth,[458] is greater in women than in men, particularly in the follicular phase of the menstrual cycle,[459] and may be blunted in older men,[414,454,455] but these are not consistent findings.[460] On the average, the magnitude of the response is greater at 11 PM than at 11 AM,[452] in accordance with the diurnal pattern of the basal TSH level, which correlates to its response to TRH. Repetitive administration of TRH to the same subject at daily intervals gradually obtunds the TSH response,[453] presumably due to increased thyroid hormone concentration[461] and also in part to TSH "exhaustion."[462] However, more than 1 hour must elapse between the increase in thyroid hormone concentration and TRH administration for inhibition of the TSH response to occur. A number of drugs (see Table 5-4) and nonendocrine diseases (see Chapter 5) may affect to various extents the magnitude of the response.

TRH-induced secretion of TSH is followed by a release of thyroid hormone that can be detected by direct measurement of serum TT$_4$ and TT$_3$ concentrations.[160] Peak levels are normally reached approximately 4 hours after the administration of TRH and are accompanied by an increase in serum TG concentration. The incremental rise in serum TT$_3$ is relatively greater, and the peak is on the average 50 percent above the basal level. Measurement of changes in serum thyroid hormone concentration after TRH administration has been proposed as an adjunctive test and is useful for evaluating the integrity of the thyroid gland or bioactivity of endogenous TSH.[463] Increase in RAIU is minimal and occurs only with high doses of TRH given orally.[455]

Side effects from the intravenous administration of TRH, in decreasing order of frequency, include nausea, flushing or a sensation of warmth, desire to micturate, peculiar taste, light-headedness or headache, dry mouth, urge to defecate, and chest tightness. They are usually mild, begin within a minute after the injection of TRH, and last for a few seconds to several minutes. A transient rise in blood pressure has been observed on occasion, but there are no other changes in vital signs, urine analysis, blood count, or routine blood chemistry tests.[456,464] The occurrence of circulatory collapse is exceedingly rare.[465]

The test provides a means to distinguish between secondary (pituitary) and tertiary (hypothalamic) hypothyroidism (Fig. 6-9). Although the diagnosis of primary hypothyroidism can be easily confirmed by the presence of elevated basal serum TSH levels, secondary and tertiary hypothyroidism are typically associated with TSH levels that are low or normal. On occasion the serum TSH concentration may be slightly elevated due to the secretion of biologically less potent molecules,[397] but it remains inappropriately low for the degree of thyroid hormone deficiency. Differentiation between secondary and tertiary hypothyroidism cannot be made with certainty without the TRH test. A TSH response suggests a hypothalamic disorder, and a failure to respond is compatible with intrinsic pituitary dysfunction.[466] Furthermore, the typical TSH response curve in hypothalamic hypothyroidism shows a delayed peak with a prolonged elevation of serum TSH before return to the basal value (Fig. 6-9). The lack of a TSH response in association with normal prolactin stimulation may be due to isolated pituitary TSH deficiency.[467] Test results should be interpreted cautiously after withdrawal of thyroid hormone replacement or after treatment of thyrotoxicosis when, despite a low serum thyroid hormone concentration, TSH may remain low and not respond to TRH for several weeks.[404,433,436,468]

In the most common forms of thyrotoxicosis, the mechanism of feedback regulation of TSH secretion is intact but is appropriately suppressed by the excessive amounts of thyroid hormone. Thus both the basal TSH level and its response to TRH are suppressed unless thyrotoxicosis is TSH induced.[404,407,417] With the development of more sensitive TSH assays, the TRH test is generally not needed to evaluate a thyrotoxic patient with an undetectable TSH.[407] Differential diagnosis of conditions leading to inappropriate secretion of TSH may be aided by the TRH test result. Elevated basal TSH values that do not respond to a further increase to TRH are typical of TSH-secreting pituitary adenomas.[439,441] Patients with inappropriate secretion of TSH due to resistance to thyroid hormone have a normal or exaggerated TSH response to TRH that, in most instances, is suppressed with supraphysiologic doses of thyroid hormone.[442]

Because of the high sensitivity of the pituitary gland to feedback regulation by thyroid hormone, small changes in the latter profoundly affect the response of TSH to TRH. Thus patients with non-TSH-induced thyrotoxicosis of the mildest degree have a reduced TSH response to TRH, whereas those with primary hypothyroidism exhibit an accentuated response that is prolonged (Fig. 6-9). These changes may occur in the absence of clinical or other laboratory evidence of thyroid dysfunction.

The TSH response to TRH is subnormal or absent in one-third of apparently euthyroid patients with autoimmune thyroid disease, and even members of their family may not respond to TRH.[469,470] Most, but not all, patients with reduced TSH response to TRH also show thyroid activity that is nonsuppressible by thyroid hormone. A common dissociation between these two tests is typified by a normal TRH response in a nonsuppressible patient. This finding is not surprising, since patients with nonsuppressible thyroid glands often have limited capacity to synthesize and secrete thyroid hormone due to prior therapy or partial destruction of their glands by the disease process. Clinically, euthyroid patients who do not respond to TRH admittedly have a slight excess of thyroid hormone. It is less easy to reconcile the rare occurrence of TRH unresponsiveness in a patient who is suppressible by exogenous thyroid hormone. It should be remembered, however, that a suppressed pituitary may take a variable amount of time to recover, a phenomenon that may be the basis of such discrepancies.[404,436,468] Despite discrepancies between the results of the TRH and T_3 suppression tests,[469,470] the use of the former is much preferred, particularly in elderly patients in whom administration of T_3 can produce untoward effects.

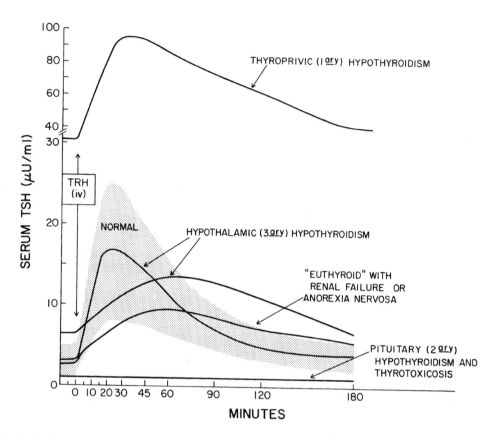

Fig. 6-9. Typical serum TSH responses to the administration of a single intravenous bolus of TRH at time 0 in various conditions. The normal response is represented by the shaded area. Data used for this figure represent the average of several studies. (From S. Refetoff, Endocrinology, L.J. DeGroot (ed). 1979, Grune & Straton Inc.)

Other Tests of TSH Reserve

It has been reasoned that by virtue of different mechanisms of action, testing the TSH response by means other than TRH may provide information of diagnostic value not obtainable from the stimulation and suppression of the pituitary by TRH and thyroid hormone, respectively.[393] Many trials using a variety of drugs such as metoclopramide, L-dopa, and dexamethasone have been carried out but so far have provided only limited additional information and thus have not found a place in clinical practice. These tests have a limited application in the study of patients with inappropriate secretion of TSH, in whom the distinction of autonomous secretion of TSH as compared to a selective unresponsiveness to thyroid hormone inhibition is of diagnostic value.[65]

Other tests indirectly measure pituitary TSH reserve during the "rebound" period after suppression of thyroid hormone synthesis or pituitary TSH secretion. Assessment of thyroid gland activity following withdrawal of antithyroid drugs or T_3 replacement has been proposed.[471,472]

Thyroid Stimulation Test

The thyroid stimulation test, also known as the *TSH stimulation test*, measures the ability of thyroid tissue to respond to exogenous TSH by increased iodide accumulation and/or hormone release. Formerly used to differentiate hypothyroidism due to thyroid gland failure from that due to TSH deficiency, the test is now almost exclusively done in conjunction with a scintiscan to localize areas of suppressed thyroid tissue. It requires the intramuscular administration of one or three 5 to 10-U doses of bovine TSH.

The response is assessed from the change in the 24-hour RAIU or the incremental change in serum TT_4 or TT_3 measured before and after the course of TSH treatment.[473,474] The presence of normal but non-functioning thyroid tissue suppressed by excess hormone from a functioning thyroid nodule, ectopic thyroid tissue, or hormone administration is best demonstrated by scanning after a 3-day course of TSH.

The test may cause discomfort, and some of the reactions to the heterologous TSH may be serious.[474] Repeated administration of bovine TSH can also lead to the production of antibodies that may neutralize its action,[475] which is the main reason for not recommending the routine use of exogenous TSH in the search for functioning metastases in patients with thyroid cancer. The introduction of recombinant human TSH is likely to eliminate these untoward effects and increase the use of this test.

Thyroid Suppression Test

The maintenance of thyroid gland activity that is independent of TSH can be demonstrated by the thyroid suppression test. Under normal conditions, administration of thyroid hormone in quantities sufficient to satisfy the body requirement suppresses endogenous TSH, resulting in reduced thyroid hormone synthesis and secretion. Since thyrotoxicosis due to excessive secretion of hormone by the thyroid gland implies that the feedback control mechanism is not operative or has been perturbed, it is easy to understand why under such circumstances the supply of exogenous hormone would also be ineffective in suppressing thyroid gland activity. The test is of particular value in patients who are euthyroid or only mildly thyrotoxic but suspected of having abnormal thyroid gland stimulation or autonomy.

Usually the test is carried out with 100 μg of L-T_3 (liothyronine) given daily in two divided doses over a period of 7 to 10 days; 24-hour RAIU is obtained before and during the last 2 days of T_3 administration.[476] Healthy persons show a suppressed RAIU that is at least 50 percent of the pre-L-T_3 treatment value. No change or lesser reduction is not only typical of Graves' disease but also other forms of endogenous thyrotoxicosis, including toxic adenoma, functioning carcinoma, and thyrotoxicosis due to trophoblastic diseases. The presence of nonsuppressibility indicates thyroid gland activity independent of TSH but not necessarily thyrotoxicosis. Euthyroid patients with autonomous thyroid function have a normal TSH response to TRH before the administration of L-T_3. However, inhibition of TSH secretion by the exogenous T_3 does not suppress the autonomous activity of the thyroid gland. This is the most commonly encountered discrepancy between the results of the two related tests. When the T_3 suppression test is used in conjunction with the scintiscan, localized areas of autonomous function can be identified. The test can be carried out without the administration of radioisotopes by measuring serum T_4 before and 2 weeks following the ingestion of L-T_3. Although total suppression of T_4 secretion never occurs, even after prolonged treatment with L-T_3, a reduction by at least 50 percent is normal.[477]

A return to thyroid gland suppressibility in patients with autoimmune thyroid disease under treatment with antithyroid drugs can be demonstrated by the suppression of the 20-minute thyroidal uptake of $^{99m}TcO_4^-$ or $^{123}I^-$ during the administration of L-T_3.[478] Unfortunately, the test has limited prognostic value in relation to long-term remission or outcome of therapy.[469,479]

Variants of the test have been proposed to reduce the potential risks of L-T_3 administration in elderly patients and in those with angina pectoris or congestive heart failure. With the availability of sensitive TSH determinations and the TRH test, which are less dangerous, thyroid suppression tests are used infrequently.

Specialized Thyroid Tests

A number of specialized tests are available for evaluating specific aspects of thyroid hormone biosynthesis, secretion, turnover, distribution, and absorption. Their primary application is investigative. Some are rather simple; others are complex. They are only briefly mentioned here for the sake of completeness. Most of these tests require in vivo administration of radioisotopes.

Iodotyrosine Deiodinase Activity

The test involves the intravenous administration of tracer MIT or DIT labeled with radioiodide. Urine, collected over a period of 4 hours, is analyzed by chromatography or resin column separation. Normally, only 4 to 8 percent of the radioactivity is excreted as such; the remainder appears in the urine in the form of iodide.[480] Excretion of larger amounts of the parent compound indicates inability to deiodinate iodotyrosine. The test is useful in the diagnosis of a dehalogenase defect (see Chapter 16).

Test for Defective Hormonogenesis

After administration of RAI, the isotopically labeled compounds synthesized in the thyroid gland and those secreted into the circulation can be analyzed by immunologic, chromatographic, electrophoretic, and density gradient centrifugation techniques.[481] Such tests evaluate the synthesis and release of thyroid hormone and delineate the formation of abnormal iodoproteins.

Iodine Kinetic Studies

The iodine kinetic procedure is used to evaluate overall iodide metabolism and to elucidate the pathophysiology of thyroid diseases. The analysis involves follow-up of the fate of administered radioiodide tracer by measuring thyroidal accumulation, secretion into blood, and excretion in the urine and feces.[482] Double tracer techniques and programs for computer-assisted analysis of data are available.

Absorption of Thyroid Hormone

Failure to achieve normal serum thyroid hormone concentration after administration of replacement doses of thyroid hormone is usually due to poor compliance, occasionally to the use of inactive preparations, and rarely, if ever, to malabsorption. The last can be evaluated by the simultaneous oral and intravenous administration of the hormone labeled with two different iodine isotope tracers. The ratio of the two isotopes in blood is proportional to the net absorbed fraction of the orally administered hormone.[483,484] Under normal circumstances, approximately 80 percent of T_4 and 95 percent of T_3 administered orally are absorbed. Hypothyroidism and a variety of other unrelated conditions have little effect on the intestinal absorption of thyroid hormones. Absorption may be diminished in patients with steatorrhea, in some cases of hepatic failure, during treatment with cholestyramine, and with diets rich in soybeans. The absorption of thyroid hormone can also be evaluated by administering a single oral dose of 100 μg T_3 or 1 mg T_4, followed by their measurement in blood sampled at various intervals.[485,486]

Turnover Kinetics of T_4 and T_3

Turnover kinetic studies require the intravenous administration of isotope-labeled tracer T_4 or T_3.[487–491] The half-time (T1/2) of disappearance of the hormone is calculated from the rate of decrease in serum trichloroacetic acid–precipitable, ethanol-extractable, or antibody-precipitable isotope counts. Compartmental analysis can be used to calculate the turnover parameters.[488,489] The calculated daily degradation (D) or production rate (PR) is the product of the fractional turnover rate (K), the extrathyroidal distribution space (DS), and the average concentration of the hormone in serum. Noncompartmental analysis may be used to calculate kinetic parameters.[488] The metabolic clearance rate (MCR) is defined as the dose of the injected labeled tracer divided by the area under its curve of disappearance. The PR is then calculated from the product of the MCR and the average concentration of the respective nonradioactive iodothyronine measured in serum over the period of the study. Simultaneous studies of the T_4 and T_3 turnover kinetics can be carried out by injection of both hormones, labeled with different iodine isotopes.[488,490,491]

Average normal values in adults for T_4 and T_3, respectively, are: T1/2 = 7.0 and 0.8 days; K = 10 and 90 percent per day; DS = 11 and 30 L of serum equivalent; MCR = 1.1 and 25 L/day; and PR = 90 and 25 μg/day.

The hormonal PR is accelerated in thyrotoxicosis and diminished in hypothyroidism.[487] In euthyroid patients with TBG abnormalities, the PR remains normal, since changes in the serum hormone concentration are accompanied by compensatory changes in the fractional turnover rate and the extrathyroidal hormonal pool.[492] A variety of nonthyroidal illnesses may alter hormone kinetics[491,493] (see Chapter 5).

Metabolic Kinetics of Thyroid Hormones and Their Metabolites

The production kinetics of various metabolites of T_4 and T_3 in peripheral tissues and their further metabolism has been studied. Most methods use radiolabeled iodothyronine tracers injected intravenously.[19,135,137,489–491] Their disappearance is followed in serum samples obtained at various intervals after injection of the tracers by chromatographic and immunologic techniques of separation.[20,137] Kinetic parameters can be calculated by noncompartmental analysis[488,490] or by two- or multiple-compartment analysis.[487,489] Estimates have been made by the differential measurement in urine of isotopes derived from the precursor and its metabolite. They are in agreement with measurements carried out in serum.[494] Conversion rates of iodothyronines, principally generated in peripheral tissues, can be calculated from the ratio of their PR and that of their respective precursors. Some iodothyronines, such as T_3, are secreted by the thyroid gland as well as generated in peripheral tissues. Studies to calculate the CR require administration of thyroid hormone to block thyroidal secretion.[493]

On the average, 35 and 45 percent of T_4 are converted to T_3 and rT_3, respectively, in peripheral tissues. The conversion of T_4 to T_3 is greatly diminished in a variety of illnesses (see Ch. 5) of nonthyroidal origin and in response to many drugs (Table 5-3). Degradation and monodeiodination of iodothyronines can be estimated without administering isotopes; however, the estimates are less accurate. The conversion of T_4 to T_3 can be estimated semiquantitatively by measuring serum TT_3 concentration after treatment with replacement doses of T_4.[493] Data can be also derived by measuring the iodothyronine in serum after administering its precursor to athyreotic patients.[136,142] Measurements of an iodothyronine in samples of serum obtained at intervals after its administration as a single large intravenous or oral dose have also been used to estimate the MCR.[150]

Measurement of the Production Rate and Metabolic Kinetics of Other Compounds

The metabolism and PRs of a variety of compounds related to thyroid physiology can be studied using their radiolabeled congeners and applying the general principles of turnover kinetics. Studies of TSH have demonstrated changes related not only to thyroid dysfunction but also associated with age, kidney, and liver disease.[495,496] Studies of the turnover kinetics of TBG have shown that the slight increases and decreases of serum TBG concentration associated with hypothyroidism and thyrotoxicosis, respectively, are due to changes in the degradation rate of TBG rather than synthesis.[492]

Transfer of Thyroid Hormone from Blood to Tissues

Transfer of hormone from blood to tissues can be estimated in vivo by two techniques. A direct method follows the accumulation of the administered labeled hormone tracer by surface counting over the organ of interest.[497] An indirect method follows the early disappearance from plasma of the simultaneously administered hormone and albumin, labeled with different radioisotope tracers.[498] The difference between the rates of disappearance of the hormone and albumin represents the fraction of hormone that has left the vascular (albumin) space and presumably has entered the tissues.

Applications of Molecular Biology in the Diagnosis of Thyroid Diseases

Recombinant technology has already produced new, highly purified reagents for the detection of anti-TSH receptor[330,331] and peroxidase antibodies.[299] Human TSH has also been made by recombinant techniques and is being tested as a diagnostic agent.[362] Restriction fragment length polymorphisms (RFLP) have proven useful in the identification of inherited defects linked to chromosome 3 in kindred with RTH[499] and linked to chromosome 10 in patients having increased risk for the inheritance of medullary cancer as part of the MEN 2A syndrome.[500] A variety of techniques has been used to identify individuals with specific gene abnormalities such as qualitative TBG abnormalities,[501] RTH as the result of an abnormal thyroid receptor,[65] and somatic and germ line mutations in patients with nonautoimmune thyrotoxicosis[344,345] (see also Chapter 16). Gene sequencing has elucidated TSH and Pit 1 defects giving rise to severe neonatal secondary hypothyroidism.[502] With the characterization of specific gene abnormalities, it will be possible to identify individuals likely to develop the inherited form of medullary carcinoma and to enhance the diagnostic value of fine-needle aspirates of thyroid lesions.

REFERENCES

1. Mercer RD: Pseudo-goiter. The Modigliani syndrome. 42:319, 1975
2. Brown-Grant K: Extrathyroidal iodide concentrating mechanisms. Physiol Rev 41:189, 1961

3. Modan B, Mart H, Baidatz D: Radiation-induced head and neck tumors. Lancet 1:277, 1974

4. Bland EP, Crawford JS, Docker MF, Farr RF: Radioactive iodine uptake by thyroid of breast-fed infants after maternal blood-volume measurements. Lancet 2:1039, 1969

5. Quimby EH, Feitelberg S, Gross W: Radioactive Nuclides in Medicine and Biology. 3rd Ed. Lea & Febiger, Philadelphia, 1970

6. MIRD: Dose estimate report no. 5. Summary of current radiation dose estimates to humans from ^{123}I, ^{124}I, ^{126}I, ^{130}I, ^{131}I, and ^{132}I as sodium iodide. J Nucl Med 16:857, 1975

7. MIRD: Dose estimate report no. 8. Summary of current radiation dose estimates to normal humans from ^{99m}Tc as sodium pertechnetate. J Nucl Med 17:74, 1976

8. Pittman JA Jr, Dailey GE III, Beschi RJ: Changing normal values for thyroidal radioiodine uptake. N Engl J Med 280:1431, 1969

9. Gluck FB, Nusynowitz ML, Plymate S: Chronic lymphocytic thyroiditis, thyrotoxicosis, and low radioactive iodine uptake: Report of four cases. N Engl J Med 293:624, 1975

10. Savoie JC, Massin JP, Thomopoulos P, Leger F: Iodine-induced thyrotoxicosis in apparently normal thyroid glands. J Clin Endocrinol Metab 41:685, 1975

11. Higgins HP, Ball D, Estham S: 20-min ^{99m}Tc thyroid uptake: a simplified method using the gamma camera. J Nucl Med 14:907, 1973

12. Baschieri L, Benedetti G, deLuca F, Negri M: Evaluation and limitations of the perchlorate test in the study of thyroid function. J Clin Endocrinol Metab 23:786, 1963

13. Morgans ME, Trotter WR: Defective organic binding of iodine by the thyroid in Hashimoto's thyroiditis. Lancet 1:553, 1957

14. Ford HC, Cooke RR, Keightley EA, Feek CM: Serum levels of free and bound testosterone in hyperthyroidism. Clin Endocrinol 36:187, 1992

15. Gray HW, Hooper LA, Greig WR, McDougall IR: A twenty-minute perchlorate discharge test. J Clin Endocrinol Metab 34:594, 1972

16. Suzuki H, Mashimo K: Significance of the iodide-perchlorate discharge test in patients with ^{131}I-treated and untreated hyperthyroidism. J Clin Endocrinol Metab 34:332, 1972

17. Harden RM, Alexander WD, Chisholm CJS, Shimmins J: The salivary iodide trap in nontoxic goiter. J Clin Endocrinol Metab 28:117, 1968

18. Chopra IJ, Fisher DA, Solomon DH, Beall GN: Thyroxine and triiodothyronine in the human thyroid. J Clin Endocrinol Metab 36:311, 1973

19. Engler D, Burger AG: The deiodination of iodothyronines and of their derivatives in man. Endocr Rev 5:151, 1984

20. Pittman CS, Shimizu T, Burger A, Chambers JB Jr: The nondeiodinative pathways of thyroxine metabolism: 3,5,3′,5′-tetraiodothyroacetic acid turnover in normal and fasting human subjects. J Clin Endocrinol Metab 50:712, 1980

21. Gavin LA, Livermore BM, Cavalieri RR et al: Serum concentration, metabolic clearance, and production rates of 3,5,3′-triiodothyroacetic acid in normal and athyreotic man. J Clin Endocrinol Metab 51:529, 1980

22. Chopra IJ, Wu S-Y, Teco GNC, Santini F: A radioimmunoassay for measurement of 3,5,3′-triiodothyronine sulfate: Studies in thyroidal and nonthyroidal diseases, pregnancy, and neonatal life. 75:189, 1992

23. deVijlder JJM, Veenboer GJM: Thyroid albumin originates from blood. Endocrinology 131:578, 1992

24. Surks MI, Oppenheimer JH: Formation of iodoprotein during the peripheral metabolism of 3,5,3′-triiodo-L-thyroxine-^{125}I in the euthyroid man and rat. J Clin Invest 48:685, 1969

25. Refetoff S, Matalon R, Bigazzi M: Metabolism of L-thyroxine (T_4) and L-triiodothyronine (T_3) by human fibroblasts in tissue culture: Evidence for cellular binding proteins and conversion of T_4 to T_3. Endocrinology 91:934, 1972

26. Koerner D, Surks MI, Oppenheimer JH: In vitro formation of apparent covalent complexes between L-triiodothyronine and plasma protein. J Clin Endocrinol Metab 36:239, 1973

27. Trevorrow V: Studies on the nature of the iodine in blood. J Biol Chem 127:737, 1939

28. Barker SB: Determination of protein-bound iodine. J Biol Chem 173:715, 1948

29. Refetoff S: Principles of competitive binding assay and radioimmunoassay. p. 215. In Gottschalk A, Potchen EJ (eds): Diagnostic Nuclear Medicine (Golden's Diagnostic Radiology), Williams & Wilkins, Baltimore, 1976

30. Mitsuma T, Colucci J, Shenkman L, Hollander CS: Rapid simultaneous radioimmunoassay for triiodothyronine and thyroxine in unextracted serum. Biochem Biophys Res Commun 46:2107, 1972

31. O'Connor JF, Wu GY, Gallagher TF, Hellman L: The 24-hour plasma thyroxin profile in normal man. J Clin Endocrinol Metab 39:765, 1974

32. Fang VS, Refetoff S: Radioimmunoassay for serum triiodothyronine: Evaluation of simple techniques to control interference from binding proteins. Clin Chem 20:1150, 1974

33. Larsen PR, Dockalova J, Sipula D, Wu FM: Immunoassay of thyroxine in unextracted human serum. J Clin Endocrinol Metab 37:117, 1973

34. Sterling K, Milch PO: Thermal inactivation of thyroxine-binding globulin for direct radioimmunoassay of triiodothyronine in serum. J Clin Endocrinol Metab 38:866, 1974

35. Mitsuma T, Nihei N, Gershengorn MC, Hollander CS: Serum triiodothyronine: Measurements in human serum by radioimmunoassay with corroboration by gas-liquid chromatography. J Clin Invest 50:2679, 1971

36. Lieblich J, Utiger RD: Triiodothyronine radioimmunoassay. J Clin Invest 51:157, 1972

37. Gaitan JE, Wahner HW, Gorman CA, Jiang NS: Measurement of triiodothyronine in unextracted urine. J Lab Clin Med 86:538, 1975

38. Ikekubo K, Konishi J, Endo K et al: Anti-thyroxine and anti-triiodothyronine antibodies in three cases of Hashimoto's thyroiditis. Acta Endocrinol 89:557, 1978

39. Sakata S, Nakamura S, Miura K: Autoantibodies against thyroid hormones or iodothyronine. Implications in diagnosis, thyroid function, treatment, and pathogenesis. Ann Intern Med 103:579, 1985

40. Canadian Task Force on the periodic health examination: Periodic health examination, 1990 Update. 1. Early detection of hyperthyroidism and hypothyroidism in adults and screening of newborns for congenital hypothyroidism. J Can Med Assoc 142:955, 1990

41. Murphy BEP, Pattee CJ: Determination of thyroxine utilizing the property of protein-binding. J Clin Endocrinol Metab 24:187, 1964

42. Schuurs AWM, Van Weemen BK: Enzyme-immunoassay. Clin Chim Acta 81:1, 1977

43. Galen RS, Forman D: Enzyme immunoassay of serum thyroxine with AutoChemist" multichannel analyzer. Clin Chem 23:119, 1977

44. Schall RF, Fraser AS, Hausen HW, et al: A sensitive manual enzyme immunoassay for thyroxine. Clin Chem 24:1801, 1978

45. Miyai K, Ishibashi K, Kawashima M: Enzyme immunoassay of thyroxine in serum and dried blood samples on filter paper. Endocrinol Jpn 27:375, 1980

46. Nihei NN, Gershengorn MC, Mitsuma T et al: Measurements of triiodothyronine and thyroxine in human serum by gas-liquid chromatography. Anal Biochem 43:433, 1971

47. Hoch FL, Kuras RA, Jones JD: Iodine analysis of biological samples by neutron activation of ^{127}I with scintillation counting of Cerenkov radiation. Anal Biochem 40:86, 1971

48. Hagen GA, Diuguid LI, Kliman B, Stanbury JB: Double-isotope derivative assay of serum iodothyronines. III. Triiodothyronine. Biochem Med 7:191, 1973

49. Hay ID, Annesley TM, Jiang NS, Gorman CA: Simultaneous determination of D- and L-thyroxine in human serum by liquid chromatography with electrochemical detection. J Chromatogr 226:383, 1981

50. Refetoff S: Inherited thyroxine-binding globulin (TBG) abnormalities in man. Endocr Rev 10:275, 1989

51. Abuid J, Klein AH, Foley TP Jr, Larsen PR: Total and free triiodothyronine and thyroxine in early infancy. J Clin Endocrinol Metab 39:263, 1974

52. Roger M, Soldat MC, Laffi E et al: La thyroxine plasmatique chez l'enfant: Variations du taux avec l'âge et applications au diagnostique des dysthyroïdies. Ann Pediatr 22:27, 1975

53. Westgren U, Burger A, Ingemanssons S et al: Blood levels of 3,5,3'-triiodothyronine and thyroxine: Differences between children, adults, and elderly subjects. Acta Med Scand 200:493, 1976

54. Nishikawa M, Inada M, Naito K et al: Age-related changes in serum 3,3'-diiodothyronine, 3',5',-diiodothyronine, and 3,5-diiodothyronine concentrations in man. J Clin Endocrinol Metab 52:517, 1981

55. Herrmann J, Rusche HJ, Kröll HJ: Free triiodothyronine (T_3) and thyroxine (T_4) serum levels in old age. Horm Metab Res 6:239, 1974

56. DeCostre P, Buhler U, DeGroot LJ, Refetoff S: Diurnal rhythm in total serum thyroxine levels. Metabolism 20:782, 1971

57. Bartalena L: Recent achievements in studies on thyroid hormone-binding proteins. Endocr Rev 11:47, 1990

58. Stockigt JR, Topliss DJ, Barlow JW et al: Familial euthyroid thyroxine excess: an appropriate response to abnormal thyroxine binding associated with albumin. J Clin Endocrinol Metab 53:353, 1981

59. Sunthornthepvarakul T, Angkeow P, Weiss RE et al: A missense mutation in the albumin gene produces familial disalbuminemic hyperthyroxinemia in 8 unrelated families. Biochem Biophys Res Commun 202:781, 1994

60. Sterling K, Refetoff S, Selenkow HA: T_3 toxicosis: Thyrotoxicosis due to elevated serum triiodothyronine levels. JAMA 213:571, 1970

61. Sterling K, Brenner MA, Newman ES et al: The significance of triiodothyronine (T_3) in maintenance of euthyroid status after treatment of hyperthyroidism. J Clin Endocrinol Metab 33:729, 1971

62. Delange F, Camus M, Ermans AM: Circulating thyroid hormones in endemic goiter. J Clin Endocrinol Metab 34:891, 1972

63. Fish LH, Schwartz HL, Cavanaugh MD et al: Replacement dose, metabolism, and bioavailability of levothyroxine in the treatment of hypothyroidism. N Engl J Med 316:764, 1987

64. Saberi M, Utiger RD: Serum thyroid hormone and

thyrotropin concentrations during thyroxine and triiodothyronine therapy. J Clin Endocrinol Metab 39: 923, 1974

65. Refetoff S, Weiss RE, Usala SJ: The syndromes of resistance to thyroid hormone. Endocr Rev 14:348, 1993

66. Luft R, Ikkos D, Palmieri G et al: A case of severe hypermetabolism of nonthyroid origin with a defect in the maintenance of mitochondrial respiratory control: a correlated clinical, biochemical, and morphological study. J Clin Invest 41:1776, 1962

67. Olsen T, Laurberg P, Weeke J: Low serum triiodothyronine and high serum reverse triiodothyronine in old age: an effect of disease not age. J Clin Endocrinol Metab 47:1111, 1978

68. Welle S, O'Conell M, Danforth D Jr, Campbell R: Decreased free fraction of serum thyroid hormones during carbohydrate over-feeding. Metabolism 33: 837, 1984

69. Portnay GI, O'Brian JT, Bush J, et al: The effect of starvation on the concentration and binding of thyroxine and triiodothyronine in serum and on the response to TRH. J Clin Endocrinol Metab 39:191, 1974

70. Azizi F: Effect of dietary composition on fasting-induced changes in serum thyroid hormones and thyrotropin. Metabolism 27:935, 1978

71. Scriba PC, Bauer M, Emmert D et al: Effects of obesity, total fasting and realimentation of L-thyroxine (T_4)), 3,5,3'-L-triiodothyronine (T_3), 3,3',5'-L-triiodothyronine (rT_3), thyroxine binding globulin (TBG), cortisol, thyrotrophin, cortisol binding globulin (CBG), transferrin, α_2-haptoglobin and complement C'3 in serum. Acta Endocrinol 91:629, 1979

72. Larsen PR: Triiodothyronine. Review of recent studies of its physiology and pathophysiology in man. Metabolism 21:1073, 1972

73. Hollander CS, Stevenson C, Mitsuma T et al: T_3 toxicosis in an iodide-deficient area. Lancet 2:1276, 1972

74. Takamatsu J, Kuma K, Mozai T: Serum triiodothyronine/thyroxine ratio: a newly recognized predictor of the outcome of hyperthyroidism due to Graves' disease. J Clin Endocrinol Metab 62:980, 1986

75. Rösler A, Litvin Y, Hage C, Gross J, Cerasi E: Familial hyperthyroidism due to inappropriate thyrotropin secretion successfully treated with triiodothyronine. J Clin Endocrinol Metab 54:76, 1982

76. Maxon HR, Burman KD, Premachandra BN et al: Familial elevation of total and free thyroxine in healthy, euthyroid subjects without detectable binding protein abnormalities. Acta Endocrinol 100:224, 1982

77. Chopra IJ, Williams DE, Orgiazzi J, Solomon DH: Opposite effects of dexamethasone on serum concentrations of 3,3',5'-triiodothyronine (reverse T_3) and 3,3',5-triiodothyronine (T_3). J Clin Endocrinol Metab 41:911, 1975

78. Cavalieri RR, Sung LC, Becker CE: Effects of phenobarbital on thyroxine and triiodothyronine kinetics in Graves' disease. J Clin Endocrinol Metab 37:308, 1973

79. Wenzel KW: Pharmacological interference with in vitro tests of thyroid function. Metabolism 30:717, 1981

80. Busnardo B, Vangelista R, Girelli ME et al: TSH levels and TSH response to TRH as a guide to the replacement treatment of patients with thyroid carcinoma. J Clin Endocrinol Metab 42:901, 1976

81. Hamolsky MW, Stein M, Freedberg AS: The thyroid hormone–plasma protein complex in man. II. A new in vitro method for study of "uptake" of labeled hormonal components by human erythrocytes. J Clin Endocrinol Metab 17:33, 1957

82. Sterling K, Tabachnick M: Resin uptake of I^{131} triiodothyronine as a test of thyroid function. J Clin Endocrinol Metab 21:456, 1961

83. Refetoff S, Hagen S, Selenkow HA: Estimation of the T_4 binding capacity of serum TBG and TBPA by a single T_4 load ion exchange resin method. J Nucl Med 13:2, 1972

84. Braverman LE, Foster AE, Arky RA: Oragrafin and the triiodothyronine uptake test of thyroid function. J Nucl Med 8:209, 1967

85. Schatz DL, Sheppard RH, Steiner G et al: Influence of heparin on serum free thyroxine. J Clin Endocrinol Metab 29:1015, 1969

86. Elzinga KE, Carr EA Jr, Beierwaltes WH: Adaptation of standard Durrum-type cell for reverse-flow electrophoresis. Am J Clin Pathol 36:125, 1961

87. Miyai K, Ito M, Hata N: Enzyme immunoassay of thyroxine-binding globulin. Clin Chem 28:2408, 1982

88. Refetoff S, Murata Y, Vassart G et al: Radioimmunoassays specific for the tertiary and primary structures of thyroxine-binding globulin (TBG): Measurement of denatured TBG in serum. J Clin Endocrinol Metab 59:269, 1984

89. Freeman T, Pearson JD: The use of quantitative immunoelectrophoresis to investigate thyroxine-binding human serum proteins. Clin Chim Acta 26:365, 1969

90. Nielsen HG, Buus O, Weeke B: A rapid determination of thyroxine-binding globulin in human serum by means of the Laurell Rocket immunoelectrophoresis. Clin Chim Acta 36:133, 1972

91. Mancini G, Carbonara AO, Heremans JF: Immunochemical quantitation of antigens by single radial immunodiffusion. Immunochemistry 2:235, 1965

92. Chopra IJ, Solomon DH, Ho RS: Competitive ligand-binding assay for measurement of thyroxine-binding globulin (TBG). J Clin Endocrinol Metab 35:565, 1972

93. Marshall JS, Levy RP, Steinberg AG: Human thyroxine-binding globulin deficiency: a genetic study. N Engl J Med 274:1469, 1966

94. Ekins R: Measurement of free hormones in blood. Endocr Rev 11:5, 1990

95. Ekins R: The free hormone hypothesis and measurement of free hormones. Clin Chem 38:1289, 1992

96. Sterling K, Brenner MA: Free thyroxine in human serum: Simplified measurement with aid of magnesium precipitation. J Clin Invest 45:153, 1966

97. Nelson JC, Tomel RT: Direct determination of free thyroxin in undiluted serum by equilibrium dialysis/radioimmunoassay. Clin Chem 34:1737, 1988

98. Surks MI, Hupart KH, Pan C, Shapiro LE: Normal free thyroxine in critical nonthyroidal illnesses measured by ultrafiltration of undiluted serum and equilibrium dialysis. J Clin Endocrinol Metab 67:1031, 1988

99. Melmed S, Geola FL, Reed AW et al: A comparison of methods for assessing thyroid function in nonthyroidal illness. J Clin Endocrinol Metab 54:300, 1982

100. Wong TK, Pekary E, Hoo GS et al: Comparison of methods for measuring free thyroxin in nonthyroidal illness. Clin Chem 38:720, 1992

101. Chopra IJ, Chopra U, Smith SR et al: Reciprocal changes in serum concentration of 3,3',5'-triiodothyronine (reverse T_3) and 3,3',5-triiodothyronine (T_3) in systemic illnesses. J Clin Endocrinol Metab 41:1043, 1975

102. Oppenheimer JH, Squef R, Surks MI, Hauer H: Binding of thyroxine by serum proteins evaluated by equilibrium dialysis and electrophoretic techniques. Alterations in nonthyroidal illness. J Clin Invest 42:1769, 1963

103. Snyder SM, Cavalieri RR, Ingbar SH: Simultaneous measurement of percentage free thyroxine and triiodothyronine: Comparison of equilibrium dialysis and Sephadex chromatography. J Nucl Med 17:660, 1976

104. Nelson JC, Bruce WR, Pandian MR: Dependence of free thyroxine estimates obtained with equilibrium tracer dialysis on the concentration of thyroxine-binding globulin. Clin Chem 38:1294, 1992

105. Van der Sluijs Veer G, Vermes I, Bonte HA, Hoorn RKJ: Temperature effects on free-thyroxine measurements: Analytical and clinical consequences. Clin Chem 38:1327, 1992

106. Larsen PR, Alexander NM, Chopra IJ et al: Revised nomenclature for test of thyroid hormones and thyroid-related proteins in serum. Clin Chem 33:2114, 1987

107. Felicetta JV, Green WL, Mass LB et al: Thyroid function and lipids in patients with chronic liver disease treated by hemodialysis with comments on the free thyroxine index. Metabolism 28:756, 1979

108. Konno N: Evaluation of free triiodothyronine index as a measure of thyroid function. Folia Endocrinol Jpn 50:711, 1974

109. Glinoer D, Fernandez-Deville M, Ermans AM: Use of direct thyroxine-binding globulin measurement in the evaluation of thyroid function. J Endocrinol Invest 1:329, 1978

110. Attwood EC: The T_3/TBG ratio and the biochemical investigation of thyrotoxicosis. Clin Biochem 12:88, 1979

111. Nuutila P, Koskinen P, Irjala K et al: Two new two-step immunoassays for free thyroxin evaluated: Solid-phase radioimmunoassay and time-resolved fluoroimmunoassay. Clin Chem 36:1355, 1990

112. Hay ID, Bayer MF, Kaplan MM et al: American Thyroid Association assessment of current free thyroid hormone and thyrotropin measurements and guidelines for future clinical assays. Clin Chem 37:2002, 1991

113. Wilkins TA, Midgley JEM, Barron N: Comprehensive study of a thyroxin-analog-based assay for free thyroxin ("Amerlex FT4"). Clin Chem 31:1644, 1985

114. John R: Autoantibodies to thyroxin and interference with free-thyroxin assay. Clin Chem 29:581, 1983

115. Ashkar FS, Buehler RJ, Chan T, Hourani M: Radioimmunoassay of free thyroxine with prebound anti-T_4 microcapsules. J Nucl Med 20:956, 1979

116. Sarne DH, Refetoff S, Murata Y et al: Variant thyroxine-binding globulin in serum of Australian aborigines: a comparison with familial TBG deficiency in Caucasians and American Blacks. J Endocrinol Invest 8:217, 1985

117. Murata Y, Refetoff S, Sarne DH et al: Variant thyroxine-binding globulin in serum of Australian Aborigines: Its physical, chemical and biological properties. J Endocrinol Invest 8:225, 1985

118. Pardridge WM, Slag MF, Morley JE et al: Hepatic bioavailability of serum thyroid hormones in nonthyroidal illness. J Clin Endocrinol Metab 53:913, 1981

119. Kaptein EM, Macintyre SS, Weiner JM et al: Free thyroxine estimates in nonthyroidal illness: Comparison of eight methods. J Clin Endocrinol Metab 52:1073, 1981

120. Lehotay DC, Weight CW, Seltman JH et al: Free thyroxin: a comparison of direct and indirect methods and their diagnostic usefulness in nonthyroidal illness. Clin Chem 28:1826, 1982

121. Oppenheimer JH, Schwartz HL, Mariash CN, Kaiser FE: Evidence for a factor in the sera of patients with nonthyroidal illness which inhibits iodothyronine binding by solid matrices, serum proteins, and rat hepatocytes. J Clin Endocrinol Metab 54:757, 1982

122. Woeber KA, Maddux BA: Thyroid hormone binding in nonthyroidal illness. Metabolism 30:412, 1981

123. Chopra IJ, Solomon DH, Teco GNC, Eisenberg JB: An inhibitor of the binding of thyroid hormones to serum proteins is present in extrathyroidal tissues. Science 215:407, 1982

124. Chopra IJ, Chua Teco GN, Mead JF et al: Relationship between serum free fatty acids and thyroid hormone binding inhibitor in nonthyroidal illnesses. J Clin Endocrinol Metab 60:980, 1985

125. Sarne DH, Refetoff S: Measurement of thyroxine uptake from serum by cultured human hepatocytes as an index of thyroid status: Reduced thyroxine uptake from serum of patients with non-thyroidal illness. J Clin Endocrinol Metab 61:1046, 1985

126. Chopra IJ: An assessment of daily production and significance of thyroidal secretion of 3,3',5'-triiodothyronine (reverse T_3) in man. J Clin Invest 58:32, 1976

127. Nicod P, Burger A, Staeheli V, Vallotton MB: A radioimmunoassay for 3,3',5'-triiodo-L-thyronine in unextracted serum: Method and clinical results. J Clin Endocrinol Metab 42:823, 1976

128. Chopra IJ: A radioimmunoassay for measurement of 3,3',5'-triiodothyronine (reverse T_3). J Clin Invest 54:583, 1974

129. O'Connell M, Robbins DC, Bogardus C et al: The interaction of free fatty acids in radioimmunoassays for reverse triiodothyronine. J Clin Endocrinol Metab 55:577, 1982

130. Burman KD, Dimond RC, Wright FD et al: A radioimmunoassay for 3,3',5'-L-triiodothyronine (reverse T_3): Assessment of thyroid gland content and serum measurements in conditions of normal and altered thyroidal economy and following administration of thyrotropin releasing hormone (TRH) and thyrotropin (TSH). J Clin Endocrinol Metab 44:660, 1977

131. Kirkegaard C, Faber J, Cohn D et al: Serum 3'-monoiodothyronine levels in normal subjects and in patients with thyroid and non-thyroid disease. Acta Endocrinol 97:454, 1981

132. Weiss RE, Angkeow P, Sunthornthepvarakul T et al: Linkage of familial dysalbuminemic hyperthyroxinemia to the albumin gene in a large Amish family. J Clin Endocrinol Metab 80:1995

133. Chopra IJ: A radioimmunoassay for measurement of 3'-monoiodothyronine. J Clin Endocrinol Metab 51:117, 1980

134. Chopra IJ, Sack J, Fisher DA: Circulating 3,3',5'-triiodothyronine (reverse T_3) in the human newborn. J Clin Invest 55:1137, 1975

135. Engler D, Markelbach U, Steiger G, Burger AG: The monodeiodination of triiodothyronine and reverse triiodothyronine in man: a quantitative evaluation of the pathway by the use of turnover rate techniques. J Clin Endocrinol Metab 58:49, 1984

136. Pangaro L, Burman KD, Wartofsky L et al: Radioimmunoassay for 3,5-diiodothyronine and evidence for dependence on conversion from 3,5,3'-triiodothyronine. J Clin Endocrinol Metab 50:1075, 1980

137. Faber J, Kirkegaard C, Lumholtz IB et al: Measurements of serum 3',5'-diiodothyronine and 3,3'-diiodothyronine concentrations in normal subjects and in patients with thyroid and nonthyroid disease: Studies of 3',5'-diiodothyronine metabolism. J Clin Endocrinol Metab 48:611, 1979

138. Geola F, Chopra IJ, Geffner DL: Patterns of 3,3',5'-triiodothyronine monodeiodination in hypothyroidism and nonthyroidal illnesses. J Clin Endocrinol Metab 50:336, 1980

139. Chopra IJ, Geola F, Solomon DH, Maciel RMB: 3',5'-diiodothyroxine in health and disease: Studies by a radioimmunoassay. J Clin Endocrinol Metab 47:1198, 1978

140. Burman KD, Wright FD, Smallridge RC et al: A radioimmunoassay for 3',5'-diiodothyronine. J Clin Endocrinol Metab 47:1059, 1978

141. Jaedig S, Faber J: The effect of starvation and refeeding with oral versus intravenous glucose on serum 3,5-,3,3'- and 3',5'-diiodothyronine and 3'-monoiodothyronine. Acta Endocrinol 100:388, 1982

142. Smallridge RC, Wartofsky L, Green BJ et al: 3'-L-monoiodothyronine: Development of a radioimmunoassay and demonstration of in vivo conversion from 3',5'-diiodothyronine. J Clin Endocrinol Metab 48:32, 1979

143. Corcoran JM, Eastman CJ: Radioimmunoassay of 3-L-monoiodothyronine: Application in normal human physiology and thyroid disease. J Clin Endocrinol Metab 57:66, 1983

144. Nakamura Y, Chopra IJ, Solomon DH: An assessment of the concentration of acetic acid and proprionic acid derivatives of 3,5,3'-triiodothyronine in human serum. J Clin Endocrinol Metab 46:91, 1978

145. Burger A, Suter P, Nicod P et al: Reduced active thyroid hormone levels in acute illness. Lancet 1:163, 1976

146. Pittman CS, Suda AK, Chambers JB Jr et al: Abnormalities of thyroid hormone turnover in patients with diabetes mellitus before and after insulin therapy. J Clin Endocrinol Metab 48:854, 1979

147. Dlott RS, LoPresti JS, Nicoloff JT: Evidence that triiodoacetate (TRIAC) is the autocrine thyroid hormone in man. Thyroid Suppl 2:S94, 1992

148. Nelson JC, Weiss RM, Lewis JE et al: A multiple ligand-binding radioimmunoassay of diiodothyrosine. J Clin Invest 53:416, 1974

149. Nelson JC, Lewis JE: Radioimmunoassay of iodotyrosines. p. 705. In Abraham GE (ed): Handbook of Radioimmunoassay, Marcel Dekker, New York, 1979

150. Meinhold H, Beckert A, Wenzel W: Circulating diiodotyrosine: Studies of its serum concentration, source, and turnover using radioimmunoassay after immunoextraction. J Clin Endocrinol Metab 53:1171, 1981

151. Van Herle AJ, Uller RP, Matthews NL, Brown J: Radioimmunoassay for measurement of thyroglobulin in human serum. J Clin Invest 52:1320, 1973

152. Schneider AB, Pervos R: Radioimmunoassay of human thyroglobulin: Effect of antithyroglobulin antibodies. J Clin Endocrinol Metab 47:126, 1978

153. Schneider AB, Favus MJ, Stachura ME et al: Plasma thyroglobulin in detecting thyroid carcinoma after childhood head and neck irradiation. Ann Intern Med 86:29, 1977

154. Pacini F, Pinchera A, Giani C et al: Serum thyroglobulin in thyroid carcinoma and other thyroid disorders. J Endocrinol Invest 3:283, 1980

155. Black EG, Cassoni A, Gimlette TMD et al: Serum thyroglobulin in thyroid cancer. Br Med J 3:443, 1981

156. Pezzino V, Filetti S, Belfiore A et al: Serum thyroglobulin levels in the newborn. J Clin Endocrinol Metab 52:364, 1981

157. Penny R, Spencer CA, Frasier D, Nicoloff JT: Thyroid-stimulating hormone and thyroglobulin levels decrease with chronological age in children and adolescents. J Clin Endocrinol Metab 56:177, 1983

158. Refetoff S, Lever EG: The value of serum thyroglobulin measurement in clinical practice. JAMA 250:2352, 1983

159. Izumi M, Kubo I, Taura M et al: Kinetic study of immunoreactive human thyroglobulin. J Clin Endocrinol Metab 62:400, 1986

160. Uller RP, Van Herle AJ, Chopra IJ: Comparison of alterations in circulating thyroglobulin, triiodothyronine and thyroxine in response to exogenous (bovine) and endogenous (human) thyrotropin. J Clin Endocrinol Metab 37:741, 1973

161. Lever EG, Refetoff S, Scherberg NH, Carr K: The influence of percutaneous fine needle aspiration on serum thyroglobulin. J Clin Endocrinol Metab 56:26, 1983

162. Uller RP, Van Herle AJ: Effect of therapy on serum thyroglobulin levels in patients with Graves' disease. J Clin Endocrinol Metab 46:747, 1978

163. Smallridge RC, DeKeyser FM, Van Herle AJ et al: Thyroid iodine content and serum thyroglobulin: Clues to the national history of destruction-induced thyroiditis. J Clin Endocrinol Metab 62:1213, 1986

164. Mariotti S, Martino E, Cupini C et al: Low serum thyroglobulin as a clue to the diagnosis of thyrotoxicosis factitia. N Engl J Med 307:410, 1982

165. Van Herle AJ, Uller RP: Elevated serum thyroglobulin: a marker of metastases in differentiated thyroid carcinoma. J Clin Invest 56:272, 1975

166. Schneider AB, Line BR, Goldman JM, Robbins J: Sequential serum thyroglobulin determinations, ^{131}I scans, and ^{131}I uptakes after triiodothyronine withdrawal in patients with thyroid cancer. J Clin Endocrinol Metab 53:1199, 1981

167. Colacchio TA, LoGerfo P, Collachio DA, Feind C: Radioiodine total body scan versus serum thyroglobulin levels in follow-up of patients with thyroid cancer. Surgery 91:42, 1982

168. Barsano CP, Skosey C, DeGroot LJ, Refetoff S: Serum thyroglobulin in the management of patients with thyroid cancer. Arch Intern Med 142:763, 1982

169. Kawamura S, Kishino B, Tajima K et al: Serum thyroglobulin changes in patients with Graves' disease treated with long term antithyroid drug therapy. J Clin Endocrinol Metab 56:507, 1983

170. Black EG, Bodden SJ, Hulse JA, Hoffenberg R: Serum thyroglobulin in normal and hypothyroid neonates. Clin Endocrinol 16:267, 1982

171. Heinze HJ, Shulman DI, Diamond FB Jr, Bercu BB: Spectrum of serum thyroglobulin elevation in congenital thyroid disorders. Thyroid 3:37, 1993

172. Czernichow P, Schlumberger M, Pomarede R, Fragu P: Plasma thyroglobulin measurements help determine the type of thyroid defect in cogenital hypothyroidism. J Clin Endocrinol Metab 56:242, 1983

173. Burke CW, Shakespear RA, Fraser TR: Measurement of thyroxine and triiodothyronine in human urine. Lancet 2:1177, 1972

174. Chan V, Landon J: Urinary thyroxine excretion as index of thyroid function. Lancet 1:4, 1972

175. Chan V, Besser GM, Landon J, Ekins RP: Urinary tri-iodothyronine excretion as index of thyroid function. Lancet 2:253, 1972

176. Burke CW, Shakespear RA: Triiodothyronine and thyroxine in urine. II. Renal handling, and effect of urinary protein. J Clin Endocrinol Metab 42:504, 1976

177. Sack J, Fisher DA, Hobel CJ, Lam R: Thyroxine in human amniotic fluid. J Pediatr 87:364, 1975

178. Chopra IJ, Crandall BF: Thyroid hormones and thyrotropin in amniotic fluid. N Engl J Med 293:740, 1975

179. Burman KD, Read J, Dimond RC et al: Measurement of 3,3′,5′-triiodothyronine (reverse T$_3$), 3,3′-L-diiodothyronine, T$_3$, and T$_4$ in human amniotic fluid

and in cord and maternal serum. J Clin Endocrinol Metab 43:1351, 1976

180. Siersbaek-Nielsen K, Hansen JM: Tyrosine and free thyroxine in cerebrospinal fluid in thyroid disease. Acta Endocrinol 643:126, 1970

181. Hagen GA, Elliot WJ: Transport of thyroid hormones in serum and cerebrospinal fluid. J Clin Endocrinol Metab 37:415, 1973

182. Nishikawa M, Inada M, Naito K et al: 3,3',5'-triiodothyronine (reverse T_3) in human cerebrospinal fluid. J Clin Endocrinol Metab 53:1030, 1981

183. Mallol J, Obregón MJ, Morreale de Escobar G: Analytical artifacts in radioimmunoassay of L-thyroxin in human milk. Clin Chem 28:1277, 1982

184. Varma SK, Collins M, Row A et al: Thyroxine, triiodothyronine, and reverse tri-iodothyronine concentrations in human milk. J Pediatr 93:803, 1978

185. Jansson L, Ivarsson S, Larsson I, Ekman R: Tri-iodothyronine and thyroxine in human milk. Acta Paediatr Scand 72:703, 1983

186. Riad-Fahmy D, Read GF, Walker RF, Griffiths K: Steroids in saliva for assessing endocrine function. Endocr Rev 3:367, 1982

187. Elson MK, Morley JE, Shafer RB: Salivary thyroxine as an estimate of free thyroxine: Concise communication. J Nucl Med 24:700, 1983

188. Reichlin S, Bollinger J, Nejad I, Sullivan P: Tissue thyroid hormone concentration of rat and man determined by radioimmunoassay: Biologic significance. Mt Sinai J Med 40:502, 1973

189. Ochi Y, Hachiya T, Yoshimura M et al: Determination of triiodothyronine in red blood cells by radioimmunoassay. Endocrinol Jpn 23:207, 1976

190. Lim VS, Zavata DC, Flanigan MJ, Freeman RM: Basal oxygen uptake: a new technique for an old test. J Clin Endocrinol Metab 62:863, 1986

191. Becker DV: Metabolic indices. p. 524. In Werner SC, Ingbar SH (eds): The Thyroid: a Fundamental and Clinical Text. Harper & Row, New York, 1971

192. Waal-Manning HJ: Effect of propranolol on the duration of the Achilles tendon reflex. Clin Pharmacol Ther 10:199, 1969

193. Rodbard D, Fujita T, Rodbard S: Estimation of thyroid function by timing the arterial sounds. JAMA 2010:884, 1967

194. Nuutila P, Irjala K, Saraste M et al: Cardiac systolic time intervals and thyroid hormone levels during treatment of hypothyroidism. Scand J Clin Lab Invest 52:467, 1992

195. Lewis BS, Ehrenfeld EN, Lewis N, Gotsman MS: Echocardiographic LV function in thyrotoxicosis. Am Heart J 97:460, 1979

196. Tseug KH, Walfish PG, Persand JA, Gilbert BW: Concurrent aortic and mitral valve echocardiography permits measurements of systolic time intervals as an index of peripheral tissue thyroid functional status. 69:633, 1989

197. Vesell ES, Shapiro JR, Passananti GT et al: Altered plasma half-lives of antipyrine, propylthiouracil, and methimazole in thyroid dysfunction. Clin Pharmacol Ther 17:48, 1975

198. Brunk SF, Combs SP, Miller JD et al: Effects of hypothyroidism and hyperthyroidism on dipyrone metabolism in man. J Clin Pharmacol 14:271, 1974

199. Kekki M: Serum protein turnover in experimental hypo- and hyperthyroidism. Acta Endocrinol, suppl. 91:1, 1964

200. Walton KW, Scott PJ, Dykes PW, Davies JWL: The significance of alterations in serum lipids in thyroid dysfunction. II. Alterations of the metabolism and turnover of ^{131}I-low-density lipoproteins in hypothyroidism and thyrotoxicosis. Clin Sci 29:217, 1965

201. Hellman L, Bradlow HL, Zumoff B, Gallagher TF: The influence of thyroid hormone on hydrocortisone production and metabolism. J Clin Endocrinol Metab 21:1231, 1961

202. Gallagher TF, Hellman L, Finkelstein J et al: Hyperthyroidism and cortisol secretion in man. J Clin Endocrinol Metab 34:919, 1972

203. Kiely JM, Purnell DC, Owen CA Jr: Erythrokinetics in myxedema. Ann Intern Med 67:533, 1967

204. Das KC, Mukherjee M, Sarkar TK et al: Erythropoiesis and erythropoietin in hypo- and hyperthyroidism. J Clin Endocrinol Metab 40:211, 1975

205. Rivlin RS, Melmon KL, Sjoerdsma A: An oral tyrosine tolerance test in thyrotoxicosis and myxedema. N Engl J Med 272:1143, 1965

206. Bélanger R, Chandramohan N, Misbin R, Rivlin RS: Tyrosine and glutamic acid in plasma and urine of patients with altered thyroid function. Metabolism 21:855, 1972

207. Lamberg BA, Gräsbeck R: The serum protein pattern in disorders of thyroid function. Acta Endocrinol 19:91, 1955

208. Anderson DC: Sex-hormone-binding globulin. Clin Endocrinol 3:69, 1974

209. DeNayer P, Lambot MP, Desmons MC et al: Sex hormone–binding protein in hypothyroxinemic patients: a discriminator for thyroid status in thyroid hormone resistance and familial dysalbuminemic hyperthyroxinemia. J Clin Endocrinol Metab 62:1309, 1986

210. Macaron CI, Macaron ZG: Increased serum ferritin levels in hyperthyroidism. Ann Intern Med 96:617, 1982

211. Takamatsu J, Majima M, Miki K et al: Serum ferritin as a marker of thyroid hormone action on peripheral tissues. J Clin Endocrinol Metab 61:672, 1985

212. Graninger W, Pirich KR, Speiser W et al: Effect of thyroid hormones on plasma protein concentration in man. J Clin Endocrinol Metab 63:407, 1986

213. Oppenheimer JH: Role of plasma proteins in the binding, distribution, and metabolism of the thyroid hormones. N Engl J Med 278:1153, 1968

214. Shah JH, Cechio GM: Hypoinsulinemia of hypothyroidism. Arch Intern Med 132:657, 1973

215. Levy LJ, Adesman JJ, Spergel G: Studies on the carbohydrate and lipid metabolism in thyroid disease: Effects of glucagon. J Clin Endocrinol Metab 30:372, 1970

216. Chopra IJ, Tulchinsky D: Status of estrogen-androgen balance in hyperthyroid men with Graves' disease. J Clin Endocrinol Metab 38:269, 1974

217. Seino Y, Matsukura S, Miyamoto Y et al: Hypergastrinemia in hyperthyroidism. J Clin Endocrinol Metab 43:852, 1976

218. Bouillon R, DeMoor P: Parathyroid function in patients with hyper- or hypothyroidism. J Clin Endocrinol Metab 38:999, 1974

219. Castro JH, Genuth SM, Klein L: Comparative response to parathyroid hormone in hyperthyroidism and hypothyroidism. Metabolism 24:839, 1975

220. Kojima N, Sakata S, Nakamura S et al: Serum concentrations of osteocalcin in patients with hyperthyroidism, hypothyroidism and subacute thyroiditis. J Endocrinol Invest 15:491, 1992

221. Body JJ, Demeester-Mirkine N, Borkowski A et al: Calcitonin deficiency in primary hypothyroidism. J Clin Endocrinol Metab 62:700, 1986

222. Hauger-Klevene JH, Brown H, Zavaleta J: Plasma renin activity in hyper- and hypothyroidism: Effect of adrenergic blocking agents. J Clin Endocrinol Metab 34:625, 1972

223. Ogihara T, Yamamoto T, Miyai K, Kumahara Y: Plasma renin activity and aldosterone concentration of patients with hyperthyroidism and hypothyroidism. Endocrinol Jpn 20:433, 1973

224. Stoffer SS, Jiang NS, Gorman CA, Pikler GM: Plasma catecholamines in hypothyroidism and hyperthyroidism. J Clin Endocrinol Metab 36:587, 1973

225. Christensen NJ: Plasma noradrenaline and adrenaline in patients with thyrotoxicosis and myxedema. Clin Sci Mol Med 45:163, 1973

226. Zimmerman RS, Gharib H, Zimmerman D et al: Atrial natriuretic peptide in hypothyroidism. J Clin Endocrinol Metab 64:353, 1987

227. Rolandi E, Santaniello B, Bagnasco M et al: Thyroid hormones and atrial natriuretic hormone secretion: Study in hyper- and hypothyroid patients. Acta Endocrinol 127:23, 1992

228. Distiller LA, Sagel J, Morley JE: Assessment of pituitary gonadotropin reserve using luteinizing hormone-releasing hormone (LRH) in states of altered thyroid function. J Clin Endocrinol Metab 40:512, 1975

229. Refetoff S, Fang VS, Rapoport B, Friesen HG: Interrelationships in the regulation of TSH and prolactin secretion in man: Effects of L-DOPA, TRH and thyroid hormone in various combinations. J Clin Endocrinol Metab 38:450, 1974

230. Honbo KS, Van Herle AJ, Kellett KA: Serum prolactin levels in untreated primary hypothyroidism. Am J Med 64:782, 1978

231. Brauman H, Corvilain J: Growth hormone response to hypoglycemia in myxedema. J Clin Endocrinol Metab 28:301, 1968

232. Rosenfield PS, Wool MS, Danforth E Jr: Growth hormone response to insulin-induced hypoglycemia in thyrotoxicosis. J Clin Endocrinol Metab 29:777, 1969

233. Hamada N, Uoi K, Nishizawa Y et al: Increase of serum GH concentration following TRH injection in patients with primary hypothyroidism. Endocrinol Jpn 23:5, 1976

234. Kung AEC, Hui WM, Ng ESK: Serum and plasma epidermal growth factor in thyroid disorders. Acta Endocrinol 127:52, 1992

235. Graig FA, Smith JC: Serum creatine phosphokinase activity in altered thyroid states. J Clin Endocrinol Metab 25:723, 1965

236. Fleisher GA, McConahey WM, Pankow M: Serum creatine kinase, lactic dehydrogenase, and glutamic-oxalacetic transaminase in thyroid diseases and pregnancy. Mayo Clin Proc 40:300, 1965

237. Doran GR, Wilkinson JH: Serum creatine kinase and adenylate kinase in thyroid disease. Clin Chim Acta 35:115, 1971

238. Stolk JM, Hurst JH, Nisula BC: The inverse relationship between serum dopamine-β-hydroxylase activity and thyroid function. J Clin Endocrinol Metab 51:259, 1980

239. Talbot NB, Hoeffel G, Shwachman H, Tuohy EL: Serum phosphatase as an aid in the diagnosis of cretinism and juvenile hypothyroidism. Am J Dis Child 62:273, 1941

240. Lieberthal AS, Benson SG, Klitgaard HM: Serum malic dehydrogenase in thyroid disease. J Clin Endocrinol Metab 23:211, 1963

241. Yotsumuto H, Imai Y, Kuzuya N et al: Increased levels of serum angiotensin-converting enzyme activity in hyperthyroidism. Ann Intern Med 96:326, 1982

242. Gow SMG, Caldwell G, Toft AD et al: Relationship between pituitary and other target organ responsiveness in thyroid patients receiving thyroxine replacement. J Clin Endocrinol Metab 64:364, 1987

243. Beckett GJ, Kellett HA, Gow SM et al: Elevated

plasma glutathione S-transferase concentrations in hyperthyroidism and in hypothyroid patients receiving thyroxine replacement: Evidence for hepatic damage. Br Med J 2:427, 1985

244. Ogura F, Morii H, Ohmo M et al: Serum coenzyme Q_{10} levels in thyroid disorders. Horm Metab Res 12: 537, 1980

245. Bouillon R, Muls E, DeMoor P: Influence of thyroid function on the serum concentration of 1,25-dihydroxy vitamin D_3. J Clin Endocrinol Metab 51:793, 1980

246. Walton KW, Campbell DA, Tonks EL: The significance of alterations in serum lipids in thyroid function. I. The relation between serum lipoproteins, carotenoids, and vitamin A in hypothyroidism and thyrotoxicosis. Clin Sci 29:199, 1965

247. Karlberg BE, Henriksson KG, Andersson RGG: Cyclic adenosine 3′,5′-monophosphate concentration in plasma, adipose tissue and skeletal muscle in normal subjects and in patients with hyper- and hypothyroidism. J Clin Endocrinol Metab 39:96, 1974

248. Peracchi M, Bamonti-Catena F, Lombardi L et al: Plasma and urine cyclic nucleotide levels in patients with hyperthyroidism and hypothyroidism. J Endocrinol Invest 6:173, 1983

249. Rivlin RS, Wagner HN Jr: Anemia in hyperthyroidism. Ann Intern Med 70:507, 1969

250. Feldman DL, Goldberg WM: Hyperthyroidism with periodic paralysis. Can Med Assoc J 101:667, 1969

251. Pettinger WA, Talner L, Ferris TF: Inappropriate secretion of antidiuretic hormone due to myxedema. N Engl J Med 272:362, 1965

252. Jones JE, Deser PC, Shane SR, Flink EB: Magnesium metabolism in hyperthyroidism and hypothyroidism. J Clin Invest 45:891, 1966

253. Baxter JD, Bondy PK: Hypercalcemia of thyrotoxicosis. Ann Intern Med 65:429, 1966

254. Weldon AP, Danks DM: Congenital hypothyroidism and neonatal jaundice. Arch Dis Child 47:469, 1972

255. Greenberger NJ, Milligan FD, DeGroot LJ, Isselbacher KJ: Jaundice and thyrotoxicosis in the absence of congestive heart failure: a study of four cases. Am J Med 36:840, 1964

256. Kuhlbäch B: Creatine and creatinine metabolism in thyrotoxicosis and hypothyroidism. Acta Med Scand, suppl. 331:1, 1957

257. Adlkofer F, Armbrecht U, Schleusener H: Plasma lecithin: Cholesterol acyltransferase activity in hypo- and hyperthyroidism. Horm Metab Res 6:142, 1974

258. Pykälistö O, Goldberg AP, Brunzell JD: Reversal of decreased human adipose tissue lipoprotein lipase and hypertriglyceridemia after treatment of hypothyroidism. J Clin Endocrinol Metab 43:591, 1976

259. De Bruin TWA, Van Barlingen H, Van Linde-Sibenius Trip M et al: Lipoprotein (a) and apolipoprotein B plasma concentrations in hypothyroid, euthyroid, and hyperthyroid subjects. J Clin Endocrinol Metab 76:121, 1993

260. Inui T, Ochi Y, Chen W et al: Increased serum concentration of type IV collagen peptide and type III collagen peptide in hyperthyroidism. Clin Chim Acta 205:181, 1992

261. Rich C, Bierman EL, Schwartz IL: Plasma nonesterified fatty acids in hyperthyroid states. J Clin Invest 38:275, 1959

262. Amino N, Kuro R, Yabu Y et al: Elevated levels of circulating carcinoembryonic antigen in hyperthyroidism. J Clin Endocrinol Metab 52:457, 1981

263. Tucci JR, Kopp L: Urinary cyclic nucleotide levels in patients with hyper- and hypothyroidism. J Clin Endocrinol Metab 43:1323, 1976

264. Guttler RB, Shaw JW, Otis CL, Nicoloff JT: Epinephrine-induced alterations in urinary cyclic AMP in hyper- and hypothyroidism. J Clin Endocrinol Metab 41:707, 1975

265. MacFarlane S, Papadopoulos S, Harden RM, Alexander WD: [131]I and MIT-^{131}I in human urine, saliva and gastric juice: a comparison between euthyroid and thyrotoxic patients. J Nucl Med 9:181, 1968

266. Hellström K, Schuberth J: The effect of thyroid hormones on the urinary excretion of taurine in man. Acta Med Scand 187:61, 1970

267. Maebashi M, Kawamura N, Sato M et al: Urinary excretion of carnitine in patients with hyperthyroidism and hypothyroidism: Augmentation by thyroid hormone. Metabolism 26:351, 1977

268. Levine RJ, Oates JA, Vendsalu A, Sjoerdsma A: Studies on the metabolism of aromatic amines in relation to altered thyroid function in man. J Clin Endocrinol Metab 22:1242, 1962

269. Copinschi G, Leclercq R, Bruno OD, Cornil A: Effects of altered thyroid function upon cortisol secretion in man. Horm Metab Res 3:437, 1971

270. Harvey RD, McHardy KC, Reid IW et al: Measurement of bone collagen degradation in hyperthyroidism and during thyroxine replacement therapy using pyridinium cross-links as specific urinary markers. J Clin Endocrinol Metab 72:1189, 1991

271. Kivirikko KI, Laitinen O, Lamberg BA: Value of urine and serum hydroxyproline in the diagnosis of thyroid disease. J Clin Endocrinol Metab 25:1347, 1965

272. Askenasi R, Demeester-Mirkine N: Urinary excretion of hydroxylysyl glycosides and thyroid function. J Clin Endocrinol Metab 40:342, 1975

273. Golden AWG, Bateman D, Torr S: Red cell sodium in hyperthyroidism. Br Med J 2:552, 1971

274. Weinstein M, Sartorio G, Stalldecker GB et al: Red cell zinc in thyroid dysfunction. Acta Endocrinol 20: 147, 1972

275. Pearson HA, Druyan R: Erythrocyte glucose-6-phosphate dehydrogenase activity related to thyroid activity. J Lab Clin Med 57:343, 1961

276. Vuopio P, Viherkoski M, Nikkïla E, Lamberg BA: The content of reduced glutathione (GSH) in the red blood cells in hypo- and hyperthyroidism. Ann Clin Res 2:184, 1970

277. Kiso Y, Yoshida K, Kaise K et al: Erythrocyte carbonic anhydrase-I concentrations in patients with Graves' disease and subacute thyroiditis reflect integrated thyroid hormone levels over the previous few months. J Clin Endocrinol Metab 72:515, 1991

278. Dube MP, Davis FB, Davis PJ et al: Effects of hyperthyroidism and hypothyroidism on human red blood cells Ca^{2+}-ATPase activity. J Clin Endocrinol Metab 62:253, 1986

279. Gwinup G, Ogundip O: Decreased leukocyte alkaline phosphatase in hyperthyroidism. Metabolism 62:253, 1974

280. Jemelin M, Frei J, Scazziga B: Production of ATP in leukocyte mitochondria from hyperthyroid patients before and after treatment with a β-adrenergic blocker and antithyroid drugs. Acta Endocrinol 66: 606, 1971

281. Strickland AL: Sweat electrolytes in thyroid disorders. J Pediatr 82:284, 1973

282. Goolamali SK, Evered D, Shuster S: Thyroid disease and sebaceous function. Br Med J 1:432, 1976

283. Christensen J, Schedl HP, Clifton JA: The basic electrical rhythm of the dudodenum in normal human subjects and in patients with thyroid disease. J Clin Invest 43:1659, 1964

284. Levy G, MacGillivray MH, Procknal JA: Riboflavin absorption in children with thyroid disorders. Pediatrics 50:896, 1972

285. Singhelakis P, Alevizaki CC, Ikkos DG: Intestinal calcium absorption in hyperthyroidism. Metabolism 23: 311, 1974

286. Thomas FB, Caldwell JH, Greenberger NJ: Steatorrhea in thyrotoxicosis: Relation to hypermotility and excessive dietary fat. Ann Intern Med 78:669, 1973

287. Wegener M, Wedmann B, Langhoff T et al: Effect of hyperthyroidism on the transport of a solid-liquid meal through the stomach, intestine, and the colon in man. J Clin Endocrinol Metab 75:745, 1992

288. Scherrer M, König MP: Pulmonary gas exchange in hypothyroidism. Pneumonologie 151:105, 1974

289. Zwillich CW, Pierson DJ, Hofeldt FD et al: Ventilatory control in myxedema and hypothyroidism. N Engl J Med 292:662, 1975

290. Lawson JD: The free Achilles reflex in hypothyroidism and hyperthyroidism. N Engl J Med 259:761, 1958

291. Hall R, Owen SG: Thyroid antibodies in cerebrospinal fluid. Br Med J 2:710, 1960

292. Hoffman I, Lowrey RD: The electrocardiogram in thyrotoxicosis. Am J Cardiol 6:893, 1960

293. Lee JK, Lewis JA: Myxoedema with complete A-V block and Adams-Stokes disease abolished with thyroid medication. Br Heart J 24:253, 1962

294. Wilkins L: Epiphysial dysgenesis associated with hypothyroidism. Am J Dis Child 61:13, 1941

295. Bonakdarpour A, Kirkpatrick JA, Renzi A, Kendall N: Skeletal changes in neonatal thyrotoxicosis. Radiology 102:149, 1972

296. Mariotti S, Anelli S, Ruf J et al: Comparison of serum thyroid microsomal and thyroid peroxidase autoantibodies in thyroid diseases. J Clin Endocrinol Metab 65:987, 1987

297. Portmann L, Hamada N, Neinrich G, DeGroot LJ: Antithyroid peroxidase antibody in patients with autoimmune thyroid disease: Possible identity with anti-microsomal antibody. J Clin Endocrinol Metab 61:1001, 1985

298. Rinke R, Seto P, Rapoport B: Evidence for the highly conformational nature of the epitope(s) on human thyroid peroxidase that are recognized by sera from patients with Hashimoto's thyroiditis. J Clin Endocrinol Metab 71:53, 1990

299. Kaufman KD, Filetti S, Seto P, Rapoport B: Recombinant human thyroid peroxidase generated in eukaryotic cells: a source of specific antigen for the immunological assay of antimicrosomal antibodies in the sera of patients with autoimmune thyroid disease. J Clin Endocrinol Metab 70:724, 1990

300. Trotter WR, Belyavin G, Waddams A: Precipitating and complement fixing antibodies in Hashimoto's disease. Proc R Soc Med 50:961, 1957

301. Boyden SV: The adsorption of proteins on erythrocytes treated with tannic acid and subsequent hemagglutination by antiprotein sera. J Exp Med 93:107, 1951

302. Holborrow EJ, Brown PC, Roitt IM, Doniach D: Cytoplasmic localization of complement-fixing auto-antigen in human thyroid epithelium. Br J Exp Pathol 40:583, 1959

303. Hamada N, Jaeduck N, Portmann L et al: Antibodies against denatured and reduced thyroid microsomal antigen in autoimmune thyroid disease. J Clin Endocrinol Metab 64:230, 1987

304. Mori T, Kriss JP: Measurements by competitive binding radioassay of serum anti-microsomal and anti-thyroglobulin antibodies in Graves' disease and other thyroid disorders. J Clin Endocrinol Metab 33: 688, 1971

305. Mariotti S, Pinchera A, Vitti P et al: Comparison of radioassay and haemagglutination methods for anti-thyroid microsomal antibodies. Clin Exp Immunol 34:118, 1978

306. Amino N, Hagen SR, Yamada N, Refetoff S: Measurement of circulating thyroid microsomal antibodies by the tanned red cell haemagglutination technique: Its usefulness in the diagnosis of autoimmune thyroid disease. Clin Endocrinol 5:115, 1976

307. Ohtaki S, Endo Y, Horinouchi K, al. e: Circulating thyroglobulin-antithyroglobulin immune complex in thyroid diseases using enzyme-linked immunoassays. J Clin Endocrinol Metab 52:239, 1981

308. Roitt IM, Doniach D: Thyroid auto-immunity. Br Med Bull 16:152, 1960

309. Anderson JW, McConahey WM, Alcarón-Segovia D et al: Diagnostic value of thyroid antibodies. J Clin Endocrinol Metab 27:937, 1967

310. Loeb PB, Drash AL, Kenny FM: Prevalence of low-titer and "negative" antithyroglobulin antibodies in biopsy-proved juvenile Hashimoto's thyroiditis. J Pediatr 82:17, 1973

311. Tamaki H, Katsumaru H, Amino N, Nakamoto H, Ishikawa E, Miyai K: Usefulness of thyroglobulin antibody detected by ultrasensitive enzyme immunoassay: a good parameter for immune surveillance in healthy subjects and for prediction of postpartum thyroid dysfunction. Clin Endocrinol (Oxf) 37:266, 1992

312. Volpé R, Row VV, Ezrin C: Circulating viral and thyroid antibodies in subacute thyroiditis. J Clin Endocrinol Metab 27:1275, 1967

313. Balfour BM, Doniach D, Roitt IM, Couchman KG: Fluorescent antibody studies in human thyroiditis: Auto-antibodies to an antigen of the thyroid distinct from thyroglobulin. Br J Exp Pathol 42:307, 1961

314. Staeheli V, Vallotton MB, Burger A: Detection of human anti-thyroxine and antitriiodothyronine antibodies in different thyroid conditions. J Clin Endocrinol Metab 41:669, 1975

315. Bastenie PA, Bonnyns M, Vanhaelst L, Nève P: Diseases associated with autoimmune thyroiditis. In Bastenie PA, Ermans A (eds): Thyroiditis and Thyroid Function. Pergamon Press, Oxford, 1972

316. Bech K, Nerup J, Larsen JH: *Yersinia enterocolitica* infection and thyroid diseases. Acta Endocrinol 84:87, 1977

317. Gupta MK: Thyrotropin receptor antibodies: Advances and importance of detection techniques in thyroid disease. Clin Biochem 25:193, 1992

318. McKenzie JM: The bioassay of thyrotropin in serum. Endocrinology 63:372, 1958

319. Furth ED, Rathbun M, Posillico J: A modified bioassay for the long-acting thyroid stimulator (LATS). Endocrinology 85:592, 1969

320. Kriss JP, Pleshakov V, Rosenblum AL et al: Studies on the pathogenesis of the ophthalmopathy of Graves' disease. J Clin Endocrinol Metab 27:582, 1967

321. Sunshine P, Kusumoto H, Kriss JP: Survival time of circulating long-acting thyroid stimulator in neonatal thyrotoxicosis: Implications for diagnosis and therapy of the disorder. Pediatrics 36:869, 1965

322. Onaya T, Kotani M, Yamada T, Ochi Y: New in vitro tests to detect the thyroid stimulator in sera from hyperthyroid patients by measuring colloid droplet formation and cyclic AMP in human thyroid slices. J Clin Endocrinol Metab 36:859, 1973

323. Hinds WE, Takai N, Rapoport B et al: Thyroid-stimulating activity and clinical state in antithyroid treatment of juvenile Graves' disease. Acta Endocrinol 94:46, 1981

324. Leedman PJ, Frauman AG, Colman PG, Michelangeli VP: Measurement of thyroid-stimulating immunoglobulins by incorporation of tritiated-adenine into intact FRTL-5 cells: a viable alternative to radioimmunoassay for the measurement of cAMP. Clin Endocrinol (Oxf) 37:493, 1992

325. Takata I, Suzuki Y, Saida K, Sato T: Human thyroid-stimulating activity and clinical state in antithyroid treatment of juvenile Graves' disease. Acta Endocrinol 94:46, 1980

326. Kendall-Taylor P, Atkinson S: A biological method for the assay of TSAb in serum. p. 763. In Stockigt R, Nagataki S (eds): Thyroid Research VII, Australian Academy of Science, Canberra, 1980

327. Petersen V, Rees Smith B, Hall R: A study of thyroid-stimulating activity in human serum with the highly sensitive cytochemical bioassay. J Clin Endocrinol Metab 41:199, 1975

328. Libert F, Lefort A, Gerard C et al: Cloning, sequencing and expression of the human thyrotropin (TSH) receptors: Evidence for binding of autoantibodies. Biochem Biophys Res Commun 165:1250, 1989

329. Nagayama Y, Kaufman KD, Seto P, Rapoport B: Molecular cloning, sequence and functional expression of the cDNA for the human thyrotropin receptor. Biochem Biophys Res Commun 165:1184, 1989

330. Ludgate M, Perret J, Parmentier M et al: Use of the recombinant human thyrotropin receptor (TRHr) expressed in mammalian cell lines to assay TSHr autoantibodies. Molec Cell Endocrinol 73:R13, 1990

331. Filetti S, Foti D, Costante G, Rapoport B: Recombinant human thyrotropin (TSH) receptor in a radioreceptor assay for the measurement of TSH receptor antibodies. J Clin Endocrinol Metab 72:1096, 1991

332. Vitti P, Elisei R, Tonacchera M et al: Detection of thyroid-stimulating antibody using Chinese hamster ovary cells transfected with cloned human thyrotropin receptor. J Clin Endocrinol Metab 76:499, 1993

333. Adams DD, Kennedy TH: Occurrence in thyrotoxicosis of a gamma globulin which protects LATS from neutralization by an extract of thyroid gland. J Clin Endocrinol Metab 27:173, 1967

334. Shishiba Y, Shimizu T, Yoshimura S, Shizume K: Direct evidence for human thyroidal stimulation by LATS-protector. J Clin Endocrinol Metab 36:517, 1973

335. Rapoport B, Greenspan FS, Filetti S, Pepitone M: Clinical experience with a human thyroid cell bioassay for thyroid-stimulating immunoglobulins. J Clin Endocrinol Metab 58:332, 1984

336. Smith BR, Hall R: Thyroid-stimulating immunoglobulins in Graves' disease. Lancet 2:427, 1974

337. Zakarija M, McKenzie JM, Munro DS: Evidence of an IgG inhibitor of thyroid-stimulating antibody (TSAb) as a cause of delay in the onset of neonatal Graves' disease. J Clin Invest 72:1352, 1983

338. Shewring G, Smith BR: An improved radioreceptor assay for TSH receptor antibodies. Clin Endocrinol 17:409, 1982

339. Endo K, Amir SM, Ingbar SH: Development and evaluation of a method for the partial purification of immunoglobulin specific for Graves' disease. J Clin Endocrinol Metab 52:1113, 1981

340. Kosugi S, Ban T, Akamizu T, Konh LD: Identification of separate determinants on the thyrotropin receptor reactive with Graves' thyroid stimulation antibodies and with thyroid stimulating blocking antibodies in idiopathic myxedema: these determinants have no homologous sequence on gonadotropin receptor. 6:166, 1992

341. Drexhage HA, Bottazzo GF, Doniach D: Thyroid growth stimulating and blocking immunoglobulins. p. 153. In Chayen J, Bitensky L (eds): Cytochemical Bioassays, Marcel Dekker, New York, 1983

342. Valente WA, Vitti P, Rotella CM et al: Autoantibodies that promote thyroid growth: a distinct population of thyroid stimulating antibodies. N Engl J Med 309:1028, 1983

343. Grove AS Jr: Evaluation of exophthalmos. N Engl J Med 292:1005, 1975

344. Parma J, Duprez L, van Sande J et al: Somatic mutations in the thyrotropin receptor gene cause hyperfunctioning thyroid adenomas. Nature 365:649, 1993

345. Duprez L, Parma J, Van Sande J et al: Germline mutations in the thyrotropin receptor gene cause non-autoimmune autosomal dominant hyperthyroidism. Nature Genet 7:396, 1994

346. McKenzie JM, Zakarija M: Fetal and neonatal hyper- and hypothyroidism due to maternal TSH receptor antibodies. Thyroid 2:155, 1992

347. Cho Y, Shong MH, Yi KH et al: Evaluation of serum basal thyrotrophin levels and thyrotrophin receptor antibody activities as prognostic markers for discontinuation of antithyroid drug treatment in patients with Graves' disease. Clin Endocrinol (Oxf) 36:585, 1992

348. Hershman JM: Hyperthyroidism induced by trophoblastic thyrotropin. Mayo Clin Proc 47:913, 1972

349. Greenspan FS, Kriss JP, Moses LE, Lew W: An improved bioassay method for thyrotropin hormone using thyroid uptake of radiophosphorus. Endocrinology 58:767, 1956

350. Nisula BC, Ketelslegers JM: Thyroid-stimulating activity and chorionic gonadotropin. J Clin Invest 54:494, 1974

351. Sobonya RE, Dobyns BM: Comparison of the responses of native Ohio fish and two species of saltwater Fundulus to the exophthalmos-producing substance (EPS) of the pituitary gland. Endocrinology 80:1090, 1967

352. Singh SP, McKenzie JM: ^{35}S-sulfate uptake by mouse harderian gland: Effect of serum from patients with Graves' disease. Metabolism 20:422, 1971

353. Winand RJ, Kohn LD: Stimulation of adenylate cyclase activity in retro-orbital tissue membranes by thyrotropin and an exophthalmogenic factor derived from thyrotropin. J Biol Chem 250:6522, 1975

354. Kodama K, Sikorka H, Bandy-Dafoe P et al: Demonstration of a circulating antibody against a soluble eye-muscle antigen in Graves' ophthalmopathy. Lancet 2:1353, 1982

355. Ryo UY, Arnold J, Colman M et al: Thyroid scintigram: Sensitivity with sodium pertechnetate Tc 99m and gamma camera with pinhole collimator. JAMA 235:1235, 1976

356. Atkins HL, Klopper JF, Lambrecht RM, Wolf AP: A comparison of technetium 99m and iodine 123 for thyroid imaging. Am J Roentgenol Radium Ther Nucl Med 117:195, 1973

357. Nishiyama H, Sodd VJ, Berke RA, Saenger EL: Evaluation of clinical value of ^{123}I and ^{131}I in thyroid disease. J Nucl Med 15:261, 1974

358. Tong ECK, Rubenfeld S: Scan measurements of normal and enlarged thyroid glands. Am J Roentgenol Radium Ther Nucl Med 115:706, 1972

359. Miller JM, Hamburger JI: The thyroid scintigram. I. The hot nodule. Radiology 84:66, 1965

360. Becker FO, Economou PG, Schwartz TB: The occurrence of carcinoma in "hot" thyroid nodules: Report of two cases. Ann Intern Med 58:877, 1963

361. Miller JM, Hamburger JI, Mellinger RC: The thyroid scintigram. II. The cold nodule. Radiology 85:702, 1965

362. Meier CA, Braverman LE, Ebner SA et al: The rhTSH Study Group. Diagnostic use of recombinant

human thyrotropin in patients with thyroid carcinoma. Thyroid, suppl. 2:35, 1992

363. Chen JJS, LaFrance ND, Allo MD et al: Single photon emission computed tomography of the thyroid. J Clin Endocrinol Metab 66:1240, 1988

364. Corstens F, Huysmans D, Kloppenborg P: Thallium-210 scintigraphy of the suppressed thyroid: an alternative for iodine-123 scanning after TSH stimulation. J Nucl Med 29:1360, 1988

365. Fairweather DS, Bradwell AR, Watson-James SF et al: Deletion of thyroid tumours using radiolabeled thyroglobulin. Clin Endocrinol 18:563, 1983

366. Hoffer HP: Fluorescent thyroid scanning. Am J Roentgenol 105:721, 1969

367. Hoffer PB, Gottschalk A, Refetoff S: Thyroid scanning technics: the old and the new. Curr Probl Radiol 2:1, 1972

368. Barki Y: Ultrasonographic evaluation of neck masses-sonographic pattern in differential diagnosis. Isr J Med Sci 28:212, 1992

369. Watters DAK, Ahuja AT, Evans RM et al: Role of ultrasound in the management of thyroid nodules. Am J Surg 164:654, 1992

370. Scheible W, Leopold GR, Woo VL, Gosink BB: High resolution real-time ultrasonography of thyroid nodules. Radiology 133:413, 1979

371. Sostre S, Reyes MM: Sonographic diagnosis and grading of Hashimoto's thyroiditis. J Endocrinol Invest 14:115, 1991

372. Brander A, Viikinkoski P, Nickels J, Kivisaari L: Thyroid gland: US screening in a random adult population. Radiology 81:683, 1991

373. Jensen F, Rasmussen SN: The treatment of thyroid cysts by ultrasonically guided fine needle aspiration. Acta Chir Scand 142:209, 1976

374. Szebeni A, Beleznay EJ: New simple method for thyroid volume determination by ultrasonography. Clin Ultrasound 20:329, 1992

375. Jarlov AE, Hegedus L, Gjorup T, Hansen JEM: Accuracy of the clinical assessment of thyroid size. Dan Med Bull 38:87, 1991

376. Paracchi A, Ferrari C, Livraghi T et al: Percutaneous intranodular ethanol injection: a new treatment for autonomous thyroid adenoma. J Endocrinol Invest 15:353, 1992

377. Yamada T, Tsukui T, Ikerjiri K et al: Volume of sella turcica in normal subjects and in patients with primary hypothyroidism and hyperthyroidism. J Clin Endocrinol Metab 42:817, 1976

378. Blum M, Reede DL, Seltzer TF, Burroughs VJ: Computerized axial tomography in the diagnosis of thyroid and parathyroid disorders. Am J Med Sci 287:34, 1984

379. Brown LR, Aughenbaugh GL: Masses of the anterior mediastinum: CT and MR imaging. Am J Radiol 157:1171, 1991

380. Damascelli B, Cascinelli N, Terno G et al: Second thoughts on the value of selective thyroid angiography. Am J Roentgenol Radium Ther Nucl Med 114:822, 1972

381. Matoba N, Kikuchi T: Thyroidolymphography: a new technic for visualization of the thyroid and cervical lymph nodes. Radiology 92:339, 1969

382. Chamla-Soumenkoff J, Frühling J, Mahaux JE: Mise eń evidence des ganglions de drainage lymphatique de la thyroïde par la camérà a scintillation aprés injection intrathyroïdienne d'un microcolloïde de 198 Au. Communication préliminaire. Ann Endocrinol 32:203, 1971

383. Clark H, Greenspan FS, Coggs GC, Goldman L: Evaluation of solitary cold thyroid nodules by echography and thermography. Am J Surg 130:206, 1975

384. Wang C, Vickery AL Jr, Maloof F: Needle biopsy of the thyroid. Surg Gynecol Obstet 143:365, 1976

385. Ashcraft MW, Van Herle AJ: Management of thyroid suppressive therapy, and fine needle aspiration. Head Neck Surg 3:297, 1981

386. Crill C Jr: The danger of surgical dissemination of papillary carcinoma of the thyroid. Surg Gynecol Obstet 102:161, 1956

387. Crill G Jr, Esselstyn CB, Hawk WA: Needle biopsy in the diagnosis of thyroid nodules appearing after radiation. N Engl J Med 301:997, 1979

388. Matos-Godilho L, Kocjan G, Kurtz A: Contribution of fine needle aspiration cytology to diagnosis and management of thyroid disease. J Clin Pathol 45:391, 1992

389. Hamberger B, Gharib H, Melton LJ 3rd et al: Fine-needle aspiration biopsy of thyroid nodules: Impact on thyroid practice and cost of care. Am J Med 73:381, 1982

390. Odell WD, Wilber FJ, Utiger RD: Studies on thyrotropin physiology by means of radioimmunoassay. Recent Prog Horm Res 23:47, 1967

391. Jackson IMD: Thyrotropin-releasing hormone. N Engl J Med 306:145, 1982

392. Wilber JF: Thyrotropin releasing hormone: Secretion and actions. Ann Rev Med 24:353, 1973

393. Scanlon MF, Rees Smith B, Hall R: Thyroid-stimulating hormone: Neuroregulation and clinical applications. Clin Sci Mol Med 55:1, 1978

394. Brown JR: The measurement of thyroid stimulating hormone (TSH) in body fluids: a critical review. Acta Endocrinol 32:289, 1959

395. Bakke JL: Assay of human thyroid-stimulating hormone by 18 different assay laboratories using 12 different methods. J Clin Endocrinol Metab 25:545, 1965

396. Ambesi-Impiombato FS, Parks LAM, Coons HG: Culture of hormone dependent epithelial cells from rat thyroids. Proc Natl Acad Sci USA 77:3444, 1980

397. Beck-Peccoz P, Amr S, Menezes-Ferreira M et al: Decreased receptor binding of biologically inactive thyrotropin in central hypothyroidism. Effect of treatment with thyrotropin-releasing hormone. J Clin Endocrinol Metab 312:1085, 1985

398. Beck-Peccoz P, Piscitelli G, Amr S et al: Endocrine, biomedical, and morphological studies of a pituitary adenoma secreting growth hormone thyortropin (TSH), and α-subunit: Evidence for secretion of TSH with increased bioactivity. J Clin Endocrinol Metab 62:704, 1986

399. Pierce JG: The subunits of pituitary thyrotropin: Their relation to other glycoprotein hormones. Endocrinology 89:1331, 1971

400. Spitz IM, LeRoith D, Hirsch H et al: Increased high-molecular-weight thyrotropin with impaired biologic activity in a euthyroid man. N Engl J Med 304:278, 1981

401. Miyai K, Fukuchi M, Kumahara Y: Correlation between biological and immunological potencies of human serum and pituitary thyrotropin. J Clin Endocrinol Metab 29:1438, 1969

402. Gendrel D, Feinstein MC, Grenier J et al: Falsely elevated serum thyrotropin (TSH) in newborn infants: Transfer from mothers to infants of a factor interfering in the TSH radioimmunoassay. J Clin Endocrinol Metab 52:62, 1981

403. Chaussain JL, Binet E, Job JC: Antibodies to human thyreotrophin in the serum of certain hypopituitary dwarfs. Rev Eur Etud Clin Biol 17:95, 1972

404. Nicoloff JT, Spencer CA: The use and misuse of the sensitive thyrotropin assays. J Clin Endocrinol Metab 71:553, 1990

405. Kricka LJ: Chemiluminescent and bioluminescent techniques. Clin Chem 37:1472, 1991

406. Klee GG, Hay ID: Assessment of sensitive thyrotropin assays for an expanded role in thyroid function testing: Proposed criteria for analytic performance and clinical utility. J Clin Endocrinol Metab 64:461, 1987

407. Spencer CA, LoPresti JS, Patel A: Applications of a new chemiluminometric thyrotropin assay to subnormal measurement. J Clin Endocrinol Metab 70:453, 1990

408. Ross DS, Ardisson LJ, Meskell MJ: Measurement of thyrotropin in clinical and subclinical hyperthyroidism using a new chemiluminescent assay. J Clin Endocrinol Metab 69:684, 1989

409. Brennan MD, Klee GG, Preissner CM, Hay ID: Heterophilic serum antibodies: a cause for falsely elevated serum thyrotropin levels. Mayo Clin Proc 62:894, 1987

410. Wood JM, Gordon DL, Rudinger AN, Brooks MM: Artifactual elevation of thyroid-stimulating hormone. Am J Med 90:261, 1991

411. Zweig MH, Csako G, Reynolds JC, Carrasquillo JA: Interference by iatrogenically induced anti-mouse IgG antibodies in a two-site immunometric assay for thyrotropin. Arch Pathol Rad Metab 1165:164, 1991

412. Kourides IA, Heath CV, Ginsberg-Fellner F: Measurement of thyroid-stimulating hormone in human amniotic fluid. J Clin Endocrinol Metab 54:635, 1982

413. Fisher DA, Kleinm AH: Thyroid development and disorders of thyroid function in the newborn. N Engl J Med 304:702, 1981

414. Snyder PJ, Utiger RD: Response to thyrotropin releasing hormone (TRH) in normal man. J Clin Endocrinol Metab 34:380, 1972

415. Hershman JM, Pittman JA Jr: Utility of the radioimmunoassay of serum thyrotropin in man. Ann Intern Med 74:481, 1971

416. Brabant G, Prank K, Ranft U et al: Physiological regulation of circadian and pulsatile thyrotropin secretion in normal man and woman. J Clin Endocrinol Metab 70:403, 1990

417. Bartalena L, Martino E, Falcone M et al: Evaluation of the nocturnal serum thyrotropin (TSH) surge, as assessed by TSH ultrasensitive assay, in patients receiving long term L-thyroxine suppression therapy and in patients with various thyroid disorders. J Clin Endocrinol Metab 65:1265, 1987

418. Ria AG, Brabant K, Prank E, Endert E, Wiersinga WM: Circadian changes in pulsatile TSH release in primary hypothyroidism. Clin Endocrinol 37:504, 1992

419. Brabant G, Prank C, Hoang-Vu C, Hesch RD, von zur Muhlen A: Hypothalamic regulation of pulsatile thyrotropin secretion. J Clin Endocrinol Metab 72:145, 1991

420. Romijn JA, Adriaanse G, Brabant K et al: Pulsatile secretion of thyrotropin during fasting: a decrease of thyrotropin pulse amplitude. J Clin Endocrinol Metab 70:1631, 1990

421. Bartalena L, Pacchiarotti A, Palla R et al: Lack of nocturnal serum thyrotropin (TSH) surge in patients with chronic renal failure undergoing regular maintenance hemofiltration: a case of central hypothyroidism. Clin Nephrol 34:30, 1990

422. Romijn JA, Wiersinga WM: Decreased nocturnal surge of thyrotropin in nonthyroidal illness. J Clin Endocrinol Metab 70:35, 1990

423. Van Cauter E, Golstein J, Vanhaelst L, Leclercq R: Effects of oral contraceptive therapy on the circadian patterns of cortisol and thyrotropin (TSH). Eur J Clin Invest 5:115, 1975

424. Brabant G, Brabant A, Ranft U et al: Circadian and pulsatile thyrotropin secretion in euthyroid man under the influence of thyroid hormone and glucocorticoid administration. J Clin Endocrinol Metab 65:83, 1987

425. Simoni M, Velardo A, Montanini V et al: Circannual rhythm of plasma thyrotropin in middle-aged and old euthyroid subjects. Horm Res 33:184, 1990

426. Wilber JF, Baum D: Elevation of plasma TSH during surgical hypothermia. J Clin Endocrinol Metab 31:372, 1970

427. Vagenakis AG, Rapoport B, Azizi F et al: Hyper-response to thyrotropin-releasing hormone accompanying small decreases in serum thyroid hormone concentration. J Clin Invest 54:913, 1974

428. Snyder PJ, Utiger RD: Inhibition of thyrotropin response to thyrotropin releasing hormone by small quantities of thyroid hormones. J Clin Invest 51:2077, 1972

429. Ehrmann DA, Weinberg M, Sarne DH: Limitations to the use of a sensitive assay for serum thyrotropin in the assessment of thyroid status. Arch Intern Med 149:369, 1989

430. Ridgway EC, Cooper DS, Walker H et al: Peripheral responses of thyroid hormone before and after L-thyroxine therapy in patients with subclinical hypothyroidism. J Clin Endocrinol Metab 53:1238, 1981

431. Aizawa T, Koizumi Y, Yamada T et al: Difference in pituitary-thyroid feedback regulation in hypothyroid patients, depending on the severity of hypothyroidism. J Clin Endocrinol Metab 47:560, 1978

432. Spencer CA: Clinical utility and cost-effectiveness of sensitive thyrotropin assays in ambulatory and hospitalized patients. Mayo Clin Proc 63:1214, 1988

433. Surks MI, Chopra IJ, Mariash CN et al: American Thyroid Association guidelines for use of laboratory tests in thyroid disorders. JAMA 263:1529, 1990

434. Delange F, Dodion J, Wolter R et al: Transient hypothyroidism in the newborn infant. J Pediatr 92:974, 1978

435. Brown ME, Refetoff S: Transient elevation of serum thyroid hormone concentration after initiation of replacement therapy in myxedema. Ann Intern Med 92:491, 1980

436. Sanchez-Franco F, Cacicedo GL, Martin-Zurro A et al: Transient lack of thyrotropin (TSH) response to thyrotropin-releasing hormone (TRH) in treated hyperthyroid patients with normal or low serum thyroxine (T_4) and triiodothyronine (T_3). J Clin Endocrinol Metab 38:1098, 1974

437. Spencer CA, Elgen A, Shen D et al: Specificity of sensitive assays of thyrotropin (TSH) used to screen for thyroid disease in hospitalized patients. Clin Chem 33:1301, 1987

438. Sunthornthepvarakul T, Gottschalk ME, Hayashi Y, Refetoff S: Resistance to thyrotropin caused by mutations in the thyrotropin receptor gene. N Engl J Med (in press)

439. Weintraub BD, Gershengorn MC, Kourides IA, Fein H: Inappropriate secretion of thyroid stimulating hormone. Ann Intern Med 95:339, 1981

440. Mihailovic V, Feller MS, Kourides IA, Utiger RD: Hyperthyroidism due to excess thyrotropin secretion: Follow-up studies. J Clin Endocrinol Metab 50:1135, 1980

441. Kourides IA, Ridgway EC, Weintraub BD et al: Thyrotropin-induced hyperthyroidism: Use of alpha and beta subunit levels to identify patients with pituitary tumors. J Clin Endocrinol Metab 45:534, 1977

442. Sarne DH, Sobieszczyk S, Ain KB, Refetoff S: Serum thyrotropin and prolactin in the syndrome of generalized resistance to thyroid hormone: Responses to thyrotropin-releasing hormone stimulation and short term triiodothyronine suppression. J Clin Endocrinol Metab 70:1305, 1990

443. Brent GA, Hershman JM, Braunstein GD: Patients with severe nonthyroidal illness and serum thyrotropin concentrations in the hypothyroid range. Am J Med 81:463, 1986

444. Topliss DJ, White EL, Stockigt JR: Significance of thyrotropin excess in untreated primary adrenal insufficiency. J Clin Endocrinol Metab 50:52, 1980

445. Wehmann RE, Gregerman RI, Burns WH et al: Suppression of thyrotropin in the low-thyroxine state of severe nonthyroidal illness. N Engl J Med 312:546, 1985

446. Bacci V, Schussler GC, Kaplan TB: The relationship between serum triiodothyronine and thyrotropin during systemic illness. J Clin Endocrinol Metab 54:1229, 1982

447. Kourides IA, Weintraub BD, Ridgway EC, Maloof F: Pituitary secretion of free alpha and beta subunit of human thyrotropin in patients with thyroid disorders. J Clin Endocrinol Metab 40:872, 1975

448. Oliver C, Charvet JP, Codaccioni J-L, Vague J: Radioimmunoassay of thyrotropin-releasing hormone (TRH) in human plasma and urine. 39:406, 1974

449. Emerson CH, Frohman LA, Szabo M, Thakker I: TRH immunoreactivity in human urine: Evidence for dissociation from TRH. 45:392, 1977

450. Mitsuma T, Hiraoka Y, Nihei N: Radioimmunoassay of thyrotropin-releasing hormone in human serum and its application. 83:225, 1976

451. Mallik TK, Wilber JF, Pegues J: Measurements of thyrotropin-releasing hormone-like material in human peripheral blood by affinity chromatography and radioimmunoassay. 54:1194, 1982

452. Weeke J: The influence of the circadian thyrotropin

rhythm on the thyrotropin response to thyrotropin-releasing hormone in normal subjects. Scand J Clin Lab Invest 33:17, 1974

453. Haigler ED Jr, Hershman JM, Pittman JA Jr, Blaugh CM: Direct evaluation of pituitary thyrotropin reserve utilizing thyrotropin releasing hormone. J Clin Endocrinol Metab 33:573, 1971

454. Azizi F, Vagenakis AG, Portnay GE et al: Pituitary-thyroid responsiveness to intramuscular thyrotropin-releasing hormone based on analyses of serum thyroxine, tri-iodothyronine and thyrotropin concentration. N Engl J Med 292:273, 1975

455. Haigler ED Jr, Hershman JM, Pittman JA Jr: Response to orally administered synthetic thyrotropin-releasing hormone in man. J Clin Endocrinol Metab 35:631, 1972

456. Ormston BJ, Kilborn JR, Garry R et al: Further observations on the effect of synthetic thyrotropin-releasing hormone in man. Br Med J 2:199, 1971

457. Hershman JM, Kojima A, Friesen HG: Effect of thyrotropin-releasing hormone on human pituitary thyrotropin, prolactin, placental lactogen, and chorionic thyrotropin. J Clin Endocrinol Metab 36:497, 1973

458. Jacobsen BB, Andersen H, Dige-Petersen H, Hummer L: Thyrotropin response to thyrotropin-releasing hormone in fullterm, euthyroid and hypothyroid newborns. Acta Paediatr Scand 65:433, 1976

459. Sanchez-Franco F, Garcia MD, Cacicedo L et al: Influence of sex phase of the menstrual cycle on thyrotropin (TSH) response to thyrotropin-releasing hormone (TRH). J Clin Endocrinol Metab 37:736, 1973

460. Harman SM, Wehmann RE, Blackman MR: Pituitary-thyroid hormone economy in healthy aging men: Basal indices of thyroid function and thyrotropin responses to constant infusions of thyrotropin releasing hormone. J Clin Endocrinol Metab 58:320, 1984

461. Wilber J, Jaffer A, Jacobs L et al: Inhibition of thyrotropin releasing hormone (TRH) stimulated thyrotropin (TSH) secretion in man by a single oral dose of thyroid hormone. Horm Metab Res 4:508, 1972

462. Wartofsky L, Dimond RC, Noel GL et al: Effect of acute increases in serum triiodothyronine on TSH and prolactin responses to TRH, and estimates of pituitary stores of TSH and prolactin in normal subjects and in patients with primary hypothyroidism. J Clin Endocrinol Metab 42:443, 1976

463. Shenkman L, Mitsuma T, Suphavai A, Hollander CS: Triiodothyronine and thyroid-stimulating hormone response to thyrotrophin-releasing hormone: a new test of thyroidal and pituitary reserve. Lancet 1:111, 1972

464. Anderson MS, Bowers CY, Kastin AJ et al: Synthetic thyrotropin-releasing hormone: a potent stimulator of thyrotropin secretion in man. N Engl J Med 285:1279, 1971

465. McFarland KF, Strickland AL, Metzger WT, Smith JS: Thyrotropin-releasing hormone test: an adverse reaction. Arch Intern Med 142:132, 1982

466. Fleischer N, Lorente M, Kirkland J et al: Synthetic thyrotropin releasing factor as a test of pituitary thyrotropin reserve. J Clin Endocrinol Metab 34:617, 1972

467. Sachson R, Rosen SW, Cuatrecasas P et al: Prolactin stimulation by thyrotropin-releasing hormone in a patient with isolated thyrotropin deficiency. N Engl J Med 287:972, 1972

468. Vagenakis AG, Braverman LE, Azizi F et al: Recovery of pituitary thyrotropic function after withdrawal of prolonged thyroid-suppression therapy. N Engl J Med 293:681, 1975

469. Tamai H, Nakagawa T, Ohsako N et al: Changes in thyroid function in patients with euthyroid Graves' disease. J Clin Endocrinol Metab 50:108, 1980

470. Tamai H, Suematsu H, Ikemi Y et al: Responses to TRH and T_3 suppression tests in euthyroid subjects with a family history of Graves' disease. J Clin Endocrinol Metab 47:475, 1978

471. Stein RB, Nicoloff JT: Triiodothyronine withdrawal test—a test of thyroid-pituitary adequacy. J Clin Endocrinol Metab 32:127, 1971

472. Mornex R, Berthezene F: Comments on a proposed new way of measuring thyrotropin (TSH) reserve. J Clin Endocrinol Metab 31:587, 1970

473. Taunton OD, McDaniel HG, Pittman JA Jr: Standardization of TSH testing. J Clin Endocrinol Metab 25:266, 1965

474. Burke G: The thyrotropin stimulation test. Ann Intern Med 69:1127, 1968

475. Hays MT, Solomon DH, Beall GN: Suppression of human thyroid function by antibodies to bovine thyrotropin. J Clin Endocrinol Metab 27:1540, 1967

476. Werner SC, Spooner M: A new and simple test for hyperthyroidism employing L-triiodothyronine and the twenty-four hour I-131 uptake method. Bull NY Acad Med 31:137, 1955

477. Duick DS, Stein RB, Warren DW, Nicoloff JT: The significance of partial suppressibility of serum thyroxine by triiodothyronine administration in euthyroid man. J Clin Endocrinol Metab 41:229, 1975

478. Alexander WD, Harden RM, McLarty D, Shimmins J: Thyroidal suppressibility after stopping long-term treatment of thyrotoxicosis with anti-thyroid drugs. Metabolism 18:58, 1969

479. Lowry RC, Lowe D, Hadden DR et al: Thyroid suppressibility: Follow-up for two years after antithyroid treatment. Br Med J 2:19, 1971

480. Stanbury JB, Kassenaar AAH, Meijer JWA: The metabolism of iodotyrosines. I. The fate of mono- and di-iodotyrosine in normal subjects and in patients with various diseases. J Clin Endocrinol Metab 16: 735, 1956

481. Lissitzky S, Codaccioni JL, Bismuth J, Depieds R: Congenital goiter with hypothyroidism and iodoserum albumin replacing thyroglobulin. J Clin Endocrinol Metab 27:185, 1967

482. DeGroot LJ: Kinetic analysis of iodine metabolism. J Clin Endocrinol Metab 26:149, 1966

483. Hays MT: Absorption of oral thyroxine in man. J Clin Endocrinol Metab 28:749, 1968

484. Hays MT: Absorption of triiodothyronine in man. J Clin Endocrinol Metab 30:675, 1970

485. Valente WA, Goldiner WH, Hamilton BP et al: Thyroid hormone levels after acute L-thyroxine loading in hypothyroidism. J Clin Endocrinol Metab 53:527, 1981

486. Ain KB, Refetoff S, Fein HG, Weintraub BD: Pseudomalabsorption of levothyroxine. JAMA 266:2118, 1991

487. Sterling K, Chodos RB: Radiothyroxine turnover studies in myxedema thyrotoxicosis and hypermetabolism without endocrine disease. J Clin Invest 35: 806, 1956

488. Oppenheimer JH, Schwartz HL, Surks MI: Determination of common parameters of iodothyronine metabolism and distribution in man by noncompartmental analysis. J Clin Endocrinol Metab 41:319, 1975

489. Curti GI, Fresco GF: A theoretical five-pool model to evaluate triiodothyronine distribution and metabolism in healthy subjects. Metabolism 41:3, 1992

490. Bianchi R, Mariani G, Molea N et al: Peripheral metabolism of thyroid hormones in man. I. Direct measurement of the conversion rate of thyroxine to 3, 5,3'-triiodothyronine (T_3) and determination of the peripheral and thyroidal production of T_3. J Clin Endocrinol Metab 56:1152, 1983

491. Faber J, Heaf J, Kirkegaard C et al: Simultaneous turnover studies of thyroxine, 3,5,3'- and 3,3',5-triiodothyronine, and 3'-monoiodothyronine in chronic renal failure. J Clin Endocrinol Metab 56:211, 1983

492. Refetoff S, Fang VS, Marshall JS, Robin NI: Metabolism of thyroxine-binding globulin (TBG) in man: Abnormal rate of synthesis in inherited TBG deficiency and excess. J Clin Invest 57:485, 1976

493. Lim VS, Fang VS, Katz AI, Refetoff S: Thyroid dysfunction in chronic renal failure: a study of the pituitary-thyroid axis and peripheral turnover kinetics of thyroxine and triiodothyronine. J Clin Invest 60: 522, 1977

494. LoPresti JS, Warren DW, Kaptein EM et al: Urinary immunoprecipitation method for estimation of thyroxine and triiodothyronine conversion in altered thyroid states. J Clin Endocrinol Metab 55:666, 1982

495. Ridgway EC, Weintraub BD, Maloof F: Metabolic clearance and production rates of human thyrotropin. J Clin Invest 895, 1974

496. Cuttelod S, Lemarchand-Beraud T, Magnenat P et al: Effect of age and role of kidneys and liver on thyrotropin turnover in man. Metabolism 23:101, 1974

497. Cavalieri RR, Searle GL: The kinetics of distribution between plasma and liver of ^{131}I-labeled L-thyroxine in man: Observations of subjects with normal and decreased serum thyroxine-binding globulin. J Clin Invest 45:939, 1966

498. Oppenheimer JH, Bernstein G, Hasen J: Estimation of rapidly exchangeable cellular thyroxine from the plasma disappearance curves of simultaneously administered thyroxine-^{131}I and albumin-[125]I. J Clin Invest 46:762, 1967

499. Usala SJ, Tennyson GE, Bale AE et al: A base mutation of the c-erbAβ thyroid hormone receptor in a kindred with generalized thyroid hormone resistance. Molecular heterogeneity in two other kindreds. J Clin Invest 85:93, 1990

500. Lairmore TC, Howe JR, Korte JA et al: Familial medullary thyroid carcinoma and multiple endocrine neoplasia type 2B map to the same region of chromosome 10 as multiple endocrine neoplasia type 2A. Genomics 9:181, 1991

501. Janssen OE, Bertenshaw R, Takeda K et al: Molecular basis of inherited thyroxine-binding globulin defects. Trends Endocrinol Metab 3:49, 1991

502. Tatsumi K, Miyai K, Notomi T et al: Cretinism with combined hormone deficiency caused by a mutation in the PIT1 gene. 1:56, 1992

Autoimmunity to the Thyroid Gland

7

A BRIEF REVIEW OF IMMUNOLOGIC REACTIONS

Immune System Development and Function-Associated Antigens

The human immune system is comprised of about 2×10^{12} lymphocytes containing approximately equal ratios of T and B cells. B lymphocytes synthe- size immunoglobulins that are first expressed on their membranes as clonally distributed antigen-specific receptors and then secreted as antibodies following antigenic stimulation. The ability of the immune system to recognize antigens is remarkable. A human being can produce more than 10^7 antibodies with different specificities. The concentration of antibodies in human serum is 15 mg/ml, which represents about 3×10^{20} immunoglobulin molecules per person! Since each B cell has approximately 10^5 antibody molecules of identical specificity on its surface, the human humoral immune system scans the antigenic universe with about 10^{17} cell-bound receptors. To maximize the chances of encountering antigen, lymphocytes recirculate from blood to lymphoid tissues and back to the blood. The 10^{10} lymphocytes in human blood have a mean residence time of approximately 30 minutes, thus an exchange rate of almost 50 times per day.

T lymphocytes develop from precursor stem cells in fetal liver and bone marrow and differentiate into mature cell types during residence in the thymus.[1] Mature T lymphocytes (antigen-responding, response-control, and response-mediating cells) are present in thymus, spleen, lymph nodes, throughout skin and other lymphatic organs, and in the bloodstream. B lymphocytes (immunoglobulin-producing cells) develop from precursor cells in fetal liver and bone marrow and are found in all lymphoid organs and in the bloodstream. The ontogeny and functions of these cells have been identified in a variety of ways, including morphologic and functional criteria, and by antibodies identifying surface proteins that correlate to a varying extent with specific functions.[2] Lymphocytes develop through stages leading to pools of cells that can be operationally defined and be recognized by acquisition of specific antigenic determinants[3,4] (Fig. 7-1; Table 7-1). Human B and T cells normally express class I (HLA-A, HLA-B, HLA-C) major histocompatibility complex (MHC) antigens on their surface, and B cells express class II antigens (HLA-DR, HLA-DP, HLA-DQ). "Activated" T cells also express class II antigens on their surface and are then described as DR^+ (or sometimes as Ia^+).[5]

Lymphocyte Surface Molecules

On their surface T cells have T cell antigen receptors (TCR), which recognize an antigen-HLA complex; accessory molecules, which recognize HLA determinants; and adhesion molecules, which recognize their counterpart ligands on antigen-presenting cells (APCs). After activation, T cells also have new receptors for cytokines, the hormone products mainly produced by macrophages, T cells, and B cells, which control other T or B cells[6,7] (Table 7-2). The T cell antigen recognition complex, or receptor, consists of disulfide-linked heterodimers, usually the TCRα and TCRβ chains, plus five or more associated peptides making up the CD3 complex.[8,9] A small proportion of T cells have TCRγ and TCRδ chain instead of α and β chains.[10] TCRα and β peptides and γ/δ peptides are derived from rearranged genes coding for proteins that are unique in each cell clone. The germline TCR genes are very large, containing 40 to 100 different V (variable) segments, D (diversity) segments (in β genes), many J (junctional) segments, and one or two C (constant) segments[11,12] (Fig. 7-2). During development of each T cell, segments of the germline gene are rearranged so that one TCR gene V segment becomes associated with one D (in the case of TCRβ), one J, and one C segment to produce a unique gene sequence. This random combination of different V, D, and J, and C segments, and additional variations in DNA sequence introduced in the J and D region during recombination, provides the enormous diversity of specific TCRs required to recognize the entire universe of T cell antigens. This process is described as "instructive," rather than "educational," in the sense that antigen-specific TCRs develop because of intrinsic genetic instructions, rather than in response to exposure to antigens. This process, for example, means that all individuals can (before clonal deletion) have preformed TCRs able to recognize thyroid antigens as well as thousands of other antigens.

The set of V, D, and J segments present in one individual's inherited (germline) TCR α, β, γ, and δ chains differs from those comprising another individual's genes. This variation can be recognized by the process of Southern blotting, in which DNA is digested by restriction enzymes that cut the DNA at specific infrequently occurring sequences. The fragments are separated by electrophoresis and identified using radioactive-labeled cDNA probes. Variations in cutting patterns—restriction fragment length polymorphisms (RFLPs), which must correlate with inheritance of certain sets of V, D, or J segments—are sometimes associated with specific disease susceptibility and have been related to thyroid disease (see discussion below).

Each individual T cell and its progeny have a "rearranged" gene with one unique combination of V, D, and J segments. Current technology makes it possible to clone individual T cells that respond to a specific antigen, to expand the progeny of a single cell manyfold, and then to determine the DNA sequence of the V, D, and J regions that provide the unique recognition function of the TCR. Based on

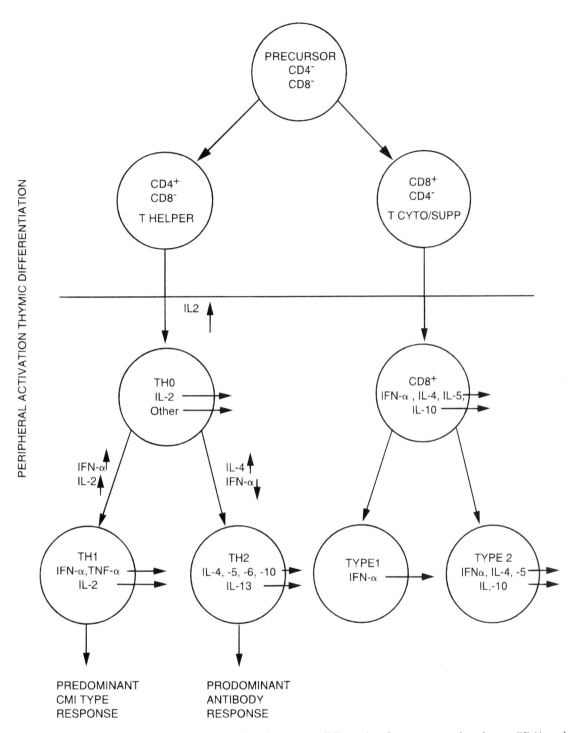

Fig. 7-1. Development of T cell subsets. In the thymus, undifferentiated precursors give rise to CD4+ and CD8+ cells. In the peripheral lymphoid tissues CD4+ cells (TH0) differentiate following activation by exposure to cognate antigen into two subsets (TH1 and TH2), which are well characterized in the mouse, less so in humans. Development of these cells is to some extent reciprocally controlled by cytokines, and the cytokines secreted are also distinct. CD8+ cells similarly mature after antigenic stimulation into less well-defined subsets. ↑ or ↓ = effect on subset proliferation. → = cytokines produced.

TABLE 7-1. Differentiation Antigens That Characterize Specific Lymphocyte Subsets

Antigen	Synonyms	Primary Distribution	Comment
CD2	LFA-2	T cells NK cells	Cytoadhesion molecule; cognate to LFA-3
CD3	T3, Leu 4	All peripheral T cells	T cell receptor complex
CD4	T4, Leu 3 (L3T4 in mice)	Class II restricted T cells (55%–70% of peripheral T cells)	CD4 binds to MHC class II
CD8	T8, Leu 2, Lyt 2	Class I restricted T cells (25%–40% of peripheral T cells)	CD8 binds to MHC class I
CD11a	LFA-1-α chain	Leukocytes	LFA-1-α chain adhesion molecule, binds to ICAM-1
CD14	LPS receptor	Monocytes	Marker for monocytes
CD16	Fc-γ, R111	NK cells, granulocytes	Low affinity Fc-γ receptor
CD20	B1	B cells	Marker for B cells
CD25	TAC, IL-2 α chain	Activated T and B cells and monocytes	Complexes with β, α chain; T cell growth
CD28	Tp44	Most T cells	T cell receptor for B7-1 and B7-2
CD29	β Chain of β-1 "integrin"	40%–45% of CD4$^+$ and CD8$^+$ cells	β-1 chain of VLA protein, an "integrin" type of adhesion molecule
CD40	—	B cells	B cell activation
CD45RO	—	25%–40% of peripheral T cells	Expressed on naive T cell subsets
CD54	ICAM-1	T and B cells	Cognate to LFA-1
CD56	NKH1	NK cells, some T cells	Neural cell adhesion molecule; NK marker

(Adapted from Knapp et al.,[3] with permission.)

such studies, it is now evident that specific V segments are preferentially used in the response to certain antigens.[12] We may thus infer that the availability of such a favored V segment in an individual's TCR repertoire must favor an immune response to a specific antigen, including an autoantigen.

Each TCR recognizes one specific antigenic peptide sequence,[13] which may consist of 8–9 amino acids for class I restricted T cells, and 13–17 amino acids for class II restricted T cells. However, some T cells respond to various portions (epitopes) of one antigen; these may represent overlapping peptide segments of the epitope. Thus the response of each individual T (and B) cell is extremely specific, but the combined effect of many T (and B) cells acting together is observed in the typical final "polyclonal" response.

T cells recognize antigen in association with ("presented by") a major histocompatibility complex (MHC) molecule; CD4$^+$ T cells (often functioning as helper cells) recognize class II molecules + antigen, and CD8$^+$ T cells (often functioning as cytotoxic/suppressor cells) recognize class I molecules + antigen.[14] Recent studies indicate that the antigen (a small peptide; see below) fits within a cleft in the HLA-DR molecule[15] (Fig. 7-3). The TCR functions to recognize the antigenic peptide on the MHC molecule (Fig. 7-3). The five associated peptides of the CD3 complex are believed to be signal transducers and to initiate intracellular events[8,9] following antigen recognition. The normal response proceeds via TCR antigen recognition, then activation of the T cell through the combined effect of antigen recognition and interleukin-1 (IL-1) action, leading to T cell IL-2 secretion and IL-2 receptor expression, followed by proliferation of the T cell into an active clone.

Lymphocyte development is controlled by cytokines (hormones) that are released by macrophages, lymphocytes, and other cells. Both T and B cells release a large array of cytokines, which carry out their affector functions and alter the function of other cells (Fig. 7-1, Table 7-2). As lymphocytes mature in the thymus and become activated on exposure to antigen, the types of cytokines to which they respond—and that they produce—become altered. In animals, and to a lesser extent in humans, types of lymphocytes can be operationally defined by the cytokines produced. For example, Th1 T cells produce IL-2, interferon-α (IFN-α) and tumor necrosis factor-α (TNF-α) and are predominant in delayed hypersensitivity type reactions, whereas Th2 T cells pro-

TABLE 7-2. Cytokines

Cytokine	Cell Source	Targets	Primary Effects On Targets
Type 1 IFN	Mononuclear phagocyte, fibroblast	All	Antiviral, antiproliferative, increased class I MHC expression
Tumor necrosis factor	Mononuclear phagocyte, T cell	Neutrophil	Inflammation
		Liver	Acute phase reactants
		Muscle	Catabolism
		Hypothalamus	Fever
Interleukin-1	Mononuclear phagocyte	Thymocyte	Costimulator
		Endothelial cell	Inflammation
		Hypothalamus	Fever
		Liver	Acute phase reactants
		Muscle, fat	Catabolism (cachexia)
Interleukin-6	Mononuclear phagocyte, endothelial cell, T cell	Thymocyte	Costimulator
		Mature B cell	Growth
		Liver	Acute phase reactants
Interleukin-2	T cells	T cell	Growth; cytokine production
		NK cell	Growth, activation
		B cell	Growth, antibody synthesis
Interleukin-4	CD4$^+$ T cell, mast cell	B cell	Isotype switching
		Mononuclear phagocyte	Inhibit activation
		T cell	Growth
Transforming growth factor-β	T cells, mononuclear phagocyte, other	T cell	Inhibit activation
		Mononuclear phagocyte	Inhibit activation
		Other cell types	Growth regulation
γ-Interferon	T cell, NK cell	Mononuclear phagocyte	Activation
		Endothelial cell	Activation
		NK cell	Activation
		All	Increased class I and class II MHC
Lymphotoxin	T cell	Neutrophil	Activation
		Endothelial cell	Activation
		NK cell	Activation
Interleukin-10	T cell	Mononuclear phagocyte	Inhibition
		B cell	Activation
Interleukin-5	T cell	Eosinophil	Activation
		B cell	Growth and activation
Interleukin-12	Macrophages	NK cells	Activation
		T cells	Activation

(Adapted from Abbas AK, Lichtman AH, and Pober JS,[418] with permission.)

duce IL-4 and IL-10, stimulate B cells, and are involved especially in antibody-mediated reactions.

Each B cell produces a unique immunoglobulin (Ig) programmed by an Ig gene that has also been "rearranged" from the germline V, D, J, and C segments (as for the TCR).[16] The TCR and immunoglobulin genes are, not surprisingly, members of one gene superfamily. Further diversity is provided by antigen-driven somatic mutations that occur during amplification of the progeny of a stimulated B cell, causing the production of a family of immunoglobulins with slightly different sequences. Some of these immunoglobulins may be better antibodies, and others might recognize other antigens, including "self."

B cells secrete their unique immunoglobulins into surrounding fluids, and some normally remain on the B cell surface, where they can bind the antigen that is recognized by (fits the structure of) the specific immunoglobulin (Fig. 7-4). The surface Ig is therefore a B cell receptor for antigen, having a specific face, or idiotype, which fits the conformation of the antigen (Ag) molecule epitope. The recognition process involves the shape of the epitope, i.e., it is conformational, and for B cells probably normally involves unprocessed or native antigen. This implies that B cell and T cell epitopes for the same antigen are usually different segments or forms of the molecule.

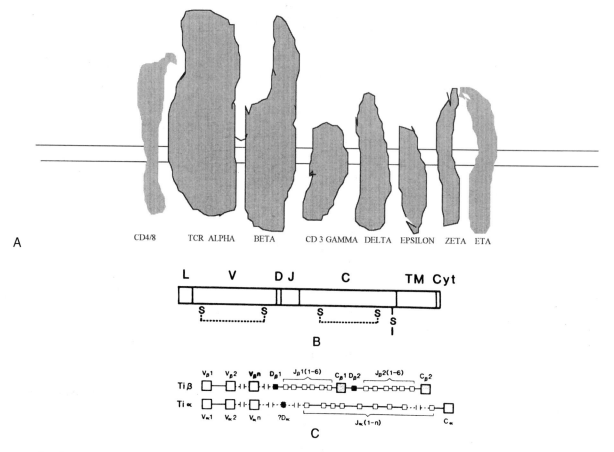

Fig. 7-2. Diagram of the human T cell receptor and its subunits. **(A)** Subunit composition of the human T cell receptor. The TCR subunits are held together by–S–S–bonds and are closely associated with either the CD4 or CD8 molecule and chains of the CD3 complex. The subunits are anchored in the cell membrane. The CD3 complex consists of three subunits referred to as gamma, delta, and epsilon. Associated in the TCR complex is another pair of 16 kD homodimer (32 kD nonreduced) subunits existing as homodimers of zeta or heterodimers of zeta and eta. **(B)** The structure of the Ti subunits. The predicted primary structure of the α-chain subunit after translation from the cDNA sequence is depicted, as are the variable region leader (L), V, D, and J segments, a hydrophobic transmembrane segment (TM) and cytoplasmic part (Cyt) in the C region, potential intrachain sulfhydryl bonds (S-S), and the single SH group (S) that can form a sulfhydryl bond with the subunit. **(C)** A scheme of the genomic organization of human α- and β-chain genes. In the locus, V indicates the V gene pool located 5′ at an unknown distance from the D_1 element, the J_1 cluster, and the C_1 constant-region gene. Further downstream, a second D_2 element, J_2 cluster, and C_2 constant-region gene are indicated. A similar nomenclature is used for the Ti-α locus, in which only a single constant region is found. ?D indicates the uncertainty about the existence of a putative Ti-diversity element. (From Janeway et al.,[4] with permission.)

Antigen Presentation on Major Histocompatibility Complex Molecules

Antigen is normally recognized by the T cell receptor complex only when presented in association with a class I or class II MHC molecule. Typically $CD8^+$ T cells recognize antigen with class I (HLA-A, HLA-B, HLA-C) proteins, and $CD4^+$ T cells are restricted in their recognition to antigen presented with class II (HLA-DR, HLA-DP, HLA-DQ) proteins. Antigens that originate within the cell are preferentially presented by class I molecules to $CD8^+$ cells.

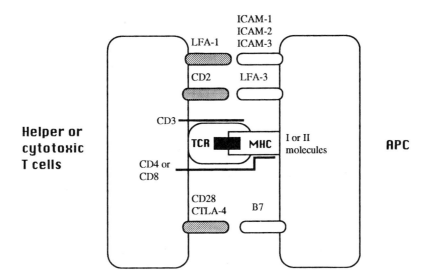

Fig. 7-3. In this diagram the antigen is depicted in a cleft of the HLA-DR molecule on an APC, being recognized by the T cell TCR. "Adhesive" peptide segments may augment close contact. A CD4 molecule is associated with the TCR. Presumably the APC surface is normally covered with many DR molecules, each studded with an antigen. T cells must somehow scan these complexes in order to find the one that best fits their TCR.

This indicates an orientation of CD8$^+$ cells toward destroying cells invaded by viruses or producing abnormal antigens. Class II molecules are directed toward presentation of external or alloantigens to CD4$^+$ helper cells.

The genes for the HLA-A, HLA-B, HLA-C and HLA-DR, HLA-DP, HLA-DQ molecules are on chromosome 6 and comprise some of the genes in a large immune response control complex. Each cell surface HLA molecule is made up of two peptide chains; an α and β 2 microglobulin for class I molecules, and α and β chains for class II. Each individual inherits from each parent one HLA-A, HLA-B, and HLA-C, one DRα and 3 DRβ genes, a pair each of DP and DQα and β genes, and other related genes that are not expressed, including DX and DO. β2 microglobulin polypeptides are the same for all individuals (Fig. 7-5). The genes are expressed in a codominant manner and, in contrast to TCR and Ig molecules, are invariant in individuals. However, the genes are

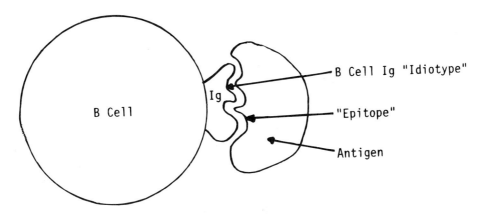

Fig. 7-4. The B cell surface is studded with specific Ig molecules that function as high-affinity receptors for specific antigen epitopes that match the shape of the Ig recognition idiotype.

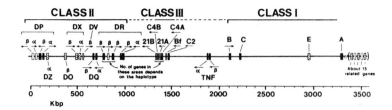

Fig. 7-5. Partial map of the short arm of human chromosome 6 showing the molecular organization of the area containing the MHC loci, with details of the HLA class I, II, and III genes. Map distances in kilobases were determined by pulsed-field gel electrophoresis. Genes are not drawn to scale. Expressed genes are designated by black boxes; pseudogenes by white boxes; and genes of undefined status by cross-hatched boxes. (From Trowsdale J, Campbell RD,[419] with permission.)

all highly polymorphic; that is, many alleles may exist for each gene. At least 16 DR variants, 9 DQβ alleles, and 6 DPβ alleles, have been recognized by allogeneic mixed lymphocyte reactions, specific antibodies and, more recently, by DNA analysis. The actual evolutionary drive for this diversity is unknown. We may note that different HLA molecules will presumably present different epitopes and thus lead to selection of a unique T cell repertoire for each HLA allele. While TCR gene rearrangement provides the T cell repertoire to respond to individual antigens, HLA diversity guarantees that different individuals will have different T cell repertoires. We may theorize that this is beneficial for survival of some members of the species when all are attacked by a pathogen, for example, the plague.

The HLA molecules play a central role in T cell clonal selection during fetal development, in normal immune responses, and in presentation of self-antigens. In many instances—including autoimmune thyroid disease (AITD) as detailed below—inheritance of a specific HLA gene correlates with increased susceptibility to a specific disease. In some cases this can now be related to a gene coding for a specific amino acid in the HLA molecule, which is believed to control epitope selection and thus be associated with disease susceptibility.

Antigen can be presented to T cells by conventional (or professional) APCs such as macrophages and dendritic cells, by B cells and activated T cells and, less effectively, by a variety of other cells (fibroblasts, glial cells, thyrocytes), when these normally HLA-DR cells are altered and express HLA molecules on their surfaces.[17,18] Extracellular (usually foreign protein) antigen is endocytosed by macro-phages (APCs). B cells collect the antigen by binding it to cognate surface Ig, and internalizing the Ig-antigen complex. Inside these cells the antigen molecule is broken down to peptides, which are 13 to 17 amino acids long.[17] Many of these peptides are destroyed, but some are retained to reappear on the cell surface as T cell antigen epitopes. These peptides, possibly in a Golgi-like organelle,[17] become associated with HLA-DR, HLA-DP, or HLA-DQ molecules, are transported to the cell surface, and there can be "presented" to a T cell (as in Fig. 7-3). Possibly the initial response to antigen proceeds via the antigen–APC–T cell route. Secondary T cell responses may follow the same route or may more frequently follow the antigen–B cell–T cell route. This is because the surface Ig of the B cell allows it to collect specific antigen circulating at a very low level and concentrate it for presentation to a T cell.

Proteins produced within the cell (including normal proteins or products encoded by invading viruses) are processed by a separate pathway and appear on the cell surface as peptides of eight to nine amino acids associated with HLA class I molecules.

T and B Cell Responses

Antigen presentation to T cells leads to a variety of responses, which include proliferative or suppressive functions, development of cell cytotoxic responses, control of Ig secretion, and many more. In addition, under specific circumstances, antigen presentation may cause the T cell to become nonresponsive—anergized.

Presumably the APC, with its surface covered by HLA-DR antigen complexes, is met by T cells having the correct receptor (idiotype) matching the processed antigen exposed on the surface of the HLA molecule. T cell and APC adhere by segments of HLA-DR and CD4 molecules, which are effectively "sticky" (Fig. 7-5B), fostering close contact of APC and T cells.[19] Costimulation is provided by other adhesion molecules on the APCs, which also pair with their counterparts on T cells. Specifically, LFA-1 on T cells binds to ICAM-1 on the APC, and CD2 binds to ICAM-2. Binding of B7 to T cell receptor CD28 or CTLA-4 is especially important. These reactions dramatically increase the bond between APC and T cell, ensure close approximation, and provide the additional, or second signal, needed to activate the T cell.[19,20] Presentation of antigen and the accompanying second signal are required to activate a naive T cell and initiate an immune response. Antigen recognition and APC-produced IL-1 (Table 7-2) stimulate the T cell. This activates the T cell to express IL-2 receptors and to secrete IL-2 itself. Increased T-cell-secreted IL-2 induces the responding T cell and nearby (bystander) T cells to proliferate.[19] T-cell-secreted IL-2 and IL-4 stimulate B cells to proliferate.[21,22,23] Intimate T cell to B cell contact may account for antigen-specific help for T cell and B cell responses, whereas the effect of T cell–secreted lymphokines on bystander T or B cells may account for stimulation of non-antigen-specific responses by these lymphocytes.[24]

T cell–B cell interaction usually occurs as T cells percolate through lymph nodes. The T cell receptors must in some way "scan" the exposed DR-antigen combinations on B cells, until by chance the T cell finds a B cell presenting the antigen epitope recognized by the TCR.

Responding lymphocytes can be segregated into groups based on whether they are naive or memory cells, CD4+ helper cells, or CD8+ cytotoxic/suppressor cells. Although not providing a clear separation as in a murine system, a functional separation based on lymphokine secretion seems to provide an important categorization. Th1 cells secreting IL-2, IFN γ, and TNF α function as "inflammatory" cells, typical of a delayed hypersensitivity type reaction. T cells secreting IL-4 and IL-5 (Th2 cells) are more specifically helper cells for B cell immunoglobulin synthesis.[22] Some CD4+ and some CD8+ cells appear to provide suppressor signals.[25,26] The nature of the recognition process in the suppressor function and of the putative affector molecules is not clear. It may involve TCR recognition of T cell or B cell idiotype,

secreted molecules representing part of the TCR receptor, or lymphokines such as IFN γ.[27] The suppressive response could also involve formation via B cells of antibodies directed to a specific T cell idiotype causing destruction of the T cell.[28] Activation, by class I molecules + antigen, of CD8+CD11−TP44+ cells, leads to cytotoxic destruction of cells bearing the cell surface HLA-ABC molecules + antigen.[29]

Since T cells stimulate or suppress other T or B cells, they may develop feedback circuits to limit responses to antigens.[30] Similarly, the specific Ig idiotype on B cells functions as an antigen and causes proliferation of other B cells to secrete anti-idiotypic antibodies, completing a B cell regulatory circuit.[31] Other such circuits have been described, including development of contrasuppressor T cells.[32]

It must be noted that the complexity of T cell function is much greater than suggested by this brief outline. There is evidence that T cells have the innate capacity to carry out either help or suppression, depending on the state of maturation of the cell, the nature of the stimulus involved, or the lymphokines produced.[33–35] For example, CD4+ T cells can function as suppressor or cytotoxic cells[33,34] and can function as suppressor or helper cells at different times in their life cycle. Some workers contest the very concept of suppressor cells. In fact an important generalization is that the T cell antigens so far defined only rarely identify unique functional sets of cells. On the other hand, functions of T cells to help T or B responses, to suppress such responses, and to kill target cells under certain conditions can be *operationally* defined, and these functions often correlate with expression of specific T cell antigens. While recognizing the inherent simplifications we have employed, it remains useful to discuss T cell subsets in relation to surface antigens and function, since so much work has been published using these concepts.

Killer and Natural Killer Cells

In addition to the standard T cell function described above, other cells participate in immune responses. Macrophages may destroy cells having immune complexes on their surface through recognition of the Fc portion of bound Ig. A subset of T cells bearing different TCR peptides (TCR γ and TCR δ proteins) has been recently recognized. This

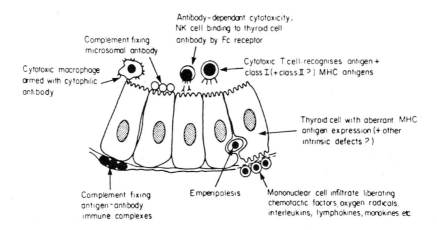

Fig. 7-6. Some of the proposed mechanisms that could produce thyroid damage in AITD. Emperipolesis is the movement of lymphocytes and macrophages between epithelial cells and occurs in many organs such as gut, bronchus, and thyroid. The existence of interepithelial cells with immunoreactive potential is obviously relevant to an understanding of how autoantigens at the luminal surface of the thyroid cells may be exposed to allow recognition. (From Logtenberg et al.,[136] with permission.)

set is of unknown function, but some of these cells are CD3[+] and function as natural killer (NK) cells. Other cells that do not bear the CD3 marker of T cell lineage exist (NK cells) and have the ability to spontaneously kill other cells (especially those expressing HLA antigens).[36] Natural killer cells are detected by specific monoclonal antibodies (anti-leu7 and anti-CD16) and are recognized as large granular lymphocytes. Macrophages, T cells, killer cells, natural killer cells, or other cells also kill cells coated with immune complexes in the process of antibody-dependent cell cytotoxicity (ADCC) (Fig. 7-6).

Self-Non-Self Discrimination

The immune system, which evolved to defend us from invading foreign proteins, normally tolerates (does not develop recognizable responses to) self-antigens. The level of this control is variable. For example, self-reactivity to serum albumin is not seen. However, antibodies to thyroid antigens exist in up to 36 percent of adult women, and their presence must be considered effectively normal.

The development of tolerance is closely associated with the restriction of TCRs to recognizing an antigen only when presented by an HLA molecule. The process, which for T cells occurs in the fetal thymus, eliminates some T cells and retains others with TCRs having desirable features. Self-antigens are believed to be presented on HLA molecules to T cells developing in the thymus. This implies that antigen must be in the thymus or in the circulation for tolerance to develop. T cells bearing TCRs that react strongly to HLA molecules not bearing antigen (autoreactive cells) are largely inactivated or destroyed. T cells that have the capacity to react with foreign antigens presented by self-MHC molecules are somehow retained. Most T cells with TCRs that bind strongly to class I or class II molecules bearing self-antigen are also clonally deleted[37] (Fig. 7-7). Presumably some T cells that react with MHC molecules + self antigen are not deleted, since otherwise an excessive number of T cells would be lost, leaving a hole in the available TCR repertoire that would compromise its ability to mount a future immune defense. This fine discrimination between perfection in clonal deletion and repertoire maintenance allows a limited number of autoreactive and self-antigen-reactive T cells to survive and thus sets the stage for autoimmune disease. It is not clear how tolerance relates to selection of cells of the CD8[+] lineage that function as suppressor cells, and it is also unclear how this mechanism produces tolerance to antigens not present in the fetal thymus or circulation, especially antigens that may be expressed only in the mature individual. It is presumed that a mechanism working outside the thymus—peripheral tolerance—completes T cell selection.

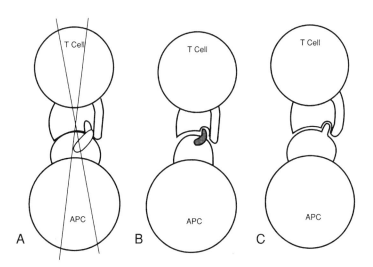

Fig. 7-7. (A): Fetal thymus; T cells strongly activated by DR alone, or strongly reactive to self-antigen presented by HLA molecules, are selectively destroyed. T cells, with a weak or absent response to DR alone, or to DR⁺ self-antigen, survive. **(B)**: Normal adult immune reaction; T cell TCR and APC-DR interaction is normally a weak or neutral signal. The presence of alloantigen switches the signal to positive. **(C)**: Allo-MLR; allogeneic DR is sufficiently different from autologous DR to act as a positive signal with or without antigen present.

During maturation in the thymus, probably 95 percent or more of the lymphocytes produced are negatively selected and die through a process described as programmed cell death, or apoptosis. This process involves several genes, including those required for apoptosis, such as Fas[37a] and NGF1-B/Nur77/Nak1, or inhibitory, such as BCL2. A similar process is thought to ensue whenever a T cell is stimulated by its cognate antigen but does not receive a second signal and during induction of anergy by some mechanisms. Defects in Fas led to preservation of autoreactive T cells in some models of animal autoimmune disease.[37a] Whether defective Fas, Nak1, or BCL2 gene function is involved in human autoimmunity is a question of great current interest.

B cells undergo a similar selection process in fetal bone marrow or liver, except for the participation of MHC molecules. If exposed to antigen during this early stage of development, B cells are somehow permanently inactivated. As for T cells, the selection process is not perfect and leaves some B cells having the ability to make antibodies directed to self-antigens in the adult. However, B cells require T cell help in order to proliferate and differentiate into mature Ig-secreting cells. In the effective absence of self-reactive T cells to help such B cells, these B cells remain dormant, and expanding clones do not develop.

Tolerance to self-antigen can be overcome (broken) in animals by injecting the antigen in an unusual site on the body, especially in the presence of adjuvant compounds such as tubercule bacillus fragments and oil, or alum, or by slightly altering the antigen structure, or by altering the responding immune system (for example, by whole body irradiation or depletion of suppressor T cells).[38,39] It is clear that some degree of recognition of self-antigens is normal, but is also normally well controlled by suppressor circuits in the immune system. Factors that may lead to amplification of the normal small number of self-reactive T cells, and thus produce "autoimmune" disease, are described subsequently.

In contrast to this low reactivity to normal self-antigens, cells bearing nonidentical class II molecules (for example, in the mixture of T cells from two individuals, the allogeneic mixed lymphocyte reaction [allo-MLR]) react vigorously to each other, and 10 to 20 percent of all T cells may respond.[40] The physiologic meaning of this response is not obvious. It must originate quite independently from the setting of organ transplantation and rejection, in which it is clinically a major issue. Presumably T cells recognize allogeneic class II molecules as if they represented autologous DR+ antigens (Fig. 7-7). The allo-MLR is often compared to the autologous mixed lymphocyte reaction (AMLR), in which previously separated T and B cells from one individual, when recombined, induce a proliferative response of the T cells. The biologic meaning of this response is, however, also best described as unknown. One school of thought perceives it to be an in vitro artifact. Alternatively, it may represent a low level of physiologic self-reactivity, perhaps mediated by T cells with low affinity for self-MHC that escaped negative selection in the thymus.

SYNDROMES OF THYROID AUTOIMMUNITY

The syndromes comprising autoimmune thyroid disease are three intimately related illnesses: (1) Graves' disease with goiter, exophthalmos, and hyperthyroidism; (2) Hashimoto's thyroiditis with goiter and euthyroidism or hypothyroidism; and (3) primary thyroid failure, or myxedema. Many variations of these syndromes are also recognized, including transient hyperthyroidism occurring independently of pregnancy and in 5 to 6 percent of postpartum women, neonatal hyperthyroidism, and neonatal hypothyroidism. The syndromes are bound together by their similar thyroid pathology, similar immune mechanisms, co-occurrence in family groups, and transition from one clinical picture to the other within the same individual over time. The immunologic mechanisms involved in these three diseases must be closely related, while the phenotypes probably differ because of the specific type of immunologic response that occurs. For example, if immunity leads to production of thyroid-stimulating antibodies, Graves' disease is produced, whereas if thyroid-stimulating hormone blocking antibodies TSBAG are formed or a cell-destructive process occurs, the result is Hashimoto's thyroiditis or primary myxedema.

Associated with autoimmune thyroid disease in some patients are other organ-specific autoimmune syndromes, including pernicious anemia, vitiligo, myasthenia gravis, primary adrenal autoimmune disease, ovarian insufficiency, pituitary insufficiency rarely, alopecia, and sometimes Sjögren's syndrome or rheumatoid arthritis or lupus, as manifestations of non-organ-specific autoimmunity.

ANTIGENS IN AUTOIMMUNE THYROID DISEASE

The three important antigens involved in thyroid autoimmunity are clearly defined. First to be recognized was thyroglobulin (TG), the 670-kD protein synthesized in thyroid cells and in which triiodothyronine (T_3) and thyroxine (T_4) are produced. Although considered to be a single unique protein, the proteins prepared from different thyroid glands, especially those with Graves' disease and thyroid malignancy, react differently with polyvalent rabbit anti-TG antisera,[41,42] suggesting that the fine structure of TG differs from person to person. Four to six B cell epitopes of TG are known to be involved in the human autoimmune responses. Animal studies suggest that antigenicity of the molecule is related to iodine content, but studies on human antisera do not bear this out.[42] Antibodies appear to recognize conformation of large fragments of TG, whereas T cells recognize peptide segments and their primary structure.[42]

The cDNA for TG has recently been cloned, and it is of considerable interest that it includes a motif analogous to the enzyme acetylcholinesterase.[43] This in a way may tie AITD to the related autoimmune disease myasthenia gravis, although the antibodies in myasthenia are directed not to acetylcholinesterase but to acetylcholine receptors. Antibodies that react with human TG do cross-react with acetylcholinesterase.[44]

The second antigen to be identified was the TSH receptor (TSH-R). TSH-R is a 764 aa glycoprotein protein. Antibodies to TSH-R mimic the function of TSH and cause disease by binding to the TSH-R and stimulating (or inhibiting) thyroid cells, as described later. Human antisera containing TSH-R antibodies immunoprecipitate 100, 90, and 75 kD thyroid epithelial cell (TEC) membrane proteins representing forms of receptor,[45] or possibly smaller peptides held together by -S-S-bonds, but the receptor is most certainly comprised of a single chain.

The human TSH-R has been cloned and sequenced in several laboratories and is known to be a member of a family of cell surface hormone receptors characterized by an extramembraneous portion, seven transmembrane loops, and an intracellular domain that binds the G_S subunit of adenyl cyclase.[46,47] Segments of the extracellular domain, including aa 12–30 and 324–344, may be involved in binding of

TSH.[48] The Ig molecules in Graves' patients are reported to bind to two specific sequences in the extracellular domain,[49] and much effort is being directed to define the B and T cell epitopes.[50] TSH-R epitopes are nonlinear conformational, perhaps composed of different segments of the protein. Antibodies recognizing the H_2 terminal area (38–45) are stimulatory (48a), whereas those binding nearer the cell surface, in the region of aa 388–403, appear to function as thyrotropin-binding inhibitory antibodies (TBIAb).[51] Antibodies raised in rabbits to the peptide forming the third extracellular loop of the transmembrane domain of the receptor are also cell stimulatory,[52] as are rabbit antibodies binding to aa 12–39 of the extracellular domain.[53] Apparent hTSH-R mRNA transcripts have been identified in retrobulbar ocular tissue, lymphocytes, and fat cells,[54–56] suggesting alternative sites that could be involved in the development of autoimmunity. A variant sequence of 1.3 kb, which includes most of the extracellular domain but does not include the transmembrane domain, also occurs in the thyroid[57] and is probably released to blood.[58]

The third thyroid antigen was described as microsomal antigen for more than three decades, since antisera from humans with thyroid autoimmunity reacted with an easily denatured protein present on the surface of thyroid cells and in cell cytoplasm.[59] Our laboratory demonstrated that human antisera reacting to microsomal antigen precipitated human thyroid peroxidase (TPO) prepared from Graves' disease thyroid tissue[60] (Fig. 7-8). By Western blot–SDS-polyacrylamide electrophoresis of thyroid epithelial cell (TEC) membrane proteins, a pair of 101 and 107 kD bands, which were the antigen, were identified.[61,62] Monoclonal antibodies developed to this antigen cross-reacted with TPO.[63] The cDNA was cloned and sequenced in several laboratories.[64–66] Czarnocka et al.[67] have also shown the identity of microsomal antigen and TPO. Alternative splicing of the mRNA probably provides the explanation for the two forms of the protein.[68] As yet a functional difference for the two forms has not been described. It is clear that there are multiple B cell epitopes present in human TPO, since different antisera recognize native, denatured, or denatured and reduced protein.[69] The interaction of human anti-TPO antisera and monoclonal antibodies also indicates the presence of several B cell epitopes.[70] Two of these have been further defined by cloning frag-

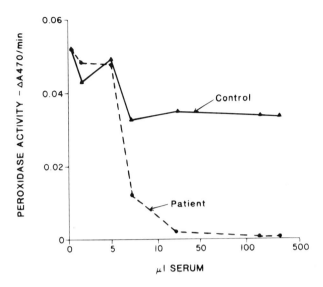

Fig. 7-8. Precipitation of peroxidase activity by sera from a patient with autoimmune thyroid disease and positive "microsomal" antibodies and from a control subject without circulating antibodies. TPO was precipitated by primary incubation with human sera, and removal of TPO-Ig complexes was achieved by adding protein H-Sepharose CL-4B. Residual hTPO activity in the supernatant was assayed in a guaiacol assay.

ments of the TPO molecule.[71] Investigation of linear epitopes of TPO recognized by T cells from patients with AITD has produced conflicting results to date. Kawakami et al.[77] found epitopes composed of amino acids 110–129, 211–230, 842–861, and 882–901 to be most reactive. Dayan et al.[73] found sequences 535–551 and 632–645 to be involved, and Tandon et al.[74] report sequences 415–432, 439–457, and 463–481 to be reactive.

Chazenbalk et al.[75] have shown that TSH stimulates production of the mRNA for the microsomal antigen-TPO protein.[76] Khoury et al.[77] have shown that microsomal antigen/TPO is expressed on the thyroid cell surface, as well as in the cytoplasm, and may represent the cell surface antigen recognized in some studies. Expression of the antigen is also increased by incubation of thyroid cells with lectins, and this response is augmented by interferon-γ (IFN-γ).[78] IFN-γ alone does not stimulate production of the antigen. Exposure of the thyroid cells to antithyroid drugs does not alter cell expression of the antigen,[79] although antithyroid drugs clearly are used primarily because they inhibit function of TPO. Surprisingly, TPO and TG are reported by some workers to share common epitopes.[80] There are small areas of amino acid sequence homology, but it is uncertain that these are important B cell epitopes.[81]

It is of considerable interest that the three major antigens involved in AITD are unique to the thyroid, and all are involved in producing thyroid hormone. On the other hand, perhaps this is circuitous reasoning, since clearly it is sensible that autoimmunity to unique thyroid antigens would produce thyroid disease. If autoimmunity cross-reacted with a variety of other organs, the disease produced would present as a different syndrome. These antigens are unique to the thyroid gland, and cross-reactivity of antibodies with proteins in other organs is extremely limited. Anti-TSH-R antibodies do cross-react with guinea pig[82] fat cell membrane receptors, and some anti-TPO antibodies cross-react with myeloperoxidase.[83]

It is believed that the antigens are not abnormal in autoimmune disease and, in fact, no specific abnormal antigen has been demonstrated in any instance. Antibodies from an individual with AITD cross-react with antigen from a "normal" person. Hamada et al.[84] have shown that thyroid peroxidase (TPOs) from Graves' or normal thyroid do not differ in 2-D SDS gels, after protease digestion, or in immunologic function. However, as noted above for TG, in some instances there are variations in the structure of the antigens. A recent report of a point mutation in TSH-R[85] actually demonstrates a common allelism.

In AITD, antibodies to a variety of other thyroid cell components are also occasionally present, including antibodies that react with T_4 or T_3,[86] antibodies reacting with tubulin and calmodulin, antibodies reacting to DNA or DNA-associated proteins[87,88] and several other thyroid cell constituents.

IMMUNE REACTION IN AUTOIMMUNE THYROID DISEASE

Humoral Immunity

Table 7-3 lists the principal autoantibodies identified in AITD and the methods for detecting them. Antibodies to the TSH receptor are discussed in detail in Chapter 11.

Observation of a factor in serum of patients with Graves' disease causing long-acting stimulation of

TABLE 7-3. Antibodies Reacting with Thyroid Autoantigens in AITD and Techniques for Detection

Antigen	Test Used To Identify Antibody
TG	Precipitin
	Hemagglutination assay
	Immunofluorescence on fixed sections of thyroid tissue: colloid localization
	Solid-phase RIA
	Immunoradiometric assay
	Hemolytic plaque assay
Colloid component other than TG	Immunofluorescence on fixed sections: colloid localization
Microsomal antigen/TPO	Complement fixation
	Immunofluorescence on unfixed sections; thyroid tissue cell localization
	Cytotoxic effect on cultured thyroid cells
	Hemagglutination assay
	ELISA
	Solid-phase RIA
	TPO activity inhibition
TSH-R	Bioassay in mice
	cAMP production by thyroid cells or membranes
	Iodide uptake by thyroid cells
	Thymidine incorporation by thyroid cells
	Inhibition of TSH action on thyroid cells
	Inhibition of TSH binding to cells or membranes
Nuclear component	Immunofluorescence on unfixed sections of tissue: nuclear localization

thyroid hormone release from an animal's thyroid (in contrast to the short-acting stimulation produced by TSH) led directly to our knowledge of anti-TSH-R antibodies. We briefly summarize here a huge amount of clinical and laboratory research. The antibodies directed to the TSH-R are currently separated into three types. Some antibodies presumably bind to an important epitope in TSH-R and activate the receptor, producing the same effects as TSH. These antibodies may be referred to as TSI (thyroid-stimulating immunoglobulins). Other antibodies bind to different epitopes and interfere with TSH binding in certain assays; thus they are known as thyrotrophin-binding inhibitory immunoglobulins, or TBII. Still others bind and prevent the action of

TSH, thus thyrotrophin-stimulation blocking anti-bodies (TSBAb). Numerous other names are used. TSI cause non-TSH-dependent (often called autonomous) stimulation of thyroid function, which if of sufficient intensity is thyrotoxicosis. TBII can produce hypothyroidism and can block the action of TSH or TSI. Predominance of TSI characterizes Graves' disease, and TSBAb are often present in Hashimoto's disease. Probably a combination is present in most patients with AITD. TSI directly cause thyroid overactivity, their level correlates roughly with disease intensity, and a drop in levels correlates loosely with disease remission. The intact TSH-R epitopes recognized by B cells remain uncertain, in large part because the epitope or epitopes are probably conformational and are made up of discontinuous but contiguous portions of the extracellular domain of the receptor.

Precipitating antibodies to TG were first detected by mixing antibody and antigen in equivalent concentrations or by agar gel diffusion, as in the Ouchterlony plate technique. Subsequently, much more sensitive methods were developed, such as solid-phase RIA[89] and the tanned red cell hemagglutination test (TGHA) of Boyden.[90] In the latter, TG is absorbed on the surface of red cells that have been treated with dilute tannic acid. Agglutination of these treated cells occurs in the presence of antibody to TG. By this method, antibody can be detected at a concentration that is 1/40,000 of that required for a positive precipitin reaction. Current RIAs for TGAb are as sensitive, or more sensitive, than TGHA. Immunoradiometric assays (IRMA) used currently involve binding of serum Ab to solid-phase antigen and secondary quantitation of antibody by binding labeled monoclonal anti-human Ig antibody. These tests are also reported to be very sensitive and specific. Hemagglutination titers of up to 1 in 5 million have been obtained with sera from patients with chronic thyroiditis. A high anti-TG titer (1/1,250 or more) is strong evidence of AITD and helps to distinguish it from multinodular goiter and thyroid carcinoma.

In some instances, TG is released into the circulation to form circulating antigen-antibody complexes that prevent the detection of free antibodies unless a special technique is used, as reported by Kriss.[91] Immune complexes thus formed can significantly reduce TG antibody levels when TG is introduced into the circulation by thyroid biopsy or operation.[92]

Antibodies directed against TG are rarely present in children without evidence of thyroid disease. The prevalence in "well" persons increases with age, and low levels are present in up to 34 percent of "normal" adult women and 4 percent of "normal" adult men.[93,94] The greatest frequency occurs in women aged 40 to 60 years. The frequency of antibodies in well persons correlates with the incidence of lymphocytic infiltration found on microscopic examination of "normal" thyroids,[95] and antibody levels correlate well with the presence of lymphocyte infiltration in the thyroid.[96] Over 90 percent of patients with Hashimoto's thyroiditis have these antibodies. Low to moderate titers (< 1/2500) are found in half of patients with Graves' disease. High antibody levels in this disease are often found in patients who become hypothyroid after thyroidectomy[97] and iodine–131 treatment.[98] Almost all patients with idiopathic hypothyroidism have high titers. Antibody levels are either absent or low in patients with subacute (De Quervain's) thyroiditis, who may be similar clinically to patients with Hashimoto's thyroiditis. Complement-fixing antibodies to purified TG have been detected in Hashimoto's disease[99] but are not extensively studied. Human TG and its autoantibody bind complement weakly.[100]

The second important antigen-antibody system was originally recognized by antibodies that by immunofluorescence were observed to bind to nondenatured thyroid cytoplasm, to fix complement in the presence of human thyroid membranes (microsomes), or to bind to microsome-coated red cells (the MCHA assay). We now know this antigen is TPO but will in discussions refer to it both as microsomal antigen, since this conforms to many original reports, and as TPO, the designation used in recent studies (Fig. 7-8). TPO is a glycoprotein present in the plasma membrane, present in two forms of 107 and 101 kD derived by different splicing of the primary mRNA. Almost all patients with Hashimoto's thyroiditis have antibodies. At least 6 percent of "normal" subjects also have such antibodies, usually in low titer, and peripheral blood mononuclear cells (PBMC) of "normal" subjects can produce anti-TPO antibodies when cultured in vitro.[101] Current assay techniques include MCHA, RIA, ELISA, and IRMA and use of purified TPO[102] or recombinant human TPO. Although all antibodies reacting with microsomes may not be directed to TPO, it is likely that TPO antibodies constitute the very major portion of "antimicrosomal" activity.[103] These antibodies also bind to and inhibit the enzymatic function of TPO, as shown by Okamoto et al.[104] This effect is probably limited in vivo by inability of the antibodies to penetrate the thyroid and reach TPO on the surface of the cells facing the colloid space.

Antibodies detected by these techniques are believed to be similar to antibodies that fix complement in the presence of extracts from a thyrotoxic gland[105] and to a cytotoxic antibody found in the serum of patients with Hashimoto's thyroiditis.[106–108] Sera from patients with Hashimoto's thyroiditis usually have high cytotoxic activity.[107–109] Complement-mediated injury probably occurs in vivo since complement-containing complexes have been identified in thyroid tissue of patients with Graves' disease and Hashimoto's thyroiditis.[110] Thyroid cell expression of a membrane protein CD59 helps prevent complement-mediated lysis,[111] and this protein is upregulated by IL-1 and IFN.

When investigated with the fluorescent antibody technique, the sera of certain patients with Hashimoto's thyroiditis show a reaction that is localized to the nuclei of the thyroid slice.[112] This antinuclear antibody is also fixed by the nuclei of other tissues. There is uncertainty as to whether these antibodies react with double-stranded DNA, as do SLE antibodies, or are less specific antibodies reacting with single-stranded DNA.[113]

In early studies, TG antibodies were demonstrated by the passive cutaneous anaphylaxis technique and by a skin test in which an extract of human thyroid gland was injected intradermally.[114] Positive skin reactions were found in patients with Hashimoto's thyroiditis and primary myxedema, and these conditions were closely correlated with the presence of circulating thyroid precipitins. The tissue change at the reaction site was that of Arthus response. This type of study obviously carries a risk of viral transmission, and thus is not now acceptable (or necessary).

The frequency of autoantibodies detected by the TGHA and MCHA tests in various thyroid disorders appears in Fig. 7-9.[115] When both systems are considered, 95 percent of the series gave positive test results in Hashimoto's thyroiditis. The figures in diffuse toxic goiter and nontoxic nodular goiter were 87 and 25 percent, respectively. The highest antibody titers are found in Hashimoto's thyroiditis and diffuse toxic goiter.

Thyroid-stimulating antibodies (TSAb), TSH-

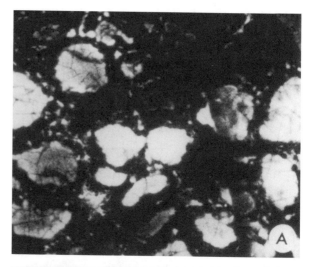
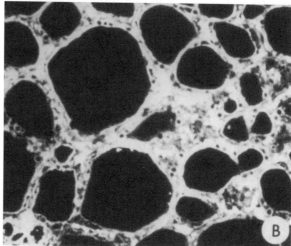

Fig. 7-9. Autoantibodies to thyroid in sera of reovirus-infected mice detected by indirect immunofluorescence. **(A)** Frozen section of normal mouse thyroid incubated with sera obtained from mice 21 days after infection, showing staining of colloid characteristic of antithyroglobulin antibody (original magnification, ×200). **(B)** Section of normal mouse thyroid (fixed in Bouin's solution) incubated with sera obtained from mice 21 days after infection, showing staining of thyroid acinar cells (original magnification, ×200). (From Okayasu I, Hatokeyama S,[420] with permission.)

blocking antibodies (TSBAb), and thyrotropin-binding inhibiting antibodies (TBIAb)[116,117] are present in Graves' disease, as described in Chapter 11. These are γ-globulins and are usually IgG.

Sera from some patients can contain a γ-globulin that has T$_4$ and T$_3$ binding activity.[118] This activity represents another antibody response to the TG antigen. The antibodies do not alter thyroid function significantly but can cause confusion in diagnosis due to artefacts in the T_4 and T_3 RIA.

The cytotoxicity of circulating antibodies has also been explored using systems in which nonimmunized lymphocytes or macrophages are coated with antibody. Exposure of these cells to antigen-coated target cells destroys the latter cells.[119,120] This reaction does not require complement.

The circulating antibodies are normal Ig molecules and can be of all types (IgM, IgA, IgG), but are primarily IgG. The IgG molecules are predominantly class I and II, with proportionally lower amounts of class III and increased amounts of class IV.[121] The specific relation of such types or classes to specific disease is not clear, although it may be noted that IgG_1, IgG_2, and IgG_3 subclass antibodies readily bind complement and might therefore be active in ADCC. Furthermore, most or all of the TSAb is found in the IgG_1 class.[112] The distribution of antibodies within specific classes appears to be characteristic of an individual and remains constant over years. Antibody titers obviously increase during the process of development of AITD, but this is not clearly documented. After first observation, they tend to be stable over months. RAI therapy augments antibody levels in Graves' disease,[122] and acute viral infections, or exposure to high levels of IFN-γ[123] or IL-2[124] also does so. With treatment of Graves' disease or replacement therapy in Hashimoto's thyroiditis or myxedema, there is characteristically a gradual reduction in antibody levels over months or years, and some patients with total destruction of thyroid tissue eventually lose detectable antibody titers.

Information is beginning to emerge on the specific B cell epitopes for TG and TPO. Most TG epitopes are located between aa 1097–1560, and antibodies from many individuals recognize an epitope between aa 1149–1250.[125,126] Using monoclonal antibodies interacting with polyvalent human serum, seven epitopic domains of TPO are recognized, and animals are known to react with a further 40 to 50 domains. The exact positions of the domains to which human autoantibodies form are not known. Similar studies on TPO have indicated at least eight major domains for human autoantibodies that are probably conformational epitopes. Using recombinant proteins and synthetic peptides, human anti-

TPO antibodies are found to recognize apparently linear epitopes in the area of aa 590–622 and 710–722.[127]

Some TPO antibodies cross-react with TG,[128] suggesting that a common epitope could play a role in initial development of autoimmunity.

Peripheral blood mononuclear cells and thyroid lymphocytes from patients with AITD have among them activated cells that spontaneously secrete anti-TG and anti-McAg/TPO antibodies.[129,130] B cell production of antibodies to McAg/TPO and TG is most easily shown using cells incubated with mitogens. Specific antibody secretion in response to PBMC stimulation by TG or purified TPO is more difficult to demonstrate.[130–135] In patients with AITD, approximately 50 B cells secreting anti-TG antibodies are found per 10^6 PBMC (~2 percent of total Ig-secreting cells) by using plaque-forming assays after stimulation of PBMC with pokeweed mitogen. Fewer are found on stimulation with TG.[131] Synthesis of anti-TG antibodies by PBMC can also be detected by enzyme-linked immunosorbent assay.[133] B cells from AITD patients synthesize antibodies in response to insolubilized TG bound to Sepharose,[136] which appears to function as an especially good antigen. There are reports of production of anti-TSH-R antibodies in vitro, but in general this response has been difficult to verify.

During initiation of AITD, thyroid autoantibody formation presumably occurs in lymph nodes draining the thyroid. In fully developed AITD, the thyroid is clearly an important source of autoantibody. In fact, since there are relatively few circulating specific autoantibody-secreting B cells,[137] it has been suggested that autoantibody formation occurs mainly or uniquely in the thyroid, where autoantibody-secreting cells are more easily demonstrated.[134] However, lymph nodes or other organs also contribute to autoantibody production, since patients with apparently destroyed thyroid tissue, or those with resected thyroids,[138] continue to have circulating thyroid autoantibodies. The total number of B cells among PBMC has been reported to be increased in Graves' disease.[132]

Cell-mediated Immunity

Techniques for identifying T lymphocyte reactivity to foreign or autologous antigens depend on culturing mixed peripheral leukocytes or semipurified

thyroid or blood lymphocytes with an antigen to which the cells may have been presensitized. Upon re-exposure to antigen, the sensitized cells change to a blastlike immature form, synthesize new protein, RNA, and DNA, and directly or through liberated effector molecules alter the function of target cells. Different end points characterize the various assays, including measurement of [³H]-thymidine uptake, assay of migration inhibitory factor (MIF), or leukocyte migration inhibition (LMI),[139] mobility of lymphocytes, and lymphokine assay. Lymphocytes and antigen are cocultured, and the supernatant is assayed for its content of lymphokine such as IL-1, IL-2, or IFN-γ by bioassay or RIA.

Other assays have also been employed. The ability of circulating B lymphocytes to bind TG-coated red blood cells[140] or to destroy TG-coated target cells[141] can be measured. Lymphocytes binding antigen (B cells) can be detected by radioautography of smears of peripheral leukocytes exposed to ¹²⁵I-labeled human TG.

Numerous reports have shown that T cell immunity can be detected in Graves' disease, thyroiditis, and primary myxedema, although responsivity of T cells to thyroid antigens is much less than to exogenous antigens such as tetanus toxoid or tuberculin. Thyroid and peripheral blood T cells from patients with AITD cultured with mitogens and APCs direct B cells to produce anti-TG or antimicrosomal antibodies.[142] PBMC, or thyroid T cells + B cells + APCs, respond to TG and microsomal antigen with antibody production, although the response is usually weak and not present in many patients. Peripheral blood T cells respond to incubation with TG by thymidine incorporation.[143] T cells secrete lymphotoxin in response to incubation with thyroid particulate membrane material, which presumably includes microsomal antigen.[144] Thyroid T cells responding to TG were reported to be of the CD4+ or 5/9 positive T helper type[145], or occasionally CD8+ cells.[146] T cells also respond to crude thyroid antigen, possibly microsomal antigen, in LMI.[147] T cell lines and T cell clones from patients with AITD respond to microsomal antigen by [³H]-thymidine incorporation.[148] T cell lines and short-term T cell clones (CD4+) are stimulated during coculture with thyroid epithelial cells (TECs) to incorporate [³H]-thymidine; DR+ TECs are especially effective stimulators.[149–151] The identity of the antigen recognized on TECs is unknown.

The specific peptide epitope fragments of TPO recognized by lymphocytes of patients with Hashimoto's thyroiditis were noted previously. Identification of T cell epitopes present within the extracellular domain of the TSH-R is now underway in several laboratories. Our studies indicate that peptides bearing sequences of aa 119–176, 158–176, 237–252, and 248–263 are especially important.[152]

In patients with Graves' disease and Hashimoto's thyroiditis, T cell–mediated immunity directed against antigens present in liver mitochondria has been detected using the lymphotoxin and LMI assays.[153] Similar responses are characteristic of primary biliary cirrhosis. The significance of this finding in thyroid disease is obscure, but such antimitochondrial immunity is present in most organ-specific autoimmune diseases.

T cell responses to an antigenic stimulus may use a wide variety of variable (V) TCR gene segments, or the response may involve (be restricted to) a few V segments. Restriction to V-β 8 segments has been found in some experimental autoimmune models. Restricted V-α and V-β usage has been reported by Davies and co-workers[154,155] and denied by Weetman's group.[156]

While T cell immunization is conventionally recognized by a stimulatory effect of antigen, direct T cell cytotoxicity of thyroid cells has been recognized in a few studies. For example, Davies and co-workers developed a CD8+ T cell clone that was cytotoxic to autologous TEC and was appropriately class I restricted.

Immune Complexes

In addition to the antibody and T cell responses, circulating immune complexes are found in patients with autoimmune thyroid disease as would be anticipated, although their pathogenic importance appears minimal. In a certain sense this is most fortuitous. Since many individuals have circulating TG antibodies and antigen, if the immune complexes caused serious disease, a plaque would ensue. Fortunately the immune complexes of TG and its antibody bind complement weakly and do not cause serious illness such as immune-complex nephritis, except in rare instances.[157–159] Immune complexes can be recognized around the basement membrane of thyroid follicular cells.[160,161] Immune complexes can be identified by specific assays in patients with Graves' disease and in thyroid cancer patients but usually not in Hashimoto's thyroiditis. Binding of antibodies to antigen on TECs could lead to their destruction by macrophages or K cells.[162-165] Release of thyroglobulin into the circulation can cause formation of immune complexes, which are rapidly removed from the circulation, and the process ultimately depletes circulating antibody levels.[92] It is possible that this antigen-dependent antibody depletion is the explanation of the lower levels of anti-TG antibody found in Graves' disease, compared to Hashimoto's thyroiditis, since the thyroid of Graves' disease releases more TG than that of Hashimoto's thyroiditis.

Killer and Natural Killer Cell Responses

Many studies have reported on natural killer cell activity and antibody-dependent cell-mediated cytotoxicity (ADCC); their conclusions vary. Endo et al.[163] found natural killer cells were decreased in Graves' disease and Hashimoto's thyroiditis and presented evidence that this was due to saturation of their Fc receptors by immune complexes. Normal natural killer and ADCC activity were found in Hashimoto's thyroiditis PBMC[166] in one study. Amino et al.[167] found decreased natural killer cells in Graves' disease, and increased natural killer cells in Hashimoto's thyroiditis. ADCC of thyroid cells, mediated by normal PBMC, was induced by anti-McAg antibody positive sera.[168] ADCC was increased in Hashimoto's thyroiditis and in postpartum thyroiditis and thought to be related to thyroid cell destruction.[169] Iwatani et al.[170] found decreased large granular lymphs in Graves' disease and interpreted this to be due to decreased natural killer cells, which might help perpetuate Graves' disease. IL-2, known to activate thyroiditis, may do this in part by activating natural killer cells, which then become cytotoxic for TECs.

Cytokines

IFN-γ is produced in the thyroid by infiltrating lymphocytes. It increases HLA class I and II expression on the surface of TECs. It also directly inhibits TEC iodination and thyroglobulin synthesis.[170,171] IL-2 can activate lymphocytes to produce IFN-γ and activate natural killer cells. TNF-α is produced by infiltrating macrophages and is potentially cytotoxic to TEC. TEC can produce IL-1, which may activate T cells, and IL-6, which stimulates B cells.[172]

To summarize, augmented pools of activated and resting T and B cells reactive to thyroid antigen exist in patients with AITD. The time course of development of these reactive cells, before clinical disease is apparent, has not been established. The cells respond to "normal" antigen, and some reactive cells exist in "normal" individuals. Immune complex formation appears to be of limited importance in the disease process. Killer and natural killer activity may be reduced in Graves' disease and increased in Hashimoto's thyroiditis and may contribute to the course of the disease—proliferative in Graves' disease and destructive in Hashimoto's thyroiditis.

EXPERIMENTAL THYROIDITIS IN ANIMALS

Chronic thyroiditis histologically identical to that in Hashimoto's thyroiditis occurs spontaneously in obese strain (OS) chickens,[173] beagles,[174] mice, and rats. It can be induced in dogs,[175] mice, rats, hamsters, guinea pigs, rabbits, monkeys,[176] and baboons[177] by immunization with autologous or allogenic thyroid homogenate mixed with adjuvants or by using heterologous TG,[178] or TG that has been arsenylated or otherwise chemically modified.[1] An important thyroiditogenic epitope includes thyroxine residue (aa 2553) in human TG.[179] Induced thyroiditis leads to formation of humoral antibodies and T cell–mediated immunity. Usually the histologic pattern conforms to that of T cell–mediated immunity.[180-181] Antibody titers are reduced and thyroiditis is intensified by splenectomy of immunized monkeys. This result suggests that circulating antibodies may inhibit T cell–mediated immunity. Thyroiditis is prevented by pretreatment with immunosuppressive agents such as cyclophosphamide or antilymphocyte serum.[182,183] In the Buffalo rat, spontaneous thyroiditis is enhanced by neonatal thymectomy,[184] perhaps because this depletes suppressor cells that are still resident in the thymus. In most studies, the intensity of the thyroiditis correlates better with T cell–mediated immunity than with antibody levels and can be transferred by T cells but not antibodies; both CD4+ and CD8+ T cells are usually needed for transfer.[85] In normal mice, thyroiditis can be produced by immunization with mouse TG in adjuvant and transferred to isogenic animals by sensitized Ly-1+ T cells. The same cells, given before immunization, vaccinate against the development of thyroiditis during subsequent immunization.[186] A specific peptide sequence from pig TPO (aa 774–788) has been found to produce thyroiditis when used to immunize C57BL/6 mice.[187] Experimental immunity typically subsides when exposure to immunizing antigen is discontinued.[188]

Spontaneous thyroiditis in OS chickens seems to differ significantly from that in most of the experimental models discussed above. For example, it is dependent on bursal cells and is intensified by thymectomy, and the extent of thyroiditis does not correlate closely with antibody production. The disease can be transferred by thymocytes of neonatal OS chicks, so abnormal T cells are involved in the pathogenesis. Some evidence suggests that the thyroid of the newly hatched chick is intrinsically abnormal, since its function is partially nonsuppressible by thyroid hormone.[189–191]

Lymphocytic thyroiditis occurs spontaneously in the BB/W rat strain and the NOD mouse line. In both instances, there are associated abnormalities in the animals' immune system. In the BB/W rat, administration of excess iodine augments the incidence of thyroiditis.[192] The mechanism for the effect of iodine is uncertain, but a similar action in the OS chicken (see above) is correlated with increased iodination and increased immunogenicity of TG.[193] Antithyroid drugs suppress the thyroiditis, perhaps because of diminished iodination of TG or through some action such as an antioxidant.

The important studies of Weigle et al.[194,195] found that after rabbits were first immunized with a heterologous or chemically modified isogenic TG, they responded immunologically to administration of unaltered TG. Apparently a variety of antibodies (isoantibodies) are produced, some of which have determinants cross-reacting with determinants on normal rabbit TG (isoantigens). Reaction to normal TG can apparently continue the immune process once it has been initiated by altered TG. Weigle et al. postulate that antibody reacting with normal TG removes it from the circulation, thus removing the normal low-dose suppression of T cells by TG, allowing them to provide help in anti-TG synthesis.[196]

Aging cats have a high incidence of hyperthyroidism, apparently due to autonomously functioning nodules.[197] To date autoimmunity has not been demonstrated in these animals, so the process does not appear to be a model for Graves' disease.

One general concept derived from these studies is that a balance of helper and suppressor T cell function is needed to prevent autoimmunity and that a variety of perterbations lead to onset of the disease.

RELATION OF THE IMMUNE RESPONSE TO THYROID CELL STIMULATION AND DESTRUCTION

We know for certain that autoantibodies can stimulate the thyroid and cause overactivity in Graves' disease and can in select circumstances inhibit thyroid function and cause hypothyroidism in neonates and some adults. Whether anti-TG or anti-McAg/TPO antibodies are primary cytotoxic agents in AITD remains an unsettled issue. TG antibodies are probably not normally cytotoxic, but antimicrosomal antibodies can certainly mediate complement-dependent thyroid cell cytotoxicity. However, the frequently reproduced natural experiment of transplacental antibody passage from a mother with AITD to her fetus, without evidence of thyroid damage, suggests that antibodies alone are not destructive to the thyroid. Cell-mediated immunity is thought to be important in thyroid cell destruction, and T cells have been shown to be reactive to thyroid epithelial cells. In a few studies, T cell lines or clones have been shown to react to thyroid epithelial cells.[151,198] The nature of the antigen recognized is unknown. One CD8+ T cell clone was shown to be cytotoxic specifically to autologous thyroid epithelial cells,[199] confirming the belief that cell-mediated TEC destruction could be an important process. In animals it is clearly shown that there can be a marked dissociation between the extent of histologic thyroiditis and the levels of antibodies, again suggesting that T cells rather than antibodies mediate cell destruction.

POSSIBLE EXPLANATIONS FOR AUTOIMMUNITY

Many reasons for the development of autoimmunity have been advanced, and several of these are briefly catalogued below. Some of these have been examined in relation to AITD and are discussed more extensively in the following sections. Currently cross-reacting epitopes, aberrant T or B cell regulatory mechanisms, inheritance of specific immune response–related genes, and aberrant HLA-DR expression on TECs are considered important for development of antithyroid immunity.

1. Abnormal presentation of antigen could occur due to cell destruction or viral invasion, thus liberating large amounts of antigen or cell fragments into lymphatics. Excessive levels of antigen are produced, thereby overwhelming the usual low dose tolerance mechanism.

2. Abnormal antigen could be produced by a malignancy, cell damage from viral attack, or other means. This antigen could be, for example, a partially degraded or denatured normal antigen.

3. Cross-reacting epitopes[200]: Bacterial epitopes, e.g., *Yersinia enterocolitica*, could induce immune responses that happen to cross-react with a self-antigen having identical conformation.

   Cross-reacting idiotypic responses: An extension of the above concept, in that the normal anti-idiotypic control response happens to produce an Ig or T cell that cross-reacts with self-antigen. For example, experimentally produced anti-idiotypic monoclonal antibodies directed to anti-TSH antibodies bind to and stimulate the TSH-R.[201]

4. Somatic mutation of a TCR gene[202] could lead to a clone of self-reactive cells. However, somatic mutation of TCR genes is believed to occur rarely, and such monoclonal or oligoclonal activation has not been documented in autoimmune disease.

   Somatic mutation of a B cell Ig gene is, as described above, a normal phenomenon during an antigen-driven proliferative response. Such an event could occur by chance during response to any antigen. However, this does not effectively introduce any new variable, since B cells capable of producing Ig molecules that can react with self-antigen are already normally present.

5. Inheritance of specific HLA-DR, HLA-DQ, HLA-DP, HLA-ABC,[203] TCR, or other genes that code for proteins having especially effective ability to process or present antigen.

6. T cell or B cell feedback control mechanisms[204,205] could be aberrant due to hereditary or environmental factors.

7. Lack of clonal deletion[206] could leave self-reactive T cells present in the adult. In fact, to some extent this is clearly normal, as described above.

8. Failure of normal maturation[207] of the immune system could allow autoreactive and widely specific fetal T and B cells to exist.

9. Polyclonal activation[208] of T or B cells could, by some unknown stimulus, lead to B cells producing self-reactive Ig in the apparent absence of antigenic stimulus. This theory is in a sense impossible to disprove but would need to coexist with other abnormalities to explain disease remission, genetic associations, associated diseases, and so on. Polyclonal activation is not typical of peripheral lymphocytes of patients with AITD.[209]

10. Normal DR$^-$ cells could become DR$^+$ and then could function as APCs for antigens, including those on their cell surface.

11. Environmental factors could distort normal control; for example, stress or steroids may alter T or B cell populations and excess IL-2 or IFN may be produced and activate thyroiditis.

Abnormal Exposure to Thyroid Antigens

Damage to the thyroid might release normally segregated antigens, inducing an immune response. Damage to thyroid cells does indeed occur in viral thyroiditis, as in association with mumps or in subacute thyroiditis of unknown cause, but autoantibodies appear only transiently at low titer, and progressive lesions of the thyroid do not usually occur. The few cases of myxedema after mumps thyroiditis reported by Eyquem et al.[210] had a high antibody titer from the start, and stimulation of a preexisting thyroid lesion cannot be excluded. It seems unlikely that a limited period of TG release, such as occurs in subacute thyroiditis, could lead to a progressive autoimmune process, since this condition is not a known sequela of subacute thyroiditis or of subtotal thyroidectomy or ^{131}I therapy for the normal thyroid, situations in which TG is released transiently into the circulation. However, up to 50 percent of patients with thyroid cancer can be shown to have blastogenic responses to TG, and in this instance continued exposure to high levels of antigen may play a role.[211] External irradiation to the thyroid also leads to a marked increase in Graves' disease and ophthalmopathy.[212]

Attention was given in past years to a possible lesion of the thyroid basement membrane that could permit a low but persistent escape of antigen from the thyroid follicles and set the stage for autoimmunization.[213] Basement membrane defects appear in experimental thyroiditis, which strongly suggests that they are a secondary phenomenon.

An argument against the hidden antigen hypothesis is that TG is a normal component of circulating plasma. It is present in sera from parturient women, in newborn infants, and in sera derived from cross-sections of adult populations, including patients with AITD.[214] TSH stimulation normally causes discharge of TG into lymph and plasma.[215] One might turn the first argument around and suggest that thyroiditis results from a lack of exposure to TG at some period, an exposure that is necessary to depress continuously an otherwise inevitable immune response. This suggestion has no clinical or experimental support, and the available evidence indicates that TG is present in the plasma of patients with active immunity.

An abnormal presentation of a normal antigen is possible. Animals and humans will develop antibodies against feeble tumor antigens if these are given by intracutaneous administration or mixed with an adjuvant.[216] This fact may imply a modification of antigenic structure or unusual contact of antigen with tissue macrophages attracted to the adjuvant. Since TG is present in both plasma and lymph, it is not obvious what this hypothetical abnormal mode of appearance could be.

Abnormal Antigens

An abnormal antigen might also serve to produce an immune reaction. The protein abnormality could be either congenital or acquired by an injury such as a virus infection. To date no evidence indicates that TG, TPO, or other proteins of the thyroid of a patient with autoimmunity are abnormal. Minor allelic differences apparently do occur. TPO exists in two forms of 107 and 105 kD, and the TSH-R gene apparently gives rise to a full-length and amino-terminal variant. However, it is not known that these lead to autoimmunity. An abnormal protein, or more likely an abnormal concentration of a normal protein, has been described in Hashimoto's thyroiditis. Patients with this illness typically have increased peptide-bound butanol-insoluble iodine in their plasma. This substance, once thought to be synthesized in the thyroid,[217] appears to be serum albumin iodinated in the gland[218] and represents a dramatic increase of a normal thyroid and plasma constituent.

Mutations that alter TPO and TG have been described (Chapter 16) but not in association with AITD. Bahn et al.[85] reported a point mutation in the TSH-R of two patients with Graves' ophthalmopathy (PRO52THR), but this is apparently actually a fairly common allele rather than a mutation.

Cross-Reacting Antigens

The theory that immune reactivity to an environmental antigen could lead to antibodies that cross-react with thyroid antigens has been bolstered by studies that show a relationship between Graves' disease and antibodies to the common enteropathogen *Y. enterocolitica*. An increased incidence of antibodies to *Yersinia* is found by some, but not all authors, in patients who have Graves' disease,[219,220] and patients with Graves' disease have positive LMI tests to *Yersinia* antigens. There are saturable binding sites for TSH on *Yersinia* proteins.[221] After infection by *Yersinia*, human sera contain Ig molecules that bind to TEC cytoplasm[200] and molecules that appear to compete with TSH for binding to thyroid membrane TSH receptors.[222] Wenzel et al.[223] have shown that the antigens involved are actually proteins encoded by plasmids present in *Yersinia*, rather than intrinsic *Yersinia* proteins, but that does not alter the general concept. A related hypothesis is that *Yersinia* antibodies lead to production of anti-idiotype antibodies that cross-react with thyroid antigens. There is no evidence for this hypothesis so far.

Obviously a question to be addressed, if *Yersinia* infection does prove to be somehow related to AITD, is why only a portion of the individuals who have contact with *Yersinia* develop Graves' disease. And it is also possible that the increased prevalence of antibodies to *Yersinia* represents a secondary phenomenon occurring because of enhanced immunity in Graves' disease.

Other recent studies suggest a relation between bacterial antigen and self-reactivity. Staphylococcal enterotoxins are very potent mitogens for human T lymphocytes. Concentrations less than 10^{-9} M activate T cells polyclonally in the presence of APC expressing HLA-D molecules. It has not been demonstrated that staphylococcal enterotoxins play a role in thyroid or other human autoimmune processes. In mice, staphyloccal enterotoxins are also highly mitogenic for T cells and behave like "superantigens" that stimulate T cells expressing certain families of TCRs. Thus in the murine system there is a link between reactivity to these potent bacterial products and the repertoire of TCRs expressed by inbred strains of mice. It will be of interest to find out whether a similar relationship exists between human TCR families and reactivity to staphylococcal enterotoxins. A second development concerns the role of heat shock proteins (HSPs) in immunity to infectious agents and possibly autoimmunity. HSPs are produced by prokaryotic and eukaryotic cells in response to heat and other forms of cellular injury. Because their structure is highly conserved in all cells studied, the potential cross-reactivity between HSPs from pathogens and humans is great. A number of pathogenetic organisms have presented HSPs as antigens in animal and human models. It is therefore possible that immunization against HSP from pathogen may lead to cross-reactivity with autologous HSPs released from damaged tissues. It is of some interest that the HLA region contains genes for the major HSP70, and polymorphisms in the HSP70 gene are associated with Graves' disease.[224] This finding could provide another link between HLA and susceptibility to infection and autoimmunity. HSPs are expressed at a high level in thyroid cells from patients with Graves' disease and in fibroblasts from patients with exophthalmos.[225] These changes may be secondary to cytokine stimulation but may be involved in an immune response.

Antibodies to TG sometimes also recognize TPO.[226] The exact reason for this is uncertain, but may—or may not—relate to short stretches of shared peptide sequence. In theory an initial response to one antigen might proceed by reacting to the other antigen and thereby spread and augment the autoimmune process.

Virus Infection

Virus infection has for years been a suspected etiologic factor in most autoimmune diseases. Proposed mechanisms include causing cell destruction and liberating antigens, forming altered antigens, inducing DR expression, or inducing $CD8^+$ T cell responses to viral antigens expressed on the cell surface. Antithyroid antibodies are elevated transiently after subacute thyroiditis, which is thought to be a virus-associated syndrome, but no clear evidence of virus-induced autoimmune thyroiditis in humans has been presented. In this regard it is of great interest that persistent, apparently benign virus infection of the thyroid can be induced in mice[227] and that infection of neonatal mice with reovirus induces a polyendocrine autoimmunity (Fig. 7-9). Cell destruction by other means can also lead to antithyroid immunization in animals. For example, iodide-induced necrosis of the thyroid, accompanied by administration of lipopolysaccharide, causes antithyroid immunization in mice.[228] These agents could work by liberating thyroid antigens. Virus infection might also augment autoimmunity by causing nonspecific secretion of IL-2 or by inducing DR expression on TEC. Insertion of retroviral sequences into thyroid cell DNA was reported to be a feature of Graves' disease,[229] but current evidence suggests this was probably an error.[230]

Lymphocyte Mutation and Oligoclonality

Some researchers have suggested that mutation of a B cell Ig gene or T cell receptor gene could play an important role in the pathogenesis of AITD by forming clones of cells producing autoantibodies.[202] A B cell Ig gene mutation could, as noted above, develop normally during the course of antigen-driven clonal expansion and add one more clone of cells to the already present pool of cells and thus make antithyroid antibodies. This event would not seem too crucial, since it would not lead to a significant antibody response unless T cell help was also induced. Also, in every circumstance in AITD the antibodies are polyclonal,[231] although in some antibody responses (such as to the TSH-R), there is evidence for favored utilization of λ-light chains.[232] Ig gene rearrangement in lymphocytes from patients with AITD has been shown to be polyclonal,[233] although there is no study on the specific B cells producing antithyroid antibodies.

Benign T cell mutation producing a clone of self-reactive T cells was suggested by Volpe[196] as a cause of AITD, but there is no evidence for somatic mutation of TCRs. The fact that so many diverse autoimmune responses are associated with thyroid disease also argues against this kind of event, which would theoretically induce a very narrow spectrum of autoimmune responses.

T cell receptor gene rearrangement has been shown to be polyclonal in AITD,[233] but this study did not examine T cells specifically reacting to thyroid antigens.

Genetic Predisposition

The role of heredity in AITD is striking, since there is a markedly augmented incidence of AITD among family members, first-degree relatives, and twins of patients with the illness.[234] For example, the incidence of thyroid abnormalities in children of parents with Graves' disease is nearly double that in control children.[235]

Hashimoto's thyroiditis, Graves' disease, and myxedema all occur in families.[236-238] In an investigation of the relatives of a group of *propositi* with high circulating antibody levels and clinical thyroid disease, approximately half of the siblings and parents (first-order relatives) were found to have significant titers of thyroid antibodies, many being without clinical thyroid disease. The results of antibody tests in other relatives were also consistent with the transmission of the tendency to thyroid autoimmunity from either parent[239,240] by a codominant[241] or possibly a dominant[242] mechanism. Forbes et al.[243] found a similar high incidence of complement-fixing antibodies in the relatives of patients with Hashimoto's thyroiditis. A study by Hall and colleagues[244] of the parents of a group of children with histologically proven Hashimoto's thyroiditis disclosed that in almost all cases one or both of the parents had overt thyroid disease or there were close relatives with thyroid disorders or circulating antibodies. Hashimoto's thyroiditis has been reported in both members of two pairs of identical twins.[245] TSAb is also reported to occur in relatives of patients with Graves' disease.[246]

Hashimoto's thyroiditis may occur in kindred also displaying Graves' disease, myxedema, or nontoxic goiter. This finding suggests that these diseases have a common genetic defect.

The important hereditary risk factor so far recognized is the inheritance of certain MHC class II genes. Inheritance of HLA-DR3 causes up to sixfold increased risk for the occurrence of Graves' disease or atrophic thyroiditis, and inheritance of HLA-DR5 has been found in some studies to increase the incidence of goitrous hypothyroidism[203,247-250] (that is, Hashimoto's thyroiditis). In postpartum painless thyroiditis[251,252] association is found with both HLA-DR4 and DR5. In our study, Graves' disease is strongly associated with a specific subtype of DR3

and equally associated with a subtype of DQw2; the dual association occurs because of the linkage of the two genes.[249] Recent studies have identified HLA-DQA1*0501, which is often linked to DR3, as having an even more pronounced predisposing effect in Caucasians.[253] This is especially important in males, in whom the presence of DQA1*0501 increases the risk of Graves' disease 11-fold[254] and may be related to the presence of arginine at position 51 of DQA1 alleles.[254a] The HLA genes, conferring increased risk, are not unique alleles but rather appear to be the same gene expressed in healthy individuals. At least the sequence of the important first extracellular domain is the same in controls and patients with AITD carrying DR3.[255] The HLA linkages found in Caucasians are not found in American blacks, and different associations are found in other ethnic groups such as Koreans, Chinese, and Japanese.[256]

Many studies have attempted to relate DR3 (or DR5) inheritance to clinical features of the disease; possibly DR3 does correlate with refractoriness to induced remission with antithyroid drug treatment. Inheritance of specific Gm allotypes (V gene constant region alleles that can be recognized by specific antisera) also confers susceptibility to Graves' disease,[250,256,257] and an association with complement genes has been found.[258] Inheritance of a specific HLA-DR and Gm haplotype can predict the occurrence of Graves' disease within a family with high accuracy.[250] There is no information on how Gm specificities relate to AITD in humans. However, it is known that in animals Gm specificities are linked to development of antibody responses to particular antigens and thus may identify a particular B cell repertoire. Identifying Gm linkage to thyroid disease, and sequencing the antigen-specific Ig genes, may demonstrate specific variable segments that are "effective" in the immune response and predispose to disease.

Recent studies by Morel and co-workers[259] have for the first time provided information on how inheritance of a specific HLA molecule may induce autoimmune disease susceptibility. They found that homozygosity for HLA genes that do not have aspartic acid at residue 57 of the DQ-β chain carries a 100-fold increased risk for insulin-dependent diabetes mellitus (IDDM). Similar observations have been made for inheritance of diabetes in NOD mice. A study of molecular models indicates that aspartic acid-57 may be situated so that it points into the

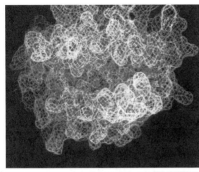

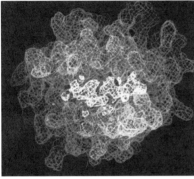

Fig. 7-10. Van der Waals surface representation of the top of the HLA-A2 molecule **(A)** showing the deep groove identified as the antigen recognition site and the electron density **(B)** found in this site. The molecule is shown from the top. Van der Waals surface of the domains show a deep groove running between the helical regions in the domains. This groove has been identified as the recognition site for processed antigens. The extra electron density found in one crystal form is shown superimposed on the Van der Waals surface. The extra density represents a bound molecule or mixture of molecules that copurified and cocrystalized. Some regions of the extra density may be wide enough to accommodate a peptide in an α-helical conformation, but without knowing its composition or whether it is one species or a mixture, it is not possible to interpret its structure unambiguously. (From Bjorkman et al.,[259a] with permission.)

"cleft" of the DQ molecule, where it can form an ionic bond with an antigen presented in the cleft (Fig. 7-10). This could affect the function of the DQ molecule by altering its ability to present an alloantigen such as a virus or an autoantigen or could, for example, limit its ability to present self-antigen in the normal process of clonal selection (Fig. 7-7) We may postulate that the inheritance of HLA-DR3 molecules that have an especially good or bad "fit" for presentation of a thyroid antigen may similarly act

by influencing the selection of the TCR repertoire or antigen presentation.

Although the observations on DQ-β aspartic acid-57 have provided a dramatic new explanation of the hereditary influence in autoimmunity, certain problems exist in the theoretical construct. For example, if the unique HLA-DQ molecule should function on an APC as an especially good presenter of autoantigen, then T cells recognizing this fit should be clonally deleted in the fetus and absent in the adult. Contrariwise, if aspartic acid-57 in the cleft prevents presentation of specific self-antigen, T cells having receptors for this antigen would survive but, logically, poor antigen presentation would also exist in adult life and prevent development of an immune response. Fitting this observation correctly into the general picture of immune regulation awaits more information.

We also must note that linkage of AITD to specific DR genes is relatively weak, that most individuals with DR3 or DR5 do not have AITD, and that linkage is found in Oriental and black American populations to other DR specificities. However, it remains possible that a common structural similarity exists in the HLA-D genes of AITD patients and will be exposed as this work progresses. HLA-DR3[+] patients have also been shown to be defective in clearing immune complexes.[261] At a minimum these studies certainly establish that inherited differences in the immune system are extremely, if not overwhelmingly, important in allowing development of autoimmune thyroid disease.

Recent studies may link specific T cell receptor genes to inheritance of Graves' disease. Demaine et al.[262] found a heterozygosity for a specific RFLP of the TCR-β chain to be increased in Graves' disease patients, especially those who are HLA-DR3[+]. Other workers[263] have reported that a different RFLP for the TCRα chain V region is increased in frequency in patients with primary hypothyroidism. Inheritance of a specific RFLP for a TCR gene would imply inheritance of a certain set of TCR, V, D, or J gene segments. It is, in a sense, a gross view of the repertoire of TCRs present in one individual.

Since it has been demonstrated that unique TCR gene variable segments are dominant in the T cell response occurring in experimental allogeneic encephalitis, it becomes interesting to analyze TCR genes present in CD4[+] and CD8[+] antigen-specific T cell clones developed from thyroid tissue or blood of patients with AITD and to determine whether one or a few TCR variable gene segments dominate in the response to thyroid antigens. If so, inheritance of this gene would predispose to AITD. Data presented by Davies[264] suggest usage of a restricted set of TCR-α variable segments by intrathyroidal lymphocytes in AITD, but information on thyroid antigen-specific clones is not available, and other workers fail to find this selective V gene usage.[265]

A reported weak association of an RFLP of the McAg-TPO gene with Graves' disease[266] implies that a specific variation in TPO antigen expression or structure could provide yet another genetic influence on development of AITD.

Abnormalities of Immune Regulation

Co-occurrence of Autoimmune Disease

The coexistence of AITD and other diseases possibly of autoimmune cause has often been reported and suggests some intrinsic abnormality in immune regulation[267–287]. The most striking association is with pernicious anemia. Perhaps 45 percent of patients with autoimmune thyroiditis have circulating anti-gastric antibodies,[267] and the reverse association is almost as strong.[268] Up to 14 percent of patients with pernicious anemia have primary myxedema, and pernicious anemia is increased in prevalence in patients with hypothyroidism.[260] The association of Sjögren's syndrome and thyroiditis is not uncommon. Precipitating antibodies to salivary and lacrimal gland proteins have been described in Sjögren's syndrome.[269] Because of the association of Sjögren's syndrome with rheumatoid arthritis and systemic lupus erythematosus (SLE), it has been suggested that the syndrome is a manifestation of SLE.[270] Rheumatoid arthritis and Hashimoto's thyroiditis are also probably significantly associated,[270] but this association has also been denied.[271]

Some reports associate Hashimoto's thyroiditis with SLE.[272,273] Holborow found a small subset of patients with thyroiditis to have antinuclear antibodies. Claims of a high incidence of positive tests for antibodies to double-stranded DNA in active Graves' disease[274] have been denied by others,[275] who find the antibody to be directed to a nuclear antigen that is neither single-stranded DNA or double-stranded DNA. The result of this test for antinuclear factor is almost invariably positive in SLE, and high titers are found. It is less frequently detected in rheumatoid

arthritis and Sjögren's syndrome. Notoriously, patients with SLE have a strong tendency to form antibodies, even to the weak erythrocyte antigens C and N, as well as to many other body components.

Addison's disease, which is most commonly an autoimmune illness, and autoimmune thyroid disease occasionally coexist.[276] Bloodworth et al.[277] reported the results of 12 autopsies on patients with proven Addison's disease. In four the thyroid was absent or almost completely destroyed, and in another four extensive lymphocytic infiltration, fibrosis, and atrophy of thyroid acini occurred. In patients who have both Hashimoto's thyroiditis and Addison's disease, as well as circulating antibodies directed against both organs,[278] one presumes that the adrenal failure is a result of an autoimmune process.[279] Addison's disease is associated with other presumed autoimmune disorders, including hypophysitis[280] and premature ovarian failure.[281] Occasionally, patients are found with remarkable combinations, such as idiopathic hypothyroidism, hypoparathyroidism, hypoadrenalism, moniliasis, and pernicious anemia.[282] Karlish and MacGregor[283] have reported a group of 10 patients with thyroiditis and Graves' disease or with thyroiditis and Addison's disease, possibly triggered by sarcoidosis.

Cirrhosis of the liver with extensive lymphocytic and plasma cell infiltration of the portal tracts has been reported in Hashimoto's thyroiditis.[284] In some patients with this syndrome, there are complement-fixing autoantibodies that react with thyroid, liver, and sometimes kidney tissue, and lupus erythematosus cells can occasionally be found. The condition may fall under the heading of lupoid hepatitis, described by Mackay and colleagues.[288] Patients with AITD react with increased frequency to liver mitochondrial antigen, as do patients with biliary cirrhosis.

Further evidence for an abnormal immune mechanism is found in the work of Blizzard et al.,[289] who encountered a high incidence of penicillin sensitivity and penicillin antibodies in patients with Hashimoto's thyroiditis. Beare[284] has also commented on the frequency of a history of allergic disease in these patients. Functional abnormalities of the thyroid, possibly related to autoimmunity[290] and antithyroid antibodies are frequent in the mothers of patients with Down's syndrome.[291,292]

Thyroid antibodies, thyroiditis, and primary thyroid failure occur with increased frequency among patients with diabetes.[293] The association is primarily with IDDM, in which anti-islet cell immunity is believed to play an etiologic role.[294] Other associations include idiopathic thromobytopenic purpura and Graves' disease, vitiligo and Graves' disease,[295,296] and thyroiditis,[297] thyroid antibodies in leprosy,[298] and the long-recognized co-occurrence of myasthenia and Graves' disease.

Together these data provide convincing proof of an association of other autoimmune phenomena with AITD. Most typically, this immunity is organ specific, but in one subset of patients, antithyroid immunity develops in association with the non-organ-specific collagen diseases. A syndrome, or running together, of course, does not prove a causal association. Nevertheless, the plethora of associations indicates that a defect in the immune system may be more likely than primary defects in each organ.

Phenomena and Mechanisms

Possible abnormalities in immunoregulation have been addressed in hundreds of studies. The basic hypothesis of this work is that a deficiency of functional T suppressor cells—either antigen-specific or nonspecific—may allow uncontrolled T and B cell immune responses to thyroid (or other) antigens. As noted above, this concept is a major theme in experimentally induced or naturally occurring thyroiditis in animal models.

Immune regulation is extremely complex and only partially understood. The studies described below have been reported over a decade, during which time our understanding of lymphocyte function, terminology, and methods of analysis have continually changed. Most of these studies define immunoregulatory responses in relation to an in vitro assay done in unique conditions or a group of cells bearing a specific surface antigen (e.g., CD4, CD8). As we have previously noted, T cell antigen expression and function can vary depending on stimulating event, culture, or other conditions. Further, whether a unique group of "suppressor cells" actually exists is uncertain. Thus we present these observations as reported (by us and others) and in the terms used by the authors.

Sridama and DeGroot found decreased suppressor cells, defined as CD8+ peripheral blood T cells, in patients with Graves' disease.[204,205] These results have been challenged, and some investigators have

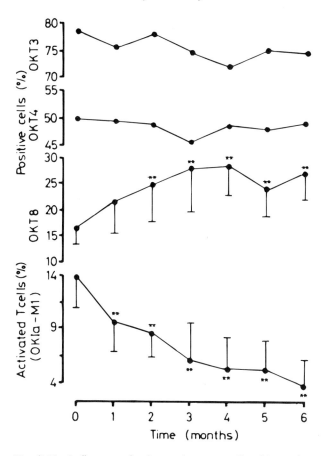

Fig. 7-11. Influence of a 6-month course of carbimazole on peripheral blood T cell subsets of 29 patients with hyperthyroid Graves' disease (Mean ± SD). OKT_4 = CD4+; OKT_3 = CD3+; OKT_8 = CD8+. ** = $P < .001$ vs. zero time value (From Ludgate et al.,[300] with permission.)

reported depression of CD4+ cells in AITD.[299] However, overall there is now clear agreement that in thyrotoxic patients with Graves' disease, a decrease in CD8+ T cell number[300–303] and function[205] is characteristically present, and that a similar abnormality exists in the thyroid. CD8+ cells return gradually toward normal during therapy and are usually but not always normal at the end of therapy[204,300] (Fig. 7-11). The phenomenon is present but less evident in Hashimoto's thyroiditis patients. It has been attributed by some workers to increased thyroid hormone levels,[304] although this issue is clouded, since there are reports suggesting and disproving the idea that hyperthyroidism per se induces suppressor cell abnormalities in humans, and reduced suppressor T cells (T_s) are found long after thyrotoxicosis is cured.[305] Our interpretation is that the abnormality is not due specifically to excess T_4 in blood but is a manifestation of ongoing active autoimmunity. Reduced nonspecific "suppressor" T cell function may be in part an inherited abnormality and is probably also a manifestation of the augmented immune reactivity ongoing in toxic Graves' disease patients. It may be largely a secondary phenomenon, but one which augments and continues the immunologic disease.

The mechanism causing reduced T_s number and function is unclear. T_s could be reduced during an active immune response by binding immune complexes on their surface, which could inactivate the lymphocytes or cause them to be removed from circulation. T_s could also be removed by cytotoxic antibodies. Antilymphocyte antibodies, relatively specific for T_s, have been found in patients with AITD.

T cells from patients with Graves' disease are unable to suppress Ig synthesis when mixed with B cells, in comparison to T cells from normal individuals.[205] Okita et al.[306] have suggested that this is due to a low number of histamine H2 receptor-positive CD8+ cells in Graves' disease patients. Another possibly related phenomenon is the decreased pokeweed mitogen (PWM) responsivity of PBMC found in Graves' disease patients during illness[307] and also when cured of disease.[308]

An alteration in helper T/suppressor T (Th/Ts) ratio may also predispose to the occurrence of postpartum transient thyrotoxicosis. We have shown a decrease in CD4+ cells in normal pregnancy,[309] possibly representing one of the factors causing the diminished immunoreactivity typically found in pregnancy. A rebound increase in CD4+ cells, which occurs during the first two or three months following delivery, may lead to a recrudescence of immunoreactivity, including antibody levels, the occurrence of postpartum transient thyrotoxicosis in some women,[310,311] and possibly other immunologic exacerbations that occur at this time, such as flaring of lupus activity.

Thyrotoxic Graves' disease patients and those with active Hashimoto's thyroiditis have a high proportion of DR+ T cells in their peripheral circulation,[312] which indicates the presence of activated T cells. It is unlikely that these cells (> 20 percent of circulating T cells) are all related to thyroid antigens, so they must include DR+ T cells with TCRs for many other antigens. There is also a marked increase in

circulating soluble IL-2 receptors in thyrotoxic Graves' disease, but this appears to be typical of thyrotoxicosis per se, and not specifically Graves' disease.[313] Nevertheless, there is no evidence for a generalized ongoing immune hyperresponsiveness in thyrotoxic patients. Perhaps these T cells (for many different specificities) are stimulated by IL-2 or IFN-γ, but in the absence of the required "second signal" provided by antigen exposure do not induce B cell proliferation or cytotoxic responses. These alterations return to normal during therapy.[300]

Totterman et al.[301] showed that when Graves' disease patients receive antithyroid drugs (which appear to have an immunosuppressive effect, see below) their DR+CD4+ cell level falls and DR+CD8+ cell level transiently increases in the circulation. Over three or six months, during continued treatment, the DR+CD8+ cells return to their original levels (Fig. 7-12). The mechanism for this drop in activated CD4+ cells and transient and presumed beneficial rise in suppressor cells is not clear. Totterman et al.[301] propose that it is induced by some factor secreted by the thyroid gland in response to treatment.

Diminished, nonspecific suppressor cell function is observed in many autoimmune diseases, including lupus and multiple sclerosis.[314,315] Takeuchi[315] has suggested that in SLE, there is an abnormality in the ability of T cells to express CD45RA antigen during the allogeneic mixed lymphocyte reaction and that this may be an intrinsic defect.

Functional assays attempting to show a deficiency in antigen-specific suppressor cells have been reported by Noma et al.,[316] Mori et al.,[317] Iitaka et al.,[318] Tao et al.,[319] Vento et al.,[320] and Yoshikawa et al.[321] A relative deficiency of TG antigen-specific suppressor cells was found using a plaque-forming cell assay. The defect was partial and was not present in all patients. Iitaka et al.[318] showed decreased ability of CD8+ cells from patients with Graves' disease or thyroiditis to diminish PWM driven anti-McAg/TPO antibody synthesis.

Biassoni reported fewer T suppressor cells in patients with thyrotoxic Graves' disease and showed that the defect was restricted to patients with active Graves' disease and was not apparent in their normal first-degree relatives.[322] How et al.[305] found that decreased thyroid antigen-specific suppressor cell function persisted for years after therapy of Graves' disease, suggesting it was an heritable and not in-

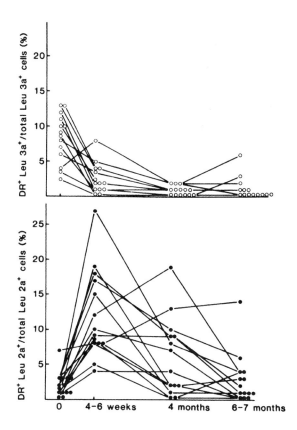

Fig. 7-12. Effect of methimazole therapy on lymphocyte subsets in six patients with Graves' disease. *Upper panel:* % DR$^+$ of all CD8$^+$ cells (activated suppressor cells). *Lower panel:* % DR$^+$ of all CD4$^+$ cells (activated helper cells). (From Mariotti et al.,[162] with permission.)

duced abnormality. While one would like to believe that an antigen-specific suppressor-cell defect might be an inherited abnormality in AITD, augmented by a nonspecific suppressor cell defect during active disease, only a few studies support this conclusion.

Many studies have examined T cell subsets in thyroid tissue of patients with active AITD.[312,323] For example, Margolick et al.[323] found increased cytotoxic/suppressor cells (Leu 2a$^+$) lacking the T cell marker Leu 1, and also increased T helper (Leu 3a$^+$) cells and a normal Th/Ts ratio. Canonica et al.[324] found increased proportions of cytotoxic/suppressor T cells in thyroids of Hashimoto's thyroiditis patients. Infiltrating cytotoxic/suppressor cells in Hashimoto's thyroiditis were found usually to be activated and to express DR antigen, whereas this response was not so obvious in Graves' disease.[317,325]

Canonica et al.[324] reported an increased proportion of activated T helper/inducer cells in both Graves' disease and Hashimoto's thyroiditis and increased cells thought to represent cytotoxic T cells in Hashimoto's thyroiditis.

Increased CD8$^+$CD11B$^-$ cells, presumed to be cytotoxic cells, were found in Graves' disease thyroids (in comparison to PBMC of Graves' disease or normal subjects), whereas "dull" CD8$^+$CD11B$^+$ natural killer cells were diminished.[326] Other studies have suggested a reduction in natural killer cells in Graves' disease and an increase in Hashimoto's thyroiditis. Tezuka et al.[327] found decreased natural killer cells in Graves' disease thyroid tissue, no differences in the natural killer activity of PBMC between Graves' and normal patients, and that the natural killer cells in Graves' disease did not kill autologous thyroid epithelial cells.[327] We have already indicated other reports of normal natural killer and ADCC in Hashimoto's PBMC and of increased ADCC in Hashimoto's thyroiditis. Most reports that have looked at Graves' disease tissues also indicate an increased proportion of B cells compared to peripheral blood subsets.

Cell cloning has also been used to examine thyroid and peripheral blood lymphocyte subsets. Bagnasco et al.[328] found a predominance of cytolytic clones releasing IFN in Hashimoto's thyroiditis but not in Graves' disease. Del Prete et al.[329] found a high proportion of cytolytic cells with the CD8$^+$ phenotype in clones from thyroid tissue and thought these results might relate to autoimmune destruction of TEC. MacKenzie et al.[330] cloned thyroidal T cells from AITD patients and found the majority to be autoreactive. Small numbers of CD4$^+$ helper/inducer cells were cloned from Graves' disease patients and CD8$^+$ cytotoxic/suppressor clones were developed from Hashimoto's thyroiditis patients. Two of the latter clones were cytotoxic to autologous TEC. We have cloned T cells from thyroid tissue of Graves' disease using McAg or TG stimulation to develop the clones. In Graves' disease the clones were predominantly CD4$^+$4B4$^+$ cells of a phenotypic helper subset.[331]

A general summary of these data is difficult. The data probably at least indicate there are increased B cells, increased DR$^+$ T cells, increased CD4$^+$DR$^+$ T helper cells, decreased CD8$^+$DR$^+$ T suppressor/cytotoxic cells, and possibly fewer natural killer cells in Graves' disease tissue and in blood than among normal subjects' PBMCs. The studies are primarily based on patients with well-developed and often treated disease and do not bear directly on early stages of the disease, or whether the changes represent primary or secondary phenomena.

To date there has been no certain indication that a nonspecific or specific suppressor cell defect exists in patients who are genetically predisposed to have AITD or in most patients who have recovered from the illness. Rather, the data suggest, at least for the better studied changes in antigen-nonspecific T cell subsets, that the changes may be a secondary although important part of disease pathology. They may play a role in disease augmentation and continuation, rather than initiation. This topic has recently been reviewed in detail.[332]

Anti-idiotype Antibodies

Whereas anti-idiotypic antibodies are thought to play a physiologic role in immunoregulation, little evidence indicates participation in, or abnormality of, this function in AITD. Immunoglobulins from some patients with Graves' disease bind TSH.[333] This suggests that anti-idiotypes to TSH antibodies are present and might theoretically function as thyroid-stimulating immunoglobulins or, conversely, that anti-idiotypes to thyroid-stimulating antibody exist and can bind TSH. One recent study indicates that these antibodies are not actually anti-idiotypic, and thus probably not disease producing.

Sikorska[334] demonstrated the presence of antibodies in sera of AITD patients that inhibit binding of TG to monoclonal anti-TG antibodies and interpreted these as anti-idiotypes. We have looked very carefully for anti-TG anti-idiotypes in patients with autoimmune thyroid disease and failed to find them.[335] Although one could postulate that a failure to produce anti-idiotype antibodies could be a feature of AITD, a more likely hypothesis is that anti-idiotypic antibodies are simply rarely produced at a detectable level. Since anti-idiotype antibodies raised in animals will suppress in vitro anti-TG antibody production, the theory that lack of anti-idiotype control is causal in AITD remains attractive, but data to support it are scant.

Aberrant Expression of Class II Antigens on Thyroid Cells

Aberrant expression of HLA-DR on thyroid epithelial cells from patients with Graves' disease was first reported by Hanafusa et al.[336] and was proposed as the cause of autoimmunity by Botazzo.[337] These workers suggest that aberrant expression of DR on these cells, which are normally DR⁻, allows them to function as APCs. Numerous reports show that lymphocyte-produced IFN-γ can augment the expression of HLA-DR (also HLA-DP and HLA-DQ) on thyroid epithelial cells[338–341] and that TSH further increases the induction caused by IFN-γ.[342,343] TNF-α also can augment (in vitro) the induction of DR by IFN-γ.[338] HLA-DR⁺ cells definitely can stimulate T cells.[344] TEC aberrantly expressing DR can present antigens to T cells.[345] However, HLA-DR is aberrantly expressed on TECs in multinodular goiter and in many benign and malignant thyroid tumors, and this does not appear to induce thyroid autoimmunity.[346] Aberrant DR expression has not been shown to develop before autoimmunity. Normal animal thyroids not expressing class II molecules can become the focus of induced thyroiditis and then express class II proteins. DR expression on Graves' disease thyroid tissue is lost when tissue is transplanted to nude mice.[347] Thus a consensus position is that DR expression could be important but is a secondary phenomenon in AITD. It also may be noted that some cells—such as normal human adrenal cells—constitutively express DR, but this does not lead to autoimmunity.[348]

Aberrant—and high level—HLA-D antigen expression on TEC could theoretically introduce other factors into the immune response. HLA-DR (or HLA-DP and HLA-DQ) molecules present antigen to CD4⁺ T cells, which are generically of the "helper" phenotype. Thus a relative increase in class II versus class I expression on TEC could alter the balance of immune reactivity toward a CD4⁺-mediated helper response and away from a CD8-mediated—class I associated—suppressor response.

It also must be considered that DR expression may be a defense mechanism against immunologic attack. For example, Caspi et al.[349] have shown in experimental retinitis that expression of DR on retinal cells gives them an immunorepressive function when added to immunized T cells stimulated by Ag in vitro. A similar phenomenon occurs in animals experimentally immunized to keratinocytes.[350] A mechanism for this response is not certain, but it might be mediated by a product secreted by the DR⁺ cells. For example, they might secrete TGF-γ or other products that could suppress immune responses.

Several remarkable studies on the etiology of

IDDM have examined the role of MHC class I or II gene expression on pancreatic beta cells by making mice transgenic for Ia genes (the murine equivalent of DR) expressed under control of the insulin gene promoter. In these mice the pancreatic beta cells become Ia$^+$ and progressively die, but there is no evidence of immunologic attack.[351] In this model "aberrant" expression of MHC molecules does not appear to cause autoimmune disease. On the other hand, MHC expression does cause death of the cells, and this may be relevant to the pathogenesis of autoimmunity. The mechanism relating MHC expression and cell death is obscure but could be secondary to altered secretory functions, altered surface receptors, transcription factors, or other metabolic effects. A similar analysis should be conducted in animal models of AITD by producing animals transgenic for MHC class II molecules expressed in the thyroid under the control of human TG or human TPO gene promoters.

Environmental Factors

IL-2 administration for cancer therapy leads to the production of antithyroid antibodies and hypothyroidism (and possibly a better tumor response).[352] IFN-α (or probably γ) administration[353] has a similar effect. Administration of IL-2[354] or IFN-γ to animals can induce thyroid autoimmunity. Thus one might hypothesize that endogenous production of IL-2 or IFN-γ for some nonrelated reason, as in response to infection, could augment antithyroid immunity. Since IFN increases lymphocyte and TEC DR expression[355] and activates natural killer cells, and IL-2 activates lymphocytes, it is easy to theorize that any nonspecific elevation of their levels could augment thyroid immunity. Cigarette smoking is associated with Graves' disease and with ophthalmopathy.[355a] The mechanism is uncertain and is doubtless more complex than a local irritative effect.

It has been reported that thyrotoxicosis tends to recur following attacks of allergic rhinitis.[356] A factor such as IL-2 or IFN could be involved.

Normal Autoimmunity

"Normal" people express antithyroid immunity, and this must be important in understanding the overall mechanism of AITD. Using sensitive assays, 36 percent of women and 15 percent of men are found to have circulating TG antibodies.[357] The prevalence of antibodies goes up with age.[358] Many people with low levels of antibodies but without clinical disease can be shown to have lymphocyte infiltrates in the thyroid at autopsy. B cells from normal individuals can be induced to secrete anti-TG antibody in vitro. These observations clearly show that incomplete deletion of clonal self-reactive T cells is indeed the normal (and indeed perhaps necessary) circumstance and provide strong support for the idea that disordered control of this low-level immunity may be important in the etiology of AITD.

Effect of Antithyroid Drugs on the Immune Response

Antithyroid drugs are used in Graves' disease to decrease production of thyroid hormone; they also diminish thyroid-stimulating antibody and other antibody levels. Direct inhibitory effects of antithyroid drugs on B cell antibody synthesis have been reported[359] but primarily at unrealistically high drug levels. Signore et al.[360] reported that at 60 mM concentration, antithyroid drugs reduced the expression of IL-2 receptors on T cells. Clinical studies show that antithyroid drug administration also diminishes antibody production in thyroxine-replaced Hashimoto's thyroiditis patients,[361] proving that their effect is not simply due to control of hyperthyroidism in Graves' disease. Surprisingly,[362] administration of KC10$_4$ to patients with Graves' disease leads to diminished serum antibodies, suggesting (contrariwise) that the effect of treatment is not specific for thionamide drugs and could be due to control of thyrotoxicosis or to formation of poorly iodinated TG with low antigenicity. Antithyroid drugs inhibit macrophage function by interfering with myeloperoxidase.[363] Following antithyroid drug treatment of active Graves' disease, there is a prompt short-term increase of DR$^+$CD8$^+$ T (suppressor?) cells in the bloodstream. Antithyroid drugs do not (directly) prevent expression of DR[364] or of TPO on the surface of thyroid epithelial cells[365] but may reduce DR expression through inhibition of lymphocyte function. They could theoretically interact chemically with antigen (TPO) and alter its immune function. Propylthiouracil or methimazole administration inhibits experimental thyroiditis in rats. This is associated with a decrease in class II molecule expression on TEC. Antibody levels are little affected, and the mechanism is unclear. Which one of

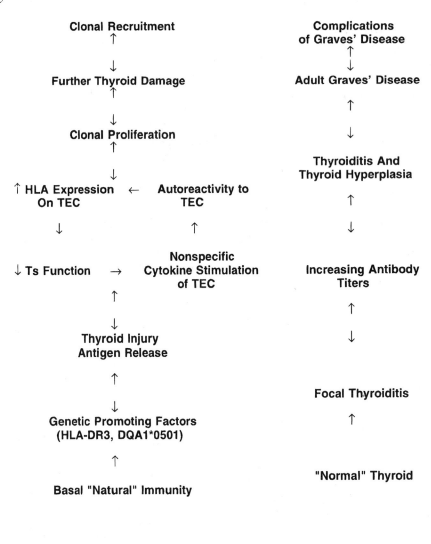

IMMUNE RESPONSE

CLINICAL RESPONSE

Fig. 7-13. Theoretical sequence of development of AITD.

these many responses, if any, produces the immuno-suppressive effect of antithyroid drugs remains uncertain.

AITD As A Consequence of a Multifactoral Process (Fig. 7-13)

Thus one is led to the uncomfortable position that AITD is probably not caused by a factor but rather by many interacting factors (Table 7-4). We have divided the roles of these potential disease-producing factors into a series of stages, emphasizing the predisposing events, antigen-driven responses, and

then the secondary and nonspecific amplification that ensues.

Stage 1

In the basal state, stage 1, immune reactivity to autologous antigen occurs as a normal process. This probably exists at a physiologically insignificant level, since not all T or B cells reacting with TPO or TG are clonally deleted, and Ag is normally present in the circulation. If assays become sensitive enough, we probably will find some level of antibodies to TPO and TG in all persons, increasing in prevalence and

TABLE 7-4. Development of Autoimmune Thyroid Disease

Stage 1: Basal state

  Normal exposure to antigen such as TG and normal low levels of antibody response

  Inherited susceptibility via HLA-DR, HLA-DQ, or TCR genes

Stage 2a: Initial thyroid damage and low level immune response

  Viral or other damage with release of normal or altered TG, TPO, or TSH-R

  Increased antibody levels in genetically susceptible host with high effeciency HLA-DR, HLA-DQ, TCR molecules

  Infection-induced elevation of IL-2 or IFM

  IL-2 stimulation of antigen specific or nonspecific Th

  IFN stimulation of DR expression and NK activation

  Glucocorticoid-induced alterations in lymphocyte function during stress

Stage 2b: Spontaneous regression of immune response

  Diminished antigen exposure

  Anti-idiotype feedback

  Antigen-specific Ts induction

Stage 3: Antigen-driven thyroid cell damage (or stimulation)

  Complement-dependent antibody-mediated cytotoxicity

  Fc receptor + cell ADCC by T, NK, or macrophage cells

  NK cell attack

  Direct CD4+ or CD8+ T cell cytotoxicity

  Antibody-mediated thyroid cell stimulation

Stage 4: Secondary disease-augmenting factors

  Thyroid cell DR, DQ expression—(?) APC function

  Immune complex binding and removal of Ts

  (?) Thyroid hormone–induced Ts reduction

Stage 5: Antigen-independent disease progression

  Recruitment of nonspecific Th or autoreactive Th

  Autoreactive Th bind DR+ TEC or B cells

  Activated DR+ T cells "self-present" antigen

  IL-2 activation of bystander Th

Stage 6: Clonal expansion with development of associated diseases

  Antigen release and new Th and B recruitment

  (?) Cross-reactivity with orbital antigen

  IL-2, IFN augmentation of normal immune response to intrinsic factor, acetylcholine receptor, DNA, melanocytes, hair follicles, etc.

---

concentration with age, and especially in women, since "femaleness" somehow augments antithyroid immunity manyfold. Patients who have inherited specific Gm allotypes, TCR molecules, or DR3 or DR5 MHC molecules will be especially prone to develop increased antibody levels because their T and B cell repertoire includes cells recognizing self-anti-

gen, or their immunocytes are especially good at collecting, presenting, and responding to antigen, or are unable to effectively clear immune complexes from their circulation.

Stage 2

Possibly viral infection, other causes of cell damage, or cross-reacting antibodies present after *Yersinia* (or other) infection leads to release of increased amounts of, or abnormal, thyroid antigens, which in genetically prone individuals develop into an increased but still low-level immune response. Nonspecific production of IL-2 and IFN-γ in response to any infection may augment DR expression on thyroid cells, allow these cells to function as APCs, and increase production of the normally occurring low levels of antibodies. The process may be affected by stress, although the mechanism remains quite uncertain.

The process may go on over years, and wax and wane, as it has been shown that thyroiditis can be clinically apparent and then disappear. Factors involved in temporary or permanent suppression of the response may include diminished thyroidal release of antigen, B cell anti-idiotype feedback, or the normal autoregulatory induction of CD8+ T cells with a suppressor function. In some individuals, thyroid cells may be unable to express DR or may secrete TGF-β and suppress immune responses. Glucocorticoid administration can also temporarily prevent the expression of nascent autoimmunity.

Stage 3

If suppressive factors do not control the developing immune response, the disease progresses to a new intensity, now driven by specific antigens, inducing cell hyperfunction (thyroid-stimulating antibody), or hypofunction (TSH-blocking antibody), or cell destruction. Direct T cell cytolysis, ADCC, and killer or natural killer cell attack presumably play an important role at this stage, and now the disease becomes clinically evident.

Stage 4

As the disease develops, a variety of secondary factors comes into play and augment antithyroid immunoreactivity. Any stimulus that causes increased DR expression on thyroid cells, such as T cell release of

IFN-γ, combined with increased TSH stimulation, may allow TECs to function as APCs. Although perhaps poor in this function, they are large in number and localized in one area. Some patients may inherit diminished antigen-specific suppressor cell function. Development of hyperthyroidism, or more likely the ongoing immune reaction itself, may lead to nonspecific suppressor cell dysfunction, further augmenting immunoreactivity. Antigen-"nonspecific," and antigen-specific suppressor T cells may be reduced by binding immune complexes.

Stage 5

T cell–secreted lymphokines may nonspecifically induce bystander antigen-specific T and B cells to be activated and produce antibody. Autoreactive cells will now accumulate in thyroid tissue because of the many strongly DR$^+$ positive lymphocytes and TECs and augment the developing response by lymphokine secretion or cytolysis in a manner independent of thyroid antigens. Activated T cells may self-present antigen, in a further escalation of the response. At this stage in the disease, nonspecific autoreactive immune processes may dominate a disease process that no longer depends upon antigen for its continuation.

Stage 6

As the concentration of activated T and B cells builds in thyroid tissue, and autoreactive and antigen nonspecific T cells become progressively involved, cell destruction may lead to release of new antigens. Cross-reacting epitopes, and nonspecific stimulation of T cells in genetically prone individuals, may cause the addition of new immunologic syndromes (exophthalmos, pretibial myxedema, atrophic gastritis) typical of older patients with more long-standing and florid disease.

THYROIDITIS, MYXEDEMA, AND GRAVES' DISEASE AS AUTOIMMUNE DISEASES

Hashimoto's Thyroiditis (Fig. 7-14)

How well do the changes of Hashimoto's thyroiditis fulfill the criteria of an immunologic reaction? Neither the presence of autoantibodies in the serum of patients with Hashimoto's thyroiditis nor the demonstration in vitro of cytotoxicity of the serum constitutes definitive evidence that autoimmunity is the cause of the disease. Rarely, if ever, is there a well-defined initial immunizing event, and accordingly a shortened latent period after a secondary stimulus has not been observed. Further, experimental passive transfer of the immune state in healthy recipients has not yet been attempted and has failed when human sera have been transfused into monkeys. This experiment is conducted by nature during pregnancy, since maternal antibodies cross the placenta. Transplacental passage of TSAb can produce neonatal thyrotoxicosis, and TSBAb can produce transient neonatal hypothyroidism. Usually, passage of TG antibody or TPO antibody has no detectable cytotoxic effect, but in rare families there is evidence of fetal thyroid damage and hypothyroidism.[366] Perhaps the lack of response to passive transfer of antibody is not surprising, since living syngeneic cells must usually be transferred for the development of experimental thyroiditis. Also, there is no report of desensitization of humans by thyroid antigens. Improvement of a disease process during glucocorticoid therapy is, at best, only indirect evidence for the participation of an immune factor in the disease. Blizzard et al.[367] have shown that steroids temporarily mask manifestations of the disease. In spite of these objections, there are compelling reasons for thinking that immunologic reactions are the pathogenesis of AITD.

The role of humoral antibodies in the development of the thyroid lesions of lymphocytic thyroiditis is unclear. They could be marker antibodies, indicating immunity, although not actively pathogenic. The evidence supporting this belief comes from studies in animals and observations in patients.[368] Both in animals and in humans there is an incomplete correlation between the extent of thyroid lesions and the presence or concentration of circulating antibodies. Failure of transfused human serum to induce disease in animals was noted above. Similarly, infusions of Hashimoto's serum containing high levels of cytotoxic factor did not influence the pulmonary metastases in a patient with advanced carcinoma of the thyroid.

If thyroid antibodies themselves are able to induce thyroid lesions, one might expect to find thyroiditis or cretinism in the offspring of women with high concentrations of humoral antibody during preg-

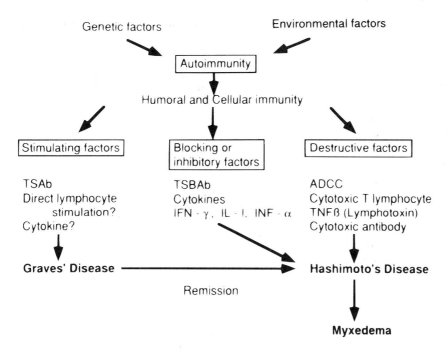

Fig. 7-14. Balance of immune reactions favoring Graves' or Hashimoto's disease.

nancy. Blizzard and co-workers[369,370] reported a higher than normal incidence of thyroid antibodies in the mothers of some cretins. These workers demonstrated the transplacental passage of antibodies and showed that they disappear over the first few months of life.[370] Thyroid damage does not usually result from the effect of maternal autoantibodies,[371–373] but Sutherland et al.[374] reported the birth of two cretinous infants to a hypothyroid mother and attributed the entire sequence to antithyroid antibody damage to the maternal and fetal thyroids. This family was extensively restudied by Goldsmith et al.,[366] who also concluded that transplacental passage of a cytotoxic factor may have been responsible for hypothyroidism in this unusual family.

In contrast to these ideas, some recent studies suggest that antibodies may play a much more important role in immunologic responses. Circulating antibodies are able to bind to certain lymphocytes or macrophages, rendering them cytotoxic against appropriate target cells.[375] Calder et al.[119] report that anti-TG antibodies will bind to nonimmune lymphocytes and render them cytotoxic when exposed to antigen-coated target cells. Also, some reports indicate transfer of thyroiditis with serum[376] and state

that the histologic picture of experimental thyroiditis develops with the humoral response before detectable T cell–mediated immunity is seen.[377] We have already mentioned the dependence of spontaneous fowl thyroiditis upon B rather than T cells. Thus, circulating antibodies are considered by some investigators to play a role as important as or more important than that of cell-mediated immunity in experimental and spontaneous thyroiditis.

Coexistence of antigen and circulating antibody may lead to immune complex formation. Deposits of immune complexes have been detected in Graves' disease and thyroiditis along the thyroid follicular basement membrane.[378] These may represent antibody reacting with TG escaping from the thyroid cell. Circulating immune complexes have been detected by tests that are dependent upon complement binding in 35 to 78 percent of patients with thyroiditis.[379–382] Using TG immune-complex-specific assays (Raji cell and the Takeda-Kriss[383] method), low levels of TG immune complexes were found in 5 percent of patients with thyroiditis and 38 percent of patients with Graves' disease.[384] Release of TG after surgery in patients with antithyroglobulin antibody leads to formation of immune complexes and temporary depression or obliteration of the antibody titer.[385] These immune complexes only rarely cause kidney damage,[386–389] probably because they bind complement poorly. There is clearly little evidence that immune complexes play an important role in the development of Hashimoto's thyroiditis or other AITD.

The evidence is overwhelming that an immune reaction mediated by T lymphocytes is involved in the development of experimental thyroiditis in animals.[390,391] Lymphocytes presensitized to antigens of the thyroid are present in most if not all patients. Since T-cell-mediated immunity is frequently lethal to cells, it is logical to assume that the T-cell-mediated immune response in thyroiditis could cause first a goiter, with lymphocyte infiltration and compensatory thyroid cell hyperplasia, and then gradual cell death and gland atrophy. The circulating antibodies may also be a functional part of this reaction. We can probably accept the idea that T-cell-mediated immunity is a pathogenic factor in thyroiditis.

Idiopathic Myxedema

Even before the present era of immunologic study, the basic unity of Hashimoto's thyroiditis and myxedema was realized. To quote from Crile, writing in 1954[392]: "Struma lymphomatosa is responsible not only for large lymphadenoid goiters, but also for fibrosis and atrophy of the thyroid. The clinical spectrum of struma lymphomatosa extends from spontaneous myxedema with no palpable thyroid tissue to a rapidly growing goiter associated with no clinical evidence of thyroid failure."

Hubble[393] has also drawn attention to the occurrence of syndromes intermediate between those of myxedema and Hashimoto's thyroiditis, in which a small, firm thyroid gland can be felt on careful palpation. Lerman found that the thyroid was palpable in one-fifth of his large series of patients with idiopathic myxedema. The histologic studies of Bastenie[394] and Douglass and Jacobson[395] revealed a close similarity in appearance of the thyroid remnant in myxedema and the Hashimoto gland. The immunologic studies of Owen and Smart,[396] and the experience in most thyroid laboratories, indicate a similar incidence and titer of antibodies in myxedema and Hashimoto's thyroiditis. A few patients have been reported in whom thyroiditis was observed to pass from the hypothyroid and goitrous condition to thyroid atrophy and idiopathic myxedema.[354] A familial association of myxedema and thyroiditis was described earlier.

Thus, idiopathic myxedema is the end result of Hashimoto's thyroiditis, in which the phase of thyroid enlargement was minimal or was overlooked. We may assume that in idiopathic myxedema the cell-destructive T-cell-mediated immune response is an important pathogenic factor in the illness, and that cytotoxic antibodies and TSH receptor stimulation inhibiting antibodies contribute to the development of hypothyroidism.

Graves' Disease

Graves' disease is equally associated with thyroid autoimmunity, since most hyperthyroid patients have circulating antibodies. High antibody levels are found in a small group of hyperthyroid patients, and histologic examination of their glands shows changes of both cell stimulation and focal thyroiditis.[397] Some patients with clinical Graves' disease have tissue changes in the thyroid that are typical of thyroiditis.[398] This type of patient with Graves' disease most often becomes hypothyroid after operation,[399] after ^{131}I therapy,[400] or possibly spontaneously.[401] Patients with progressive exophthalmos have a high incidence of antibodies and tend to have high antibody titers.[402] The association of symptoms suggestive of thyrotoxicosis in some patients with Hashimoto's thyroiditis is also noted.

The humoral (B cell) response in Graves' disease leads to production of anti-TG and antimicrosomal antibodies. In addition, as described in Chapter 10, these cells produce TSAb and TSH-binding inhibitory antibody,[403] TSBAb, and probably other factors. These factors are antibodies to TSH-R. TSAb stimulates thyroid release of hormone and acts on the thyroid cell membrane by binding to the TSH-R,[404] initiating all of the responses characteristic of TSH. TSAb is a true cell stimulators and can even induce experimental goiter. TSBAb, which prevents absorption of TSAb by thyroid cell microsomes, may be thought of as a blocking antibody, although it has cell stimulatory activity in humans.[405] Other potentially important blocking antibody activities have been described. For example, antimicrosomal antibody has been shown to block in part the stimulatory effect of TSH and LATS, possibly by preventing attachment of the stimulators to their receptors.[406]

Evidence supports a role for T-cell-mediated immunity to thyroid antigens in Graves' disease and possibly against orbital antigens in patients with exophthalmos. We speculate that Graves' disease may be a condition representing a semistable balance between stimulatory, blocking, and cell-lethal immune responses. Thus, TSAb could cause thyroid hyperplasia and produce hyperthyroidism. Other serum factors might block the action of TSAb and prevent this hyperplastic response in some patients. Cytotoxic T cells could gradually destroy cells and produce hypothyroidism either spontaneously or after therapy. Both circulating antibodies[407,408] and T-cell-mediated immunity may be involved in exophthalmos.

RELATION TO OTHER THYROID DISEASES

Thyroid Cancer

Thyroid antibodies are present in increased prevalence (up to 32 percent) in patients with carcinoma of the thyroid and usually are at low titer. Histologic evidence of thyroiditis is found in 26 percent of tumors.[409,410] Histologic changes range from diffuse thyroiditis to focal collections of lymphocytes around the tumor or reactive lymphoid hyperplasia. Release of antigens possibly leads to increased antithyroid immunity. Some evidence suggests that patients who have thyroid antibodies have a better prognosis than antibody-negative patients (Ch. 18).

Lymphoma and lymphosarcoma of the thyroid are associated with Hashimoto's thyroiditis[411–413] or antithyroid antibodies,[414] and there is evidence that thyroiditis may precede development of the tumor.

An increased frequency of carcinoma, especially of the papillary type, has been reported in Hashimoto's thyroiditis.[415] Our experience does not indicate an association greater than that dictated by chance. Woolner et al.,[412] in a study of 600 cases, reached the same conclusion. It is also possible that focal thyroiditis in thyroid cancer represents a secondary immune response to the tumor.

Adolescent Goiter

Enlargement of the thyroid during the second decade, accompanied by normal results of function tests, usually is labeled adolescent goiter. If the examination includes needle biopsy, an appreciable incidence of Hashimoto's thyroiditis is found[416]—up to 65 percent. Eighty percent of these children with thyroiditis have a positive thyroid antibody test result. The parents of many of them have either overt thyroid disease or circulating thyroid antibodies. Hyperplasia, in response to an increased demand for thyroid hormone, and colloid involution are at the root of some of these goiters, but Hashimoto's thyroiditis is the most frequent explanation of adolescent goiter.

Transient Thyrotoxicosis, Painless Thyroiditis, Postpartum Thyroiditis, and Related Syndromes

These illnesses, all similar, involve an acute exacerbation of thyroid autoimmunity occurring independent of or following pregnancy in women and also occurring in men. They are characterized by sequential inflammation-induced T_4 and TG release and transient hypothyroidism; they usually return to euthyroidism and are discussed in Chapters 8 and 14. They are considered subtypes of Hashimoto's thyroiditis and, in the postpartum period appear to result from release of the immunoinhibitory effects of normal pregnancy.

Focal Thyroiditis

Focal lymphocytic infiltrations are frequently seen in Graves' disease, nodular goiter, nontoxic or colloid goiter, and thyroid carcinoma. The significance of these changes is not precisely known, but they correlate with positive antibody titers and may represent variations that do not differ qualitatively from thyroiditis.

Reproduction Problems

An association between the occurrence of maternal antithyroid antibodies and recurrent abortion has been reported.[417] Whether this observation will be supported in future studies is unknown. One possibility is that the antibodies are effectively markers for other immune responses responsible for fetal death.

SUMMARY

While the preceding construction cannot yet be supported in each detail by direct observations, it may be of value in helping to direct future studies on the pathogenesis of thyroid autoimmunity. It stresses the normal occurrence of immune self-reactivity, the genetic and environmental forces that may amplify such responses, the role of the antigen-driven immune attack, secondary disease-enhancing factors, and the important contributory role of antigen-independent immune reactivity. Least understood is the last area, that of clonal expansion involved in development of the associate immunologic syndromes. Research on thyroid autoimmunity has benefited greatly by knowledge of the specific target antigens and easy access to blood cells and involved target tissue. As research moves into the realm of molecular immunology, we may look for rapid progress in understanding and controlling these common illnesses.

REFERENCES

1. Fink PJ: Stop and go in the thymus. Immunol Today 9:377, 1988
2. Rich RR, El Masry MN, Fox EJ: Human suppressor T cells: Induction, differentiation, and regulatory functions. Human Immunol 17:369, 1986
3. Knapp W, Stockinger H, Majdic O, Shevach EM: The CD system of leukocyte surface molecules. Monoclonal antibodies to human cell-surface antigens. Current Protocols Immunol p. A.4.1., 1991
4. Janeway CA, Carding S, Jones B et al: CD4$^+$ T cells: specificity and function. Immunol Rev 101:39, 1988
5. Blackman MA, Kappler JW, Marrack P: T-cell specificity and repertoire. Immunol Rev 101:5, 1988
6. Allison JP: Structure, function, and serology of the T-cell antigen receptor complex. Ann Rev Immunol 5:503, 1987
7. Kronenberg M, Siu G, Hood LE, Shastri N: The molecular genetics of the T-cell antigen receptor and T-cell antigen recognition. Ann Rev Immunol 4:529, 1986
8. Goldsmith MA, Weiss A: New clues about T-cell antigen receptor complex function. Immunol Today 9:220, 1988
9. Isakov N: Cell activation and signal initiation. Immunol Today 9:251, 1988
10. Bonneville M, Janeway CA, Ito K et al: Intestinal intraepithelial lymphocytes are a distinct set of gamma delta T cells. Nature 336:479, 1988
11. Yoshikai Y, Anatoniou D, Clark SP et al: Sequence and expression of transcripts of the human T-cell receptor beta-chain genes. Nature 312:521, 1984
12. Zamvil SS, Mitchell DJ, Lee NE et al: Predominant expression of a T cell receptor V beta gene subfamily in autoimmune encephalomyelitis. J Exp Med 167:1586, 1988
13. Cresswell P: Antigen recognition by T lymphocytes. Immunol Today, 8:67, 1987
14. Meuer SC, Schlossman SF, Reinherz EL: Clonal analysis of human cytotoxic T lymphocytes: T4$^+$ and T8$^+$ effector T cells recognize products of different major histocompatibility complex regions. Proc Natl Acad Sci USA 79:4395, 1982
15. Bjorkman PJ, Saper MA, Samaroui B et al: The foreign antigen binding site and T cell recognition regions of class I histocompatibility antigens. Nature 329:512, 1987
16. Hozumi N, Tonegawa S: Evidence for somatic rearrangement of immunoglobulin genes coding for variable and constant regions. Proc Natl Acad Sci USA 73:3628, 1976
17. Lanzavecchia A: Clonal sketches of the immune response. EMBO J 7:2945, 1988
18. Hewitt CRA, Feldman M: Human T cell clones present antigen. Immunology 142:1429, 1989
19. Janeway CA Jr, Bottomly K: Signals and signs for lymphocyte responses. Cell 76:275, 1994
20. Springer TA: Adhesion receptors of the immune system. Nature 346:425, 1990
21. Singer A, Hodes RJ: Mechanisms of T cell-B cell interactions. Ann Rev Immunol 1:211, 1983
22. O'Garra A, Umland S, De France T, Christiansen J: 'B-cell factors' are pleiotropic. Immunol Today 9:45, 1988
23. Hawrylowicz CM, Unanue ER: Regulation of antigen-presentation-I. IFN-γ induces antigen-presenting properties on B cells. J Immunol 141:4083, 1988
24. Swain SL, Dutton RW: Consequences of the direct interaction of helper T cells with B cells presenting antigen. Immunol Rev 99:263, 1987
25. Mohagheghpour N, Damle NK, Moonka DK et al: A human alloreactive inducer T cell clone that selectively activates antigen-specific suppressor T cells. J Immunol 133:133, 1984
26. Takeuchi T, Schlossman SF, Morimoto C: Development of an antigen-specific CD8 suppressor effector clone in man. J Immunol 141:3010, 1988
27. Zheng H, Boyer M, Fotedar A et al: An antigen-specific helper T cell hybridoma produces an antigen-specific suppressor inducer molecule with identical antigenic fine specificity. Implications for the antigen recognition and function of helper and suppressor inducer T cells. J Immunol 140:1351, 1988
28. Pacini F, Sridama V, Pressendo J et al: Binding of immunoglobulin-G from patients with thyroid autoimmune disease in normal T-lymphocytes. Clin Endocrinol 18:29, 1983
29. Damle NK, Mohagheghpour N, Engleman EG: Solu-

ble antigen-primed inducer T cells activate antigen-specific suppressor T cells in the absence of antigen-pulsed accessory cells: Phenotypic definition of suppressor-inducer and suppressor-effector cells. J Immunol 132:644, 1984

30. Janeway CA, Broughton B, Smith LA et al: Direct receptor: receptor interactions between T and B lymphocytes: idiotypic restriction in the antibody response to a cloned helper T cell receptor. J Molec Cell Immunol 3:83, 1987

31. Jerne NK: Towards a network theory of the immune system. Ann Immunol (Paris) 125C:373, 1974

32. Kelly CJ, Mok H, Neilson EG: The selection of effector T cell phenotype by contrasuppression modulates susceptibility to autoimmune injury. J Immunol 141:3022, 1988

33. Morimoto C, Letvin NL, Boyd AW et al: The isolation and characterization of the human helper inducer T cell subset. J Immunol 134:3762, 1985

34. Kotani H, Mitsuya H, Jarrett RF et al: An autoreactive T cell clone that can be activated to provide both helper and suppressor function. J Immunol 136: 1951, 1986

35. Patel SS, Duby AD, Thiele DL, Lipsky PE: Phenotypic and functional characterization of human T cell clones. J Immunol 141:3726, 1988

36. Hercend T, Schmidt RE: Characteristics and uses of natural killer cells. Immunol Today 9:291, 1988

37. Marrack P, Kappler J: The T-cell repertoire for antigen and MHC. Immunol Today 9:308, 1988

37a. Mountz JD, Edwards CK: Murine models of autoimmunity: T-cell and B-cell defects. Current Opinion Rheumatol 4:612, 1992

38. Sakaguchi S, Fukuma K, Kuribayashi K, Masuda T: Organ-specific autoimmune diseases induced in mice by elimination of T cell subset. I. Evidence for the active participation of T cells in natural self-tolerance: deficit of a T cell subset as a possible cause of autoimmune disease. J Exp Med 161:72, 1985

39. Sugihara S, Izumi Y, Yoshioka T et al: Autoimmune thyroiditis induced in mice depleted of particular T cell subsets. I. Requirement of Lyt-1^{dull} L3T4^{bright} normal T cells for the induction of thyroiditis. J Immunol 141:105, 1988

40. Bach FH, Van Rood JJ: The major histocompatibility complex: Genetics and biology. N Engl J Med 295: 806, 1976

41. Kim PS, Dunn AD, Dunn JT: Altered immunoreactivity of thyroglobulin in thyroid disease. J Clin Endocrinol Metab 67:161, 1988

42. Shimojo N, Saito K, Kohno Y et al: Antigenic determinants on thyroglobulin: comparison of the reactivities of different thyroglobulin preparations with serum antibodies and T cells of patients with chronic thyroiditis. J Clin Endocrinol Metab 66:689, 1988

43. Mercken L, Simons M-J, Swillens S et al: Primary structure of bovine thyroglobulin deduced from the sequence of its 8,431-base complementary DNA. Nature 316:647, 1985

44. Hurel S, Wilkin TJ: Thyroglobulin antibodies cross-react with acetyl cholinesterase: a role in Graves' ophthalmopathy? Book of Abstracts for the 17th Annual Meeting of the European Thyroid Association, No. 80, Montpellier, France, September 11–16, 1988

45. Heyma P, Harrison LC: Precipitation of the thyrotropin receptor and identification of thyroid autoantigens using Graves' disease immunoglobulins. J Clin Invest 74:1090, 1984

46. Libert F, Lefort A, Gerard C et al: Cloning, sequencing, and expression of the human thyrotropin (TSH) receptor: Evidence for binding of autoantibodies. Biochem Biophys Res Commun 165:1250, 1989

47. Nagayama Y, Kaufman KD, Seto P, Rapoport B: Molecular cloning, sequence and functional expression of the cDNA for the human thyrotropin receptor. Biochem Biophys Res Commun 165:1184, 1989

48. Atassi MZ, Manshouri T, Sakata S: Localization and synthesis of the hormone-binding regions of the human thyrotropin receptor. Proc Natl Acad Sci USA 88:3613, 1991

49. Murakami M, Mori M: Identification of immunogenic regions in human thyrotropin receptor for immunoglobulin G of patients with Graves' disease. Biochem Biophys Res Commun 171:512, 1990

50. Nagayama Y, Rappaport B: The thyrotropin receptor 25 years after its discovery: New insight after its molecular cloning. Molecul Endocrinol 6:145, 1992

51. Kosugi S, Ban T, Akamizu T, Kohn LD: Further characterization of a high affinity thyrotropin binding site on the rat thyrotropin receptor which is an epitope for blocking antibodies from idiopathic myxedema patients but not thyroid stimulating antibodies from Graves' patients. Biochem Biophys Res Commun 180:1118, 1991

52. Endo T, Ohmori M, Ikeda M, Onaya T: Rabbit antibodies toward extracellular loops of the membrane spanning region of human thyrotropin receptor possess thyroid stimulating activities. Biochem Biophys Res Commun 181:1035, 1991

53. Matsui I, Sakata S, Ogawa T et al: Biological activities of rat antisera raised against synthetic peptides of human thyrotropin receptor. Endocr J 40:607, 1993

54. Francis T, Burch HB, Cal WY et al: Lymphocytes express thyrotropin receptor-specific mRNA as detected by the PCR technique. Thyroid 1:223, 1991

55. Endo T, Ohno M, Kotani S et al: Thyrotropin receptor in non-thyroid tissues. Biochem Biophys Res Commun 190:774, 1993

56. Rosselli-Rehfuss L, Robbins LS, Cone RD: Thyrotropin receptor messenger ribonucleic acid is expressed in most brown and white adipose tissues in the guinea pig. Endocrinology 130:1857, 1992

57. Graves PN, Tomer Y, Davies TF: Cloning and sequencing of a 1.3 kb variant of human thyrotropin receptor mRNA lacking the transmembrane domain. Biochem Biophys Res Commun 187:1135, 1992

58. Murakami M, Miyashita K, Yamada M et al: Characterization of human thyrotropin receptor-related peptide-like immunoreactivity in peripheral blood of Graves' disease. Biochem Biophys Res Commun 186:1074, 1992

59. McLachlan SM, Rapoport B: The molecular biology of thyroid peroxidase: Cloning, expression, and role as autoantigen in autoimmune thyroid disease. Endocr Rev 13:192, 1992

60. Portmann L, Hamada N, Heinrich G, DeGroot LJ: Antithyroid peroxidase antibody in patients with autoimmune thyroid disease: Possible identity with anti-microsomal antibody. J Clin Endocrinol Metab 61:1001, 1985

61. Hamada N, Grimm C, Mori H, DeGroot LJ: Identification of a thyroid microsomal antigen by Western blot and immunoprecipitation. J Clin Endocrinol Metab 61:120, 1985

62. Hamada N, Portmann L, DeGroot LJ: Characterization and isolation of thyroid microsomal antigen. J Clin Invest 79:819, 1987

63. Portmann L, Fitch F, Havran W et al: Characterization of the thyroid microsomal antigen, and its relationship to thyroid peroxidase, using monoclonal antibodies. J Clin Invest 81:1217, 1988

64. Libert F, Ruel J, Ludgate M et al: Thyroperoxidase, an autoantigen with a mosaic structure made of nuclear and mitochondrial gene modules. EMBO J, 6: 4193, 1987

65. Kimura S, Kotani T, McBride OW et al: Human thyroid peroxidase: Complete cDNA and protein sequence, chromosome mapping, and identification of two alternately spliced mRNAs. Proc Natl Acad Sci USA 84:5555, 1987

66. Magnusson RP, Chazenbalk GD, Gestautas J et al: Molecular cloning of the complementary deoxyribonucleic acid for human thyroid peroxidase. Molec Endocrinol 1:856, 1987

67. Czarnocka B, Ruf J, Ferrand M et al: Purification of the human thyroid peroxidase and its identification as the microsomal antigen involved in autoimmune thyroid diseases. FEBS Letters 190:147, 1985

68. Kimura S, Kotani T, McBride OW et al: Human thyroid peroxidase: Complete cDNA and protein sequence, chromosome mapping, and identification of two alternately spliced mRNAs. Proc Natl Acad Sci USA 84:5555, 1987

69. Hamada N, Jaeduck N, Portmann L et al: Antibodies against denatured and reduced thyroid microsomal antigen in autoimmune thyroid disease. J Clin Endocrinol Metab 64:230, 1987

70. Ruf J, Toubert M-E, Czarnocka B et al: Relationship between immunological structure and biochemical properties of human thyroid peroxidase. Endocrinology 125:1211, 1989

71. Ludgate M, Mariotti S, Libert F et al: Antibodies to human thyroid peroxidase in autoimmune thyroid disease: Studies with a cloned recombinant complementary deoxyribonucleic acid epitope. J Clin Endocrinol Metab 68:1091, 1989

72. Kawakami Y, Fisfalen M-E, DeGroot LJ: Proliferative responses of peripheral blood mononuclear cells from patients with autoimmune thyroid disease to synthetic peptide epitopes of human thyroid peroxidase. Autoimmunity 13:17, 1992

73. Dayan CM, Londei M, Corcoran AE et al: Autoantigen recognition by thyroid-infiltrating T cells in Graves' disease. Proc Natl Acad Sci USA 88:7415, 1991

74. Tandon N, Freeman M, Weetman AP: T cell responses to synthetic thyroid peroxidase peptides in autoimmune thyroid disease. Clin Exp Immunol 86: 56, 1991

75. Chazenbalk G, Magnusson RP, Rapoport B: Thyrotropin stimulation of cultured thyroid cells increases steady state levels of the messenger ribonucleic acid for thyroid peroxidase. Molec Endocrinol 1:913, 1987

76. Chiovato L, Vitti P, Lombardi A et al: Expression of the microsomal antigen on the surface of continuously cultured rat thyroid cells is modulated by thyrotropin. J Clin Endocrinol Metab 61:12, 1985

77. Khoury EL, Hammond L, Bottazzo GF, Doniach D: Presence of the organ-specific "microsomal" autoantigen on the surface of human thyroid cells in culture: its involvement in complement-mediated cytotoxicity. Clin Exp Immunol 45:316, 1981

78. Iwatani Y, Iitaka M, Gerstein HC et al: Separate induction of MHC and thyroid microsomal antigen (McAg) expression on thyroid cell monolayers: enhancement of lectin-induced McAg expression by interferon-γ. J Clin Endocrinol Metab 64:1302, 1987

79. Aguayo J, Michaud P, Iitaka M et al: Lack of effect of methimazole on thyrocyte cell-surface antigen expression. Autoimmunity 2:133, 1989

80. Kohno Y, Naito N, Hiyama Y et al: Thyroglobulin and thyroid peroxidase share common epitopes recognized by autoantibodies in patients with chronic autoimmune thyroiditis. J Clin Endocrinol Metab 67:899, 1988

81. Henry M, Zanelli E, Malthiery Y: Antihuman thyroid peroxidase and antihuman thyroglobulin antibodies present no cross-reactivity on recombinant peptides. Clin Exp Immunol 86:478, 1991

82. Shinozawa T, Villadolid MC, Ingbar SH: Detection and measurement of fat cell-binding immunoglobulins: a new method applicable to the diagnosis and study of Graves' disease. J Clin Endocrinol Metab 62:1, 1986

83. Banga JP, Doble N, Tomlinson RWS, Odell E, McGregor AM: Cross-reactivity of autoantibodies to the thyroid peroxidase antigen with myeloperoxidase, lactoperoxidase and horseradish peroxidase. Book of Abstracts for the 17th Annual Meeting of the European Thyroid Association, No. 130, Montpellier, France, September 11–16, 1988

84. Hamada N, DeGroot LJ, Portmann L et al: Thyroid microsomal antigen in Graves' thyroid is not different from that in normal thyroid. Endocrinol Japan 38:471, 1991

85. Bahn RS, Dutton CM, Heufelder AE, Sarkar G: A genomic point mutation in the extracellular domain of the thyrotropin receptor in patients with Graves' ophthalmopathy. J Clin Endocrinol Metab 78:256, 1994

86. Benvenga S, Trimarchi F, Robbins J: Circulating thyroid hormone autoantibodies. J Endocrinol Invest 10:605, 1987

87. Tachi J, Amino N, Iwatani Y et al: Increase in antideoxyribonucleic acid antibody titer in postpartum aggravation of autoimmune thyroid disease. J Clin Endocrinol Metab 67:1049, 1988

88. Katakura M, Yamada T, Aizawa T et al: Presence of antideoxyribonucleic acid antibody in patients with hyperthyroidism of Graves' disease. J Clin Endocrinol Metab 64:405, 1987

89. Ekins DI, Wilkin TJ: A clinical comparison of the enzyme-linked immunosorbent assay (ELISA) and hemagglutination (TRC) in the routine detection of antithyroglobulin antibodies. Acta Endocrinol 103:216, 1983

90. Boyden SV: The adsorption of proteins on erythrocytes treated with tannic acid and subsequent hemagglutination by antiprotein sera. J Exp Med 93:107, 1951

91. Takeda Y, Kriss JP: Radiometric measurement of thyroglobulin-antithyroglobulin immune complex in human serum. J Clin Endocrinol Metab 44:46, 1977

92. Mariotti S, Kaplan EL, Medof ME, DeGroot LJ: Circulating thyroid antigen antibody immune complexes. Proceedings of the Eighth International Thyroid Congress, Sydney, Australia, February 3–8, 1980

93. Dingle PR, Ferguson A, Horn DB et al: The incidence of thyroglobulin antibodies and thyroid enlargement in a general practice in northeast England. Clin Exp Immunol 1:277, 1966

94. Yoshida H, Amino N, Yagawa K et al: Association of serum antithyroid antibodies with lymphocytic infiltration of the thyroid gland. Studies of seventy autopsied cases. J Clin Endocrinol Metab 46:859, 1978

95. Williams ED, Doniach I: Post-mortem incidence of focal thyroiditis. J Pathol Bact 83:255, 1962

96. Schade R, Owen SG, Smart GA, Hall R: The relation of thyroid autoimmunity to round-cell infiltrations of the thyroid gland. J Clin Pathol 13:499, 1960

97. Hjort T, Jeppesen F, Okholm K, Temler J: The prognostic significance of thyroid autoantibodies in the development of postoperative myxedema. Dan Med Bull 10:159, 1963

98. Lundell G, Jonsson J: Thyroid antibodies and hypothyroidism in ^{131}I therapy for hyperthyroidism. Acta Radiol 12:443, 1973

99. Anderson JR, Goudie RB, Gray KG: Complement-fixing autoantibody to thyroglobulin in Hashimoto's disease. Lancet 1:644, 1959

100. Mariotti S, DeGroot LJ, Scarborough D, Medof ME: Study of circulating immune complexes in thyroid diseases. Comparison of Raji cell radioimmunoassay and specific thyroglobulin-antithyroglobulin radioassay. J Clin Endocrinol Metab 49:679, 1979

101. Iitaka M, Aguayo JF, Iwatani Y et al: In vitro induction of antithyroid microsomal antibody-secreting cells in peripheral blood mononuclear cells from normal subjects. J Clin Endocrinol Metab 67:749, 1988

102. Roman SH, Korn F, Davies TF: Enzyme-linked immunosorbent microassay and hemagglutination compared for detection of thyroglobulin and thyroid microsomal autoantibodies. Clin Chemistry 30:246, 1984

103. Mariotti S, Anelli S, Ruf J et al: Comparison of serum thyroid microsomal and thyroid peroxidase autoantibodies in thyroid disease. J Clin Endocrinol Metab 65:987, 1987

104. Okamoto Y, Hamada N, Saito H et al: Thyroid peroxidase activity-inhibiting immunoglobulins in patients with autoimmune thyroid disease. J Clin Endocrinol Metab 68:730, 1989

105. Trotter WR, Belvayin G, Waddams A: Precipitating and complement-fixing antibodies in Hashimoto's disease. Proc R Soc Med 50:961, 1957

106. Pulvertaft RJV, Doniach D, Roitt IM, Hudson RV: Cytotoxic effects of Hashimoto serum on human thyroid cells in tissue culture. Lancet 2:214, 1959

107. Khoury EL, Hammond L, Bottazzo GF et al: Presence of organ-specific "microsomal" autoantigen on

the surface of human thyroid cells in culture: its involvement in complement-mediated cytotoxicity. Clin Exp Immunol 45:316, 1981

108. Fenzi GF, Bartalena L, Chiovato L et al: Studies on thyroid cell surface antigens using cultured human thyroid cells. Clin Exp Immunol 47:336, 1982

109. Chiovato L, Bassi P, Santini F et al: Antibodies producing complement-mediated thyroid cytotoxicity in patients with atrophic or goitrous autoimmune thyroiditis. J Clin Endocrinol Metab 77:1700, 1993

110. Weetman AP, Cohen SB, Oleesky DA, Morgan BP: Terminal complement complexes and Cl/Cl inhibitor complexes in autoimmune thyroid disease. Clin Exp Immunol 77:25, 1989

111. Weetman AP, Freeman MA, Morgan BP: Thyroid follicular cell function after non-lethal complement membrane attack. Clin Exp Immunol 82:69, 1990

112. Holborow EJ: Serum antinuclear factor and autoimmunity. Proc R Soc Med 53:625, 1960

113. McDermott MT, West SG, Emlen JW, Kidd GS: Antideoxyribonucleic acid antibodies in Graves' disease. J Clin Endocrinol Metab 71:509, 1990

114. Buchanan WW, Anderson JR, Goudie RB, Gray KG: A skin test in thyroid disease. Lancet 2:928, 1958

115. Amino N, Hagen SR, Yamada N, Refetoff S: Measurement of circulating thyroid microsomal antibodies by the tanned red cell-hemagglutination technique. Its usefulness in the diagnosis of autoimmune thyroid disease. Clin Endocrinol 5:115, 1976

116. Adams DD, Kennedy TH: Evidence to suggest that LATS protector stimulates the human thyroid gland. J Clin Endocrinol Metab 33:47, 1971

117. Smith BR, McLachlan SM, Furmaniak J: Autoantibodies to the thyrotropin receptor. Endocr Rev 9:106, 1988

118. Premachandra BN, Blumenthal HT: Abnormal binding of thyroid hormone in sera from patients with Hashimoto's disease. J Clin Endocrinol Metab 27:931, 1967

119. Calder EA, Penhale WJ, McCleman D et al: Lymphocyte dependent antibody-mediated cytotoxicity in Hashimoto's thyroiditis. Clin Exp Immunol 14:153, 1973

120. Suzuki S, Mitsunaga M, Miyoshi M: Cytophilic antithyroglobulin antibody and antibody-dependent monocyte-mediated cytotoxicity in Hashimoto's thyroiditis. J Clin Endocrinol Metab 51:446, 1980

121. Weetman AP, Yateman ME, Ealey PA et al: Thyroid-stimulating antibody activity between different immunoglobulin G subclasses. J Clin Invest 86:723, 1990

122. Fenzi G, Hashizume K, Roudebush CP, DeGroot LJ: Changes in thyroid-stimulating immunoglobulins during antithyroid therapy. J Clin Endocrinol Metab 48:572, 1979

123. Kaplan MM: Hypothyroidism after treatment with interleukin-2 and lymphokine-activated killer cells. N Engl J Med 318:1557, 1988

124. Burman P, Totterman TH, Oberg K, Karlsson FA: Thyroid autoimmunity in patients on long term therapy with leukocyte-derived interferon. J Clin Endocrinol Metab 63:1086, 1986

125. Bouanani M, Piechaczyk M, Pau B, Bastide M: Significance of the recognition of certain antigenic regions on the human thyroglobulin molecules by natural autoantibodies from healthy subjects. J Immunol 143:1129, 1989

126. Henry M, Zanelli E, Piechaczyk M et al: A major human thyroglobulin epitope defined with monoclonal antibodies is mainly recognized by human autoantibodies. Eur J Immunol 22:315, 1992

127. Libert F, Ludgate M, Dinsart C, Vassart G: Thyroperoxidase, but not the thyrotropin receptor, contains sequential epitopes recognized by autoantibodies in recombinant peptides expressed in the pUEX vector. J Clin Endocrinol Metab 73:857, 1991

128. Martin A, Davies RF: T cell and human autoimmune thyroid disease: Emerging data show lack of a need to invoke suppressor T cell problems. Thyroid 2:247, 1992

129. Benveniste P, Wenzel BE, Khalil A et al: Spontaneous secretion of thyroid autoantibodies by cultured peripheral blood lymphocytes from patients with Hashimoto's thyroiditis detected by micro-ELISA techniques. Clin Exp Immunol 58:273, 1984

130. McLachlan SM, Pegg CAS, Atherton MC et al: Subpopulations of thyroid autoantibody secreting lymphocytes in Graves' and Hashimoto thyroid glands. Clin Exp Immunol 65:319, 1986

131. Petersen J, Feldt-Rasmussen U, Larsen F, Siersbaek-Nielsen K: Autoreactive lymphocytes in thyroid disorders. Quantitation of anti-thyroglobulin antibody formation by a specific hemolytic plaque forming cell (PFC) assay. Acta Endocrinol (Copenh) 113:50, 1986

132. Mori H, Amino N, Iwatani Y et al: Increase of peripheral B lymphocytes in Graves' disease. Clin Exp Immunol 42:33, 1980

133. Iitaka M, Aguayo JF, Iwatani Y et al: In vitro induction of antithyroid microsomal antibody-secreting cells in peripheral blood mononuclear cells from normal subjects. J Clin Endocrinol Metab 67:749, 1988

134. McLachlan SM, Dickinson AM, Malcolm A et al: Thyroid autoantibody synthesis by cultures of thyroid and peripheral blood lymphocytes. I. Lymphocyte markers and response to pokeweed mitogen. Clin Exp Immunol 52:45, 1983

135. Weetman AP, Gunn C, Hall R, McGregor AM: Thyroid autoantigen-induced lymphocyte proliferation

in Graves' disease and Hashimoto's thyroiditis. J Clin Lab Immunol 17:1, 1985

136. Logtenberg T, Kroon A, Gmelig-Meyling FHJ, Ballieux RE: Production of anti-thyroglobulin antibody by blood lymphocytes from patients with autoimmune thyroiditis, induced by the insolubilized autoantigen. J Immunol 136:1236, 1986

137. McLachlan SM, Fawcett J, Atherton MC et al: Thyroid autoantibody synthesis by cultures of thyroid and peripheral blood lymphocytes. II. Effect of thyroglobulin on thyroglobulin antibody synthesis. Clin Exp Immunol 52:620, 1983

138. Weetman AP, McGregor AM, Lazarus JH, Hall R: Thyroid antibodies are produced by thyroid-derived lymphocytes. Clin Exp Immunol 48:196, 1982

139. Okita N, Kidd A, Row VV, Volpe R: Sensitization of T-lymphocytes in Graves' and Hashimoto's diseases. J Clin Endocrinol Metab 51:316, 1980

140. Perruder-Badoux A, Frei PC: On the mechanism of "rosette" formation in humans and experimental thyroiditis. Clin Exp Immunol 5:117, 1969

141. Podleski WK: Cytotoxic lymphocytes in Hashimoto's thyroiditis. Clin Exp Immunol 11:543, 1972

142. Fisfalen ME, Quintans J, Kawakami Y et al: Regulation of antibody production by CD4+/CDW29+ T cell clones (TCC) in autoimmune thyroid disease (AITD). Abstract presented at the 71st Annual Meeting of the Endocrine Society, Seattle, Washington, June 21–24, 1989

143. Aoki N, DeGroot LJ: Lymphocyte blastogenic response to human thyroglobulin in Graves' disease, Hashimoto's thyroiditis, and metastatic thyroid cancer. Clin Exp Immunol 38:523, 1979

144. Amino N, DeGroot LJ: Insoluble particulate antigen(s) in cell-mediated immunity of autoimmune thyroid disease. Metabolism 24:45, 1975

145. Canonica GW, Cosulich ME, Croci R et al: Thyroglobulin-induced T-cell in vitro proliferation in Hashimoto's thyroiditis: identification of the responsive subset and effect of monoclonal antibodies directed to Ia antigens. Clin Immunol Immunopathol 32:132, 1984

146. Canonica GW, Caria M, Bagnasco M et al: Proliferation of T8-positive cytolytic T lymphocytes in response to thyroglobulin in human autoimmune thyroiditis: analysis of cell interactions and culture requirements. Clin Immunol Immunopathol 36:40, 1985

147. Lamki L, Row VV, Volpe R: Cell-mediated immunity in Graves' disease and in Hashimoto's thyroiditis as shown by the demonstration of migration inhibition factor (MIF). J Clin Endocrinol Metab 36:358, 1973

148. Fisfalen ME, Quintans J, Kawakami Y et al: Regulation of antibody production by CDr+/CDW29+ T cell clones (TCC) in autoimmune thyroid disease (AITD). Abstract submitted to the 71st Annual Meeting of the Endocrine Society, Seattle, Washington, June 21–24, 1989

149. Davies TF: Cocultures of human thyroid monolayer cells and autologous T cells: impact of HLA class II antigen expression. J Clin Endocrinol Metab 61:418, 1985

150. Weetman AP, Volkman DJ, Burman KD et al: The production and characterization of thyroid-derived T-cell lines in Graves' disease and Hashimoto's thyroiditis. Clin Immunol Immunopathol 39:139, 1986

151. Londei M, Bottazzo GF, Feldmann M: Human T-cell clones from autoimmune thyroid glands: specific recognition of autologous thyroid cells. Science 228: 85, 1985

152. Soliman M, Guimaraes V, Fisfalen M-E, DeGroot LJ: Definition of T cell epitopes of thyrotropin receptor by testing T cell reactivity to human recombinant thyrotropin extracellular domain and its synthetic peptides in AITD patients. 76th Annual Meeting of the Endocrine Society, Anaheim, California, June 15–18, 1994

153. Ling NR, Acton AB, Roitt IM, Doniach D: Interaction of lymphocytes from immunized hosts with thyroid and other cells in culture. Br J Exp Pathol 66: 348, 1965

154. Davies TF, Martin A, Concepcion ES et al: Evidence for selective accumulation of intrathyroidal T lymphocytes in human autoimmune thyroid disease based on T cell receptor V gene usage. J Clin Invest 89:157, 1992

155. Davies TF, Concepcion ES, Ben-Nun A et al: T-cell receptor V gene use in autoimmune thyroid disease: Direct assessment by thyroid aspiration. J Clin Endocrinol Metab 76:660, 1993

156. McIntosh RS, Watson PF, Pickerill AP et al: No restriction of intrathyroidal T cell receptor Vα families in the thyroid of Graves' disease. Clin Exp Immunol 91:147, 1993

157. Ploth DW, Fitz A, Schnetzler D et al: Thyroglobulin-anti-thyroglobulin immune complex glomerulonephritis complicating radioiodine therapy. Clin Immunol Immunopathol 9:327, 1978

158. O'Regan S, Fong JSC, Kaplan BS et al: Thyroid antigen-antibody nephritis. Clin Immunol Immunopathol 6:341, 1976

159. Matsuura M, Kikkawa Y, Akashi K et al: Thyroid antigen-antibody nephritis: Possible involvement of fucosyl-GMl as the antigen. Endocrinol Japon 34:587, 1987

160. Kalderon AE, Bogaars HA: Immune complex deposits in Graves' disease and Hashimoto's thyroiditis. Am J Med 63:729, 1977

161. Fujiwara H, Torisu M, Koitabashi Y et al: Immune complex deposits in thyroid glands of patients with Graves' disease. Clin Immunol Immunopathol 19: 98, 1981

162. Mariotti S, DeGroot LJ, Scarborough D, Medof ME: Study of circulating immune complexes in thyroid diseases. Comparison of Raji cell radioimmunoassay and specific thyroglobulin antithyroglobulin radioassay. J Clin Endocrinol Metab 49:679, 1979

163. Endo Y, Aratake Y, Yamamoto I et al: Peripheral K cells in Graves' disease and Hashimoto's thyroiditis in relation to circulating immune complexes. Clin Endocrinol 18:187, 1983

164. Calder EA, Irvine WJ: Cell-mediated immunity and immune complexes in thyroid disease. Clin Endocrinol Metab 4:287, 1975

165. Suzuki S, Mitsunaga M, Miyoshi M et al: Cytophilic antithyroglobulin antibody and antibody-dependent monocyte-mediated cytotoxicity in Hashimoto's thyroiditis. J Clin Endocrinol Metab 51:446, 1980

166. Sack J, Baker JR, Jr, Weetman AP et al: Killer cell activity and antibody-dependent cell-mediated cytotoxicity are normal in Hashimoto's disease. J Clin Endocrinol Metab 62:1059, 1986

167. Amino N, Mori H, Iwatani Y et al: Peripheral K lymphocytes in autoimmune thyroid disease: decrease in Graves' disease and increase in Hashimoto's disease. J Clin Endocrinol Metab 54:587, 1982

168. Bogner U, Schleusener H, Wall JR: Antibody-dependent cell mediated cytotoxicity against human thyroid cells in Hashimoto's thyroiditis but not Graves' disease. J Clin Endocrinol Metab 59:734, 1984

169. Hidaka Y, Amino N, Iwatani Y et al: Increase in peripheral natural killer cell activity in patients with autoimmune thyroid disease. Autoimmunity 11:239, 1992

170. Iwatani Y, Amino N, Kabutomori O et al: Decrease of peripheral large granular lymphocytes in Graves' disease. Clin Exp Immunol 55:239, 1984

170a. Kung AWC, Lau LMA, Lau KS: The role of interferon-γ in lymphocytic thyroiditis: Its functional and pathological effect on human thyrocytes in culture. Clin Exp Immunol 87:261, 1992

171. Sato K, Yamazaki K, Shizume K et al: Pathogenesis of autoimmune hypothyroidism induced by lymphokine-activated killer (LAK) cell therapy: in vitro inhibition of human thyroid function by interleukin-2 in the presence of autologous intrathyroidal lymphocytes. Thyroid 3:179, 1993

172. Nagataki S, Eguchi K: Cytokines and immune regulation in thyroid autoimmunity. Autoimmunity 13: 27, 1992

173. Kite JH, Witebsky E: Hereditary autoimmune thyroiditis in the fowl. Science 160:1357, 1968

174. Beierwaltes WH, Nishyama RH: Dog thyroiditis. Occurrence and similarity to Hashimoto's struma. Endocrinology 83:501, 1968

175. Evans TC, Beierwaltes WH, Nishyama RH: Experimental canine Hashimoto's thyroiditis. Endocrinology 84:641, 1969

176. Kite JH, Argue H, Rose NR: Experimental thyroiditis in the rhesus monkey. I. Cytotoxic, mixed-agglutinating and complement-fixing antibodies. Clin Exp Immunol 1:139, 1966

177. Beall GN, Daniel PM, Pratt OE, Solomon DH: Effects of immunization of baboons with human thyroid tissue. J Clin Endocrinol Metab 29:1460, 1969

178. Weigle WO, Nakamura RM: The development of autoimmune thyroiditis in rabbits following injection of aqueous preparations of heterologous thyroglobulins. J Immunol 99:223, 1967

179. Champion BR, Page KR, Parish N et al: Identification of a thyroxine-containing self-epitope of thyroglobulin which triggers thyroid autoreactive T cells. J Exp Med 174:363, 1991

180. Mieschner P, Gorstein F, Benacerraf B, Gell PGH: Studies on the pathogenesis of experimental immune thyroiditis. Proc Soc Exp Biol Med 107:12, 1961

181. Ringertz B, Wasserman J, Packalen TH, Perlmann P: Cellular and humoral immune responses in experimental autoimmune thyroiditis. Int Arch Allergy Appl Immunol 40:917, 1971

182. Salvin SB, Liauw HL: Immunologic unresponsiveness to allergic thyroiditis in guinea pigs. J Immunol 98:432, 1967

183. MacSween RNM, Ono K, Bell PRF et al: Experimental allergic thyroiditis in rats: Suppression by heterologous (rabbit) anti-lymphocyte sera to lymph node, thymic, and splenic lymphocytes. Clin Exp Immunol 6:273, 1970

184. Silverman DA, Rose NR: Neonatal thymectomy increases the incidence of spontaneous and methyl-cholanthrene-enhanced thyroiditis in rats. Science 184:162, 1974

185. Flynn JC, Conaway DH, Cobbold S et al: Depletion of L3T4⁺ and Lyt-2⁺ cells by rat monoclonal antibodies alters the development of adoptively transferred experimental autoimmune thyroiditis. Cell Immunol 122:377, 1989

186. Maron R, Zerubavel R, Friedman A, Cohen IR: T lymphocyte line specific for thyroglobulin produces or vaccinates against autoimmune thyroiditis in mice. J Immunol 131:2316, 1983

187. Kotani T, Umeki K, Yagihashi S et al: Identification of thyroiditogenic epitope on porcine thyroid peroxidase for C57BL/6 mice. J Immunol 148:2084, 1992

188. Rose NR, Skelton FR, Kite JH, Witebsky E: Experi-

mental thyroiditis in the rhesus monkey. III. Course of the disease. Clin Exp Immunol 1:171, 1966

189. Nilsson LA, Wick G, Kite J: Demonstration of thyroglobulin in the thyroid glands of obese strain and normal white leghorn chicken embryos. Clin Exp Immunol 11:83, 1972

190. Sundick RS, Bagchi N, Livezey MD et al: Abnormal thyroid regulation in chickens with autoimmune thyroiditis. Endocrinology 105:493, 1979

191. Sundick RS, Wick G: Increased iodine uptake by obese strain thyroid glands transplanted to normal chick embryos. J Immunol 116:1319, 1976

192. Allen EM, Appel MC, Braverman LE: Iodine-induced thyroiditis and hypothyroidism in the hemithyroidectomized BB/W rat. Endocrinology 121:481, 1987

193. Sundick RS, Herdegen DM, Brown TR, Bagchi N: The incorporation of dietary iodine into thyroglobulin increases its immunogenicity. Endocrinology 120:2078, 1987

194. Nakamura RM, Weigle WO: Isoantigens of thyroglobulin and their significance in experimental autoimmune thyroiditis. J Immunol 101:876, 1968

195. Weigle WO, High GJ: The behavior of autologous thyroglobulin in the circulation of rabbits immunized with either heterologous or altered homologous thyroglobulin. J Immunol 98:1105, 1967

196. Weigle WO, Romball CG: Humoral and cell-mediated immunity in experimental progressive thyroiditis in rabbits. Clin Exp Immunol 21:351, 1975

197. Peter HJ, Gerber H, Studer H et al: Autonomous growth and function of cultured thyroid follicles from cats with spontaneous hyperthyroidism. Thyroid 1:331, 1991

198. MacKenzie WA, Schwartz AE, Friedman EW, Davies TF: Intrathyroidal T cell clones from patients with autoimmune thyroid disease. J Clin Endocrinol Metab 64:818, 1987

199. MacKenzie WA, Davies TF: An intrathyroidal T-cell clone specifically cytotoxic for human thyroid cells. Immunology 61:101, 1987

200. Lidman K, Eriksson U, Norberg R, Fagraeus A: Indirect immunofluorescence staining of human thyroid by antibodies occurring in *Yersinia enterocolitica* infections. Clin Exp Immunol 23:429, 1976

201. Costagliola S, Ruf J, Durand-Gorde M-J, Carayon P: Monoclonal anti-idiotypic antibodies interact with the 93 kilodalton thyrotropin receptor and exhibit heterogeneous biological activities. Endocrinology 128:1555, 1991

202. Volpe R, Farid NR, Westarp CV, Row VV: The pathogenesis of Graves' disease and Hashimoto's thyroiditis. Clin Endocrinol 3:239, 1974

203. Stenzky V, Kozma L, Balazs CS et al: The genetics of Graves' disease: HLA and disease susceptibility. J Clin Endocrinol Metab 61:735, 1985

204. Sridama V, Pacini F, DeGroot LJ: Decreased suppressor T-lymphocytes in autoimmune thyroid diseases detected by monoclonal antibodies. J Clin Endocrinol Metab 54:316, 1982

205. Pacini F, DeGroot LJ: Studies of immunoglobulin synthesis in cultures of peripheral T and B lymphocytes: reduced T-suppressor cell activity in Graves' disease. Clin Endocrinol 18:219, 1983

206. Nakamura M, Burastero SE, Ueki Y et al: Probing the normal and autoimmune B cell repertoire with Epstein-Barr virus. Frequency of B cells producing monoreactive high affinity autoantibodies in patients with Hashimoto's disease and systemic lupus erythematosus. J Immunol 141:4165, 1988

207. Marcos MAR, Toribio M-L, de la Hera A et al: Mutual cell interactions and the selection of immune repertoires: Implication in autoimmunity. Immunol Today 9:204, 1988

208. Bottazzo GF, Todd I, Mirakian R et al: Organ-specific autoimmunity: a 1986 overview. Immunol Rev 94:137, 1986

209. Dziarski R: Autoimmunity: polyclonal activation or antigen induction? Immunol Today 9:340, 1988

210. Eyquem A, Calmettes C, Decourt J: Immunological studies on Hashimoto's goiter consecutive to mumps thyroiditis. Rev Fr Etudes Clin Biol 4:1039, 1959

211. Aoki N, DeGroot LJ: Lymphocyte blastogenic response to human thyroglobulin in Graves' disease, Hashimoto's thyroiditis, and metastatic thyroid cancer. Clin Exp Immunol 38:523, 1979

212. Hancock SL, Cox RS, McDougall IR: Thyroid diseases after treatment of Hodgkin's disease. N Engl J Med 325:599, 1991

213. Sommers SC, Meissner WA: Basement membrane changes in chronic thyroiditis. Am J Clin Pathol 24:434, 1954

214. Van Herle AJ, Uller RP, Mathews NL, Brown J: Radioimmunoassay for measurement of thyroglobulin in human serum. J Clin Invest 52:1320, 1973

215. Roitt IM, Torrigiani G: Identification and estimation of undergraded thyroglobulin in human serum. Endocrinology 81:421, 1967

216. Smith RT: Possibilities and problems of immunologic intervention in cancer. N Engl J Med 287:439, 1972

217. Jonckheer MH: Presence d'un albumine comme constituant normal des proteines thyroidiennes. Ann Endocrinol 24:756, 1963

218. Shimoda K, Thompson B: Radioiodine labelling of serum albumin in vivo. Endocrinology 76:570, 1965

219. Shenkman L, Bottone EJ: Antibodies to *Yersinia enterocolitica* in thyroid disease. Ann Intern Med 85:735, 1976

220. Resetkova E, Notenboom R, Arreaza G et al: Seroreactivity to bacterial antigens is not a unique phenomenon in patients with autoimmune thyroid diseases in Canada. Thyroid 4:269, 1994

221. Weiss M, Ingbar SH, Winblad S, Kasper DL: Demonstration of a saturable binding site for thyrotropin in *Yersinia enterocolitica.* Science 219:1331, 1983

222. Wolf MW, Misaki T, Bech K et al: Immunoglobulins of patients recovering from yersinia enterocolitica infections exhibit Graves' disease-like activity in human thyroid membranes. Thyroid 1:315, 1991

223. Wenzel BE, Heesemann J, Wenzel KW, Scriba PC: Patients with autoimmune thyroid diseases have antibodies to plasmid encoded proteins of enteropathogenic Yersinia. J Endocrinol Invest 11:139, 1988

224. Ratanachaiyavong S, Demaine AG, Campbell RD, McGregor AM: Heat shock protein 70 (HSP70) and complement C4 genotypes in patients with hyperthyroid Graves' disease. Clin Exp Immunol 84:48, 1991

225. Heufelder AE, Wenzel BE, Gorman CA, Bahn RS: Detection, cellular localization, and modulation of heat shock proteins in cultured fibroblasts from patients with extrathyroidal manifestations of Graves' disease. J Clin Endocrinol Metab 73:739, 1991

226. Ruf J, Feldt-Rasmussen U, Hegedus L et al: Bispecific thyroglobulin and thyroperoxidase autoantibodies in patients with various thyroid and autoimmune diseases. J Clin Endocrinol Metab 79:1404, 1994

227. Klavinskis LS, Notkins AL, Oldstone MBA: Persistent viral infection of the thyroid gland: alteration of thyroid function in the absence of tissue injury. Endocrinology 122:567, 1988

228. Okayasu I, Hatakeyama S: A combination of necrosis of autologous thyroid gland and injection of lipopolysaccharide induces autoimmune thyroiditis. Clin Immunol Immunopathol 31:344, 1984

229. Lagaye S, Vexiau P, Morozov V et al: Human spumaretrovirus-related sequences in the DNA of leukocytes from patients with Graves' disease. Proc Natl Acad Sci USA 89:10070, 1992

230. Tominaga T, Katamine S, Namba H et al: Lack of evidence for the presence of human immunodeficiency virus type 1–related sequences in patients with Graves' disease. Thyroid 1:307, 1991

231. Doble ND, Banga JP, Pope R et al: Autoantibodies to the thyroid microsomal/thyroid peroxidase antigen are polyclonal and directed to several distinct antigenic sites. Immunology 64:23, 1988

232. Knight J, Laing P, Knight A et al: Thyroid-stimulating autoantibodies usually contain only lambda-light chains: evidence for the "forbidden clone" theory. J Clin Endocrinol Metab 62:342, 1986

233. Kaulfersch W, Baker JR Jr, Burman KD et al: Immunoglobulin and T cell antigen receptor gene arrangements indicate that the immune response in autoimmune thyroid disease is polyclonal. J Clin Endocrinol Metab 66:958, 1988

234. Bartels ED: Heredity in Graves' disease. Copenhagen, Enjnar Munksgaards Forlag, 1941

235. Carey C, Skosey C, Pinnamaneni KM et al: Thyroid abnormalities in children of parents who have Graves' disease; possible pre-Graves' disease. Metabolism 29:369, 1980

236. Dunning EJ: Struma lymphomatosa: a report of three cases in one family. J Clin Endocrinol Metab 19:1121, 1959

237. DeGroot LJ, Hall R, McDermott WV Jr, Davis AM: Hashimoto's thyroiditis, a genetically conditioned disease. N Engl J Med 267:267, 1962

238. Roitt IM, Doniach D: A reassessment of studies on the aggregation of thyroid autoimmunity in families of thyroiditis patients. Clin Exp Immunol 2:727, 1967

239. Hall R, Owen SG, Smart GA: Evidence for genetic predisposition to formation of thyroid auto-antibodies. Lancet 2:187, 1960

240. Hall R, Dingle PR, Roberts DF: Thyroid antibodies: a study of first degree relatives. Clin Genet 3:319, 1972

241. Phillips D, McLachlan S, Stephenson A et al: Autosomal dominant transmission of autoantibodies to thyroglobulin and thyroid peroxidase. J Clin Endocrinol Metab 70:742, 1990

242. Phillips D, Prentice L, Upadhyaya M et al: Autosomal dominant inheritance of autoantibodies to thyroid peroxidase and thyroglobulin—studies in families not selected for autoimmune thyroid disease. J Clin Endocrinol Metab 72:973, 1991

243. Forbes IJ, Roitt IM, Doniach D, Solomon IL: The thyroid cytotoxic autoantibody. J Clin Invest 41:996, 1962

244. Hall R, Saxena K, Owen SG: A study of the parents of patients with Hashimoto's disease. Lancet 2:1291, 1962

245. Irvine WJ, MacGregor AG, Stuart AE, Hall GH: Hashimoto's disease in uniovular twins. Lancet 2:850, 1961

246. Bonnyns M, Vanhaelst L, Golstein J et al: Long-acting thyroid stimulator and thyroid function in relatives of patients with Graves' disease. Clin Endocrinol 2:277, 1973

247. Evans AWH, McDougall CDM, Woodrow JC, Chew AR: Antibodies in the families of thyrotoxic patients. Lancet 1:636, 1967

248. Weetman AP, McGregor AM: Autoimmune thyroid disease: Developments in our understanding. Endocr Rev 5:309, 1984

249. Mangklabruks A, Cox N, DeGroot LJ: Genetic factors in autoimmune thyroid disease analyzed by restriction fragment length polymorphisms of candidate genes. J Clin Endocrinol Metab 73:236, 1991

250. Tamai H, Uno H, Hirota Y et al: Immunogenetics of Hashimoto's and Graves' diseases. J Clin Endocrinol Metab 60:62, 1985

251. Pryds O, Lervang HH, Ostergaard-Kristensen HP et al: HLA-DR factors associated with postpartum hypothyroidism: an early manifestation of Hashimoto's thyroiditis? Tissue Antigens 30:34, 1987

252. Volpe R: Autoimmune thyroid disease: a perspective. Molec Biol Med 3:25, 1986

253. Yanagawa T, Mangklabruks A, Chang Y-B et al: Human histocompatibility leukocyte antigen-DQA1*0501 allele associated with genetic susceptibility to Graves' disease in a Caucasian population. J Clin Endocrinol Metab 76:1569, 1993

254. Yanagawa T, Mangklabruks A, DeGroot LJ: Strong association between HLA-DQA1*0501 and Graves' disease in a male Caucasian population. J Clin Endocrinol Metab, 79:227, 1994

254a. Badenhoop K, Walfish PG, Rav H et al: Susceptibility and resistance alleles of human leukocyte antigen (HLA) DQA1 and HLA DQB1 are shared in endocrine autoimmune disease. J Clin Endocrinol Metab 870:2112, 1995

255. Hu R, Beck C, Chang Y-B, DeGroot LJ: HLA Class II genes in Graves' disease. Autoimmunity 12:103, 1992

256. Nakao Y, Matsumoto H, Miyazaki T et al: IgG heavy chain allotypes (Gm) in autoimmune diseases. Clin Exp Immunol 42:20, 1980

256a. Cho BY, Chung JH, Shong YK et al: A strong association between thyrotropin receptor-blocking antibody-positive atrophic autoimmune thyroiditis and HLA-DR8 and HLA-DQB1*0302 in Koreans. J Clin Endocrinol Metab 77:611, 1993

257. Uno H, Sasazuki T, Tamai H, Matsumoto H: Two major genes, linked to HLA and Gm, control susceptibility to Graves' disease. Nature 292:768, 1981

258. Skanes V, Larsen B, Sampson-Murphy L, Farid NR: Polymorphism of the fourth component of complement in Graves' disease and type I diabetes mellitus. Clin Invest Med 8:126, 1985

259. Morel PA, Dorman JS, Todd JA et al: Aspartic acid at position 57 of the HLA-DQ beta chain protects against type I diabetes: a family study. Proc Natl Acad Sci USA 85:8111, 1988

259a. Bjorkman PJ, Saper MA, Samaroui B, Bennett WS, Strominger JL, Wiley DC: The foreign antigen binding site and T cell recognition regions of class I histocompatibility antigens. Nature 329:512, 1987

260. Tudhope GR, Wilson GM: Deficiency of vitamin B$_{12}$ in hypothyroidism. Lancet 1:703, 1962

261. Lawley TJ, Hall RP, Fauci AS et al: Defective Fc-receptor functions associated with the HLA-B8/DRw3 haplotype. N Engl J Med 304:185, 1981

262. Demaine A, Welsh KI, Hawe BS, Farid NR: Polymorphism of the T cell receptor beta-chain in Graves' disease. J Clin Endocrinol Metab 55:643, 1987

263. Weetman AP, So AK, Roe C et al: T-cell receptor α chain V region polymorphism linked to primary autoimmune hypothyroidism but not Graves' disease. Human Immunol 20:167, 1987

264. Davies TF, Martin A, Concepcion ES et al: Evidence for selective accumulation of intrathyroidal T lymphocytes in human autoimmune thyroid disease based on T cell receptor V gene usage. J Clin Invest 89:157, 1992

265. McIntosh RS, Watson PF, Pickerill AP et al: No restriction of intrathyroidal T cell receptor Vα families in the thyroid of Graves' disease. Clin Exp Immunol 91:147, 1993

266. Mangklabruks A, Correa Billerbeck A-E, Wajchenberg B et al: Genetic linkage studies of thyroid peroxidase (TPO) gene in families with TPO deficiency. J Clin Endocrinol Metab 72:471, 1991

267. Irvine WJ, Davies SH, Teitelbaum S et al: The clinical and pathological significance of gastric parietal cell antibody. Ann NY Acad Sci 124:657, 1965

268. Doniach D, Roitt IM, Taylor KB: Autoimmune phenomena in pernicious anemia. Serological overlap with thyroiditis, thyrotoxicosis, and systemic lupus erythematosus. Br Med J 1:1374, 1963

269. Jones BR: Lacrimal and salivary precipitating antibodies in Sjögren's syndrome. Lancet 2:773, 1958

270. Buchanan WW, Crooks J, Alexander WD et al: Association of Hashimoto's thyroiditis and rheumatoid arthritis. Lancet 1:245, 1961

271. Mulhern LM, Masi AT, Shulman LE: Hashimoto's disease: a search for associated disorders in 170 clinically detected cases. Lancet 2:508, 1966

272. White RG, Bass BH, Williams E: Lymphadenoid goiter and the syndrome of systemic lupus erythematosus. Lancet 1:368, 1961

273. Larsen RA, Godal T: Family studies in systemic lupus erythematosus (SLE). IX. Thyroid diseases and antibodies. J Chronic Dis 25:225, 1972

274. Katakura M, Yamada T, Aizawa T et al: Presence of antideoxyribonucleic acid antibody in patients with hyperthyroidism of Graves' disease. J Clin Endocrinol Metab 64:405, 1987

275. Baethge BA, Levine SN, Wolf RE: Antibodies to nuclear antigens in Graves' disease. J Clin Endocrinol Metab 66:485, 1988

276. Carpenter CCJ, Solomon N, Silverberg SG et al: Schmidt's syndrome (thyroid and adrenal insufficiency): a review of the literature and a report of

fifteen new cases including ten instances of coexistent diabetes mellitus. Medicine 43:153, 1964

277. Bloodworth JMB, Karkendall WM, Carr TL: Addison's disease associated with thyroid insufficiency and atrophy (Schmidt syndrome). J Clin Endocrinol Metab 14:540, 1954

278. Mead RK: Autoimmune Addison's disease. N Engl J Med 266:583, 1962

279. Irvine WJ: Clinical and immunological associations in adrenal disorders. Proc R Soc Med 61:271, 1968

280. Goudie RB: Anterior hypophysitis associated with autoimmune disease. Proc R Soc Med 61:275, 1968

281. Editorial: Autoimmunity in idiopathic Addison's disease. Lancet 1:1040, 1967

282. Kenny FM, Holliday MA: Hypoparathyroidism, moniliasis, Addison's and Hashimoto's diseases. N Engl J Med 271:708, 1964

283. Karlish AJ, MacGregor GA: Sarcoidosis, thyroiditis, and Addison's disease. Lancet 2:330, 1970

284. Beare RLB: Lymphadenoid goiter (Hashimoto's disease): a clinicopathological study. Br Med J 1:480, 1958

285. Neufeld M, Maclaren NK, Blizzard RM: Two types of autoimmune Addison's disease associated with different polyglandular autoimmune (PGA) syndromes. Medicine 60:355, 1981

286. Muir A, Schatz DA, MacLaren NK: Polyglandular failure syndromes. p. 3013. In DeGroot LJ (ed): Endocrinology, 3rd Ed. WB Saunders Co, Philadelphia, 1994

287. McConkey B, Callaghan P: Thyroiditis and cirrhosis of the liver. Lancet 1:939, 1960

288. Mackay IR, Taft LI, Cowling DC: Lupoid hepatitis. Lancet 2:1323, 1956

289. Blizzard RM, Hamwi GJ, Skillman TG, Wheeler WE: Thyroglobulin antibodies in multiple thyroid disease. N Engl J Med 260:112, 1959

290. McHardy-Young S, Doniach D, Polani PE: Thyroid function in Turner's syndrome and allied conditions. Lancet 2:1161, 1970

291 Vallotton MB, Forbes AP: Autoimmunity in gonadal dysgenesis and Klinefelter's syndrome. Lancet 1:648, 1967

292. Fialkow PJ, Hecht F, Uchida IA, Motulsky AG: Increased frequency of thyroid autoantibodies in mothers of patients with Down's syndrome. Lancet 2:868, 1965

293. Irvine WJ, Scarth L, Clarke BF et al: Thyroid and gastric autoimmunity in patients with diabetes mellitus. Lancet 2:7665, 1970

294. Faustman D, Li X, Lin HY et al: Linkage of faulty major histocompatibility complex class I to autoimmune diabetes. Science 254:1756, 1991

295. Marshall J: ITP and Graves' disease. Ann Intern Med 67:411, 1967

296. Ochi Y, DeGroot LJ: Vitiligo in Graves' disease. Ann Intern Med 71:935, 1969

297. MacKay IR: Autoimmune aspects of three skin diseases. Pemphigus, cutaneous lupus erythematosus, and vitiligo. Austral J Dermatol 9:113, 1967

298. Bonomo L, Dammacco F: Characterization studies of thyroglobulin antibodies in leprosy: an immunological study of diethylaminoethylcellulose chromatographic fractions. Immunology 13:565, 1967

299. Fournier C, Chen H, Leger A, Charreire J: Immunological studies of autoimmune thyroid disorders: abnormalities in the inducer T cell subset and proliferative responses to autologous and allogeneic stimulation. Clin Exp Immunol 54:539, 1983

300. Ludgate ME, McGregor AM, Weetman AP et al: Analysis of T cell subsets in Graves' disease: Alterations associated with carbimazole. Br Med J 288:526, 1984

301. Totterman TH, Karlsson FA, Bengtsson M, Mendel-Harvig IB: Induction of circulating activated suppressor-like T cells by methimazole therapy for Graves' disease. N Engl J Med 316:15, 1987

302. Misaki T, Konishi J, Iida Y et al: Altered balance of immunoregulatory T lymphocyte subsets in autoimmune thyroid diseases. Acta Endocrinol 105:200, 1984

303. Di Mario U, Scardellato A, Irvine WJ et al: Immunity in Graves' disease at diagnosis: correlation between activated T cells and humoral immune factors. Acta Endocrinol (Copenh) 113:493, 1986

304. Volpe R, Karlsson A, Jansson R, Dahlberg PA: Evidence that antithyroid drugs induce remissions in Graves' disease by modulating thyroid cellular activity. Clin Endocrinol 25:453, 1986

305. How J, Topliss DJ, Strakosch C et al: Lymphocyte sensitization and suppressor T lymphocyte defect in patients long after treatment for Graves' disease. Clin Endocrinol 18:61, 1983

306. Okita N, How J, Topliss D et al: Suppressor T lymphocyte dysfunction in Graves' disease: role of the H-2 histamine receptor-bearing suppressor T lymphocytes. J Clin Endocrinol Metab 53:1002, 1981

307. Goldrath N, Shoham J, Bank H, Eisenstein Z: Antithyroid drugs and lymphocyte function. II. The in vivo effect on blastogenesis and suppressor cell activity in Graves' disease. Clin Exp Immunol 50:62, 1982

308. Hallengren B, Forsgren A: Suppressor T lymphocyte function in Graves' disease. Acta Endocrinol 101:354, 1982

309. Sridama V, Pacini F, Yang S-L et al: Decreased levels of helper T cells: a possible cause of immunodeficiency in pregnancy. N Engl J Med 307:352, 1982

310. Jansson R, Bernander S, Karlsson A et al: Autoimmune thyroid dysfunction in the postpartum period. J Clin Endocrinol Metab 58:681, 1984

311. Amino N, Tamaki H, Aozasa M et al: Postpartum onset of Graves' disease. p. 231. In Pinchera A, Ingbar SH, McKenzie JM, Fenzi GF (eds): Thyroid Autoimmunity, Plenum Press, New York, 1987

312. Jackson RA, Haynes BF, Burch WM et al: IA⁺ T cells in new onset Graves' disease. J Clin Endocrinol Metab 59:187, 1984

313. Koukkou E, Panayiotidis P, Alevizou-Terzaki V, Thalassinos N: High levels of serum soluble interleukin-2 receptors in hyperthyroid patients: Correlation with serum thyroid hormones and independence from the etiology of the hyperthyroidism. J Clin Endocrinol Metab 73:771, 1991

314. Morimoto C, Hafler DA, Weiner HI et al: Selective loss of the suppressor-inducer T-cell subset in progressive multiple sclerosis: Analysis with anti-2H4 monoclonal antibody. N Engl J Med 316:67, 1987

315. Takeuchi T, Tanaka S, Steinberg AD et al: Defective expression of the 2H4 molecule after autologous mixed lymphocyte reaction activation in systemic lupus erythematosus patients. J Clin Invest 82:1288, 1988

316. Noma T, Yata J, Shishiba Y, Inatsuki B: In vitro detection of anti-thyroglobulin antibody forming cells from the lymphocytes of chronic thyroiditis patients and analysis of their regulation. Clin Exp Immunol 49:565, 1982

317. Mori H, Hamada N, DeGroot LJ: Studies on thyroglobulin-specific suppressor T cell function in autoimmune thyroid disease. J Clin Endocrinol Metab 61:306, 1985

318. Iitaka M, Aguayo JF, Iwatani Y et al: Studies of the effect of suppressor T lymphocytes on the induction of antithyroid microsomal antibody secreting cells in autoimmune thyroid disease. J Clin Endocrinol Metab 66:1988

319. Tao T-W, Gatenby PA, Leu S-L et al: Helper and suppressor activities of lymphocyte subsets on anti-thyroglobulin production in vitro. J Clin Endocrinol Metab 61:520, 1985

320. Vento S, Hegarty JE, Bottazzo G et al: Antigen specific suppressor cell function in autoimmune chronic active hepatitis. Lancet 2:1200, 1984

321. Yoshikawa N, Morita T, Resetkova E et al: Reduced activation of suppressor T lymphocytes by specific antigens in autoimmune thyroid disease. J Endocrinol Invest 15:609, 1992

322. Biassoni P, Ciprandi G, Ferrini S et al: Incidence of T cell subset imbalance in relatives of Graves' disease patients. J Endocrinol Invest 7:141, 1984

323. Margolick JB, Hsu S-M, Volkman DJ et al: Immuno-histochemical characterization of intrathyroid lymphocytes in Graves' disease. Interstitial and intraepithelial populations. Am J Med 76:815, 1984

324. Canonica GW, Caria M, Torre G et al: Autoimmune thyroid disease: Purification and phenotypic analysis of intrathyroid T cells. J Endocrinol Invest 7:641, 1984

325. Misaki T, Konishi J, Arai K et al: HLA-DR antigen expression on intrathyroidal lymphocytes and thyrocytes in Hashimoto's thyroiditis and Graves' disease: an immunohistological study. Endocrinol Japan 34:257, 1987

326. Ueki Y, Eguchi K, Otsubo T et al: Phenotypic analyses and Concanavalin-A-induced suppressor cell dysfunction of intrathyroidal lymphocytes from patients with Graves' disease. J Clin Endocrinol Metab 67:1018, 1988

327. Tezuka H, Eguchi K, Fukuda T et al: Natural killer and natural killer-like cell activity of peripheral blood and intrathyroidal mononuclear cells from patients with Graves' disease. J Clin Endocrinol Metab 66:702, 1988

328. Bagnasco M, Venuti D, Prigione I et al: Graves' disease: phenotypic and functional analysis at the clonal level of the T-cell repertoire in peripheral blood and in thyroid. Clin Immunol Immunopathol 47:230, 1988

329. Del Prete GF, Maggi E, Mariotti S et al: Cytolytic T lymphocytes with natural killer activity in thyroid infiltrate of patients with Hashimoto's thyroiditis: analysis at clonal level. J Clin Endocrinol Metab 62:52, 1986

330. MacKenzie WA, Schwartz AE, Friedman EW, Davies TF: Intrathyroidal T cell clones from patients with autoimmune thyroid disease. J Clin Endocrinol Metab 64:818, 1987

331. Fisfalen ME, DeGroot LJ, Quintans J et al: Microsomal antigen-reactive lymphocyte lines and clones derived from thyroid tissue of patients with Graves' disease. J Clin Endocrinol Metab 66:776, 1988

332. Volpe R: Suppressor T lymphocyte dysfunction is important in the pathogenesis of autoimmune thyroid disease: a perspective. Thyroid 3:345, 1993

333. Raines KB, Baker JR, Lukes YG et al: Antithyrotropin antibodies in the sera of Graves' disease patients. J Clin Endocrinol Metab 61:217, 1985

334. Sikorska HM: Anti-thyroglobulin anti-idiotypic antibodies in sera of patients with Hashimoto's thyroiditis and Graves' disease. J Immunol 137:3786, 1986

335. Hara Y, Sridama V, DeGroot LJ: Auto-anti-idiotype antibody against antithyroglobulin auto-antibody in humans. J Clin Lab Immunol 26:13, 1988

336. Hanafusa T, Chiovato L, Doniach D et al: Aberrant expression of HLA-DR antigen on thyrocytes in Graves' disease: relevance for autoimmunity. Lancet 2:1111, 1983

337. Bottazzo GF, Pujol-Borrell R, Hanafusa T, Feldman

F: Role of aberrant HLA-DR expression and antigen presentation in induction of endocrine autoimmunity. Lancet 2:1115, 1983

338. Buscema M, Todd I, Deuss U et al: Influence of tumor necrosis factor-α on the modulation by interferon-γ of HLA class II molecules in human thyroid cells and its effect on interferon-γ binding. J Clin Endocrinol Metab 69:433, 1989

339. Matsunaga M, Eguchi K, Fukuda T et al: Class II major histocompatibility complex antigen expression and cellular interactions in thyroid glands of Graves' disease. J Clin Endocrinol Metab 62:723, 1986

340. Weetman AP, Volkman DJ, Burman KD et al: The in vitro regulation of human thyrocyte HLA-DR antigen expression. J Clin Endocrinol Metab 61:817, 1985

341. Piccinini LA, MacKenzie WA, Platzer M, Davies TF: Lymphokine regulation of HLA-DR gene expression in human thyroid cell monolayers. J Clin Endocrinol Metab 64:543, 1987

342. Aguayo J, Iitaka M, Row VV, Volpe R: Studies of HLA-DR expression on cultured human thyrocytes: Effect of antithyroid drugs and other agents on interferon-γ-induced HLA-DR expression. J Clin Endocrinol Metab 66:903, 1988

343. Chiovato L, Lapi P, Mariotti S et al: Simultaneous expression of thyroid peroxidase and human leukocyte antigen-DR by human thyroid cells: Modulation by thyrotropin, thyroid-stimulating antibody, and interferon-γ. J Clin Endocrinol Metab 79:653, 656, 1994

344. Davies TF, Bermas B, Platzer M, Roman SH: T-cell sensitization to autologous thyroid cells and normal nonspecific suppressor T-cell function in Graves' disease. Clin Endocrinol 22:155, 1985

345. Eguchi K, Otsubo T, Kawabe Y et al: Synergy in antigen presentation by thyroid epithelial cells and monocytes from patients with Graves' disease. Clin Exp Immunol 72:84, 1988

346. Fisfalen M-E, Franklin WA, DeGroot LJ et al: Expression of HLA-ABC and -DR antigens in thyroid neoplasia and correlation with mononuclear leukocyte infiltration. J Endocrinol Invest 13:41, 1990

347. Leclere J, Bene MC, Duprez A et al: Behavior of thyroid tissue from patients with Graves' disease in nude mice. J Clin Endocrinol Metab 59:175, 1984

348. Mhost J, Knapp W, Wick G: Class II antigens in Hashimoto's thyroiditis. I. Synthesis and expression of HLA-DR and HLA-DQ by thyroid epithelial cells. Clin Immunol Immunopathol 41:165, 1986

349. Caspi RR, Roberge FG, Nussenblatt RB: Organ-resident, nonlymphoid cells suppress proliferation of autoimmune T-helper lymphocytes. Science 237:1029, 1987

350. Gaspari AA, Jenkins MK, Katz SI: Class II MHC-bearing keratinocytes induce antigen-specific unresponsiveness in hapten-specific TH1 clones. J Immunol 141:2216, 1988

351. Lo D, Burkly LC, Widera G et al: Diabetes and tolerance in transgenic mice expression class II MHC molecules in pancreatic beta cells. Cell 53:159, 1988

352. Kaplan MM: Hypothyroidism after treatment with interleukin-2 and lymphokine-activated killer cells. N Engl J Med 318:1557, 1988

353. Burman P, Totterman TH, Oberg K, Karlsson FA: Thyroid autoimmunity in patients on long term therapy with leukocyte-derived interferon. J Clin Endocrinol Metab 63:1086, 1986

354. Kawakami Y, Kuzuya N, Yamashita K: A new model of autoimmune thyroiditis in mouse. Abstract (No. 12-18-021) presented at the 8th International Congress of Endocrinology, Kyoto, Japan, July 17–23, 1988

355. Otsubo T, Eguchi K, Shimomura C et al: In vitro cellular interactions among thyrocytes, T cells, and monocytes from patients with Graves' disease. Acta Endocrinol (Copenh) 117:282, 1988

355a. Bertelsen JB, Hegedus L: Cigarette smoking and the thyroid. Thyroid 4:327, 1994

356. Hidaka Y, Amino N, Iwatani Y et al: Recurrence of thyrotoxicosis after attack of allergic rhinitis in patients with Graves' disease. J Clin Endocrinol Metab 77:1667, 1993

357. Ericsson UB, Christensen SB, Thorell JI: A high prevalence of thyroglobulin autoantibodies in adults with and without thyroid disease as measured with a sensitive solid-phase immunosorbent radioassay. Clin Immunol Immunopathol 37:154, 1985

358. Dingle PR, Ferguson A, Horn DB et al: The incidence of thyroglobulin antibodies and thyroid enlargement in a general practice in northeast England. Clin Exp Immunol 1:277, 1966

359. McLachlan SM, Pegg CAS, Atherton MC et al: The effect of carbimazole on thyroid autoantibody synthesis by thyroid lymphocytes. J Clin Endocrinol Metab 60:1237, 1985

360. Signore A, Pozzilli P, Di Mario U et al: Inhibition of the receptor for interleukin-2 induced by carbimazole: relevance for the therapy of autoimmune thyroid disease. Clin Exp Immunol 60:111, 1985

361. McGregor AM, Ibbertson HK, Smith BR, Hall R: Carbimazole and autoantibody synthesis in Hashimoto's thyroiditis. Br Med J 281:968, 1980

362. Wenzel KW, Lente JR: Similar effects of thionamide drugs and perchlorate on thyroid-stimulating immunoglobulins in Graves' disease: Evidence against an immunosuppressive action of thionamide drugs. J Clin Endocrinol Metab 58:62, 1984

363. Weetman AP, Holt ME, Campbell AK et al: Methimazole and generation of oxygen radicals by monocytes: potential role in immunosuppression. Br Med J 288:518, 1984

364. Aguayo J, Iitaka M, Row VV, Volpe R: Studies of HLA-DR expression on cultured human thyrocytes: effect of antithyroid drugs and other agents on interferon-γ-induced HLA-DR expression. J Clin Endocrinol Metab 66:903, 1988

365. Davies TF, Yang C, Platzer M: The influence of antithyroid drugs and iodine on thyroid cell MHC class II antigen expression. Clin Endocrinol 31:125, 1989

366. Goldsmith RE, McAdams AJ, Larsen PR et al: Familial autoimmune thyroiditis: Maternal-fetal relationship and the role of generalized autoimmunity. J Clin Endocrinol Metab 37:265, 1973

367. Blizzard RM, Hung M, Chandler RW et al: Hashimoto's thyroiditis: Clinical and laboratory response to prolonged cortisone therapy. N Engl J Med 267: 1015, 1962

368. Roitt IM, Doniach D: Human autoimmune thyroiditis. Serological studies. Lancet 2:1027, 1958

369. Blizzard RM, Chandler RW, Landing BH et al: Maternal autoimmunization to thyroid as a probable cause of athyreotic cretinism. N Engl J Med 263:327, 1960

370. Chandler RW, Blizzard RM, Hung W, Kyle M: Incidence of thyrotoxic factor and other antithyroid antibodies in the mothers of cretins. N Engl J Med 267: 376, 1962

371. Hill OW: Thyroglobulin antibodies in 1,297 patients without thyroid disease. Br Med J 1:1793, 1961

372. Parker RH, Beierwaltes WH: Thyroid antibodies during pregnancy and in the newborn. J Clin Endocrinol Metab 21:792, 1961

373. Dussault JH, Letarte J, Guyda H, Laberge C: Lack of influence of thyroid antibodies on thyroid function in the newborn infant and on a mass screening program for congenital hypothyroidism. J Pediatr 96:385, 1980

374. Sutherland JM, Esselborn VM, Burket RL et al: Familial non-goitrous cretinism apparently due to maternal antithyroid antibody. N Engl J Med 263:336, 1960

375. Mitchell MS, Mokyr MB, Aspres GT, McIntosh S: Cytophilic antibodies in man. Ann Intern Med 79: 333, 1973

376. Nakamura RM, Weigle WO: Transfer of experimental autoimmune thyroiditis by serum from thyroidectomized donors. J Exp Med 130:263, 1969

377. Clinton BA, Weigle WO: Cellular events during the induction of experimental thyroiditis in the rabbit. J Exp Med 136:1605, 1972

378. Kalderon A, Boggars H: Immune complex deposits in Graves' disease and Hashimoto's thyroiditis. Am J Med 63:729, 1977

379. Calder EA, Penhale WJ, Barnes EW, Irvine WJ: Evidence for circulating immune complexes in thyroid disease. Br Med J 2:30, 1974

380. Al-Khateeb SF, Irvine WJ: Detection, quantitation and characterization of soluble immune complexes in sera of patients with thyroid disorders. J Clin Lab Immunol 1:55, 1978

381. Brohee D, Delespesse G, Debisschop MJ, Bonnyns M: Circulating immune complexes in various thyroid diseases. Clin Exp Immunol 36:379, 1979

382. Cano P, Chertman MM, Jerry LM, McKenzie JM: Circulating immune complexes in Graves' disease. Endocr Res Commun 3:307, 1976

383. Takeda Y, Kriss JP: Radiometric measurement of thyroglobulin-antithyroglobulin immune complex in human serum. J Clin Endocrinol Metab 44:46, 1977

384. Mariotti S, DeGroot LJ, Scarborough D, Medof ME: Study of circulating immune complexes in thyroid diseases. Comparison of Raji cell radioimmunoassay and specific thyro-globulin-antithyroglobulin radioassay. J Clin Endocrinol Metab 49:679, 1979

385. Mariotti S, Kaplan EL, Medof ME, DeGroot LJ: circulating thyroid-antigen-antibody immune complexes. p. 696. In Stockigt JR, Nagataki S (eds): Thyroid Research VII, Australian Academy of Science, Canberra, 1980

386. Jordan SC, Buckingham B, Sakai R, Olsen D: Studies of immune-complex glomerulonephritis mediated by human thyroglobulin. N Engl J Med 304:1212, 1981

387. Horvath F, Teague P, Gaffney EF et al: Thyroid antigen associated immune complex glomerulonephritis in Graves' disease. Am J Med 67:901, 1979

388. Ploth DW, Fitz A, Schnetzler D et al: Thyroglobulin-anti-thyroglobulin immune complex glomerulonephritis complicating radioiodine therapy. Clin Immunol Immunopathol 9:327, 1978

389. O'Regan S, Fong JC, Kaplan BS et al: Thyroid-antigen-antibody nephritis. Clin Immunol Immunopathol 6:341, 1976

390. Felix-Davies D, Waksman BH: Passive transfer of experimental immune thyroiditis in the guinea pig. Arthritis Rheum 4:416, 1961

391. Rose NR, Molotchnikoff MF, Twarog FJ: Factors affecting transfer of experimental autoimmune thyroiditis in rats. Immunology 24:859, 1973

392. Crile G Jr: The treatment of diseases of the thyroid gland. Ann R Coll Surg Engl 14:158, 1954

393. Hubble D: The diagnosis and treatment of auto-immunizing thyroiditis. Scott Med J 4:55, 1959

394. Bastenie PA: Contribution a l'etiologie du myxo-

deme spontane de l'adulte. Bull Acad Med Belg 9: 179, 1944

395. Douglass RC, Jacobson SD: Pathologic changes in adult myxedema. Survey of necropsies. J Clin Endocrinol Metab 17:1354, 1957

396. Owen SG, Smart GA: Thyroid antibodies in myxedema. Lancet 2:1034, 1958

397. Buchanan WW, Alexander WD, Crooks J et al: Association of thyrotoxicosis and autoimmune thyroiditis. Br Med J 1:843, 1961

398. Fatourechi V, McConahey WM, Woolner LB: Hyperthyroidism associated with histologic Hashimoto's thyroiditis. Mayo Clin Proc 46:682, 1971

399. Whitesell FB, Black BM: Statistical study of clinical significance of lymphocytic and fibrocytic replacements in hyperplastic thyroid gland. J Clin Endocrinol 9:1202, 1949

400. Blagg CR: Antibodies to thyroglobulin in patients with thyrotoxicosis treated with radioactive iodine. Lancet 2:1364, 1960

401. Eason J: Correlation of Graves' disease and thyroiditis. Edinburgh Med J 35:169, 1928

402. Hales IB, Myhill J, Rundle FF et al: Relation of eye signs in Graves' disease to circulating antibodies to thyroglobulin. Lancet 1:468, 1961

403. Wall JR, Good BF, Forbes IJ, Hetzel BS: Demonstration of the production of the long acting thyroid stimulator (LATS) by peripheral lymphocytes cultured in vitro. Clin Exp Immunol 14:555, 1973

404. Fayet G, Verrier B, Giraud A et al: Effects of long-acting thyroid stimulator on the reorganization into follicles of isolated thyroid cells and on the binding of radioiodinated thyrotropin to reassociated cells. FEBS Lett 32:299, 1973

405. Shishiba Y, Shimizu T, Yoshimura S, Shizume K: Direct evidence for human thyroidal stimulation by LATS-protector. J Clin Endocrinol Metab 36:517, 1973

406. Foldes J, Tako J, Banos C et al: Reduced sensitivity of the thyroid to thyrotropic hormone and LATS following treatment with antimicrosomal antibodies. Acta Endocrinol 74:675, 1973

407. Konishi J, Herman MM, Kriss JP: Binding of thyroglobulin and thyroglobulin-antithyroglobulin im-mune-complex to extraocular muscle membrane. No. T-22. Forty-ninth Meeting of the American Thyroid Association, September, Seattle, Washington, 1973

408. Winand RJ, Kohn LD: The binding of [s3H] thyrotropin and an ^{3}H-labeled exophthalmogenic factor by plasma membranes of retro-orbital tissue. Proc Natl Acad Sci USA 69:1711, 1972

409. DeGroot LJ, Hoye K, Refetoff S et al: Serum antigens and antibodies in the diagnosis of thyroid cancer. J Clin Endocrinol Metab 45:1220, 1977

410. DeGroot LJ, Paloyan E: Thyroid carcinoma and radiation: a Chicago endemic. JAMA 225:487, 1973

411. Walt AJ, Woolner LB, Black BM: Small cell malignant lesions of the thyroid gland. J Clin Endocrinol Metab 17:45, 1957

412. Woolner LB, McConahey WM, Beahrs OH: Struma lymphomatosa and related thyroidal disorders. J Clin Endocrinol Metab 19:53, 1959

413. Holmes HB, Kreutner A, O'Brien PH: Hashimoto's thyroiditis: Its relationship to other thyroid diseases. Surg Gynecol Obstet 144:887, 1977

414. Fujimoto Y, Suzuki H, Abe K: Autoantibodies in malignant lymphoma of the thyroid gland. N Engl J Med 276:380, 1967

415. Dailey ME, Lindsay S, Skahen R: Relation of thyroid neoplasms to Hashimoto's disease of the thyroid gland. Arch Surg 70:291, 1955

416. Gribetz D, Talbot NB, Crawford JD: Goiter due to lymphocytic thyroiditis (Hashimoto's struma): Its occurrence in preadolescent and adolescent girls. N Engl J Med 250:555, 1954

417. Pratt DE, Kaberlein G, Dudkiewicz A et al: The association of antithyroid antibodies in euthyroid nonpregnant women with recurrent first trimester abortions in the next pregnancy. Fertil Steril, 60:1001, 1993

418. Abbas AK, Lichtman AH, Pober JS: Cellular and Molecular Immunology. 2nd Ed. WB Saunders, Philadelphia, 1992

419. Trowsdale J, Campbell RD: Physical map of the human HLA region. Immunol Today 9:34, 1988

420. Okayasu I, Hatokeyama S: Clin Immunol Immunopathol 31:334, 1984

Hashimoto's Thyroiditis

8

HISTORICAL REVIEW

In 1912 Hashimoto described four patients with a chronic disorder of the thyroid, which he termed *struma lymphomatosa.* The thyroid glands of these patients were characterized by diffuse lymphocytic infiltration, fibrosis, parenchymal atrophy, and an eosinophilic change in some of the acinar cells.[1] Clinical and pathologic studies of this disease have appeared frequently since Hashimoto's original description. The disease has been called Hashimoto's thyroiditis, chronic thyroiditis, lymphocytic thyroiditis, lymphadenoid goiter and, recently, autoimmune thyroiditis. Classically, the disease occurs as a painless, diffuse enlargement of the thyroid gland in a young or middle-aged woman. It is often associated with hypothyroidism. The disease was thought to be uncommon for many years, and the diagnosis was usually made by the surgeon at the time of operation or by the pathologist after thyroidectomy. The increasing use of the needle biopsy and serologic tests for antibodies has led to much more frequent recognition, and there is reason to believe that its incidence may be increasing.[2] It is now one of the most common thyroid disorders.

The first indication of an immunologic abnormality in this disease was an elevation of the plasma γ-globulin (1gG) fraction detected by Fromm et al.[3] This finding, together with abnormalities in serum flocculation test results,[4] indicated that the disease might be related to a long-continued autoimmune reaction. Rose and Witebsky[5] showed that immunization of rabbits with extracts of rabbit thyroids produced histologic changes in the thyroid glands resembling those seen in Hashimoto's thyroiditis. They also found antithyroglobulin antibodies in the blood of the animals. Subsequently, Roitt et al.[6] observed that a precipitate formed when an extract of human thyroid gland was added to serum from a patient with Hashimoto's thyroiditis. It thus appeared that the serum contained antibodies to a constituent of the human thyroid and that these antibodies might be responsible for the disease process. These original observations led directly to entirely new concepts of the causation of disease by autoimmunization.

PATHOLOGY

The goiter is generally symmetric, often with a conspicuous pyramidal lobe. Grossly, the tissue involved in Hashimoto's thyroiditis is pinkish-tan to frankly yellowish and tends to have a rubbery firmness. The capsular surface is gently lobulated and nonadherent to perithyroid structures. Microscopically, there is a diffuse process consisting of a combination of epithelial cell destruction, lymphoid cellular infiltration, and fibrosis. The thyroid cells tend to be slightly larger and assume an acidophilic staining character; they are then called Hürthle or Askanazy cells and are packed with mitochondria. The follicular spaces shrink, and colloid is absent or sparse. Clusters of macrophagelike cells may be seen within the follicles. The lymphoid infiltration in the inter-

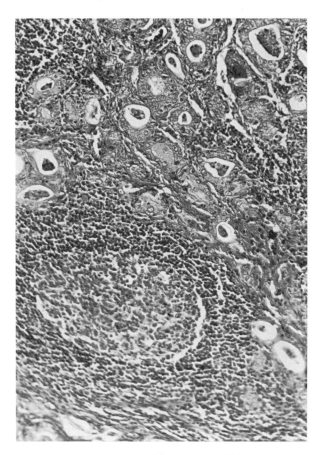

Fig. 8-1. Pathology of Hashimoto's thyroiditis. In this typical view of severe Hashimoto's thyroiditis, the normal thyroid follicles are small and greatly reduced in number, and with the hematoxylin-eosin stain are seen to be eosinophilic. There is marked fibrosis. The dominant feature is a profuse mononuclear lymphocytic infiltrate and lymphoid germinal center formation.

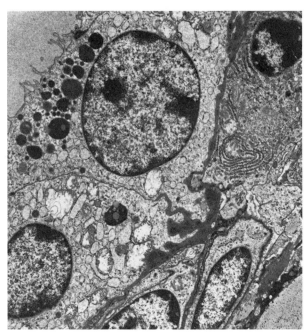

Fig. 8-2. Electron microscopy image of thyroid tissue from a patient with Hashimoto's thyroiditis, showing electron-dense deposits of IgG and TG along the basement membrane of follicular cells.

stitial tissue is accompanied by actual follicles and germinal centers (Fig. 8-1). Plasma cells are prominent. Totterman has studied the characteristics of the lymphocytes in the thyroid and reports that they are made up of equal proportions of T and B cells.[7] Thyroglobulin-binding lymphocytes were increased in percentage relative to their occurrence in blood. Fibrosis may be completely absent or present in degrees ranging from slight to moderate; it may be severe, as observed in subacute or Riedel's thyroiditis. Foreign body giant cells and granulomas are not features of Hashimoto's thyroiditis, in contrast to subacute thyroiditis. In children, oxyphilia and fibrosis are less prominent, and hyperplasia of epithe-

lial cells may be marked. Deposits of dense material representing IgG are found along the basement membrane on electron microscopy (Fig. 8-2).

The quantity of parenchymal tissue left in the thyroid varies. In some instances it is actually increased, perhaps as a compensatory hyperplastic response to inefficient iodide metabolism.

Typically, the pathologic process involves the entire lobe or gland. Focal thyroiditis, which is microscopically similar, may be found in thyroid glands with diffuse hyperplasia of Graves' disease, in association with thyroid tumors, or in multinodular thyroid glands. The thymus, which is frequently enlarged in thyroiditis, as it is in Graves' disease, does not present the picture of enhanced immunologic activity.[8,9]

Pathogenesis

The putative causes of autoimmune thyroid disease (AITD) are reviewed in Chapter 7, and the basic concepts reviewed there apply of course to Hashimoto's thyroiditis. In Hashimoto's thyroiditis, the immunologic attack appears to be typically aggressive and destructive, rather than stimulatory, as in Graves' disease, and the difference is most likely due to the characteristics of the immune response. Hashimoto's thyroiditis is reported to occur in two varieties: an atrophic variety, perhaps associated with HLA-DR3 gene inheritance, and a goitrous form associated with HLA-DR5.

High titers of antibody against thyroglobulin (TG) and thyroid peroxidase (TPO) are present in most patients with Hashimoto's thyroiditis.[10] TPO antibodies are complement fixing and may be cytotoxic. However, the evidence for cytotoxicity is scant, especially since normal transplacental antibody passage of anti-TPOAb to the human fetus does not usually induce thyroid damage. Thus recent studies suggest that cytotoxic T cells, or killer or natural killer cells, may play an important role. A few reports do show T cell line or clone cytotoxicity toward isologous thyroid epithelial cells, and experimental thyroiditis can be transferred by lymphocytes. T cells from patients with Hashimoto's disease proliferate when exposed to TG and TPO. These responses are known to be directed to specific sequences in the TPO molecule, including epitopes at aa 110-129, 210-230, 420-439, and 842-861.[11] Increased killer cell and natural killer cell function has been reported in Hashimoto's thyroiditis. Despite the lack of understanding of the primary cause or causes, it is certain that thyroid autoimmunity drives the lymphocyte collection in the thyroid and is responsible for thyroid epithelial cell damage. Progressive thyroid cell damage can change the apparent clinical picture from goitrous hypothyroidism to that of primary hypothyroidism, or "atrophic" thyroiditis. Primary hypothyroidism is considered to be the end stage of Hashimoto's thyroiditis.

An alternative cause of atrophic hypothyroidism is the development of thyroid-stimulation-blocking antibodies (TSBAb), which, as the name implies, prevent TSH binding to TSH-R but do not stimulate thyroid cells and produce hypothyroidism. It has been proposed that TSBAb bind to epitopes near the carboxly end of the TSH-R extracellular domain, in contrast to thyroid-stimulating antibodies (TSAb), which bind to epitopes near aa 40 at the amino terminus.[12] This syndrome occurs in neonates, children, and adults. However, in contrast to the usual progressive and irreversible thyroid damage, these blocking antibodies tend to follow the course of TSAb; that is, they decrease or disappear over time, and the patient may become euthyroid again.[13] A change from a predominant TSAb response to a predominant TSBAb response can cause patients to have sequential episodes of hyper- and hypothyroid function.[14]

Apparent de novo development of antibodies, augmentation of preexisting thyroid autoimmunity, goiter, and hypothyroidism are induced in some cancer patients receiving courses interleukin-2 (IL-2), interleukin-2α (IL-2α), plus lymphokine-activated killer cells and/or interferon-γ (IFN-γ). The phenomenon may reflect activation of lymphocytes by the lymphokine and secretion of tumor necrosis factor-α (TNF-α) and IFN-γ, which can injure or suppress TEC function. IFN-γ may also augment thyrocyte HLA-DR expression, which could enable the thyrocyte to present self-antigens.

Smoking has also been identified as a risk factor for hypothyroidism, but the reason for the association is unknown.[16]

INCIDENCE AND DISTRIBUTION

The incidence of Hashimoto's thyroiditis is unknown but is roughly equal to that of Graves' disease (on the order of 0.3 to 1.5 cases per 1,000 population per year.)[17–19] The disease is 15 to 20 times as frequent in women as in men. It occurs especially from ages 30 to 50 but may be seen in any age group, including children. It certainly exists with a much higher frequency than is diagnosed clinically, and its frequency seems to be increasing. Family studies always bring to light a number of relatives with moderate enlargement of the thyroid gland suggestive of Hashimoto's thyroiditis. Many of these persons have TG and TPO antibodies, and most are entirely asymptomatic. Inoue et al. found 3 percent of Japanese children aged 6 to 18 to have thyroiditis.[20] In most instances, biopsy revealed focal rather than diffuse thyroiditis.

In addition to overt thyroiditis, roughly 10 percent of most populations have positive TG and TPO antibody test results[17–19] even when physical examination reveals no thyroid disease. In a classic study of an entire community, Tunbridge et al.[19] found that 1.9 to 2.7 percent of women had present or past thyrotoxicosis, 1.9 percent had overt hypothyroidism, 7.5 percent had elevated TSH levels, 10.3 percent had test results positive for TPOAb (microsomal antigen) measured by hemagglutination assay (MCHA), and about 15.0 percent had goiter. Men had ten- to fourfold lower incidence of thyroid abnormalities. In a study of children whose parents had no history of thyroid disease, Carey et al.[21] found a 24 percent incidence of thyroid "abnormalities," including an incidence of 6.9 percent abnormal thyroids, and 9.3 percent with positive TGAb measured by hemagglutination assay (TGHA) and 7.8 percent positive MCHA assays. Gordin et al.[17] found that 8 percent of adult Finns had positive TGHA results, and 26 percent had positive MCHA results. TSH levels were elevated in 30 percent of these persons. On the basis of positive antibody titers and elevated TSH levels, 2 percent to 5 percent were believed to have asymptomatic thyroiditis. These test results correlate with focal collection of lymphocytes on histologic examination of the thyroid glands, are frequently associated with elevated levels of TSH,[22] and probably represent one end of a spectrum of thyroid damage. Women with both positive antibody test results and raised TSH levels become hypothyroid at the rate of 5 percent per year.[23] A reasonable approximation of the incidence of positive antibody tests in women is greater than 10 percent and of clinical disease is at least 2 percent. Men have one-tenth this incidence.

COURSE OF THE DISEASE

Hashimoto's thyroiditis begins as a gradual enlargement of the thyroid gland and gradual development of hypothyroidism. It is often discovered by the patient, who finds a fullness of the neck or a new lump while examining herself because of a vague discomfort in the neck. Perhaps most often, it is found by the physician during the course of an examination for some other complaint.

In some instances the thyroid gland may enlarge rapidly; rarely, it is associated with dyspnea or dysphagia from pressure on structures in the neck or with mild pain and tenderness. Rarely, pain is persistent and unresponsive to medical treatment and requires medical therapy or surgery. The goiter of Hashimoto's thyroiditis may remain unchanged for decades,[19] but usually it gradually increases in size. Occasionally the course is marked by symptoms of mild thyrotoxicosis, especially during the early phase of the disease. Symptoms and signs of mild hypothyroidism may be present in 20 percent of pa-

TABLE 8-1. Presentations of Hashimoto's Thyroiditis

Euthyroidism and goiter
Subclinical hypothyroidism and goiter
Primary thyroid failure
Hypothyroidism
Adolescent goiter
Postpartum painless thyroiditis
Transient thyrotoxicosis
Alternating hypo- and hyperthyroidism

tients when first seen[22] or commonly develop over a period of several years. Progression from subclinical hypothyroidism (normal free thyroxine [FT_4] but elevated TSH) to overt hypothyroidism occurs in a certain fraction (perhaps 3 to 5 percent) each year. Eventually thyroid atrophy and myxedema may occur.[24] This assertion is based on the clinical observation that patients with Hashimoto's thyroiditis often develop myxedema and the knowledge that patients with myxedema due to atrophy of the thyroid have a high incidence of thyroglobulin antibodies (TGAb) in their serum. The disease frequently produces goitrous myxedema in young women, and we have occasionally observed a goitrous and hypothyroid patient who went on to develop thyroid atrophy.

Generally the progression from euthyroidism to hypothyroidism has been considered an irreversible process due to thyroid cell damage and loss of thyroidal iodine stores (Fig. 8-3 and Table 8-1). However, it is now clear that up to one-fourth of patients who are hypothyroid may spontaneously return to normal function over the course of several years. This sequence may reflect the initial effect of high titers of TSBAb, which fall with time and allow thyroid function to return.[14]

Within the past few years, some studies have described unusual syndromes believed to be associated with or part of the clinical spectrum of Hashimoto's thyroiditis. Occasionally a patient develops amyloid deposits in the thyroid.[25] Shaw et al.[26] described five patients with a relapsing steroid-responsive encephalopathy including episodes like stroke and seizures, high cerebrospinal fluid (CSF) protein, abnormal electroencephalogram (EEG), and normal computed tomography (CT) scans. Khadori et al.[27] described a steroid-responsive lymphocytic interstitial pneumonitis in four patients. It remains uncertain how these illnesses relate to lymphocytic thyroi-

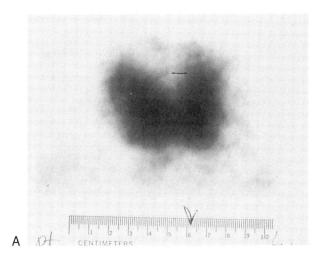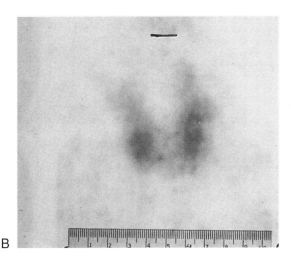

Fig. 8-3. Fluorescent thyroid scan in thyroiditis. (A) The normal thyroid scan allows identification of a thyroid with normal stable (^{127}I) stores throughout both lobes. (B) A marked reduction in ^{127}I content is apparent throughout the entire gland involved with Hashimoto's thyroiditis.

ditis, which until now has been largely identified as an organ-specific disease.

Hashimoto's thyroiditis and hypothyroidism are associated with Addison's disease, diabetes mellitus, hypogonadism, hypoparathyroidism, and pernicious anemia. Such combinations are described as the polyglandular failure syndrome. Two forms of polyglandular autoimmunity have been recognized.[28] In the type I syndrome patients have hypoparathyroidism, mucocutaneous candidiasis, Addison's disease, and occasionally hypothyroidism. Type II, which is more frequent, often includes familial associations of diabetes mellitus, hypothyroidism, hypoadrenalism, and occasionally gonadal or pituitary failure. In these syndromes, antibodies reacting with the affected end organs are characteristically present. Vitiligo, hives, and alopecia are associated with thyroiditis. There is also a clear association with primary and secondary Sjögren syndrome.[29] Some patients appear to start with Hashimoto's thyroiditis and progress with time to Riedel's thyroiditis, including the frequently associated retroperitoneal fibrosis.[30]

Musculoskeletal symptoms, including chest pain, fibrositis, and rheumatoid arthritis, occur in one-quarter of patients,[31] and of course, any of the musculoskeletal symptoms of hypothyroidism may likewise occur.

Some studies suggest that thyroiditis predisposes to vascular disease and coronary occlusion. Abnor-mally elevated titers of thyroid autoantibodies and the morphologic changes of thyroiditis are said to occur with increased frequency among patients with coronary artery disease. Mild hypothyroidism[32] associated with asymptomatic atrophic thyroiditis could predispose patients to heart disease. Others have failed to find increased TGAb in patients with coronary artery disease[33] or increased coronary disease. in association with thyroiditis.

In children, retarded growth, retarded bone age, decreased hydroxyproline excretion, and elevated cholesterol levels may be seen (Fig. 8-4).

*Hashimoto's Thyroiditis in Identical Twin Boys**

D.L. was seen at age 12 for failure to grow over the past 4 years. The patient had an identical twin, whose development up to age 8 had been entirely normal. Pubertal changes had developed at age 11. No goiter had been noted (Fig. 8-4).

On physical examination, he was a short, cooperative, pubertal boy of normal intelligence, 129 cm in height and 35 kg in weight. The thyroid gland was smooth and firm and of normal size. The skin was dry, cool, and mottled. Reflex relaxation was delayed. Estimated T_4 levels were < 4 gmg/dl, and the 24-hour radioactive iodide uptake (RAIU) was 4 percent. Thyroid scan showed a normal thyroid gland. Bone age was 8 years. The potassium thiocyanate discharge test result

---

* These patients were studied in cooperation with Dr. William H. Milburn, to whom we are greatly indebted.

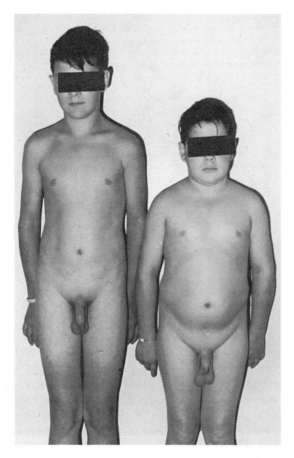

Fig. 8-4. Identical male twins with Hashimoto's thyroiditis were photographed at age 12. At age 8, they had the same height and appearance. During the intervening 4 years, small goiters developed and the growth of the twin on the right almost stopped. Biopsy indicated Hashimoto's thyroiditis in each twin's thyroid.

was negative. Thyroid biopsy showed a moderately diffuse lymphocytic infiltrate with lymphoid germinal centers and a diffuse, dense fibrous reaction.

R.L. was seen simultaneously with D.L. and was an active, healthy-appearing boy with early pubertal changes. His height was 149 cm, and his weight was 39.7 kg. His pulse was 104, and his skin was normal. The thyroid gland was enlarged to about three times the normal size and was not nodular. Protein-bound iodine (PBI) levels were 6.4 and 7.2 μg/dl, and the 24-hour RAIU was 21 percent. Bone age was 11 years. A potassium thiocyanate discharge test caused no decrease in neck radioactivity. Biopsy showed diffuse lymphocytic infiltration, lymphoid follicles and germinal centers, atrophy of thyroid follicles, oxyphilic cytoplasm, and dense fibrosis.

Similar fingerprints, similar lip and ear shapes, and identity of 15 blood factors indicated that they were identical twins. There was no family history of thyroid disease.

Iodide kinetic studies showed rapid turnover of thyroid iodide and production of excess quantities of plasma butanol–insoluble iodine. Hemagglutination test results for TGAb were negative, but an immunofluorescence assay showed a strongly positive reaction against a cytoplasmic antigen. Bioassay of the serum for thyroid-stimulating activity gave a TSH-type response.

When goiter is induced by iodine administration, lymphocytic thyroiditis is frequently found and thyroid autoantibodies are often present.[34]

Remission of Hashimoto's thyroiditis, with loss of goiter, hypothyroidism, and serum thyroid autoantibodies, has been reported during pregnancy, with relapse after delivery.[35] Antibody levels usually fall during pregnancy.[36] These phenomena may reflect the immunosuppressive effects of pregnancy. After delivery, thyroid autoantibody levels rise, and after 1 to 5 months goiter and hypothyroidism may suddenly return.[37]

Of course, maternal antibodies cross the placenta, and as in Graves' disease, may affect the fetus and neonate. TPO and TGAb typically appear to have no adverse effect. Some evidence suggests cytotoxic antibodies, which are thought to be different from TPOAb or TGAb, could cause fetal hypothyroidism.[38] However, TSBAb can rarely produce neonatal hypothyroidism, which is self-limiting over 4 to 6 weeks as the maternal IgG is metabolized.

Not-So-Transient Postpartum Hypothyroidism

Y.L.C., a 22-year-old patient had had menarche at age 16 and had regular periods. She married at age 24 and was not able to conceive. After receiving danazol therapy for 7 months for treatment of extensive endometriosis, she became pregnant and delivered after 36 weeks' gestation. During the course of this pregnancy, her thyroid gland was noted to be normal; no thyroid function tests were done. After delivery, she nursed the infant for 1 week. She then stopped nursing, but galactorrhea and amenorrhea continued for the next 5 months. After the fourth month, she was noted to have an enlarged thyroid gland; the FT$_4$I was found to be 3.4 (normal, 6.0 to 10.5) and TSH level 27 μU/ml. There were symptoms of mild hypothyroidism, with some lowering of the voice and increased fatigue. A sister had an overactive thyroid and mild exophthalmos.

Her thyroid was estimated to weigh about 40 g, with

a smooth surface and an enlarged lobe. Her skin was dry, and there was some delay in the reflex relaxation. TGAb were present at a titer of 1/160 and TPOAb at 1/20480. Serum T_3 level was 123 ng/dl, and the RAIU was 16 percent at 4 hours and 32 percent at 24 hours. The thyroid scan was within normal limits. Prolactin level was elevated at 43 ng/ml. Sella turcica x-ray films and a CT scan of the head were normal.

It was hypothesized that the patient had postpartum hypothyroidism due to transient exacerbation of thyroiditis and that this condition might resolve spontaneously. Whether the hyperprolactinemia, amenorrhea, and galactorrhea were secondary to the hypothyroidism or were independent problems was unclear. The patient was treated expectantly, since she appeared to be in no distress and there was no evidence of pituitary tumor. One month after the initial observations, the TSH level had fallen to 13.5 μU/ml and the T_3 level remained at 126 ng/dl. Eight weeks later, the FT_4I had risen to 5.8, the T_3 level was 113 ng/dl, TSH 9.1 μU/ml, and the prolactin level remained at 66 ng/ml. Later, all test results became normal.

Postpartum Thyroid Disease

In the last decade several syndromes involving clinically significant but self-limited exacerbations of AITD have been delineated.[34–39] Women who have had preexisting Graves' disease, Hashimoto's thyroiditis, or only serum thyroid autoantibodies (39), are prone to develop the following conditions 2 to 4 months after delivery: (1) transient thyroid enlargement, (2) hypothyroidism, or (3) most classically, transient thyrotoxicosis followed by transient hypothyroidism (Fig. 8-5). Up to 6% of postpartum women have one of these syndromes. A predisposition to this syndrome has been associated with inheritance of the HLA-DRβ5 or HLA-DRβ4 gene.[39] Transient thyrotoxicosis (described more fully elsewhere) is typically of mild severity, associated with a small goiter, absence of eye signs, low levels of TPOAb and TGAb, and a zero to low RAIU.[40–46] It is believed to be due to autoimmune-induced damage to the thyroid that causes excess hormone release; for this reason it is not responsive to antithyroid drugs, potassium iodide, (KI), or $KClO_4$, but does respond, if treatment is necessary, to prednisone.[44] Obviously, with low RAIU, therapy with iodine (^{131}I) is not possible, nor would it be appropriate. The disease tends to run its course with or without treatment in 3 to 6 months and is then frequently followed by a period of hypothyroidism over 3 to 4 months; the thyroid then returns to normal

function. In some women—perhaps 5%—hypothyroidism may be permanent. The syndrome can recur after subsequent pregnancies. A similar syndrome unrelated to pregnancy also occurs in women or men. The histologic picture of the thyroid in these patients is that of lymphocyte infiltration and fibrosis compatible with chronic thyroiditis, both during and after the acute episode, or the thyroid may appear normal after recovery.[45] Some patients have had alternating episodes of typical high-uptake thyrotoxicosis and episodes of transient low-uptake thyrotoxicosis.[46]

Iodide Metabolism

Many patients with Hashimoto's thyroiditis do not respond to injected TSH with the expected increase in RAIU or release of hormone from the gland.[47] These findings probably mean that the gland is partially destroyed by the autoimmune attack and is unable to augment iodine metabolism further. Further, the thyroid gland of the patient with Hashimoto's disease does not organify iodide normally[48] (Fig. 8-3). Administration of 400 mg potassium perchlorate 1 hour after giving a tracer iodide releases 20 to 60 percent of the glandular radioactivity. Also, a fraction of the iodinated compounds in the serum of patients with Hashimoto's thyroiditis is not soluble in butanol, as are the thyroid hormones, but is an abnormal peptide-linked iodinated component. This low-weight iodoprotein is probably serum albumin that has been iodinated in the thyroid gland. A similar iodoprotein is also found in several other kinds of thyroid disease, including carcinoma, Graves' disease, and one form of goitrous cretinism. It may be formed as part of the hyperplastic response. TG is also detectable in serum in these conditions.

The thyroid gland of Hashimoto's thyroiditis is especially sensitive to administered iodide. In this respect, it mimics the response of the thyroid in Graves' disease and iodide goiter. Thus, Paris et al.[48] found that administration of 2 mg iodide, together with a tracer ^{131}I, resulted in an average 84 percent decrease in thyroidal uptake. In healthy persons there was only a 25 percent fall in uptake when this loading dose of potassium iodide was given.

Buchanan et al.[49,50] have studied iodide metabolism in Hashimoto's thyroiditis. They found that ^{131}I uptake and clearance rates were variable. Plasma in-

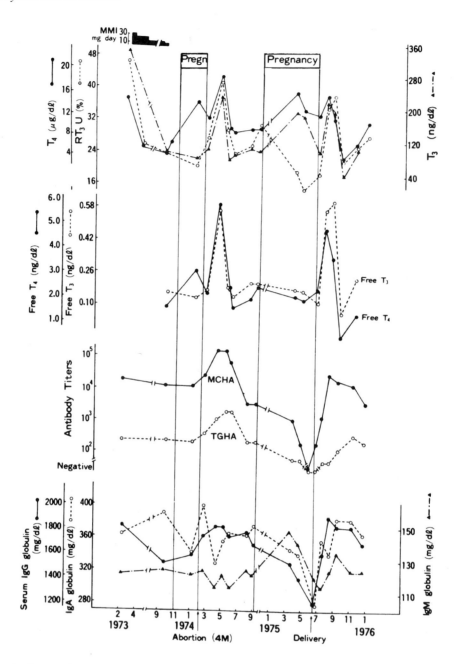

Fig. 8-5. Episodes of postpartum thyroid dysfunction occurred following two pregnancies associated with elevated antibodies and T_4 levels. (From Amino,[36] with permission.)

organic iodide was normal, as was uptake of stable iodide. The intrathyroid-exchangeable iodine and the efficiency of use of trapped iodide by the thyroid both tended to be low. The plasma ^{131}PBI concentration varied from below normal to an elevated value, whereas the plasma PBI concentration tended to be low. An increased proportion of plasma organic iodide was butanol insoluble.

An iodide kinetic analysis[51] demonstrated a marked increase of thyroid iodide clearance in some patients, but a diminished thyroid iodine pool with accelerated turnover and an increased rate of release of tracer as iodide, hormone, and iodoprotein. The reduced iodine pool in the thyroid is presumably a result of fibrosis and destruction of acini, as well as diminished binding efficiency. The iodine depletion of the gland is also apparent on fluorescent scans (which quantify stable iodine content).

Iodide metabolism is not entirely homogeneous in this group of patients, but the data fit the concept that the diseased gland releases some trapped iodide back to plasma without incorporating it into organic form, has a diminished ability to maintain normal thyroid iodine stores, and has a high turnover rate if the iodine pool of the gland is low. It also releases nonhormonal organic iodine into the circulation. Because of this inefficient use of iodine and the consequent decrease in T_4, TSH rises.

DIAGNOSIS

Diagnosis involves two considerations: the differential diagnosis of the thyroid lesion and the determination of the metabolic status of the patient.

A diffuse, firm goiter with pyramidal lobe enlargement and without signs of thyrotoxicosis should suggest the diagnosis of Hashimoto's thyroiditis. Most often the gland is bosselated or "nubbly." It is usually symmetric, although much variation in symmetry (as well as consistency) can occur. The trachea is rarely deviated or compressed. The association of goiter with hypothyroidism is almost diagnostic of this condition, but is also seen in certain syndromes due to defective hormone synthesis or hormone response, as described in Chapter 12. Pain and tenderness are unusual but may be present. A rapid onset is also unusual, but the goiter may rarely grow from normal to several times the normal size in a few weeks. Most commonly the gland is two to four times normal size. Satellite lymph nodes may be present, especially the Delphian node above the isthmus.

The T_4 concentration and the FT_4 range from low to high but are most typically in the normal or low range.[52] The RAIU (rarely required) is variable and ranges from below normal to elevated values, depending on such factors as TSH levels, the efficiency of use of iodide by the thyroid, and the nature of the components being released into the circulation. γ-Globulin levels may be elevated, although usually they are normal.[53] This alteration evidently reflects the presence of high concentrations of circulating antibodies to TG, for an antibody concentration as high as 5.2 mg/ml has been reported.

T_4 and FTI are normal or low.[52] Serum TSH reflects the patient's metabolic status. However, some patients are clinically euthyroid, with normal FTI and T_3 levels, but have mildly elevated TSH. Whether this "subclinical hypothyroidism" represents partial or complete compensation is a matter of debate. TPOAb and, less frequently, TGAb are present in serum. High levels are diagnostic of autoimmune thyroid disease. TGAb are positive in about 80% of patients, and if both TGAb and TPOAb are measured, 97% are positive. Young patients tend to have lower and occasionally negative levels. In this age group, even low titers signify the presence of thyroid autoimmunity. Typically total immunoglobulin levels are normal.[53] Rarely sera contain proteins (antibodies ?) that appear to inhibit hemagglutination assays for antibody.[54] RAIU (rarely done) is variable from below normal to elevated levels, and may be nonsuppressible because of the presence of TSAb.

Fine needle aspiration (FNA) can be a useful diagnostic procedure but is infrequently required. FNA typically reveals lymphocytes, macrophages, scant colloid, and a few epithelial cells that may show Hürthle cell change. Biopsy results are less frequently diagnostic in children.[55]

Thyroid isotope scan is not usually necessary but can be helpful. The image is characteristically that of a diffuse or mottled uptake in an enlarged gland, in striking contrast to the focal "cold" and "hot" areas of multinodular goiter. Focal loss of isotope accumulation may occur in severely diseased portions of the thyroid.

A useful (but rarely available) development has been the *fluorescence thyroid scan,*[56,57] which images the content and distribution of stable iodine. The thyroid iodine content decreases progressively as the disease continues, and in well-developed Hashimoto's thyroiditis the gland is often devoid of iodine, although the result of the regular isotopic scan may appear quite normal (Fig. 8-3).

DIFFERENTIAL DIAGNOSIS

Hashimoto's thyroiditis is to be distinguished from nontoxic nodular goiter or Graves' disease. The presence of gross nodularity is strong evidence against Hashimoto's thyroiditis, but differentiation on this basis is not infallible (Fig. 8-6). In multinodular goiter, thyroid function test results are usually normal, and the patient is only rarely clinically hypo-

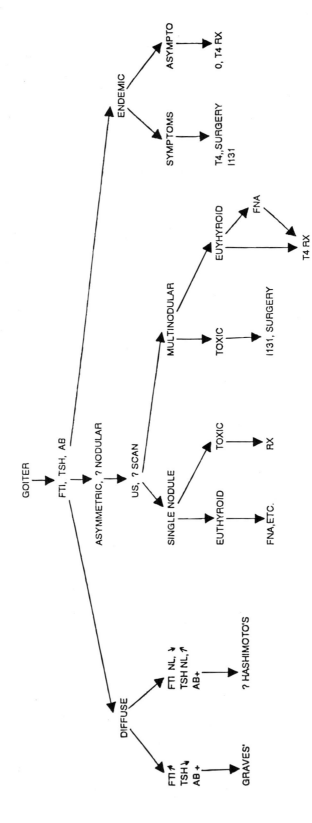

Fig. 8-6. Diagnostic approach to common types of thyroid enlargement. Diffuse goiter, positive antibody assays, normal or reduced T_4, and normal or elevated TSH characterize Hashimoto's thyroiditis.

thyroid. Thyroid autoantibodies tend to be absent or to occur in low titers, and the scan result is typical. FNA can resolve the question but is usually unnecessary. In fact, the two conditions quite commonly occur together in adult women. Whether this is by chance, or due to the effect of thyroid growth-stimulating antibodies (or other causes) is unknown.

Moderately and diffusely enlarged thyroid glands in teenagers are usually the result of thyroiditis, but some enlargements may result from adolescent goiters; that is, the enlargement may result from moderate hyperplasia of the thyroid gland in response to a temporarily increased demand for hormone. This condition is more often diagnosed than proved. Thyroid function test results should be normal. Antibody assays may resolve the issue. The diagnosis can be settled with certainty only by a biopsy disclosing normal or hyperplastic thyroid tissue and absence of findings of thyroiditis. The possibility of colloid goiter may be entertained in the differential diagnosis. Colloid goiter is a definite pathologic entity, as described in Chapter 15. Presumably it is the resting phase after a period of thyroid hyperplasia.

Tumor must also be considered in the differential diagnosis, especially if there is rapid growth of the gland or persistent pain. The diffuse nature of autoimmune thyroiditis, characteristic hypothyroidism, and involvement of the pyramidal lobe are usually sufficient for differentiation. FNA is indicated if there is uncertainty. However, it must be remembered that lymphoma or a small cell carcinoma of the thyroid can be and has been mistaken for Hashimoto's thyroiditis. Clusters of nodes at the upper poles strongly suggesting papillary cancer may disappear after thyroid hormone replacement therapy. However, we have seen a sufficient number of patients with both thyroiditis and tumor to know that one diagnosis in no way excludes the other. Thyroid lymphoma must always be considered if there is continued (especially asymmetric) enlargement of a Hashimoto's gland or if pain, tenderness, hoarseness, or nodes develop. Thyroiditis is a risk factor for thyroid lymphoma, although the incidence is very low. Thyroid lymphoma usually develops in glands that harbor thyroiditis. This condition and its management are discussed in Chapter 18.

Occasionally the picture of Hashimoto's thyroiditis blends rather imperceptibly into that of thyrotoxicosis. Some patients have symptoms of mild thyrotoxicosis but then develop typical Hashimoto's thyroiditis. In fact, it is best to think of Graves' disease and Hashimoto's thyroiditis as two closely related syndromes produced by thyroid autoimmunity. Categorization depends on associated eye findings and the metabolic level, but the pathogenesis, histologic findings, and function may overlap.

Likewise, we have seen patients who appear to have a mixture of Hashimoto's thyroiditis and subacute thyroiditis, with goiter, positive thyroid autoantibodies, normal or low FT_4, and biopsies that have suggested Hashimoto's on one occasion and included giant cells on another. A form of painful chronic thyroiditis with amyloid infiltration has also been described and is probably etiologically distinct from Hashimoto's thyroiditis.[58]

THERAPY

Many patients need no treatment, for frequently the disease is asymptomatic and the goiter is small. This approach is justified by studies showing that clinically and pathologically the disease may remain static and the clinical condition unchanged over many years.

If the goiter is a problem because of local pressure symptoms of is unsightly, thyroid hormone therapy is indicated. Thyroid hormone often causes a gratifying reduction in the size of the goiter after several months of treatment.[58] We have been especially impressed with this result in young people. It seems likely that in older patients there may be more fibrosis and therefore less tendency for the thyroid to shrink. In young patients the response often occurs within 2 to 4 weeks, but in older ones the thyroid decreases in size more gradually. Thyroid hormone in a full replacement dose is, of course, indicated if hypothyroidism is present. Therapy is probably indicated if the TSH level is elevated and the FT_4 is low-normal, since the onset of hypothyroidism is predictable in such patients. There is no evidence that thyroid replacement actually halts the ongoing process of thyroiditis, but in some patients receiving treatment, antibody levels gradually fall over many years.[59]

The dosage of thyroxine should normally be that required to bring the serum TSH level to the low-normal range, such as 0.3 to 1 μU/ml. This is typically achieved with 1 μg thyroxine/lb body weight/day and ranges from 75 to 125 μg/day, in women and 125 to 200 μg/day in men. It is sensible to initiate therapy with a partial dose, since in some instances the thyroid gland may be nonsuppressible even though functioning at a level below normal. Once thyroxine treatment is initiated, it is required indefinitely in most patients. However, it has been found that up to 20% of initially hypothyroid individuals will later recover and have normal thyroid function if challenged by replacement hormone withdrawal. This may represent subsidence of cytotoxic antibodies, modulation of TSBAb, or some other mechanism.[13] These individuals can be identified by administration of thyrotropin-releasing hormone (TRH), which will induce an increase in serum T_4 and T_3 if the thyroid has recovered.[60] Replacement T_4 therapy should be taken several hours before or after medications such as cholesterol-binding resins, Carafate, and $FeSO_4$, which can reduce absorption.[61] (See Ch. 5.)

In some instances the acute onset of the disease, in association with pain, has prompted therapy with glucocorticoids. This treatment alleviates the symptoms and improves the associated biochemical abnormalities, and in some studies has been shown to increase plasma T_3 and T_4 levels by suppressing the autoimmune process.[62] Blizzard and co-workers[63] have given steroids over several months to children in an attempt to suppress antibody production and possibly to achieve a permanent remission. The adrenocortical hormones dramatically depress clinical activity of the disease and antibody titers, but all return to pretherapy levels when treatment is withdrawn. We cannot recommend steroid therapy for this condition because of the undesirable side effects of the drug. Chloroquine has been reported in one study to reduce antibody titers.[64] Because of toxicity, its use is not advised.

X-ray therapy also results in a decrease in goiter size—frequently in myxedema—but should not be used because of the possible induction of thyroid carcinoma.

Surgery has been used in therapy. This treatment, of course, removes the goiter but usually results in hypothyroidism. We believe that it is not indicated unless significant pain or cosmetic or pressure symptoms remain after a fair trial of thyroid therapy.

Some patients do not fit easily into the usual diagnostic categories; accordingly, choosing an appropriate course of therapy for them is more difficult. Frequently, it is impossible to differentiate Hashimoto's thyroiditis from multinodular goiter without performing an open biopsy. In these cases, if no suggestion of carcinoma exists, it is logical to treat such patients with hormone replacement and to observe them closely. A reduction in the goiter justifies continuation of the therapy, even in the absence of a diagnosis.

In some patients, especially teenagers, the examination discloses perithyroidal lymph nodes or an apparent discrete nodule, in addition to the diffusely enlarged thyroid of Hashimoto's thyroiditis. Such nodules should be evaluated by FNA, ultrasound, and possibly scintiscan. Thyroid hormone treatment may cause regression of the nodes or nodule. If uncertainty persists after full evaluation, if nodes remain present, or if a nodule grows, surgical exploration is indicated.

Occasionally, symptoms of serositis or arthritis suggest the coincident occurrence of another autoimmune disorder. We have given thyroid hormone to decrease thyroid activity and possibly reduce a tendency to antibody formation and have treated the generalized disorder independently as indicated.

SUMMARY

Hashimoto's thyroiditis is characterized clinically as a commonly occurring, painless, diffuse enlargement of the thyroid gland occurring predominantly in middle-aged women. The patients are often euthyroid, but hypothyroidism may develop. The thyroid parenchyma is diffusely replaced by a lymphocytic infiltrate and fibrotic reaction; frequently, lymphoid germinal follicles are visible. Attention has been focused on this process because of the demonstration of autoimmune phenomena in most patients. Persons with Hashimoto's thyroiditis have serum antibodies reacting with TG, TPO, and against an unidentified protein present in colloid. In addition, many patients have cell-mediated immunity directed against thyroid antigens, demonstrable by several techniques. Cell-mediated immunity is also a feature of experimental thyroiditis induced in animals by injection of thyroid antigen with adjuvants.

All theories of thyroiditis also emphasize a basic abnormality in the immune surveillance system, which in some way allows autoimmunity to develop against thyroid antigens, as well as against other tissues, including stomach, adrenal, glands, and ovaries in many patients.

We suggest that Hashimoto's thyroiditis, primary myxedema, and Graves' disease are different expressions of a basically similar autoimmune process and that the clinical appearance reflects the spectrum of the immune response in each patient. This response may include cytotoxic antibodies, stimulatory antibodies, blocking antibodies, or cell-mediated immunity. Thyrotoxicosis is viewed as an expression of the effect of circulating thyroid stimulatory antibodies. Hashimoto's thyroiditis is predominantly the clinical expression of cell-mediated immunity leading to destruction of thyroid cells, which in its severest form produces thyroid failure and idiopathic myxedema.

The clinical disease is probably equal in frequency to Graves' disease. The incidence is on the order of three to six cases per 10,000 population per year, and prevalence among women is at least 2%.

The gland involved by thyroiditis tends to lose its ability to store iodine, produces and secretes iodoproteins that circulate in plasma, and is inefficient in making hormone. Thus, the thyroid gland is under increased TSH stimulation, fails to respond to exogenous TSH, and has a rapid turnover of thyroidal iodine.

Diagnosis is made by the finding of a diffuse, smooth, firm goiter in a young woman, with strongly positive titers of TGAb and/or TPOAb and a euthyroid or hypothyroid metabolic status.

A patient with a small goiter and euthyroidism does not require therapy unless the TSH level is elevated. The presence of a large gland, progressive growth of the goiter, or hypothyroidism indicates the need for replacement thyroid hormone. Surgery is rarely indicated. Development of lymphoma, though very unusual, must be considered if there is growth or pain in the involved gland.

REFERENCES

1. Hashimoto H: Zur Kenntniss der lymphomatosen Veranderung der Schilddruse (struma lymphomatosa). Arch Klin Chir 97:219, 1912
2. McConahey WM, Keating FR Jr, Beahrs OH, Woolner LB: On the increasing occurrence of Hashimoto's thyroiditis. J Clin Endocrinol Metab 22:542, 1962
3. Fromm GA, Lascano EF, Bur GE, Escalenta D: Tiroiditis cronica inespecifica. Rev Assoc Med Arg 67:162, 1953
4. Luxton RW, Cooke RT: Hashimoto's struma lymphomatosa: Diagnostic value and significance of serum-flocculation reactions. Lancet 2:105, 1956
5. Rose NR, Witebsky E: Studies on organ specificity. V. Changes in thyroid glands of rabbits following active immunization with rabbit thyroid extracts. J Immunol 76:417, 1956
6. Roitt IM, Doniach D, Campbell PN, Hudson RV: Auto-antibodies in Hashimoto's thyroiditis (lymphadenoid goiter). Lancet 2:820, 1956
7. Totterman TH: Thyroid-infiltrating immunocompetent cells in human autoimmune thyroid disease (thesis). University of Helsinki, Helsinki, Finland, 1978
8. Gunn A, Michie W, Irvine WJ: The thymus in thyroid disease. Lancet 2:776, 1964
9. Michie W, Beck JS, Mahaffy RG et al: Quantitative radiological and histological studies of the thymus in thyroid disease. Lancet 1:691, 1967
10. Mori T, Kriss JP: Measurements by competitive binding radioassay of serum antimicrosomal and anti-thyroglobulin antibodies in Graves' disease and other thyroid disorders. J Clin Endocrinol Metab 33:688, 1971
11. Kawakami Y, Fisfalen M-E, DeGroot LJ: Proliferative responses of peripheral blood mononuclear cells from patients with autoimmune thyroid disease to synthetic peptide epitopes of human thyroid peroxidase. Autoimmunity 13:17, 1992
12. Kosugi S, Ban T, Akamizu T, Kohn LD: Identification of separate determinants on the thyrotropin receptor reactive with Graves' thyroid-stimulating antibodies and with thyroid-stimulating blocking antibodies in idiopathic myxedema: These determinants have no homologous sequence on gonadotropin receptors. Molec Endocrinol 6:168, 1992
13. Okamura K, Sato K, Yoshinari M et al: Recovery of the thyroid function in patients with atrophic hypothyroidism and blocking type TSH binding inhibitor immunoglobulin. Acta Endocrinol (Copenh) 122:107, 1990
14. Takasu N, Yamada T, Takasu M et al: Disappearance of thyrotropin-blocking antibodies and spontaneous recovery from hypothyroidism in autoimmune thyroiditis. N Engl J Med 326:513, 1992
15. Atkins MB, Mier JW, Parkinson DR et al: Hypothyroidism after treatment with interleukin-2 and lymphokine-activated killer cells. N Engl J Med 318:1557, 1988
16. Nystrom E, Bengtsson C, Lapidus L et al: Smoking—A risk factor for hypothyroidism. J Endocrinol Invest 16:129, 1993
17. Gordin A, Maatela J, Miettinen A et al: Serum thyrotrophin and circulating thyroglobulin and thyroid microsomal antibodies in a Finnish population. Acta Endocrinol 90:33, 1979

18. Ling SM, Kaplan SA, Weitzman JJ et al: Euthyroid goiters in children. Correlation of needle biopsy with other clinical and laboratory findings in chronic lymphocytic thyroiditis and simple goiter. Pediatrics 44:695, 1969

19. Tunbridge WMG, Evered DC, Hall R et al: The spectrum of thyroid disease in a community. The Whickham Survey. Clin Endocrinol 7:481, 1977

20. Inoue M, Taketani N, Sato T, Nakajima H: High incidence of chronic lymphocytic thyroiditis in apparently healthy school children: Epidemiological and clinical study. Endocrinol Jpn 22:483, 1975

21. Carey C, Skosey C, Pinnamaneni KM et al: thyroid abnormalities in children of parents who have Graves' disease. Possible pre-Graves' disease. Metabolism 29:369, 1980

22. Gordin A, Saarinen P, Pelkonen A, Lamberg B-A: Serum thyroglobulin and the response to thyrotropin releasing hormone in symptomless autoimmune thyroiditis and in borderline and overt hypothyroidism. Acta Endocrinol 75:274, 1974

23. Tunbridge WMG, Brewis M, French JM et al: Natural history of autoimmune thyroiditis. Br Med J 282:258, 1981

24. Buchanan WW, Harden RM: Primary hypothyroidism and Hashimoto's thyroiditis. Arch Intern Med 115:411, 1965

25. Moriuchi A, Yokoyama S, Kashima K et al: Localized primary amyloid tumor of the thyroid developing in the course of Hashimoto's thyroiditis. Acta Pathologica Japonica 42:210, 1992

26. Shaw PJ, Walls TJ, Newman PK et al: Hashimoto's encephalopathy: A steroid-responsive disorder associated with high antithyroid antibody titers—report of five cases. Neurology 41:228, 1991

27. Khardori R, Eagleton LE, Soler NG, McConnachie PR: Lymphocytic interstitial pneumonitis in autoimmune thyroid disease. Am J Med 90:649, 1991

28. Eisenbart GS, Wilson PW, Ward F et al: The polyglandular failure syndrome. Disease inheritance, HLA type, and immune function. Ann Intern Med 91:528, 1979

29. Loviselli A, Mathieu A, Pala R et al: Development of thyroid disease in patients with primary and secondary Sjögren's syndrome. J Endocrinol Invest 11:653, 1988

30. Best TB, Munro RE, Burwell S, Volpe R: Riedel's thyroiditis associated with Hashimoto's thyroiditis, hypoparathyroidism, and retroperitoneal fibrosis. J Endocrinol Invest 14:767, 1991

31. Becker KL, Ferguson RH, McConahey WM: The connective-tissue diseases and symptoms associated with Hashimoto's thyroiditis. N Engl J Med 268:277, 1963

32. Bastenie PA, Vanhaelst L, Golstein J et al: Asymptom-atic autoimmune thyroiditis and coronary heart-disease. Lancet 1:155, 1977

33. Heinonen OP, Aho K, Pyorala K et al: Symptomless autoimmune thyroiditis in coronary heart disease. Lancet 1:785, 1972

34. Hall R, Turner-Warwick M, Doniach D: Autoantibodies in iodide goiter and asthma. Clin Exp Immunol 1:285, 1966

35. Amino N, Miyai K, Onishi T et al: Transient hypothyroidism after delivery in autoimmune thyroiditis. J Clin Endocrinol Metab 42:296, 1976

36. Amino N, Kuro R, Tanizawa O et al: Changes of serum antithyroid antibodies during and after pregnancy in autoimmune thyroid diseases. Clin Exp Immunol 31:30, 1978

37. Amino N, Miyai K, Kuro R et al: Transient postpartum hypothyroidism. Fourteen cases with autoimmune thyroiditis. Ann Intern Med 87:155, 1977

38. Bogner U, Gruters A, Sigle B et al: Cytotoxic antibodies in congenital hypothyroidism. J Clin Endocrinol Metab 68:671, 1989

39. Roti E, Emerson CH: Clinical Review 29. Postpartum thyroiditis. J Clin Endocrinol Metab 74:3, 1992

40. Gluck FB, Nusynowitz ML, Plymate S: Chronic lymphocytic thyroiditis, thyrotoxicosis, and low radioactive iodine uptake: Reports of four cases. N Engl J Med 292:624, 1975

41. Nikolai TF, Brosseau J, Kettrick MA et al: Lymphocytic thyroiditis with spontaneously resolving hyperthyroidism (silent thyroiditis). Arch Intern Med 140:478, 1980

42. Dorfman SG, Copperman MT, Nelson RL et al: Painless thyroiditis and transient hyperthyroidism without goiter. Ann Intern Med 86:24, 1977

43. Woolf PD: Transient painless thyroiditis with hyperthyroidism. A variant of lymphocytic thyroiditis. Endocr Rev 1:411, 1980

44. Nikolai TF, Coombs GJ, McKenzie AK et al: Treatment of lymphocytic thyroiditis with spontaneously resolving hyperthyroidism (silent thyroiditis). Arch Intern Med 142:2281, 1982

45. Inada M, Nishikawa M, Naito K et al: Reversible changes of the histological abnormalities of the thyroid in patients with painless thyroiditis. J Clin Endocrinol Metab 52:431, 1981

46. Taylor HC, Sheeler LR: Recurrence and heterogeneity in painless thyrotoxic lymphocytic thyroiditis. Report of five cases. JAMA 248:1085, 1982

47. Skillern PG, Crile G Jr, McCullaugh EP et al: Struma lymphomatosa: Primary thyroid failure with compensatory thyroid enlargement. J Clin Endocrinol Metab 16:35, 1956

48. Paris J, McConahey WM, Tausie WN et al: The effect of iodides on Hashimoto's thyroiditis. J Clin Endocrinol Metab 21:1037, 1961

49. Buchanan WW, Koutras DA, Alexander WD et al: Iodine metabolism in Hashimoto's thyroiditis. J Clin Endocrinol Metab 21:806, 1961

50. Buchanan WW, Harden RM, Koutras DA, Gray KG: Abnormalities of iodine metabolism in euthyroid, nongoitrous women with complement-fixing antimicrosomal thyroid autoantibodies. J Clin Endocrinol Metab 25:301, 1965

51. DeGroot LJ: Kinetic analysis of iodine metabolism. J Clin Endocrinol Metab 26:149, 1966

52. McConahey WM, Keating FR, Butt HR, Owen CA: Comparison of certain laboratory tests in the diagnosis of Hashimoto's thyroiditis. J Clin Endocrinol Metab 21:879, 1961

53. Glynne A, Thomson JA: Serum immunoglobulin levels in thyroid disease. Clin Exp Immunol 12:71, 1972

54. Wilkin, TJ, Beck JS, Hayes PC et al: A passive hemagglutination (TRC) inhibitor in thyrotoxic serum. Clin Endocrinol 10:507, 1979

55. Monteleone JA, Davis RK, Tung KSK et al: Differentiation of chronic lymphocytic thyroiditis and simple goiter in pediatrics. J Pediatr 83:381, 1973

56. Hoffer PB, Gottschalk A, Refetoff S: Thyroid scanning techniques. The old and the new. Curr Probl Radiol 2:5, 1972

57. Jonckheer MH, VanHaelst L, DeConinck F, Michotte Y: Atrophic autoimmune thyroiditis. Relationship between the clinical state and intrathyroidal iodine as measured in vivo in man. J Clin Endocrinol Metab 53:476, 1981

58. McConahey WM, Woolner LB, Black BM, Keating FR Jr: Effect of desiccated thyroid in lymphocytic (Hashimoto's) thyroiditis. J Clin Endocrinol Metab 19:45, 1959

59. Papapetrou PD, MacSween RNM, Lazarus JH, Harden R McG: Long-term treatment of Hashimoto's thyroiditis with thyroxine. Lancet 2:7786, 1972

60. Takasu N, Komiya I, Asawa T et al: Test for recovery from hypothyroidism during thyroxine therapy in Hashimoto's thyroiditis. Lancet 336:1084, 1990

61. Campbell NRC et al: Effect of ferrous sulfate on thyroid hormone replacement in hypothyroidism. Ann Intern Med 117:1010, 1992

62. Yamada T, Ikejiri K, Kotani M, Kusakabe T: An increase of plasma triiodothyronine and thyroxine after administration of dexamethasone to hypothyroid patients with Hashimoto's thyroiditis. J Clin Endocrinol Metab 46:784, 1981

63. Blizzard RM, Hung M, Chandler RW et al: Hashimoto's thyroiditis. Clinical and laboratory response to prolonged cortisone therapy. N Engl J Med 267:1015, 1962

64. Ito S, Tamura T, Nishikawa M: Effects of desiccated thyroid, prednisolone and chloroquine on goiter and antibody titer in chronic thyroiditis. Metabolism 17:317, 1968

Adult Hypothyroidism

9

In this initial chapter on the various hypothyroid states, adult hypothyroidism and myxedema are considered together. Attention is focused on the full-blown expression of hypothyroidism, myxedema (Gull's disease), with the tacit assumption that qualitatively similar anomalies exist in lesser degrees of hypothyroidism.

A hypothyroid state may arise as a result of intrinsic disease of the thyroid gland, such as Hashimoto's thyroiditis, after total thyroidectomy, after complete blocking of thyroid function by an antithyroid drug, or after destruction of the gland by irradiation. Failure of thyrotropic function on the part of the pituitary, because of disease, removal, or destruction of that gland, or because thyrotropin-releasing hormone (TRH) from the hypothalamus is not secreted, may also give a complete picture of myxedema.

Hypothyroidism may exist in utero or may develop in infancy, in childhood, or in adult life. Since the thyroid hormones play a role in growth and maturation, a lack of them during the period of growth produces different and far more serious effects than would a deficiency occurring after maturity has been attained. If the lack is not corrected early by adequate substitution therapy, developmental failure occurs that no amount of later treatment can completely overcome. This condition is called *congenital hypothyroidism,* and in some aspects resembles endemic cretinism (see Chs. 15 and 20). Fagge,[1] at Guy's Hospital in 1871, was the first to suspect that a deficiency of the thyroid might be the cause of this disorder.

Adult myxedema escaped serious attention until Gull described it in 1874.[2] That it was a state resembling the familiar endemic cretinism, but coming on in adult life, was what chiefly impressed Gull. Ord[3] invented the term *myxedema* in 1873. The disorder arising from surgical removal of the thyroid gland (*cachexia strumipriva*) was described in 1882 by Reverdin[4] of Geneva and in 1883 by Kocher of Berne.[5]

After Gull's description, myxedema aroused enormous interest, and in 1883 the Clinical Society of London appointed a committee to study the disease and report its findings.[6] The committee's report, published in 1888, contains a significant portion of what is known today about the clinical and pathologic aspects of myxedema. It is referred to in the following discussion as the *Report on Myxoedema.*

The final conclusions of the 200-page volume are penetrating. They are as follows:

1. That myxedema is a well-defined disease.
2. That the disease affects women much more frequently than men, and that the subjects are for the most part of middle age.
3. That clinical and pathological observations, respectively, indicate in a decisive way that the one condition common to all cases is destructive change of the thyroid gland.
4. That the most common form of destructive change of the thyroid gland consists in the substitution of a delicate fibrous tissue for the proper glandular structure.
5. That the interstitial development of fibrous tissue is also observed very frequently in the skin, and, with much less frequency, in the viscera, the appearances presented by this tissue being suggestive of an irritative or inflammatory process.
6. That pathological observation, while showing

cause for the changes in the skin observed during life, for the falling off of the hair, and the loss of the teeth, for the increased bulk of body, as due to the excess of subcutaneous fat, affords no explanation of the affections of speech, movement, sensation, consciousness, and intellect, which form a large part of the symptoms of the disease.

7. That chemical examination of the comparatively few available cases fails to show the general existence of an excess of mucin in the tissues adequately corresponding to the amount recorded in the first observation, but that this discrepancy may be, in part, attributed to the fact that tumefaction of the integuments, although generally characteristic of myxedema, varies considerably throughout the course of the disease, and often disappears shortly before death.
8. That in experiments made upon animals, particularly on monkeys, symptoms resembling in a very close and remarkable way those of myxedema have followed complete removal of the thyroid gland, performed under antiseptic precautions, and with, as far as could be ascertained, no injury to the adjacent nerves or to the trachea.
9. That in such experimental cases a large excess of mucin has been found to be present in the skin, fibrous tissues, blood, and salivary glands; in particular the parotid gland, normally containing no mucin, has presented that substance in quantities corresponding to what would be ordinarily found in the submaxillary gland.
10. That following removal of the thyroid gland in man in an important proportion of the cases, symptoms exactly corresponding with those of myxedema subsequently develop.
11. That in a considerable number of cases the operation has not been known to have been followed by such symptoms, the apparent immunity being in many cases probably due to the presence and subsequent development of accessory thyroid glands, or to accidentally incomplete removal, or to insufficiently long observation of the patients after operation.
12. That, whereas injury to the trachea, atrophy of the trachea, injury of the recurrent laryngeal nerves, injury of the cervical sympathetic, and endemic influences, have been by various ob-

servers supposed to be the true cases of experimental or of operative myxedema (cachexia strumipriva), there is, in the first place, no evidence to show that, of the numerous and various surgical operations performed on the neck and throat, involving various organs and tissues, any, save those in which the thyroid gland has been removed, have been followed by the symptoms under consideration; that in many of the operations on man, and in most, if not all, of the experimental operations made by Professor Horsley on monkeys and other animals, this procedure avoided all injury of surrounding parts, and was perfectly antiseptic; that myxedema has followed removal of the thyroid gland in persons neither living in nor having lived in localities the seat of endemic cretinism; that, therefore, the positive evidence on this point vastly outweighs the negative; and that it appears strongly proved that myxedema is frequently produced by the removal, as well as by the pathological destruction, of the thyroid gland.

13. That whereas, according to Clause 2, in myxedema women are much more numerously affected than men, in the operative form of myxedema no important numerical difference is observed.

14. That a general review of symptoms and pathology leads to the belief that the disease described under the name of myxedema, as observed in adults, is practically the same disease as that named sporadic cretinism when affecting children; that myxedema is probably identical with cachexia strumipriva; and that a very close affinity exists between myxedema and endemic cretinism.

15. That while these several conditions appear, in the main, to depend on, or to be associated with, destruction or loss of the function of the thyroid gland, the ultimate cause of such destruction or loss is at present not evident.

CAUSES OF ADULT HYPOTHYROIDISM AND MYXEDEMA

A variety of functional or structural disorders may lead to hypothyroidism, the severity of which depends on the degree and duration of thyroid hor-

TABLE 9-1. Causes of Hypothyroidism

Primary (thyropivic) hypothyroidism
    Primary idiopathic hypothyroidism (probably end-stage Hashimoto's disease)
    Postablative (iatrogenic) [131]I or surgery or after therapeutic irradiation for nonthyroidal malignancy
    Sporadic athyreotic hypothyroidism (agenesis or dysplasia)
    Endemic cretinism (less common agoitrous form)
    Unresponsiveness to TSH
Goitrous
    Hashimoto's (chronic lymphocytic) thyroiditis
    Reidel's struma
    Endemic iodine deficiency
    Iodine-induced hypothyroidism
    Antithyroid agents (thionamides, thiourylenes, thiocyanate, perchlorate, lithium, resorcinol, *p*-aminosalicylic acid, cyanogenic glucosides, plants from the *Brassica* genus, etc.; see Chapter 5)
    Inherited defects of hormone synthesis
    amyloidosis, cystinosis, sarcoidosis, hemochromatosis, and scleroderma
Transient
    Thyroid hormone treatment withdrawal
    Removal of toxic adenoma or a portion of the thyroid gland for Graves' disease
    DeQuervain's (subacute) thyroiditis
    Postpartum thyroiditis
    Post ^{131}I treatment for Graves' disease
Secondary (pituitary) hypothyroidism
    Panhypopituitarism (Sheehan's syndrome, tumors, infiltrative disorders)
    Isolated idiopathic TSH deficiency
    TSH synthentic defect
    Defect in TSH receptor
Tertiary (hypothalamic) hypothyroidism (idiopathic, traumatic, tumors, infiltrative disorders)
Peripheral tissue resistance to thyroid hormone action

mone deprivation. A classification according to etiology appears in Table 9-1. The two principal categories of hypothyroidism are primary, or thyroprivic, caused by an inherent inability of the thyroid gland to supply a sufficient amount of the hormone, and trophoprivic hypothyroidism, due to inadequate stimulation of an intrinsically normal thyroid gland resulting from a defect at the level of the pituitary (secondary hypothyroidism) or the hypothalamus (tertiary hypothyroidism). In a third (uncommon) form of hypothyroidism, regulation and function of the thyroid gland are intact. Instead, manifestations of hormone deprivation arise from a defect in the target tissues that reduces their responsiveness to the hormone (peripheral tissue resistance to thyroid hormone).

The most common cause of hypothyroidism is destruction of the thyroid gland by disease or as a consequence of vigorous ablative therapies to control thyrotoxicosis. Primary hypothyroidism may also result from inefficient hormone synthesis caused by inherited biosynthetic defects (see Ch. 16), a deficient supply of iodine (see Ch. 20), or inhibition of hormonogenesis by various drugs and chemicals (see Ch. 5). In such instances, hypothyroidism is typically associated with thyroid gland enlargement (goitrous hypothyroidism).

Idiopathic Thyroid Atrophy: Relation to Hashimoto's Thyroiditis

Atrophy of the thyroid gland is the most common finding in adult spontaneous hypothyroidism, being present in one series of 80 patients in over half the cases.[7]

Extensive studies, documented in Chapter 8 on Hashimoto's thyroiditis, have demonstrated in the serum of patients with myxedema due to "spontaneous atrophy" a high incidence of antibodies against homologous thyroid antigens. That there is progression in some cases of Hashimoto's thyroiditis from the metabolically normal stage to hypothyroidism has become well established, although in most cases we have seen the thyroid gland remain palpable. Also, in most patients high titers of antithyroid antibodies indicate chronic lymphocytic thyroiditis. Some have elevated plasma thyroid-stimulating hormone (TSH) levels but are entirely euthyroid otherwise.[8,9] They appear to be on their way to thyroid atrophy but are in a compensated state. Others are decompensated in that they have clinical and laboratory evidence of hypothyroidism.[10] Thus, hypothroidism associated with "spontaneous atrophy" of the thyroid gland may be accepted as, in general, an expression of the end state of Hashimoto's thyroiditis. No doubt this is not the whole story, but probably it is a large part of it.

Atrophy of the thyroid gland is also known to occur rarely after subacute thyroiditis.[11] and it has been reported as the spontaneous end result of Graves' disease.[12] Hypothyroidism in association with classic features of Graves' disease, such as exophthalmos and pretibial myxedema, may develop in patients having no evidence of previous thyrotoxicosis. Michaelson and Young[13] have described one such patient with a high titer of long-acting thyroid

stimulator (LATS). Thyroid biopsy showed thyroiditis, presumably an extension of the usual focal lymphocytic involvement of the thyroid gland in Graves' disease. Thus, Graves' disease, Hashimoto's disease, and idiopathic hypothyroidism have overlapping clinical expression and pathologic manifestations, as described in Chapter 8. The findings in one of our patients also suggest this course of events.

Postablative (Iatrogenic) Hypothyroidism

A leading cause of hypothyroidism or myxedema today is radioactive iodine (RAI) treatment of Graves' disease. The frequency with which hypothyroidism supervenes RAI therapy is dependent on multiple factors, the principal one being the dose of RAI administered. The incidence of hypothyroidism 5 years after treatment is variously reported as 7 to 50 percent. Hypothyroidism may appear within a few months of therapy in some patients, but it may not be manifest until years later in others. Its cumulative occurrence continues to rise with time, and it has been suggested that virtually all patients treated in this way will eventually become hypothyroid. Various treatment schedules have been devised with the hope of diminishing the incidence of RAI-induced hypothyroidism,[15,18] but in general, a lower incidence of hypothyroidism is invariably associated with a higher prevalence of persistent thyrotoxicosis that requires either retreatment or control with antithyroid drugs or iodide.[14-18] Inadvertent administration of RAI during gestation may cause neonatal hypothyroidism when given to the mother during the last two trimesters and also occasionally in the first trimester of pregnancy.[19] Hypothyroidism is a rare consequence of iodine Q131 treatment of toxic adenomas.

Hypothyroidism may supervene after therapeutic irradiation of the neck for any of a number of malignant diseases. It is particularly common after irradiation for Hodgkins' and non-Hodgkins' lymphoma and after radiotherapy for laryngeal carcinoma, particularly after partial thyroidectomy, which usually precedes radiation x-ray therapy in this condition.[20] Mild hypothyroidism may also occur after x-ray treatment in preparation for bone marrow transplantation.[21]

Another important cause of hypothyroidism is surgical removal of the gland. From 5 to 43 percent of patients who undergo thyroidectomy for Graves' disease develop hypothyroidism.[17,22,23] The frequency depends on the zeal of the surgeon and on other factors, such as the function of the thyroid remnant or the presence of active thyroiditis. The recorded frequency also depends on the thoroughness of follow-up. However, in general, the incidence of hypothyroidism after surgery is lower than that observed after RAI treatment.[17,23] Hypothyroidism after subtotal thyroidectomy for Graves' disease may become apparent shortly after surgery, or it may not appear for years. Its occurrence correlates with the presence of antibodies to thyroid antigens. Thus, progressive destruction of residual tissue by thyroiditis may be the pathogenic mechanism. Hypothyroidism after surgical removal of multinodular goiter is infrequent. Myxedema occurs almost invariably after subtotal thyroidectomy for Hashimoto's thyroiditis and after removal of lingual thyroids.

Goitrous Hypothyroidism

In the adult, goitrous hypothyroidism is most commonly an expression of Hashimoto's thyroiditis. Reidel's struma is a rare cause. In endemic goiter (see Ch. 20) hypothyroidism may be seen in association with multinodular goiter, and rare patients with sporadic multinodular goiter are hypothyroid.[24] Goitrous hypothyroidism accompanies the more severe forms of inherited defects of hormone synthesis (see Ch. 16). The production of hypothyroidism by sarcoid, amyloidosis, lymphoma, tuberculosis, and metastatic tumors must also be mentioned for completeness, despite the rarity of these conditions. Among the extremely rare causes of primary hypothyroidism are those associated with sarcoidosis, amyloidosis, tuberculosis, scleroderma, and cystinosis.[25]

The association of hypothyroidism with several apparently unrelated diseases appears to be too frequent to be attributable to chance. Most of these associated disorders are autoimmune. Their higher prevalence in patients with hypothyroidism is related not to the hormone deficiency but to Hashimoto's thyroiditis, itself an autoimmune disease that is responsible for the great majority of spontaneous hypothyroidism in the adult.[26]

Hashimoto's thyroiditis and hypothyroidism are increased in prevalence in patients with certain chromosomal abnormalities such as trisomy 21, Kleinfelter and Turner syndromes (see also Ch. 8 and 15).[27]

The manifestations related to hypothyroidism, but not to the chromosomal abnormality may be corrected by hormone therapy. For more details, see Chapters 8 and 15.

Drug-Induced Hypothyroidism

A variety of therapeutic drugs can lead to moderate or even severe hypothyroidism (see also Ch. 5). The common antithyroid drugs (carbimazole, methimazole, and propylthiouracil) if given in sufficient quantity will cause hypothyroidism. This is also theoretically possible with agents that can block the uptake of iodide by the thyroid, such as perchlorate or thiocyanate, although these are rarely given. In susceptible individuals, primarily those with a history of autoimmune thyroid disease such as Hashimoto's or Graves' disease or in patients who have had either radiation or surgical trauma to the thyroid gland, large doses of iodide can cause goitrous hypothyroidism.[28,29] While this is now less common, since iodides are no longer given for chronic pulmonary disease and lipid-soluble contrast agents are no longer used in diagnostic procedures, the problem may arise with patients taking iodine supplements or natural foods with high iodine content. Lithium has similar effects to those of iodide; it inhibits thyroid hormone release as well as hormone synthesis.[30] While lithium-induced hypothyroidism is more common in patients with underlying autoimmune disease, it has been reported in individuals with apparently normal thyroid glands. There are a large number of organic compounds that may impair thyroid function in animals. These include phenol derivatives such as resorcinol, benzoic acid compounds such as para-aminosalicylic acid, the oral sufonylurea compounds, phenylbutazone, aminoglutethimide, and a number of other agents that are no longer in common use.

Transient Hypothyroidism

Provision of thyroid hormone in physiologic or supraphysiologic doses suppresses serum TSH and thyroid gland function. Recovery of the hypothalamic-pituitary-thyroid axis may take up to 12 weeks, but on average 3 to 4 weeks are required. Thus, transient hypothyroidism occurs during the recovery phase after hormone withdrawal.[31,32] Transient hypothyroidism is also characteristic of the recovery phase following either granulomatous (painful) or lymphocytic (painless) thyroiditis, whether this occurs spontaneously or in the postpartum period (see Ch. 19) It may also appear in some patients with Graves' disease during the second or third month following radioactive iodine treatment due to the prolonged suppression of TSH synthesis that is a consequence of the hyperthyroidism.

Hypothalamic and Pituitary Hypothyroidism

Hypothyroidism may occur because the pituitary secretes TSH in sufficient quantities or with an abnormal glycosylation pattern. Hypothalamic disorders cause reduced TSH secretion generally by impairing the production or transport of TRH to the pituitary gland. Pathologic processes include tumors of the pituitary-hypothalamic areas such as pituitary adenoma, craniopharyngioma, meningioma, and rare metastatic tumors. Radiation therapy can induce TRH deficiency, as can histiocytosis or sarcoidosis. Certain of the same tumors can destroy the pituitary gland (pituitary adenomas, craniopharyngiomas, or metastatic tumors). In addition, surgery or radiation therapy, postpartum pituitary necrosis (Sheehan's syndrome) and a number of infiltrative conditions such as sarcoidosis, histiocytosis, and hemochromatosis have been associated with TSH deficiency.[33] Uncommonly, the pituitary gland may be affected in the polyglandular autoimmune syndromes leading to TSH deficiency.[34]

There are two hereditary causes of TSH deficiency that are of interest from a molecular biologic viewpoint. One of these is a deficiency of the pituitary-specific transcription factor Pit-1 due to a mutation in the gene encoding this protein.[35] Families with this condition generally have combined deficiencies of TSH and growth hormone. A second hereditary form of TSH deficiency has been identified in certain Japanese families in which there is a single base substitution in the 29th codon of the TSH β-subunit gene.[36] This causes synthesis of TSH β-subunit with a glycine for arginine substitution that impairs the capacity of the α- and β-subunits to dimerize to form the intact TSH molecule. Further discussion of the causes, manifestations, diagnosis, and treatment of hypothyroidism due to TRH or TSH deficiency is provided in a subsequent section. (See also Ch. 4 and 15.)

TSH Receptor Abnormalities

In theory, hypothyroidism will also occur if the thyroid cell does not respond to TSH. To date this has been identified as a cause of hypothyroidism in only a few patients. In one group, patients with pseudohypoparathyroidism, there is a mutation in the G_s protein that couples the TSH receptor to adenylate cyclase.[39] This defective protein does not transduce TSH receptor occupancy to an increase in thyroid cell cyclic AMP. Thus, these patients do not respond to TSH and usually have mild congenital hypothyroidism (see Ch. 15).

A second type of abnormality has been described recently in a family in which the propositus has congenital hypothyroidism. In this patient, a mutation in the TSH receptor causes a decrease in the capacity of the receptor to activate adenylate cyclase.[40] Hypothyroidism occurs due to failure of the thyroid to respond to TSH. A similar defect has been identified in the congenitally hypothyroid (hyt/hyt) mouse.[41]

FREQUENCY AND DISTRIBUTION

Spontaneous myxedema is an uncommon disease. As a proportion of total hospital admissions, it varies from 0.01 to 0.08 percent. In our clinics, it has been one-eighth as frequent as thyrotoxicosis. In keeping with the general pattern of thyroid disease, it occurs four to seven times as frequently in women as in men.

Hypothyroidism of various degrees, short of myxedema, occurs frequently, usually as a by-product of the treatment of Graves' disease or as a result of Hashimoto's thyroiditis. In a careful survey of 2,779 persons carried out in County Durham, England, hypothyroidism was detected in 1.9 percent of women and was overt in 1.4 percent. The prevalence of hypothyroidism among men was less than 0.1 percent. One-third to one-fourth of the cases were of iatrogenic cause.[37]

Recent surveys show thyroid dysfunction in elderly patients to be more prevalent than in the population in general. In a study of the Framingham population, 5.9 percent of women and 2.4 percent of men over the age of 60 had serum TSH concentrations greater than 10 mU/L.[38] In this study a significant fraction of such patients have antibodies directed against thyroglobulin or microsomal antigen, indicating the presence of subclinical autoimmune thyroiditis as the cause for mild hypothyroidism.

PATHOLOGY

The pathologic changes of primary hypothyroidism have been well described. Among the reported cases, the thyroid usually shows dense fibrosis. Often focal lymphocyte and plasma cell infiltrations and multinucleated giant cells are seen. Scattered follicles or separate thyroid cells may persist, some showing Hürthle cell or squamous metaplasia. The follicles may persist as clumps of cells without a lumen.

In the pituitary in primary myxedema there is an increase in a class of cells that can be identified by the iron-periodic, acid-Schiff, or aldehyde fuchsin staining techniques.[42] These are referred to variously as gamma cells, sparsely granulated basophils, or amphophils. Presumably they are derived from basophilic cells or chromophobes and are active in secreting TSH. Acidophilic cells are decreased. Patients who are congenitally hypothyroid and those who are hypothyroid during childhood may develop pituitary enlargement and pituitary fossa enlargement. Occasionally prolonged hypothyroidism leads to sella enlargement in the adolescent and adult, and pituitary tumors have been described.[43] In these glands acidophils are virtually absent. In pituitary hypothyroidism the pituitary may be replaced by fibrous and cystic structures, granulomas, or neoplasia. Occasionally hypothyroidism due to deficient TSH secretion occurs in patients having the empty sella syndrome or because of isolated TSH or TRH deficiency.

The adrenals may be normal or their cortex may be atrophied. The combination of adrenal cortical atrophy and hypothyroidism is known as Schmidt's syndrome and is thought to be of autoimmune etiology. Bloodworth found clinical evidence for hypothyroidism in 9 of 35 patients with Addison's disease; in 8 there was fibrosis of the thyroid, with atrophy in 4. The adrenal medulla appeared normal.[44]

The ovaries and parathyroids have shown no definite abnormalities. The testes may show Leydig cells with involutionary nucleus and cytoplasm, hyalinization, or involution of the tubular cells, and proliferation of intertubular connective tissue in hypothyroidism with onset before puberty. Onset after maturity, in one case, led to similar changes that were restricted to the tubules.

The pancreatic islets are usually normal, although hyperplasia was present in one of our autopsied cases.

The skin is distinctly abnormal. There is hyperkeratotic plugging of sweat glands and hair follicles. The dermis is edematous, and the collagen fibers are separated, swollen, and frayed. Extracellular material that appears eosinophilic or basophilic in hematoxylin and eosin stains, or that appears pink (metachromatic) with toluidine blue, or takes the periodic acid–Schiff (PAS) stain for mucopolysaccharides is much increased in the dermis. A sparse mononuclear cell infiltrate may be found about the blood vessels.

Skeletal muscle cells are swollen and appear grossly to be pale and edematous. Frequently microscopic examination reveals no significant abnormality. Alternatively, the normal striations are lost, and degenerative foci are seen in the cells. The fibers are separated in these degenerative foci by accumulations of a basophilic, PAS-positive homogeneous infiltrate. This infiltrate may appear as a semilunar deposit under the sarcolemma.

The heart may be dilated and hypertrophied. Interstitial edema and an increase in fibrous tissue are present. The individual muscle cells may show the same changes seen in skeletal muscle.

The serous cavities may all contain abnormal amounts of fluid with a normal or high protein content.

The liver may appear normal or may show evidence of edema. Central congestive fibrosis in the absence of congestive heart failure has been described. The mitochondria tend to be spherical and their limiting membranes smooth, whereas those of the liver in thyrotoxicosis vary in shape and have wrinkled outer membranes.[45]

The skeleton may be unusually dense on radiographic examination. In children, bone maturation is usually retarded, and typical epiphyseal dysgenesis of hypothyroidism is present.[46]

The brain may show atrophy of cells, gliosis, and foci of degeneration. Deposition of mucinous material and round bodies containing glycogen (neural myxedematous bodies) has been found in the cerebellum of patients with long-standing myxedema and ataxia.[47] In uncorrected congenital hypothyroidism, the brain retains infantile characteristics. There is neuronal hypoplasia, retarded myelination, and decreased vascularity[48] (see Ch. 15).

The blood vessels often show prominent atherosclerosis. Whether this condition is more severe than might be anticipated on the basis of the patient's age and sex remains an unsettled question and is discussed below.

In the intestinal tract there is an accumulation of mast cells and interstitial mucoid material, especially near the basement membrane. The smooth muscle cells may show lesions similar to those seen in skeletal muscle. The mucosa of the stomach, small bowel, and large bowel may be atrophic. The rest of the gastrointestinal tract, especially the colon, may be very dilated (myxedema megacolon).

The uterus typically has a proliferative or atrophic endometrium in premenopausal women.

The kidney is grossly normal. Light and electron microscopic studies of renal biopsy samples have demonstrated thickening of the glomerular and tubular basement membranes, proliferation of the endothelial and mesangial cells, intracellular inclusions, and extracellular deposition of amorphous material with characteristics of acid mucopolysaccharides.[49,50]

COURSE OF THE DISEASE

Although technologically dated, one of the most charming and clear descriptions of a typical case of myxedema is that given by William M. Ord[51] in Allbutt's *System of Medicine*, published first in 1897. It is as follows:

The Picture of the Disease

Thirty years ago the writer of this article had occasion to investigate the case of a lady suffering from myxoedema in a most definite form, and therefore offering complete opportunity of studying the symptoms and the relations of the disease. The patient, a lady of thirty-five, who had several children, presented an appearance suggestive of Bright's disease, yet, although she was greatly swollen on the whole of her body, on careful examination the swelling did not appear to be due to an ordinary dropsy. There was nowhere any pitting on pressure, and there was no albuminuria in the slightest amount. The diagnosis of chronic Bright's disease without albuminuria at first suggested itself, but on further examination many symptoms not known to be related with Bright's disease came under the eye. The face, very much swollen in all parts, was particularly swollen in the eyelids, upper and lower, in the lips, and in the alae nasi. There was a flush, very limited, over the malar bones, contrasting with a complete pallor over the orbital regions. The eyebrows were greatly raised by the effort to keep the lids apart. The skin of the face, and indeed of the whole body, was completely dry, rough and harsh to the touch; not exactly doughy, but giving a sensation of the loss of all elasticity or resilience. The hair was scanty, had no proper gloss, and was much broken. In the absence of all signs of visceral disease the condition of the nervous system was such as to attract much attention. The physiognomy was singularly placid at most times, less frequently heavy, with signs of somnolence, very rarely alert. In interviews the patient was imperturbably garrulous to a degree that could not fail to attract attention. For many minutes she would talk without cessation until obliged to stop and take a good breath. What she said was not altogether relevant, but it had to be said. All interrupting questions were disregarded. If, at the end of a small pause, she was asked to put out her tongue, she ignored the request, but at the end of a varying time, when her breath became short, she would put out her tongue for a long time. She dealt in the same way with questions put to her in respect of the points raised by her statements. Her letters were frequent, voluminous, and, as regarded handwriting, very good. Her speech was slow and laboured. There was some difficulty in it, evidently due to the swelling of the lips, but there was more than this: the words hung in a way that indicated nervous as well as physical difficulty, and inflexions of the voice were wanting. The tones of the voice were leathery, and suggested rather those of an automaton. The proper timbre was quite lost. Doubtless this was in part, again, due to obvious thickenings in the fauces and the larynx; but it did not in any way resemble the character of voice observed in ordinary swellings of those parts. Her temper was singularly equable, she was the most tender and solicitous of mothers, and in a long course of years during which she was under the writer's observation no word of unkindness or suspicion fell from her lips. Lethargy was an impressive part of her mental condition. Memory was slow, but correct. She thought slowly, performed all movements slowly, and was slow in receiving impressions. Her toilet, and she was no fashionable person, occupied hours. Her household duties could never be overtaken, and she had to seek assistance. Her gait presented a distinct ataxic quality. As her bulky body moved across a room, there occurred at each step forward a quiver running from the legs upwards, such as may be seen in people under the influence of great emotion, as in Lady Macbeth. This appeared to be due to a want of complete concert in the action of the flexors and extensors of the body, the flexors acting for the most part in advance. The interval between the action of the two sets of muscles was at some times extreme enough to determine falls, not in any way produced by obstacles. She fell forward on her knees, and, as a result, she sustained fracture of the patella on one side, and of the patellar tendon on the other. Similar conditions existing in the head and neck produced excessive distress. From time to time the head would fall forward in spite of all voluntary effort to prevent it. The chin would then rest on the upper part of the sternum, as is seen in cretins. Sometimes by prolonged exertion of the will, sometimes with the assistance of the hands, the head would be raised, not always to good effect; for unless great care were exercised the head would fall backwards with a suddenness that was alarming. There was no obvious defect of the sense of touch, but it must be admitted that the speed of the reception of tactile sensations was not noted. After the establishment of the disease she bore two children; on both occasions severe postpartum haemorrhage occurred. She had no other haemorrhages. The first impression was, as I said above, that the case was one of Bright's disease without albuminuria. The urine was examined regularly for years without detection of albumin, and there were no such changes in the heart and arteries as belong to Bright's disease. After ten years, however, albumin appeared in the urine, and the patient died ultimately with symptoms of contracting granular kidney. A postmortem examination could not be obtained, and therefore the condition of the thyroid gland and of the kidneys cannot be recorded.

Onset of the Disease

The onset of naturally occurring hypothyroidism is insidious. The patient is often unaware of it, as may be friends and relations. As the gland is gradually replaced by fibrous tissue, lymphocytic infiltration, or both, the serum hormone levels and metabolic rate begin slowly to fall. The first symptoms may be a decrease in sweating and dislike of cold. They may be present alone for a period of years before dramatic events occur. One of our patients gave a story of marked hypersensitivity to cold for 12 years, at the end of which time the picture of full-blown myxedema developed. Sometimes the presenting symptom may be a demand for a warmer room or more clothing. Sometimes a mere decrease in activity due to listlessness, lack of energy, or fatigue, is the first change noted. In other patients, mental dullness or drowsiness may be observed. We have also seen the opposite change, namely, nervousness and irritability, or even peevishness in the exceptional case. Progressive constipation or increase in menstrual flow may occasionally be the first event. So, too, may any of the following: deafness, falling hair, thick speech,

dizziness, puffiness of the face, headache, pallor, weight gain, or fatigue.

When hypothyroidism occurs more suddenly, as after surgical thyroidectomy or RAI therapy, the symptoms may not be so insidious, and indeed may be quite upsetting to the patient. Musculoskeletal symptoms such as frequent cramps may be distressing, and acute depression or acute anxiety may appear. Thus, the clinical course may be much influenced by the cause of the hypothyroid state.

Obvious symptoms and signs usually appear as the thyroxine (T_4) level falls below normal. Of these symptoms, nonpitting edema, from which myxedema derives its name, is pathognomonic. It is a specific thyroprival sign, and when it develops, the disease is in the full-blown state. There may be little apparent change in the patient's appearance or condition for several years. During such a period the patient may be well off subjectively. The increased sensitivity to cold can be met by maintaining the living area at an unduly warm temperature. The decreased energy makes the person content to do little or nothing. The myxedematous state is characterized by an amazing placidity. The terminal stage may be called *myxedematous cachexia*.

Myxedematous Cachexia

Myxedematous cachexia is characterized by an intensification of all the symptoms and signs. There is great thickening of the tongue, thickness, dryness, and coarseness of the skin, thickening and brittleness of the nails, falling and brittleness of the hair, progressive decrease in activity and responsiveness, and a closer and closer approach to a purely vegetative existence. Although the mucous edema persists—and indeed tends to increase—body fat may disappear, so that actual wasting takes place. After this stage has persisted for an indefinite period of months or even years, death takes place because of intercurrent infection, congestive heart failure, or both. The final symptom is coma, which may last for days.

In the untreated patient, the length of time between the first symptoms and death may be as long as 15 years. It is, fortunately, seldom nowadays that one witnesses the natural termination of the disease. It is seen only when the patient is already moribund when he or she comes to the physician, the diagnosis previously having been overlooked or where severe myxedema is present in association with another serious illness. In the *Report on Myxoedema*, which was published before the discovery of the cure of the disease, the duration is given as 10 years or more.

The evolution of the symptoms of myxedema is slowly progressive. If one compares patients with myxedema of 3, 6, or 12 years' duration, although all may have classic symptoms and identical thyroid function test results, the clinical picture will be more intense at 6 years than at 3 and still more at 12. The mental manifestations, and the integumentary changes in particular, intensify as the years pass. Such severe manifestations of hypothyroidism are rarely seen in the current era.

Patients and their friends and relatives are often strangely unaware of evidence of myxedema. Often patients are identified during treatment for some entirely unrelated disorder. Myxedema has been called a "consultant's diagnosis," because the changes that appear as the disease develops are so subtle and gradual that they are often overlooked by the patient's family physician. This fact is becoming less true with the ready availability of objective diagnostic tests.

SIGNS, SYMPTOMS, AND ASSOCIATED FUNCTIONAL PATHOLOGY

Facies and Integument

In the *Report on Myxoedema* there is a detailed analysis of the symptoms of 109 patients described as "cretinoid," "expressionless," "heavy," "apathetic," "masklike," "vacant," "stolid," "good-tempered," "blunted," and "large-featured." The face is expressionless when at rest, but it is not masklike, as in Parkinson's disease. When spoken to, the person with myxedema usually responds with a smile, which spreads after a latent period very slowly over the face. The patient is good-tempered but not entirely apathetic. The face is not vacant, as that of a psychopathic patient may be. The features (except for the tongue) are not large, as in acromegaly. The face is expressionless at rest, puffy, pale, and often with a yellowish or old ivory tint. It is seldom as puffy as the classic facies of chronic renal failure. The skin of the face is parchmentlike. In spite of the swelling it may be traced with fine wrinkles, particularly in

pituitary myxedema. The swelling sometimes gives it a round or moonlike appearance (Fig. 9-1).

The eyelids are often edematous. The palpebral fissure may be narrowed because of blepharoptosis, due to diminished tone of the sympathetic nervous fibers to Müller's levator palpebral superious muscle and is the opposite of the lid retraction seen in thyrotoxicosis. The modest measurable exophthalmos seen in some patients with myxedema is presumably related to accumulation of the same mucous edema in the orbit as is seen elsewhere. It is not progressive and carries no threat to vision, as in the ophthalmopathy of Graves' disease. The central visual fields may be restricted in primary myxedema, probably because of the associated pituitary hyperplasia, which also is commonly associated with enlargement of the sella turcica.[52]

The tongue is usually large, occasionally to the point of clumsiness. Sometimes a patient will complain of this problem. Sometimes it is smooth, as in pernicious anemia (of course, pernicious anemia may coexist). Patients do not usually complain of soreness of the tongue, as they may in pernicious anemia. When anemia is marked, the tongue may be pale, but more often it is red, in contrast to the pallid face.

The voice is husky, low-pitched, and coarse. The speech is deliberate and slow. Often there is difficulty in articulation. Certain words are stumbled over and slurred, much as they are during alcoholic intoxication. The enlargement of the tongue, and possibly some thickness of the lips, may be responsible.

The hair, both of the head and elsewhere, is dry, brittle, and sparse, and lacks shine. It varies in texture from coarse to normal. Its growth is retarded and it falls out readily. The eyebrows often are practically gone. Their disappearance begins at the lateral margin, giving rise to Queen Anne's sign. It should be noted, however, that this sign is not uncommon in elderly euthyroid women. In men the beard becomes sparse, and its rate of growth becomes greatly retarded. Haircuts are necessary only at long intervals. A shave a week is sufficient. The scalp is dry and scaly.

The skin is cool as a result of decreased metabolism as well as cutaneous vasoconstriction. It is dry due to reduced secretion by sweat and sebaceous glands. Scaling is common but rarely assumes the appearance characteristic of ichthyosis. The tissues

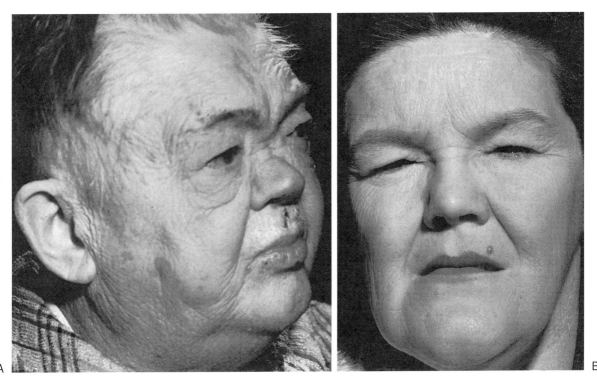

Fig. 9-1. **(A)** The classic torpid facies of severe myxedema in a man. The face appears puffy, and the eyelids are edematous. The skin is thickened and dry. **(B)** The facies in pituitary myxedema is often characterized by skin of normal thickness, covered by fine wrinkles. Puffiness is usually less than in primary myxedema.

beneath it seem thick, but usually do not pit on pressure. In the lower extremities, pitting edema is not uncommon. Subcutaneous fat may be increased, with the formation of definite fat pads, especially above the clavicles, but is conspicuously absent in the more advanced form of the disease (myxedematous cachexia).

Retardation in the rate of healing of surgical wounds and of ulcerations, such as leg ulcers, has been described in myxedema.

The nails are thickened and brittle. These changes are probably dependent, as are those of skin and hair, on retardation in growth. Nails require paring only at greatly lengthened intervals.

The hands and feet have a broad appearance, due to thickening of subcutaneous tissue. However, there is no bony overgrowth, so that they bear no resemblance to the extremities in acromegaly. Unusual coldness of the arms and legs is sometimes a subject of complaint. The palms are cool and dry.

The characteristic skin changes are due to an increased amount of normal glycosaminoglycans and protein. The glycosaminoglycans are demonstrated by metachromasia after staining with toluidine blue. An increased concentration of glycosaminoglycans, composed principally of hyaluronic acid and chondroitin sulfuric acid, occurs in histologically similar skin lesions found in hyperthyroidism (pretibial myxedema: see Chapter 12). This excess accumulation of normal intercellular material represents not only an alteration in steady-state equilibrium but an actual increase in the synthesis and accumulation of glycosaminoglycan.[53]

The glycosaminoglycans are long-chain polymers of D-glucuronic acid and N-acetyl-D-glucosamine, forming hyaluronic acid, or of L-iduronic acid and N-acetyl-D-galactosamine sulfate, forming chondroitin sulfate B. They exist free and in ionic or covalent linkage to protein. These mucoproteins comprise part of the normal nonfibrillar intercellular matrix, the ground substance holding cells together. As they are characteristically hygroscopic, they presumably hold in bound form the nonpitting water comprising the mucous edema. Aikawa[54] showed that the total amount of exchangeable sodium was increased in myxedema despite a slight reduction in its plasma concentration. The sodium was extravascular and probably in the interstitial spaces. The diuresis seen after giving thyroid hormone to a hypothyroid subject occurs coincidentally with a decrease in tissue metachromasia and a temporary negative nitrogen balance,[55] and with this condition the extravascular sodium is mobilized and excreted.

Studies with human skin fibroblasts have suggested that thyroid hormone inhibits the synthesis of hyaluronate. The mechanism for this effect has not been identified, but the thyroid hormone levels required to produce it *in vitro* are in the physiologic range.[53,56]

Although similar deposits of mucopolysaccharides are found in the orbits of patients with the ophthalmopathy of Graves' disease and in the areas of localized myxedema, this striking observation has unfortunately not provided any basic understanding of the phenomenon, either in this condition or in primary myxedema.

Cardiovascular System

Pulse rate and stroke volume are diminished in hypothyroidism, and cardiac output is accordingly decreased, often to one-half the normal value.[57] Myocardial contractility is reduced, but there is also a steep decline in the circulatory load, so that the circulation rarely fails until very late in the disease.[58] The speed of shortening is slowed, but the total force is not much modified.[59] Myocardial adenyl cyclase levels are reduced.[60] The decrease in pulse rate occurs more or less in parallel with that of the metabolism. Stroke volume is reduced more than pulse rate at any given level, and is therefore the major determinant of the low cardiac output. Since the reduction in cardiac output is usually proportional to the decreased oxygen consumption by the tissues, the arteriovenous (AV) oxygen difference is normal or may be slightly increased. Slow peripheral circulation, and therefore more complete extraction of oxygen, as well as anemia, may be responsible for the increased AV oxygen difference. Myocardial oxygen consumption is decreased, usually more than blood supply to the myocardium, so that angina is infrequent. In some patients a reduction in cardiac output greater than the decline in oxygen consumption indicates specific cardiac damage from the myxedema.[9,61]

Venous pressure is normal, but peripheral resistance is increased. Cerebrovascular resistance is increased, and blood flow and oxygen are reduced.[62,63] Arterial blood pressure is often mildly increased. It varies widely, but is usually restored to normal after treatment.[62] The incidence of hypertension is higher than in the general population, but it must be recognized that hypothyroidism most frequently occurs in middle-aged or elderly women who already tend to have a high incidence of hypertension. Induced hypothyroidism lowers the blood pressure of experimentally hypertensive rats to normal.[64]

The heart in hypothyroidism has been a focus of much controversy. The term Myxodemherz was introduced by Zondek in 1918.[65] It embraced dilatation of the left and right sides of the heart, slow, indolent heart action with normal blood pressure, and lowering of the P and T waves of the electrocardiogram. Zondek found that after treatment with thyroid hormone there was a return of the dilated heart to somewhere near normal size, a more rapid pulse without change in blood pressure, and gradual return of the P and T waves to normal. These findings have been confirmed and extended. Indeed, occasional severely hypothyroid patients without underlying heart disease have congestive heart failure or low cardiac output reversed by thyroid hormone administration.[63,66,67] Therefore, congestive heart failure or impaired cardiac output relative to metabolic needs can be caused by hypothyroidism. Microscopic examination discloses myxedematous changes of the myocardial fibers, as described above.

The cause of the cardiac enlargement has been disputed. Clearly, it is not due to hypertrophy alone, since it would not disappear so rapidly with treatment. One factor may be a decrease in contractility of the heart muscle. This decrease would require a lengthening of muscle fibers in order to perform the required work. Disappearance of interstitial fluid alone could account for only part of the observed shrinkage. Altered myosin synthesis (see Chapter 3) is also important.

Gordon[68] long ago called attention to the occurrence of pericardial effusions in myxedema and explained the increase in the transverse diameter of the heart shadow on this basis. Effusion must frequently play a role in the increase in the size of the heart shadow, but it has amazingly little effect on cardiodynamics. The presence of fluid may be reflected in the right ventricular pressure contour, but tamponade, although reported, is rare.[69,70] Effusions of the pericardium, pleura, and peritoneum are common findings in hypothyroidism.[71] The protein of the effusion may be high or in the range of transudates. In 11 patients with tamponade studied, pericardial fluid protein ranged from 2.2 to 7.6 g/dl.[69] Occasionally, the fluid is high in cholesterol, with a "gold paint" appearance.[70]

The hypothyroid heart responds normally to exercise.[9,61,63] Graettinger et al.[57] found that after exercise the low resting cardiac output increased normally with an increase of stroke volume and, usually, of pulse rate. Their patients had slightly elevated resting pulmonary artery and right ventricular pressures and a diastolic dip in right ventricular pressure, all compatible with pericardial effusion. They doubt that myxedema alone can ever produce congestive heart failure, and believe that the recorded abnormalities represent not myocardial disease but pericardial effusion. The heart, in experimental hypothyroidism, also responds to norepinephrine with a rise in cAMP, but less so than does the normal heart, although the response in contractility is the same.

Plasma catecholamines in hypothyroid patients are elevated rather than reduced, even though circulating cyclic AMP is lower.[63] This may be explained by a decrease in cyclic AMP generation in response to catecholamines only in certain tissues. There is a decrease in the number of β-adrenergic receptors in the myocardium of hypothyroid rats, but there are no data with respect to human myocardium.[60,61,63,67]

Since the treatment of myxedema restores the hypothyroid heart to normal, there is apparently little permanent structural damage.[66,67]

Cardiac glycosides will not improve the function of the heart in uncomplicated myxedema. Although the drug is efficacious if heart failure has been produced by coincident organic disease, myxedematous patients with coincident heart disease and congestive heart failure may tolerate digoxin poorly, just as they do morphine. This poor tolerance probably represents delayed metabolism, rather than myocardial sensitivity to the drug. The plasma concentration of digoxin is higher than in the normal subject at the same dose level, and smaller doses are required. When the heart in myxedema does not return to a normal size under thyroid hormone administration,

hypertrophy due to some other disease is present as a complication. The return in size to normal under treatment is slow and progressive, requiring between 3 weeks and 10 months for completion. This decrease in size, like the progressive elevation of the T waves (described below), is of diagnostic value.

The electrocardiogram reveals characteristic changes.[61,63,67,72–76] The rate is slow and the voltage is low. The T waves are flattened or inverted. Axis deviation, an increased P-R interval, and widened QRS complexes and prolonged Q1 interval are seen, but these signs are not diagnostic of myxedema. The pattern reverts toward normal with treatment, but the final pattern depends on the presence or absence of intrinsic myocardial disease. The rare occurrence of complete heart block complicated by Adams-Stokes attacks, with reversion to sinus rhythm after treatment with thyroid hormone, has been reported as has ventricular tachycardia.[75,76] Changes resembling those of ischemic heart disease may be found during exercise: they may indicate an intrinsic anoxia rather than organic narrowing of the coronary vessels.[61,63,67,74]

The ECG changes have usually been attributed to the histologic changes in the myocardium. However, removal of pericardial fluid may immediately reverse the pattern toward normal, suggesting that the effusion may in part be responsible for the abnormalities.

The systolic time intervals are prolonged in hypothyroidism.[9,61,63,67] They can be measured by several techniques and have been expressed as the ratio of the pre-ejection period and the left ventricular ejection time or the interval between the onset of the QRS complex of the ECG and the onset of the Korotkoff sound.[77,78]

It is frequently suggested that accelerated atherosclerosis occurs in hypothyroidism. Hypothyroidism accelerates atheromatous changes when these are induced experimentally in animals, but data in humans are not complete enough to justify this assertion. Most autopsied myxedematous subjects have severe atherosclerosis, but they are also usually 60 years or more of age. Arterial disease did not appear to be accelerated in patients rendered hypothyroid for therapy of angina pectoris or congestive heart failure,[78] but they have been observed over a relatively short period. Increased coronary arteriosclerosis is found in myxedematous patients with hypertension, but not if they are normotensive.[79]

Unfortunately, observations of young persons with hypothyroidism of several years' duration are not available. It must be concluded that at present this issue is unresolved, although Bastenie et al. have presented strong clinical and pathologic evidence supporting a relationship between atherosclerotic disease and hypothyroid states.[80,81] Other results dispute this relationship.[82,83]

Occasionally angina pectoris is encountered in myxedema under two sets of circumstances. The less common is that in which angina or anginalike pain is present before treatment.[82,84,85] This generally indicates the presence of significant coronary artery compromise since there is inadequate myocardial oxygenation despite reduced cardiac output and O_2 utilization. Although improvement sometimes occurs with therapy,[84] this should not be undertaken until angiographic evaluation of the coronary arteries has been performed (see below). Angina may also appear for the first time after therapy has been initiated, indicating that coronary flow is inadequate for resumption of normal cardiac function.[82,84,85] Again, this may indicate the presence of a structural lesion (see below).

Because the serum creatine phosphokinase (CPK) levels in myxedema are often elevated,[86–88] chest pain occurring during the initiation of hormone replacement therapy may be erroneously interpreted as indicating a recent myocardial infarction. This problem can be avoided by measuring the serum CPK level before instituting hormone therapy in elderly myxedematous patients.

Pulmonary Function

Dyspnea is a frequent complaint of myxedematous patients, but it is also a common symptom among well persons. Congestive heart failure of separate origin, pleural effusion, anemia, obesity, or pulmonary disease may be responsible.

Some information on pulmonary function in hypothyroidism is available.[89–93] Wilson and Bedell[89] found a normal vital capacity and arterial PCO_2 and PO_2 in 16 patients. They also found a decreased maximal breathing capacity, decreased diffusion capacity, and decreased ventilatory response to carbon dioxide.

Decreased ventilatory drive is present in about one-third of hypothyroid patients, and the response to hypoxia returns rapidly within a week after beginning therapy. The severity of hypothyroidism parallels the incidence of impaired ventilatory drive. The role of CO_2 retention in myxedema coma is not clear, although the two conditions may be associated. Often myxedema coma is precipitated by a complicating illness or overmedication with sedatives. These studies suggest that while the decreased ventilatory response of the hypothyroid patient may contribute to the CO_2 retention it is generally not the only cause for this problem.[90–93]

Weakness of the respiratory muscles has also been implicated as a cause of alveolar hypoventilation. Patients with myxedema may develop carbon dioxide retention, and carbon dioxide narcosis may be a cause of myxedema coma.[91,92] Myxedematous patients are more subject to respiratory infections. Obstructive sleep apnea has been documented in myxedema and is reversible with therapy.[93]

Gastrointestinal System

The symptoms from the digestive system are essentially the expression of the slow rate at which the living machinery is turning over. Anorexia, which is common, can reasonably be interpreted as the reflection of a lowered food requirement, and constipation, which is frequently present, is the result of a lowered food intake and decreased peristaltic activity. Although two-thirds of patients have reported weight gain, it is of modest degree and due largely to the accumulation of fluid rather than fat. Contrary to popular belief, obesity is decidedly not a feature of myxedema.

Complete achlorhydria occurs in more than half of myxedematous patients.[94] As many as 25 percent of patients with myxedema, like those with Hashimoto's thyroiditis, have circulating antibodies directed against the gastric parietal cells. This finding explains, at least in part, the frequency of achlorhydria and impaired absorption of vitamin B_{12} described later. It is reported that up to 14 percent of patients with idiopathic myxedema have coincident pernicious anemia.[95]

Gaseous distention may be a persistent and troublesome symptom. It responds slowly to thyroid therapy. Fecal impaction may occur. The syndrome of ileus may be seen occasionally,[96] and a megacolon may be evident on radiography.[97,98] Intestinal absorption is slowed. Galactose and glucose tolerance curves show a delayed rise to a lower peak than normal and a delayed return to baseline. Xylose absorption is impaired.[99]

Symptoms or signs of disturbed liver or exocrine pancreatic function are usually not encountered, but chemical examination may suggest disease. Serum glutamine-oxaloacetic transaminase (GOT), lactate dehydrogenase (LDH), and CPK levels are elevated in patients with hypothyroidism.[86] The enzymes return to normal over 2 to 4 weeks during treatment. These findings are thought to represent altered metabolism of the enzymes (akin to changes in cholesterol or uric acid) and not liver damage, although one report suggests that central lobular congestive fibrosis may occur in myxedematous patients in the absence of heart failure.[100] Urinary amylase levels may be increased. CEA levels are also increased and drop with therapy.[101] Gallbladder motility is decreased, and the gallbladder may appear distended on x-ray examination.[102]

Renal Function, Water, and Electrolytes

Hypothyroid patients tend to drink small amounts of water and to have diminished urinary output. Clinical evidence of renal failure is not often found, but laboratory examination may disclose certain departures from normal renal function. Because of decreased cardiac output and blood volume, renal blood flow is decreased, but it remains the same percentage of cardiac output. The glomerular filtration rate and effective renal plasma flow are decreased, but the filtration fraction is normal or variably altered.[103–105]

The response to water loading is variable. Moses et al.[106] reported that deficient diuresis after water loading is a sign of pituitary myxedema, but others, notably Crispell and co-workers,[107] have found that severe primary myxedema may be associated with a delay in water excretion that is not corrected by cortisone but rather by replacement with thyroid hormone. Perhaps the difference in opinion arises from interpretation of the normal response to water loading. This possibility is suggested by the data of Bleifer et al.,[108] who found a decrease in maximal diuresis in some patients with primary myxedema to below the normal lower limit of urine flow (3ml/min), but not down to the 1 to 3 ml/min seen in panhypopituitarism. The role of antidiuretic hormone and of solute excretion in producing the decreased response to water loading is unknown.

The defect is usually attributed to a decreased glomerular filtration rate, but in some patients inappropriately high levels of serum vasopressin have been demonstrated.[109–112] Since urinary hydroxycorticoid excretion is decreased, the adrenals might be incriminated as responsible for delayed water excretion. Other evidence suggests (see below) that the tissue supply of adrenal cortical hormones is usually normal in myxedema.

Occasionally, minimal proteinuria is seen. This condition could be due to congestive heart failure or to the increased capillary transudation of protein typical of hypothyroidism. Other causes of proteinuria, such as pyelonephritis or vascular disease, often coexist.

The total body sodium content is increased. The excessive sodium is presumably bound to extracellular mucopolysaccharides. In spite of reduced renal blood flow and blood volume, the sodium retention is probably not a reflection of altered renal function. In fact, salt loads are usually excreted readily and serum sodium concentrations tend to be low, in contrast to other clinical situations associated with sodium retention, such as congestive heart failure.[109] The dilutional syndrome may be a result of inappropriate secretion of ADH,[110–112] but not in all patients. Thus, the dilutional syndrome in severe myxedema may be due to a resetting of the osmolar receptor, which causes water to be retained at a lower level of plasma osmotic pressure. The various changes in renal function may not return to normal at the same rate after treatment.

The serum uric acid level is elevated in hypothyroid men and postmenopausal women, apparently as a consequence of a decrease in renal blood flow characteristic of the disease.[113]

No consistent changes in plasma potassium levels have been reported. Total magnesium levels may be elevated, and the bound fraction and urinary excretion are reduced.[114] A modest hypocalcemia has been observed in some patients.

Pituitary Function

Thyrotroph hyperplasia caused by primary hypothyroidism may result in sellar enlargement, particularly when the condition has remained untreated for a long period of time.[43,115] Rarely, such hyperplasia may give rise to a tumor or replace the normal pituitary tissue enough to produce insufficiency.[116]

The serum prolactin concentration is elevated in approximately one-third of patients with primary hypothyroidism.[117] The hyperprolactinemia is modest in degree and is rarely associated with galactorrhea.[118] When present, it subsides with thyroid hormone replacement in conjunction with the reduction in the serum prolactin level. From experiments using rat prolactin producing pituitary tumors in culture, it appears that the hyperprolactinemia is due to increased synthesis and secretion of prolactin caused by an increase in the number of TRH receptors on prolacting-secreting cells associated with thyroid hormone deprivation.[119] Alternatively, since thyroid hormone decreases the mRNA for pre-proTRH in the paraventricular nuclei, it is conceivable that hypothyroidism leads to increased TRH secretion, unopposed by thyroid hormones, with consequent hyperprolactinemia.

In contrast, the growth hormone response to insulin-induced hypoglycemia is blunted in hypothyroidism.[120] Animal experiments in vivo and in vitro have shown that thyroid hormone plays an important role in the regulation of growth hormone synthesis by increasing the cytoplasmic accumulation of its mRNA.[121,122]

A thyroid hormone response element (see Ch. 3) has been identified in the 5′ flanking region of the rat growth hormone (rGH) gene.[123] It is possible to confirm triiodothyronine (T_3) response of the rGH promoter in transfection experiments using chimeric rate promoter-CAT-reporter gene constructs.[124] Of considerable interest is the fact that the human GH (hGH) 5′ flanking region does not contain a T_3 response element (TRE), and this promoter does not confer T_3 responsiveness to reporter genes.[125] Thus, the mechanism by which thyroid hormone influences hGH secretion remains unknown. The area under the curve of growth hormone secretion after various stimuli is attenuated in children with primary hypothyroidism.[126,127] This attenuation is associated with a reduction in insulin-like growth factor (IGF-I) concentrations.[128] These studies raise the possibility that hypothyroidism impairs growth in part by blocking production of IGF-I from the liver. However, it should be noted that in some patients receiving growth hormone treatment for hypopituitarism, concomitant thyroid deficiency impairs the growth response, suggesting that there may also be adverse effects of hypothyroidism di-

rectly at the cartilage level. Thus, deficiency of thyroid hormone may impair the action of IGF-I as well as its production.

Reproductive Function

In both sexes libido is usually, but not invariably, decreased. The man may be impotent. The testicles are histologically immature if hypothyroidism preceded puberty and show tubular involution if onset was after puberty.[129] Although infertility may be a problem in either sex, the literature contains many reports of pregnancy in untreated myxedematous women.[130,131] When treatment has been started during pregnancy, more often than not a normal child is produced, but abortion is frequent in the myxedematous woman, and even with treatment the incidence of various congenital abnormalities may be increased.[130–134] This finding may possibly be attributed to secondary factors such as poor placental development, rather than an inadequate transplacental supply of maternal hormone. The independent function of the fetal pituitary–thyroid axis is discussed in Chapters 14 and 15.

Women who develop the disease before menopause usually have menorrhagia, which may be severe.[135] Menorrhagia is sufficiently impressive in ordinary myxedema so that in several cases that have come to our attention, patients have actually had dilatation and curettage or hysterectomy for it, the diagnosis of myxedema having been missed. The endometrium in premenopausal patients is typically proliferative or, less commonly, atrophic. The proliferative endometrium and low urinary pregnanetriol levels suggest failure of luteinizing hormone (LH) production and of ovulation.[136] In some patients, amenorrhea rather than menorrhagia occurs, with a reinstitution of a normal menstrual pattern after therapy. In children, hypothyroidism sometimes induces precocious puberty with menstruation and breast development, for reasons yet unknown but thought to be a result of altered hypothalamic-pituitary regulation.[137] On rare occasions, precocious testicular enlargement with early seminiferous tubular maturation has also been reported.[138] These abnormalities promptly subside with the correction of the hypothyroid state. Although less frequent, amenorrhea and galactorrhea are occasionally found in adult hypothyroidism and are reversible with treatment.[139]

Thyroid has been widely used for the empirical treatment of infertility in both sexes and for irregularity of menses, dysmenorrhea, and habitual abortion in patients without clinically evident hypothyroidism. Despite testimonies to the efficacy of thyroid hormone in these situations, no convincing documentation has been presented. However, in the presence of a clear-cut elevation in serum TSH despite the absence of classic symptoms, a therapeutic trial of levothyroxine therapy is certainly indicated.

Alterations in both androgens and estrogens associated with hypothyroidism are rather complex and are due to the consequences of thyroid hormone deprivation on the production, metabolic pathways, and serum transport of these steroids. The concentrations of both testosterone and estradiol in serum are decreased, predominantly due to a diminution in the concentration of the carrier sex hormone–binding globulin (SHBG),[140] but because of the concomitant increase in the unbound fraction of the steroids, their absolute free concentration remains normal.

In sharp contrast to cortisol and aldosterone, the metabolic clearance rate of testosterone increases in hypothyroidism.[141,142] The conversion ratio of testosterone to androstenedione increases and that to androsterone decreases.[141,143] It has been postulated that this shift of testosterone metabolism toward etiocholanolone rather than androsterone may be responsible for the hypercholesterolemia associated with hypothyroidism, since administration of the androsterone metabolite has a cholesterol-lowering effect.[144] Dihydrotestosterone, a hormone derived predominantly from peripheral tissue conversion of testosterone, mediates the intracellular androgenic action in certain target tissues. It also binds more tightly to SHBG, and important alterations may be anticipated in association with thyroid dysfunction. However, precise information about this important and potent androgen in hypothyroidism is not available.

The reduction of the amount of 2-hydroxyestrone in myxedema supports the hypothesis that thyroid hormone regulates reciprocally the hydroxylation of carbons 2 and 6 of estrone.[141]

Serum follicle-stimulating hormone (FSH) and LH values are usually normal, but the midcycle FSH and LH surge may fail to appear.

Adrenal Cortex

Adrenal steroid hormone production and metabolism are considerably affected. Serum cortisol levels are normal, but the turnover time is slowed. This slowing is principally due to a decrease in the rate of cortisol oxidation as a result of reduced 11-β-hydroxysteroid dehydrogenase activity.[141] Conjugation with glucuronic acid in the liver is normal.[145] Reflecting these alterations, urinary 17-hydroxycorticoid (as well as 17-ketosteroid) excretion is reduced.[141,142]

The turnover rate of aldosterone is also decreased in hypothyroidism.[141] This reduction is probably due to an alteration in steroid reductases that tends to diminish the proportion of androsterone formed and reciprocally increases the level of the etiocholanolone metabolite.[144] The serum concentration of aldosterone is low or normal.[146] Renin activity is also often reduced, as is the sensitivity to angiotensin II.[147]

Adrenal responsiveness to adrenocorticotrophic hormone (ACTH) may be reduced, or the response may be delayed until the second and third days of the standard ACTH test, with an actual augmentation of the total response.[148] The adrenal glands often atrophy. Pituitary responsiveness to the metyrapone test has been variable. Normal but delayed peak response,[149] impaired response,[150] or even lack of response[150] has been reported. Grossly impaired responses to the stimulation with lysine-8-vasopressin and a delayed increase in serum cortisol levels after insulin-induced hypoglycemia have also been observed.[151,152,153]

A general picture of adrenal function in the hypothyroid patient who is not under stress seems clear. Adrenal steroid metabolism and production decrease. The decreased production is accomplished automatically by the pituitary through decreased ACTH secretion. The result is a normal concentration of free cortisol in the serum. Presumably, sufficient hormone is produced for the reduced needs of the hypothyroid subject. Whether steroid production can be augmented sufficiently in times of stress is not clear, but the provocative test results suggest that these patients usually have a mildly impaired hypothalamic-pituitary adrenal axis.[154,155]

Primary hypothyroidism may be associated with either the type I or type II polyglandular autoimmune syndrome. The specific association of primary hypothyroidism and primary adrenal cortical insufficiency without pituitary insufficiency is known as *Schmidt's syndrome*.[156] However, this combination may also be accompanied by abnormalities of other endocrine glands. There are two major forms of polyglandular autoimmune syndrome. In type I, mucocutaneous candidiasis, hypoparathyroidism, Addison's disease, alopecia, chronic active hepatitis, malabsorption syndrome, and gonadal failure are the most common features. Autoimmune thyroid disease is reported in 10 to 12 percent of these patients. Type I polyglandular autoimmune syndrome presents more commonly in childhood, and there are no HLA associations. The type II syndrome is more common and presents in adult life in association with HLA-B8, D3 and DR3 haplotypes. Addison's disease, Hashimoto's disease, and diabetes are the most common endocrine deficiencies found in these patients, although gonadal failure, pernicious anemia, and vitiligo are observed in a significant percentage.[157] Hypoparathyroidism, chronic mucocutaneous candidiasis, chronic active hepatitis, and sprue are not part of this syndrome. Rarely a combination of primary and pituitary hypothyroidism or ACTH deficiency occurs, presumably also on an autoimmune basis.[34] Thus, it is important to recognize the possibility that other glands are affected with increased frequency in patients with autoimmune thyroid disease.

Another aspect of the interrelationship between the adrenal and thyroid in patients with autoimmune disease occurs in individuals with primary adrenal insufficiency who have modest decreases in serum T_4 and elevated serum TSH levels.[158] When the hypoadrenalism is corrected, TSH and thyroid function normalizes. It is not certain whether this represents a subtle autoimmune thyroid disease that is suppressed by administration of physiologic doses of cortisol or whether the lack of glucocorticoid leads to TSH hypersecretion. As mentioned in Chapter 4, glucocorticoids suppress TSH release, and it is conceivable that hypoadrenalism leads to release of tonic inhibition by this hormone. Nonetheless, an unequivocal diagnosis of permanent primary hypothyroidism should not be made in a patient with primary adrenal insufficiency until after glucocorticoid supplementation begins.

Because of the metabolic clearance of cortisol is reduced in patients with hypothyroidism, primary adrenal insufficiency may not be obvious in patients with concomitant hypothyroidism. Just as in patients with hypopituitarism, where glucocorticoid replacement should precede thyroid hormone replacement, thyroid treatment of patients with apparent primary hypothyroidism may uncover adrenal insufficiency. Likewise, severely hypothyroid patients receiving therapeutic glucocorticoids will have excessive sensitivity to its effects due to impaired clearance of the steroid. Appropriate adjustments need to be made in glucocorticoid replacement when thyroid status is altered.

Adrenal Medulla and Catecholamines

The plasma concentration of norepinephrine in hypothyroid humans is elevated and returns to normal with treatment.[159,160] The epinephrine concentration is normal. Excretion of catecholamines in the urine is normal.[161] The circulatory response to injected epinephrine decreases in hypothyroidism but returns rapidly to normal after small doses of thyroid hormone.[162-164] Hypothyroidism appears to be a state of a sympathetic nervous system overactivity. It can be speculated that this is compensation for the hypometabolism associated with the hypothyroid state; certainly a good case can be made for this in the case of the experimental animal. In the rat, brown adipose tissue, a principal thermogenic organ, is activated in the hypothyroid state by enhanced sympathetic nerve tone.[165] Brown adipose tissue per se is not nearly as localized in the adult human, and recent evidence has identified a wide spread distribution of the brown fat specific β_3-adrenergic receptor in various white fat depots in humans.[166] This suggests that brown fat cells may be interspersed in white adipose tissue in humans as opposed to their concentrated locations in the interscapular and periaortic regions in rodents. As such, they may contribute to oxygen consumption and heat production when catecholamine secretion is enhanced. While there is evidence of increased tone of the sympathetic nervous system in hypothyroidism, there is also evidence of impaired responsiveness to β-adrenergic stimulation, at least in some cells. However, the marked differences between mechanisms by which hypothyroidism reduces catecholamine responsiveness between species (reducing cyclic AMP generation in response to β-adrenergic stimuli in some while reducing receptor number in other tissues) makes it difficult to extrapolate with confidence to the situation in humans.

Taken together, these results suggest a curious paradox in hypothyroidism in which the heart rate is slow, cardiac output is reduced, and yet catecholamines and peripheral vascular resistance are elevated. While cardiac responsiveness to exogenous catecholamines may be attenuated, it is not clear whether this is secondary to the excessive sympathetic nervous system tone or to hypothyroidism per se. Patients with myxedema coma or vascular instability secondary to severe myxedema do not respond to catecholamines in terms of vascular support, suggesting maximum vasoconstriction is already present. Thus, volume expansion and glucocorticoid and thyroid hormone administration are the first lines of therapy for hypotension in these circumstances. Nonetheless, the fact that propranolol appropriately reduces heart rate in hypothyroidism indicated that the β-adrenergic receptors are functional in this organ even though reduced in number.

Muscles

The strength and tone of muscles may be normal or reduced. Movements are slowed. Transient pain, stiffness, and cramps in the muscles are frequent complaints. One may reasonably infer that these manifestations are an expression of the separation of the fibers by the mucoedema and perhaps of actual changes in the sarcoplasm. The symptoms are often intensified when therapy begins and are aggravated by exposure to cold. They are also prominent during the rapid onset of hypothyroidism after surgery or ^{131}I therapy. One patient with disabling muscle cramps was found to have reduced α-glucosidase activity in a muscle biopsy; after therapy with T_4, the symptoms disappeared and the muscle enzyme activity returned to normal.[167]

Some patients manifest a "myoedema," a transient local swelling of a muscle elicited by percussion with a reflex hammer. This condition is best demonstrated on the biceps.

The myotonic phenomenon occurs rarely in myxedema and disappears after appropriate therapy.[168] Cases have been described in which incapacitating myotonia followed the onset of hypothyroidism and was completely relieved by treatment. There was no family history of myotonia to suggest a simple coincidence of the two diseases.

The electromyogram in myxedema may be normal or may demonstrate abnormalities distinct from those seen in myotonia or other muscle disease.[169] Polyphasic action potentials, hyperirritability, repetitive discharge, and low-voltage, short-duration motor unit potentials have been described. In the hypothyroid rat the rate of isometric relaxation is slow, and tension is less than in euthyroid or hypothyroid rat muscle at the same frequency of stimulation.[170]

Generalized muscular hypertrophy, accompanied by easy fatigue and slowness of movements, occurs in some cretins and myxedematous children or adults. It has been referred to as the *Kocher-Debré-Sémélaigne syndrome* in children[171] and as *Hoffmann's syndrome* in adults.[172] These patients do not have the classic electromyographic findings of myotonia. The myopathy of hypothyroidism is in some patients associated with weakness even though the muscles are hypertrophied. Type II muscle fibers are atrophic and type I predominate.[173]

Reflex contraction and relaxation time is prolonged mainly because of the intrinsic alterations in muscle contractility. Nerve conduction time may also be prolonged. Delayed reflex relaxation is characteristic and has been developed into a diagnostic test of thyroid function.[174] As with many other tests, there is considerable overlap between normal and mildly hypothyroid ranges. It should be noted that the myxedema reflex is not identical to the myotonic reflex. In the latter, the relaxation phase is not prolonged, despite the prolonged relaxation time occurring in myotonia after voluntary muscular activity. The rate-limiting step in muscle relaxation is the reuptake of calcium by the sarcoplasmic reticulum. In skeletal muscle, this process is dependent on the content of calcium ATPase. Recent studies have indicated that calcium ATPase activity of the fast twitch variety (SrCa1) is markedly reduced in hypothyroidism,[175] and there is an accompanying impairment of calcium reuptake as a consequence. This probably occurs at a transcriptional level, since thyroid hormone response elements have been identified in the 5′ flanking region of the mouse SerCaI calcium ATPase gene.[176] It is the mirror image of the events occurring in hyperthyroidism, where relaxation of skeletal muscle is much more rapid than normal. Nonetheless, the reduction in calcium ATPase would appear to explain one of the most obvious clinical manifesta-

TABLE 9-2. Manifestations of Hypothyroidism in the Skeletal System

Clinical Symptoms and Signs
    Arthralgias, joint stiffness
    Joint effusions and pseudogout
    Carpal tunnel syndrome
    Polymyalgia
    Delayed linear bone growth in children
Laboratory
    Normal ionized calcium, phosphate, and bone density
    Increased serum PTH, $1\alpha25$ $(OH)_2$-vitamin D_3
    Normal 25–OH vitamin D_3
    Reduced urine calcium, hydroxyproline, serum alkaline phosphatase, osteocalcin, and IGF1
    Epiphyseal dysgenesis or delayed ossification in children

tions of hypothyroidism, namely, delayed relaxation of the deep tendon reflexes.

Skeletal System and Calcium Homeostasis

Hypothyroidism may impact the skeletal system at clinical and biochemical levels. Table 9-2 summarizes the effects of hypothyroidism on this tissue. At the clinical level, patients with hypothyroidism may present with many manifestations, suggesting rheumatic disease such as arthralgias, joint stiffness, effusions, and carpal tunnel syndrome.[177,178] On the other hand, the symptoms may also suggest polymyalgia rheumatica, or primary myositis. In children, delayed linear growth or short stature are well-recognized signs suggesting the possibility of hypothyroidism. The similarity of the symptoms of hypothyroidism to those of rheumatoid arthritis or osteoarthritis, especially when these are combined with the paresthesias of more severe hypothyroidism, should automatically lead to a consideration of hypothyroidism in any patient presenting with these symptoms. For example, in 5 to 10 percent of patients with carpal tunnel syndrome, primary hypothyroidism may be the cause, due to the accumulation of the hygroscopic glycosaminoglycan in the interstitial space with compression of the median nerve.

While calcium, phosphate, and bone density are generally normal in hypothyroidism, there is evidence of reduced bone turnover and resistance to the action of parathyroid hormone (PTH).[179–186] Thus, serum (PTH) levels are elevated.[181] This is presumably the cause of the elevation in $1\alpha,$

$25(OH)_2$-vitamin D_3.[184] 25-OH-vitamin D_3 levels are normal. The increase in PTH and vitamin D in turn increases calcium absorption. The reduction in glomerular filtration rate (GFR) and reduced bone turnover reduce urinary calcium and hydroxyproline levels and cause subnormal alkaline phosphatase, osteocalcin, and IGF-I levels.[180] The alkaline phosphatase reduction is particularly important in children, in whom this enzyme is normally elevated due to bone growth. In addition, it is well recognized that epiphyseal dysgenesis and the delayed appearance of calcification centers are characteristic of hypothyroidism in infants and children. This subject is discussed in greater detail in Chapter 15.

Nervous System

Table 9-3 lists the numerous symptoms suggesting either neurologic or psychiatric disorders in patients with moderate to severe hypothyroidism. We are aware of no characteristic *motor* phenomena other than those due to weakness and to syndromes that seem to represent cerebellar dysfunction. A tendency to poor coordination was noted originally by the Myxoedema Commission. Jellinek and Kelly[187] described a series of myxedematous patients with ataxia, intention tremor, nystagmus, and dysdiadochokinesia. Ataxia has been noted in 8 percent of a large series of hypothyroid patients.[188] The delayed relaxation phase of the deep tendon reflexes has

TABLE 9-3. Neurologic and Psychiatric Manifestations of Hypothyroidism

Neurologic Symptoms or Signs
    Headache
    Paresthesias
    Carpal tunnel syndrome
    Cerebellar ataxia
    Deafness: nerve or conduction type
    Vertigo or tinnitus
    Delayed relaxation of deep tendon reflexes
    Cognitive deficits: calculation, memory, reduced attention span
    Low-amplitude theta and delta waves on EEG
    Prolonged evoked potentials
    Sleep apnea
    Myxedema coma
    Elevated CSF protein concentration
Psychiatric Syndromes
    Depression: akinetic or agitated
    Schizoid or affective psychoses
    Biopolar disorders

been mentioned previously as a manifestation of abnormal muscle calcium dynamics.

Patients may have intention tremor, nystagmus, and an inability to make rapid alternating movements. In fact, this inability has long been used as a test for myxedema. The cause of this syndrome is not apparent, although deposition of mucinous material in the cerebellar tissue may be of pathogenetic importance. Round bodies containing glycogen and termed *neural myxedema bodies* have been found in the cerebellum of a patient with long-standing myxedema and ataxia.[47] An edematous infiltrate may occupy the endoneurium and perineurium of the spinal nerves. The neurologic manifestations of myxedema have been thoroughly reviewed by Sanders.[188] Whatever the cause is, it is important that these symptoms show a prompt and definite decrease after replacement therapy with thyroid hormone.[189]

Sensory phenomena are common. Numbness, tingling, and painful paresthesias are frequent[190] and are especially common in hypothyroidism after surgery or ^{131}I therapy. Paresthesias were present in 79 percent of one series of 109 patients. A metachromatic infiltrate has been found in the lateral femoral cutaneous nerve and sural nerve, together with axon cylinder degeneration.[191] Nerve conduction time is usually normal. Murray and Simpson[192] found that in some hypothyroid patients signs of median nerve pressure were present, apparently because of encroachment on the nerve by myxedematous infiltrates in the carpal tunnel.[177,178]

Deafness is a very characteristic and troublesome symptom of hypothyroidism. Both nerve and conduction deafness and combinations of the two have been reported, and vestibular abnormalities have also been demonstrated. Serous otitis media is not uncommon.

Two-thirds of patients complain of dizziness, vertigo, or tinnitus occasionally: these problems again suggest damage to the eighth nerve or labyrinth, or possibly to the cerebellum. Whatever type of deafness is present, there is marked improvement after thyroid therapy. Acquired hearing loss in association with adult-onset hypothyroidism should be distinguished from the sensorineural deafness of Pendred's syndrome. In the latter, treatment of hypothyroidism does not correct the hearing defect (see Ch. 16).

Night blindness is not uncommon. It is caused by a deficiency in the pigment retinene, which is required for the adaptation to dark.

Uncorrected deficiency of thyroid hormone during neonatal life causes not only more profound neurologic abnormalities but also irreversible damage. Nystagmus is prominent[193] and mental retardation typical (see Ch. 15).

Mental Symptoms

The mental picture usually is one of extreme complacency. Memory is undoubtedly impaired, and attention and the desire to think are reduced. The emotional level seems definitely low, and irritability is decreased. Except in the terminal stage, reasoning power is preserved. Questions are answered intelligently, but slowly and without enthusiasm, and often with evidence of amusement. In a minority of patients, nervousness and apprehension are present. Psychosis may occur in untreated myxedema or during the initiation of therapy. This problem is discussed below.

Depression is so often associated with hypothyroidism that thyroid function tests should be performed in the evaluation of any patient presenting with this symptom. At times, this manifestation of hypothyroidism is more severe than are many of the other clinical manifestations of the disease. Because hypothyroidism is so readily treated, it is an especially important cause to eliminate. Cognitive tests of patients with moderate to severe hypothyroidism indicate difficulties in performing calculations, recent memory loss, reduced attention span, and slow reaction time.[194] EEG abnormalities are also present, again depending on the severity and duration of the hypothyroidism. There may be absence of a waves and presence of low-amplitude theta and delta waves. Visual and auditory evoked potentials may be delayed as a consequence of abnormal cerebral cortical metabolism. Sleep apnea is not uncommon. It has been difficult to assign a causal role for the myopathy versus the coexistent obesity in some of the reported cases. However, the muscular dysfunction may extend to the diaphragm and intercostal muscles, thus impairing the ventilatory mechanism.

The most extreme CNS manifestation of hypothyroidism is myxedema coma. This is a rare condition but continues to occur, usually in conjunction with intercurrent illness such as infection, sedative administration, hypothermia, or other stress. The protein concentration of the cerebrospinal fluid may be normal or remarkably increased in hypothyroidism. If such an observation is made in a comatose patient, the possibility of hypothyroidism should be evaluated if it has not already been. The typical somnolence of severe hypothyroidism may suggest the psychiatric diagnosis of depression or dementia.[98] Patients are generally akinetic, though isolated case reports appear of patients who become hypomanic and agitated or garrulous (myxedema wit) as manifestations of this condition. Bipolar affective disorders and schizoid or paranoid ideations may also occur. These may so dominant the clinical picture that the signs of hypothyroidism may be obscured or pass unnoticed. Accordingly, it is critical to evaluate thyroid function in any patient presenting with such functional disorders before instituting other forms of therapy. If the condition is due to hypothyroidism, it will resolve with time and appropriate treatment.[195]

Cerebral blood flow, oxygen consumption, and glucose consumption have been reported to be diminished in proportion to the drop in metabolism in the rest of the body,[196] but most studies find unaltered glucose and oxygen use by the brain in either hypo- or hyperthyroid animals or humans.[197] In one study, cerebral cortical perfusion was little changed with treatment, but there was a decided fall in cerebrovascular resistance.[198]

Cerebrospinal fluid (CSF) protein levels are elevated, and the γ-globulin fraction is increased out of proportion to the total. In one series the CSF protein averaged 49 mg/dl, but values up to 300 mg/dl have been recorded. The relationship of neurologic development and cretinism to congenital hypothyroidism is discussed in Chapter 15.

Hematopoietic System

In hypothyroidism, plasma volume and RBC mass are both diminished, and blood volume is decreased. Anemia of mild degree is commonly present, and the the hemoglobin level may be as low as 8 to 9 g/dl. In two reports on a large series of patients with hypothyroidism from various causes, the incidence of anemia ranged from 32 percent[199] to as high as 84 percent.[200] The anemia may be a result of a specific depression of marrow that lacks thyroid hormone[201] or may be due to blood loss from menorrhagia, to decreased iron absorption because of gastric achlor-

hydria, to coincident true Addisonian pernicious anemia, or to a decreased absorption of vitamin B_{12} which has been found to occur in certain patients with myxedema as a result of diminished intrinsic factor or possibly diminished production of erythropoietin by the kidney. Experiments with mice indicate that the erythro-poietic effect of thyroid hormone is mediated through erythropoietin.[202] This substance increases RBC production by stimulating the erythroid differentiation of the bone marrow, and its secretion by the kidney appears to be inversely related to the oxygen tension of the tissue. A rise in the tension would be expected in hypothyroidism as a result of the lowered metabolic rate and the lowered oxygen consumption by the tissue.

Anemia caused by hypothyroidism per se may be normocytic or macrocytic and responds to thyroid therapy. If iron deficiency develops from menorrhagia, a hypochromic and microcytic anemia may occur. This condition usually responds to iron alone, but may respond optimally only to combined iron and thyroid hormone.[203] Hypothyroidism per se causes diminished blood cell formation probably as a response to decreased oxygen demand.[204] Plasma and RBC iron turnover are decreased, and the bone marrow is frequently hypoplastic.[204] There is a positive correlation between the metabolism of the lean body mass and the RBC mass.

The thromboplastin time is frequently prolonged, and the level of serum thromboplastin is reduced. The level of antihemophilic factor is also reduced.[98,205,206] The megakaryocytes of the marrow are normal relative to the other marrow elements. These coagulation defects disappear after administration of thyroid hormone and apparently are related to its effect on protein synthesis.[207] Hypothyroidism may also be associated with increased fibrinolytic activity that reverts to normal as the euthyroid state is restored.[208] The clinical relevance of this finding remains to be established. Capillary fragility is decreased but reverts to normal if the skin is warmed.[209] Erythropoiesis is diminished, and RBC turnover slowed.[210]

The relationship between hypothyroidism and pernicious anemia has been well established. Patients have been reported who developed pernicious anemia while hypothyroid, and who lost their need for parenteral vitamin B_{12} when hypothyroidism was treated. It is also known that some hypothyroid patients absorb oral vitamin B_{12} poorly, and the defect is sometimes corrected by intrinsic factor.[211,212] After thyroid therapy, the absorption defect may disappear or may persist.[212] The incidence of pernicious anemia is higher than normal in myxedematous persons.[157,203,212] In Tudhope and Wilson's series of 73 patients with spontaneous primary hypothyroidism, 12.3 percent had true Addison's anemia that responded to vitamin B_{12}.[212] They believe that macrocytic anemia in hypothyroidism should not be accepted as a manifestation of thyroid hormone lack per se, but that it is due instead to the increased coincidence of Addison's anemia. Half of the patients with Addisonian anemia have serum antibodies against the thyroid gland and half of the patients with Hashimoto's thyroiditis have antibodies against gastric cell cytoplasm, parietal cells, or intrinsic factor.

Megaloblastic anemia due to folic acid deficiency has also been demonstrated in hypothyroidism. Reduced intestinal absorption secondary to hypothyroidism may be responsible for this deficiency, as suggested by the changes observed in a patient given tritiated pteroylglutamate before and after treatment with thyroid hormone.[213] Also, a peculiar RBC abnormality has been described in patients with untreated hypothyroidism[214]; a small number of irregularly contracted RBCs resembling burr cells are present. The significance of this condition, which may be reversed by the administration of thyroid hormone, is unknown.

If iron deficiency or vitamin B_{12} deficiency clearly exists, appropriate oral or parenteral therapy with the required hematopoietic agent is in order. If there is no obvious explanation for the anemia other than hypothyroidism, therapy with the thyroid hormone will ordinarily restore the hemoglobin level to normal.

The white blood cell count is normal, as is the platelet level. The erythrocyte sedimentation rate may be elevated in uncomplicated hypothyroidism[215]

Frequency of Symptoms

Table 9-4 lists the relative frequency of symptoms and signs accumulated by Lerman in a study of 77 myxedematous patients in one thyroid clinic and by Murray in a study of 100 patients with primary hypothyroidism, 15 pituitary hypothyroid patients, and 100 normal control subjects.[216]

This analysis identifies the cardinal manifestations of the disease. It also discloses that a certain number of manifestations are occasionally found in overt myxedema that are somewhat more suggestive of hypothyroidism than of hypothyroidism. Under this heading may be listed dyspnea, nervousness, palpitations, precordial pain, loss of weight, and emotional instability. These symptoms are also found in normal control subjects in nearly the same frequency. In most patients they are far outweighed by the obvious signs of myxedema, so that there is no probability of confusion.

Many symptoms typical of primary hypothyroidism are not commonly found in pituitary hypothyroidism—for example, coarse skin, thick tongue, coarseness of hair, peripheral edema, hoarseness, and paresthesias.

Metabolic Rate

Perhaps the most constant functional departure from normal is the lowering of the basal metabolic rate (BMR), a test rarely performed in the present era. In patients with complete athyreosis it falls between 35 and 45 percent below normal. In Addison's disease, the BMR may fall to -25 or -30 percent and, in hypopituitarism to below -50 percent. The failure to find a metabolic rate as low as -35 percent, when the clear-cut picture of myxedema is present is very unusual.

Protein Metabolism

The effect of hypothyroidism on protein metabolism is complex, and its effect on the concentration of a given protein difficult to predict. In general, both the synthesis and the degradation of proteins are reduced, but hypothyroid patients are in positive nitrogen balance. However, results of feeding excess food to hypothyroid animals indicates that positive nitrogen balance can be induced, but this is not nearly so positive as it is in euthyroid animals. Lewallen et al.[217] showed that for albumin, despite both a decrease in the rate of synthesis and degradation, the total exchangeable albumin pool increases in myxedema. The albumin was distributed in a much larger volume, suggesting enhanced permeability of capillary walls. A synthesis of thyroid hormone–responsive proteins is clearly reduced in the hypothyroid state, whereas that of proteins such as TSH or glycosaminoglycans may be increased under the

TABLE 9-4. Incidence of Symptoms and Signs in Hypothyroidism

Symptoms and Signs	Lerman's Series: Percent of 77 Cases of Primary Hypothyroidism	Murray's Series		
		Percent of 100 Cases of Primary Hypothyroidism	Percent of 15 Cases of Pituitary Hypothyroidism	Percent of 100 Normal Control Subjects
Weakness	99	98	100	21
Dry skin	97	79	47	26
Coarse skin	97	70	7	10
Lethargy	91	85	80	17
Slow speech	91	56	67	7
Edema of eyelids	90	86	40	28
Sensation of cold	89	95	93	39
Decreased sweating	89	68	80	17
Cold skin	83	80	60	33
Thick tongue	82	60	20	17
Edema of face	79	95	53	27
Coarseness of hair	76	75	40	43
Cardiac enlargement (on x-ray film)	68	—	—	—
Pallor of skin	67	50	87	14
Impaired memory	66	65	67	31
Constipation	61	54	33	10
Gain in weight	59	76	47	36
Loss of hair	57	41	13	21
Pallor of lips	57	50	—	—
Dyspnea	55	72	73	52
Peripheral edema	55	57	0	2
Hoarseness	52	74	33	18
Anorexia	45	40	—	15
Nervousness	35	51	53	42
Menorrhagia[a]	32	33	—	—
Deafness	30	40	26	15
Palpitations	31	23	13	20
Poor heart sounds	30	—	—	—
Precordial pain	25	16	7	9
Poor vision	24	—	—	—
Fundus oculi changes	20	—	—	—
Dysmenorrhea	18	—	—	—
Loss of weight	13	9	26	23
Atrophic tongue	12	—	—	—
Emotional instability	11	—	—	—
Choking sensation	9	—	—	—
Fineness of hair	9	—	—	—
Cyanosis	7	—	—	—
Dysphagia	3	—	—	—
Brittle nails	—	41	13	20
Depression	—	60	73	41
Muscle weakness	—	61	73	21
Muscle pain	—	36	13	17
Joint pain	—	29	26	24
Paresthesia	—	56	13	15
Heat intolerance	—	2	0	12
Slow cerebration	—	49	67	9
Slow movements	—	73	60	14
Exophthalmos	—	11	0	4
Sparse eyebrows	—	81	80	58

[a] Premenopausal patients.

same circumstances.[53,56] Comparative studies of protein translation by hepatic ribosomes from T_3-treated hypothyroid rats shows that the mRNAs from some proteins are increased and others are decreased. Most of these proteins have not been identified. Treatment of myxedema is accompanied by mobilization of extracellular protein and a marked but temporary negative nitrogen balance, reflecting the mobilization of extracellular protein.[218] In a later phase there is an increase in urinary potassium and phosphorus together with nitrogen in amounts suggesting that cellular protein is also being metabolized.[219]

Lipid Metabolism

The plasma concentrations of cholesterol, low-density lipoproteins (LDL), and triglycerides are significantly elevated in hypothyroidism and bear in general a reciprocal relationship to the level of thyroid activity.[82,220–226] The elevation in triglyceride level is less than that of cholesterol or LDL.[226] Type 3 hyperlipoproteinemia may be aggravated by hypothyroidism.[227] The free fatty acid concentration is usually normal. Diet has a marked effect on the hypercholesterolemia and hypertriglycerdemia of myxedema.[228] Low levels of postheparin lipolytic activity are found, and this condition may be one cause of the hypertriglyceridemia[225,229,230]

The relationships between cholesterol and other lipids in myxedema have been studied often. The increased serum cholesterol level may represent an alteration in a substrate steady-state level caused by a transient proportionally greater retardation in degradation than in synthesis.[220,231,232] LDL catabolism is similarly reduced in hypothyroidism.[233–236] Free fatty acid mobilization in response to fasting is decreased.[237] Serum carotene levels are also increased because of impaired conversion to vitamin A, which accounts for the characteristic yellowness of the skin.[238]

Carbohydrate Metabolism

Glucose is absorbed from the intestine at a slower rate than normal. Fasting plasma glucose values are on average lower than normal.[120,239] The oral glucose tolerance test usually produces a low peak value that remains elevated at 2 hours. This response does not resemble that encountered in diabetes mellitus and is probably related to slow gastric motility and delayed absorption. However, the glucose disappearance rate is also prolonged when the sugar is given intravenously, although, the peak value is normal in magnitude and in time of occurrence.[240] Insulin release in response to an oral glucose load may be variable due to the absorptive abnormalities associated with hypothyroidism. The insulin response to intravenous glucose is blunted and slightly delayed.[240] In contrast to adult-onset diabetes, there is no evidence of resistance to insulin. In fact, the prolonged hypoglycemic effect of exogenous insulin in hypothyroid patients suggests increased sensitivity to insulin action.[239,241] This response, as well as the decrease in appetite, accounts for the diminished insulin requirement for the control of hypothyroid diabetics.

DIAGNOSIS

Clinical Evaluation

The diagnosis of severe hypothyroidism is relatively straightforward on clinical grounds. All of the manifestations mentioned in the above discussion are present, and laboratory testing merely confirms the high index of clinical suspicion.[242] However, severe hypothyroidism has become increasingly rare in the United States due to physicians' raised level of consciousness about the relatively high prevalence of this disease in women and the ease of making a laboratory diagnosis. Rather it is the more subtle or unusual presentations of hypothyroidism that may present difficulties to the primary care physician. Since laboratory confirmation of hypothyroidism is straightforward, the critical factor in successful diagnosis is maintaining a high degree of suspicion. If the diagnosis is not suspected in a patient with some of the typical manifestations of hypothyroidism at the first encounter, it may be several months before the physician reconsiders this explanation for the patient's complaints. Thus, hypothyroidism may be more readily diagnosed by a consultant who has not seen the patient before, since both the patient and the regular physician may have assumed that the many nonspecific symptoms are insignificant or at least unrelated to a specific organic disease.

There are certain symptoms or signs that should, irrespective of other factors, lead to a biochemical evaluation for possible hypothyroidism. In the child or adolescent, growth retardation is one of these.

The presence of an enlarged thyroid should trigger a similar response. However, more subtle, less specific complaints, including depression or other organic mental syndromes, muscle cramps, paresthesias, carpal tunnel syndrome, hoarse voice, elevated cholesterol, elevated CPK and CSF protein levels, pericardial effusion, arthritis, yellow skin (carotenemia), hyperkeratosis of the palms or soles, or menorraghia, can be manifestations of hypothyroidism. In addition, certain constellations of autoimmune disease occur in concert with hypothyroidism, including primary adrenal insufficiency, type I diabetes, and pernicious anemia. The presence of any of these should lead to a search for primary thyroid dysfunction. Comatose patients should be evaluated for hypothyroidism as a routine matter.

Laboratory Evaluation

The diagnosis, particularly of primary hypothyroidism, is one of the simplest to establish in medicine. (See also Ch. 4 and 6.) The presence of a low serum free T_4 estimate and an elevation in serum TSH is highly sensitive and specific. Most of the material in Table 9-5 is provided to deal with the relatively small percentage of instances in which this pattern of test results is not present or in situations in which there is a discordance between the serum TSH and the serum T_4 concentrations. As an initial evaluation we recommend a combination of serum TSH, a free T_4 estimate, and determination of antibodies directed against a thyroidal antigen such as thyroid peroxidase (TPO) (anti-TPO or antithyroid microsomal antibody) or thyroglobulin (TG). It could be argued that if the clinical index of suspicion is low, only a serum TSH determination is required. Although, this may be a cost-effective screening strategy, it is not sufficient for those in whom a diagnosis of hypothyroidism is suspected on clinical grounds because it will not identify the approximately 1 percent of patients with hypothyroidism who have hypothalamic or pituitary dysfunction. One could argue that if the serum TSH and T_4 do not indicate primary thyroid disease that quantitation of TPO antibodies is not necessary. However, for most endocrinologists, the possibility of thyroid dysfunction is often already a major consideration and justifies this approach. The TSH assay and free T_4 estimates have been discussed in Chapters 4 and 6, which should be reviewed, particularly with respect to potential artifacts in these assays that may explain discordant results of serum TSH and free T_4 indices.

Table 9-5 organizes an evaluation of biochemical results starting with the level of serum TSH. The prominence given to this test is justified by its specificity and by the rare instances in which artifactual results occur. The test has become especially useful as second-and third-generation immunometric TSH assays have been developed. In terms of sensitivity, however, first-generation "radioimmunoassays" were adequate to discriminate between a normal and an elevated serum TSH.

If the serum TSH is greater than 10 mU/L and the free T_4 estimate is low, the diagnosis of primary hypothyroidism is established. The presence of TPO or thyroglobulin (TG) antibodies points to the diagnosis of autoimmune thyroid disease as the cause of the thyroid gland impairment and is necessary to terminate a search for other rare causes of primary thyroid disease alluded to above, such as tuberculosis, sarcoidosis, or drug-induced hypothyroidism. It should be noted that measurements of serum T_3 or determination of the radioactive iodine uptake or thyroid scan are generally not required for the accurate diagnosis of the hypothyroid patient. Serum T_3 concentrations remain in the normal range in patients with primary hypothyroidism until thyroid function becomes severely affected. This fact, together with the common finding of reduced serum T_3 concentrations in patients with nonthyroidal illness, make the determination of serum T_3 in simple primary hypothyroidism an unnecessary expense.

Patients with adrenal insufficiency may present with a similar constellation of laboratory results, which are reversed upon treatment with glucocorticoids.[158,243,244] Whether this indicates that glucocorticoid deficiency leads to the transient appearance of cryptic autoimmune thyroid dysfunction or is due to adverse effects of gluccocorticoid defficiency on thyroid function remains to be determined. It is not universally found in patients with adrenal insufficiency, suggesting that it occurs primarily in patients who will eventually develop autoimmune primary hypothyroidism.

If the serum TSH is elevated but the free T_4 estimate is in the low-normal range and TPO antibodies are present, an earlier stage of autoimmune thyroid impairment is present than in the first group. If such patients are not symptomatic (which is usually the case) the term *subclinical hypothyroidism* has been used to characterize them. In fact, if the serum TSH is less than 10 mU/L, it is quite likely that any clinical symptoms that led to the suspicion of thyroid dys-

TABLE 9-5. Laboratory Evaluation of Patients with Suspected Hypothyroidism or Thyroid Enlargement

Initial Tests
  Serum TSH
  Serum free T_4 estimate
  TPO or TG Antibodies

Possible Outcome Keyed to TSH Result	TPO or TGAb	Diagnosis
TSH > 10 mU/L		
Free T_4 estimate		
Low	+	Primary hypothyroidism due to autoimmune thyroid disease
Low-normal	+	Primary "subclinical" hypothyroidism (autoimmune)
Low or low-normal	−	Recovery from systemic illness
		External irradiation, drug-induced, congenital hypothyroidism
		Iodine deficiency
		Seronegative autoimmune thyroid disease
		Rare thyroid disorders (amyloidosis, sarcoidosis, etc.)
		Recovery from subacute granulomatous thyroiditis
Normal	+, −	Consider TSH or T_4 assay artifacts
Elevated	−	Thyroid hormone resistance
		Blockade of T_4 to T_3 conversion (amiodarone), congenital
		Consider assay artifacts
TSH 5–10 mU/L		
Free T_4 estimate		
Low, low-normal	+	Early primary autoimmune hypothyroidism
Low, low-normal	−	Milder forms of nonimmune hypothyroidism (see above)
		Central hypothyroidism with impaired TSH bioactivity
Elevated	− (+)	Consider thyroid hormone resistance
		T_4 to T_3 conversion blockade
TSH 0.5–5 mU/L		
Free T_4 estimate		
Low, low-normal	− (+)	Central hypothyroidism
		Salicylate or phenytoin therapy
		Desiccated thyroid or T_3 replacement
TSH < 0.5 mU/L		
Free T_4 estimate		
Low, low-normal	− (+)	"Post hyperthyroid" hypothyroidism (^{131}I or surgery)
		Central hypothyroidism
		T_3 or desiccated thyroid excess
		Post excess thyroxine withdrawal

function in the first instance may not be explained by hypothyroidism, even though some functional thyroid impairment is present. In general, they will not improve with treatment. If the symptoms or signs that led to the suspicion of hypothyroidism are severe (such as pericardial effusion or coma), then the detection of relatively minor abnormalities in thyroid function should not stop the search for the cause of the primary symptom.

Rarely the constellation of elevated serum TSH and low or low-normal free T_4 estimate is not accompanied TPO antibodies. A seronegative form of auto-immune thyroiditis has been reported, although this has not been re-evaluated with the more sensitive TPO antibody testing techniques now available. Seronegative primary hypothyroidism may also occur in patients with TSH receptor blocking antibodies but without TPO antibodies.[245] Such patients will usually have a normal or small atrophic thyroid gland. Other conditions that may present with such a pattern include iodine deficiency (virtually unheard of in North America), congenital hypothyroidism of various causes, drug-induced hypothyroidism (though again this is rare, since drugs such as phenylbutazone and para-aminosalicylic acid are rarely given in sufficient quantities), or rare primary thyroid diseases. External irradiation-induced hypothyroidism is another cause of this constellation of abnormalities and is particularly common in patients with Hodgkin's disease, breast carcinoma, or in combination with subtotal thyroidectomy as part of therapy for laryngeal carcinoma.[20,21,246] Certain patients with granulomatous (postviral) thyroiditis may present with elevated TSH, low thyroid hormone, and negative TPO antibodies during the recovery phase from this illness; a history of prior hyperthyroidism or neck pain symptoms should be sought (see Ch. 19). Furthermore, in the normal recovery from acute illness there is an interval—between the period of illness-induced TSH suppression with reduced thyroid function that accompanies the re-establishment of normal thyroid function and clinical recovery—during which serum TSH is modestly elevated but serum but serum thyroid hormone levels remain low.[247]

Two types of discordant results may be seen in patients evaluated for potential hypothyroidism. The first is an extreme elevation in TSH in the presence of a normal free T_4 and a euthyroid state. The second is an elevated TSH accompanied by an elevated free T_4 estimate. In the former case, it is possible that TSH is artifactually elevated due to the presence of an anti-mouse Ig in the serum, which can cause a false-positive assay. The antibody does this by serving as a bridge between the first and second TSH antibodies. In most assays, the effects of such antibodies are neutralized by the inclusion of mouse immunoglobulin in the assay matrix. However, in some sera the levels of the heterophilic antibodies exceed those that are neutralized by this technique. One approach to eliminate the issue of an artifactual TSH result is to request that the laboratory assay the TSH after serial dilution of the patient's serum with normal serum to determine if there is a linear response. Most such artifactually elevated TSH results will not pass this test. Other less direct approaches to eliminating this factor are to perform a TRH stimulation test or to administer replacement thyroxine to suppress TSH temporarily and re-assay the TSH. The artifactually elevated TSH will not change in a physiologically appropriate fashion. Lastly, a standard TSH radioimmunoassay (as opposed to an immunometric assay) will not be affected by mouse immunoglobulins.

A second discordancy that may occur is in the quantitation of serum T_4. Depending on how the total T_4 or free T_4 estimate is measured, certain sera containing abnormally avid albumin or transthyretin (TTR) or endogenous anti-T4 antibodies may give false estimates of the total or free T_4. The direction in which T_4 deviates from normal depends on the technique used to separate the bound and free tracer T_4 in the assay or on the analog used in the free T_4 estimate when using this methodology. Whichever way the result deviates, if the serum TSH is normal, the patient is euthyroid. If an abnormal serum albumin or transthyretin is suspected, measurements of total and free T_4 values in family members should be performed, since these abnormalities are inherited in a dominant fashion. Also, albumin or TTR T_4 binding can be evaluated directly.[248,249]

Rarely, an elevated TSH and T_4 may be found in a patient with autoimmune thyroiditis. This can be explained by the presence of anti-T_4 antibodies. This occurs using methods of T_4 RIA that employ T_4 antibody complexed to the side of a test tube or encapsulated in a semipermeable membrane. Such methods assume that the unlabeled T_4 present in the patient's sera will compete with tracer T_4 for binding sites on the immobilized antibody. Since the endogenous T_4 antibody will bind the tracer T_4, the tracer bound to the immobilized antibodies is reduced and is interpreted as a high serum T_4. Since this is a condition often, although not always, associated with autoimmune thyroiditis, it is the serum TSH, not the serum free T_4 estimate, which is correct. This discordance can usually be resolved by demonstrating tracer T_4-endogenous antibody binding using IgG precipitation or by performing a dialyzable or ultra-filtrable free T_4 determination. Anti-T_3 antibodies can interfere with serum T_3 assay in the same way.

Nonartifactual discrepancies are found between the serum free T_4 estimate and the TSH concentrations in thyroid hormone resistance and in patients in whom conversion of T_4 to T_3 is chronically inhibited, as by amiodarone.[250] The history will usually lead to recognition of the explanation, or an evaluation of the family will confirm a diagnosis of dominantly inherited generalized resistance to thyroid hormone. It should be recognized that TSH is not usually greater than 10 mU/L in patients with thyroid hormone resistance unless these individuals are severely affected or have had prior (inappropriate) thyroidectomy or[131] I therapy (see Ch. 16). Such a result may also be a manifestation of early primary hypothyroidism, which is usually confirmed by the presence of positive antibodies directed against TPO or TGO. Some patients with normal serum T_4 values may have transient TSH elevations in the 5 to 10mU/L range for unknown reasons. In the absence of TPO antibodies, thyroid tests should be repeated several months later to establish that the TSH elevation is permanent.

Patients with low free T_4 estimates and normal or slightly elevated (up to 20 mU/L) TSH may have central hypothyroidism. This is due to the fact that the TSH secreted in patients with TRH deficiency due to pituitary tumor or hypothalamic disease does not have normal bioactivity (see Ch. 4).[251–253] Such patients can be recognized by the discrepancy between a modest elevation of TSH and a significant decrease in the serum free T_4 estimate below the level that would be expected to be associated with that serum TSH concentration in a patient with primary thyroid disease. More typical patients with central hypothyroidism have normal TSH but low or low normal free T_4 estimates. Before considering a diagnosis of central hypothyroidism, however, it is important to eliminate the possibility of salicylate or phenytion ingestion. Therapy with either of these compounds can cause reductions in the serum free T_4 estimate of 20 to 40 percent with no change in TSH (see Ch. 5). The possibility of surreptitious T_3 (or desiccated thyroid) administration also needs to be considered in this group of patients, especially if they have access to pharmaceutical agents. In such patients, measurement of serum T_3 concentrations is justified, since it may unravel the paradox of the combined suppression of T_4 and TSH.

The final diagnostic group to be considered consists of patients in whom the TSH is suppressed below normal (0.5 mU/L) who have a low or low-normal free T_4 estimate. In addition to central hypothyroidism and T_3 ingestion, this pattern may be found in a patient with a history of hyperthyroidism who has had either surgical or radioiodine therapy with a relatively rapid resolution of the elevated T_4 secretion.[254–256] Some 6 to 12 weeks may be required for recovery of the hypothalamic-pituitary axis after prolonged suppression due to conditions such as Graves' disease or autonomously functioning thyroid adenomas. Patients with subacute or painless thyroiditis may have a similar problem in the postdestructive phase of the disease. In addition, patients who have received chronic excess T_4 replacement for many years in whom replacement is stopped to test for potential thyroid dysfunction may also develop transient central hypothyroidism.[31] The laboratory evaluation of patients suspected of hypothalamic hypothyroidism is discussed later in this chapter.

The patient who is severely ill may present with a similar constellation of laboratory results for reasons discussed in Chapters 4 and 5. The differentiation of these thyroid test abnormalities from those due to central hypothyroidism can be challenging and involves careful clinical and historical evaluation and tests for the presence of ACTH, gonadotropin, and growth hormone deficiency. To make the issue more complex, sick patients receiving dopamine may have a previously elevated TSH due to primary hypothyroidism suppressed into the normal range by this agent (see Ch. 4). Sick patients with this pattern of test results must be evaluated for both possibilities, and in some cases empirical therapy is begun with levothyroxine until the cause of the abnormalities can be definitively resolved.

TREATMENT OF THE PATIENT WITH PRIMARY HYPOTHYROIDISM.

Pharmacology of Thyroid Hormone Replacement Preparations

The use of thyroxine has recently been reviewed by several authorities.[257–259] Levothyroxine, levotriiodothyronine (T_3), liotrix (combinations of T_3 and T_4), and desiccated thyroid (thyroid USP) are all available for thyroid hormone replacement therapy. These preparations function equally well biologically, but L-thyroxine is preferred due to its long half-life, its ready quantitation in the blood, ease of absorption, and the availability of multiple tablet strengths. Administration of prohormone also is most similar to the physiologic circumstances in humans with respect to the complex processes regulating conversion of T_4 to T_3 in various tissues (see Ch. 3).[260,261] Desiccated thyroid is still used in a minority of patients with primary hypothyroidism; for this reason it is important to recognize that one grain of desiccated thyroid is stipulated to contain about 44 μg T_4 and 9 μg of T_3.[262,263] The hormones are in the form of thyroglobulin, which may be of porcine or bovine origin. The only liotrix preparation currently available in the United States contains 12.5 μg T$_3$ and 50 μg T$_4$/1 grain equivalent but is *biologically* equivalent to a 65 mg (1 grain) tablet of desiccated thyroid. In our experience, the biologic potency of a 1-grain desiccated thyroid tablet is about 75 to 88 μg T$_4$ and treatment with 1.5 grains causes subnormal TSH values in a significant fraction of female patients. Because of the relatively high ratio of T$_3$ to T$_4$ in desiccated thyroid or liotrix, patients receiving an amount of this medication adequate to normalize serum TSH generally have serum T$_4$ concentrations in the lower half of the normal range. Serum T$_3$ concentrations will vary in such patients, depending on the interval between ingestion of the medication and the time of blood sampling. The time course of the absorption of T$_3$ is similar whether it is contained in thyroglobulin or free in the tablet, with peak levels reached approximately 2 to 4 hours after oral administration.[264] Because the penetration of T$_3$ into its large volume of distribution (~30 to 35 L) is slow relative to its rate of absorption (see Chapter 3), the serum T$_3$ concentration reaches supraphysiologic levels after ingestion of 50 and sometimes even after only 25 μg of T$_3$. The latter approximates the amount contained either in 2 grains of desiccated thyroid or the liotrix 2 (2 grain equivalent) mixtures. While L-thyroxine is the preferred replacement, there are patients who have taken desiccated thyroid for many decades and are reluctant to consider a change. This is not a problem as long as the physician recognizes that the end point of therapy should be normalization of the serum TSH rather than of the serum free T$_4$ index. Whether there are any thyroid hormone–sensitive systems that respond to the transient serum T$_3$ elevations that occur during desiccated thyroid therapy is not known but seems unlikely. It has been shown, for example, that serum TSH remains constant throughout a 24-hour period during once daily T$_3$ administration. The difficulties that led to the development of levothyroxine as a replacement preparation, namely inconstant and subpotent desiccated thyroid tablets, have been largely obviated by new USP standards for quantitation of T$_3$ and T$_4$ in desiccated thyroid tablets. These guidelines require digestion of the desiccated thyroid prior to HPLC assay of T$_3$ and T$_4$ and are a marked improvement over the previous standard, which depended only on quantitation of organic iodine in the tablet.[265] The latter standard did not distinguish between iodotyro-

sines and iodothyronines and thus led to the potential problem of a tablet meeting USP specifications with respect to organic iodine but not containing appropriate quantities of thyroid hormones.[262]

The thyroxine content of levothyroxine tablets is stipulated to be between 90 and 110 percent of their stated amount. Thyroxine is readily absorbed by most patients; absorption occurs along the entire small intestine.[266,267] Serum T$_4$ concentrations peak 2 to 4 hours after an oral dose and remain above normal for approximately 6 hours in patients receiving daily replacement therapy.[268,269] However, serum T$_3$ concentrations increase so slowly after thyroxine absorption that with daily levothyroxine administration, no significant changes in circulating free T$_3$ are detectable. In North America, levothyroxine tablets are available from several manufacturers in tablet strengths of 25, 50, 75, 88, 100, 112, 125, 137, 150, 175, 200 and 300 μg. The availability of so many different strengths reflects the increased attention paid to optimizing therapy to maintain serum TSH concentrations in the normal range in patients with primary hypothyroidism. This can usually be accomplished with a single daily tablet.

Goals of Therapy with Levothyroxine

The goal of levothyroxine therapy is to normalize the thyroid status of the patient regardless of the cause of hypothyroidism. As has been discussed, most tissues are thyroid hormone responsive, and there are multiple physiologic abnormalities in the hypothyroid individual. However, the most sensitive and readily quantified reflection of thyroid status in the patient with primary hypothyroidism is the serum TSH concentration. Supplying sufficient thyroxine to reduce the serum TSH concentration to between 0.5 and 3 mU/L is the proper goal of therapy. If this is done, other biologic abnormalities related to low thyroid function will be corrected. Normalization of TSH will also prevent overtreatment of patients with levothyroxine, a situation that may lead to adverse affects on the myocardium and, especially, may contribute to a decrease in cortical bone density in postmenopausal women.[270–272] Thus, optimal treatment of the patient with primary hypothyroidism requires use of at least a second-generation TSH immunometric assay with usable limits of 0.5 to 5 mU/L.

Because TSH is employed as the criterion for thyroxine replacement, it is important to recognize that in certain situations serum TSH concentrations are suppressed. These have been reviewed in Chapter 4 (Table 4-3). Serum TSH concentrations cannot be used to monitor therapy in patients with central hypothyroidism in whom the free T_4 index should be used as an end point. If serum TSH concentrations are normalized in patients with primary hypothyroidism, then serum free T_4 concentrations will generally be above the middle of the normal range mildly elevated, and serum T_3 concentrations will be slightly below the mean normal value. This is because of the dual regulation of TSH by both plasma T_4 and T_3, as discussed in Chapter 4. Since about 80 (not 100) percent of serum T_3 in humans derives from peripheral T_4 to T_3 conversion (see Ch. 3), serum T_3 concentrations will be slightly lower for any given T_4 in patients on T_4 replacement than in those with intact thyroid function. It has not been possible to document biochemical or physiologic evidence of hypothyroidism in association with this situation, although studies sufficiently rigorous to detect very subtle differences have not been performed.

Institution of Therapy

The rapidity with which normal thyroid hormone levels should be restored depends on a number of factors, including the age of patient, the duration and severity of the hypothyroidism, and the presence or absence of other disorders, particularly those of the cardiovascular system. Most patients under the age of 60 can immediately begin a complete replacement dose of 1.6 to 1.8 μg levothyroxine/kg *ideal* body weight (about 0.7 to 0.8 μg/1b). Requirements for children and infants are discussed separately and are higher than those for adults between the ages of 20 and 70. In patients in the eighth and ninth decades, thyroid hormone requirements are decreased by 20 to 30 percent.[273] The cause of hypothyroidism also influences replacement in that patients with total thyroidectomy or severe primary hypothyroidism have slightly higher requirements than do patients who become hypothyroid after radioiodine or surgical treatment for Graves' disease.[274,275] The latter group may have some residual thyroid function that is autonomous, and thus a complete replacement dose is excessive. For most women, a complete replacement dose will be be-

tween 100 and 150 μg per day and, for most men, between 125 and 200 μg per day.

Full replacement doses should not be administered initially to patients over the age of 60, to patients who have a history of coronary artery disease, or to patients with long-standing severe hypothyroidism unless they are comatose. While levothyroxine improves cardiac function in patients with hypothyroidism and increases cardiac output and decreases systemic vascular resistance and end-diastolic volume, it also increases myocardial oxygen consumption. In the classic study of Keating et al. of 1,500 hypothyroid patients, 2 percent developed new-onset angina during thyroid therapy.[84] However, anginal symptoms disappeared in 40 percent and were unchanged in 45 percent, worsening only in 16 percent of those with pre-existing angina. Thus, while patients with coronary artery disease and angina may benefit from reversal of their hypothyroid state, to avoid precipitating acute myocardial ischemia, the dose should be titrated, starting with 25 μg a day and increased by increments of 25 μg at 8-week- intervals until serum TSH falls to normal or symptoms of angina worsen or appear. The approach to the patient with pre-existing symptomatic coronary disease and hypothyroidism is discussed below. A similar slow approach is prudent in patients with long-standing, severe hypothyroidism.

In the patient given what is thought to be a complete replacement dose of levothyroxine, a TSH and free T_4 index should be measured about 2 months after therapy begins to establish that the estimated dose is appropriate for the patient. At that time, serum TSH may be still elevated, indicating the need for a modest increase in dose, or TSH may be suppressed, indicating that a reduction is in order. This is usually done in 12- to 25-μg increments, depending on the patient.[276] These studies should be repeated again in 2 months to titrate proper dosage. After proper dosage has been achieved, the tests should be repeated yet again after the patient has been euthyroid for approximately 6 months. This is because in certain patients, normalization of thyroxine clearance may require more than 8 weeks, and a dose of levothyroxine that is adequate when the patient is metabolizing thyroxine more slowly may be inadequate when the patient is euthyroid. This dose should be continued and monitored on an annual basis. In patients with severe primary hypothyroidism, few adjustments will be required after the initial titration until the eighth decade. However, patients with Graves' disease who have had radioactive iodine may require dosage adjustments up to as long as 5 to 10 years after treatment is begun. A similar course may be followed by patients who have had subtotal thyroidectomy for Graves' disease due to the slow deterioration of residual thyroid function.

Therapy should be monitored with TSH measurements (using an immunometric assay) and estimates of free T_4. On occasion, patients will be irregularly compliant and ingest several extra tablets shortly before their visit. This is reflected in an elevation of both free T_4 and TSH in the same sample. Because compliance may be difficult for a life-long medication, a practical remedy is for the patient to isolate a week's supply of the drug in a separate container once weekly. On the last day of the week, up to two or three remaining tablets can be taken as a single dose. The onset of the effects of thyroxine is so slow in the euthyroid subject that this small bolus will not produce clinical manifestations.

Situations in Which Levothyroxine Requirements May Change

Table 9-6 lists a number of circumstances in which dosage requirements for levothyroxine may change in *compliant* patients. Patients who develop clinical malabsorptive disorders may require a change in dosage. In some, changing brands may suffice, since the dissolution time of some brands is longer than for others. For example, one study reported that T_4 absorption was higher with Levoxine (now Levoxyl) than with Synthroid.[277] Since T_3 is more readily absorbed than is T_4 (about 100 percent for T_3 and 80 percent for T_4), patients who cannot absorb thyroxine may be given replacement liothyronine to avoid the requirement for parenteral levothyroxine therapy. Malabsorption may also occur in patients who ingest large quantities of bran; the timing of the dose should be adjusted to take this into account. There is a 50 to 100 percent increase in thyroxine requirement in pregnant patients with primary hypothyroidism.[275,278] Patients with hypothyroidism planning to become pregnant should be instructed to report to their physician when pregnancy is confirmed, and the serum TSH and/or free T_4 estimate should be monitored and the levothyroxine dose adjusted upward as indicated. The increase in thyrox-

TABLE 9-6. Circumstances in Which Levothyroxine Requirements May Be Altered

Increased levothyroxine requirements
Malabsorption
Gastrointestinal disorders
Mucosal diseases of the small bowel (for example, sprue)
After jejunoileal bypass and small bowel resection
Diabetic diarrhea
Cirrhosis
Pregnancy
Therapy with certain pharmacologic agents
Drugs that block absorption
Cholestyramine
Sucralfate
Aluminum hydroxide
Ferrous sulfate
Possibly lovastatin
Drugs that increase nondeiodinative T_4 clearance
Rifampin
Carbamazepine
Phenytoin
Drugs that block T_4 to T_3 conversion
Amiodarone
Selenium deficiency
Decreased levothyroxine requirements
Aging (65 years and older)
Androgen therapy in women

(Modified from Mandel et al.[258])

ine dose may not occur until as late as the sixth month but is often apparent by the second month of gestation.[275] This subject is discussed further in Chapter 14. The dosage may be reinstituted at its pregestational level immediately after delivery.

Levothyroxine should be administered several hours after the patient takes any of the agents listed that can block its absorption, but the dosage or preparation used may still have to be increased during therapy with some of these agents.[279–283] Several drugs (e.g., carbamezepine) induce enzymes of the cytochrome P450 class, which can accelerate thyroxine clearance via pathways that do not lead to T_3 production.[284–288] Under these circumstances, dosage must be increased to compensate for this. Lastly, amiodarone and, theoretically at least, selenium deficiency may also block T_4 to T_3 conversion.[250,289,290] In patients over the age of 70 levothyroxine requirements are reduced about 25 percent.[273] Androgen therapy in women with breast cancer has also recently been shown to reduce levothyroxine requirements by 25 to 50 percent.[291] The mechanism is not known, but thyroxine-binding globulin (TBG) levels are significantly reduced.

Treatment of the Patient With Coexisting Coronary Artery Disease

As mentioned, most patients with coronary artery disease and primary hypothyroidism improve during therapy due to improved myocardial function and reduced peripheral vascular resistance as the hypothyroid state is corrected.[61,63,67,84] However, patients with preexisting angina should be evaluated for obstructive coronary lesions before thyroxine therapy begins. Retrospective studies suggest that the possibility of myocardial infarction is greater than is the possibility of an adverse event during angiography or angioplasty.[292–295] However, it is quite surprising that major surgery, such as coronary artery bypass grafting, can be very easily withstood by the patient with even moderate hypothyroidism as long as attention is paid to reducing the level of analgesics, maintaining adequate ventilation, and controlling the administration of free water.[294] In a few patients, remediable lesions will not be present or, even with bypass grafting, complete correction of the hypothyroid state will not be possible. In such patients, submaximal amounts of levothyroxine supplemented by other agents to enhance myocardial function may be helpful in allowing the reestablishment of normal thyroid function.[85]

Potential Adverse Effects of Treatment

While interventional T_4 therapy to suppress TSH is recognized to lead to loss of cortical bone in postmenopausal patients,[270] it has been assumed that replacement therapy with maintenance of TSH in the normal range would not. In two cross-sectional studies divergent conclusions were drawn. In one, there was no effect of replacement therapy on cortical bone density in patients maintained on replacement rather than a TSH-suppressive amount of levothyroxine.[271] In a second study, however, there was evidence of cortical bone density decreases even though serum TSH was normal.[296] The critical factor missing from both studies was the longitudinal follow-up of patients from diagnosis through several years of therapy to establish whether the results in these relatively small series represented typical changes. It is clear that what is true for all women, namely that

optimal calcium intake should be maintained to maximize bone density, is also true for patients with primary hypothyroidism. Further studies are needed to determine whether the unexpected result of loss of cortical bone during physiologic thyroxine replacement will be substantiated in other studies.

Chronic supraphysiologic T_4 treatment sufficient to suppress TSH will cause left ventricular hypertrophy,[297] another reason to monitor patients on a regular basis. Occasionally a patient may develop psychoses or agitation during the initial phase of replacement if hypothyroidism is severe and long-standing.[298–300] For this reason, patients who are thought to have been hypothyroid for many years or who are, in fact, myxedematous should be given only one-half the replacement dose as initial therapy. In addition, such patients may also be given replacement glucocorticoids until such time as their pituitary-adrenal axis has normalized. Pseudotumor cerebri has been described in several pediatric patients during initiation of therapy for primary hypothyroidism.[301]

Clinical Response

In general, serum thyroxine normalizes before serum TSH, and both may normalize before the disappearance of all of the symptoms of hypothyroidism. In the severely hypothyroid patient with long-standing disease, a number of profound alterations may occur as the hypothyroid state is corrected. Thus, loss of weight, primarily due to mobilization of interstitial fluid as the glycosaminoglycans are degraded, is prominent. The moon facies, coarse nasal voice, puffy fingers, deafness, and sleep apnea will all diminish. Many of nonspecific symptoms, such as fatigue or cold intolerance, will eventually reverse as well. Hair and skin abnormalities take longer to improve. Despite weight loss due to fluid loss, the obese patient should not expect more than a 10-pound weight change, particularly if serum TSH values are only modestly elevated. Virtually all of the weight loss in hypothyroidism is associated with mobilization of fluid, and significant decreases in body fat rarely occur. While metabolic rate increases, in general, appetite increases as well, and a new equilibrium is established.

Treatment Failures

There are few compliant patients whose symptoms and signs do not resolve after thyroid hormone administration. Patients with thyroid hormone resistance sometimes present in this fashion, but presently such patients are usually recognized before treatment, since they can present with mild symptoms of hypothyroidism associated with elevations in serum thyroid hormones. However, a rare hypothyroid patient may have been treated inappropriately with radioiodine for mistakenly diagnosed hyperthyroidism and will require excessive thyroxine to normalize TSH levels.[302,303] This is true thyroid hormone resistance, and investigation of the thyroid receptor β gene will generally reveal an abnormality in the ligand-binding domain that is inherited in a dominant fashion (see Ch. 16). Very rarely a patient may be resistant even to large quantities of T_3. Kaplan et al.[304] reported one such patient, who requires 300 μg per day of T_3 to normalize many of the biochemical and physical parameters of hypothyroidism. However, it should be noted that despite a serum T_3 concentration 10 fold the mean normal, this patient did not have tachycardia, indicating that she was truly thyroid hormone resistant. Her β thyroid hormone receptor gene has been sequenced and is entirely normal.[305] The cause of her resistance remains unknown.

In patients whose symptoms do not improve with levothyroxine therapy, the first step is to establish that they are taking and absorbing the medication and that it is physiologically effective in reducing TSH. If TSH and free T_4 estimates are normal, then it is quite likely that the symptoms are not due to hypothyroidism but related to another system. These could be psychiatric, and the patient should be evaluated by a specialist in that discipline. In exceptional patients, special studies to establish peripheral, but not central, thyroid hormone resistance will be needed, including measurements of BMR at various replacement doses together with urinary hydroxyproline, prolacting, and TRH response tests to document the nature of the resistance.[304]

Subclinical Hypothyroidism

This condition is usually diagnosed in a patient with an elevation in TSH (usually modest) but in whom the serum free T_4 index is still in the normal range. It should be stated at the outset that the term is a misnomer, since it is not usually defined by any clinical criteria. Nonetheless it is in common parlance. Should such patients be treated for their biochemical abnormalities? For example, is subclinical hypothyroidism associated with an abnormal lipid profile and would this be corrected by treatment? This is considerable disagreement in the literature on this subject. Most studies show no significant impact or only modest results.[306–309] For example, a reduction in mean serum TSH from 16.6 to 3.1 decreased LDL concentrations 22 percent.[309] Increases in high-density lipoprotein (HDL) have also been reported.[308] On the other hand, other studies report no significant change in HDL and a number of other parameters.[306] Modest improvement in certain indices of cardiac function have been observed by some[310,311] but not all observers.[306] At the present time data are not sufficient to allow the conclusion that lipid abnormalities in a given patient will respond satisfactorily to treatment of subclinical hypothyroidism. Since the sense of well-being may be improved by levothyronine therapy in about 25 percent of patients with subclinical hypothyroidism,[312] a replacement trial is reasonable. Adequate levothyroxine to normalize TSH should be given for 6 to 12 months, and the clinical state, as well as the serum lipid profile cholesterol, should be reassessed at 4-month intervals following institution of therapy. If there is persistent improvement in the clinical state or in the lipid profile, replacement should be continued permanently; otherwise it can be discontinued.

MYXEDEMA COMA

The natural evolution to complete athyreosis is a process that extends over many years. Gradually, all the functions of the body become progressively slowed. Ultimately the untreated patient ends in coma. The subject has been thoroughly reviewed.

There is nothing distinctive about the clinical picture of myxedema coma, aside from the advanced picture of athyreosis. The patient may be entirely obtruded or may be roused by stimuli. Usually lethargy and sleepiness have been present for many months. Sleep may have occupied 20 hours or more of the day and may have interfered even with eating. There may actually have been transient episodes of coma at home before a more complete variety developed. Convulsions may have occurred.

Usually coma comes on during the winter months. The severely myxedematous patient becomes essentially poikilothermic. With cold weather the body temperature may drop sharply. Often another disease, such as cellulitis, pneumonia, or pyelonephritis, appears to destroy a tenuous equilibrium and precipitate a final episode of coma. Coma may also be precipitated with tranquilizers, sedatives, analgesics, or anesthetic agents that patients with myxedema metabolize poorly.

The patient has the classic signs of severe, long-standing hypothyroidism. The temperature is subnormal, often much depressed: a temperature of 74°F (23.3°C) has been recorded. A thermometer reading lower than the usual 97°F must be used, or hypothermia may be missed. The pulse is slow, and blood pressure may be at the level of shock. The skin is cold, dry, and coarse, and the reflexes are markedly prolonged.

Diagnosis on clinical grounds is relatively easy once the possibility is considered. Any patient with hypothermia and obtundation should be considered as having potential myxedema coma, especially if chronic renal insufficiency and hypoglycemia can be ruled out. The diagnosis can be confirmed by finding a reduced free T_4 estimate and marked elevation of serum TSH. Cholesterol should be elevated but may not be so if the patient has been anorectic. Creatine phosphokinase and transaminases are often elevated. Serum sodium is often reduced, as is serum osmolality, but the urine may not be dilute due to inappropriate ADH secretion. Both hypoxia and hypercarbia may be present.[313]

Myxedema coma is a medical emergency. It is sufficiently rare that it has been difficult to perform randomized studies to resolve the issue of whether T_4 or T_3 is the most appropriate treatment. The mortality rate, with the current treatment regimen, is estimated to be approximately 20 percent.[314] There are advocates of T_4 therapy alone,[315] T_3 therapy alone,[316,317] and combinations thereof.[318] If T_4 alone is used, it should be given parenterally in doses of 300 to 500 μg to replace the calculated T_4 deficit.[319] Since the average volume of distribution of T_4 in a 70-kg human is approximately 7 L, 420 μg should cause an increase of 77 nM/L in the serum T_4 concentration. Following this, 75 μg/day are given intravenously. Advocates of T_3 therapy point to the impairment of T_4 to T_3 conversion characteristic of hypothyroidism that is due to a combination of the low levels of type I deiodinase as well as the generalized illness and inadequate caloric intake. Parenteral preparations of T_3 are now commercially available. Replacement should be given at a dose of 25 μg

intravenously every 12 hours. The patient can be switched to oral therapy when the circulatory system is stabilized and the patient is receiving other oral medications. Other authorities recommend a combination of T_4 and T_3 giving 200 to 300 μg of T_4 and 25 μg T_3 intravenously as an initial dose.[318] The T_3 is repeated 12 hours later and 100 μg of T_4 24 hours later. This is followed by 50 μg T_4 daily from the third day until the patient regains consciousness. While death associated with T_3 treatment in higher doses has been reported,[318] it is difficult to know whether this reflects a direct effect of this form of treatment or individual factors in the patients' illnesses. In addition to replacement of T_4, intravenous glucocorticoids (hydrocortisone 10 mg/hr) should also be administered during the first days of therapy, since in severe hypothyroidism pituitary-adrenal function is impaired, and the cortisol production rate is lower. While this low production is adequate when cortisol metabolism is reduced, as it is in hypothyroidism, the rapid restoration of a normal metabolic rate from the above treatment may precipitate transient adrenal insufficiency.

In addition, the patient should be intubated and measures taken to retain body heat. Central warming may be attempted but peripheral warming should not, since it may lead to vasodilatation and shock. The cutaneous blood flow is markedly reduced in the hypothyroid patient in order to conserve body heat. Warming blankets will defeat this mechanism. Mechanical ventilation may be needed, particularly when obesity and myxedema are combined. The thoracic and abdominal adipose tissue puts an added burden on the respiratory musculature and may lead to hypoxia, cardiac arrhythmia, and death. Hyponatremia is characteristic and free water restriction and the use of isotonic sodium chloride will usually restore normal serum sodium, as will improved cardiovascular function, which is one cause of the impaired free water clearance. Serum glucose should be monitored. Supplemental glucose may be necessary, especially if adrenal insufficiency is present. Carbohydrate is also required for conversion of T_4 to T_3; at least 100 g/day IV should be supplied to the comatose patient. Hypotension may develop, particularly if myxedema is severe. Volume expansion is usually required to remedy this, since patients are usually maximally vasoconstricted. Dopamine should be added if fluid therapy does not restore efficient circulation.

Concomitantly, a vigorous search for precipitating factors should be instituted. Determining whether an infection is present should be a priority, since as many as 35 percent of patients with myxedema coma have infection. Since hypothyroid patients cannot mount an adequate temperature response, the usual signs of infection, including tachycardia, fever, and elevated white blood count, may be absent. Prophylactic antibiotics are indicated until infection can be ruled out; upper respiratory infection should be eliminated.

Unfortunately, most patients with myxedema coma develop it in the hospital in response to the stress of a complicating illness. While the hypothyroid patient withstands the stress of surgery in general very well,[294] inadvertently excessive narcotics, sedatives, and hypnotics can tip a severely hypothyroid patient into coma.

Response to Therapy

Most patients begin to show increases in body temperature within the first 24 hours of treatment. The absence of an increase in body temperature within 48 hours should lead to consideration of more aggressive therapy, specifically T_3 therapy if it has not already been initiated. Most patients regain consciousness within a few days. As mentioned, the institution of intensive medical care and monitoring has considerably reduced the mortality rate, although in the elderly patient the prognosis is still grave.

PITUITARY AND HYPOTHALAMIC HYPOTHYROIDISM (CENTRAL HYPOTHYROIDISM)

In most instances of pituitary (secondary) hypothyroidism, thyroid hormone deficiency is only one component of a more generalized hormonal failure, or panhypopituitarism. Thus, evidence of hypogonadism, growth hormone (GH) deficiency, and hypocortisolism accompanies the hypothyroidism. The generalized pituitary insufficiency usually spares the lactotrophic function for several reasons. First, prolactin (PRL)-producing tumors are often responsible for the destruction of the pituitary. Second, PRL reserve may be unimpaired even if the residual normal pituitary tissue is reduced to a bare minimum. Third, because of the physiologic inhibitory influence of the hypothalamus on PRL secretion, interruption of the hypothalamic-pituitary communication by the disease process actually enhances PRL release.

Although tumors of pituitary origin constitute the principal cause of secondary hypothyroidism, postpartum necrosis of the pituitary (Sheehan's syndrome), metastatic tumors, infiltrative diseases, or idiopathic atrophy of the hypophysis may also give rise to trophoprivic hypothyroidism. Rarely, TSH deficiency may be isolated or unitropic. The cause is usually undetermined (idiopathic),[33,320,321] and rarely caused by a tumor. A syndrome of familial unitropic TSH deficiency has also been described.[322]

TSH deficiency may also arise from impairment of hypothalamic function resulting in tertiary hypothyroidism.[33,323] It can be caused by suprasellar tumors, including craniopharyngioma, and inflammatory processes such as sarcoidosis. Idiopathic hypothalamic hypothyroidism is more common in children.

The clinical manifestations of trophoprivic hypothyroidism are often mixed with symptoms and signs related to other hormone deficiencies. Amenorrhea, loss of libido, loss of body hair, atrophy of the skin, and hypoglycemia are commonly found. Cachexia may occur. Although the appearance is usually distinct from that of primary myxedema, the features of hypothyroidism may dominate the clinical picture to such an extent as to make the two very similar.

Certain clinical findings may aid in the differentiation. There may be a history of premature menopause after a postpartum hemorrhage (Sheehan's syndrome). This condition is especially noteworthy if hot flashes did not occur or if the patient was unable to nurse her infant. Headaches or visual field defects may suggest a suprasellar lesion. Hypopituitary patients usually lose weight. The skin tends to be cool but not as coarse as in primary myxedema, and the face is covered by tiny wrinkles. Pubic, axillary, and facial hair may be lost and the eyebrows thinned. There is a fineness rather than a coarseness of the residual hair. The tongue is not so obviously enlarged, nor is the voice so coarse as in primary myxedema. The heart is small. In the male, the testes may show signs of atrophy.

In general, the symptoms of hypothyroidism associated with hypopituitarism are less severe than are those of primary hypothyroidism.[33] This is because central hypothyroidism is rarely as severe as is primary hypothyroidism due to the presence of a modest degree of TSH-independent thyroid function. Thus, only rarely are patients with pituitary hypothyroidism myxedematous. The diagnosis is generally made when evaluating patients for complaints related to hypopituitarism. Laboratory confirmation consists of a reduced free T_4 index not associated with an appropriate elevation in serum TSH (Table 9-5). As mentioned, some patients with central hypothyroidism may have TSH values as high as 15 to 20 mU/L, but these are not appropriate for the decrease in serum T_4.[251–253] It is thought that the TSH of the patient with central hypothyroidism may be poorly glycosylated and therefore biologically less effective (see Ch. 4).

If hypothyroidism is the first manifestation of hypopituitarism, a thorough endocrine evaluation for both gonadal and adrenal dysfunction should be undertaken to document the extent of the pituitary disease. A serum prolactin should be obtained to determine whether or not a prolactinoma is present, which could lead to treatment with the dopaminergic agonists. Pituitary magnetic resonance imaging (MRI) and/or computed tomography (CT) scanning is indicated to elucidate structural abnormalities together with neurologic and ophthalmologic problems. Therapy should be directed at correcting the pituitary abnormality and the hormonal deficit. Thyroid hormone replacement should not begin until glucocorticoid replacement has been established, since acceleration of the metabolic clearance of glucocorticoid may precipitate adrenal crisis if ACTH secretion is compromised. In addition, appropriate gonadal steroid replacement should be instituted. Replacement doses of levothyroxine should be adjusted to result in a free T_4 estimate in the upper half of the normal range. Serum TSH concentrations cannot be used as a guideline under these circumstances. The usual calculation for T_4 replacement of 1.6 μg T_4/kg is appropriate.

SUMMARY

This chapter has discussed hypothyroidism, a condition caused by a deficient supply of thyroid hormone from whatever cause. Myxedema is the term applied to the most severe expression of hypothyroidism. The condition may follow thyroid surgery or RAI therapy for hyperthyroidism, but it also occurs spontaneously as so-called idiopathic myx-

edema (Gull's disease), which is now thought to be the end result of an autoimmune process similar or identical to that in Hashimoto's thyroiditis. Numerous other causes, including drug-induced goitrous hypothyroidism and myxedema of hypothalamic and pituitary origins, must be remembered in the differential diagnosis.

The prevalence of symptomatic hypothyroidism is 2 percent in the general female population but less than 1 percent in men. Approximately one-third of the cases are of iatrogenic origin. The disease is, however, infrequently the cause of hospital admission because the occurrence of full-blown myxedema is rare. The pathogenesis seems to be almost entirely explicable on the basis of a deficiency of thyroid hormone action at the peripheral tissue level. The most prominent feature in the pathology is deposition of glycosaminoglycans in the intercellular spaces, especially in the skin and muscle.

Prominent clinical features include a puffy face, a pleasant personality, nonpitting myxedema, marked cold intolerance, and coarse, dry skin and hair. Cardiac output is decreased. Enlargement of the heart shadow is frequently due to a pericardial effusion, and effusions are found in the other serous spaces. 17-Ketosteroid and hydroxycorticoid excretion is decreased, which appears to represent a balanced decrease in adrenal function due to decreased tissue demands for, or metabolism, of, the adrenal hormones. The body is less sensitive to catecholamines. Reflex relaxation time is markedly prolonged; frequently this finding can be used as a diagnostic sign. Certain features, including a decreased metabolic rate and increased concentrations of blood cholesterol and other lipid fractions, are also well recognized. The alteration in cholesterol level is due to a decreased rate of synthesis characteristic of hypothyroidism.

The diagnosis of hypothyroidism may be overlooked for several years because the onset of symptoms is so insidious. The diagnosis of primary hypothyroidism is confirmed by finding an elevation of serum TSH accompanied by a reduced free T_4 index. The hypothalamic-pituitary axis is so sensitive that it is often possible to detect TSH elevation indicating thyroid damage before the patient notices symptoms and while the serum free T_4 index is still within the normal, albeit low-normal, range. This condition is termed *subclinical hypothyroidism*. The serum TSH level is not usually elevated in trophoprivic hypothyroidism. Therapy of primary hypothyroidism should be instituted with levothyroxine at a dose that takes into account the age of the patient, the severity and duration of the hypothyroidism, and the presence of coexisting medical conditions, particularly symptomatic coronary artery disease. In younger patients, with no complicating illnesses, a complete levothyrorine replacement dose of 0.6 to 0.7 μg/1b ideal body weight (1.6 to 1.8 μg/kg) can be given immediately. Lower doses should be used in elderly patients or those with illnesses that may compromise the capacity of the cardiorespiratory system to respond to an increased metabolic demand. Patients who present with hypothyroidism and symptomatic angina should be evaluated prior to treatment for the presence of a readily treated obstructive lesion of the coronary arteries. The biochemical end point of therapy is normalization of the serum TSH, which may require several months to achieve. Chronic therapy should be monitored on an annual basis by measurements of TSH using an assay capable of accurately measuring the lower limit of the normal range (usually 0.3 to 0.5 μU/L), depending on the specific test used.

Patients with hypothyroidism due to pituitary or hypothalamic causes (*trophoprivic hypothyroidism*) should be evaluated for deficiencies of other trophic hormones, especially ACTH, and should receive glucocorticoid replacement prior to the institution of levothyroxine treatment. They should also be evaluated for anatomical abnormalities by appropriate imaging of the hypothalamic-pituitary region. The biochemical endpoint of levothyroxine replacement in these individuals is a free T_4 index or equivalent in the high normal range.

The coexistence of certain conditions such as pregnancy or malabsorption will increase levothyroxine requirements, as will administration of cholesterol or potassium-binding resins, $FeSO_4$, anticonvulsants, certain antacids, and amiodarone. Levothyroxine requirements are decreased in the elderly and in women receiving androgens. Appropriate adjustments and more frequent monitoring are necessary when such conditions are present.

Myxedema coma represents the ultimate expression of progressively lowered body metabolism due to thyroid hormone deficit. Whether massive or minute doses of hormone should be used in the institution of therapy is not clear; large doses are favored. Steroids should be given concurrently, and if the circulation and oxygenation are not well maintained, vasopressor drugs and intubation should be used. Ancillary measures include internal readministration of fluids while keeping in mind the impaired free H_2O clearance of the hypothyroid patient.

REFERENCES

1. Fagge CH: On sporadic cretinism, occurring in England. Medico-Chir Trans 54:155, 1871
2. Gull WW: On a cretinoid state supervening in adult life in women. Trans Clin Soc London 7:180, 1874
3. Ord WM: On myxoedema, a term proposed to be applied to an essential condition in the "cretinoid" affection occasionally observed in middle-aged women. Medico-Chir Trans 61:57, 1878
4. Reverdin JL: In discussion. Société médicale de Genève. Rev Med Suisse Romande 2:539, 1882
5. Kocher T: Ueber Kropfexstirpation und ihre Folgen. Arch Klin Chir 29:254, 1883
6. Report of a Committee of the Clinical Society of London to Investigate the Subject of Myxoedema. London, Longmans. Green & Co. Ltd. 1888
7. Bloomer HA. Kyle LH: Myxedema. Arch Intern Med 104:234, 1959
8. Bonnyns M. Bastenie PA: Serum thyrotrophin in myxedema and in asymptomatic atrophic thyroiditis. J Clin Endocrinol Metab 27:849, 1967
9. Crowley WF, Ridgway EC, Bough EW et al: Noninvasive evaluation of cardiac function in hypothyroidism: Response to gradual thyroxine replacement. N Engl J Med 296:1, 1977
10. Evered DC, Ormston BJ. Smith PA et al: Grades of hypothyroidism. Br Med J 1:657, 1973
11. Ivy H.K: Permanent myxedema: an unusual complication of granulomatous thyroiditis. J Clin Endocrinol Metab 21:1384, 1961
12. Wood LC, Peterson M, Ingbar SH: Delayed thyroid failure and decreased reserve following antithyroid therapy in Graves' disease, presented at the 48th Meeting of the American Thyroid Association, Chicago, Illinois, September 20–23, 1972
13. Michaelson ED, Young RL: Hypothyroidism with Graves' disease. JAMA 23:1351, 1970
14. Smith RN, Wilson GN: Clinical trial of different doses of ^{131}I in treatment of thyrotoxicosis. Br Med J 1:129, 1967
15. Hagen GA, Ouellette RP, Chapman EM: Comparison of high and low dosage levels of ^{131}I in the treatment of thyrotoxicosis. N Engl J Med 277:559, 1967
16. Hershman JM: Treatment of hyperthyroidism. Mod Treat 6:497, 1969
17. Ito K, Nishikawa N, Harada T et al: A comparative

evaluation of the treatment of hyperthyroidism. Endocrinol Jpn 21:131, 1974

18. Roudebush CP, Hoye KE, DeGroot LJ: Compensated low-dose ^{131}I therapy of Graves' disease. Ann Intern Med 87:441, 1977

19. Stoffer SS, Hamburger JI: Inadvertent ^{131}I therapy for hyperthyroidism in the first trimester of pregnancy. J Nucl Med 17:146, 1976

20. Glastein E, McHardy-Young S, Brast N et al: Alterations in serum thyrotropin (TSH) and thyroid function following radiotherapy in patients with malignant lymphoma. J Clin Endocrinol Metab 32:833, 1971

21. Kaplan MM, Garnick MB, Gelber R et al: Risk factors for thyroid abnormalities after neck irradiation for childhood cancer. Am J Med 74:272, 1983

22. Beahrs OH, Sakulsky SB: Surgical thyroidectomy in the management of exophthalmic goiter. Arch Surg 96:512, 1968

23. Hedley AJ, Flemming CJ, Chesters MI et al: Surgical treatment of thyrotoxicosis. Br Med J 1:519, 1970

24. Cassidy CE, Eddy RL: Hypothyroidism in patients with goiter. Metabolism 19:751, 1970

25. Chau AM, Lynch MJG, Bailey JD et al: Hypothyroidism in cystinosis: a clinical, endocrinologic and histologic study involving sixteen patients with cystinosis. Am J Med 48:678, 1970

26. Bastenie PA, Bonnyns M, Vanhaelst L, Neve P: Diseases associated with autoimmune thyroiditis. p. 261. In Bastenie PA, Ermans EM (eds): Thyroiditis and Thyroid Function. Oxford. Pergamon Press, 1972

27. Vanhaelst L, Bonnyns M, Bastenie PA: Thyroiditis and chromosomal anomalies. p. 289. In Bastenie PA, Ermans AM (eds): Thyroiditis and Thyroid Function. Oxford, Pergamon Press, 1972

28. Braverman LE, Woeber KA, Ingbar SH: Induction of myxedema by iodide in patients euthyroid after radioiodine or surgical treatment of diffuse toxic goiter. N Engl J Med 281:816, 1969

29. Braverman LE, Ingbar SH, Vagenakis AG et al: Enhanced susceptibility to iodide myxedema in patients with Hashimoto's thyroiditis. J Clin Endocrinol 32:515, 1971

30. Berens SC, Bernstein RS, Robbins J, Wolff J: Antithyroid effects of lithium. J Clin Invest 49:1357, 1970

31. Vagenakis AG, Braverman LE, Azizi F et al: Recovery of pituitary thyrotropic function after withdrawal of prolonged thyroid-suppression therapy. N Engl J Med 293:681, 1975

32. Carpi A, Iervasi G, Nicolini A et al: Serum thyroid hormone concentrations and recovery of TSH secretion after excision of autonomously functioning thyroid nodules. Metabolism 31:417, 1982

33. Emerson CH: Central hypothyroidism and hyper-thyroidism. p. 1019. In Kaplan MM, Larsen PR (eds): The Medical Clinics of North America, Philadelphia, WB Saunders, 1985

34. Lack EE: Lymphoids "hypophysitis" with end organ insufficiency. Arch Pathol 99:215, 1975

35. Radovick S, Nations M, Du Y et al: A mutation in the POU-homeodomain of Pit-1 responsible for combined pituitary hormone deficiency. Science 257:1115, 1992

36. Hayashizaki Y, Hiraoka Y, Tatsumi K: Deoxyribonucleic acid analyses of five families with familial inherited thyroid stimulating hormone deficiency. J Clin Endocrinol Metab 71:792, 1990

37. Tunbridge WMG, Evered DC, Hall R et al: The spectrum of thyroid disease in a community: the Whickham Survey, Clin Endocrinol 7:481, 1977

38. Sawin CT, Castelli WP, Hershman JM et al: The aging thyroid. Thyroid deficiency in the Framingham study. Arch Intern Med 145:1386, 1985

39. Levine MA, Downs RW, Moses AM: Resistance to multiple hormones in patients with pseudohypoparathyroidism: association with deficient activity of guanine nucleotide regulatory protein. Am J Med 74:545, 1983

40. Sunthornthepvarakul T, Gottschalk ME, Hayashi Y, Refetoff S: Brief report: Resistance to thyrotropin caused by mutations in the thyrotropin-receptor gene. N Engl J Med 332:155, 1994

41. Stein SA, Zakarija M, McKenzie JM et al: The site of the molecular defect in the thyroid gland of the hyt/hyt mouse: Abnormalities in the TSH receptor-G protein complex. Thyroid 1:257, 1991

42. Ezrin C, Swanson HE, Humphrey JG et al: The cells of the human adenohypophysis in thyroid disorders. J Clin Endocrinol Metab 19:958, 1959

43. Yamada T, Tsukui T, Ikejiri K et al: Volume of sella turcica in normal subjects and in patients with primary hypothyroidism and hyperthyroidism. J Clin Endocrinol Metab 42:817, 1976

44. Bloodworth JMB, Kirkendall WM, Carr TL: Addison's disease associated with thyroid insufficiency and atrophy (Schmidt syndrome). J Clin Endocrinol Metab 14:540, 1954

45. Klion FM, Segal R, Schaffner F: The effect of altered thyroid function on the ultrastructure of the human liver. Am J Med 150:137, 1971

46. Wilkins L: Epiphysial dysgenesis associated with hypothyroidism. Am J Dis Child 61:13, 1941

47. Price TR, Netsky MG: Myxedema and ataxia: Cerebellar alterations and "neural myxedema bodies." Neurology 16:957, 1966

48. Rossman NP: Neurological and muscular aspects of thyroid dysfunction in childhood. Pediatr Clin North Am 23:575, 1976

49. Naeye RL: Capillary and venous lesions in myxedema. Lab Invest 12:465, 1963

50. Salomon MI, DiScala V, Grishman E et al: Renal lesions in hypothyroidism: a study based on kidney biopsies. Metabolism 16:846, 1967

51. Ord WM: In Allbutt TC (ed): System of Medicine. New York. The Macmillan Co, 1897

52. Yamamoto K, Saito K, Takai T et al: Visual field defects and pituitary enlargement in primary hypothyroidism. J Clin Endocrinol Metab 57:283, 1983

53. Smith TJ, Murata Y, Horwitz AL et al: Regulation of glycosaminoglycan accumulation by thyroid hormone in vitro. J Clin Invest 70:1066, 1982

54. Aikawa JK: The nature of myxedema: Alterations in the serum electrolyte concentrations and radiosodium space and in the exchangeable sodium and potassium contents. Ann Intern Med 44:30, 1956

55. Crispell KR, Williams GA, Parson W, Hollifeld G: Metabolic studies in myxedema following administration of 1-triiodothyronine: (1) Duration of negative nitrogen balance: (2) effect of testosterone proprionate: (3) comparison with nitrogen balance in a healthy volunteer. J Clin Endocrinol Metab 17:221, 1957

56. Smith TJ, Horwitz AL, Refetoff S: The effect of thyroid hormone on glycosaminoglycan accumulation in human skin fibroblasts. Endocrinology 108:2397, 1981

57. Graettinger JS, Muenster JJ, Checchia CS et al: A correlation of clinical and hemodynamic studies in patients with hypothyroidism. J Clin Invest 37:502, 1958

58. DeGroot WJ, Leonard JJ: The thyroid state and the cardiovascular system. Mod Concepts Cardiovasc Dis 38:23, 1969

59. Buccino RA, Spann JF Jr, Sonnenblock EH, Braunwald E: Effect of thyroid state on myocardial contractility. Endocrinology 82:191, 1968

60. Levey GS, Skelton L, Epstein SE: Decreased myocardial adenyl cyclase activity in hypothyroidism. J Clin Invest 48:2244, 1969

61. Santos AD, Miller RP, Puthenpurakal KM et al: Echocardiographic characterization of the reversible cardiomyopathy of hypothyroidism. Am J Med 68:675, 1980

62. Fuller H Jr, Spittell JA Jr, McConahey WM. Schirger A: Myxedema and hypertension. Postgrad Med 40:425, 1966

63. Polikar R, Burger AG, Scherrer U, Nicod P: The thyroid and heart. Circulation 87:1435, 1993

64. Fregly MJ: Effects of prophythiouracil on development and maintenance of renal hypertension in rats. Am J Physiol 194:149, 1958

65. Zondek H: Das Myxödemherz. Muenchen Med Wochenschr 65:1180, 1918

66. Ladenson PW, Sherman SI, Baughman KL et al: Reversible alterations in myocardial gene expression in a young man with dilated cardiomyopathy and hypothyroidism. Proc Natl Acad Sci USA 89:5251, 1992

67. Ladenson PW: Recognition and management of cardiovascular disease related to thyroid dysfunction. Am J Med 88:638, 1990

68. Gordon AH: Pericardial effusion in myxedema. Trans Assoc Am Physicians 50:272, 1935

69. Smolar EN, Rubin JE, Avramides A, Carter AC: Cardiac tamponade in primary myxedema and review of the literature. Am J Med Sci 272:345, 1976

70. Davis PJ, Jacobson S: Myxedema with cardiac tamponade and pericardial effusion of "gold paint" appearance. Arch Intern Med 120:615, 1967

71. Hardisty CA, Naik DR, Munro DS: Pericardial effusion in hypothyroidism. Clin Endocrinol 13:349, 1980

72. Zondek H: The electrocardiogram in myxoedema. Br Heart J 26:227, 1964

73. Lee JK, Lewis JA: Myxoedema with complete A-V block and Adams-Stokes disease abolished with thyroid medication. Br Heart J 24:253, 1962

74. Cohen RD, Lloyd-Thomas HG: Exercise electrocardiogram in myxoedema. Br Med J 2:327, 1966

75. Fredlund B-O, Olsson SB: Long QT interval and ventricular tachycardia of "torsade de pointe" type in hypothyroidism. Acta Med Scand 213:231, 1983

76. Nesher G, Zion MM: Recurrent ventricular tachycardia in hypothyroidism—report of a case and review of the literature. Cardiology 75:301, 1988

77. Rodbard D, Fujita T, Rodbard S: Estimation of thyroid function by timing the arterial sounds. JAMA 201:884, 1967

78. Blumgart HL, Freedberg AS, Kurland GS: Hypercholesterolemia, myxedema, and atherosclerosis. Am J Med 14:665, 1953

79. Steinberg AD: Myxedema and coronary artery disease—a comparative autopsy study. Ann Intern Med 68:338, 1968

80. Bastenie PA, Neve P, Bonnyns M et al: Clinical and pathological significance of asymptomatic atrophic thyroiditis: a condition of latent hypothyroidism. Lancet 1:915, 1967

81. Bastenie PA, Vanhaelst L, Bonnyns M et al: Preclinical hypothyroidism: a risk factor for coronary heart disease. Lancet 1:203, 1971

82. Becker C: Hypothyroidism and atherosclerotic heart disease: pathogenesis, medical management, and the role of coronary artery bypass surgery. Endocr Rev 6:432, 1985

83. Tunbridge WMG, Evered DC, Hall R et al: Lipid profiles and cardiovascular disease in the Whickham

area with particular reference to thyroid failure. Clin Endocrinol 7:495, 1977

84. Keating FR, Parkin TW, Selby JB, Dickinson LS: Treatment of heart disease associated with myxedema. Prog Cardiovasc Dis 3:364, 1961

85. Levine HD: Compromise therapy in the patient with angina pectoris and hypothyroidism: a clinical assessment. Am J Med 69:411, 1980

86. Fleisher G, McConahey W, Pankow M: Serum creatine kinase, lactic dehydrogenase, and glutamic-oxalacetic transaminase in thyroid diseases and pregnancy. Mayo Clinic Proc 40:300, 1965

87. Hickman PE, Silvester W, McLellan GH et al: Cardiac enzyme changes in myxedema coma. Clin Chem 33:622, 1987

88. Klein I, Mantell P, Parker M, Levy GS: Resolution of abnormal muscle enzyme studies in hypothyroidism. Am J Med Sci 279:159, 1980

89. Wilson WR, Bedell GN: The pulmonary abnormalities in myxedema. J Clin Invest 39:42, 1960

90. Zwillich CW, Pierson DJ, Hofeldt FD et al: Ventilatory control in myxedema and hypothyroidism. N Engl J Med 292:662, 1975

91. Nordqvist P, Dhunér KG, Stenberg K, Örndahl G: Myxoedema coma and CO_2 retention. Acta Med Scand 166:189, 1960

92. Weg JG, Calverly JR, Johnson C: Hypothyroidism and alveolar hypoventilation. Arch Intern Med 115:302, 1965

93. Orr WC, Males JL, Imes NK: Myxedema and obstructive sleep apnea. Am J Med 70:1061, 1981

94. Lerman J. Means JH: The gastric secretion in exophthalmic goitre and myxoedema. J Clin Invest 11:167, 1932

95. Donaich D, Roitt IM: An evaluation of gastric and thyroid auto-immunity in relation to hematologic disorders. Semin Hematol 1:313, 1964

96. Hohl RD, Nixon RK: Myxedema ileus. Arch Intern Med 115:145, 1965

97. Nickerson JF, Hill SR, McNeil JH, Barker SB: Fatal myxedema with and without coma. Ann Intern Med 53:475, 1960

98. Tachman ML, Guthrie GP Jr: Hypothyroidism: diversity of presentation. Endocr Rev 5:456, 1984

99. Broitman SA, Bondy DC, Yachnin I et al: Absorption and disposition of D-xylose in thyroxtoxicosis and myxedema. N Engl J Med 270:333, 1964

100. Baker A, Kaplan M, Wolfe H: Central congestive fibrosis of the liver in myxedema ascites. Ann Intern Med 77:927, 1972

101. Amino N, Kuro R, Yabu Y et al: Elevated levels of circulating carcinoembryonic antigens in hypothyroidism. J Clin Endocrinol Metab 52:457, 1981

102. Lorenzo y Losade H Jr, Staricco EC, Cerviño JM et al: Hypotonia of the gallbladder, of myxedematous origin. J Clin Endocrinol Metab 17:133, 1957

103. Yount E, Little JM: Renal clearance in patients with myxedema. J Clin Endocrinol Metab 15:343, 1955

104. Discala VA, Kinney MJ: Effects of myxedema on the renal diluting and concentrating mechanism. Am J Med 50:325, 1971

105. Ford RV, Owens JC, Curd GW Jr et al: Kidney function in various thyroid states. J Clin Endocrinol Metab 21:548, 1961

106. Moses AM, Gabrilove JL, Soffer LJ: Simplified water loading test in hypoadrenocorticism and hypothyroidism. J Clin Endocrinol Metab 18:1413, 1958

107. Crispell KR, Parson W, Sprinklle P: A cortisone-resistant abnormality in the diuretic response to ingested water in primary myxedema. J Clin Endocrinol Metab 14:640, 1954

108. Bleifer KH, Belsky JL, Saxon L, Papper S: The diuretic response to administered water in patients with primary myxedema. J Clin Endocrinol Metab 20:409, 1960

109. Davies CE, MacKinnon J, Platts MM: Renal circulation and cardiac output in "low-output" heart failure and in myxoedema. Br Med J 2:595, 1952

110. Pettinger WA, Tálner L, Ferris TF: Inappropriate secretion of antidiuretic hormone due to myxedema. N Engl J Med 272:361, 1965

111. Showsky WR, Kikuchi TA: The role of vasopressin in the impaired water excretion of myxedema. Am J Med 64:613, 1978

112. Iwasaki Y, Oiso Y, Yamauchi K et al: Osmoregulation of plasma vasopressin in myxedema. J Clin Endocrinol Metab 70:534, 1990

113. Leeper RD, Benua RS, Brener JL, Rawson RW: Hyperuricemia in myxedema. J Clin Endocrinol Metab 20:1457, 1960

114. Jones JE, Desper PC, Shane SR, Flink EB: Magnesium metabolism in hyperthyroidism and hypothyroidism. J Clin Invest 45:891, 1966

115. Yamamoto K, Saito K, Takai T et al: Visual field defects and pituitary enlargement in primary hypothyroidism. J Clin Endocrinol Metab 57:283, 1983

116. Vagenakis AG, Dole K, Braverman LE: Pituitary enlargement, pituitary failure, and primary hypothyroidism. Ann Intern Med 85:195, 1976

117. Honbo KS, Van Herle AJ, Kellett KA: Serum prolactin levels in untreated primary hypothyroidism. Am J Med 64:782, 1978

118. Onishi T, Miyai K, Aono T et al: Primary hypothyroidism and galactorrhea. Am J Med 63:373, 1977

119. Hinkle PM, Perrone MH, Schonbrunn A: Mechanism of thyroid hormone inhibition of thyrotropin-releasing hormone action. Endocrinology 108:199, 1981

120. Brauman H, Corvilain J: Growth hormone response to hypoglycemia in myxedema. J Clin Endocrinol Metab 28:301, 1968

121. Seo H, Vassart G, Brocas H, Refetoff S: Triiodothyronine stimulates specifically growth hormone mRNA in rat pituitary tumor cells. Proc Natl Acad Sci USA 74:2054 1977

122. Seo H, Refetoff S, Martino E et al: The differential stimulatory effect of thyroid hormone on growth hormone synthesis and estrogen on prolactin synthesis due to accumulation of specific messenger ribonucleic acid. Endocrinology 194:1083, 1979

123. Koenig RJ, Brent GA, Warne RL et al: Thyroid hormone receptor binds specifically to a site in the rat growth promoter required for response to thyroid hormone. Proc Natl Acad Sci USA 84:5670, 1987

124. Larsen PR, Harney JW, Moore DD: Sequences required for cell-type-specific thyroid hormone regulation of the rat growth hormone promoter activity. J Biol Chem 261: 14373, 1986

125. Brent GA, Harney JW, Moore DD, Larsen PR: Multihormonal regulation of the human, rat, and bovine growth hormone promoters: differential effects of 3′, 5′-cyclic adenosine monophosphate, thyroid hormone, and glucocorticoids. Molec Endocrinol 2:792, 1988

126. Chernausek SD, Underwood LE, Utiger RD, Van Wyk JJ: Growth hormone secretion and plasma somatomedin-c in primary hypothyroidism. Clin Endocrinol 19:337, 1983

127. Chernausek SD, Turner R: Attenuation of spontaneous nocturnal growth hormone secretion in children with hypothyroidism and its correlation with plasma insulin-like growth factor I concentrations. J Pediatr 114:968, 1989

128. Miell JP, Taylor AM, Zini M et al: Effects of hypothyroidism and hyperthyroidism on insulin-like growth factors (IGFs) and growth hormone- and IGF-binding proteins. J Clin Endocrinol Metab 76:950, 1993

129. de la Balze FA, Arrillaga F, Mancini RE et al: Male hypogonadism in hypothyroidism: a study of six cases. J Clin Endocrinol Metab 22:212, 1962

130. Davis LE, Leveno KJ, Cunningham FG: Hypothyroidism complicating pregnancy. Obstet Gynecol 72: 108, 1988

131. Potter JD: Hypothyroidism and reproductive failure. Surg Gynecol Obstet 150:251, 1980

132. Montoro M, Collea JV, Frasier SD, Mestman JH: Successful outcome of pregnancy in women with hypothyroidism. Ann Intern Med 94:31, 1981

133. Liu H, Momotani N, Noh JY et al: Maternal hypothyroidism during early pregnancy and intellectual development of progeny. Arch Intern Med 154:785, 1994

134. Man EB, Brown JF, Serunian SA: Maternal hypothyroxinemia: Psychoneurological deficits of progeny. Ann Clin Lab Ser 21:227, 1991

135. Ross GT, Scholz DA, Lamberg EH, Geraci JE: Severe uterine bleeding and degenerative skeletal-muscle changes in unrecognized myxedema. J Clin Endocrinol Metab 18:492, 1958

136. Goldsmith RE, Sturgis SH, Lerman J, Stanbury JB: The menstrual pattern in thyroid disease. J Clin Endocrinol Metab 12:846, 1952

137. Costin G, Kershnar AK, Kogut MD, Turkington RW: Prolactin activity in juvenile hypothyroidism and precocious puberty. Pediatrics 50:881, 1972

138. Hopwood NJ, Lockhart LH, Bryan GT: Acquired hypothyroidism with muscular hypertrophy and precocious testicular enlargement. J Pediatr 85:233, 1974

139. Ross F, Nusynowitz ML: A syndrome of primary hypothyroidism, amenorrhea and galactorrhea. J Clin Endocrinol 28:591, 1968

140. Anderson DC: Sex-hormone-binding globulin. Clin Endocrinol 3:69, 1974

141. Gordon GG, Southren AL: Thyroid-hormone effects on steroid-hormone metabolism. Bull NY Acad Med 53:241, 1977

142. Copinschi G, Leclercq R, Bruno OD, Cornil A: Effects of altered thyroid function upon cortisol secretion in man. Horm Metab Res 3:437, 1971

143. Gordon GG, Southern AL, Tochimoto S et al: Effect of hyperthyroidism and hypothyroidism on the metabolism of testosterone and androstenedione in man. J Clin Endocrinol Metab 29:164, 1969

144. Hellman L, Bradlow HL, Zumoff B et al: Thyroid-androgen interrelations and the hypocholesteremic effect of androsterone. J Clin Endocrinol Metab 19: 936, 1959

145. Brown H, Englert E, Wallach S: Metabolism of free and conjugated 17-hydroxycorticosteroids in subjects with thyroid disease. J Clin Endocrinol Metab 18:167, 1958

146. Ogihara T, Yamamoto T, Miyai K, Kumahara Y: Plasma renin activity and aldosterone concentration of patients with hyperthyroidism and hypothyroidism. Endocrinol Jpn

147. Saruta T, Kitajima W, Hayashi M et al: Renin and aldosterone in hypothyroidism: relation to excretion of sodium and potassium. Clin Endocrinol 12:483, 1980

148. Felber JP, Reddy WJ, Selenkow HA, Thorn GW: Adrenocortical response to the 48-hour ACTH test in myxedema and hyperthyroidism. J Clin Endocrinol Metab 19:895, 1959

149. Liddle GW, Estep HL, Kendall JW Jr et al: Clinical application of a new test of pituitary reserve. J Clin Endocrinol Metab 19:875, 1959

150. Gold EM, Kent JR, Forsham PH: Clinical use of a new diagnostic agent, methopyrapone (SU-4885), in pituitary and adrenocortical disorders. Ann Intern Med 54:175, 1961

151. Lessof MH, Maisey MN. Lyne C, Sturge RA: Effect of thyroid failure on the pituitary-adrenal axis. Lancet 1:642, 1969

152. Ridgway EC, McCammon JA, Benotti J, Maloof F: Acute metabolic responses in myxedema to large doses of intravenous L-thyroxine. Ann Intern Med 77:549, 1972

153. Bigos ST, Ridgway EC, Kourides IA, Maloof F: Spectrum of pituitary alterations with mild and severe thyroid impairment. J Clin Endocrinol Metab 46: 317, 1978

154. Kamilaris TC, DeBold CR, Pavlou SN et al: Effect of altered thyroid hormone levels on hypothalamic-pituitary-adrenal function. J Clin Endocrinol Metab 65:994, 1987

155. Clausen N, Lins PE, Adamson U et al: Counterregulation of insulin-induced hypoglycemia in primary hypothyroidism. Acta Endocrinol 111:516, 1986

156. Carpenter CCJ, Solomon N, Silverberg SG et al: Schmidt's syndrome (thyroid and adrenal insufficiency): a review of the literature and a report of fifteen new cases including ten instances of coexistent diabetes mellitus. Medicine 43:153, 1964

157. Salvi M, Fukazawa H, Bernard N et al: Role of autoantibodies in the pathogenesis and association of endocrine autoimmune disorders. Endocr Rev 9:450, 1988

158. Gharib H, Gastineau CF, Hodgson SF et al: Reversible hypothyroidism in Addison's disease. Lancet 2: 734, 1972

159. Christiansen CJ: Increased levels of plasma noradrenalin in hypothyroidism. J Clin Endocrinol 35: 359, 1972

160. Stoffer SS, Jiang N-S, Gorman CA, Pikler GM: Plasma catecholamines in hypothyroidism and hyperthyroidism. J Clin Endocrinol Metab 36:587, 1973

161. Lee, WY, Morimoto PK, Bronsky D, Waldstein SS: Studies of thyroid and sympathetic nervous system interrelationships: I. The biepharoptosis of myxedema. J Clin Endocrinol Metab 21:1402, 1961

162. Raab W: Epinephrine tolerance of the heat altered by thyroxine and thiouracil. J Pharmacol Exp Ther 82:330, 1944

163. Raab W: Diminution of epinephrine sensitivity of the normal human heart through thiouracil. J Lab Clin Med 30:774, 1945

164. Schneckloth RE, Kurland GS, Freedberg AS: Effect of variation in thyroid function on the pressor response to norepinephrine in man. Metabolism 2: 546, 1953

165. Leonard JD, Mellen SA, Larsen PR: Thyroxine 5′-deiodinase activity in brown adipose tissue. Endocrinology 112:1153, 1982

166. Krief S, Lonnqvist F, Raimbault S et al: Tissue distribution of β3-adrenergic receptor mRNA in man. J Clin Invest 91:344, 1993

167. Hurwitz LJ, McCormick D, Allen IV: Reduced muscle α-glocosidase (acid-maltase) activity in hypothyroid myopathy. Lancet 1:67, 1970

168. Goldstone H, Ford FR: Severe myotonia as a complication of postoperative thyroid deficiency: Complete relief of myotonia by thyroid extract: Report of two cases. Bull Johns Hopkins Hosp 97:53, 1957

169. Waldstein SS, Bronsky D, Shrifter HB, Oester YT: The electromyogram in myxedema. Arch Intern Med 101:97, 1958

170. Gold HK, Spann JF Jr. Graunwald E: Effect of alternations in the thyroid state on the intrinsic contractile properties of isolated rat skeletal muscle. J Clin Invest 49:849, 1970

171. Debré. R, Sémélaigne G: Syndrome of diffuse muscular hypertrophy in infants causing athletic appearance: Its connection with congenital myxedema. Am J Dis Child 50:1351, 1935

172. Thomasen E: Myotonia, Thomsen's Disease, Paramyotonia, Dystrophia Myotonica, Aahrus, Denmark, Universitetsforlaget, 1948

173. Khaleeli AA, Griffith DG, Edwards RHT: The clinical presentation of hypothyroid myopathy. Clinical Endocriminology 19:365, 1983

174. Lambert EH, Underdahl LO, Beckett S, Mederos LO: A study of the ankle jerk in myxedema. J Clin Endocrinol Metab 11:1186, 1951

175. Famulski KS, Pilarska M, Wrzosek A, Sarzala MG: ATPase activity and protein phosphorylation in rabbit fast skeletal muscle sarcolemma. Eur J Biochem 171:363, 1988

176. Simonides WS, van Hardeveld C, Larsen PR: Identification of sequences in the promoter of the fast isoform of sarcoplasmic reticulum Ca-ATPase (SERCA1) required for transcriptional activation by thyroid hormone, abstracted. Thyroid 2:S-102, 1992

177. Bland JH, Frymoyer JW: Rheumatoid syndrome of myxedema. N Engl J Med 282:1171, 1970

178. Frymoyer JW, Bland JH: Carpal-tunnel syndrome in patients with myxedematous arthropathy. J Bone Joint Surg 55A:78, 1973

179. Bonakdarpour A, Kirkpatrick JA, Renzi A, Kendall N: Skeletal changes in neonatal thyrotoxicosis. Radiology 102:149, 1972

180. Krane SM, Bronwell GL, Stanbury JB, Corrigan H: The effect of thyroid disease on calcium metabolism in man. J Clin Invest 35:874, 1956

181. Bouillon R, DeMoor P: Parathyroid function in pa-

tients with hyper- or hypothyroidism. J Clin Endocrinol Metab 38:999, 1974

182. Lever EG: Primary hyperparathyroidism masked by hypothyroidism. Am J Med 74:144, 1983

183. Lave CE, Bird ED, Thomas WC: Hypercalcemia in myxedema. J Clin Endocrinol Metab 22:261, 1962

184. Bouillon R, Muls E, DeMoor P: Influence of thyroid function on the serum concentration of 1.25-dihydroxy vitamin D₃. J Clin Endocrinol Metab 51:793, 1980

185. Mundy GR, Shapiro JL, Bandelin JG et al: Direct stimulation of bone resorption by thyroid hormones. J Clin Invest 58:529, 1976

186. Eriksen EF: Normal and pathological remodeling of human trabecular bone: Three dimensional reconstruction of the remodeling sequence in normals and in metabolic bone disease. Endocr Rev 7:379, 1986

187. Jellinek EH, Kelly RE: Cerebellar syndrome in myxoedema. Lancet 2:225, 1960

188. Sanders V: Neurological manifestations of myxedema. N Engl J Med 266:577, 599, 1962

189. Cremer GM, Goldstein NP, Paris J: Myxedema and ataxia. Neurology 19:37, 1969

190. Crevasse LE, Logue RB: Peripheral neuropathy in myxedema. Ann Intern Med 50:1433, 1959

191. Nickel SN, Frame B: nervous and muscular systems in myxedema. J Chronic Dis 14:570, 1961

192. Murray IPC, Simpson JA: Acroparaesthesia in myxoedema. Lancet 1:1360, 1958

193. Schulman JD, Crawford JD: Congenital nystagmus and hypothyroidism. New Eng J Med 280:708, 1969

194. Murray IPC: The reaction time in myxoedema. Lancet 2:384, 1956

195. Loosen PT: Thyroid function in affective disorders and alcoholism. Endocrinol Metab Clin North Am 17:55, 1988

196. Scheinberg P, Stead EA, Braman ES, Warren JV: Correlative observations on cerebral metabolism. J Clin Invest 29:1139, 1950

197. Sensenbach W, Madison L, Eisenberg S, Ochs L: The cerebral circulation and metabolism in hyperthyroidism and myxedema. J Clin Invest 33:1434, 1954

198. O'Brien MD, Harris PWR: Cerebral-cortex perfusion rates in myxedema. Lancet 1: 1170, 1965

199. Watanakunakorn C, Hodges RE, Evans TC: Myxedema: a study of 400 cases. Arch Intern Med 116:183, 1965

200. Stern B. Altshule MD: Hematological studies in hypothyroidism following total thyroidectomy. J Clin Invest 15:633, 1936

201. Bomford R: Anaemia in myxoedema: and the role of the thyroid gland in erythropoiesis. Q J Med 7:495, 1938

202. Shalet M, Coe D, Reismann KR: Mechanism of erythropoietic action of thyroid hormone. Proc Soc Exp Biol Med 123:443, 1966

203. Tudhope GR, Wilson GM: Anemia in hypothyroidism. Q J Med 29:513, 1960

204. Muldowney FP, Crooke J, Wayne EJ: The total red cell mass in thyrotoxicosis and myxoedema. Clin Sci 16:309, 1957

205. Simone JV, Abildgaard CF, Schulman I: Blood coagulation in thyroid dysfunction. N Engl J Med 273:1057, 1965

206. Rogers JS, Shane SR, Jencks FS: Factor VIII activity and thyroid function. Ann Intern Med 97:713, 1982

207. Hoak JC, Wilson WR, Warner ED et al: Effects of triiodothyronine induced hypermetabolism on factor VIII and fibrinogen in man. J Clin Invest 48:768, 1969

208. Bennett NB, Ogston CM, McAndrew JM: The thyroid and fibrinolysis. Br Med J 4:147, 1967

209. Thomson JA: Alterations in capillary fragility in thyroid disease. Clin Sci 26:55, 1964

210. Kiely JM, Purnell DC, Owen CA Jr: Erythrokinetics in myxedema. Ann Intern Med 67:533, 1967

211. Leithold SL. David D, Best WR: Hypothyroidism with anemia demonstrating abnormal vitamin B₁₂ absorption. Am J Med 24:535, 1958

212. Tudhope GR, Wilson GM: Deficiency of vitamin B₁₂ in hypothyroidism. Lancet 1:703, 1962

213. Hines JD. Halstead CH, Griggs RC, Harris JW: Megaloblastic anemia secondary to folate deficiency associated with hypothyroidism. Ann Intern med 68:792, 1968

214. Wardrop C. Hutchinson HE: Red cell shape in hypothyroidism. Lancet 1:1243, 1969

215. Lillington GA, Gastineau CF, Underdahl LO: The sedimentation rate in primary myxedema. Proc Staff Meetings Mayo Clinic. 34:605, 1959

216. Murray IPC: Personal communication.

217. Lewallen CG, Rall JE, Berman M: Studies of iodoalbumin metabolism. II. The effects of thyroid hormone. J Clin Invest 38:88, 1959

218. Crispell KR, Parson W, Hollifield G: A study of the rate of protein synthesis before and during the administration of L-triiodothyronine to patients with myxedema and healthy volunteers using N-15 glycine. J Clin Invest 35:164, 1956

219. Lamberg BA, Gräsbeck R: The serum protein pattern in disorders of thyroid function. Acta Endocrinol 19:91, 1955

220. Abrams JJ, Grundy SM: Cholesterol metabolism in hypothyroidism and hyperthyroidism in man. J Lipid Res 22:323, 1981

221. Muls E, Rosseneu M, Blaton V et al: Serum lipids and apolipoprotein AI, AII and B in primary hypothyroidism before and during treatment. Eur J Clin Invest 14:12, 1984

222. Dullaart RPF, Hoogenberg K, Groener JEM et al: The activity of cholesteryl ester transfer protein is decreased in hypothyroidism: a possible contribution to alterations in high-density lipoproteins. Eur J Clin Invest 20:581, 1990

223. Aviram M, Luboshitzky R, Brook J: Lipid and lipoprotein patter in thyroid dysfunction and the effect of therapy. Clin Biochem 15:62, 1982

224. Agdeppa D, Macaron C, Mallik T, Schuda ND: Plasma high density lipoprotein cholesterol in thyroid disease. J Clin Endocrinol Metab 49:476, 1979

225. Lithell H, Boberg J, Hellsing K et al: Serum lipoprotein and apoprotein concentrations and tissue lipoprotein-lipase activity in overt and subclinical hypothyroidism: the effect of substitution therapy. Eur J Clin Invest 11:3, 1981

226. Kuusi T, Taskinen M-R, Nikkila EA: Lipoproteins, lipolytic enzymes, and hormonal status in hypothyroid women at different levels of substitution. J Clin Endocrinol Metab 66:51, 1988

227. Hazzard WR, Bierman EL: Aggravation of broad-β disease (type 3 hyperlipoproteinemia) by hypothyroidism. Arch Intern Med 130:822, 1972

228. O'Hara D, Porte D Jr, Williams RH: The effect of diet and thyroxin on plasma lipids in myxedema. Metabolism 15:123, 1966

229. Porte D Jr, O'Hara DD, Williams RH: The relation between postheparin lipolytic activity and plasma triglyceride in myxedema. Metabolism 15:107, 1966

230. Abrams JJ, Grundy SM, Ginsberg H: Metabolism of plasma triglycerides in hypothyroidism and hyperthyroidism in man. J Lipid Res 22:307, 1981

231. Kritchevsky D: Influence of thyroid hormones and related compounds on cholesterol biosynthesis and degradation: a review. Metabolism 9:984, 1960

232. Kurland GS, Lucas JL, Freedberg AS: The metabolism of intravenously infused ^{14}C-labeled cholesterol in euthyroidism and myxedema. J Lab Clin Med 57:574, 1961

233. Walton KW, Scott PJ, Dykes PW, Davies JWL: The significance of alterations in serum lipids in thyroid dysfunction. II. Alterations of the metabolism and turnover of ^{131}I low-density lipoproteins in hypothyroidism and thyrotoxicosis. Clin Sci 29:217, 1965

234. Chait A, Bierman EL, Albers JJ: Regulatory role of triiodothyronine in the degradation of low density lipoprotein by cultured human skin fibroblasts. J Clin Endocrinol Metab 48:887, 1979

235. Scarabottolo L, Trezzi E, Roma P, Catapano AL: Experimental hypothyroidism modulates the expression of the low density lipoprotein receptor by the liver. Atherosclerosis 59:329, 1986

236. Thompson GR, Soutar AK, Spengel FA et al: Defects of receptor mediated low density lipoprotein catabolism in homozygous familial hypercholesterolemia and hypothyroidism in vivo. Proc Natl Acad Sci USA 78:2591, 1981

237. Valdermarsson S: Plasma lipoproteins alterations in thyroid dysfunction. Roles of lipoprotein lipase, hepatic lipase and LCAT. Acta Endocrinol (Copenh) 103:1, 1983

238. Escamilla RF: Carotenemia in myxedema: Explanation of the typical slightly icteric tint. J Clin Endocrinol Metab 2:33, 1942

239. Shah JH, Motto GS, Papagiannes E, Williams GA: Insulin metabolism in hypothyroidism. Diabetes 24:922, 1975

240. Shah JH, Cerchio GM: Hypoinsulinemia of hypothyroidism. Arch Intern Med 132:657, 1973

241. Hecht A, Gershberg H: Diabetes mellitus and primary hypothyroidism. Metabolism 17:108, 1968

242. Means JH, Lerman J: Symptomatology of myxedema: Its relation to metabolic levels, time intervals, and rations of thyroid. Arch Intern Med 55:1, 1935

243. Topliss DJ, White EL, Stockigt JR: Significance of thyrotropin excess in untreated primary adrenal insufficiency. J Clin Endocrinol Metab 50:52, 1980

244. Farah DA, Boag D, Moran F, McIntosh S: High concentrations of thyroid-stimulating hormone in untreated glucocorticoid deficiency: Indications of primary hypothyroidism? Br Med J 172:285, 1982

245. Konishi J, Iida Y, Kasagi K et al: Primary myxedema with thyrotrophin-binding inhibitor immunoglobulins. Ann Intern Med 103:26, 1985

246. Buisset E, Leclerc L, Lefebure JL et al: Hypothyroidism following combined treatment for hypotpharyngeal and laryngeal carcinoma. Am J Surg 162:345, 1991

247. Bacci V, Schussler GC, Kaplan TB: The relationship between serum triiodothyronine and thyrotropin during systemic illness. J Clin Endocrinol Metab 54:1229, 1982

248. Bartalena L: Recent achievements in studies on thyroid hormone-binding proteins. Endocr Rev 11:47, 1990

249. Bartalena L: Thyroid hormone-binding proteins: Update 1994. Endocr Rev 3:140, 1994

250. Figge J, Dluhy RG: Amiodarone-induced elevation of thyroid stimulating hormone in patients receiving levothyroxine for primary hypothyroidism. Ann Intern Med 113:553, 1990

251. Beck-Peccoz P, Amir S, Menezes-Ferreira MM et al: Decreased receptor binding of biologically inactive thyrotropin in central hypothyroidism: Effect of treatment with thyrotropin-releasing hormone. N Engl J Med 312:1085, 1985

252. Faglia G, Bitensky L, Pinchera A et al: Thyrotropin

secretion in patients with central hypothyroidism: Evidence for reduced biological activity of immuno-reactive thyrotropin. J Clin Endocrinol Metab 48: 989, 1979

253. Petersen VB, McGregor AM, Belchetz PE et al: The secretion of thyrotrophin with impaired biological activity in patients with hypothalamic-pituitary disease. Clin Endocrinol 8:397, 1978

254. Sanchez-Franco F, Cacicedo GL, Martin-Zurro A et al: Transient lack of thyrotropin (TSH) response to thyrotropin-releasing hormone (TRH) in treated hyperthyroid patients with normal or low serum thyroxine (T_4) and triiodothyronine (T_3). J Clin Endocrinol Metab 38:1098, 1974

255. Toft AD, Irvine WJ, Hunter WM et al: Anomalous plasma TSH levels in patients developing hypothyroidism in the early months after ^{131}I therapy for thyrotoxicosis. J Clin Endocrinol Metab 39:607, 1974

256. Toft AD, Irvine WJ, McIntosh D et al: Temporary hypothyroidism after surgical treatment of thyrotoxicosis. Lancet 2:817, 1976

257. Roti E, Minelli R, Gardini E, Braverman LE: The use and misuse of thyroid hormone. Endocr Rev 14: 401, 1993

258. Mandel SJ, Brent GA, Larsen PR: Levothyroxine therapy in patients with thyroid disease. Ann Intern Med 199:492, 1993

259. Toft AD: Thyroxine therapy. N Engl J Med 331:174, 1994

260. Braverman LE, Ingbar SH, Sterling K: Conversion of thyroxine (T_4) to triiodothyronine (T_3) in athyreotic subjects. J Clin Invest 49:855, 1970

261. Larsen PR, Silva JE, Kaplan MM: Relationships between circulating and intracellular thyroid hormones: Physiological and clinical implications. Endocr Rev 2:87, 1981

262. Rees-Jones RW, Rolla AR, Larsen PR: Hormone content of thyroid replacement preparations. JAMA 243:549, 1980

263. Rees-Jones RW, Larsen PR: Triiodothyronine and thyroxine content of desiccated thyroid tablets. Metabolism 26:1213, 1977

264. LeBoff MS, Kaplan MM, Silva JE, Larsen PR: Bioavailability of thyroid hormones from oral replacement preparations. Metabolism 31:900, 1982

265. Blumberg KR, Mayer WJ, Parikh DK, Schnell LA: Liothyronine and levothyroxine in Armour thyroid. J Pharm Sci 76:346, 1993

266. Hays MT: Localization of human thyroxine absorption. Thyroid 3:241, 1991

267. Hays MT: Thyroid hormone and the gut. Endocr Res 14:203, 1988

268. Wennlund A: Variation in serum levels of T_3, T_4, FT_4, and TSH during thyroxine replacement therapy. Acta Endocrinol 113:47, 1986

269. Browning MCK, Bennet WM, Kirkaldy AJ, Jung RT: Intra-individual variation of thyroxine, triiodothyronine, and thyrotropin in treated hypothyroid patients: Implications for monitoring replacement therapy. Clin Chem 34:696, 1988

270. Faber J, Galloe AM: Changes in bone mass during prolonged subclinical hyperthyroidism due to L-thyroxine treatment: a meta-analysis. Eur J Endocrinol 130:350, 1994

271. Greenspan SL, Greenspan FS, Resnick NM et al: Skeletal integrity in premenopausal and postmenopausal women receiving long-term L-thyroxine therapy. Am J Med 91:5, 1991

272. Stall GM, Harris S, Sokoll LF, Dawson-Hughes B: Accelerated bone loss in hypothyroid patients overtreated with L-thyroxine. Ann Intern Med 113:265, 1990

273. Rosenbaum RL, Barzel US: Levothyroxine replacement dose for primary hypothyroidism decreases with age. Ann Intern Med 96:53, 1982

274. Bearcroft CP, Toms GC, Williams SJ et al: Thyroxine replacement in post-radioiodine hypothyroidism. Clin Endocrinol 34:115, 1991

275. Kaplan MM: Monitoring thyroxine treatment during pregnancy. Thyroid 2:147, 1992

276. Carr K, Mcleod DT, Parry G, Thornes HM: Fine adjustment of thyroxine replacement dosage: Comparison of the thyrotrophin releasing hormone tests using a sensitive thyrotrophin assay with measurement of free thyroid hormones and clinical assessment. Clin Endocrinol 28:325, 1988

277. Berg JA, Mayor GH: A study in normal human volunteers to compare the rate and extent of levothyroxine absorption from Synthroid and Levoxine. J Clin Pharmacol 33:1135, 1993

278. Mandel SJ, Larsen PR, Seely EW: Increased need for thyroxine during pregnancy in women with primary hypothyroidism. N Engl J Med 323:91, 1990

279. Harmon SM, Seifert CF: Levothyroxine-cholestyramine interaction reemphasized. Ann Intern Med 115:658, 1991

280. Havrankova J, Lahaie R: Levothyroxine binding by sucralfate. Ann Intern Med 117:445, 1992

281. Sperber AD, Liel Y: Evidence for interference with the intestinal absorption of levothyroxine sodium by aluminum hydroxide. Arch Intern Med 152:183, 1992

282. Campbell NRC, Hasinoff BB, Stalts H et al: Ferrous sulfate reduces thyroxine efficacy in patients with hypothyroidism. Ann Intern Med 117:1010, 1992

283. McLean M, Kirkwood I, Epstein M et al: Cation-exchange resin and inhibition of intestinal absorption of thyroxine. Lancet 341:1286, 1993

284. DeLuca F, Arrigo T, Pandullo E et al: Changes in thyroid function tests induced by 2 month carbamazepine treatment in L-thyroxine-substituted hypothyroid children. Eur J Pediatr 145:77, 1986

285. Faber J, Lumholtz IB, Kirkegaard C et al: The effects of phenytoin on the extrathyroidal turnover of thyroxine, 3,5,3′-triiodothyronine, 3,3′,5′-triiodothyronine, and 3′,5′-diiodothyronine in man. J Clin Endocrinol Metab 61:1093, 1985

286. Isley WL: Effect of rifampin therapy on thyroid function tests in a hypothyroid patient on replacement L-thyroxine. Ann Intern Med 107:517, 1987

287. Demke DM: Drug interaction between thyroxine and lovastatin. N Engl J Med 321:1341, 1989

288. Curran PG, DeGroot LJ: The effect of hepatic enzyme-inducing drugs on thyroid hormones and the thyroid gland. Endocr Rev 12:135, 1991

289. Burger A, Dinchert D, Nirod P et al: Effect of amiodarone on serum triiodothyronine, reverse triiodothyronine, thyroxine, and thyrotropin. J Clin Invest 58:255, 1976

290. Contempre B, Dumont JE, Bebe N et al: Effect of selenium supplementation in hypothyroid subjects of an iodine and selenium deficient area: the possible danger of indiscriminate supplementation of iodine-deficient subjects with selenium. J Clin Endocrinol Metab 73:213, 1991

291. Arafah BM: Decreased levothyroxine requirement in women with hypothyroidism during androgen therapy for breast cancer. Ann Intern Med 121:247, 1994

292. Hay ID, Duick DX, Vlietstra RE et al: Thyroxine therapy in hypothyroid patients undergoing coronary revascularization: a retrospective analysis. Ann Intern Med 95:456, 1981

293. Weinberg AD, Brennan MD, Gorman CA et al: Outcome of anesthesia and surgery in hypothyroid patients. Arch Intern Med 143:893, 1983

294. Ladenson PW, Levin AA, Ridgway EC, Daniels GH: Complications of surgery in hypothyroid patients. Am J Med 77:261, 1984

295. Takasu N, Komiya I, Asawa T et al: Test for recovery from hypothyroidism during thyroxine therapy in Hashimoto's thyroiditis. Lancet 336:1084, 1990

296. Kung AW, Pun KK: Bone mineral density in premenopausal and postmenopausal women receiving long-term physiological doses of levothyroxine. JAMA 265:2688, 1991

297. Biondi B, Fazio S, Carella C et al: Cardiac effects of long term thyrotropin-suppressive therapy with levothyroxine. J Clin Endocrinol Metab 77:334, 1993

298. Hall RCW: Psychiatric effects of thyroid hormone disturbance. Psychosomatics 24:7, 1983

299. Josephson AM, Mackenzie TB: Thyroid-induced mania in hypothyroid patients. Br J Psychiatr 137:222, 1980

300. Josephson AM, Mackenzie TB: Appearance of manic psychosis following rapid normalization of thyroid status. Am J Psychiatr 136:846, 1979

301. Van Dop C, Conte FA, Koch TK et al: Pseudotumor cerebri associated with initiation of levothyroxine therapy for juvenile hypothyroidism. N Engl J Med 308:1076, 1983

302. Refetoff S, Weiss RE, Usala SJ: The syndromes of resistance to thyroid hormone. Endocr Rev 14:348, 1993

303. Refetoff S, Weiss RE, Usala SJ, Hayashi Y: The syndromes of resistance to thyroid hormone: Update 1994. Endocr Rev 3:336, 1994

304. Kaplan MM, Swartz SL, Larsen PR: Partial peripheral resistance to thyroid hormone. Am J Med 70:1115, 1981

305. Usala SJ: Molecular diagnosis and characterization of thyroid hormone resistance syndromes. Thyroid 1:361, 1991

306. Cooper DS, Halpern R, Wood LC et al: L-thyroxine therapy in subclinical hypothyroidism: a double-blind, placebo-controlled trial. Ann Intern Med 101:18, 1984

307. Althaus BU, Staub J-J, Ryff-De-Leche A et al: LDL/HDL-changes in subclinical hypothyroidism: Possible risk factors for coronary heart disease. Clin Endocrinol 28:157, 1988

308. Caron P, Calazel C, Parra HJ et al: Decreased HDL cholesterol in subclinical hypothyroidism: the effect of L-thyroxine therapy. Clin Endocrinol 33:519, 1990

309. Arem R, Patsch W: Lipoprotein and apolipoprotein levels in subclinical hypothyroidism. Arch Intern Med 150:2097, 1990

310. Bell GM, Todd WTA, Forfar JC et al: End-organ responses to thyroxine therapy in subclinical hypothyroidism. Clin Endocrinol 22:83, 1985

311. Forfar JC, Wathen CG, Todd WTA et al: Left ventricular performance in subclinical hypothyroidism. Q J Med 224:857, 1985

312. Nystrom E, Caidahl K, Fager G, et al: A double-blind cross-over 12-month study of L-thyroxine treatment of women with "subclinical" hypothyroidism. Clin Endocrinol 29:63, 1988

313. Nicoloff JT, LoPresti JS: Myxedema coma: a form of decompensated hypothyroidism. p. 279. In Endocrinology and Metabolism Clinics of North America, WB Saunders, Philadelphia, 1993

314. Jordan RM: Myxedema coma: the prognosis is improving. Endocrinologist 3:149, 1993

315. Holvey DN, Goodner CJ, Nicoloff JT, Dowling JT:

Treatment of myxedema coma with intravenous thyroxine. Arch Intern Med 113:139, 1964

316. Blackburn CM, McConahey WM, Keating RF, Albert A: Calorigenic effects of single intravenous doses of L-triiodothyronine and L-thyroxine in myxedematous persons. J Clin Invest 33:819, 1954

317. MacKerrow SD, Osborn LA, Levy H et al: Myxedema-associated cardiogenic shock treated with intravenous triiodothyronine. Ann Intern Med 117:1014, 1992

318. Hylander B, Rosenquist U: Treatment of myxedema coma-factors associated with fatal outcome. Acta Endocrinol 108:65, 1985

319. Arlot S, Debussche X, Lalau JD et al: Myxedema coma: Response of thyroid hormones with oral and intravenous high-dose L-thyroxine treatment. Intensive Care Med 17:16, 1991

320. Odell WD: Isolated deficiencies of anterior pituitary hormones. JAMA 197:1006, 1966

321. Lee HB, Faiman C: Isolated thyrotropin deficiency due to a pituitary tumor. Can Med Assoc J 116:520, 1977

322. Miyai K, Azukizawa M, Kumahara Y: Familial isolated thyrotropin deficiency with cretenism. N Engl J Med 285:1043, 1971

323. Patel YC, Burger HG: Serum thyrotropin (TSH) in pituitary and/or hypothalamic hypothyroidism: Normal or elevated basal levels and paradoxical responses to thyrotropin-releasing hormone. J Clin Endocrinol Metab 37:190, 1973

Graves' Disease and the Manifestations of Thyrotoxicosis

10

This chapter reviews Graves' disease, its pathogenesis, and the general pathophysiologic changes caused by the action of excess thyroid hormone. The clinical syndrome produced by excess thyroid hormone is usually referred to as thyrotoxicosis, or as hyperthyroidism if the source of excess hormone is the thyroid.

The eponym *Graves' disease*[1] is used in the English and American literature for this disturbance, caused by autoimmunity to thyroid antigens, characterized in its classic form by hypertrophy and hyperplasia of the thyroid, hyperthyroidism (or thyrotoxicosis), by a unique type of ophthalmopathy, and occasionally by specific dermopathy. Cases will rarely exhibit

371

all these signs and symptoms. The thyrotoxicosis of Graves' disease, for example, may exist without the ophthalmopathy, and conversely, the ophthalmopathy may be present and even severe without evidence of thyrotoxicosis.

The English physician Caleb H. Parry (1755–1822), first described the clinical syndrome. Later, Karl A. von Basedow (1799–1854) described the illness in the German language. *Basedow's disease* is the eponym usually given to the illness in continental Europe.

Thyrotoxicosis is a condition characterized by a distorted and accelerated metabolism in most tissues of the body. It is usually caused by the uncontrolled formation of hormone in the diffuse hyperplastic thyroid of Graves' disease. It may also be caused by toxic multinodular goiter, by the release of thyroid hormone in the wake of thyroiditis or radiation injury to the gland, or by uncontrolled release of hormones from toxic thyroid adenomas, carcinomas, and ectopic thyroid tissue. Thyrotoxicosis arises only rarely from pituitary resistance to feedback control, thyrotropin-secreting pituitary tumors, and thyroid-stimulating substances secreted by hydatidiform moles, choriocarcinomas, and seminomas. Thyrotoxicosis may have an exogenous cause, such as administration of thyroid-stimulating hormone or too much thyroid hormone, or ingestion of excess iodine. In each instance, the final common pathway is the excess circulating thyroid hormone, and the pathophysiologic changes resulting from the thyrotoxicosis are identical. Thus, the clinical and metabolic changes due to thyrotoxicosis, described in this chapter, are also seen in response to any other source of hormone beyond physiologic need.

Because of its clinical importance, Graves' disease is covered in detail in this chapter, and the manifestations of thyrotoxicosis in general are considered as they present in Graves' disease. Thyrotoxicosis from other causes is discussed in Chapter 13 or treated in relation to the parent syndromes; toxic nodular goiter, for example, is discussed with multinodular goiter.

Special terms are used for certain variations from the typical clinical picture. *Euthyroid Graves' disease* usually refers to a patient with Graves' ophthalmopathy but without other clinical evidence of the classic syndrome. *Apathetic hyperthyroidism* is used to describe certain patients, usually elderly, in whom the symptoms are mild or veiled, although the illness may be severe. The term *masked hyperthyroidism* is somewhat analogous. *Recurrent thyrotoxicosis* is a self-explanatory term. One may have recurrences after spontaneous recovery or after treatment, surgical or otherwise. The term *toxic goiter* is not specific; it may be applied to toxic nodular goiter or to Graves' disease. Graves' disease is also caused occasionally by hyperfunctioning paranodular tissue adjacent to functioning thyroid nodules. This is called the *Marine-Lenhart syndrome*.[2] A specific subset of autoimmune hyperthyroidism, often occurring in the postpartum period, is referred to as *transient thyrotoxicosis* or *painless thyroiditis*.

CAUSE

Although we may consider Graves' disease to be an autoimmune illness, its true cause is not established (Table 10-1). With the possible exception of an experimental syndrome induced in one study in rabbits,[3] and possibly an illness in cats (which seems more related to toxic nodular goiter) it is limited to humans. The most definite clues to its cause are its remarkable family incidence, its close relationship to Hashimoto's thyroiditis and myxedema, and the associated disturbances in the immune system. Of possible but unproven significance are observations that onset sometimes follows a severe emotional stress, and that the disease has occasionally followed a period of intentional weight reduction achieved with or without the use of thyroid hormone. Association of Graves' disease with prior ingestion of excess iodine and with radiation to the neck have also been reported.[4,5]

The possible basic cause of thyroid autoimmunity are considered in Chapter 7.

Constitutional and Hereditary Background

Heredity is a major factor in Graves' disease. In clinical practice, it is common to observe several cases of the disease in one family, and in successive

TABLE 10-1. Factors Suggested in the Etiology of Graves' Disease

Heredity
Immunologic abnormalities (See Table 10-2)
Psychic trauma
Sympathetic "overactivity"
Weight loss
Iodine
TSH

generations. Years ago, Bartels[6] found a family predisposition to Graves' disease in 60 percent of his cases of toxic diffuse goiter, Martin[7] suggested the presence of a hereditable recessive factor predisposing to exophthalmic goiter, and Harvald and Hauge[8] found a significant increase in incidence among twins.

In a study of nearly 200 children of parents with Graves' disease, we found a 50 percent higher incidence of abnormalities of the thyroid gland and thyroid function tests compared to a normal population.[9] Antithyroglobulin antibodies can be demonstrated in relatives of patients with Graves' disease in an inheritance pattern consistent with that of a codominant trait.[10] Tami et al. noted abnormal TRH responses (reduced or increased) in many apparently well relatives of patients with Graves' disease.[11] Chopra et al. demonstrated frequent abnormalities including hyper-responsiveness to TRH and failure of thyroid suppressibility in relatives lacking any other clinical or chemical stigmata of Graves' disease.[12] Although evidence of abnormal thyroid function and antithyroid antibodies is commonly present, specific thyroid-stimulating antibodies are absent in most relatives.[13]

A familial incidence could be explained on the basis of a common environment, a hereditary abnormality in personality structure (if psychological stress plays a role), an abnormality of endocrine function transmitted genetically, or a hereditary immunologic abnormality.

The predisposition to Graves' disease is now known to be related to inheritance of specific genes coding for histocompatibility antigens. Grumet et al.[14] first recognized that the HLA-B8 Class I histocompatibility antigen is present on the leukocytes of 47 percent of whites with Graves' disease versus 21 percent of control subjects. Among Japanese, an association was found with HLA-Bw35.[15] Subsequently, a more important association was observed for HLA-DR3 and DR5. Inheritance of DR3 increases the risk of Graves' disease 5.7-fold.[16] A less powerful association with DR3 is noted for autoimmune thyroid failure (idiopathic hypothyroidism), and goitrous Hashimoto's thyroiditis is found to be more associated with HLA-DR5.[17] These tissue antigens constitute part of the immune response genes on chromosome 6. HLA-B8 and DR3 factors are additive for risk. The gene HLA-DQβw2 is also associated with increased risk for Graves' disease[18,] and

the haplotype DR3-DQA*0501-DQB*0201 is specifically associated with Graves' disease.[19] The HLA-DR3 haplotype may (or may not) confer relative resistance to antithyroid drug and RAI-induced remission, and possibly a greater risk for exophthalmos.[20,21]

It must be noted that Graves' disease is not uniquely tied to these genotypes, and other hereditary factors await discovery. These factors include genes controlling IgG heavy chains, since specific Gm allotypes occur in increased frequency in family members with Graves' disease,[22] and association with certain T cell receptor genes and complement factors have been reported. These inheritable factors, which are more extensively discussed in Chapter 7, presumably are important since they predispose the individual to develop antithyroid autoimmunity.

Abnormality of the Immune System and Thyroid-Stimulating Immunoglobulins

Serious consideration of the possibility that an abnormality in the immune system might underlie Graves' disease began with the discovery of TSAb (Long-Acting Thyroid Stimulator) and its identification as an IgG immunoglobulin (Table 10-2). Many features of the disease make this concept attractive. There is general hypertrophy of the lymphoid tissue in the disease, and extensive collections of lymphocytes are found in the hyperplastic gland. Graves' disease, thyroiditis, and myxedema often occur in families, patients may progress from one illness to another, and several other organ-specific autoimmune diseases are associated with the three thyroid conditions. Antibodies directed against thyroglobulin (TG) and a thyroid peroxidase (thyroid microsomal antigen) (TPO) are present in patients (and their

TABLE 10-2. Theories on the Immunological Etiology of Graves' Disease

Persistence of autoreactive T cells and B cells
Inheritance of specific HLA and other immune-response related genes
Reduced T cells with suppressor function
Cross-reacting epitopes
Inappropriate HLA-DR expression
Mutated T or B cell clones
Activation of T cells by polyclonal stimuli
Re-exposure of antigens by thyroid cell damage

TABLE 10-3. Antibodies in Graves' Disease

Elevated levels of TSAb, TBII, and (rarely) TSBAb
Elevated levels of anti-TPOAb ($\pm 80\%$)
Elevated levels of anti-TGAb ($\pm 50\%$)
Antibodies to DNA
Antibodies to Parietal Cells (infrequent)
Antibodies binding to platelets

relatives in each of the conditions. About 86 percent of patients with previously untreated Graves' disease have antimicrosomal thyroid antibodies, and about 50 percent have anti-TG antibodies. Patients occasionally have antibodies binding specifically T_4 or T_3 (Table 10-3).[23]

TSAb, TSBAb, and Other Thyroid Stimulators

In addition to circulating anti-TG and anti-TPO antibodies, Graves' patients have circulating thyroid stimulators that are gamma globulins. In 1958, Adams announced the discovery that the serum of patients with Graves' disease contained an abnormal thyroid-activating principle.[24] This substance differed from TSH in that it caused a delayed stimulation of the thyroid of the test animal that lasted longer than did the effect of TSH, and was accordingly designated long-acting thyroid stimulator (TSAb or LATS) McKenzie independently confirmed this observation.[25] Since TSAb is an immunoglobulin, it is metabolized in a test animal much more slowly than TSH. The plasma disappearance half-time is approximately seven and a half hours, whereas that of TSH is about 30 minutes.[26] TSAb, or thyroid stimulating antibody, binds to and stimulates the TSH-receptor (TSH-R) on cell membranes.[27] TSAb are not affected by antibodies to TSH but are neutralized by antihuman gamma globulin. TSAb bind to thyroid cell membranes and can displace TSH from its binding site.[27] These antibodies stimulate cell growth, and activate expression of numerous genes including c-fos.[28] The antibodies stimulate thyroid tissue from normal or Graves' disease patients, indicating that the abnormality is in the IgG, not the thyroid.[29]

In a study of 101 patients, McKenzie found TSAb in 8 of 9 persons with exophthalmos and hyperthyroidism, 19 of 25 with hyperthyroidism alone, 19 of 23 exophthalmic patients with previous hyperthyroidism, 1 of 14 who had exophthalmos with no history of hyperthyroidism, and 1 of 25 normal persons.[30] Many other reports documented the association. Transfusions of blood from patients with Graves' disease stimulate the thyroids of recipients, presumably because of the transfer of TSAb.[31] TSAb have been reported to be produced by lymphocytes in vitro,[32,33] and soluble TSH receptor is reported to bind to blood lymphocytes of patients with Graves' disease.[34] These findings emphasize the immune production of the thyroid stimulator.

A slightly different factor that stimulates the thyroid was detected in the blood of patients with Graves' disease[35] who had no LATS. Called human thyroid stimulator (HTS), it differed from LATS in that it failed to stimulate the mouse thyroid (the test animal in the LATS assay), but stimulated colloid droplet formation in epithelial cells in tissue slices of human thyroids. It is probably identical to the serum factor called LATS protector (LATS-P), which was recognized by its stimulatory action on the thyroid[36] and by its ability to protect LATS from inactivation when LATS is in contact with human thyroid extracts. LATS-P appears to be almost always present in sera from patients with Graves' disease that show no LATS activity. The factor is an IgG immunoglobulin[37,38] and is closely related to clinical Graves' disease.

It is now accepted that LATS, LATS-P, and HTS are slightly different immunoglobulins reacting with thyroid tissue, and these activities are now referred to generically as thyroid stimulating immunoglobulins, or, here, as TSAb. The body of published work on this topic, an area of central concern to researchers for a decade, is enormous. A recent review may be consulted for more details.[39]

The serum factors can be detected by stimulation of T_3 secretion from thyroid lobes in vitro and by stimulation of adenyl cyclase activity in tissue slices, cells, or membranes,[40] or activation of lysosomes.[41] In addition to the responses that have in common some evidence of a biologic thyroid stimulatory activity (TSAb), related immunoglobulins can be detected by inhibition of binding of ^{125}I-labeled TSH to thyroid plasma membrane receptors. Such assays are plagued by a variety of eponyms, but perhaps can be generically called thyrotrophin-binding inhibitory immunoglobulin (TBIAb).[42,43] These antibodies are less closely related to in vivo thyroid stimulation.[44] Binding to the receptor may cause stimulation, or no action,[45] or may even antagonize the response to TSH and cause hypothyroidism.[46–49]

Antibodies which block the action of TSH by binding to TSH-R are often referred to as thyroid-stimulating blocking antibodies (TSBAb). It is apparent that a family of antibodies exists with specificity for varying epitopes of the TSH receptor, and also the ability to cross-react with animal TSH receptors or receptors found on fat cell membranes[50] and testes.[51] These antibodies are absorbed or neutralized by interaction with receptor components from thyroid tissue.[52] The immunoglobulins are of several classes, but usually are IgGs, and have a restricted (but not monoclonal) distribution of subtypes.[53] The immunoglobulin can be synthesized in vitro by lymphocytes stimulated by mitogens or plasma membranes.

Depending upon the assay, 80 to 90 percent of Graves' disease patients have positive test results for TSAb. The remainder may have levels too low for detection. Normal subjects rarely have such immunoglobulins. Some patients with thyroiditis have positive test results. The levels and occurrence fall over months and years during and after successful treatment by any means, but may be transiently increased after RAI therapy.[54] Failure of reduction during antithyroid therapy predicts relapse.[55] TSAbs are not usually found in toxic multinodular goiter.[56] A different type of antibody, one that causes cell growth but not hyperfunction, is reported to occur in patients with nontoxic goiter.[57]

Although thyroid-stimulating antibodies occupy center stage in Graves' disease, many other immune reactions occur. Nearly 86 percent of patients have antibodies reacting with microsomal/TPO antigen, and 50 percent have positive antithyroglobulin antibody titers. The role of these antibodies in cell-destructive processes is reviewed in Chapter 7. Occasionally antibodies are produced which specifically bind T_3 or T_4.[23,58] Circulating immune complexes occur in Graves' disease, both with specific antigens (such as thyroglobulin) and with undetermined antigens.[59] Immune complex deposits are formed along the basement membrane of the thyroid cell as well.[60]

The immunologic reactions in Graves' disease involve cell-mediated reactions as well as circulating antibodies. Leukocyte migration inhibition was demonstrated when lymphocytes from patients with Graves' disease were exposed to thyroid antigens.[61,62] Amino and DeGroot[63] showed cell-mediated immunity (CMI) against thyroid antigens in patients with Graves' disease using a lymphotoxin assay system. They observed immunity directed primarily against particulate antigens. CMI did not correlate with FTI, size of the thyroid, or antibodies, but was more severe in thyroiditis and most striking in primary hypothyroidism. Okita et al.[64] demonstrated migration inhibition of Graves' T lymphocytes when exposed to a TSH receptor preparation. Lymphocytes from patients with Graves' disease also demonstrate blastogenesis when exposed to human TG[65] or "microsomal antigen." In our laboratory we have demonstrated that the patients' lymphocytes respond to specific peptide sequences in TPO (aa 110–129, 211–230, 842–861, and 882–901), as well as in TSH-R (aa 44–62, 158–176, 237–252, and 248–263),[66,67] and as well to the extracellular domain of the TSH receptor. While lymphocytes of patients with Graves' disease appear to respond to thyroid antigens, they do not respond abnormally to agents that provoke common delayed hypersensitivity reactions, such as tuberculin,[68] suggesting there is no general hyperimmune state in Graves' disease.

The proven immunologic reactions in Graves' disease thus include potentially cell-destructive antibodies, circulating thyroid stimulatory antibodies, and CMI. We favor the view (see Ch. 7) that normally repressed anti-self-antibody and cell-mediated responses are abnormally amplified in these patients. The response, in our view, encompasses antibodies such as antithyroglobulin, thyroid-stimulating antibodies, antibody reactions affecting orbital tissues, cell-mediated immune responses, and TSH blocking antibodies. The clinical spectrum (Graves' disease, Hashimoto's thyroiditis, and primary myxedema) depends on the balance of these factors in the individual patient.

Hypotheses on the basic cause of the defect in immune homeostasis are reviewed in Chapter 7, but some observations on Graves' disease should be made here. We have recognized defective nonspecific suppressor cell function in untreated toxic Graves' disease and in patients who were thyrotoxic while receiving therapy, using four separate functional assays[69,70] (Fig. 10-1). These results have been confirmed by some groups,[71] but not others.[72,73] We, and others, have also detected in some patients a specific abnormality in antithyroglobulin suppressor cell function. Sridama et al. enumerated lymphocytes by immunofluorescent techniques and found a low suppressor/helper lymphocyte ratio in toxic Graves' patients.[74] This observation was confirmed by Thielemans et al.[75] and Ludgate et al.[76] Topliss et al.[77] have found

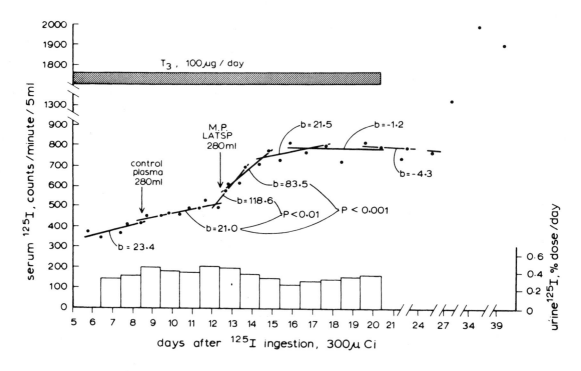

Fig. 10-1. Stimulation of thyroid secretion by LATS-P, a form of TSI. The subject's thyroid iodine was labeled by administration of ^{131}I, and serial observations were made on the appearance of ^{131}I-labeled hormone in blood (ordinate) over one month (abscissa). An infusion of 280 ml control plasma had no effect, but 280 ml plasma from a patient with Graves' disease (and without serum LATS activity) caused a marked stimulation of secretion of hormone from the thyroid. (From Adams et al,[36] with permission.)

evidence for a deficit in Graves' disease of suppressor cells specific for thyroid antigen.

Many conflicting studies of T/B cell ratios in Graves' disease have been reported. Mori et al.[78] reported an increased percentage and total number of B cells and a decreased number of IgG-Fc receptor-bearing T lymphocytes in toxic Graves' patients; both returned to normal when remission was achieved.[79] Similarly, antibody-producing B cells are increased in blood of patients with active Graves' disease.

Numerous studies have examined the status of immunocytes within the thyroid of patients with Graves' disease, usually in patients who have been appropriately prepared for therapeutic partial thyroidectomy. Such patients have increased T and B lymphocytes, which are activated (expressing DR antigens or other markers). Typically, B cells are increased more than T cells. Many reports document a relative decrease of activated "suppressor" cells and a relative increase in activated "helper" cells. The suppressor cells may have diminished function.

Patients with Graves' disease have a hereditary propensity toward making antithyroid antibodies, related to inheritance of specific histocompatibility antigens or specific V genes for B cells or T cell receptor genes, and abnormalities in suppressor cell function. Cross-reacting immunity to environmental antigens may play a role. Stress-induced alterations in suppressor/helper lymphocyte function may enhance immune responses and lead to thyrotoxicosis. Thyroid hyperplasia and thyrotoxicosis may perpetuate the abnormal immune responses by further altering the ratio of suppressor/helper lymphocytes. Lymphocyte infiltration in the thyroid may augment DR expression on thyroid cells and further increase the immune reaction (see also Ch. 7).

Psychic Trauma

Does psychic trauma cause the disease? While there is no proof of this, physicians frequently elicit a history of unusual emotional stress just before the initial symptoms of Graves' disease appear. The increased incidence of thyrotoxicosis in Denmark during World War II[80] has been attributed to psychic stress. In Belgium, on the other hand, the incidence of hyperthyroidism decreased and its severity may have diminished, events that were attributed to the modifying action of chronic undernutrition. Coincidentally, there was a significant increase in the incidence of simple goiter, which may have been the result of a poor diet, high in brassica vegetables. The incidence of thyrotoxicosis has not increased in Northern Ireland in association with the ongoing guerilla warfare during the past two decades. Most studies of the incidence of stressful episodes in lives of patients with Graves' disease do not show a greater incidence of these events than found in controls, yet some data support the association.[81] Patients with Graves' disease do not appear to have unusual pre- or post-morbid personalities. An elevated free thyroxine index (FTI) occurs in about 20 percent of patients with acute psychosis and within a few weeks falls to normal.[82] This elevation is not clearly related to prior use of psychotropic drugs, although this may be a possible explanation.

If psychic stress is involved, what is the pathway? Glucocorticoids probably depress TRH production, and clearly depress TSH secretion and pituitary responsiveness to TRH. A direct action on the thyroid is less clear (see Ch. 4). Glucocorticoids also depress T_4 deiodination to T_3. If the adrenal cortex responds normally to stress with increased production of glucocorticoids, the thyroid hormone supply and immunity should be depressed, not increased. Adrenal cortical secretion is definitely increased in Graves' disease, but this may not be true at the onset of the condition. An adrenal response to stress in a genetically susceptible subject might in theory alter the function of suppressor or helper T lymphocytes, augment a previous immune response, and initiate clinical Graves' disease. Glucocorticoids, however, are primarily immunosuppressive, although the mechanism is unclear. They appear to depress both helper and suppressor T lymphocytes, without—in most studies—clearly altering their ratio.

Sympathetic Nervous System Activation

Sympathetic nervous system stimulation may also be implicated in a stress-induced activation of the thyroid (see ref 83). In animals, α-adrenergic ago-

nists inhibit TSH secretion. This effect is variable and not present in humans. Neither α nor β agonists alter the pituitary response to TRH in humans. α-adrenergic agonists usually cause direct stimulation of thyroid hormone synthesis and release in animals in vivo and in vitro, and cervical sympathetic nerve stimulation increases hormone secretion. β-adrenergic agonists also cause thyroid hormone secretion in animals. Neither α- nor β- adrenergic blockade has been shown to alter thyroid hormone release in humans. β-adrenergic blockade inhibits peripheral tissue conversion of T_4 to T_3, lowers the serum T_3 level, and may occasionally elevate the serum T_4 level, but has not been shown to affect thyroid hormone secretion directly. The bulk of evidence indicates that the autonomic nervous system is not likely to be a route of thyroid activation in Graves' disease.

The interrelations of the sympathetic nervous system and thyroid hormone action are discussed in Chapter 4.

Strenuous Weight Reduction and Thyroid Hormone Administration

Probably related to emotional stress, thyrotoxicosis occasionally begins in the course of weight reduction programs involving severe diet restriction, psychomotor stimulants such as amphetamines, or administration of thyroid hormone. Many instances have been recorded in which patients on such a regimen continued to lose weight after stopping the diet or medication, and then proceeded to develop thyrotoxicosis.[84] Perhaps induced hypermetabolism acts on an organism already susceptible to Graves' disease, or perhaps the metabolic imbalance accompanying weight reduction regimens upsets endocrine or immune system control in a manner similar to that which initiates Graves' disease.

Jodbasedow

The only nonhormonal agent known to produce hyperthyroidism is iodine. Some patients living in endemic goiter areas develop thyrotoxicosis when iodide is administered.[85–88] This phenomenon, called Jodbasedow, occurs when iodide is added to the diet, and the increment need not be large. It is also seen after injection of iodinated oil and administration of saturated solution of KI, roentgenographic contrast media, or drugs containing iodine. The thyroid glands of patients who develop thyrotoxicosis under such circumstances most characteristically are nodular goiters. These glands presumably contain nodules which have escaped from normal control, and when sufficient substrate iodide becomes available, an excess of hormone is produced. We think that the phenomenon is usually a manifestation of a gradually developing autonomy of function in a multinodular goiter. It is also possible that some patients have Graves' disease that does not become manifest until a threshold level of iodine intake is reached. The phenomenon of Jodbasedow is not confined to subjects previously deficient in iodine; thyrotoxicosis occasionally develops after administration of iodine to patients with multinodular goiters who were not iodine deficient earlier.[88] This possibility should be remembered when examining all patients, but especially older persons with toxic nodular goiter, since the hyperthyroidism induced by excess iodide may be self-limiting.[89]

The most thoroughly documented example of epidemic Jodbasedow occurred in Tasmania after iodization of bread. Most of the patients were considered to have long-standing multinodular goiter with autonomous nodules. The iodide supply was the regulator of hormone synthesis in these glands, and when the iodide supply was increased, excess hormone was formed.[86,87,90]

While Jodbasedow is associated primarily with multinodular goiter, in Graves' disease, excess iodine typically acts to suppress hormone formation and release. But in some individuals, who appear to have started with normal thyroids, continued exposure to high levels of iodine (especially in organic form such as iodine-containing antibacterial agents or amiodarone) is followed by thyrotoxicosis which resembles Graves' disease (see Ch. 13).

TSH in Graves' Disease

Excessive TSH is not the usual cause or accompaniment of diffuse thyroid hyperplasia with thyrotoxicosis. The plasma TSH level[91] is low or undetectable in the thyrotoxicosis of Graves' disease, and the pituitary response to TRH is obliterated. When a patient with Graves' disease is made hypothyroid by antithyroid drugs, the plasma TSH level rises, and the thyroid gland undergoes hypertrophy. This reaction indicates that production of TSH is suppressed in thyrotoxicosis and is resumed when the patient becomes hypothyroid. Excessive TSH proba-

bly does cause thyrotoxicosis (although not Graves' disease) in some unusual conditions. Excessive thyrotropin secretion was detected in one patient who evidently produced too much TRH.[92] In patients with pituitary thyrotrophic tumors, thyrotoxicosis is induced by elevated plasma TSH levels.[93,94] TSH level is also elevated in patients thought to have selective pituitary thyroid hormone resistance,[95] described in Chapter 13.

Thyrotoxicosis has been reported in several patients who may be presumed to have had no functioning pituitary,[96,97] and accelerated T_4 formation and secretion, characteristic of the human thyrotoxic thyroid, may persist after the pituitary has been surgically ablated.[98,99]

Although much effort was made in the past to find a relationship, TSH does not appear to cause the ophthalmic findings of Graves' disease. In 1953, Dobyns and Steelman[100] reported the chemical separation of an exophthalmos-producing substance (EPS) from crude thyroid-stimulating hormone preparation. Other workers have corroborated their results.[101] Dutch workers,[102] as well as Dobyns' group, made many assays on normal subjects and patients with Graves' disease and found a correlation between active clinical exophthalmos and elevated serum levels of EPS. Thus, there is semi-historical evidence for a serum factor in Graves' disease that was related to exophthalmos, and was not TSH. Many recent studies suggest but do not yet prove a role for antibodies which bind to eye muscle membranes, or stimulate mucopolysaccharide formation, or are active in antibody dependent cell-mediated cytotoxicity. The cause of exophthalmos is discussed in detail in Chapter 12.

Chorionic Gonadotropin

Hyperthyroidism (but not Graves' disease) may be induced by a stimulator produced by trophoblastic tissue. Many patients with hyperthyroidism in association with hydatidiform mole and choriocarcinoma have been reported.[103,104] This trophoblastic thyrotropin is not an IgG, but weakly cross-reacts immunologically with human or bovine TSH. Much evidence indicates that it is either hCG, which shares an identical α subunit with TSH, or a desialated derivative of hCG. Some patients with hydatiform moles or choriocarcinomas have evidence of chemical thyrotoxicosis without clinical thyrotoxicosis. A factor causing peripheral resistance to thyroid hormone has been postulated in these cases. TSH-like activity and hyperthyroidism have been reported in a patient with an embryonal carcinoma of the testis. These effects are probably also due to the weak TSH-like action of hCG produced by these tumors.

Patients with hyperemesis of pregnancy typically have elevated thyroid T_4, sometimes elevated T_3, and often suppressed TSH. Some of these patients, especially with 2- to 3-fold elevated T_4 and FTI appear to be clinically toxic, although this is less obvious in patients with mildly elevated FTI levels. Those with severe elevation of FTI and clinical evidence of thyrotoxicosis require treatment with antithyroid drugs, which alleviates the thyrotoxicosis. If hyperemesis subsides, the thyroid abnormalities also cease in most instances. Considerable evidence indicates that high levels of hCG may be responsible for this syndrome.[105] The problem is examined in detail in Chapter 13.

External Irradiation to the Thyroid

A group of individuals have been reported who developed exophthalmos or thyrotoxicosis after receiving cervical radiotherapy for treatment of malignant tumors.[5] Theoretically such irradiation, which damages the thyroid and may produce hypothyroidism, could liberate antigens and initiate autoimmune thyroid disease.

In summary, the diffuse thyroid hyperplasia and thyrotoxicosis of Graves' disease are caused by one of several immunoglobulin factors circulating in the blood. CMI may also be involved in the associated changes of Graves' disease, but its role is less clear. Only rarely is thyrotoxicosis caused by an elevation of authentic TSH arising from the pituitary or by a stimulator having its origin in trophoblastic cells or other causes, as described in Chapter 13, and these conditions do not produce Graves' disease.

Numerous other theories regarding the cause of Graves' disease have been proposed in the past. For a critical review of earlier speculations and a superb bibliography, the reader is referred to the monograph by Iversen.[80]

Hereditary Familial Hyperthyroidism

Duprez and co-workers[106] have recently recognized the cause of nonautoimmune hyperthyroidism inherited in an autosomal dominant mother. In two sibships, activating germline mutations were found in the transmembrane segments of the TSH-R. The mutations cause persistent basal hyperfunction of the receptor and early onset of thyrotoxicosis.

PATHOGENESIS

Thyroid Gland Function

While the ultimate cause or causes of Graves' disease remain uncertain, the pathophysiologic mechanisms and pathogenesis are more clear. The thyroid gland is functioning at an accelerated rate. Cell membrane adenyl cyclase activity in tissue from Graves' patients is higher than in normal thyroids, and the increment coincides with TSAb in the serum,[107] which acts on TSH receptors to cause the response. Clearance of plasma iodide by the gland is increased from the normal rate of 10 to 20 ml/min to 40 to several hundred ml/min. In one patient, we have estimated iodide clearance to exceed 2 L/min. For this reason, the percentage of a tracer dose of ^{131}I found in the gland at 24 hours is characteristically elevated. Thyroid peroxidase activity is increased. Because of rapid secretion, the period of retention of iodine within the thyroid is reduced, causing the characteristic drop in RAIU between 12 and 24 hours after administration of a tracer. The total quantity of iodine in the gland is variable. In the past it tended to be reduced, but now it is often elevated because of increasing amounts of iodine in our diet. The volume of the gland is characteristically but not invariably increased. Thyroid hormones, TG, small amounts of an iodinated albumin-like protein,[108] and iodotyrosines[109] are released into the blood at increased rates. The latter two components are normally either not secreted or are released in minute amounts.

Many studies with radioiodine have confirmed the accelerated physiologic activity of the thyroid in Graves' disease. Labeled hormones appear as plasma $PB^{131}I$ more rapidly and reach higher levels than in normal persons after administration of ^{131}I. The rate of turnover of plasma hormones is also increased. Accelerated degradation is almost certainly secondary to hypermetabolism and not a primary event,[110] although it has been reported that accelerated T_4 turnover persists after therapy for thyrotoxicosis.[111]

With the general hyperactivity of the thyroid, excess TG is released and serum TG levels are elevated in active Graves' disease. After therapy the levels tend to fall, and normalization during antithyroid therapy is an excellent predictor of remission.[112] This excessive release of TG leads to formation of circulating immune complexes with anti-TG antibodies, and can lower the titer of these antibodies in the serum.

An important abnormality in thyroid function during Graves' disease is that the uptake of ^{131}I by the thyroid is not suppressed by administration of exogenous T_4 or T_3.[113,114] This holds true even if large amounts of hormone are given. Indeed, administration of T_3 may cause, on average, a slight increase in the 24-hour radioiodine uptake. This abnormal response to the administration of thyroid hormone occurs in spite of responsiveness of the thyroid to administered exogenous TSH, as measured by augmented release of thyroid hormone. It may persist after thyrotoxicosis has been ameliorated by surgery, but typically suppressibility eventually returns after treatment. Nonsuppressibility is observed so regularly that for many years it was used in doubtful cases as a criterion for diagnosis. Nonsuppressibility is caused by stimulation of the thyroid by TSAb, and independence of feedback control by TSH. There is a general, but not complete, correlation between T_3 nonsuppressibility and positive assays for TSAb.[115] Even long after apparent remission of Graves' disease, some patients show some resistance to T_3 suppression or TSH stimulation.[116] Also, some euthyroid relatives of Graves' disease patients show these abnormalities in the absence of overt thyroid disease.

The pituitary does not respond to TRH in the thyrotoxic state, either in hyperthyroid Graves' disease or when thyroid hormone is administered. Some patients with euthyroid Graves' disease respond to TRH and others do not; the responses do not correlate with the results of T_3 suppression tests.[117,118] For the diagnosis of Graves' disease, suppression of serum TSH is currently the most useful criterion, as it is more convenient than the TRH test and preferable to the T_3 suppression test in patients with heart disease. In patients with euthyroid Graves' disease, test results are not uniformly abnormal.

Effects of Iodine

Iodide affects the metabolism of the diffusely hyperplastic thyrotoxic gland in a way radically different from its action on the normal gland. Years ago,

Plummer demonstrated that Graves' disease can be temporarily or permanently controlled by the administration of iodide.[119] The amount needed is 6 mg/day or more. Administration of large doses of iodide to laboratory animals causes a temporary inhibition of iodide organification, the Wolff-Chaikoff block. High intrathyroidal iodide concentration is the crucial factor inducing this response.[120] The same phenomenon occurs in humans, and thyrotoxic patients are especially sensitive to this effect. The thyroid uptake of ^{131}I is acutely depressed in thyrotoxic patients by administration of 2 mg potassium iodide, whereas more than 5 mg is needed to depress uptake in normal subjects.[121] Concentrations of serum iodide above 5 μg/dl block binding in the thyrotoxic gland.[122]

The biochemical mechanism of the Wolff-Chaikoff block is not clear. Iodide does not prevent TSH or TSAb binding to the TSH membrane receptor, but does inhibit both TSH-stimulated adenyl cyclase production of cAMP, and cAMP actions. Since iodide inhibition of cAMP production and action is blocked by methimazole, it is hypothesized that an oxidized iodide intermediate is involved. Alternatively, the block of iodination may be caused by depression of H_2O_2 generation. It is not known if the inhibition of iodide transport and binding relate to the recognized changes in cAMP formation (see Ch. 2).

In animals the block of iodide binding is transient; during continuous iodide administration, binding recommences. This escape also occurs in most normal humans. Few individuals who take large doses of iodine continuously develop myxedema. Adaptation to excess iodine in animals involves a reduction of iodide transport into the thyroid, a lowering of intrathyroidal iodide content, and escape from the Wolff-Chaikoff block. This adaptation occurs independently of TSH action. Possibly because the Graves' gland is hyperactive under continued stimulation by TSAb, it remains blocked by administered iodide, and hormone production remains suppressed. A similar sensitivity to inhibition by iodide occurs in Hashimoto's thyroiditis, hyperfunctional adenomas, and possibly the normal gland when stimulated by exogenous TSH.[123] Myxedema can often by induced by administration of iodide to patients who have had a partial thyroidectomy for Graves' disease.[124,125] Thus, there is an inherent susceptibility of these glands to the action of iodine.

Sensitivity of the thyroid gland in Graves' disease

to iodide is also demonstrated with the iodide-perchlorate test.[124] This test shows that the dose of iodide required to block organification in Graves' disease is much smaller than that in the normal subject. The inhibition of binding by iodide is revealed by administration of perchlorate, which discharges the accumulated ^{131}I present in the gland as free iodide.

Coincident with the block in uptake, iodide also causes a marked reduction in the release of previously formed hormone from the thyrotoxic gland. This phenomenon has been repeatedly observed[126] and helps to explain the beneficial therapeutic effect of iodide in Graves' disease, as originally recognized by Plummer. Iodide administration blocks release of hormone from the gland but does not completely prevent hormone synthesis, for under these circumstances the gland gradually accumulates an increased store of organic iodine. Ochi et al.[127] have shown that chronic administration of iodide in Graves' disease blocks the stimulating effect on hormone release of both TSH and TSAb. It is this block of release, rather than a block of hormone synthesis, that is responsible for the dramatic rapid beneficial therapeutic effects of iodide administration.[128,129] The block of hormone release that occurs in the thyroid of patients with Graves' disease can be observed, although not uniformly, in the normal gland and in the normal gland made hyperactive by repeated administration of exogenous TSH. Iodide also inhibits the release of hormone from autonomous hyperfunctioning adenomas, presumably in the absence of endogenous TSH. This observation also indicates that iodide block is by a direct action on the thyroid gland.

Thus, the Graves' gland appears to be unusually sensitive to small amounts of iodide, as manifested by, first, a block of iodide uptake and binding and, second, a block of hormone release. Perhaps these are two parts of the same fundamental process. Sensitivity to iodide may be related to the TSAb dependent, hyperactive, iodide-concentrating mechanism of the Graves' gland.

A further abnormality in intrathyroid iodine metabolism of the gland was described by Slingerland and Burrows[130] and by DeGroot.[131] They demonstrated that the toxic gland continuously releases into the circulation large amounts of nonthyroxine iodide, in addition to hormone. The iodide may be a product of the deiodination of iodotyrosines released from TG during its hydrolysis.

INCIDENCE

Outside an endemic goiter region, thyrotoxicosis currently is usually equal in frequency to Hashimoto's thyroiditis, about eight times as common as myxedema, and more common than nontoxic nodular goiter. In Minnesota the incidence has recently been 0.3 cases per 1,000 population annually.[132] Iversen's data[80] suggested a rate of about 0.2 per 1,000 in pre-World War II Copenhagen. Tunbridge and co-workers[133] conducted a complete survey of an English town, examining 2,779 people for evidence of thyroid disease. The total incidence of past and present Graves' disease was 2.7 percent in women and 0.23 percent in men. In the same survey, they found hypothyroidism to be about two-thirds as common; antithyroid antibodies were present in 10.3 percent of women, and goiters in 15 percent of women. They estimate the incidence of thyrotoxicosis to be 1 to 2 cases per 1,000 per year, several-fold higher than previously recognized.

Geographic Distribution

There is not much information relating Graves' disease to geographic factors. A survey in Sweden did not suggest a relationship between the incidence of endemic goiter and Graves' disease.[134] Statistical studies have suggested that in the United States there may be a relationship between the incidence of nodular goiter and that of thyrotoxicosis (of all causes), but many of the thyrotoxic patients had toxic nodular goiter rather than the diffuse hyperplasia of Graves' disease.[135] Evidence also does not support a variation in the severity of Graves' disease among areas.

Epidemiology

A retrospective study of the incidence of Graves' disease in Olmsted County, Minnesota, from 1935 to 1967, found no noteworthy trend in the incidence of disease, which was 30.5 cases per 10^5 persons each year.[132] During World War II, occupied Denmark experienced a three- to fourfold increase in the incidence of Graves' disease. Shortly after the country was liberated from the Germans, however, the incidence returned to its peacetime value.[80] In Iversen's study, thyrotoxicosis showed a clearcut seasonal variation, with a peak hospital admission rate in the summer.

Perhaps the most carefully documented epidemic of thyrotoxicosis is the one that occurred in Tasmania, but this was not in fact an epidemic of Graves' disease. Circumstances were particularly favorable for study, because all the patients were hospitalized in only two hospitals. The epidemic started in 1966, a few months after the baking industry began using potassium iodate as a bread conditioner.[86] Surveys disclosed that this product caused an increase of 80 to 270 μg/day of iodide in the diet. Tasmania had long been known as a region of mild endemic goiter, with low average iodine intake in the population. The epidemic reached its peak about a year after it began, when there was a quadrupling of the annual admission rate. The epidemic then slowly subsided. The age distribution was skewed toward older age groups, and most of these patients had toxic nodular goiters. There was no rise in exophthalmos in the population, and most cases were mild.

Age Distribution

The age distribution of Graves' disease spreads over the entire span of human life. It is encountered from infancy to old age. The peak of the age distribution curve is in the third and fourth decade, and seems to have no relation to geographic location.

Sex Distribution

The sex distribution of Graves' disease, like that of myxedema and Hashimoto's thyroiditis, shows a decided preponderance of females: the disease is seven to ten times as frequent in females as in males. Myxedema is also more common in females, where the ratio of females to males is about 9:1. Indeed, all types of thyroid disorder, except perhaps anaplastic cancer, are more common in females. The reason for this is unknown.

Racial Incidence

The disease has been reported from all races.

Familial Incidence

The remarkable prevalence of Graves' disease in certain families has been described above, along with information relating this finding to inheritance of specific histocompatibility antigens.

PATHOLOGY

It should be noted that only the abnormalities of the thyroid, orbital contents, lymphatic system, and skin can be considered specific for Graves' disease; the other lesions may be caused by thyrotoxicosis of any cause.

The Thyroid

It is known from observations made before the introduction of iodide or antithyroid drugs that the essential lesion of Graves' disease is parenchymatous hypertrophy and hyperplasia (Fig. 10-2). The central features are increased height of the epithelium from cuboidal to columnar; and redundancy of the follicular wall, giving on section the picture of papillary infoldings, cytologic evidence of increased activity, hypertrophy of the Golgi apparatus, increased number of mitochondria, and increased vacuolization of colloid. There is probably nothing specific about the hyperplasia. Any stimulus that calls for sus-

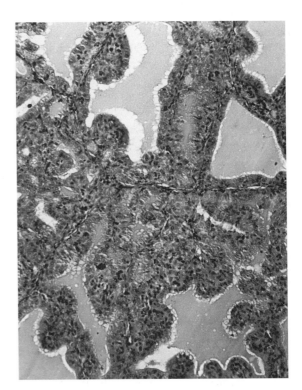

Fig. 10-2. Extreme thyroid hyperplasia found in a patient with untreated Graves' disease.

tained hyperfunction produces this picture, such as antithyroid drugs. There is also a characteristic lymphocyte and plasma cell infiltrate. This infiltrate may be mild and diffuse throughout the gland, but more typically occurs as aggregates of mononuclear cells and even lymphoid germinal centers, referred to as *focal thyroiditis*. Occasionally the histologic pattern completely overlaps that of Hashimoto's thyroiditis.

Fine structure examination discloses a rather widely varying size and shape of the follicles, with columnar cells and reduced homogeneous colloid.[136] The basement membrane is well demarcated and is 400 to 1,000 Å thick. Between the follicles is a large array of capillaries, together with lymphocytes and fibrocytes. The apical end of the follicular cell often bulges into the lumen and cuplike villi extend into the lumen. Vesicles and free ribosomes may be found in these villi. These microvilli vary in size and shape; some may enclose colloid. The nucleus is near the basal part of the cell. The mitochondria are numerous; they are mostly large, elongated structures, and some are branched. The endoplasmic reticulum is usually well developed. Ribosomes occur in great numbers. The Golgi apparatus is well developed. Vesicles are present in abundance, but vary in size and number from cell to cell. Multivesicular bodies are occasionally found near the Golgi apparatus. Droplets, globules, and dense bodies appear. Phagolysosomes are common. All these changes are similar to those of the normal thyroid chronically stimulated by TSH.

There are some data on the thyroid of persons who have recovered from Graves' disease.[137] Autopsy material from seven patients who had recovered from exophthalmic goiter and later died of other causes showed complete regression of the hyperplastic changes.

Extrathyroidal Changes

The ophthalmologic problem and pretibial myxedema, both unique to Graves' disease, are described in Chapter 11.

Abnormalities in striated muscle may be a part of Graves' disease.[138-140] Askanazy and Rutishauser[141] studied four patients with hyperthyroidism on whom autopsies were performed. They found a diffuse process in all striated muscles, including the extrinsic muscles of the eyeball, consisting of degenerative atrophy of muscle cells, fatty infiltration, loss of stria-

tion and uniform appearance, vacuolization, and proliferation or degeneration of nuclei. Cardiac and smooth muscle were not involved in this process. Not all muscle groups were equally involved, nor were the same muscles involved in different patients.

Dudgeon and Urquhart,[142] in studies of the muscles in nine postmortem cases of Graves' disease, found interstitial myositis in various skeletal muscles, characterized by plasma cells, tissue macrophages, and atrophy of fibers. Ocular muscles were more affected and cardiac muscle less affected than skeletal muscle. The lesions were spotty and were observed in only a small fraction of the sections. On the other hand, Naffziger[143] examined biopsy muscle specimens from other parts of the body in patients with the ophthalmopathy of Graves' disease and found no abnormalities. The fat content of skeletal muscle may be increased, as in the extraocular muscles.[144]

Myocardial degenerative lesions have been reported in thyrotoxicosis, with foci of cell necrosis, mononuclear infiltrates, and mucopolysaccharide deposits similar to those described in extraocular and skeletal muscles,[145] and severe damage has been found in patients dying of thyrotoxicosis[146] (Fig. 10-3).

The extraocular muscle lesions are probably specific for Graves' disease, whereas the remainder of the abnormalities may reflect the action of excess hormone.

Not surprisingly, the anterior pituitary demonstrates a dramatic decrease in identifiable thyrotro-

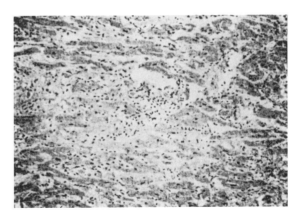

Fig. 10-3. Appearance of cardiac muscle from a patient who died from thyrotoxicosis and acute cardiovascular collapse.

pin-containing cells in patients dying in thyroid storm. This loss is found to be entirely reversed in patients who are autopsied after treatment to euthyroidism.[147–149]

Lesions specific for Graves' disease do not appear in the parathyroids, gonads, or pancreas.

Studies based on autopsies of patients with Graves' disease made years ago demonstrated focal and even diffuse liver cell necrosis,[150] atrophy, and cirrhosis, including a kind of peripheral fibrosis that was believed to be peculiar to this disease—cirrhosis Basedowiana. In more contemporary series of liver biopsy specimens obtained from thyrotoxic persons, the deviations from normal were minimal.[151,152] Some decrease in glycogen and increase in fat, and some round cell infiltrates, were noted. The lesser severity and duration of the disease in those patients studied during life partly explains the differences among these studies.

Hyperplastic changes may be found in the spleen, thymus, and lymph nodes in Graves' disease. The thymus occasionally presents as an anterior mediastinal mass[153] and has been inadvertently resected. Persistence or enlargement of the thymus was once believed to be significant in Graves' disease, and early in the century thymectomies were performed for its treatment, with apparent benefit.

Prolonged hyperthyroidism is known to cause osteoporosis.[154] The bones of patients with thyrotoxicosis have been examined in several studies. Cook et al.[155] found only osteoporosis in bone biopsy specimens, but both Askanazy and Rutishauser[141] and Follis[156] found evidence of bone destruction. Follis found osteitis fibrosa in the vertebrae of all 20 patients he examined. Four of the group also had evidence of osteoporosis, which may be a reflection in part of the predominant age and sex of the group of patients having thyrotoxicosis. Histomorphometric studies show clear evidence of excess bone formation and resorption. The high degree of exchangeability of calcium in the bones of patients with thyrotoxicosis and the high rate of loss of calcium in the urine are discussed later in this chapter. Serum ^{1,25}dihydroxycholecalciferol is decreased, probably in response to increased bone tumor.[157]

Cytologic investigations of mitochondria using the electron microscope have revealed anatomic lesions not visible by light microscopy. Schulz et al.[158] reported that the mitochondria from tissues of T_4-treated animals appeared to be swollen.

DEVELOPMENT OF THE CLINICAL PICTURE AND THE COURSE OF THE DISEASE

Graves' disease displays an array of possible clinical patterns extending from that of goiter and thyrotoxicosis, but without ophthalmopathy, to that of ophthalmopathy without goiter or thyrotoxicosis.

Onset of the Disease

In classic exophthalmic goiter, or Graves' disease, the most common onset is the simultaneous and gradual development, over a period of weeks or months, of the symptoms of thyrotoxicosis, enlargement of the thyroid, and prominence or related abnormality of the eyes (Fig. 10-3). It is quite possible for classic Graves' disease to develop in a patient with preceding (and probably unrelated) nontoxic goiter. This is common in a goitrous country.

Often the onset of symptoms is so gradual that it is difficult or impossible for the patient or physician to fix its date. The more abrupt onset may sometimes be sufficiently rapid to justify the term *fulminating*. The picture of classic full-blown exophthalmic goiter has appeared in a person apparently previously well in as short a period as two to five days. In rare cases, patients have first developed hypothyroidism and later thyrotoxicosis,[46,47] probably because the initial development of TBIAb is followed by some natural immune modulation and development of stimulatory antibodies.

In many patients, the symptoms of Graves' disease are first noted after some emotional trauma. These associations are certainly of importance in understanding the patient's background, but, as noted above, whether or not they bear a causal relationship to the development of Graves' disease remains conjectural.

As noted in Chapter 14, Graves' disease is frequently partially or totally suppressed during pregnancy, and initial or recurrent manifestations can occur in the postpartum period. Sometimes the "painless thyroiditis" characteristic of this period coexists and masks the development of Graves' disease.[48]

Weight reduction, as mentioned above, has also been linked to Graves' disease.

Course of the Disease

The natural history of the thyrotoxic process is usually altered by definitive therapy. Before the availability of good treatment, however, hyperthyroidism tended to progress through periods of exacerbation and remission. In perhaps a quarter of the patients, especially those with a mild form of the disease, the process was self-limited to one year or more, as the patients spontaneously returned to a euthyroid state.

Thyrotoxicosis with Spontaneous Remission

M.S., a 27-year-old male physician, developed tachycardia, hyperkinesis, decreased heat tolerance, slight tremor, and weight loss over 3 or 4 months. On examination, blood pressure (BP) was 150/150, pulse rate 86, and the skin was sweaty. There was a fine tremor. The eyes were entirely normal. There was a grade 1 precordial systolic murmur. The thyroid was about twice the normal size, diffusely enlarged, and firm. There were several cervical lymph nodes bilaterally. PBI was 11, and the rT_3U level was elevated. RAIU was 57 percent and BMR-10. All tests were repeated, and the results remained as indicated.

The patient was given 100 mg PTU three times daily and was maintained on this program for 18 months. During this time, the T_4 level was maintained in the range of 7.3 $\mu g/dl$ and the FTI in the range of 6; the white cell count remained normal. The TGHA titer was 1/320, and there was a borderline positive TSAb bioassay response. During the course of therapy, the 20-minute technetium uptake test was repeatedly measured while the patient received both antithyroid drugs and suppressive doses of T_3; suppressibility of the thyroid gradually fell to the normal range. Eighteen months after the initiation of therapy, the patient developed an acute gastroenteritis and was briefly hospitalized. At this time, because of the possible association of PTU with gastric irritation, the medication was discontinued.

M.S. subsequently remained well for three months, but then developed symptoms of mild hyperthyroidism. The thyroid was again found to be two to three times the normal size, the T_4 level to be 10.3 $\mu g/dl$, and the FTI to be 11.9. Since the symptoms were mild, the decision was made to observe events without therapy for a period. Initially, the symptoms, signs, and laboratory test results remained abnormal, but over several months the mild tachycardia, increased sweating, and increased nervousness gradually dissipated. Six months later, the T_4 level was 6.7 $\mu g/dl$ and the FTI 8. The TSAb bioassay result remained positive. No further treatment was given, and the patient has remained entirely well with a moderate thyroid enlargement, normal thyroid function test results, and no symptoms over the subsequent 20 years.

In one of the few documented reports of untreated thyrotoxicosis, White[159] found that of 12 patients, 7 died in an average of three and a half years and the remainder lived on without therapy. From a large series, Sattler estimated that in the past, mortality was as high as 11 percent.[160] Fortunately, death due to hyperthyroidism is now rare, but we are aware of two patients who died of severe undiagnosed and untreated thyrotoxicosis in Chicago within the past four years.[146] Deaths are attributed most frequently to cardiovascular complications such as myocardial infarction, arrythmia, or heart failure, or infections secondary to debility. Some patients become spontaneously hypothyroid, and in fact most individuals apparently cured of Graves' thyrotoxicosis demonstrate evidence of hypothyroidism decades later. Coincident autoimmune thyroiditis presumably plays a role in such thyroid atrophy. Since all current treatments of thyrotoxicosis are associated with the spontaneous reestablishment of thyroid homeostasis after a period of enforced reduction in hormone formation (by drugs, surgery, or ^{131}I treatment), it is obvious that the thyrotoxic phase of the disease tends to be self-limiting in many patients.

Toxic crisis, or thyroid storm, was also a frequent feature of Graves' disease in the past. This serious and often fatal development is an extreme instance of thyrotoxicosis, with hyperthermia, uncontrolled tachycardia, weakness, and delirium. This condition, now rarely encountered, is discussed in Chapter 12.

The ophthalmopathy of Graves' disease may follow a course quite different from that of thyrotoxicosis. This topic is also discussed in Chapter 12.

CLINICAL MANIFESTATIONS OF THYROTOXICOSIS

In patients with Graves' disease, the ocular changes, lymphoid hyperplasia, localized abnormalities of skin and connective tissue (e.g., acropachy) and the goiter itself represent parts of the autoimmune syndrome. The remainder of the changes appear to be entirely attributable to an excess of thyroid hormone. Certain systems or organs (e.g., the muscles and cardiovascular system) play paramount roles in the disease, but as far as can be determined, these changes are all fundamentally related to and dependent on the excessive serum concentration of thyroid hormones.

Symptoms and Signs

The symptoms may be any of the classic ones of hyperthyroidism. Often the presenting symptoms are weight loss, weakness, dyspnea, palpitations, increased thirst or appetite, hyperdefecation, irritability, profuse sweating, sensitivity to heat or increased tolerance to cold, or tremor. Occasionally, prominence of the eyes or diplopia is the apparent symptom, and goiter may long antedate all other manifestations. Often a relative or friend notices eye signs, goiter, or nervous phenomena before the patient is conscious of any departure from his or her usual status. This asymptomatic phase of thyrotoxicosis is more commonly found in men and children. The excess of thyroid hormone produces an intoxication that in some persons takes the form of exhilaration. They may feel not only healthy but healthier than usual while exhibiting unmistakable signs of thyrotoxicosis. In older patients particularly, the symptom or symptoms may point to the heart more than to any other part of the body, since thyrotoxicosis frequently masquerades as heart disease.

The habitus in Graves' disease shows nothing characteristic. In childhood, those afflicted are tall for their age. This association is an effect of the disease, not an etiologically related variable.

The nutritional state varies greatly. Sometimes the patient is severely emaciated, but on average the weight loss is 5 to 20 lbs. Infrequently, perhaps in 1 out of 10 instances, the patient actually gains weight while thyrotoxic.

The facies may betray very little, or it may instantly provide the diagnosis. An expression of fright or extreme anxiousness is common, largely because of the peculiar eye signs that may be present. Marked flushing is often noted. A drawn or sunken appearance may result from emaciation or dehydration. It is possible, especially in older patients, to find a considerable degree of thyrotoxicosis without any distinguishing evidence in the facies.

A change in reaction to external temperature is a good symptom. The development of a preference for cold weather, of a desire for less clothing and less bed covering, and of decreased ability to tolerate hot weather is highly suggestive of hyperthyroidism.

The tongue tends to be red and smooth; it may also exhibit a definite tremor. The tonsils, if present, are usually rather large, as is the postpharyngeal lymphoid tissue.

The neck is usually conspicuous due to the goiter. It is possible, although rare, for thyrotoxicosis to exist without a visible or palpable goiter. We note reports in the literature that up to a quarter of patients may not have a goiter,[161] but this is not our experience. In the neck, the carotids will often be seen to throb violently; this condition may contribute to the anxiety of the patient.

The eye signs characteristic of Graves' disease often constitute the most striking feature (Figs. 10-4 to 10-6, Table 10-4). Prominence of the eyes is the most important sign. A wild or staring expression is often observed. Lag of the lids behind the globes on downward rotation and lag of the globes behind the lids in upward rotation, infrequent blinking, failure to wrinkle the forehead on looking upward, and decreased ability to converge are also cardinal manifestations. Swelling of the lids is a characteristic and

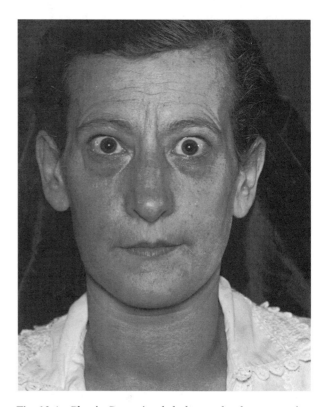

Fig. 10-4. Classic Graves' ophthalmopathy demonstrating a widened palpebral fissure, periorbital edema, proptosis, chemosis, and conjunctival injection.

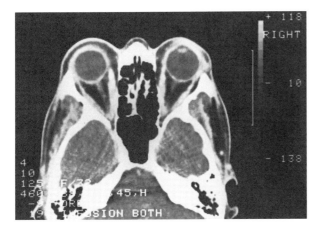

Fig. 10-5. CAT image of enlarged extraocular muscles in a patient with Graves' ophthalmopathy.

frequent eye sign. The bulbar conjunctiva may be edematous (chemosis). The insertions of the medial and lateral rectus muscles are often enlarged, inflamed, and quite obvious (Fig. 10-4). The lacrimal gland may protrude below the orbital bone margin.

For convenience, the ophthalmic phenomena may be grouped as in Table 10-1. A classification of the eye changes and a system of grading of their severity have been adopted by the American Thyroid Association[162] and is given in Chapter 12.

The eye signs may vary independently of the intensity of the thyrotoxicosis. Although it is true that in most patients with Graves' disease, eye signs, goiter, and symptoms of thyrotoxicosis appear more or less coincidentally, it is also true that in certain cases eye signs become worse when the thyrotoxicosis is subsiding. Indeed, in some patients, serious exophthalmos may develop at a time when the thyrotoxicosis has been controlled by treatment.

The eye symptoms of Graves' disease are extremely distressing. Diplopia is common, while decreased visual acuity and other visual disturbances are less so. More frequent are symptoms due to conjunctival or corneal irritation. These symptoms include burning, photophobia, tearing, pain, and a gritty or sandy sensation.

Horner's syndrome on one side is occasionally encountered when the goiter has pressed upon the trunk of the cervical sympathetic chain. This syndrome consists of unilateral enophthalmos, ptosis of the lid, and miosis, as well as decreased sweating on the homolateral face.

TABLE 10-4. Ocular Signs and Symptoms in Graves' Disease

Ophthalmic phenomena reflecting thyrotoxicosis per se and apparently resulting from sympathetic overactivity:
    Lid reaction
    Wide palpebral aperture (Dalrymple's sign)
    Lid lag (von Graefe's sign)
    Staring or frightened expression
    Infrequent blinking (Stellwag's sign)
    Absence of forehead wrinkling on upward gaze (Joffroy's sign)
Ophthalmic phenomena unique for Graves' disease and caused by specific pathologic changes in the orbit and its contents:
    Inability to keep the eyeballs converged (Mobius' sign)
    Limitation of movement of the eyeballs, especially upward
    Diplopia
    Blurred vision due to inadequate convergence and accommodation
    Swelling of orbital contents and puffiness of the lids
    Chemosis, corneal injection, or ulceration
    Irritation of the eye or pain in the globe
    Exophthalmos (also produces mechanically a wide palpebral fissure)
    Visible and palpable enlargement of the lacrimal glands
    Visible swelling of lateral rectus muscles as they insert into the globe, and injection of the overlying vessels
    Decreased visual acuity due to papilledema, retinal edema, retinal hemorrhages, or optic nerve damage

The Thyroid

The thyroid may be smooth, lobulated, or rarely nodular. In thyrotoxicosis associated with nodular goiters, the hyperfunctioning tissue may reside between the nodules,[163] which would constitute Graves' disease in a nodular goiter. Often the surface is lobulated, and the upper poles may seem to contain nodules above the site of entry of the superior thyroid artery.

The diffuse toxic goiter is usually more or less symmetric. The size is related, but not closely, to the severity of the disease. It varies from the barely palpable normal (15 to 20 g) to an enlargement of six times normal (100 g) or, rarely, even more, but averages about 45 g. The near symmetry and usually moderate size of the diffuse goiter of Graves' disease make it somewhat less unsightly than many of the nodular goiters. It is commonly stated that the gland is not palpable in 1 percent of cases, either percent

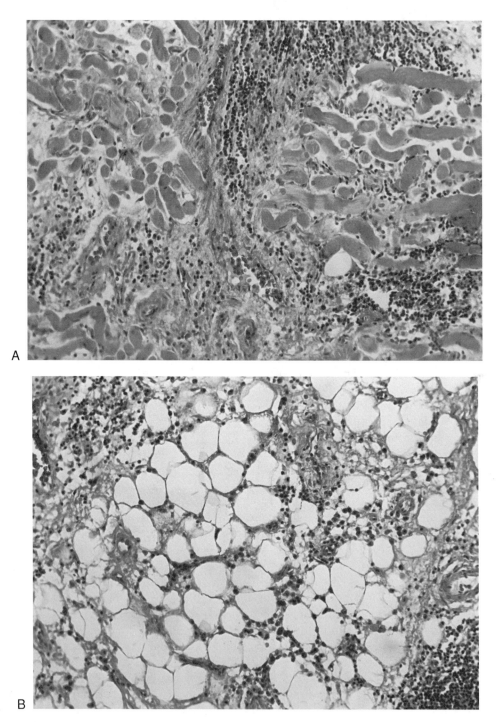

A

B

Fig. 10-6. Histologic appearance of *(A)* extraocular muscle, *(B)* retrobulbar fat, and *(C)* lacrimal gland removed during a Kronlein procedure on a patient with severe exophthalmos. *(Figure Continues.)*

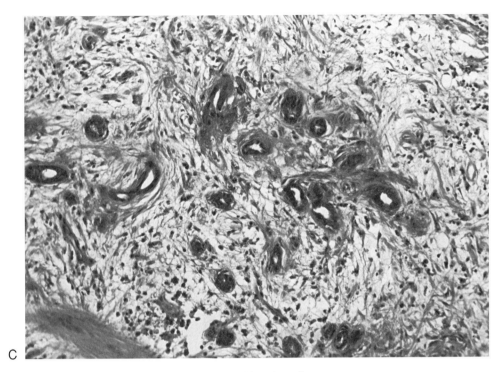

C

Fig. 10-6. (Continued).

because the thyroid is actually smaller than normal or because it is beneath the manubrium. In the presence of thyrotoxicosis, however, a small or normal-sized thyroid should alert the physician to the possibility of some other cause of the illness.

The consistency of diffuse toxic glands is firm but elastic, or very firm if iodide has been given. The borders are easily demarcated by palpation. The pyramidal lobe should always be searched for since enlargement indicates the presence of diffuse disease of the thyroid. Also, if left behind at operation, it may be the site of recurrence of the disease.

Thrills and bruits are important but often absent. Their presence usually denotes hyperfunction. A thrill is less common than a bruit. It is more likely to be felt as a systolic purr in the region of the superior poles over the superior thyroid arteries. Bruits may be continuous or systolic in time, similar to a blowing cardiac murmur. Usually they are audible over the entire thyroid, often being louder on one side than on the other. Either a thrill or a bruit is highly suggestive, but not pathognomonic, of thyrotoxicosis. If local examination of a goiter discloses either of these signs, even though other evidence

of hyperfunction may be lacking, especially careful investigation into the possibility of thyrotoxicosis is indicated. Both thrills and bruits tend to decrease in intensity as thyrotoxicosis subsides. They completely disappear in a few days under treatment with iodide.

The thrill is the palpable and the bruit the audible sign of turbulence associated with an increased rate of flow through rather tortuous vessels. The location of the thrill suggests that the larger thyroid vessels are chiefly responsible. Bruits may be distinguished from venous hums by occlusion of venous return by gentle pressure above the thyroid. A carotid or innominate thrill or bruit may be difficult to distinguish from sounds originating in the thyroid gland. Their localization over the vessel and distal transmission usually allow a distinction to be made.

Neighborhood symptoms, including dysphagia and the sensation of a lump in the neck, may be produced by toxic as well as nontoxic varieties of goiter. Sometimes the supraclavicular lymph nodes become enlarged and tender.[164]

Vocal cord palsy is encountered, but is found chiefly in cancer of the thyroid, occasionally in nodular goiter, and only rarely in Graves' disease. Occasionally it is found on routine preoperative laryngoscopic examination, having produced no symptoms such as dysphonia or hoarseness.

The Skin

Cutaneous manifestations are nearly always present when hypermetabolism is significant. The patient feels hot and prefers a cold environment. Active sweating occurs under circumstances that would provoke no response in normal persons. Hand shaking can give a nearly diagnostic impression: the hand of the thyrotoxic person is erythematous, hot, and moist (sometimes actually dripping wet). Although such hands may occasionally be found in other conditions, the finding of a cold hand—dry or moist—virtually excludes hyperfunction of the thyroid. Flushing is also common, more in younger patients than in older ones. There may be more or less continuous erythema of the face and neck, with superimposed transient blushing. Occasionally diffuse pruritis or urticaria occurs.

The vasomotor system is overactive. Many of these cutaneous manifestations may be considered expressions of or incidental to increased heat elimination.

Redness of the elbows, first noted by Plummer, is frequently present. It is probably the result of the combination of increased activity, an exposed part, and a hyperirritable vasomotor system.

Although the integument is thinned, manifestations due to alteration in the growth of the tissue are less evident. It is possible that the type of fingernail described by Plummer (onycholysis) belongs in this category (Fig. 10-7). The process may involve all fingers and toes, but typically begins on the fourth digit

of each hand. The free margin of the nail leaves the nail bed, producing a concave or wavy margin at the line of contact. The hyponychium may be ragged and dirty, despite the patient's best efforts at personal hygiene. Plummer's nails are a frequent and interesting clinical finding in Graves' disease. Occasionally the spoon-shaped fingernails of hypochromic anemia are encountered.

Patchy hyperpigmentation, especially of the face and neck, is frequently seen, and occasionally there is a general increase in pigmentation. Most dark-skinned persons detect a definite increase in pigmentation during the onset of thyrotoxicosis, which may be dramatically localized around the eyes.

Patchy vitiligo is found in 7 percent of patients with Graves' disease, and we have observed several instances of complete loss of pigmentation in association with thyrotoxicosis.[165] These changes are manifestations of associated autoimmunity directed toward melanocytes. The vitiligo, often of the hands and feet, may precede the onset of Graves' disease by years or even decades. Observation of this change is a useful clinical sign when attempting to establish the cause of thyrotoxicosis or exophthalmos.

Hair tends to be fine, soft, and straight. Women may complain that it will not retain a curl. (This complaint is also typical of patients with myxedema.) Temporary thinning of the hair is common, but alopecia is rare. Hair loss is often extreme after marked changes in metabolic rate are induced during therapy. We have seen complete or partial alopecia develop in a few patients with Graves' disease, sometimes in association with urticaria. These changes are believed to be manifestations of autoimmunity directed against the hair follicles.

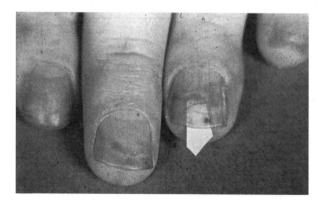

Fig. 10-7. Plummer's nail changes, showing thinning of the nail and marked posterior erosion of the hyponychium.

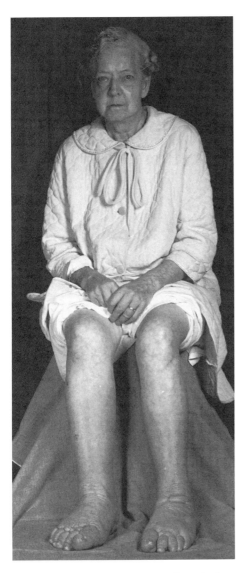

Fig. 10-8. Remarkable "pretibial myxedema", also present on feet and hands, of a patient with Graves' disease and exophthalmos.

Peripheral edema, unrelated to congestive heart failure or renal disease, is common.

Pretibial myxedema (Fig. 10-8) and the other remarkable abnormalities of "thyroid acropachy" are discussed in Chapter 12.

Neural and Mental Findings

Neural and mental findings are varied and striking. The patient complains of nervousness or irritability and appears to be restless and fidgety. It some-times seems impossible for the thyrotoxic patient to remain still for an instant. The tendon reflexes tend to be brisk, and the reflex relaxation time is shortened. The reaction to all sorts of stimuli is distinctly excessive. When asked to sit up, the patient jumps into an upright position. He or she may wish to cooperate but rather overdoes it. The patient is, so to speak, "hypercooperative."

Such behavior constitutes an almost pathognomonic pattern. In the clinic, we are familiar with what we call the "thyrotoxic entrance and exit." The thyrotoxic patient hops into the clinic room like a jack-in-in-the-box, often with staring eyes, quickly sits in the clinic chair (bolt upright), looks rapidly about the room, and does whatever is asked with pathologic alacrity. His or her exit is equally precipitous. Emotional instability is often combined with this pattern, sometimes to the point of a change in personality. The patient may be given to fits of crying, but may have sufficient insight to realize that the crying is pathologic. Some patients become hyperirritable and combative, and this can lead to accidents or even aggressive behavior.

In some patients, the emotional pattern is that of hypomania or pathologic well-being (euphoria). In others, hyperactivity seems to produce a state of exhaustion, and profound fatigue or asthenia chiefly characterizes the picture. The mind is often very active, and the patient is troubled with insomnia. Rarely, patients develop visual or auditory hallucinations or a frank psychosis. The latter may not completely clear up after thyrotoxicosis has been treated. It is probable that thyrotoxicosis makes manifest an abnormality already present rather than inducing a psychosis de novo.

Impairment of intellectual function has been found in patients with untreated hyperthyroidism. It is usually assumed that such abnormalities return to normal with therapy. Perild et al.,[166] however, report that ten years after successful therapy of thyrotoxicosis a group of patients manifested abnormal neuropsychological tests, and half had significant intellectual impairment which was apparently permanent. This surprising observation awaits confirmation. Marked increase in fatigability, or asthenia, is often prominent. This increased weariness may be combined with hyperactivity. Patients remark that they are impelled to incessant activity, which, however, causes great fatigue.

A fine, rapid tremor of the outstretched fingers is

TABLE 10-5. Neuromuscular Manifestations of Thyrotoxicosis

Tremor
Hyperactive reflexes
Accelerated reflex relaxation
Anxiety
Disorientation
Psychosis
Thyrotoxic neuropathy (rare)
Acute thyrotoxic encephalopathy (very rare)
Seizures (with or without an underlying abnormality)
Neuropathy secondary to nerve entrapment by lesions of pretibial myxedema
Corticospinal tract disease with pyramidal tract damage (rare)
Chorea and athetoid movements (rare)
Hypokalemic periodic paralysis
Myopathy
(Myasthenia gravis—associated)

classically found, and a generalized tremulousness, involving also the tongue, may be evident. Muscle fibrillations are not a usual part of the syndrome, but they may occur in chronic thyrotoxic myopathy. Polyneuropathy has also been reported.[167]

More severe neurologic problems also occur during Graves' disease (Table 10-5). Patients who are known to have a convulsive disorder may become more difficult to control with the usual medications, and seizures may appear in patients who have never previously manifested such symptoms.[168] Electroencephalography[168] reveals increased fast wave activity, and occasionally bursts of tall spike waves. In animals, excess T_4 decreases the threshold to convulsive stimuli.[169]

Psychosis with Thyrotoxicosis

C.H., a 52-year-old woman, appeared in the emergency room on December 27, 1980, in a confused and agitated state. She refused to talk, but would on occasion answer questions. She appeared to be extremely paranoid and was resistant to offers of help.

She came to the emergency room alone, and after one interview disappeared. A few hours later, she returned in the same agitated, confused, paranoid, and semimute condition. She stated that she heard voices quoting the Scripture. Although she denied that these voices directed her to harm herself or others, she believed she was somehow responsible for all the world's problems.

Relatives were contacted and indicated that the patient had been entirely well up to the previous few days, when she had become confused and agitated. It was

determined that the patient had worked for more than 20 years and had lost her position 4 years ago. She was married and had been separated from her husband intermittently since the loss of her job. She knew her address, was aware of the month and year (but not the date), and was confused about current events.

The BP was 150/80 and the pulse rate 140. The patient was disheveled, thin, and hyperactive. The eyes were normal. Results of routine blood chemistry tests, complete blood count, and urinalysis were negative.

The patient was treated initially with haloperidol, 1 mg twice a day, and gradually calmed. The diagnosis of hyperthyroidism was considered and confirmed by an FTI of 19. Antithyroid antibodies were absent.

During treatment, the patient's paranoia and anxiety subsided. She subsequently indicated that there had been a gradual increase in tiredness and weakness, weight loss of 10 lbs, heat intolerance, palpitations, and tremor over the previous 1 to 2 years. Previous medical problems included a hysterectomy for fibroids and mild hypertension treated by diuretics. There was no history of previous psychiatric illness in the patient or her family.

On further examination, the thyroid was seen to be enlarged to about 35 g and was diffusely increased in size, without nodules; there was no bruit. Propranolol was added to the therapy, and Haldol was continued. The patient rapidly became psychologically normal and entirely cooperative, and regained control of her personal affairs.

An RAIU test was 49.7 percent. The patient received 4 mCi of radioactive [131]I. After radioactive iodine therapy, the patient was given an antithyroid drug that brought her thyroid hormone levels back to normal. When this drug was discontinued, her FTI returned to 15.7. She was given 3.4 mCi of radioactive iodine again, and PTU was restarted. When last examined, her FTI was in the normal range.

There has been no return of any abnormal psychological function, and the patient has received no further psychiatric care.

This episode appeared to be an acute psychotic reaction associated with severe hyperthyroidism, occurring in a patient with no previously known psychological disease. It cleared promptly with medical therapy, including treatment of the hyperthyroidism, and the patient is now apparently well.

Thyrotoxic Neuropathy

C.J., a 43-year-old woman, was referred for evaluation in January 1980 with a history of obesity, hypertension for 2 years, prominence of the right eye for 2 years, and thyroid overactivity known for 6 months. She had gained 50 lbs during the interval preceding the examination because of excess eating. Increasing dyspnea and shortness of breath, present for the previous two years, had become worse in the previous two months. She came to the emergency room because of symptoms of asthma. Examination revealed a pulse rate of 120 and an enlarged heart. There was LVH and strain on the electrocardiogram, and on echocardiogram an enlarged left atrium and a left ventricle with decreased function, especially of the lateral and posterior inferior walls. Thyroid function tests showed a T_4 level of 17 ug/dl, an FTI of 16.8, and a T_3 level of of 357 ng/dl. She received digoxin, 0.25 mg daily, furosemide, 40 mg daily, potassium chloride, and aminophylline.

On examination in the endocrine clinic, the BP was 170/100, and the patient was obese and hyperactive. There was moderate bilateral proptosis and inflamed insertions of the extraocular muscles. There was 22 mm proptosis bilaterally. The thyroid was diffusely enlarged to about 40 g. Neurologic examination showed weakness of ocular motility with diplopia on the left lateral gaze, bilateral nystagmus, marked proximal muscle weakness without fasciculations, and decreased touch, pinprick, and vibration sense in a glove distribution of both arms, the left greater than the right. There was no significant deficit in the feet. Weakness in the left upper extremity was marked. Deep tendon reflexes were absent. The differential diagnosis included Graves' disease, cardiomyopathy and peripheral neuropathy, congestive heart failure, and hypertension.

A neurologic consultant confirmed the neuropathy and noted mild choretic movements of the left hand and arm. Other known causes of neuropathy were excluded. The patient was treated for one month with antithyroid drugs and then given 2.7 mCi [131]I. Because of continued hyperthyroidism, the patient was retreated with 3.2 mCi ^{131}I seven months after the initial treatment. Three months later the FTI was normal at 10.4, and there were no symptoms or signs of congestive heart failure. Some decreased strength and clumsiness of the left hand persisted. The diplopia and proptosis were unchanged. The neuropathy in the hands had decrease, and the patient was euthyroid.

This patient exhibited profound cardiomyopathy and skeletal myopathy, choreiform movements, and peripheral neuropathy, all apparently related to severe thyrotoxicosis. She improved rapidly with appropriate treatment of the thyrotoxicosis.

The tremor of Parkinsonism is greatly intensified during thyrotoxicosis. Signs and symptoms of cerebellar disease or pyramidal tract lesions have been seen.[170,171] Rarely, patients manifest extreme restlessness, disorientation, aphasia, grimacing, chorioathetoid movements, symptoms suggestive of encephalitis,[172] or episodes of hemiparesis or bulbar paralysis. These symptoms clear up completely after restoration of metabolism to normal. No definite lesions have been found in the brain. In rare cases, polyneuropathy has been severe enough to cause paraplegia.[173]

Interestingly, the brain of a thyrotoxic human subject does not have an elevated consumption of oxygen. Sensenbach et al.[174] found the cerebral blood flow to be increased, the cerebral vascular resistance decreased, arteriovenous (AV) oxygen difference decreased, and oxygen consumption unchanged in thyrotoxicosis. Reciprocal changes occurred in myxedema, and all reverted to normal after therapy.

Although it is possible that some of the central nervous system irritability is a manifestation of elevated sensitivity to circulating epinephrine, this has not been proved. Epinephrine levels and catecholamine excretion are actually not elevated, but propranolol, presumably acting by inhibition of α-adrenergic sympathetic activity, certainly reduces anxiety and tremulousness in a useful manner. The clinical applications of these findings are discussed in Chapters 11 and 12.

The Muscles

The muscles suffer in a peculiar way in thyrotoxicosis. The muscular symptoms vary from mild myasthenia to profound muscular weakness and atrophy, especially of proximal muscle groups. This weakness forms the basis of a useful clinical test. If a thyrotoxic patient seated in a chair is asked to hold one leg out horizontally, he or she may be able to do so for only 25 to 30 seconds; normal persons can maintain such a position for 60 to 120 seconds. Toe standing and step climbing may also bring out muscle weakness that is otherwise not apparent.

In the more extreme forms of muscular involvement, there is not only weakness but also atrophy. Wasting of the temporals and interossei may be noted in a considerable number of patients, and in a few, wasting of all skeletal muscles. This wasting may go so far as to bear a close resemblance to progressive muscular atrophy; occasionally the myopathy may develop into polymyositis. Muscle cell necrosis and lymphocyte infiltration may be visible histologically, but usually are not found even when the symptoms of weakness are severe.[175] Tremor, which is usually present, is ascribed to altered neural function. Fasciculations are unusual.

The speed of both tension development[176] and relaxation of the muscles is increased, so that the reflex time is shortened. The electromyogram is normal in most instances but may occasionally resemble that of muscular dystrophy.[177] Work efficiency, measured in terms of the calories of heat produced while performing a given amount of work, has been reported to be both decreased[178] and normal. Creatine excretion is increased. The muscles have decreased ability to take up creatine, produced in the liver, from the blood,[179] and thus there is a decreased creatine tolerance.[180–182] Creatinine excretion is initially increased by the general catabolism of hyperthyroidism, but as muscle mass diminishes, creatinine excretion in the urine is depressed.

Myasthenia gravis may simulate thyrotoxicosis, and vice versa. It has been reported that neostigmine both strengthens the muscles in thyrotoxic myopathies and is without effect. Certainly, the response is small in comparison with the immediate and striking correction of weakness seen in myasthenia gravis. Thyrotoxicosis may rarely ameliorate myasthenia gravis, but typically it is accentuated by thyrotoxicosis and is also worsened by myxedema.[183] The close relationship between these two diseases is apparent in the observation that thyrotoxicosis occurs in 3 percent of patients with myasthenia gravis. The pathogenic anti-acetylcholine receptor antibodies that occur in myasthenia gravis are clearly comparable to the anti-TSH receptor antibodies found in Graves' disease. In addition, it has been found that TG and acetylcholinesterase share epitopes recognized by B cells. Thus antibodies to either antigen can cross-react with the other. It is, however, unclear whether this plays a role in the pathogenesis of muscle disease in Graves' patients.

Periodic paralysis is precipitated and worsened by thyrotoxicosis.[184] This relationship has been extensively studied in Japan, where it is a familiar syndrome, particularly in men. The paralysis is usually associated with and due to hypokalemia. While the exact mechanism is not known, the hypokalemia is believed to be caused by a shift to the intracellular compartment. It has been demonstrated that thyrotoxicosis augments K^+ uptake and release from cells. Experimental T_4 treatment augments synthesis of membrane Na^+-K^+ activated ATPase. The episodes of paralysis tend to be infrequent and sporadic, but most commonly occur after a meal, following exercise, or start during sleep, and can be induced by administration of glucose and insulin. The onset following meals or exercise presumably relates to rapid K^+ uptake by cells. Episodes last from minutes to hours, usually involving peripheral muscles, but can cause paralysis of the diaphragm and affect the heart. Serious episodes can be associated with extensive muscle cell damage and necrosis, ECG abnormalities such as ST and T wave changes, PVCs, first degree heart block, prolonged QT intervals, and even ventricular fibrillation.[185]

Potassium treatment has some protective effect, and quickens recovery from attacks. Propranolol, for reasons not entirely clear, has prophylactic action. Therapy of the thyrotoxicosis almost always causes the rapid, and permanent disappearance of the syndrome.

Myotonia congenita and myotonia dystrophic do not occur with increased frequency with thyrotoxicosis.

Skeleton and Calcium Metabolism

Roentgenographic examination of the bones frequently discloses evidence of decalcification. Microdensitometry demonstrates this condition at all ages and in both sexes.[186,189] Patients with even mild increases in thyroid hormone lose bone mass, and those with a history of thyrotoxicosis extending over a number of years may have osteoporosis that is severe and premature. Fractures are uncommon, with the most frequent being collapsed vertebra in a chronically thyrotoxic postmenopausal woman. Skeletal mass is augmented after therapy.[187] Treatment restores the density in younger patients, but not usually in the elderly.[188] Periarthritis of the shoulder (subacromial bursitis) is occasionally associated with thyrotoxicosis. Linear bone growth may be accelerated in children. The time of epiphyseal closure may be accelerated in children, and bone age may exceed chronologic age.

Thyrotoxicosis results in an accelerated turnover of bone calcium and collagen.[190] As described in the section on pathology, the histologic picture of bones from the thyrotoxic patient may suggest osteitis fibrosa with increased osteoclastic activity, fibrosis, and an increased number of osteoblasts.[156] Histomorphometric evaluations with tetracycline labelling demonstrates accelerated bone resorption and formation, both in spontaneous hyperthyroidism and in women treated with excess thyroid hormone.[154] In bone biopsy specimens the thin trabeculae of osteoporosis are seen.[156] The serum calcium level is usually normal, but may be elevated sufficiently to produce nausea and vomiting[191] and, rarely, renal damage.[192,193] It may be made clinically evident when thyrotoxic patients become relatively immobile (for example, at bed rest during illness). In contrast to what occurs in hyperparathyroidism, the hypercalcemia can usually be corrected partially or totally by the administration of glucocorticoids,[194] but these have not been effective in all cases.[195] Phosphorus administration also lowers the concentration of calcium in serum and urine to normal.[196] The exchangeable calcium pool is remarkably increased.[197] Serum osteocalcin is increased in parallel with hormone levels.[198] The alkaline phosphatase level may be elevated, with a pattern showing the normal equal distribution of bone and liver isoenzymes. The changes in calcium and alkaline phosphatase correlate with serum T_3 levels.[199] After therapy, the alkaline phosphatase level tends to increase, and bone isoenzyme becomes predominant, probably due to skeletal repair.[200]

Fecal and urinary calcium excretion is greatly augmented. Renal stones are rarely formed since there is a concomitant increase in excretion of colloids that stabilize the calcium. Urinary hydroxyproline excretion is increased and falls to normal after therapy.[201] Serum osteocalcin levels and urinary osteocalcin secretion are increased and return to normal with therapy.[202]

The serum phosphorus level is in the normal range or depressed. Renal phosphorus resorption is in the normal range or elevated.[193,194] Although some of the observations suggest the presence of hyperparathyroidism, the changes probably reflect the direct metabolic effects of thyroid hormone. The parathyroid glands are histologically normal. In fact, parathyroid hormone (PTH) levels tend to be suppressed in hyperthyroidism, apparently in response to the elevated calcium levels[201] 1,25-dihydroxyvitamin D_3 levels are likewise about 40 percent below normal.[202]

The increased fractional tubular phosphate reabsorption characteristic of hypoparathyroidism may also occur in thyrotoxicosis, probably because of reduced PTH levels. In one reported study,[192] urinary phosphorus excretion was depressed after calcium infusion. Thus, a normal response was obtained rather than that found in hyperparathyroidism.

The hypercalcemia appears to be a manifestation of thyroid hormone action on bone metabolism,[202] and calcium absorption from the intestine is usually reduced.[203] Both catabolism and anabolism of bone are accelerated. Negative calcium balance can sometimes be corrected by administration of calcium, an observation that perhaps should be given more attention in the management of thyrotoxic patients. Hypercalcemia can be corrected by propranolol therapy in some patients.[204] Bone turnover can be reduced by pamidronate, which may therefore have a useful role in reducing thyrotoxicosis-induced osteopenia.[205]

Two exceptional cases have been reported with coincident thyrotoxicosis and hypercalcemia with elevated PTH levels. Treatment of thyrotoxicosis eliminated all abnormalities, for reasons unknown.[206]

The Respiratory System

Except for dyspnea, which may or may not represent abnormal respiratory function, symptoms deriving from the lungs are not prominent. Nevertheless, measurements show some reduction in vital capacity, expiratory reserve volume, pulmonary compliance, and airway resistance. Minute volume response to exercise is excessive for the amount of oxygen consumed.[207] Dyspnea on effort is present in a large majority of the patients. A thorough study of pulmonary function in patients without coincident congestive heart failure has demonstrated reduction in vital capacity, decreased pulmonary compliance, weakness of the respiratory muscles, increase in respiratory dead space ventilation, and normal diffusion capacity. A combination of the four abnormalities may produce dyspnea.[208] Amelioration of intractable bronchial asthma has been reported after treatment of coincident thyrotoxicosis (Table 10-6).[209]

The Circulatory System

First and foremost of the symptoms deriving from the circulatory system are palpitations and tachycardia. The heart may beat with extreme violence, which may be distressing to the patient, particularly at night or on exercise. The pulse on palpation is rapid and bounding. The systolic blood pressure is

TABLE 10-6. Cardiac Manifestation of Graves' Disease

Tachycardia
LVH and strain on EKG
Premature atrial and ventricular contractions
Atrial fibrillation
Congestive heart failure
Angina with (or without) coronary artery disease
Myocardial infarction
Systemic embolization
Death from cardiovascular collapse
Resistance to some drug effects (digoxin, coumadin)
Residual cardiomegaly

frequently elevated. The diastolic blood pressure is characteristically decreased, and the pulse pressure is elevated, usually between 50 and 80 mm Hg.

Left ventricular hypertrophy may be suggested on physical examination. A bounding precordium is so typically found that its absence is a point against the diagnosis of hyperthyroidism. In the majority of instances, however, roentgenograms show the heart to be normal in transverse diameter. A systolic murmur is usually heard over the precordium. One reason for this murmur is the development of mitral valve prolapse during thyrotoxicosis.[210] This can be detected by angiography, or more easily by echography. It is postulated that papillary muscle dysfunction due to inadequate ATP supplies may be responsible for the lesion. Prolapse is usually not clinically evident but rarely is a cause of symptomatic mitral valve insufficiency. The prolapse can revert to normal with therapy.[210]

Interpretation of physical signs in the heart, especially systolic murmur and gallop rhythm, is difficult and uncertain in the presence of thyrotoxicosis. In evaluating heart status in thyrotoxicosis, one should concentrate chiefly on the presence or absence of signs of failure rather than on physical signs in the heart itself. If no signs of failure are present, the best procedure regarding abnormal cardiac findings is to ascertain whether they persist after thyrotoxicosis has been abolished.

A grating pulmonic systolic sound ("Lerman Scratch"), which has some of the characteristics of a pericardial friction rub, is occasionally heard over the sternum in the second left interspace. It is heard best at the end of full expiration. Its intensity subsides as thyrotoxicosis improves. The diagnosis of pericarditis may be suggested on the basis of this sound. The fact that it is superficial and tends to disappear on inspiration suggests a pleuropericardial origin. It may be related to the dilated pulmonary conus often seen on radiographs in thyrotoxic patients. The sign has no prognostic significance.

Extrasystoles are frequent, and paroxysmal atrial tachycardia and atrial fibrillation, paroxysmal or continuous, occur in 6 to 12 percent of patients. Precordial pain that seems distinct from angina pectoris occurs occasionally. Cardiac enlargement and congestive heart failure may occur with or without prior heart disease[211,212] (Fig. 10-9). The electrocardiographic manifestations are confined to tachycardia, increased voltage, and sometimes a prolongation of the PR interval,[213] unless there is a dysrhythmia or an accompanying but unrelated disorder of the heart.

Patients with coronary atherosclerosis often develop angina during thyrotoxicosis. Occasionally angina develops de novo in young women with arteriography-proven normal coronary arteries. This condition has been ascribed to an imbalance between increased cardiac work and blood supply, so that a functionally deficient blood supply occurs even with a patent vessel.[214] Occasionally myocardial infarction occurs in toxic patients with normal coronary vessels.[215]

In thyrotoxicosis the heart rate, stroke volume, and cardiac output are increased. Circulation time is decreased. There is dilatation of superficial capillaries. Coronary blood flow and myocardial oxygen consumption in each stroke are increased.[216] Circulating plasma volume is increased. AV oxygen differences are variable but tend to be normal. Cardiac output in response to exercise is excessive in relation to oxygen consumed.

The relation of cardiac systolic time intervals to thyroid function has provided a valuable in vivo bioassay of hormone action. The pre-ejection period is shortened in thyrotoxicosis, and the left ventricular ejection time remains relatively normal. The interval from initiation of the QRS complex to arrival of the arterial pulse in the brachial artery is reduced.[217] Cardiac diastolic function as evaluated by echocardiography remains normal in the majority of patients.[218]

Congestive heart failure and atrial fibrillation, when due to or associated with thyrotoxicosis, are relatively resistant to the action of digoxin. Accelerated metabolism of digoxin, plus the cardiac ineffi-

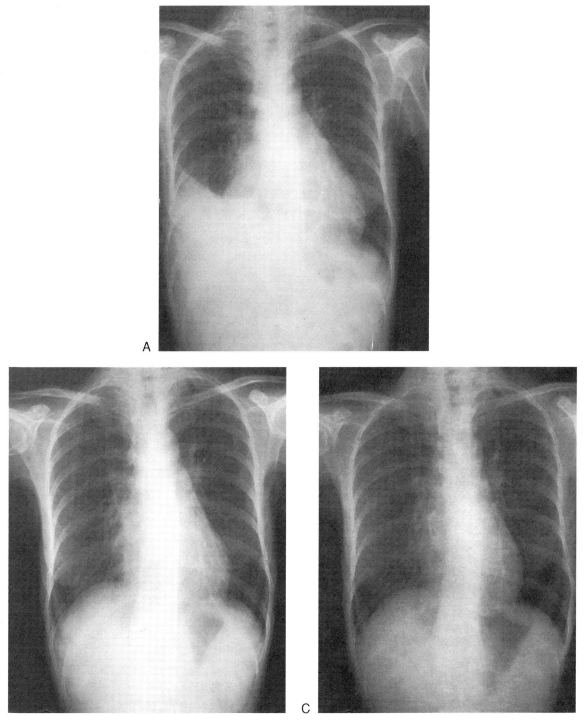

Fig. 10-9. Congestive heart failure induced in an otherwise healthy young woman *(A)*, which receded *(B)*, and returned to normal *(C)*, during and after therapy.

ciency and irritability produced by thyrotoxicosis, may be at least two of the factors producing this resistance. Although the response to the drug will be blunted, a beneficial effect will occur if a proper level of digoxin is attained. Atrial fibrillation should be treated by anticoagulation if it is persistent, since it is associated with serious embolism in 10 percent of cases. The usual contraindications of old age, HBP, bleeding tendency, recent CVA, etc. apply, and the dose of Coumadin needed is lower than normal in thyrotoxic patients. AF tends to revert spontaneously to normal when hyperthyroidism is cured, but this may not occur before 6 months, or not at all, if AF was of long standing. Therapeutic cardioversion is recommended if AF persists 6 months beyond achievement of euthyroidism. Treatment of thyrotoxic heart disease has been reviewed recently.[219]

It has been suggested that the changes in the cardiovascular system are secondary to increased demand for metabolites and to increased heat production. Dilatation of superficial capillaries for the dissipation of heat does cause increased blood flow and cardiac output. A direct action of thyroid hormone on the heart is also increased, however, since the sinus node has higher intrinsic activity, the isolated thyrotoxic heart beats faster than normal, and isolated papillary muscle from a thyrotoxic heart has a shortened contraction time.[220,221] The heart shares in the general increase in respiratory quotient found in skeletal muscle. Excess thyroid hormone increases cardiac Na^+-K^+ activated membrane ATPase, and sarcoplasmic reticulum Ca^{2+}-activated ATPase, both of which contribute to the heightened contractility of cardiac muscle. In addition excess thyroid hormone, at least in experimental animals, causes, by a direct effect on DNA transcription rates, an increased synthesis of alpha-myosin heavy chain with high ATPase activity, and decrease of beta myosin heavy chain synthesis. This alteration in α/β ratio is associated with increased contractility.[222]

The cardiovascular changes may be due in part to increased sensitivity to circulating epinephrine. Thyroid hormone administration may increase, or not alter, the catecholamine content of the heart. Guanethidine partially restores cardiac dynamics to normal, perhaps by releasing catecholamine from the heart and thus reducing the cardiac stimulation caused by this agent. Guanethidine and β-adrenergic blockers slow the tachycardia of thyrotoxicosis.

Concomitant with this slowing is an increase in stroke volume, and there may be either a decrease[223] or little change in cardiac output.[224] T_4 can increase the heart rate directly in a manner not mediated by catecholamines,[225] and presumably this direct chromatotropic effect adds to coincident sympathetic effects on the heart.

Thyrotoxicosis causes increased β-adrenergic receptors in the heart and increased responsiveness to isoproterenol.[226,227] α-adrenergic and cholinergic receptors are reduced. In animal studies, adenyl cyclase may be activated by T_3, but reduced cardiac levels of ATP limit the response through protein kinase activation. The net effect is β-adrenergic sensitization and cholinergic desensitization. Thyrotoxicosis also increased β-adrenergic receptors on a variety of tissues.[228] An increased number of β-adrenergic receptors could cause hyper-responsiveness to adrenergic agonists, and could mediate the heightened plasma cAMP levels noted in thyrotoxic patients in the basal state (in some studies) and after assumption of an upright posture or administration of glucagon and epinephrine.[229,230] Propranolol treatment normalizes the cAMP responses to these drugs and, of course, inhibits the action of β-adrenergic agonists on the heart. Possibly these actions of propranolol explain its ability to reduce somewhat the consumption of oxygen in thyrotoxicosis.

The impact of the interrelation of excess thyroid hormone and the sympathetic nervous system in humans is not finally settled.[83,231] There is clear evidence for increased β-adrenergic receptors in the heart and elsewhere in thyrotoxicosis, as inferred from animal studies. Responses of the thyrotoxic human to adrenergic agonists are probably not excessive in relation to responses in normal subjects, although this question is much debated. β-adrenergic blockade clearly reduces some pathophysiologic responses, including the increased nitrogen and oxygen consumption, toward but not to normal. Metabolism of the heart and other organs is stimulated directly by thyroid hormone, and sympathetic effects are additive. It remains possible that the sympathetic responses are in fact exaggerated; it is also clear that sympathetic responses do not mediate thyroid hormone action.

Hematologic Changes

In most patients the hemoglobin and hematocrit are in the normal or low range.[232] Blood volume is increased, and the red cell mass is actually increased in some patients. In severe thyrotoxicosis, normocytic anemia with hemoglobin concentrations as low as 8 to 9 g/dl may be observed. Hyperthyroid patients with anemia may show impaired iron use.[232,233] Malnutrition may play a role in this decrease. These anemias are unresponsive to hematinic therapy, but the blood picture returns to normal when the thyrotoxicosis controlled.[234] Iron deficiency or megaloblastic anemia is exceptional and requires a search for some explanation other than thyrotoxicosis. It is possible that thyrotoxicosis may increase the need for vitamin B_{12} as shown experimentally, and perhaps for folic acid. Also, there is an increased incidence of antigastric antibodies and mild pernicious anemia in patients with Graves' disease.

The glucose-6-phosphate dehydrogenase activity of red cells is increased in thyrotoxicosis.[235]

A relative lymphocytosis is frequently found in the peripheral blood due to neutropenia.[236] A relative and an absolute increase in the number of monocytes was noted years ago.[237] The monocyte count was between 10 and 15 percent; in only 2 of the 30 cases was it less than 10 percent. Relative lymphocytosis and relative monocytosis, with a normal or slightly low total white cell count, constitute the characteristic blood findings of Graves' disease. There is also an increase in the percentage and number of B lymphocytes[78] and, as discussed previously, an altered ratio of T lymphocyte subsets.[81]

Graves' disease is often associated with mild thrombocytopenia, and occasionally with idiopathic thrombocytopenic purpura.[238] This co-occurrence is thought to reflect the autoimmune pathogenesis of both diseases. Fourteen percent of patients with ITP are reported to have coincident Graves' disease. Mild thrombocytopenia may disappear spontaneously or with treatment of hyperthyroidism, or if severe, may respond to glucocorticoid therapy.[239] Other more severe cases are managed as typical cases of ITP. Bone marrow examination may show normal or increased megakaryocytes.[239] Hyperthyroidism also induces a shortened platelet life span, believed to be due to more rapid clearing of normal platelets by an activated reticulo-endothelial system. Both antiplatelet antibodies and shortened platelet life span could contribute to the low or low-normal levels of platelets found in Graves' patients. It is reported that all patients with Graves' disease have evidence of IgG bound to platelets.

Coagulation is usually normal in spite of mild prolongation of the prothrombin time. Antihemophilic factor is often elevated in level and returns to normal with treatment.[240] Capillary fragility is increased. Severe liver damage caused by thyrotoxicosis and secondary congestive heart failure may be associated with a hemorrhagic tendency.

The Reticuloendothelial and Lymphocytic Systems

The reticuloendothelial and lymphocytic systems undergo hyperplasia. There may be generalized lymphadenopathy, and the thymus may be enlarged. Occasionally the thymus presents as an anterior mediastinal mass, but diminishes to normal size with control of the thyrotoxicosis.[241] Some authors have reported that the spleen tip can be felt in 20 percent of patients, but in our experience this is less common.

Gastrointestinal Findings

The appetite is characteristically increased. The effect of this increase is to offset, in part (sometimes completely), the loss of weight that might be expected from the increased catabolism. Indeed, the pattern of weight loss with increased appetite is nearly pathognomonic of thyrotoxicosis, although it may occur in diabetes mellitus and malabsorption or intestinal parasitism. A minority of patients complain of anorexia, and are likely to show the greatest weight loss. Nausea and vomiting are rare, but when they occur, they are serious. They are usually features of severe thyrotoxicosis but may also reflect hypercalcemia. In the presence of hypermetabolism, vomiting leads quickly to dehydration, ketosis, and perhaps avitaminosis.

The stomach per se gives rise to no characteristic symptoms. The incidence of achlorhydria in exophthalmic goiter was found some years ago to be approximately 40 percent and slightly higher in myxedema.[242] The figures would probably be lower today. Berryhill and Williams[243] found that 73 percent showed a return of free hydrochloric acid after surgical thyroidectomy. Gastric enzyme production is decreased, and a mild chronic gastritis may be present.[244] Fasting serum gastrin levels, and responses to arginine, are increased.[245]

Abdominal pain is an occasional symptom of thyrotoxicosis. Its nature and origin are obscure. Epigastric pain may suggest ulcer, gallbladder disease, or pancreatitis. Vomiting is sometimes associated with the pain.

The rate of absorption from the gastrointestinal tract is accelerated. The glucose tolerance curve may show an abnormally rapid rise and fall. Absorption of vitamin A is enhanced, and vitamin A formation from carotene is also increased.

Increased frequency of normal bowel movements is common, and occasionally diarrhea occurs. Transit time is decreased, and fat absorption may be impaired to the point of steatorrhea if fat intake is excessive.[246]

The liver is frequently palpable in the absence of congestive heart failure, and is typically palpable with heart failure. Evidence of mild to severe liver disease may be found.[247] The plasma albumin level may be below 4 g/dl, and the globulin level above 3 g/dl. Galactose tolerance is impaired. There may be mild retention of bromsulfophthalein, if tested, and elevation of PT. The LFTs can give the impression of viral hepatitis. For example, in one survey of 81 thyrotoxic patients, three-fourths had some LFT abnormality, including 31 percent with elevated bilirubin, 24 percent with elevated SGOT, 13 percent with elevated LDH, 26 percent with elevated SGPT, and 67 percent with elevated alkaline phosphatase (which, of course, may reflect bone metabolism). Cholesterol is often depressed. The abnormalities clear with treatment.[248]

Bilirubin retention and jaundice are occasionally seen without evidence of congestive heart failure, but they are much more commonly found when this complication is also present. On hepatic biopsy the liver may be entirely normal histologically, even when there are abnormalities in chemical findings; alternatively, there may be evidence of focal collections of lymphocytes, decrease in glycogen, and occasionally death of cells. On electron microscopy, the mitochondria are increased in size and the smooth endoplasmic reticulum is hypertrophic. The glycogen level is decreased.[249] The fine stellate scarrings seen in the livers of patients with severe thyrotoxicosis and reported in the earlier literature are rarely observed today. The cause of hepatic disease has been thought to be congestive heart failure, malnutrition, intercurrent infections, and a direct toxic effect of thyroid hormone. Malnutrition must play a role. Congestive heart failure by itself certainly can induce gross abnormalities in liver function, and

presumably this insult is worsened by coincident thyrotoxicosis. The splanchnic blood flow is increased in thyrotoxicosis and the arteriovenous oxygen difference is greater than normal, but hepatic anoxia, at least in the portal areas, might occur even without circulatory failure if the metabolic demand for oxygen exceeds the supply.

Several patients who have been jaundiced without signs of congestive heart failure or other cause of hepatic dysfunction have been reported.[250] In two of these patients there was considerable elevation of the indirect-reacting bilirubin level. Studies in one patient showed that conjugation products of glucuronic acid were secreted into the urine in greatly increased quantities. This finding ruled out any absolute deficiency in the glucuronyl transferase enzyme in the liver. It was hypothesized that in certain thyrotoxic patients there is a great increase in metabolites that must be excreted by means of the glucuronyl transferase enzyme system. Since bilirubin competes relatively inefficiently in this enzyme system, it may be crowded out in the presence of an increased quantity of substrates. As a result, it may not be conjugated as rapidly as normally, and its concentration in the serum would therefore rise. All of these patients had residual abnormalities in bilirubin metabolism when euthyroid. This finding suggests that an underlying abnormality was present and was exacerbated by thyrotoxicosis. It is probable that the occasional thyrotoxic and jaundiced patient may actually suffer from an unrecognized separate abnormality, such as Gilbert's disease or posthepatitic liver dysfunction, brought to light by thyrotoxicosis.

The Urinary Tract

The urinary tract is the locus of no characteristic signs of symptoms, except polyuria and occasionally glycosuria, in uncomplicated thyrotoxicosis. Standard clinical renal function tests give normal results. Glycosuria may reflect accelerated absorption of sugar from the intestine.

In hyperthyroid animals and humans, the glomerular filtration rate and renal blood flow are on average increased, as are tubular transfer maxima for glucose and diodrast. The glomerular filtration rate and renal blood flow alterations probably are secondary to increased cardiac output, whereas the increased tubular activity may be a direct effect of thyroid hormone on renal function.[251] Polyuria does

TABLE 10-7. Changes in Endocrine Function in Graves' Disease

FTI and T_3 increased, TSH reduced
Prolactin normal
Growth hormone normal
Parathyroid hormone suppressed
Cortisol normal, urinary 17-OHCS increased, urinary free cortisol normal
Free testosterone reduced in males
Diabetic control worsened

not indicate insensitivity to vasopressin, for the kidney responds normally to vasopressin with an increase in concentration of urine.[252]

Hypercalcemia is a feature of severe thyrotoxicosis, but it rarely injures the kidneys. Occasionally hyposthenuria and uremia occur,[192,193] or more selective renal damage takes place. Huth et al.[253] reported a patient with renal tubular acidosis coincident with hyperthyroidism. Circumstantial evidence suggested that hyperthyroidism led to hypercalcemia, which in turn had damaged the renal medulla and produced acidosis (Table 10-7).

The Reproductive System

Menstruation is characteristically decreased in volume. With severe thyrotoxicosis, the menstrual cycle may be either shortened or prolonged, and finally amenorrhea develops. The relative importance of a primary action of excess thyroid hormone on the ovary or uterus, and pituitary dysfunction, are unclear. In some cases, amenorrhea with a proliferative endometrium is found. This finding suggests failure of pituitary LH production and ovulation.[254,255]

Fertility is depressed, but pregnancy, nonetheless, can develop. The incidence of miscarriage is increased.[256] Pregnancy, on the other hand, often ameliorates the symptoms of thyrotoxicosis, but relapse is prone to occur in the 3 to 4 months following delivery. This topic is discussed in Chapter 14.

Infants born to thyrotoxic mothers usually show no evidence of hyperthyroidism at birth. Fetal and neonatal thyrotoxicosis, fortunately infrequent events, are discussed in Chapter 14.

Gynecomastia, with ductal elongation and epithelial hyperplasia, occasionally occurs.[257] The circulating level of free estradiol may be elevated in these men.[258–260] Peripheral conversion of testosterone

and androstenedione to estrone and estradiol is increased in both sexes during hyperthyroidism.[261] This elevation probably accounts in part for the abnormality. In addition, the slightly elevated LH in men with gynecomastia suggests hypothalamic insensitivity to feedback control and some peripheral unresponsiveness to LH.[258] An imbalance between testosterone and estrogen may be related to gynecomastia.

Kidd et al.[262] found impotence in half of a small group of thyrotoxic men and sperm counts below 40 million in four of five tested. In these studies, the total testosterone level was elevated, but because the testosterone-estrogen binding globulin level was also high, the free testosterone level was reduced and the response to hCG was blunted. Thus, both Leydig cell and spermatogenic abnormalities may be present.

PRL probably plays no role in these reproductive abnormalities, since in hypothyroidism, its release tends to be inhibited both at the hypothalamic and pituitary level.[263] Surprisingly, galactorrhea, in women with normo-prolactinemia, occurs with increased frequency.[264]

The Adrenal Cortex

There are no obvious signs or symptoms of altered adrenal cortical function in thyrotoxicosis, but distinct changes have been detected. In thyrotoxicosis the adrenal cortex is often hyperplastic. Administered adrenal steroids disappear from the plasma at an accelerated rate.[265] Their metabolism by reduction of the steroid nucleus is accelerated, and conjugation of the reduced steroids is proportionally increased. Since plasma corticoid levels are normal and their rate of metabolism is increased, total daily metabolism and excretion of 17-ketosteroids and 17 hydroxy-corticoids are usually increased.[255,266]

Along with the accelerated plasma cortisol clearance of thyrotoxicosis, the pathways of metabolism are also altered. For example, thyrotoxicosis is associated with a relatively increased excretion of 11-oxy-corticoid metabolites.[267] The 11-oxy compounds may be biologically inactive. Because of the negative feedback control from the pituitary, this preferential channeling of steroids into the 11-oxy derivatives could be partly responsible for increased steroid production. There is increased production of steroids by the adrenal gland in order to maintain a normal concentration of active steroids in the peripheral

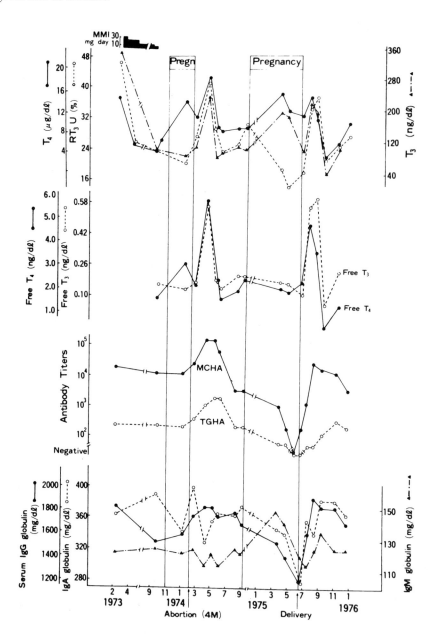

Fig. 10-10. Clinical course of a patient who had transient exacerbation of Graves' disease on two occasions shortly following delivery.

blood and in the tissues.[268] Secretion of adrenocorticotropic hormone (ACTH) by the pituitary is reported to be increased.[269] There are increases in secretory episodes during the day, but the fall to zero secretion after midnight is retained. A reduced response to exogenous ACTH[270] indicates that adrenal reserve is reduced. In fact, it has been hypothe-

sized that in severe thyrotoxicosis and in thyroid storm there may be an element of adrenal insufficiency. This contention has not been proved. There is no reason to believe that T_4 opposes the peripheral action of adrenal steroids.

An increase in the 5-α metabolite of testosterone (androsterone) and a relative decrease in the 5-β metabolite (etiocholanolone) are seen in the urine of thyrotoxic patients,[271] but no comparable change in adrenal corticoid metabolism has been observed. These interesting biochemical alterations could have physiologic significance, for the ketosteroid 5-α metabolites, such as androsterone, are biologically active. In hypothyroidism the reverse change occurs, that is, an increase in the biologically inactive 5-β metabolites such as etiocholanolone. Because administration of large amounts of androsterone depresses the level of serum lipids, Hellman and coworkers[271] have hypothesized that this change in steroid metabolism may be a way in which T_4 (or its lack) affects lipid metabolism and produces a depression or elevation in serum cholesterol concentration.

Other Metabolic Aspects

Oxygen Consumption

The basal oxygen consumption in thyrotoxicosis, as measured by the BMR, is elevated. The increase is above the level of metabolism that the person would have if he or she were not thyrotoxic. In extreme thyrotoxicosis, the BMR may be double the standard, that is, according to the usual mode of expression, $+100$. In moderately severe thyrotoxicosis it may be from $+30$ to $+60$, and in mild thyrotoxicosis from $+10$ to $+30$.

In addition to the BMR, one should consider the total metabolism, that is the basal plus the increments occasioned by work, food, or emotion. An increased cost of muscular work in thyrotoxicosis was reported many years ago by Plummer and Boothby[272] and Briard et al.,[273] among others. These studies, whose results have been disputed, suggested that the thyrotoxic subject has less efficient coupling of oxidation and energy use than either the normal subject or, for example, the hypermetabolic patient with leukemia. More recent studies indicate that the increase in energy expenditure caused by work is not altered by thyrotoxicosis.[274]

Carbohydrate Metabolism

Absorption of carbohydrate from the intestine is accelerated, as is its removal from the plasma. After a standard oral glucose load is given, the thyrotoxic patient characteristically has an early and rapid rise in blood glucose concentration in 30 to 60 minutes (possibly to more than 200 mg/dl) and a rapid fall, so that by two hours the concentration is normal. The early peak may be associated with glycosuria. Intravenous administration does not usually elevate the blood glucose level beyond the rise found in normal subjects.

Thyrotoxicosis increases the demand for insulin, perhaps by accelerating its metabolism. In addition, resistance to the action of insulin is present, since in nondiabetic thyrotoxic patients normal fasting blood glucose levels are associated with double the normal insulin concentration,[275] and resistance is found on incubation of adipocytes in vitro.[276] Diabetes may be activated or intensified, and is ameliorated or may disappear when the thyrotoxicosis is treated. In the past, experimental diabetes was shown to result from long-standing thyrotoxicosis in the presence of partial pancreatectomy.[277] The adverse effect of hyperthyroidism on glucose control in patients with noninsulin dependent diabetes is caused by increased basal hepatic glucose production and reduced ability of insulin and glucose to suppress hepatic glucose production.[278] Although hyperthyroidism increases the requirement for insulin, the effectiveness of exogenous insulin on carbohydrate metabolism is actually enhanced. If glucose is administered intravenously and continuously to a thyrotoxic subject so that blood sugar is maintained at a high level, administered insulin has an effect on glucose removal from the blood[279] that is greater than that in the normal subject.

Type I diabetes mellitus co-occurs with increased frequency in autoimmune thyroid disease. Postpartum thyroid dysfunction is especially common in patients with diabetes.[280] In recent years many similarities in immunologic phenomena have been noted in the two diseases, including insulin receptor antibodies and islet cell antibodies.

Lipid Metabolism

The serum cholesterol level is depressed in thyrotoxicosis. There is an increase both in synthesis and in degradation, but the balance results in a new lower steady-state concentration in the serum. The cholesterol pool in the body is altered by thyroid hormone in different directions, depending on the species involved, and does not necessarily parallel the serum cholesterol level. Hypocholesterolemia may be produced without a distinct decrease in total body or liver cholesterol.[281] Part of the cholesterol-lowering action of thyroid hormone may be due to the effects of malnutrition and weight loss, and part may be simply a manifestation of hypermetabolism, since agents that elevate metabolism, such as salicylates, also lower serum lipid levels. Thyroid hormone directly enhances conversion of cholesterol to bile acids and their excretion in the bile. This metabolic route accounts for the disposal of 70 to 90 percent of the cholesterol formed in the body.[282] Thyroid hormone may also affect cholesterol metabolism by directly increasing the number of membrane surface low-density lipoprotein (LDL) receptors.[283]

Levels of the other serum lipid components are lowered as well.[285-288] Plasma triglycerides are in the low normal range, and the clearance rate of infused triglycerides may be elevated. Postheparin lipolytic activity may be low or normal.[284,285]

The free tocopherol level of the plasma changes in parallel with the cholesterol alterations in thyrotoxicosis.[288]

Rich et al.[289] found the level of nonesterified fatty acids elevated in thyrotoxic patients. This response can be seen within six hours after administration of L-T$_3$ to normal subjects, and might be related to the observation that ketosis occurs more readily in thyrotoxic patients than in normal subjects.

Protein Metabolism

Protein formation and destruction are both accelerated in hyperthyroidism. Nitrogen excretion is increased, and nitrogen balance may be normal or negative, depending on whether intake meets the demands of increased catabolism. Testosterone is able to exert its anabolic effects in thyrotoxicosis.

Lewallen et al.[290] found that administration of thyroid hormone increases albumin synthesis and degradation in normal subjects, increases the fractional rate of degradation, and reduces the quantity of exchangeable albumin.

Thyroid hormone in vivo[291] or in vitro,[292] as reviewed in Chapter 2, may exert its basic action through stimulation of transcription and mRNA translation. Thyroid hormone stimulates incorporation of amino acids into protein by liver microsomes. This action is at least partially explained by increased production of mRNA and by an increased transfer of soluble tRNA-bound amino acids into microsomal protein.[293] Clinically, a great excess of thyroid hormone appears to have the opposite effect.

Crispell et al. found that protein synthesis may be depressed by feeding thyroid hormone to normal humans.[291] Catabolism of collagen is increased,[294] and urinary hypodroxyproline excretion is characteristically increased. Gluconeogenesis from alanine is stimulated by thyroid hormone.[295] The elevated somatomedin levels found in thyrotoxicosis[296] probably contribute to augmented protein synthesis.

cAMP Metabolism

Basal cAMP levels are on average elevated in serum of thyrotoxic humans (Fig. 10-8), and there is hyperresponsiveness to stimuli such as epinephrine and glucagon[297] (Fig. 10-8). Urinary cAMP is likewise increased.[298] Treatment with propranolol (in some studies) lowers basal cAMP toward, but not to, normal.[299] Opposite changes occur in hypothyroidism. β-adrenergic receptors are increased in number, and responses are enhanced as compared to the normal state (see Ch. 2).

Vitamin Metabolism

The absorption of vitamin A is increased and conversion of carotene to vitamin A is accelerated in thyrotoxicosis. The requirements of the body are likewise increased, and low blood concentrations of vitamin A may be found.

Requirements for thiamine and vitamin B$_6$ are increased.[300] Lack of the B vitamins has been implicated as a cause of liver damage in thyrotoxicosis. It has been demonstrated that vitamin B$_{12}$ requirements are increased in experimental thyrotoxicosis.

Radiosensitivity

Radiosensitivity of animal and human tumors may be enhanced by administration of L-T$_3$.[301]

CAUSES OF DEATH

Given current therapeutic resources, death from thyrotoxicosis or from its treatment should be rare. Thyroid storm, when it occurs, however, can be a lethal event. In a study from Scottish hospitals, 20 of 33 patients who died had congestive heart failure, 6 bronchial pneumonia, and 6 embolism in various sites. Nineteen had atrial fibrillation. Eight were considered to have thyroid storm.[302] One might suspect that several causes of death might be identified in any particular case, and that rarely if ever would pure thyrotoxicosis be the only assignable cause. In two recent deaths of which we are aware, in patients with fulminant thyrotoxicosis, the immediate cause was sudden cardiovascular collapse, with shock and arrhythmias including ventricular fibrillation, which was resistant to all usual resuscitative efforts.

DIFFERENCES BETWEEN THE SEXES

Over the years, we have become impressed that thyrotoxic men, considered collectively, present some striking differences from thyrotoxic women in their response to the disease. For a given rise in metabolism, the symptoms of women tend to be more conspicuous than do those of men. Of course, there are frequent exceptions. Men with moderately severe thyrotoxicosis often have few or minimal symptoms, whereas many women with much milder thyrotoxicosis often present an impressive array of symptoms.

A statistical study of symptoms and signs, chiefly circulatory, in a series of 184 thyrotoxic patients (52 men, 132 women), using 233 patients with nontoxic nodular goiter as controls,[303] the male patients were somewhat older than the females, and there were more severe cases among men than among women. Cardiac symptoms were more common in women than in men, even though the men were older and more often had a severe form of the disease. Palpitations and dyspnea are both more common and more severe in the female than in the male group.

DIFFERENCES ATTRIBUTABLE TO AGE

Certain differences in symptoms are attributable to age. Classic exophthalmic goiter is more frequent among younger patients, but severe infiltrative exophthalmos is virtually unknown before mid-adolescence. The character of the symptomatic response may be differentiated in another way. In younger patients, the nervous symptoms tend to be more evident than those in older ones; in older patients, circulatory symptoms are more in evidence.[304] In older patients, emotional instability is often hard to identify, and the symptoms and signs are manifestly circulatory. In many older patients with Graves' dis-

ease, the thyroid is not readily palpable. Anorexia in this group is fairly frequent, as is constipation. Devastating personality and emotional changes often appear in the child or adolescent with Graves' disease.

SUMMARY

This chapter considers the clinical syndrome of thyrotoxicosis, and in particular Graves' disease, its usual cause in the United States. Thyrotoxicosis may also be produced by toxic multinodular goiter, toxic adenomas, excessive thyroid hormone ingestion, or several other rare syndromes. Graves' disease includes thyrotoxicosis, goiter, toxic adenomas, excessive thyroid hormone ingestion, or several other rare syndromes. Graves' disease includes thyrotoxicosis, goiter, exophthalmos, and pretibial myxedema when fully expressed, but can occur with one or more of these features.

Graves' disease is a disease of autoimmunity, but the final cause of autoimmunity remains unclear. A strong hereditary tendency is present. Inheritance of HLA antigens B8, Dr3, DQβ2, and DQA1*0501 predispose to Graves' disease. Psychic trauma, sympathetic nervous system activation, strenuous weight reduction, and iodide administration have been associated with the onset of Graves' disease, but have not been proven to play an etiologic role. The abnormal immune response is characterized by the presence of antibodies directed against thyroid tissue antigens, including antibodies that react with the thyrotrophin receptor by binding to the receptor. Some of these antibodies act as agonists and stimulate the thyroid. The best-known of the antibodies is the serum factor *LATS*, now known as *TSAb*. Hypersecretion of TSH is not a cause of Graves' disease, and serum TSH is typically suppressed to or near zero.

It has been shown in active Graves' disease that T-lymphocyte suppressor cell function is diminished and suppressor cell number is reduced. Specific T suppressor cells controlling thyroid autoantibody production may also be diminished. It is hypothesized that an abnormality in the control of autoimmune responses is present in this disease and leads to production of high levels of autoantibodies that may stimulate the thyroid or eventually cause thyroid damage and cell death. The goiter, lymphocyte infiltrate, and antithyroid antibodies, with the exception of thyroid-stimulating antibodies, overlap with features of Hashimoto's thyroiditis.

The thyroid gland is hyperfunctioning in Graves' disease, and its action is not suppressed by administration of exogenous T_3. The pituitary response to TRH is also suppressed. The gland is unusually responsive to small doses of iodide, which both block further hormone synthesis and inhibit release of hormone from the gland.

In recent studies, the incidence of Graves' disease is reported to be 1 to 2 cases per 1,000 population per year in England. This rate is considerably higher than the rate of about 0.3 cases per 1,000 previously reported from this country. The frequency in women is much greater than in men.

Thyrotoxicosis itself is associated with pathologic changes including damage to muscles and mild damage to the liver. Graves' disease is associated with hyperplasia of and lymphoid infiltrates in the thyroid, generalized lymphoid hyperplasia, and the specific changes of infiltrative ophthalopathy and pretibial myxedema.

The classic features of thyrotoxicosis are nervousness, diminished sleep, tremulousness, tachycardia, increased appetite, weight loss, and increased perspiration. In Graves' disease these symptoms and signs are associated with goiter, occasionally with exophthalmos, and rarely with pretibial myxedema. Physical findings include fine skin and hair, tremulousness, a hyperactive heart, Plummer's nails, muscle weakness, accelerated reflex relaxation, occasional splenomegaly, and often peripheral edema. Autoimmune vitiligo or hives may coexist.

The disease typically begins gradually in adult women and is progressive unless treated. Muscle weakness is frequent, myasthenia may coexist, and hypokalemic periodic paralysis may be induced by thyrotoxicosis. Hypercalciuria is frequent, but severe osteitis fibrosa or osteomalacia and fractures are rare. Kidney stones rarely occur. Thyrotoxicosis can cause congestive heart failure. Mitral valve prolapse occurs with increased frequency in toxic patients. Atrial tachycardia and fibrillation are commonly caused by thyrotoxicosis. Normocytic anemia is found. Diarrhea occurs, but malabsorption is unusual. Minimal liver damage and hyperbilirubinemia may be induced. Amenorrhea or anovulatory cycling is common in women, and fertility is reduced.

Oxygen consumption is greatly increased, lipid production and turnover are accelerated, and plasma total lipid and cholesterol levels tend to be low.

Thyrotoxicosis in untreated cases leads to cardiovascular damage, bone loss and fractures, or inanition, and can be fatal. The long-term history also includes spontaneous remission in some cases and eventual spontaneous development of hypothyroidism if autoimmune thyroiditis coexists and destroys the thyroid gland.

REFERENCES

1. Graves RJ: Clinical lectures. London Med Surg J (pt 2):516, 1835
2. Charles DN: Graves' disease with functioning nodules (Marine-Lenhart syndrome). J Nucl Med 13: 885, 1972
3. Kracht J, Kracht U: Zum histochemischen Perosydasenachweis in der Shilddruse unter normalen und pathologischen Bedingungen. Arch Exp Pathol Pharmakol 213:429, 1951
4. Wasmich RD: Ophthalmopathy following external neck irradiation for nonthyroidal neoplastic disease. J Clin Endocrinol Metab 37:703, 1973
5. Hancock SL, Cox RS, McDougall IR: Thyroid diseases after treatment of Hodgkin's disease. N Engl J Med 325:599, 1991
6. Bartels ED: Heredity in Graves' Disease. Enjnar Munksgaards Forlag, Copenhagen, 1941
7. Martin L: The hereditary and familial aspect of exophthalmic goiter and nodular goiter. Q J Med 14: 207, 1945
8. Harvald B, Hauge M: A catamnestic investigation of Danish twins. Dan Med Bull 3:150, 1956
9. Carey C, Skosey C, Pinnamaneni KM et al: Thyroid abnormalities in children of parents who have Graves' disease: possible pre-Graves' disease. Metabolism 29:369, 1980
10. Saxena KM: Inheritance of thyroglobulin antibody in thyrotoxic children. Lancet 1:583, 1965
11. Tami H, Suematsu H, Ikemi Y et al: Responses to TRH and T_3 suppression tests in euthyroid subjects with a family history of Graves' disease. J Clin Endocrinol Metab 47:475, 1978
12. Chopra IJ, Solomon DH, Chopra U et al: Abnormalities in thyroid function in relatives of patients with Graves' disease and Hashimoto's thyroiditis: lack of correlation with inheritance of HLA-B8. J Clin Endocrinol Metab 45:45, 1977
13. Banovac K, Zakarija M, McKenzie JM et al: Absence of thyroid-stimulating antibody and long-acting thy-

roid stimulator in relatives of Graves' disease patients. J Clin Endocrinol Metab 53:651, 1981

14. Grumet FC, Payne RO, Konishi J, Kriss JP: HLA antigens as markers for disease susceptibility and autoimmunity in Graves' disease. J Clin Endocrinol Metab 39:1115, 1974

15. Yoshinobu N, Kishihara M, Baba Y et al: HLA antigens in autoimmune thyroid diseases. Arch Intern Med 138:567, 1968

16. Farid NR, Stone E, Johnson G: Graves' disease and HLA: clinical and epidemiologic associations. Clin Endocrinol 13:535, 1980

17. Farid NR (ed): HLA in Endocrine and Metabolid Disorders. Academic Press, New York, 1981

18. Mangklabruks A, Cox N, DeGroot LJ: Genetic factors in autoimmune thyroid disease analyzed by restriction fragment length polymorphisms of candidate genes. J Clin Endocrinol Metab 73:236, 1991

19. Yanagawa T, Mangklabruks A, Chang Y-B et al: Human histocompatibility leukocyte antigen-DQA1*0501 allele associated with genetic susceptibility to Graves' disease in a Caucasian population. J Clin Endocrinol Metab 76:1569, 1993

20. Irvine WJ, Gray RS, Morris PJ, Ting A: Correlation of HLA and thyroid antibodies with clinical course of thyrotoxicosis treated with antithyroid drugs. Lancet 1:898, 1977

21. Dahlberg PA, Holmlund G, Karlsson FA, Safwenberg J: HLA-A, B-C, and -DR antigens in patients with Graves' disease and their correlation with signs and clinical course. Acta Endocrinol 97:42, 1981

22. Nakao Y, Matsumoto H, Miyazaki T et al: IgG heavy chain allotypes (Gm) in autoimmune diseases. Clin Exp Immunol 42:20, 1980

23. Wang P-W, Huang M-J, Liu R-T, Chen CD: Triiodothyronine autoantibodies in Graves' disease: their changes after antithyroid therapy and relationship with the thyroglobulin antibodies. Acta Endocrinol (Copenh) 122:22, 1990

24. Adams DD: The presence of an abnormal thyroid-stimulating hormone in the serum of some thyrotoxic patients. J Clin Endocrinol Metab 18:699, 1958

25. McKenzie JM: Further evidence for a thyroid activator in hyperthyroidism. J Clin Endocrinol Metab 20:380, 1960

26. Adams DD: A comparison of the rates at which thyrotrophin and the human abnormal thyroid stimulator disappear from the circulating blood of the rat. Endocrinology 66:658, 1960

27. Smith BR, Hall R: Binding of thyroid stimulators to thyroid membranes. FEBS Lett 42:301, 1974

28. Huber GK, Safirstein R, Neufeld D, Davies TF: Thyrotropin receptor autoantibodies induce human thyroid cell growth and c-fos activation. J Clin Endocrinol Metab 72:1142, 1991

29. Jortso E, Molne J, Boeryd B et al: Effects of thyroid stimulating immunoglobulin on function and morphology of xenotransplanted toxic diffuse, toxic nodular, and normal thyroid tissue. J Endocrinol Invest 10:435, 1987

30. McKenzie JM: Studies on the thyroid activator of hyperthyroidism. J Clin Endocrinol Metab 21:635, 1961

31. Arnaud CD, Kneubuhler HA, Seiling VL et al: Responses of normal human to infusions of plasma from patients with Graves' disease. J Clin Invest 44:1287, 1965

32. Miyai K, Fukuchi M, Kumahara Y, Abe H: LATS production by lymphocyte culture in patients with Graves' disease. J Clin Endocrinol Metab 27:855, 1967

33. McKenzie JM, Gordon J: The origin of the long-acting thyroid stimulator. p. 445. In Cassano C, Andreoli M (eds): Current Topics of Thyroid Research. Academic Press, San Diego, 1965

34. Wenzel B, Wenzel KW, Kotulla P, Schleusener H: Binding of solubilized human TSH-receptor protein by peripheral blood lymphocytes of patients with Graves' disease. J Endocrinol Invest 4:161, 1981

35. Onaya T, Kotani M, Yamada T, Ochi Y: New in vitro tests to detect the thyroid stimulator in sera from hyperthyroid patients by measuring colloid droplet formation and cyclic AMP in human thyroid slices. J Clin Endocrinol Metab 36:859, 1973

36. Adams DD, Fastier FN, Howie JB et al: Stimulation of the human thyroid by infusions of plasma containing LATS protector. J Clin Endocrinol Metab 39:826, 1974

37. Adams DD, Kennedy TH: Evidence to suggest that LATS protector stimulates the human thyroid gland. J Clin Endocrinol Metab 33:47, 1971

38. Shishiba Y, Shimizu T, Yoshimura S, Shizume K: Direct evidence for human thyroidal stimulation by LATS-protector. J Clin Endocrinol Metab 36:517, 1973

39. Rees Smith B, McLachlan SM, Furmaniak J: Autoantibodies to the thyrotropin receptor. Endocr Rev 9:106, 1988

40. Orgiazzi J, Williams DE, Chopra IJ, Solomon DH: Human thyroid adenyl cyclase-stimulating activity in immunoglobulin G of patients with Graves' disease. J Clin Endocrinol Metab 42:341, 1976

41. Loveridge N, Zakarija M, Bitensky L, McKenzie JM: The cytochemical bioassay for thyroid-stimulating antibody of Graves' disease: further experience. J Clin Endocrinol Metab 49:610, 1979

42. Mukhtar ED, Smith BR, Pyle GA et al: Relation of thyroid-stimulating immunoglobulins to thyroid function and effect of surgery, radioiodine, and antithyroid drugs. Lancet 1:713, 1975

43. Doctor R, Bos G, Visser TJ, Hennemann G: Thyrotropin-binding inhibiting immunoglobulins in Graves' disease before, during, and after antithyroid therapy, and its relation to long-acting thyroid stimulator. Clin Endocrinol 12:143, 1980

44. Kuzuya N, Chiu SC, Ikeda H et al: Correlation between thyroid stimulators and 3,5,3'-triiodo-thyronine suppressibility in patients during treatment for hyperthyroidism with thionamide drugs: comparison of assays by thyroid-stimulating and thyrotropin-displacing activities. J Clin Endocrinol Metab 48:706, 1979

45. Ozawa Y, Maciel RMB, Chopra IJ et al: Relationships among immunoglobulin markers in Graves' disease. J Clin Endocrinol Metab 48:381, 1979

46. Endo K, Kasagi K, Konishi J et al: Detection and properties of TSH-binding inhibitor immunoglobulins in patients with Graves' disease and Hashimoto's thyroiditis. J Clin Endocrinol Metab 46:734, 1978

47. Irvine WJ, Lamberg B-A, Cullen DR, Gordin R: Primary hypothyroidism preceding thyrotoxicosis: a report of 2 cases and a review of the literature. J Clin Lab Immunol 2:349, 1979

48. Momotani N, Noh J, Ishikawa N, Ito K: Relationship between silent thyroiditis and recurrent Graves' disease in the postpartum period. J Clin Endocrinol Metab 79:285, 1994

49. Matusura N, Yamada Y, Nohara Y et al: Familial neonatal transient hypothyroidism due to maternal TSH-binding inhibitor immunoglobulins. N Engl J Med 303:738, 1980

50. Endo K, Amir SM, Ingbar SH: Development and evaluation of a method for the partial purification of immunoglobulins specific for Graves' disease. J Clin Endocrinol Metab 52:113, 1981

51. Trokoudes MK, Sugenoya A, Hazani E et al: Thyroid-stimulating hormone (TSH) binding to extrathyroidal human tissues: TSH and thyroid-stimulating immunoglobulin effects on adenosine 3'5'-monophosphate in testicular and adrenal tissues. J Clin Endocrinol Metab 48:919, 1979

52. Mehdi QS, Badger J, Kriss JP: Thyrotropin-binding and long-acting thyroid stimulator absorbing activities in subcellular fractions from isolated thyroid cells and thyroid homogenates. Endocrinology 101:59, 1977

53. Zakarija M, McKenzie JM: Isoelectric focusing of thyroid-stimulating antibody of Graves' disease. Endocrinology 103:1469, 1978

54. Fenzi G, Hashizume K, Roudebush CP, DeGroot LJ: Changes in thyroid-stimulating immunoglobulins during antithyroid therapy. J Clin Endocrinol Metab 48:572, 1979

55. Davies TF, Yeo PPB, Evered DC et al: Value of thyroid-stimulating antibody determinations in predicting short-term thyrotoxic relapse in Graves' disease. Lancet 1:1181, 1977

56. Bolk JH, Elte JWF, Bussemaker JK et al: Thyroid-stimulating immunoglobulins do not cause non-autonomous, autonomous, or toxic multinodular goiters. Lancet 1:61, 1979

57. Drexhage HA, Bottazzo GF, Doniach D et al: Evidence for thyroid growth-stimulating immunoglobulins in some goitrous thyroid diseases. Lancet 2:287, 1980

58. Nakamura S, Sakata S, Shima H et al: Thyroid hormone autoantibodies (THAA) in two cases of Graves' disease: effects of antithyroid drugs, prednisolone, and subtotal thyroidectomy. Endocrinol Japan 33:751, 1986

59. Mariotti S, Kaplan EL, Medof ME, DeGroot LJ: Circulating thyroid antigen antibody immune complexes. Presented at the Eighth International Thyroid Congress; February 3–8, 1980 Sydney, Australia.

60. Fujiwara H, Torisu M, Koitabashi Y et al: Immune complex deposits in thyroid glands of patients with Graves' disease. Clin Immunol Immunopathol 19:98, 1981

61. Lamki L, Row VV, Volpe R: Cell-mediated immunity in Graves' disease and in Hashimoto's thyroiditis as shown by the demonstration of migration inhibition factor (MIF). J Clin Endocrinol Metab 36:358, 1973

62. Wartenberg J, Doniach D, Brostaff J, Roitt IM: Leucocyte migration inhibition in thyroid disease. Int Arch Allergy Appl Immunol 44:396, 1973

63. Amino N, DeGroot LJ: Insoluble particulate antigen(s) in cell-mediated immunity of autoimmune thyroid disease. Metabolism 24:45, 1975

64. Okita N, Kidd A, Row VV, Volpe R: Sensitization of T-lymphocytes in Graves' and Hashimoto's diseases. J Clin Endocrinol Metab 51:316, 1980

65. Aoki N, DeGroot LJ: Lymphocyte blastogenic response to human thyroglobulin in Graves' disease, Hashimoto's thyroiditis, and metastatic cancer. Clin Exp Immunol 38:523, 1979

66. DeGroot LJ, Kawakami Y, Fisfalen M-E et al: T cell epitopes in TPO and TSH receptor. Presented at the International Hashimoto Symposium—80th Anniversary of Hashimoto's Disease; December 2–5, 1992; Fukuoka, Japan.

67. Soliman M, Guimaraes V, Fisfalen M-E, DeGroot LJ: Definition of T cell epitopes of thyrotropin receptor by testing T cell reactivity to human recombinant thyrotropin extracellular domain and its synthetic peptides in AITD patients. Presented at the 76th Annual Meeting of the Endocrine Society, June 15–18, 1994; Anaheim, CA.

68. Robinson RG, Guttler RB, Rea TH, Nicoloff JT: Delayed hypersensitivity in Graves' disease. J Clin Endocrinol Metab 38:322, 1974

69. Aoki N, Pinnamaneni KM, DeGroot LJ: Studies on suppressor cell function in thyroid diseases. J Clin Endocrinol Metab 48:803, 1979

70. Pacini F, DeGroot LJ: Studies of immunoglobulin synthesis in cultures of peripheral T and B lymphocytes. Reduced T-suppressor cell activity in Graves' disease. Clin Endocrinol 18:219, 1983

71. Topliss DJ, Okita N, Lewis M et al: Allosuppressor T lymphocytes abolish migration inhibition factor production in autoimmune thyroid disease: evidence from radiosensitivity experiments. Clin Endocrinol 15:335, 1981

72. Beall GN, Kruger SR: Antithyroglobulin production by peripheral blood leukocytes in vitro. J Clin Endocrinol Metab 48:712, 1979

73. McLachlan SM, Bird AG, Weetman AP et al: Use of plaque assays to study thyroglobulin autoantibody synthesis by human peripheral blood lymphocytes. Scand J Immunol 14:233, 1981

74. Sridama V, Pacini F, DeGroot LJ: Decreased suppressor T-lymphocytes in autoimmune thyroid diseases detected by monoclonal antibodies. J Clin Endocrinol Metab 54:316, 1982

75. Thielemans C, VanHaelst L, DeWaele M et al: Autoimmune thyroiditis: a condition related to a decrease in T-suppressor cells. Clin Endocrinol 15:259, 1981

76. Ludgate ME, McGregor AM, Weetman AP et al: Analysis of T cell subsets in Graves' disease: alterations associated with carbimazole. Br Med J 288:526, 1984

77. Topliss D, How J, Lewis M et al: Evidence for cell-mediated immunity and specific suppressor T-lymphocyte dysfunction in Graves' disease and diabetes mellitus. J Clin Endocrinol Metab 57:700, 1983

78. Mori H, Amino N, Iwatani Y et al: Increase of peripheral B lymphocytes in Graves' disease. Clin Exp Immunol 42:33, 1980

79. Mori H, Amino N, Iwatani Y et al: Decrease of immunoglobulin G-Fc receptor-bearing T lymphocytes in Graves' disease. J Clin Endocrinol Metab 55:399, 1982

80. Iversen K: Temporary rise in the frequency of thyrotoxicosis in Denmark 1941–1945. Rosenkilde and Bagger, Copenhagen, 1948

81. Winsa B, Adami HO, Bergstrom R et al: Stressful life events and Graves' disease. Lancet 338:1475, 1991

82. Spratt DI, Pont A, Miller MB et al: Hyperthyroxinemia in patients with acute psychiatric disorders. Am J Med 73:41, 1982

83. Landsberg L: Catecholamines and hyperthyroidism. Clin Endocrinol Metab 6:697, 1977

84. Bruun E: Exophthalmic goiter developing after treatment with thyroid preparations. Acta Med Scand 122:13, 1945

85. Stanbury JB, Brownell GI, Riggs DS et al: Endemic Goiter. p. 66. Harvard University Press, Cambridge, 1954

86. Connolly RJ, Vidor GI, Stewart JC: Increase in thyrotoxicosis in endemic goiter area after iodation of bread. Lancet 1:500, 1970

87. Vidor GI, Stewart JC, Wall JR et al: Pathogenesis of iodine-induced thyrotoxicosis: studies in northern Tasmania. J Clin Endocrinol Metab 37:901, 1973

88. Vagenakis AG, Wang CA, Bruger A et al: Iodide-induced thyrotoxicosis in Boston. N Engl J Med 287:523, 1972

89. Nilsson G: Self-limiting episodes of Jod-Basedow. Acta Endocrinol 74:475, 1973

90. Stewart JC, Vidor GI, Butterfield IH, Hetzel BS: Epidemic thyrotoxicosis in northern Tasmania. Studies of clinical features and iodine nutrition. Aust NZ J Med 3:203, 1971

91. Adams DD, Kennedy TH, Purves HD: Comparison of the thyroid-stimulating hormone content of serum from thyrotoxic and euthyroid people. J Clin Endocrinol Metab 29:900, 1969

92. Emerson CH, Utiger RD: Hyperthyroidism and excessive thyrotropin secretion. N Engl J Med 287:328, 1972

93. Lamberg BA, Ripatti J, Gordin A et al: Chromophobe pituitary adenoma with acromegaly and TSH-induced hyperthyroidism associated with parathyroid adenoma. Acta Endocrinol 60:157, 1969

94. Hamilton CR Jr, Maloof F: Acromegaly and toxic goiter. Cure of the hyperthyroidism and acromegaly by proton-beam partial hypophysectomy. J Clin Endocrinol Metab 35:659, 1972

95. Weintraub BD, Gershengorn MC, Kourides IA, Fein H: Inappropriate secretion of thyroid-stimulating hormone. Ann Intern Med 95:339, 1981

96. Fajans SS: Hyperthyroidism in a patient with postpartum necrosis of the pituitary: case report and implications. J Clin Endocrinol Metab 18:271, 1958

97. Werner SC, Stewart WB: Hyperthyroidism in a patient with a pituitary chromophobe adenoma and a fragment of normal pituitary. J Clin Endocrinol Metab 18:266, 1958

98. Werner SC, Becker DV, Row VV: Distribution of serum radioiodinated compounds in euthyroid and hyperthyroid patients following hypophysectomy. J Clin Endocrinol Metab 19:953, 1959

99. Beckers DV: Effects of hypophysectomy on certain parameters of thyroid function in two patients with Graves' disease. J Clin Endocrinol Metab 19:840, 1959

100. Dobyns BM, Steelman SL: The thyroid-stimulating hormone of the anterior pituitary as distinct from exophthalmos-producing substance. Endocrinology 52:705, 1953

101. Wegelius O, Naumann J, Brunish R: Uptake of ^{35}S-labeled sulfate in the harderian and the ventral lachrymal glands of the guinea pig during stimulation with ophthalmotrophic pituitary agents. Acta Endocrinol 30:53, 1959

102. der Kinderen PJ, Houstra-Lanz M, Schwarz F: Exophthalmos-producing substance in human serum. J Clin Endocrinol Metab 20:712, 1960

103. Hershman J: Hyperthyroidism induced by trophoblastic thyrotropin. Mayo Clin Proc 47:913, 1972

104. Karp PJ, Hershman JM, Richmond S et al: Thyrotoxicosis from molar thyrotropin. Arch Intern Med 132:432, 1973

105. Goodwin TM, Montoro M, Mestman JH et al: The role of chorionic gonadotropin in transient hyperthyroidism of hyperemesis gravidarum. J Clin Endocrinol Metab 75:1333, 1992

106. Duprez L, Parma J, Van Sande J et al: Germline mutations in the thyrotropin receptor gene cause non-autoimmune autosomal dominant hyperthyroidism. Nature Genetics 7:396, 1994

107. Kasagi K, Konishi J, Endo K et al: Adenylate cyclase activity in thyroid tissue from patients with untreated Graves' disease. J Clin Endocrinol Metab 51:492, 1980

108. Stanbury JB, Janssen MA: The iodinated albumin-like component of the plasma of thyrotoxic patients. J Clin Endocrinol Metab 22:978, 1962

109. Farran HEA, Shalom ES: Effect of L-tyrosine upon the protein bound iodine in thyrotoxicosis. J Clin Endocrinol Metab 26:918, 1966

110. Sterling K, Chodos RB: Radiothyroxine turnover studies in myxedema, thyrotoxicosis, and hypermetabolism without endocrine disease. J Clin Invest 35:806, 1956

111. Ingbar SH, Freinkel N: Studies on thyroid function and the peripheral metabolism of ^{131}I-labeled thyroxine in patients with treated Graves' disease. J Clin Invest 37:1603, 1958

112. Uller RP, Van Herle AJ: Effect of therapy on serum thyroglobulin levels in patients with Graves' disease. J Clin Endocrinol Metab 46:747, 1978

113. Greer MA, Smith GE: Method for increasing the accuracy of the radioiodine uptake as a test for thyroid function by the use of desiccated thyroid. J Clin Endocrinol Metab 14:1374, 1954

114. Werner SC, Spooner M: A new and simple test for hyperthyroidism employing L-triiodothyronine and the twenty-four hour ^{131}I uptake methods. Bull NY Acad Med 31:137, 1955

115. Clague R, Mukhtar ED, Pyle GA et al: Thyroid-stimulating immunoglobulins and the control of thyroid function. J Clin Endocrinol Metab 43:550, 1976

116. Lamberg BA, Ard A, Saarinen P et al: Response to TRH, serum thyroid hormone concentration, and serum markers of autoimmunity after antithyroid therapy in Graves' disease. J Endocrinol Invest 1:9, 1978

117. Chopra IJ, Chopra U, Orgiazzi J: Abnormalities of hypothalamo-hypophyseal-thyroid axis in patients with Graves' ophthalmopathy. J Clin Endocrinol Metab 37:955, 1973

118. Franco PS, Hershman JM, Haigler ED, Pittman JA Jr: Response to thyrotropin-releasing hormone compared with thyroid suppression tests in euthyroid Graves' disease. Metabolism 22:1357, 1973

119. Plummer HS: Results of administering iodine to patients having exophthalmic goiter. JAMA 80:1955, 1923

120. Raben MS: The paradoxical effects of thiocyanate and of thyrotropin on the organic binding of iodine by the thyroid in the presence of large amounts of iodide. Endocrinology 45:296, 1949

121. Feinberg WD, Hoffman DL, Owen CA: The effects of varying amounts of stable iodide on the function of the human thyroid. J Clin Endocrinol Metab 19:567, 1959

122. Stanley MM: The direct estimation of the rate of thyroid hormone formation in man: the effect of the iodide ion on thyroid iodine utilization. J Clin Endocrinol Metab 9:941, 1949

123. Paris J, McConahey WM, Tauxe WN et al: The effect of iodides on Hashimoto's thyroiditis. J Clin Endocrinol Metab 21:1037, 1961

124. Suzuki H, Mashimo K: Significance of the iodide-perchlorate discharge test in patients with ^{131}I-treated and untreated hyperthyroidism. J Clin Endocrinol Metab 34:332, 1972

125. Braverman LE, Woeber KA, Ingbar SH: Induction of myxedema by iodide in patients euthyroid after radioiodine or surgical treatment of diffuse toxic goiter. N Engl J Med 281:816, 1969

126. Greer MA, DeGroot LJ: The effect of stable iodide thyroid secretion in man. Metabolism 5:682, 1956

127. Ochi Y, Hachiya T, Yoshimura M et al: Inhibitory effect of excess iodide on Graves' disease. Iodine Metab Thyroid Function 6:127, 1973

128. Wartofsky L, Ransh BJ, Ingbar SH: Inhibition by iodine of the release of thyroxine from the thyroid glands of patients with thyrotoxicosis. J Clin Invest 49:78, 1970

129. Buhler UK, DeGroot LJ: Effects of stable iodine on thyroid iodine release. J Clin Endocrinol Metab 29:1546, 1969

130. Slingerland DW, Burrows BA: A probable abnormality in intrathyroidal iodine metabolism in hyperthyroidism. J Clin Endocrinol Metab 22:368, 1962

131. DeGroot L: Kinetic analysis of iodine metabolism. J Clin Endocrinol Metab 26:149, 1966

132. Furszyfer J, Kurland LT, McConahey WM, Elveback LR: Graves' disease in Olmsted County, Minnesota, 1935 through 1967. Mayo Clin Proc 45:636, 1970

133. Tunbridge WMG, Evered DE, Hall R et al: The spectrum of thyroid disease in a community: the Wickham Survey. Clin Endocrinol 7:481, 1977

134. Sallstrom T: Vorkommen und Verbreitung der Thyrotoxicosis in Schweden, Stockholm, 1935, abstracted. JAMA 106:216, 1936

135. Pendergrast WJ, Milmore BK, Marcus SC: Goiter, thyrotoxicosis, and cancer. J Chronic Dis 13:22, 1961

136. Heimann P: Ultrastructure of human thyroid. Acta Endocrinol, suppl. 110:5, 1966

137. Pemberton J de J: Recurring exophthalmic goiter: its relation to the amount of tissue preserved in operation on the thyroid gland. JAMA 94:1483, 1930

138. Adams RD, Denny-Brown D, Pearson CM: Diseases of Muscle. Harper & Row, New York, 1962

139. Bostrom H, Hed R: Thyrotoxic myopathy and polymyositis in elderly patients: differential-diagnostic viewpoints. Acta Med Scand 162:225, 1958

140. McEachern D, Ross WD: Chronic thyrotoxic myopathy: report of three cases with review of previously reported cases. Brain 65:181, 1942

141. Askanazy M, Rutishauser E: Die Knochen der Basedow-Kranken: Beitrag zur latenten Osteodystrophia fibrosa. Virchows Arch 291:653, 1933

142. Dudgeon LS, Urquhart AL: Lymphorrhages in the muscles in exophthalmic goiter. Grain 49:182, 1926

143. Naffziger HC: Progressive exophthalmos after thyroidectomy. West J Surg Obstet Gynecol 40:530, 1932

144. Rundle FF, Pochin EE: Orbital tissues in thyrotoxicosis: quantitative analysis relating to exophthalmos. Clin Sci 5:51, 1944

145. Wright EA: Case of malignant exophthalmos associated with fatal myocarditis. Guy's Hosp Rep 106:36, 1957

146. Terndrup TE, Heisig DG, Garceau JP: Sudden death associated with undiagnosed Graves' disease. J Emergency Med 8:553, 1990

147. Russfield AB: Histology of the human hypophysis in thyroid disease. Hypothyroidism, hyperthyroidism, and cancer. J Clin Endocrinol Metab 15:1393, 1955

148. Ezrin C, Swanson HE, Humphrey JG et al: The cells of the human adenohypophysis in thyroid disorders. J Clin Endocrinol Metab 19:958, 1959

149. Scheithauer BW, Kovacs KT, Young WF Jr, Randall RV: The pituitary gland in hyperthyroidism. Mayo Clin Proc 67:22, 1992

150. Beaver DC, Pemberton J de J: The pathologic anatomy of the liver in exophthalmic goiter. Ann Intern Med 7:687, 1933

151. Movitt ER, Gerstl B, Davis AE: Needle biopsy in thyrotoxicosis. Arch Intern Med 91:729, 1953

152. Piper J, Poulsen E: Liver biopsy in thyrotoxicosis. Acta Med Scand 127:439, 1947

153. Bergman TA, Mariash CN, Oppenheimer JH: Anterior mediastinal mass in a patient with Graves' disease. J Clin Endocrinol Metab 55:587, 1982

154. Fallon MD, Perry HM III, Bergfeld M et al: Exogenous hyperthyroidism with osteoporosis. Arch Intern Med 143:442, 1983

155. Cook PB, Nassim JR, Collins J: The effects of thyrotoxicosis upon the metabolism of calcium, phosphorus, and nitrogen. Q J Med 28:505, 1959

156. Follis RH: Skeletal changes associated with hyperthyroidism. Bull Johns Hopkins Hosp 92:405, 1953

157. MacFarlane IA, Mawer EB, Berry J, Hann J: Vitamin D metabolism in hyperthyroidism. Clin Endocrinol 17:51, 1982

158. Shulz H, Low H, Ernster L, Sjostrand FS: Electronenmikroskopische Studien an Leberschnitten von Thyroxin-behandelten Ratten. p. 134. In Sjostrand FS, Rhodin J (eds): European Regional Conference on Electron Microscopy. 1st Proceedings of the Stockholm Conference, September 1956. Academic Press, New York, 1957

159. White WH: On prognosis of secondary symptoms of exophthalmic goiter. Br Med J 2:151, 1886

160. Sattler H: Marchand GW, Marchand JF (trans): Basedow's Disease. Grune & Stratton, Orlando 1952

161. Hegedus L, Hansen JM, Karstrup S: High incidence of normal thyroid gland volume in patients with Graves' disease. Clin Endocrinol 19:603, 1983

162. Werner S: Classification of the eye changes of Graves' disease. J Clin Endocrinol Metab 29:982, 1969

163. Leblond CP, Fertman MB, Puppel ID, Curtis GM: Radioiodine autography in studies of human goitrous thyroid glands. Arch Pathol Lab Med 41:510, 1946

164. Mahaux JE, Chamla-Soumenkoff J, Delcourt R, Levin S: Painful enlargement of left subtrapezoid lymph nodes in Graves' disease. Br Med J 1:384, 1971

165. Ochi Y, DeGroot LJ: Vitiligo in Graves' disease. Ann Intern Med 71:935, 1969

166. Perrild H, Hansen JM, Arnung K et al: Intellectual impairment after hyperthyroidism. Acta Endocrinol 112:185, 1986

167. Feibel JH, Campa JF: Thyrotoxic neuropathy (Basedow's paraplegia). J Neurol Neurosurg Psychiatry 39:491, 1976

168. Condon JV, Becka DR, Gibbs FA: Electroencephalo-

graphic abnormalities in hyperthyroidism. J Clin Endocrinol Metab 14:1511, 1954

169. Woodbury DM, Hurley RE, Lewis NG et al: Effect of thyroxine, thyroidectomy, and 6-N-propyl-2-thiouracil on brain function. J Pharmacol Exp Ther 106: 331, 1952

170. Ravera JJ, Cervino JM, Fernandez G et al: Two cases of Graves' disease with signs of a pyramidal lesion: improvement in neurologic signs during treatment with antithyroid drugs. J Clin Endocrinol Metab 20: 876, 1960

171. Swanson JW, Kelly JJ Jr, McConahey WM: Neurologic aspects of thyroid dysfunction. Mayo Clin Proc 56:504, 1981

172. Waldenstrom J: Acute thyrotoxic encephalomyopathy: its cause and treatment. Acta Med Scand 121: 251, 1945

173. Feibel JH, Campa JF: Thyrotoxic neuropathy (Basedow's paraplegia). J Neurol Neurosurg Psychiatry 39:491, 1976

174. Sensenbach W, Madison L, Eisenberg S, Ochs L: The cerebral circulation and metabolism in hyperthyroidism and myxedema. J Clin Invest 33:1434, 1954

175. Whitfield AGW, Hudson WA: Chronic thyrotoxic myopathy. Q J Med 30:257, 1961

176. Gold HK, Spann JF Jr, Braunwald E: Effects of alterations in the thyroid state on the intrinsic contractile properties of isolated rat skeletal muscle. J Clin Invest 49:849, 1970

177. Sanderson KV, Adey WR: Electromyographic and endocrine studies in chronic thyrotoxic myopathy. J Neurol Neurosurg Psychiatry 15:200, 1952

178. Zurcher RM, Horber FF, Grunig BE, Frey FJ: Effect of thyroid dysfunction on thigh muscle efficiency. J Clin Endocrinol Metab 69:1082, 1989

179. Fitch CD, Coker R, Dinning JS: Metabolism of creatine I-^{14} C by vitamin E deficient and hyperthyroid rats. Am J Physiol 198:1232, 1960

180. Thorn G: Creatine studies in thyroid disease. Endocrinology 20:628, 1936

181. Kuby SA, Noda L, Lardy HA: Adenosinetriphosphate-creatine transphosphorylase, III. Kinetic studies. J Biol Chem 210:65, 1954

182. Noda L, Kuby SA, Lardy HA: Adenosinetriphosphate-creatine transphosphorylase, IV. Equilibrium studies. J Biol Chem 210:83, 1954

183. Drachman DB: Myasthenia gravis and the thyroid gland. N Engl J Med 266:330, 1962

184. Engel AG: Thyroid function and periodic paralysis. Am J Med 30:327, 1961

185. Fisher J: Thyrotoxic periodic paralysis with ventricular fibrillation. Arch Intern Med 142:1362, 1982

186. Fraser SA, Anderson JB, Smith DA, Wilson GM: Osteoporosis and fractures following thyrotoxicosis. Lancet 1:981, 1971

187. Rosen CJ, Adler RA. Longitudinal changes in lumbar bone density among thyrotoxic patients after attainment of euthyroidism. J Clin Endocrinol Metab 75: 1531, 1992

188. Toh SH, Claunch BC, Brown PH: Effect of hyperthyroidism and its treatment on bone mineral content. Arch Intern Med 145:883, 1985

189. Ettinger B, Wingerd J: Thyroid supplements: effect on bone mass. West J Med 136:473, 1982

190. Harvey RD, McHardy KC, Reid IW et al: Measurement of bone collagen degradation in hyperthyroidism and during thyroxine replacement therapy using pyridinium cross-links as specific urinary markers. J Clin Endocrinol Metab 72:1189, 1991

191. Sataline LR, Powell C, Hamwi GJ: Suppression of the hypercalcemia of thyrotoxicosis by corticosteroids. N Engl J Med 267:646, 1962

192. Sallin O: Hypercalcemic nephropathy in thyrotoxicosis. Acta Endocrinol 29:425, 1958

193. Epstein FH, Freedman LR, Levitin H: Hypercalcemia, nephrocalcinosis, and reversible renal insufficiency associated with hyperthyroidism. N Engl J Med 258:782, 1958

194. Bortz W, Eisenberg E, Bowers CY, Pout M: Differentiation between thyroid and parathyroid causes of hypercalcemia. Ann Intern Med 54:610, 1961

195. David NJ, Verner JV, Engel FL: Diagnostic spectrum of hypercalcemia: case reports and discussion. Am J Med 33:88, 1962

196. Kleeman CR, Tuttle S, Bassett SH: Metabolic observations in a case of thyrotoxicosis with hypercalcemia. J Clin Endocrinol Metab 18:477, 1958

197. Krane SM, Brownell GL, Stanbury JB, Corrigan H: The effect of thyroid disease on calcium metabolism in man. J Clin Invest 35:874, 1956

198. Lukert BP, Higgins JC, Stoskopf MM: Serum osteocalcin is increased in patients with hyperthyroidism and decreased in patients receiving glucocorticoids. J Clin Endocrinol Metab 62:1056, 1986

199. Manicourt D, Demeester-Mirkine N, Brauman H, Corvilain J: Disturbed mineral metabolism in hyperthyroidism: good correlation with triiodothyronine. Clin Endocrinol 10:407, 1979

200. Cooper DS, Kaplan MM, Ridgway EC et al: Alkaline phosphatase isoenzyme patterns in hyperthyroidism. Ann Intern Med 90:164, 1979

201. Bouillon R, DeMoor P: Parathyroid function in patients with hyper- or hypothyroidism. J Clin Endocrinol Metab 38:999, 1974

202. Bouillon R, Muls E, DeMoor P: Influence of thyroid function on the serum concentration of 1,25-dihydroxyvitamin D_3. J Clin Endocrinol Metab 51:793, 1980

202. Garrel DR, Delmas PD, Malaval L. Tourniaire J:

Serum bone Gla protein: a marker of bone turnover in hyperthyroidism. J Clin Endocrinol Metab 62: 1052, 1986

203. Peerenboom H, Keck E, Kruskemper HL, Strohmeyer G: The defect of intestinal calcium transport in hyperthyroidism and its response to therapy. J Clin Endocrinol Metab 59:936, 1984

204. Rude RK, Oldham SB, Singer FR, Nicoloff JT: Treatment of thyrotoxic hypercalcemia with propranolol. N Engl J Med 294:431, 1976

205. Rosen HN, Moses AC, Gundberg C et al: Therapy with parenteral pamidronate prevents thyroid hormone-induced bone turnover in humans. J Clin Endocrinol Metab 77:664, 1993

206. Barsotti MM, Targovnik JH, Verso TA: Thyrotoxicosis, hypercalcemia, and secondary hyperparathyroidism. Arch Intern Med 139:661, 1979

207. Massey DG, Becklake MR, McKenzie JM, Bates DV: Circulatory and ventilatory response to exercise in thyrotoxicosis. N Engl J Med 276:1104, 1967

208. Stein M, Kinbel P, Johnson RL: Pulmonary function in hyperthyroidism. J Clin Invest 40:348, 1961

209. Hamolsky MW: Asthma and hyperthyroidism. J Allergy Clin Immunol 49:348, 1972

210. Reynolds J, Woody HB: Thyrotoxic mitral regurgitation. Am J Dis Child 122:544, 1971

211. Sandler G, Wilson GM: The nature and prognosis of heart disease in thyrotoxicosis. Q J Med 28:347, 1959

212. Graettinger JS, Muenster JJ, Selverstone LA, Campbell JA: A correlation of clinical and hemodynamic studies in patients with hyperthyroidism with and without congestive heart failure. J Clin Invest 38: 1316, 1959

213. Blizzard JJ, Rupp JJ: Prolongation of the P-R interval as a manifestation of thyrotoxicosis. JAMA 173: 1845, 1960

214. Resnekov L, Falicow R: Thyrotoxicosis and lactate-producing angina pectoris with normal coronary arteries. Brit Heart J 39:1051, 1977

215. Kotler N, Kyriakos M, Bouchard J, Warbasse JR: Myocardial infarction associated with thyrotoxicosis. Arch Intern Med 132:723, 1973

216. Rowe GG, Huston JH, Weinstein AB et al: The hemodynamics of thyrotoxicosis in man with special reference to coronary blood flow and myocardial oxygen metabolism. J Clin Invest 35:272, 1956

217. Rodbard D, Fugita T, Rodbard S: Estimation of thyroid function by timing the arterial sounds. JAMA 201:884, 1967

218. Buccino RA, Spann JF Jr, Sonnenblick EH, Braunwald E: Effect of thyroid state on myocardial contractility. Endocrinology 82:191, 1968

219. Woeber KA: Thyrotoxicosis and the heart. N Engl J Med 327:94, 1992

220. Mintz G, Pizzarello R, Klein I: Enhanced left ventricular diastolic function in hyperthyroidism: noninvasive assessment and response to treatment. J Clin Endocrinol Metab 73:146, 1991

221. Valcavi R, Menozzi C, Roti E et al: Sinus node function in hyperthyroid patients. J Clin Endocrinol Metab 75:239, 1992

222. Dillmann WH: Biochemical basis of thyroid hormone action in the heart. Amer J Med 88:626, 1990

223. Pietras RJ, Real MA, Poticha GS et al: Cardiovascular response in hyperthyroidism. the influence of adrenergic-receptor blockade. Arch Intern Med 129:426, 1972

224. deGroot WJ, Leonard JJ, Paley HW et al: The importance of autonomic integrity in maintaining the hyperkinetic circulating dynamics of human hyperthyroidism. J Clin Invest 40:1033, 1961

225. McDevitt DG, Shanks RG, Hadden DR et al: The role of the thyroid in the control of the heart rate. Lancet 1:997, 1968

226. Tse J, Wrenn RW, Kuo JF: Thyroxine-induced changes in characteristics and activities of β-adrenergic receptors and adenosine 3', 5'-monophosphate and guanosine 3', 5'-monophosphate systems in the heart may be related to reputed catecholamine supersensitivity in hyperthyroidism. Endocrinology 107:6, 1980

227. Williams LT, Lefkowitz RJ, Watanabe AM et al: Thyroid hormone regulation of β-adrenergic receptor number. J Biol Chem 252:2787, 1977

228. Ginsberg AM, Clutter WE, Shah SD, Cryer PE: Triiodothyronine-induced thyrotoxicosis increases mononuclear leukocyte β-adrenergic receptor density in man. J Clin Invest 67:1785, 1981

229. Nilsson OR, Anderson RGG, Karlberg BE: Effects of propranolol and atenolol on plasma and urinary cyclic adenosine 3', 5'-monophosphate in hyperthyroid patients. Acta Endocrinol 94:38, 1980

230. Guttler RB, Croxon MS, De Quattro VL et al: Effects of thyroid hormone on plasma adenosine 3', 5'-monophosphate production in man. Metabolism 26: 1155, 1977

231. Levey GS, Klein I: Catecholamine-thyroid hormone interactions and the cardiovascular manifestations of hyperthyroidism. Amer J Med 88:642, 1990

232. Nightingale S, Vitek PJ, Himsworth RL: The hematology of hyperthyroidism. Q J Med 47:35, 1978

233. Popovic WJ, Brown JE, Adamson JW: The influence of thyroid hormones on in vitro erythropoiesis. J Clin Invest 60:907, 1977

234. Rivlin RS, Wagner HN Jr: Anemia in hyperthyroidism. Ann Intern Med 70:507, 1969

235. Viherkoski M, Lamberg BA: The glucose-6-phosphate dehydrogenase activity (G-6-PD) of the red

blood cells in hyperthyroidism and hypothyroidism. Scand J Clin Lab Invest 25:137, 1970

236. Irvine WJ, Wu FCW, Urbaniak SJ, Toolis F: Peripheral blood leukocytes in thyrotoxicosis (Graves' Disease) as studied by conventional light microscopy. Clin Exp Immunol 27:216, 1977

237. Hertz S, Lerman J: The blood picture in exophthalmic goiter and its changes resulting from iodine and operation. J Clin Invest 11:1179, 1932

238. Lamberg BA, Kivikangas V, Pelkonen R, Viopio P: Thrombocytopenia and decreased life-span of thrombocytes in hyperthyroidism. Ann Clin Res 3:98, 1971

239. Adrouny A, Sandler RM, Carmel R: Variable presentation of thrombocytopenia in Graves' disease. Arch Intern Med 142:1460, 1982

240. Simone JV, Abildgaard CF, Schulman I: N Engl J Med 273:1058, 1965

241. Bergman TA, Mariash CN, Oppenheimer JH: Anterior mediastinal mass in a patient with Graves' disease. J Clin Endocrinol Metab 55:587, 1982

242. Lerman J, Means JH: The gastric secretion in exophthalmic goiter and myxedema. J Clin Invest 11:167, 1932

243. Berryhill WR, Williams HA: A study of the gastric secretion in hyperthyroidism before and after operation. J Clin Invest 11:753, 1932

244. Siurala M, Lamberg BA: Stomach in thyrotoxicosis. Acta Med Scand 165:181, 1959

245. Seino Y, Matsukura S, Miyamoto Y et al: Hypergastrinemia in hyperthyroidism. J Clin Endocrinol Metab 43:852, 1976

246. Wegener M, Wedmann B, Langhoff T et al: Effect of hyperthyroidism on the transit of a caloric solid-liquid meal through the stomach, the small intestine, and the colon in man. J Clin Endocrinol Metab 75:745, 1992

247. Lamberg BA, Gordin R: Liver function in thyrotoxicosis. Acta Endocrinol 15:82, 1954

248. Thompson P Jr, Strum D, Boehm T, Wartofsky L: Abnormalities of liver function tests in thyrotoxicosis. Military Medicine 548, 1978

249. Klion FM, Segal R, Schaffner F: The effect of altered thyroid function on the ultrastructure of the human liver. Am J Med 50:317, 1971

250. Greenberger NJ, Milligan FD, DeGroot LJ, Isselbacher KJ: Jaundice and thyrotoxicosis in the absence of congestive heart failure. Am J Med 36:840, 1964

251. Ford RV, Owens JC, Curd GW Jr et al: Kidney function in various thyroid states. J Clin Endocrinol Metab 21:548, 1961

252. Epstein FH, Rivera MJ: Renal concentrating ability in thyrotoxicosis. J Clin Endocrinol Metab 18:1135, 1958

253. Huth EJ, Maycock RL, Kerr RM: Hyperthyroidism associated with renal tubular acidosis. Am J Med 26:818, 1959

254. Goldsmith RE, Sturgis SH, Lerman J, Stanbury JB: The menstrual pattern in thyroid disease. J Clin Endocrinol Metab 12:846, 1952

255. Bray GA, Jacobs HS: Thyroid activity and other endocrine glands. p. 413. In M. Greer (ed): Handbook of Physiology. Vol. 3. American Physiology Society, Washington, DC, 1974

256. Freedberg IM, Hamolsky MW, Freedberg AS: The thyroid gland in pregnancy. N Engl J Med 256:505, 1957

257. Becker KL, Winnacker JL, Matthews MJ, Higgins GA: Gynecomastia and hyperthyroidism. An endocrine and histological investigation. J Clin Endocrinol Metab 28:277, 1968

258. Chopra IJ, Tulchinsky D: Status of estrogen-androgen balance in hyperthyroid men with Graves' disease. J Clin Endocrinol Metab 38:269, 1974

259. Chopra IJ, Abraham GE, Chopra U et al: Alterations in circulating estradiol-17-β in male patients with Graves' disease. N Engl J Med 286:124, 1972

260. Bercovici JP, Mauvais-Jarvis P: Hyperthyroidism and gynecomastia: metabolic studies. J Clin Endocrinol Metab 35:671, 1972

261. Southren AL, Olivo J, Gordon GG et al: The conversion of androgens to estrogens in hyperthyroidism. J Clin Endocrinol Metab 38:207, 1974

262. Kidd SG, Glass AR, Vigersky RA: The hypothalamic-pituitary-testicular axis in thyrotoxicosis. J Clin Endocrinol 48:798, 1979

263. Sawers JSA, Kellett HA, Brown NS et al: Prolactin response to metoclopramide in hyperthyroidism. J Clin Endocrinol Metab 55:175, 1982

264. Kapcala LP: Galactorrhea and thyrotoxicosis. Arch Intern Med 144:2349, 1984

265. Peterson RE: The influence of the thyroid on adrenal cortical function. J Clin Invest 37:736, 1958

266. Kenny FM, Iturzaeta N, Preeyasombat C et al: Cortisol production rate, VII. Hypothyroidism and hyperthyroidism in infants and children. J Clin Endocrinol 27:1616, 1967

267. Hellman L, Bradlow HL, Zumoff B, Gallagher TF: Influence of thyroid hormone on hydrocortisone production and metabolism. 21:1231, 1961

268. Gallagher TF, Hellman L, Finkelstein J et al: Hyperthyroidism and cortisol secretion in man. J Clin Endocrinol Metab 34:919, 1972

269. Hilton JG, Black WC, Athos W et al: Increased ACTH-like activity in plasma of patients with thyrotoxicosis. J Clin Endocrinol Metab 22:900, 1962

270. Felber JP, Reddy WJ, Selenkow HA, Thorn GW: Adrenocortical response to the 48-hour ACTH test in myxedema and hyperthyroidism. J Clin Endocrinol Metab 19:895, 1959

271. Hellman L, Bradlow HL, Zumoff B et al: Thyroid-androgen interrelations and the hypocholesteremic effect of androsterone. J Clin Endocrinol Metab 19: 936, 1959

272. Plummer HS, Boothby WM: The cost of work in exophthalmic goiter. Am J Physiol 53:406, 1923

273. Briard SP, McClintock JT, Baldridge CW: Cost of work in patients with hypermetabolism due to leukemia and to exophthalmic goiter. Arch Intern Med 56:30, 1935

274. Acheson K, Jequier E, Burger A, Danforth E Jr: Thyroid hormones and thermogenesis: the metabolic cost of food and exercise. Metabolism 33:262, 1984

275. Kabadi UM, Eisenstein AB: Impaired pancreatic α cell response in hyperthyroidism. J Clin Endocrinol Metab 51:478, 1980

276. Wennlund A, Arner P, Ostman J: Changes in the effects of insulin on human adipose tissue metabolism in hyperthyroidism. J Clin Endocrinol Metab 53:631, 1981

277. Houssay BA: Thyroid and metathyroid diabetes. Endocrinology 35:158, 1944

278. Bratusch-Marrain PR, Komjati M, Waldhausal WK: Glucose metabolism in noninsulin-dependent diabetic patients with experimental hyperthyroidism. J Clin Endocrinol Metab 60:1063, 1985

279. Elrick H, Hlad CJ Jr, Arai Y: Influence of thyroid metabolism on carbohydrate metabolism and a new method for assessing response to insulin. J Clin Endocrinol Metab 21:387, 1961

280. Gerstein HO. Incidence of postpartum thyroid dysfunction in patients with type I diabetes mellitus. Annals Int Med 118:419, 1993

281. Kritchevsky D: Influence of thyroid hormones and related compounds on cholesterol biosynthesis and degradation: a review. Metabolism 9:984, 1960

282. Siperstein MD, Murray AW: Cholesterol metabolism in man. J Clin Invest 34:1149, 1955

283. Chait A, Bierman EL, Albers JJ: Regulatory role of triiodothyronine in the degradation of low-density lipoprotein by cultured human skin fibroblasts. J Clin Endocrinol Metab 48:887, 1979

284. Tulloch BR, Lewis B, Fraser RT: Triglyceride metabolism in thyroid disease. Lancet 1:391, 1973

285. Arons DL, Schreibman PH, Downs P et al: Decreased postheparin lipases in Graves' disease. N Engl J Med 286:233, 1972

286. Sachs BA, Danielson E, Isaacs MC, Weston RE: Effect of triiodothyronine on the serum lipids and lipoproteins of euthyroid and hyperthyroid subjects. J Clin Endocrinol Metab 18:506, 1958

287. Strisower B, Elmlinger P, Gofman JW, deLalla O: Effect of L-thyroxine on serum lipoprotein and cholesterol concentrations. J Clin Endocrinol Metab 19: 117, 1959

288. Postel S: Total free tocopherols in the serum of patients with thyroid disease. J Clin Invest 35:1345, 1956

289. Rich C, Bierman EL, Schwartz I: Plasma nonesterified fatty acids in hyperthyroid states. J Clin Invest 38:275, 1959

290. Lewallen CG, Rall JE, Berman M: Studies of iodoalbumin metabolism, II. The effects of thyroid hormone. J Clin Invest 38:88, 1959

291. Crispell KR, Parson W, Hollifield G: A study of the rate of protein synthesis before and during the administration of L-triiodothyronine to patients with myxedema and healthy volunteers using N-15 glycine. J Clin Invest 35:164, 1956

292. Sokoloff L, Kaufman S: Effects of thyroxine on amino acid incorporation into protein. Science 129: 569, 1959

293. Sokoloff L, Kaufman S, Gelboin HV: Thyroxine stimulation of soluble ribonucleic acid-bound amino acid transfer to microsomal protein. Biochim Biophys Acta 52:410, 1961

294. Kivirikko KI, Laitinen O, Aer J, Halme J: Metabolism of collagen in experimental hyperthyroidism and hypothyroidism in the rat. Endocrinology 80: 1051, 1967

295. Singh SP, Snyder AK: Effect of thyrotoxicosis on gluconeogenesis from alanine in the perfused rat liver. Endocrinology 102:182, 1978

296. Marek J, Schullerova M, Schreiberova O, Limanova Z: Effect of thyroid function on serum somatomedin activity. Acta Endocrinol 96:491, 1981

297. Guttler RB, Croxson MS, DeQuattro VL et al: Effects of thyroid hormone on plasma adenosine 3′, 5′-monophosphate production in man. Metabolism 26: 1155, 1977

298. Peracchi M, Bamonti-Catena F, Lombardi L et al: Plasma and urine cyclic nucleotide levels in patients with hyperthyroidism and hypothyroidism. J Endocrinol Invest 6:173, 1983

299. Nilsson OR, Andersson RGG, Karlberg BE: Effects of propranolol and atenolol on plasma and urinary cyclic adenosine 3′, 5′-monophosphate in hyperthyroid patients. Acta Endocrinol 94:38, 1980

300. Wohl MG, Levy HA, Szutka A, Maldia G: Pyridoxine deficiency in hyperthyroidism. Proc Soc Exp Biol Med 105:523, 1960

301. Stein JA, Griem ML: Effect of triiodothyronine on radiosensitivity. Nature 182:1681, 1958

302. Parker JLW, Lawson DH: Death from thyrotoxicosis. Lancet 2:894, 1973

303. Means JH, DeGroot LJ, Stanbury JB. p. 203. The Thyroid and Its Diseases. 3rd Ed. McGraw-Hill, New York, 1963

304. Davis PJ, Davis FB: Hyperthyroidism in patients over the age of 60 years. Medicine 53:161, 1974

Graves' Disease: Diagnosis and Treatment *11*

DIAGNOSIS

The diagnosis of Graves' disease is usually easily made. The combination of eye signs, goiter, and any of the characteristic symptoms of hyperthyroidism forms a picture that can hardly escape recognition (See Fig. 11-1.) It is only in the atypical cases, or with coexistence of some other disease, or in cases in which the disease is so mild or early as to be unconvincing, that the diagnosis may be in doubt.

The symptoms and signs of Graves' disease have been described in detail in the preceding chapter. For convenience, the classic findings from the history and physical examination are grouped together in Table 11-1.

These occur with sufficient regularity that clinical diagnosis can be reasonably accurate. Scoring the presence or absence and severity of particular symptoms and signs can provide a clinical diagnostic index almost as reliable a diagnostic measure as laboratory tests. The frequency of signs and symptoms, adapted from the index of Wayne et al.[1] appears in Table 11-2.

Laboratory Diagnosis

Serum Hormone Measurements

Once the question of thyrotoxicosis has been raised, laboratory data are required to verify the diagnosis, help estimate the severity of the condition, and assist in planning therapy. The numerous techniques of laboratory assessment are critically reviewed in Chapter 6. A single test such as the TSH or the FTI may be enough, but in view of the sources of error in all determinations, most clinicians prefer to assess two more or less independent measures of thyroid function. For this purpose, the FTI and sensitive TSH are suitable.

As an initial single test, a sensitive TSH assay may be most cost-effective and specific. TSH should be 0 to .1 μU/ml in significant thyrotoxicosis, although values of .1 to .3 are seen in patients with mild illness, especially with smoldering toxic multinodular goiter in older patients. TSH can be normal—or elevated—only if there are spurious test results from antibodies, or the thyrotoxicosis is TSH-driven, as in a pituitary TSH-secreting adenoma or pituitary resistance to thyroid hormone. Measurement of FTI (or any measure of free T_4) is also useful, and the degree of elevation of the FTI above normal provides an estimate of the severity of the disease. Elevations of FTI not due to thyrotoxicosis are unusual, and are given in Table 11-3. Of course the T_4 level may normally be as high as 16 or 20 μg/dl in pregnancy, and can be elevated without thyrotoxicosis in patients with familial hyperthyroxinemia due to abnormal albumin, the presence of hereditary excess TBG, the presence of antibodies binding T_4, the thy-

TABLE 11-1. Symptoms and Signs of Graves' Disease

Features	Symptoms	Physical Signs
General	Change in temperature preference Weight loss with increased appetite	Weight loss Hyperkinetic behavior, thought, and speech
Eyes	Prominence of eyes, puffiness of lids Pain or irritation of eyes Blurred or double vision, decreasing acuity Decreased motility	Prominence of eyes, lid lag, globe lag Exophthalmos, lid edema, chemosis, extraocular muscle weakness Decreased visula acuity, scotomata, papilledema, retinal hemorrhage, and edema
Neck	Goiter	Goiter Sometimes enlarged cervical nodes Thrill and bruit
Respiratory	Dyspnea	None, or tachypnea on exertion
Cardiac	Palpitations or pounding of the heart Ankle edema (without cardiac disease) Less frequently, orthopnea, paroxysmal tachycardia, anginal pain, and CHF	Tachycardia, overactive heart, widened pulse pressure, and bounding pulse Occasional cardiomegaly, signs of congestive heart failure, and paroxysmal tachycardia or fibrillation
Gastrointestinal	Increased frequency of stools	None
Genitourinary	Polyuria Decrease in menstrual flow; menstrual irregularity or amenorrhea Decreased fertility	None
Neuromuscular	Fatigue Weakness Tremulousness Occasional bursitis	Tremulousness Objective muscle wasting and weakness Quickened and hypermetric reflexes
Emotional	Nervousness, irritability Emotional lability Insomnia or decreased sleep requirement	Emotional lability
Dermatologic	Thinning of hair Loss of curl in hair Increased perspiration Change in texture of skin and nails Increased pigmentation Vertiligo Swelling over outer surface of skin	Fine, warm, moist skin Fine and often straight hair Oncholysis (Plummer's nails) Pretibial myxedema Acropachy Hyperpigmentation or vertiligo
Family History	Any thyroid disease, especially Graves' disease	—

roid hormone resistance syndrome, and conditions listed in Table 11-3. The T_4 level may be normal in thyrotoxic patients who have depressed serum levels of T_4-binding protein or because of severe illness, even though they are toxic. Thus, thyrotoxicosis may exist when the T_4 level is in the normal range; measurement of free T_4 or FTI usually obviates this source of error and is the best test. In the presence of typical symptoms, one measurement of suppressed TSH or elevated FTI is sufficient to make a definite diagnosis, although it does not identify a cause. If the FTI is normal, repetition is in order to rule out error, along with a second test such as serum T_3.

A variety of methods for FTI determination have become available, including commercial kits. Although these methods are usually reliable, assays using different kits do not always agree among themselves or with the determination of free T_4. Usually T_4 and T_3 levels are both elevated in thyrotoxicosis, as are the FTI and an index constructed using the serum T_3 and rT_3U levels, and the newer measures of "free T_4" or "free T_3."

The serum T_3 level determined by RIA is almost always elevated in thyrotoxicosis and is a useful but not commonly needed secondary test. Usually the serum T_3 test is interpreted directly without use of

TABLE 11-2. Incidence of Common Signs and Symptoms in Thyrotoxic Patients and Controls

Symptoms	Thyrotoxic Patients (%)	Controls (%)	Signs	Thyrotoxic Patients (%)	Controls (%)
Dyspnea on exertion	81	40	Goiter	87	11
Palpitations	75	26	Diffuse	49	11(slight)
Tiredness	80	31	Nodular	32	0
Preference for cold	73	41	Single adenoma	4	0
Excessive sweating	68	31	Exophthalmos	34	2
Nervousness	59	21	Lid lag	62	16
Increased appetite	32	2	Hyperkinesis	39	9
Decreased appetite	13	3	Finger tremor	66	26
Weight loss	52	2	Sweating hands	72	22
Weight gain	4	16	Hot hands	76	44
Diarrhea	8	0	Atrial fibrillation	19	0
Constipation	15	21	Regular pulse over 90	68	19
Excessive menses	3	6	Average pulse in beats/min	100	78
Scant menses	18	3			

(From Wayne,[1] with permission.)

a correction for protein binding. Alterations of TBG affect T_3 to a lesser extent than T_4. Any confusion caused by alterations in binding proteins can be avoided by use of a free T_3 assay or T_3 index calculated as for the FTI. In patients with severe illness

TABLE 11-3. Conditions Associated with Transient Elevations of the FTI

Condition	Explanation
Estrogen withdrawal	Rapid decrease in TBG level
Amphetamine abuse	Possibly induced TSH secretion[2]
Acute psychosis	Unknown
Hyperemesis gravidarum	Unknown, possibly HCG, may be associated with thyrotoxicosis
Iodide administration	Thyroid autonomy
Beginning of T_4 administration	Delayed T_4 metabolism[3]
Severe illness (rarely)	Decreased T_4 to T_3 conversion
Amiodarone treatment	Decreased T_4 to T_3 conversion, iodine load
Gallbladder contrast agents	Decreased T_4 to T_3 conversion, iodine load
Propranolol (large doses)	Inhibition of T_4 to T_3 conversion
Prednisone (rarely)	Inhibition of T_4 to T_3 conversion
High altitude exposure	Possibly hypothalamic activation
Selenium deficiency	Decreased T_4 to T_3 conversion

and thyrotoxicosis,[4,5] especially those with liver disease or malnutrition or who are taking steroids or propranolol, the serum T_3 level is not elevated, since peripheral deiodination of T_4 to T_3 is suppressed (T_4 toxicosis). A normal T_3 level has also been observed in thyrotoxicosis combined with diabetic ketoacidosis.[6] Whether or not these patients actually have tissue hypermetabolism at the time their serum T_3 is normal is not entirely certain. In these patients the rT_3 level may be elevated. If the complicating illness subsides, the normal pattern of elevated T_4, FTI, and T_3 levels may return. Elevated T_4 levels with normal serum T_3 levels are also found in patients with thyrotoxicosis produced by iodine ingestion.[7]

T_3 Toxicosis

Since 1957, when the first patient with T_3 thyrotoxicosis was identified, a number of patients have been detected who had clinical thyrotoxicosis, normal serum levels of T_4 and TBG, and elevated concentrations of T_3 and FT_3.[8] Hollander et al.[9] found that approximately 4 percent of patients with thyrotoxicosis in the New York area fit this category. These patients often have mild disease but otherwise have been indistinguishable clinically from others with thyrotoxicosis. Some have had the diffuse thyroid hyperplasia of Graves' disease, others toxic nodular goiter, and still others thyrotoxicosis with hyperfunctioning adenomas. Interestingly, in Chile, a country of generalized iodine deficiency, 12.5 percent of thyrotoxic subjects fulfilled the criteria for T_3 thyrotoxicosis.[10] Asymptomatic hypertriiodothyronemia is an occasional finding several months before the development of thyrotoxicosis with elevated T_4 levels.[11] Since T_4 is normally metabolized to T_3, and the latter hormone is predominantly the hormone bound to nuclear receptors, it makes sense that elevation of T_3 alone can produce thyrotoxicosis.

RAIU

The RAIU in patients with thyrotoxicosis at 24 hours is characteristically above normal. In the United States, which has had an increasing iodine supply in recent years, the upper limit of normal is now about 25 percent of the administered dose. This value is higher in areas of iodine deficiency and endemic goiter. The uptake value at a shorter time interval, 6 hours, for example, is as valid a test and may be more useful in the infrequent cases having such a rapid isotope turnover that uptake has fallen to normal by 24 hours. If there is reason to suspect that thyroid isotope turnover is rapid, it is wise to do both a 6- and a 24-hour RAIU determination during the initial laboratory study. Because of convenience, and since serum assays of thyroid hormones and TSH are reliable and readily available, the RAIU is infrequently determined unless ^{131}I therapy is planned. A drawback of this approach is that cases of transient thyrotoxicosis (described below) may be missed unless the typical low RAIU is recognized. To avoid errors, we recommend that the RAIU test be done in patients who are believed to be thyrotoxic but who do not have typical symptoms and/or signs such as patients with brief symptom duration, small goiter, or lacking eye signs, absent family history, or negative antibody test results.[12] Obviously other causes of a low RAIU test need to be considered and excluded.

Thyroid Scanning

Scanning of the thyroid has a limited role in the diagnosis of thyrotoxicosis, except in those patients in whom the thyroid is difficult to feel or in whom nodules are present that require evaluation, or rarely to prove the function of ectopic thyroid tissue. Nodules may be incidental, or may be the source of thyrotoxicosis (toxic adenoma), or may contribute to the thyrotoxicosis that also arises from the rest of the gland. Scanning should usually be done with ^{123}I in this situation, in order to combine it with an RAIU measurement.

Fluorescence scanning is available in some institutions and can be used to delineate the anatomy of the thyroid when the use of radioactive isotopes is contraindicated (pregnancy, lactation) or when the uptake is suppressed by excess iodides. This technique is used only as a research tool. Fluorescence scanning has also been used to quantitate the thyroidal iodine content, which is not usually elevated in Graves' disease, at least in the United States.

Antithyroid Antibodies

Determination of antibody titers provides supporting evidence for Graves' disease. More than 95 percent of patients have positive assays for TPO-microsomal antigen, and about 50 percent have positive anti-thyroglobulin antibody assays. In thyroiditis the prevalence of positive TG antibody assays is higher. Positive assays prove that autoimmunity is present, but they do not prove thyrotoxicosis. Patients with causes of thyrotoxicosis other than Graves' disease usually have negative assays. During therapy with antithyroid drugs the titers characteristically go down, and this change persists during remission. Titers tend to become more elevated after RAI treatment.

Thyroid-stimulating antibody assays have become more readily available, and a positive result supports the diagnosis. The assay is valuable as another supporting fact in establishing the cause of exophthalmos, and high levels may predict neonatal thyrotoxicosis. The test, however, is expensive, and is only rarely needed.

BMR

Determination of the BMR might be of theoretical interest, but is not a good diagnostic test and is often unreliable when done for the first time. It requires a skilled technician and appropriate equipment, both of which are not generally available.

Other Assays

General availability of assays that can reliably measure suppressed TSH has made this the gold standard to which other tests must be compared, and has effectively eliminated the need for most previously used ancillary tests. There are only rare causes of confusion in the sTSH assay. Severe illness, dopamine and steroids, and hypopituitarism, can cause low sTSH, but suppression below 1 μU/mL is uncommon and below 0.1 μU/mL is exceptional, except in thyrotoxicosis. Thyrotoxicosis is associated with normal or high TSH in patients with TSH producing pituitary tumors and selective pituitary resistance to thyroid hormone.

If these procedures do not establish the diagnosis, it may be wise to do nothing further except to observe the course of events. In patients with significant thyroid hyperfunction, the symptoms and signs will become clearer, and the laboratory measurements will fall into line (Fig. 11-1).

In past years it was common to try to resolve confusion by use of a T_3 suppression test or TRH test. It must be remembered that the T_3 suppression test may be positive in Graves' disease, in the absence of thyrotoxicosis, since it measures "thyroid autonomy" and not hyperthyroidism per se. The test result is also positive in hyperfunctioning adenomas and in some glands having the histologic picture of Hashimoto's disease. The cumbersome and occasionally dangerous T_3 suppression test was largely discarded in favor of the simpler TRH test. An increase in TSH level after TRH administration is regularly absent in patients with hyperthyroid Graves' disease; the response in those with euthyroid Graves' disease is often but not always absent. Lack of response is strong presumptive evidence of chemical, if not clinical, thyrotoxicosis. Ormston et al.[13] found the TRH test to correlate fairly closely with the T_3 suppression test in patients with exophthalmos. The response was usually exaggerated when the patient was borderline hypothyroid and low or absent when the patient was borderline thyrotoxic. Others have found a poor correlation between suppressibility, the TRH response, and the course of exophthalmos.[14] Unresponsiveness to TRH may also be found in patients with treated Graves' disease.[15]

The vast majority of patients are diagnosed by elevated FTI or T_3 levels and suppressed TSH, and TRH testing is rarely indicated. Since there is very high correlation between basal TSH levels and response to TRH, TRH testing provides no additional information.

In the past, some clinicians placed diagnostic reliance on the striking response of patients with Graves' disease to the administration of iodine. If 6 mg iodine or more is given daily to a person who has Graves' disease and is not already receiving iodine, within the succeeding 7 or 10 days there will be an amelioration in symptoms, and the FTI level will fall in parallel. Often the patient may reach a euthyroid state, at least temporarily. If iodine administration is then stopped, the signs and symptoms quickly return to their previous state. Since iodine administration interferes with treatment by antithyroid drugs and with ^{131}I therapy, this may prove to be a difficulty. The therapeutic trial with iodine is thus primarily of historical interest.

Differential Diagnosis (See Also Ch. 13)

Graves' disease must first be differentiated from other conditions in which thyrotoxicosis is present (Table 11-4). Thyrotoxicosis may be caused by taking T_4 or its analogs—thyrotoxicosis factitia. Most commonly, this is due to administration of excessive replacement hormone by the patient's physician, but hormone may be taken surreptitiously by the patient for weight loss or psychological reasons. The typical findings are a normal or small thyroid gland, an ^{131}I uptake of zero, a low serum TG, and, of course, a

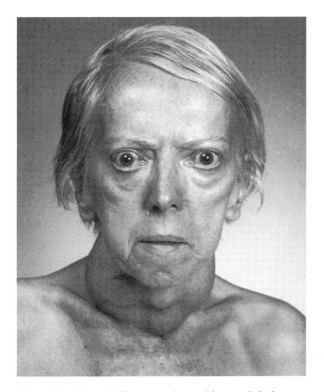

Fig. 11-1. Graves' disease patient with exophthalmos.

TABLE 11-4. Causes of Thyrotoxicosis

Cause	Course of Disease	Physical Finding	Diagnostic Finding	Treatment or Comment
Graves' disease	Familial, prolonged	Goiter	+ Ab, increased RAIU, eye signs	Antithyroids, RAI, surgery
Transient thyrotoxicosis (painless thyroiditis)	Brief	Small goiter	Low Ab, no eye signs, RAIU = 0 Normal or ↑ Tg	Possibly steroids; thyroid ablation between attacks
Subacute thyroiditis	Brief	Tender goiter	RAIU = 0, elevated ESR, recent URI Normal or ↑ Tg	Nothing, NSAID or steroids
Toxic multinodular goiter	Prolonged, mild	Nodular goiter	Typical scan result	Antithyroids, RAI, surgery
Iodide induced (including amiodarone)	Recent, mild	Nodular goiter, rarely normal	Low RAIU, abnormal scan result	Antithyroids, time, ablation, withdrawal of iodine source, $KClO_4$
Toxic adenoma	Prolonged, mild	One nodule	"Hot" nodule on scan	Surgery, RAI
Thyroid carcinoma	Recent	Variable, with metastasis	Functioning metastases	Surgery + RAI
Exogenous thyroid hormone	Variable	Small thyroid	Zero RAIU; psychiatric illness, low TG	Withdrawal, counseling
Hydatidiform mole	Recent, mild	Goiter	Pregnancy, vaginal bleeding Increased HCG	Surgery, chemotherapy
Choriocarcinoma	Recent, mild	Goiter	Increased HCG	Surgery, chemotherapy
Excess production of TRH (possibly)	?	Goiter	Poor response to TRH	Not known
TSH-producing adenoma	Prolonged	Goiter	Excess alpha subunits, ↑ TSH, pituitary adenoma	Adenomectomy, somatostatin, thyroid ablation
Pituitary T_3/T_4 resistance	Prolonged	Goiter	Elevated or normal TSH, no tumor, no α subunit, mild thyrotoxicosis	Not certain; possibly T_3, triac, somatostatin, thyroid ablation
Struma ovari	Variable	With or without goiter	Positive scan result or operation	Surgery
Thyroid destruction	Variable	Variable	Variable	Reported with ^{131}I therapy, lymphoma,[20] other causes cited above such as subacute thyroiditis
Hamburger Toxicosis	Recent, self-limiting	Small gland, No eye signs	Suppressed TSH and TG, ↓ RAIU	Avoid meat trimmings, including thyroid tissue

striking lack of response to antithyroid drug therapy. The problem can easily be confused with "painless thyroiditis," but in thyrotoxicosis factitia, the gland is typically small.

Toxic nodular goiter is usually distinguished by careful physical examination and a history of goiter for many years before symptoms of hyperthyroidism developed. The thyrotoxicosis comes on insidiously, and often, in the older people usually afflicted, symptoms may be mild, or suggest another problem such as heart disease. The thyroid scan may be diagnostic. The results of assays for TSAb[16] and other antithyroid antibodies are usually negative, but some researchers have found "growth-stimulating" antibodies in sera from these patients. A hyperfunctioning solitary adenoma is suggested on physical examination by atrophy of the remainder of the thyroid, and is proved by a scintiscan demonstrating preferential radioisotope accumulation in the nodule. This type of adenoma must be differentiated from congenital absence of one of the lobes of the thyroid. Toxic nodules typically present in adults with gradually developing hyperthyroidism and a nodule larger than 3 cm in size. Occasionally autonomous nodules produce hyperthyroidism in children.[17] Rarely, functioning thyroid carcinomas produce thyrotoxicosis. The diagnosis is made by the history, absence of the normal thyroid, and usually widespread functioning metastasis in lung or bones. Invasion of the gland by lymphoma has produced thyrotoxicosis.[18]

Thyrotoxicosis associated with subacute thyroiditis is usually mild and transient, and the patient lacks the physical findings of long-standing thyrotoxicosis. If thyrotoxicosis is found in conjunction with a painful goiter and low or absent ^{131}I uptake, this diagnosis may be entertained. Usually the erythrocyte sedimentation rate (ESR) is greatly elevated, and the leukocyte count may also be increased. Antibody titers are low or negative. Many patients have the HLA-B35 antigen, indicating a genetic predisposition to the disease.

The very rare thyrotroph tumor will be missed unless one measures the plasma TSH level, or until the enlargement is sufficient to produce deficiencies in other hormones, pressure symptoms, or expansion of the sella turcica. These patients have thyrotoxicosis with inappropriately elevated TSH levels and may/or may not secrete more TSH after TRH stimulation. The characteristic finding is an elevated TSH alpha subunit level in blood, measured by special

RIA. Thyroid stimulatory IgGs are not present. Exophthalmos, family history, and antibodies or Graves' disease are absent. Measurement of the TSH level is certainly useful, but is not required in the usual case of Graves' disease is there is a family history of Graves' disease or eye signs, or if antithyroid antibodies are present. In the absence of these features, TSH levels should be routinely assayed to exclude these rare cases.

The category of patients with thyrotoxicosis and inappropriately elevated TSH levels also includes the very rare persons with excess TRH secretion, or pituitary "T_3 resistance."[19] TRH hypersecretion, a possible cause of thyrotoxicosis,[20] is marked by an absence of pituitary tumor, elevated TSH levels, and failure to respond to TRH. The syndrome of pituitary thyroid hormone resistance[19,21] is marked by mild thyrotoxicosis, elevated TSH levels, absence of pituitary tumor, a generous response to TRH, no excess TSH alpha subunit secretion,[19] and by TSH suppression if large doses of T_3 are administered.

Administration of large amounts of iodide in medicines, for roentgenographic examinations, or in foods can occasionally precipitate thyrotoxicosis in patients with multinodular goiter or functioning adenomas. This history is important to consider since the illness may be self-limiting. Iodide induction of thyrotoxicosis has also been observed in apparently normal individuals following prolonged exposure to organic iodide containing compounds such as antiseptic soaps and amiodarone.

An increasingly recognized form of thyrotoxicosis is the syndrome described variously as painless thyroiditis, transient thyrotoxicosis, or "hyperthyroiditis."[22,23] Its hallmarks are self-limited thyrotoxicosis, small painless goiter, and low or zero RAIU. The patients usually have no eye signs, a negative family history, and low antibody titers. This condition is due to autoimmune thyroid disease. It occurs sporadically, usually in young adults. It frequently occurs 3 to 12 weeks after delivery, apparently representing the effects of immunologic rebound from the immunosuppressive effects of pregnancy in patients with Hashimoto's thyroiditis.[24,25] The course typically includes development of a painless goiter, mild to moderate thyrotoxicosis, no eye signs, remission of symptoms in 3 to 20 weeks, and often a period of hypothyroidism before return to euthyroid function. The cycle may be repeated several times. Histologic examination shows chronic thyroiditis, but it is not typical of Hashimoto's disease or subacute thyroiditis and may revert to normal after the attack.[26]

In most patients, the thyrotoxic episode occurs in the absence of circulating TSAb. This finding suggests that the pathogenesis is quite distinct from that in Graves' disease.[27] The thyrotoxicosis is caused by an inflammation-induced discharge of preformed hormone due to the thyroiditis. The T_4/T_3 ratio is higher than in typical Graves' disease,[28] and thyroid iodine stores are depleted. Since the thyrotoxicosis is due to an inflammatory process, therapy with antithyroid drugs or potassium iodide is usually to no avail, and RAI treatment of course cannot be given. Propranolol is usually helpful for symptoms. Glucocorticoids may be of help if the process—often transient and mild—requires some form of therapy. Propylthiouracil and/or ipodate can be used to decrease T_4 to T_3 conversion and will ameliorate the illness. Repeated episodes may be handled by surgery or by RAI therapy during a remission. Variants of this syndrome have been described. Shigemasa et al.[29] described patients with a similar clinical picture but painful chronic thyroid enlargement frequently ending in time with thyroid atrophy and hypothyroidism.

Hydatidiform moles, choriocarcinomas, and rarely seminomas secrete vast amounts of HCG. HCG, with an alpha subunit identical to TSHα, and β subunit related to TSHβ, binds to and activates the thyroid TSH receptor with about 1/1,000th the efficiency of TSH itself. There is controversy as to whether the "molar thyrotropin" is HCG or another distinct factor. Current evidence indicates that very elevated levels of native HCG,[30] or perhaps desialated HCG,[31] cause the thyroid stimulation, although this evidence is not universally accepted.[32] Many patients have goiter or elevated thyroid hormone levels or both, but little evidence of thyrotoxicosis, whereas others are clearly thyrotoxic.[33] Diagnosis rests on recognizing the tumor (typically during or after pregnancy) and measurement of HCG. Therapy is directed at the tumor.[33]

Two common diagnostic problems are first, the question of hyperthyroidism in patients with goiter of another cause, and, second, mild neuroses such as anxiety, fatigue states, and neurasthenia. Most patients with goiter receive a battery of examinations to survey their thyroid function at some time. Usually these tests are done more for routine assessment than because there is serious concern over the possibility of thyrotoxicosis. In the absence of significant symptoms or signs of hyperthyroidism and ophthalmologic problems, a normal FTI or sTSH determination is sufficiently reassuring to the physician and the patient. Of course, the most satisfactory conclusion of such a study is the positive identification of an alternate cause for enlargement of the thyroid.

Some patients complain of fatigue and palpitations, weight loss, nervousness, irritability, and insomnia. These patients may demonstrate brisk reflex activity, tachycardia (especially during examinations), perspiration, and tremulousness. In the absence of thyrotoxicosis, the hands are more often cool and damp rather than warm and erythematous. Serum TSH assay should be diagnostic.

Mild and temporary elevation of the FTI may occur if there is a transient depression of TBG production—for example, when estrogen administration is omitted. This problem is occasionally seen in hospital practice, usually involving a middle-aged woman receiving estrogen medication that is discontinued when the patient is hospitalized. Estrogen withdrawal leads to decreased TBG levels and a transiently elevated FTI. After two to three weeks, both the T_4 level and the FTI return to normal (Table 11-3).

It should be remembered that thyrotoxicosis is today not only a clinical but also a laboratory diagnosis. Consistent elevation of the FTI, and the T_3 level, and suppressed TSH can indicate that thyrotoxicosis is present even in the absence of clear-cut signs. These elevations themselves may be a sufficient indication for therapy.

In the differential diagnosis of heart disease, the possibility of thyrotoxicosis must always be considered. Some cases of thyrotoxicosis are missed because the symptoms are so conspicuously cardiac that the thyroid background is not perceived. This is especially true in patients with atrial fibrillation.

Many disorders may on occasion show some of the features of hyperthyroidism or Graves' disease. In malignant disease, especially lymphoma, weight loss, low grade fever, and weakness are often present. Parkinsonism in its milder forms may initially suggest thyroid disease. So also do the flushed countenance, bounding pulse, thyroid hypertrophy, and dyspnea of pregnancy. Patients with chronic pulmonary disease may have prominent eyes, tremor, tachycardia, weakness, and even goiter from therapeutic use of iodine. One should remember the weakness, fatigue, and jaundice of hepatitis and the puffy eyes of trichinosis and nephritis. Cirrhotic patients frequently have prominent eyes and lid lag, and the alcoholic patient with tremor, prominent eyes, and flushed face has not infrequently been suspected of having thyrotoxicosis, at least initially. Distinguishing between Graves' disease with extreme myopathy and myopathies of other origin can be clinically difficult. The term chronic thyrotoxic myopathy is used to designate a condition characterized by weakness, fatigability, muscular atrophy, and weight loss usually associated with severe thyrotoxicosis. Occasionally fasciculations are seen. The electromyogram result may be abnormal. If the condition is truly of hyperthyroid origin, the thyroid function tests are abnormal and the muscular disorder is reversed when the thyrotoxicosis is relieved. Usually a consideration of the total clinical picture and assessment of TSH and FTI are sufficient to distinguish thyrotoxicosis from polymyositis, myasthenia gravis, or progressive muscular atrophy. True myasthenia gravis may coexist with Graves' disease, in which case the myasthenia responds to neostigmine therapy. (The muscle weakness of hyperthyroidism may be slightly improved by neostigmine, but never relieved.) Occasionally electromyograms, muscle biopsy, neostigmine tests, and ACH-receptor antibody assays must be used to settle the problem.

Apathetic hyperthyroidism designates a thyrotoxic condition characterized by fatigue, apathy, listlessness, dull eyes, extreme weakness, often congestive heart failure, and low-grade fever.[34,35] Often such patients have small goiters, modest tachycardia, occasionally cool and even dry skin, and few eye signs. The syndrome may, in some patients, represent an extreme degree of fatigue induced by long-standing thyrotoxicosis. Once the diagnosis is considered, standard laboratory tests should confirm or deny the presence of thyrotoxicosis even in the absence of classical symptoms and signs.

TREATMENT

Three forms of primary therapy for Graves' disease are in common use today: (1) destruction of the thyroid by ^{131}I; (2) blocking of hormone synthesis by antithyroid drugs; and (3) partial surgical ablation of the thyroid. Iodine alone as a definitive form of treatment has been used in the past, but is not used today because its benefits may be transient or incomplete and because more effective methods have become available. Iodine is primarily used now in conjunction with antithyroid drugs to prepare patients for surgical thyroidectomy when that plan of therapy has been chosen. Roentgen irradiation was also used in the past.[36]

Selection of therapy depends on a multiplicity of considerations. Availability of a competent surgeon, for example, undue emotional concern about the hazards of ^{131}I irradiation, or the probability of adherence to a strict medical regimen might govern one's decision regarding one program of treatment as opposed to another. In the succeeding paragraphs, we will examine in some detail the resources available to the physician and attempt to weigh their merits. Antithyroid drug therapy offers the opportunity to avoid induced damage to the thyroid (and parathyroids or recurrent nerves), as well as radiation exposure and operation. The difficulties are the requirement of adhering to a medical schedule for many months or years, frequent visits to the physician, occasional adverse reactions, and, most importantly, a disappointingly low permanent remission rate. Therapy with antithyroid drugs is used as the initial modality in people under age 18 to 20, in many adults through age 40, and in most pregnant women.

Iodine-131 therapy is quick, easy, and relatively inexpensive, avoids surgery, and is without significant risk in adults and probably teenagers. The larger doses required to give prompt and certain control generally induce hypothyroidism, and low doses are associated with a frequent requirement for retreatment or ancillary medical management over one to two years. We use ^{131}I as the primary therapy in most persons over age 40 and in many adults over age 21, if antithyroid drugs fail to control the disease.

Surgery, which was the main therapy until 1950, has been to a major extent replaced by ^{131}I treatment. As the high frequency of ^{131}I-induced hypothyroidism became apparent, some revival of interest in thyroidectomy occurred. The major advantage of surgery is that definitive management is obtained over an 8- to 12-week period, including preoperative medical control, and the majority of adult patients are euthyroid after operation. Its well-known disadvantages include expense, surgery itself, and the risks of recurrent nerve and parathyroid damage, hypothyroidism, and recurrence. Nevertheless, if a skillful surgeon is available, surgical management may be used as the primary or secondary therapy in many young adults, as the secondary therapy in children poorly controlled on antithyroid drugs, in pregnant women requiring large doses of antithyroid drugs, and in patients with significant exophthalmos.

Two recent surveys reporting trends in therapeutic choices made by thyroidologists have been published.[37] In Europe, most physicians tended to treat children and adults first with antithyroid drugs, and adults secondarily with ^{131}I or less frequently surgery. Surgery was selected as primary therapy for patients with large goiters. [131]I was selected as the primary treatment in older patients. Most therapists attempted to restore euthyroidism by use of ^{131}I or surgery. In the United States, ^{131}I therapy is the initial modality of therapy selected by members of the American Thyroid Association for management of uncomplicated Graves' disease in an adult woman.[38] Two-thirds of these clinicians attempted to give ^{131}I in a dosage calculated to produce euthyroidism, and one-third planned for thyroid ablation.

Iodine-131 Therapy for Thyrotoxicosis

In many thyroid clinics, ^{131}I therapy is now used for most patients with Graves' disease who are beyond the adolescent years. It is used in most patients who have had prior thyroid surgery, because the incidence of complications, such as hypoparathyroidism and recurrent nerve palsy, is especially high in this group if a second thyroidectomy is performed. Likewise, it is the therapy of choice for any patient who is a poor risk for surgery because of complicating disease.

The question of an age limit below which RAI should not be used frequently arises. With lengthening experience these limits have been lowered. Several studies with average follow-up periods of 12 to 15 years attest to the safety of ^{131}I therapy in adults.[39–41] Treated persons have shown no tendency to develop thyroid cancer, leukemia, or reproductive abnormalities, and their children have had no increase in congenital defects or evidence of thyroid damage.[42–44] Although there is much less data on long term results in this age group, there is a gradual tendency to use this treatment in teenagers over age 15.

TABLE 11-5. Iodine-131 Therapy for Graves' Disease

Indications
 Any patients above a preselected age limit, especially those patients who fail to respond to antithyroid drugs
 Prior thyroid or other neck surgery
 Contraindications to surgery, such as severe heart, lung, or renal disease
General Contraindications
 Pregnancy or lactation
 Insufficient ^{131}I uptake due to prior medication or disease
 Question of malignant thyroid tumor
 Age below a preselected age limit, such as (possibly) age 15
 Patient concerns regarding radiation exposure
Questionable Contraindications
 Unusually large glands
 Active exophthalmos
 Age under 21

Certain other findings may dictate the choice of therapy. Occasionally, the ^{131}I uptake is significantly blocked by prior iodine administration. One may either wait for a few days to weeks until another ^{131}I tracer indicates that the uptake is in the toxic range or use an alternative therapeutic approach such as antithyroid drugs. Rarely a patient with thyrotoxicosis harbors a thyroid gland with a configuration suggesting the presence of a malignant neoplasm. These patients require surgical exploration. [131]I therapy causes an increase in titers of TSH-RAbs, and anti-TG or TPO antibodies, which reflects an activation of autoimmunity, and may be due to release of thyroid antigens by cell damage, or possibly destruction of intrathyroidal suppressor T cells. Although statistical proof is lacking, many thyroidologists are convinced that ^{131}I therapy can lead to exacerbation of infiltrative ophthalmopathy, perhaps because of this immunologic response. Thus, as described below, patients with significant ophthalmopathy may receive corticosteroids along with ^{131}I, or may be selected for surgical management. The indications and contraindications for ^{131}I therapy are given in Table 11-5.

Dosage

The dosage initially was worked out by a trial-and-error method and by successive approximations. The introduction of ^{131}I into therapy has been reviewed by E. M. Chapman[45], who figured importantly in the development of this treatment. By about 1950, the standard dose had become 160 uCi ^{131}I per gram of estimated thyroid weight. Of course, estimating the weight of the thyroid gland by examination of the neck is an inexact procedure. Also, marked variation in radiation sensitivity no doubt exists and cannot be estimated at all. It was gratifying that in practice this dosage scheme worked well enough. Over the years some effort was made to refine the calculation. Account was taken of uptake, half-life of the radioisotope in the thyroid, concentration per gram, and so on, but it is evident that the result in a given instance depends on factors that cannot be estimated precisely.[46,47] One factor must be the tendency of the thyroid to return to normal if a dose of radiation is given that is large enough to make the gland approach, for a time, a normal functional state; and in many patients, "cure" is associated actually with thyroid ablation.

In the early 1960s, it was recognized that a complication of RAI therapy was a high incidence of hypothyroidism. It was 20 to 40 percent in the first year after therapy and increased about 2.5 percent per year, so that by 10 years 50 to 80 percent of patients had low function.[48] In 1964, in an effort to lower the dose of RAI and possibly reduce the incidence of late hypothyroidism, Hagen and colleagues reduced the quantity of ^{131}I to 0.08 mCi per gram of estimated gland weight.[48] No increase was reported in the number of patients requiring retreatment, and there was a substantial reduction in the incidence of hypothyroidism. Most of these patients were maintained on potassium iodide for several months after therapy, in order to ameliorate the thyrotoxicosis while the radioiodine had its effect.[49,50]

Many attempts have been made to improve the therapeutic program by giving the RAI in smaller doses. Reinwein et al.[51] studied 334 patients several years after they had been treated with serial doses of less than 50 uCi ^{131}I per gram of estimated thyroid weight. One-third of these patients had increased levels of TSH, although they were clinically euthyroid. Only 3 percent were reported to be clinically hypothyroid.

Approaches to dosage adjustment usually include a factor for gland size, a standard dose in microCuries per gram, and a correction to account for ^{131}I uptake.[52]

The Thyroid Group at the University of Chicago used for many years a Low-Dose Protocol designed to compensate for the apparent radiosensitivity of small glands and resistance of larger glands.[53] Using this approach, after one year, 10 percent of patients were hypothyroid, 60 percent are euthyroid, and 30 percent remained intrinsically toxic,[53] although euthyroid by virtue of antithyroid drug treatment. After ten years, 40 percent are euthyroid and 60 percent are hypothyroid. A problem with low-dose therapy is that about 25 percent of patients require a second treatment and 5 percent require a third. Although this approach reduces early hypothyroidism, it does so at a cost in time, money, and patient convenience (Fig. 11-2). To answer these problems, we tended to retreat, if necessary, within 6 months, rather than waiting a full year, and employed propranolol and antithyroid drugs between ^{131}I doses if needed. Unfortunately, our experience and that of others shows that even low-dose ^{131}I therapy is followed by a progressive development of hypothyroidism in up to 40 to 50 percent of patients ten years after therapy.[54–57]

Impressed by the need to retreat nearly a third of patients, we have in the past 4 years utilized a Moderate-Dose Protocol (Table 11-6). This is a fairly conventional program with a mean dose of about 9 mCi. The ^{131}I dosage is related to gland weight and RAIU and is increased as gland weight increases. The calculation used is as follows:

$$\text{uCi given} = \frac{\text{estimated thyroid weight in grams} \times \text{uCi/g for appropriate weight from Table 11-6}}{\text{fractional 24-hour RAIU}}$$

For the convenience of readers who may, like us, find difficult the conversion of older units in Curies, rads, and rems to newer units of measurement, we are providing Table 11-7.

Some physicians advocate a planned complete destruction of the thyroid by ^{131}I treatment, followed by replacement therapy.[58] For example, a dose is given that will result in about 7 mCi retained at 24 hrs. They argue that the near certainty of prompt control and the inevitability of hypothyroidism make this a realistic and preferable approach. However, over 50 percent of patients given low-dose therapy remain euthyroid after ten years and can easily be surveyed at one- or two-year intervals.

Some physicians give antithyroid drugs before ^{131}I treatment in order to deplete the gland of stored

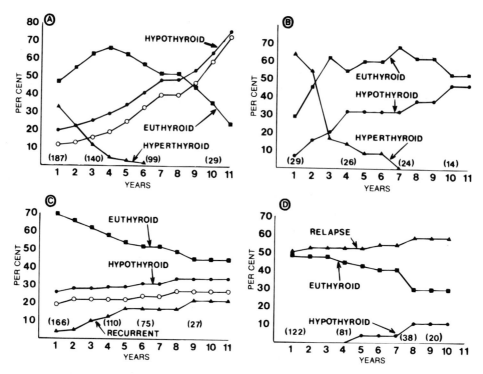

Fig. 11-2. Comparison of outcome of treatment of thyrotoxicosis by [131]I *(left upper panel)*; ^{131}I plus ATD + KI *(right upper panel)*; surgery *(left lower panel)*; and ATD *(right lower panel)*; over ten years follow-up. Surgery produced the highest final percentage of euthyroidism without therapy, followed by ATD and [131]I.

TABLE 11-6. Dosage Schedule for [131]I Therapy

Thyroid Weight (gm)	Low-Dose Protocol		Moderate-Dose Protocol	
	Desired μCi Retained Per g/Thyroid at 24 Hours	Average Dose (Rads), Assuming 5.9-Day Thyroid [131]I t 1/2	μCi/gm	RADS
10–20	40	3,310	80	6200
21–30	45	3,720	90	7440
31–40	50	4,135	100	8270
41–50	60	4,960	120	9920
51–60	70	5,790	140	11580
61–70	75	6,200	150	12400
71–80	80	6,620	160	13240
81–90	85	7,030	170	14060
91–100	90	7,440	180	14880
100 +	100	8,270	200	16540

TABLE 11-7. Conversion of International Units of Measurement

International Units	Conversion Factors
Becquerel (Bq)	2.7×10^{-11} Curies
Gray (Gy)	100 rads
Sievert (Sv)	100 rems

hormone and to restore the FTI to normal before ^{131}I therapy. The antithyroid drug is discontinued two days before RAIU and therapy. This pretreatment does not appear to reduce the efficacy of ^{131}I treatment.[59] Pretreatment is usually optional but is indicated in two circumstances. In patients with severe heart disease, an ^{131}I-induced exacerbation of thyrotoxicosis could be serious or fatal. We also have the impression, without proof, that pretreatment may reduce exacerbation of eye disease (see below). Alternatively, one may prescribe antithyroid drug (typically 10 mg methimazole q8h) beginning one day after administration of ^{131}I and add KI (2 drops q8h) after the second dose of methimazole. KI is continued for two weeks, and antithyroid drug as needed. This promotes a rapid return to euthyroidism, but by preventing recirculation of ^{131}I it can lower the effectiveness of the treatment. This method has been employed in a large number of patients at the University of Chicago, and is especially useful in patients requiring rapid control—for

example, with CHF. Typical responses are shown in Figure 11-3. It also has provided the largest proportion of patients remaining euthyroid at 10 years after therapy, in comparison to other treatment protocols. Antithyroid drugs may be given starting ten days after RAI without significantly lowering the radiation dose delivered to the gland.

As an alternative to ^{131}I, and because it might offer certain advantages, ^{125}I was tried in the treatment of thyrotoxicosis.[60] [125]I is primarily a gamma ray emitter, but secondary low-energy electrons are produced that penetrate only a few microns, in contrast to the high-energy β rays of [131]I. Thus, it might theo-

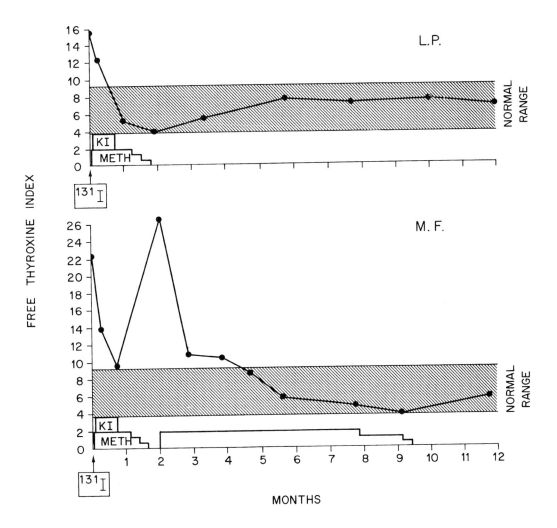

Fig. 11-3. ^{131}I-ATD-KI protocol. Twenty-four hours after ^{131}I therapy, methimazole is instituted (5-10 mg q8h), followed by KI (two drops Lugol's solution or similar q8h) at the time of each subsequent dose of ATD. KI is stopped at two weeks, and ATD continued or tapered as appropriate.

retically be possible to treat the cytoplasm of the thyroid cell with relatively little damage to the nucleus. Appropriate calculations indicated that the radiation dose to the nucleus could be perhaps one-third that to the cytoplasm, whereas this difference would not exist for ^{131}I. Extensive therapeutic trials have nonetheless failed to disclose any advantage thus far for ^{125}I. Larger doses—10 to 20 mCi—are required, increasing whole body radiation considerably.[61,62]

Course after Treatment

Usually the T_4 level falls progressively, beginning in two to three weeks, if adequate treatment has been given. Labeled thyroid hormones, iodotyrosines, and iodoproteins appear in the circulation.[63] TG is released, starting immediately after therapy. Another iodoprotein, which seems to be an iodinated albumin, is also found in plasma. This compound is similar or identical to a quantitatively insignificant secretion product of the normal gland. It comprises up to 15 percent or more of the circulating serum ^{131}I in thyrotoxic patients.[64] It is heavily labeled after ^{131}I therapy, and its proportional secretion is probably increased by the radiation. Iodotyrosine present in the serum may represent leakage from the thyroid gland, or may be derived from peripheral metabolism of TG or iodoalbumin released from the thyroid.

The return to the euthyroid state usually requires at least two months, and often the declining function of the gland proceeds gradually over six months to a year. For this reason, it is logical to avoid retreating a patient before six months have elapsed unless there is no evidence of control of the disease. While awaiting the response to ^{131}I, the symptoms may be controlled by propranolol, antithyroid drugs, or iodide. Hypothyroidism develops transiently in 10 to 20 percent of patients, but thyroid function returns spontaneously to normal in most patients in a period ranging from three to six months. These patients rarely become toxic again. Others develop permanent hypothyroidism and require replacement therapy. It is advantageous to give the thyroid adequate time to recover function spontaneously before starting permanent replacement therapy. This can be difficult for the patient unless at least partial replacement is given.

Hypothyroidism may ultimately be inescapable after any amount of radiation that is sufficient to reduce the function of the hyperplastic thyroid to normal.[65] Many apparently euthyroid patients (as many as half) have elevated serum levels of TSH long after ^{131}I therapy, with normal plasma hormone levels.[66] An elevated TSH level with a low normal T_4 level is an indicator of changes progressing toward hypothyroidism. Gordin et al.[67] found elevated TSH concentrations in 13 percent of 72 patients treated with ^{131}I 1 to 10 years previously; five of them had circulating antithyroglobulin antibodies. As expected, most of the patients with an elevated TSH level also had an exaggerated response to TRH. The hypothyroidism is doubtless also related to the continued autoimmune attack on thyroid cells. Hypofunction is a common end stage of Graves' disease independent of ^{131}I use; it occurs spontaneously as first noted in 1895[68] and in patients treated only with antithyroid drugs.[69] Just as after surgery, the development of hypothyroidism is correlated positively with the presence of antithyroid antibodies.

During the rapid development of postradiation hypothyroidism, the typical symptoms of depressed metabolism are evident, but two rather unusual features also occur. The patients may have marked aching and stiffness of joints and muscles. They may also develop severe centrally located and persistent headache. The headache responds rapidly to thyroid hormone therapy and suggests physiologic swelling of the pituitary.

In patients developing hypothyroidism rapidly, the plasma T_4 level and FTI accurately reflect the metabolic state. However, it should be noted that the TSH response may be suppressed for weeks or months by prior thyrotoxicosis; thus, the TSH level may not accurately reflect hypothyroidism in these persons and should not be used in preference to the FTI.

If permanent hypothyroidism develops, the patient is given replacement hormone therapy and is impressed with the necessity of taking the medication for the remainder of his or her life. It has been our policy not to prescribe thyroid hormone for those who develop only temporary hypothyroidism, although it is possible that patients in this group should receive replacement hormone, for their glands have been severely damaged and they may be likely to develop myxedema at a later date. Perhaps these thyroids, under prolonged TSH stimulation, may tend to develop adenomatous or malignant changes, but this has not been observed.

Permanent replacement therapy (regardless of the degree of thyroid destruction) for children who receive ^{131}I may have a better theoretical basis. In these cases, it may be advisable to prevent TSH stimulation of the thyroid and so mitigate any (unproven) tendency toward carcinoma formation.

During the period immediately after therapy, there may be a transient elevation of the T_4 or T_3 level,[70] but usually the T_4 level falls progressively toward normal. Among our treated hyperthyroid patients with Graves' disease, we have observed only rare exacerbations of the disease. These patients have had cardiac problems such as worsening angina pectoris, congestive heart failure, or disturbances of rhythm such as atrial fibrillation or even ventricular tachycardia. Radiation-induced thyroid storm and even death have unfortunately been reported.[71–73] These untoward events argue for pretreatment of selected patients who have other serious illness, especially cardiac disease, with antithyroid drugs prior to ^{131}I therapy.

RAI-Therapy-Induced Exacerbation of Thyrotoxicosis

I. W., a 48-year-old woman, developed nervousness and was told by her physician that she had a goiter, but no medication was prescribed. She subsequently experienced shaking hands, heat intolerance, palpitations, and crying. She was experiencing substantial emotional stress because of her husband's alcoholism, concern about a son who was in Vietnam, and a daughter-in-law with two young children who were living with her.

On examination, BP was 120/70, pulse rate 80, and respirations 16/min. The eyes were normal. The thyroid was about two to three times normal in size, diffusely enlarged, and rubbery. The heart was not enlarged on physical examination. The PMI was in the fifth left intercostal space at the midclavicular line. There was a grade 1 systolic murmur. There was no jugular venous distention. S-1 and S-2 were normal. The skin was warm and fine. She had 1 + pitting edema of the extremities. There was a fine tremor.

The T_4 level was 14.2 μ/dl, and the FTI was 16.2. The anti-TG antibody titer was positive at 1/5120. The electrocardiogram showed LVH and a left bundle branch block. The RAIU was elevated at 47 percent. Radiographs showed a generalized enlargement of the heart. The ESR was 3 mm. Hemogram, urinalysis, electrolyte, and blood sugar test results were normal.

The patient was treated with 4.6 mCi of radioactive [131]I. Twenty-eight days later, she experienced an episode of stabbing chest pain that woke her from sleep and caused breathlessness. She was brought to the emergency room, where an electrocardiogram revealed the changes previously described. At this time, she also described a similar episode occurring several weeks earlier, and stated that she had dyspnea after walking two or three blocks. There were no other symptoms of congestive heart failure. The BP was 120/80 and the pulse rate 120; results of the physical examination were otherwise unchanged.

While being admitted, the patient developed atrial fibrillation with a ventricular rate of 160/min. A gallop was present, and there were basilar rales. Diagnostic considerations included myocardial ischemia due to thyrotoxicosis, acute myocardial infarction, and pulmonary embolism. She was given 0.5 mg digoxin intravenously and propranolol to control her heart rate, receiving doses of up to 6 mg over 10 minutes intravenously to bring her rate to 120 BPM. She was stabilized on a dosage of propranolol of 30 mg every six hours, and was also given furosimide and potassium chloride. She was immediately started on PTU, 150 mg every six hours, and potassium iodide solution. She continued to experience episodes of stabbing chest pain and flushing. The heart rate declined with treatment to about 90, and BP was 120/80 to 140/80.

The initial T_4 level was 26.6 μg/dl, and the FT_4I was 47. Lung scan findings were unremarkable. The serum ASAT and LDH levels were normal. Serial electrocardiograms did not show evidence of myocardial infarction, and there was no evidence of pulmonary embolism. The CPK level was normal and the leukocyte count was never elevated.

During the subsequent days, while continuing to receive antithyroid drugs, potassium iodide, digoxin, propranolol, and diazepam, the patient had occasional chest pain, some shortness of breath, and sensations of flushing. She had no obvious symptoms of severe thyrotoxicosis.

The following values for T_4 and FTI were recorded:

Date	T_4 (μg/dl)	FTI (units)
March 22	12.3	12.9
March 27	(RAI therapy)	
April 23	26.6	47.3
April 27	40.2	72.8
May 2	44.6	83.8
May 3	38.4	76
May 5	34.4	58.5
May 15	22.3	29
June 7	4.4	3.2

Studies of T_4 degradation indicated a turnover half-time of four days. It was estimated that T_4 degradation exceeded 1 mg/d. On May 6, since potassium iodide

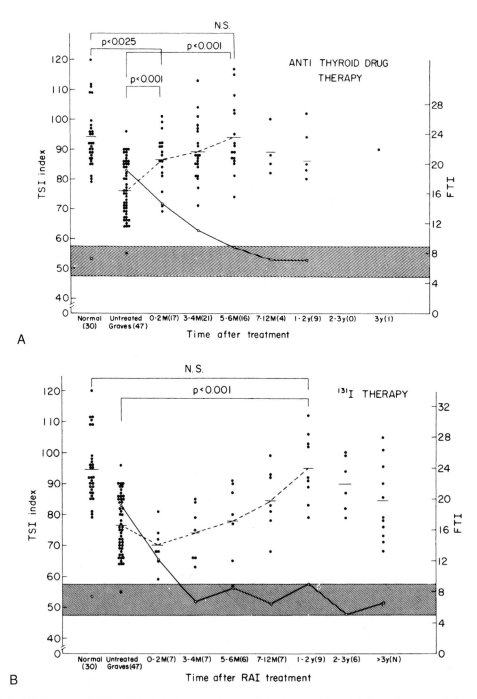

Fig. 11-4. (A) Return of TBII (TSI Index) toward normal during antithyroid drug therapy of thyrotoxicosis. **(B)** Transient increase in TBII followed by a decrease in patients treated with [131]I. (Note that in this study a lower TSI Index number means more TBII are present.)

seemed to be producing no effect, it was discontinued, and PTU was increased to 250 mg/d. The electrocardiogram eventually reverted to the pattern present before RAI therapy was instituted.

By July the patient's FTI had fallen to 1, the thyroid was normal in size, and she required replacement therapy. She continued to have occasional chest pain, but was otherwise without symptoms. Treatment during follow-up included digoxin and thyroxine.

It was believed that the patient's chest pain and atrial fibrillation represented effects of severe thyrotoxicosis induced by release of hormone from a gland damaged by radiation thyroiditis. The symptoms of thyrotoxicosis were not marked, perhaps because of the administration of propranolol and diazepam. PTU and potassium iodide treatment appeared to have little effect on the level of thyroid hormone, which reached remarkable levels. Potassium iodide was eventually discontinued, and subsequently the hormone levels returned to normal.

After ^{131}I therapy, the FTI level accurately reflects the level of circulating hormone and can be used as an index of recovery.

Problems Following [131]I Therapy

The immediate side effects of ^{131}I therapy are minimal. A few patients develop mild pain and tenderness over the thyroid and, rarely, dysphagia. Some patients develop temporary thinning of the hair, but this condition occurs two to three months after therapy rather than at two to three weeks, as occurs after ordinary radiation epilation. Hair loss also occurs after surgical therapy, so that it is a metabolic rather than a radiation effect. Permanent hypoparathyroidism has been reported very rarely as a complication of RAI therapy for heart disease and thyrotoxicosis.[74–76]

In contrast to the experience with antithyroid drugs or surgery, antithyroid antibodies including TSH-RSAb levels increase after RAI.[77,78] (Fig. 11-4). Coincident with this condition, exophthalmos may be worsened.[79,80] (Fig. 11-5). Although we believe that this change is an immunologic reaction to discharged thyroid antigens, this is conjecture, and the relationship of radiation therapy and exacerbation of exophthalmos remains uncertain.[79] Recent data indicates that there is a significant correlation.[80] Nevertheless, we consider "bad eyes" to be a relative contraindication to RAI. Pretreatment with antithyroid drugs has been used empirically in an attempt to prevent this complication. Its possible success may be related to an immunosuppressive effect of PTU, described below. Treatment with methimazole before and for three months after ^{131}I therapy has been shown to prevent the treatment-induced rise in TSH-R antibodies which is otherwise seen.[81] Also, administration of prednisone with ^{131}I may help prevent exacerbation of exophthalmos, and it has been suggested that this approach be followed in patients who have significant exophthalmos at the time of treatment.[82]

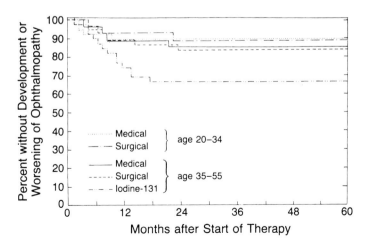

Fig. 11-5. More patients experienced worsening of exophthalmos following ^{131}I therapy than after surgery or ATD treatment. (From Tallstedt et al,[80] with permission.)

Failure of ^{131}I treatment occurs occasionally. The reason for this failure is usually not clear. The radiation effect may occur slowly. A large store of hormone in a large gland may be one cause of a slow response. Occasionally, glands having an extremely rapid turnover of ^{131}I require such high doses of the isotope that surgery is preferable to continued ^{131}I therapy and its attendant whole body radiation. If a patient fails to respond to one or two doses of ^{131}I, it is important to consider that rapid turnover may reduce the effective dose. Turnover can easily be estimated by measuring RAIU at 4, 12, 24, and 48 hours, or longer. The usual combined physical and biological half-life of ^{131}I retention is about 6 days. This may be reduced to 1 or 2 days in some cases, especially in patients who have had prior ^{131}I therapy or subtotal thyroidectomy. If this rapid release of ^{131}I is found, and ^{131}I therapy is desired, the total dose given must be increased to compensate for rapid release. A rough guide to this increment is as follows:

$$\text{Increased dose} = \text{usual dose} \times \frac{\text{usual half time of 6 days}}{\text{observed half time of ``X'' days}}$$

Most successfully treated glands return to a normal or cosmetically satisfactory size. Some large glands remain large, and in that sense may constitute a treatment failure. In such a situation secondary thyroidectomy could be done, but it is rarely required in practice.

Patients who have been treated with RAI should continue under the care of a physician who is interested in their thyroid problem for the remainder of their lives. The first follow-up visit should be made six to eight weeks after therapy. By this time, it will often be found that the patient has already experienced considerable improvement and has begun to gain weight. The frequency of subsequent visits will depend on the progress of the patient. Symptoms of hypothyroidism, if they develop, are usually not encountered until after two to four months, but one of the unfortunate facts of RAI therapy is that hypothyroidism may occur almost any time after the initial response.

Hazards of ^{131}I Treatment

In the early days of RAI treatment for Graves' disease, only patients over 45 years of age were selected for treatment because of the fear of ill effects of radiation. This age limit was gradually lowered, and some clinics, after experience extending over nearly 40 years, have now abandoned any age limitation. The major fear has been concern for induction of neoplasia, as well as the possibility that ^{131}I might induce undesirable mutations in the germ cells that would appear in later generations.

Carcinogenesis

Radiation is known to induce tumor formation in many kinds of tissues and to potentiate the carcinogenic properties of many chemical substances. Radiation therapy to the thymus or nasopharyngeal structures plays an etiologic role in thyroid carcinoma both in children and in adults.[83-85] ^{131}I radiation to the animal thyroid can produce tumors, especially if followed by PTU therapy.[86] Cancer of the thyroid has appeared more frequently in survivors of the atomic explosions at Hiroshima and Nagasaki than in control populations.[87] Thyroid nodules, some malignant, have appeared in the natives of Rongelap Island as the result of fallout after a nuclear test explosion in which the radiation cloud unexpectedly passed over the island.[88]

The experience at 26 medical centers with thyroid carcinoma after ^{131}I therapy was collected in a comprehensive study of the problem. A total of 34,684 patients treated in various ways were included. Beginning more than one year after ^{131}I therapy, 19 malignant neoplasms were found; this result did not differ significantly from the frequency after subtotal thyroidectomy. Thyroid adenomas occurred with increased frequency in the ^{131}I-treated group, and the frequency was greatest when the patients were treated in the first two decades of life.[39] Holm et al.[41] have thoroughly examined the history of a large cohort of ^{131}I-treated patients in Sweden and similarly found no evidence for an increased incidence of thyroid carcinoma or other tumors. For reasons that are unclear, the injury caused by ^{131}I therapy for Graves' disease seems to induce malignant changes infrequently, if at all. This result may occur because the damage from ^{131}I therapy is so severe that the irradiated cells are unable to undergo malignant transformations, or possibly because of the slow rate at which the dose is delivered.[89] Furthermore, in up to one-half of patients followed for 5 to 10 years, there may be no viable thyroid cells remaining. We note that reported studies extend through an average follow-up period of 15 years, but there is no data so far to suggest an increased risk at a later date. Nevertheless, this concern cannot be forgotten.

Leukemia

The incidence of leukemia among patients treated with RAI for Graves' disease has not exceeded that calculated from a control group.[90] This problem was also studied by the consortium of 26 hospitals.[91] The incidence of leukemia in this group was slightly lower than in a control group treated surgically, but slightly higher in the latter group than in the general population.

Genetic Damage

In the group of RAI-treated patients, there has been no evidence of genetic damage, although, as will shortly be seen, this problem cannot be disregarded. In the United States, about 100×10^6 children will be born to the present population of over 200×10^6 persons. Approximately 4 percent of these children will have some recognizable defect at birth. Of these, about one-half will be genetically determined or ultimately mutational, and represent the natural mutation rate in the human species. These mutations are attributed in part to naturally occurring radiation.

All penetrating radiation, from whatever sources, produces mutations. The effects may vary with rate of application, age of the subject, and no doubt many other factors, and are partially cumulative. Nearly all of these mutations behave as recessive genetic factors; perhaps 1 percent are dominant. Almost all are minor changes, and those produced by experimental radiation are the same as those produced by natural radiation.

Whether or not mutations are bad is in essence a philosophic question. Most of us would agree that the cumulative effect of mutations over past eras brought the human race to its present stage of development. Most mutations, however, at least those that are observable, are detrimental to individual human population as a whole, and detrimental mutant genes must be eliminated by the death of the carrier. We can agree that an increase in mutation rate is not desirable. It is hardly worth considering the pros and cons of the already considerable spontaneous mutation rate.

In mice, the occurrence of visible genetic mutations in any population group is probably doubled by acute exposure of each member of the group over many generations to about 30 to 40 rads and by chronic exposure to 100 to 200 rads.[92] This radiation dosage is referred to as the doubling dose. Ten percent of this increase might be expressed in the first-generation offspring of radiated parents, the remainder gradually appearing over succeeding generations. The change in mutation rate in Drosophila is in proportion to the dosage in the range above 5 rads. Data from studies of mice indicate that at low exposures (from 0.8 down to 0.0007 rads/min), the dose causing a doubling in the spontaneous rate of identifiable mutations is 110 rads.[92] Linearity, although surmised, has not been demonstrated at lower doses.

At present, residents of the United States receive about 300 mrad/year, or 9 rads before age 30, the median parental age. Roughly half of this dose is from natural sources and half from medical and, to a lesser extent, industrial exposure. The National Research Council has recommended a maximum exposure rate for the general population of less than 10 rads above background before age 30. (The present level may therefore approach this limit.)

The radiation received by the thyroid and gonads during ^{131}I therapy of thyrotoxicosis can be estimated from the following formula:

$$\text{Total } \beta \text{ radiation dose} = 73.8$$
$$\times \text{ concentration of } ^{131}\text{I in the tissue } (\mu\text{Ci/g})$$
$$\times \text{ average } \beta\text{-ray energy } (0.19 \text{ meV})$$
$$\times \text{ effective isotope half-life}$$

For illustration, we can assume a gland weight of 50 g, an uptake of 50 percent at 24 hours, a peak level of circulating protein-bound iodide (PB^{131}I) of 1 percent dose/liter, an administered dose of 5 mCi, a thyroidal iodide biologic half-life of 6 days, and a gamma dose of about 10 percent of that from β rays. On this basis, the thyroid receives almost 4,100 rads, or roughly 1,600 rads/mCi retained. The gonadal dose, being about one-half the body dose, would approximate 2 rads, or roughly 0.4 rads/mCi administered.

If the radiation data derived from *Drosophila* and lower vertebrates are applied to human radiation exposure (a tenuous but not illogical assumption), the increased risk of visible mutational defects in the progeny can be calculated. On the basis of administration to the entire population of sufficient ^{131}I to deliver to the gonads 2 rads or 2 percent of the doubling dose (assumed to be the same as in the mouse), the increase in the rate of mutational defects would ultimately be about 0.04 percent, although only one-tenth would be seen in the first generation. Obviously only a minute fraction of the population will ever receive therapeutic ^{131}I. The incidence of thyrotoxicosis is perhaps 0.03 percent per year, or 1.4 percent for the normal life span. At least one-half of these persons will have their disease after the child-bearing age has passed. Although most of them will be women, this fact does not affect the calculations after a lapse of a few generations. Assuming that the entire exposed population receives ^{131}I therapy in an average amount of 5 mCi, the increase in congenital genetic damage would be on the order of 0.02 (present congenital defect rate) × 0.04 (^{131}I radiation to the gonads as a fraction of the doubling dose) × 0.014 (the fraction of the population ever at risk) × 0.5 (the fraction of patients of childbearing age) = 0.0000056.

This crude estimate, developed from several sources, also implies that, if all patients with thyrotoxicosis were treated with ^{131}I, the number of birth defects might ultimately increase from 4 to 4.0006 percent. This increase may seem startlingly small or large, depending on one's point of view, but it is a change that would be essentially impossible to confirm from clinical experience.

Unfortunately, it is more difficult to provide a reliable estimate of the increased risk of genetic damage in the offspring of any given treated patient. Calculations such as the above simply state the problem for the whole population. Since most of the mutations are recessive, they appear in the children only when paired with another recessive gene derived from the normal complement carried by all persons. Assuming that only one parent received radiation from ^{131}I therapy amounting to 2 percent of the doubling dose, the risk of apparent birth defects in the patient's children might increase from the present 4.0 percent to 4.004 percent.

0.02 (present genetic defect rate) × 0.04 (fraction of the doubling dose) × 0.1 (fraction of defects appearing in the first generation) = 0.00008, or an increase from 4.0 percent to 4.008 percent.

Similar estimates can be derived by considering the number of visible mutations derived from experimental radiation in lower species.[92,93]

6×10^{-8} (mutations produced per genetic locus per rad of exposure) × 10^4 (an estimate of the number of genetic loci in humans) × 2 (gonadal radiation in rads as estimated above) × 0.1 (fraction of mutations appearing in the first generation) = 0.000012 or 0.012 percent

On this basis, the increase in the birth defect rate would be from 4.0 percent to 4.012 percent. One important observation stemming from these calculations is that large numbers of children born to irradiated parents must be surveyed if evidence of genetic damage is ever to be found. Reports of "no problems" among 30 to 100 such children are essentially irrelevant when one is seeking an increase in the defect rate of about 4.0 percent to about 4.004 percent.

These statistics are presented in an attempt to give some quantification to the genetic risk involved in ^{131}I therapy, and should not be interpreted as in any sense exact or final. The point we wish to stress is that radiation delivered to future parents probably will result in an increased incidence of genetic damage, but an increase so slight that it is difficult to measure. Nonetheless, the use of ^{131}I for large numbers of women who subsequently become pregnant will inevitably introduce change in the gene pool.

In considering the significance of these risks, one must remember that the radiation exposure to the gonads from the usual therapeutic dose of ^{131}I may be only one or two times that produced during a procedure such as a barium enema[94,95] and similar to the 10 rads received from a CAT scan. These examinations are ordered by most physicians without fear of radiation effect (Table 11-8).

When assessing the risks of ^{131}I therapy, one must, of course, consider the risks of any alternative choice of procedure. Surgery carries a small but finite mortality, as well as a risk of permanent hypoparathyroidism, hypothyroidism, and vocal cord paralysis. Some of these risks are especially high in children, the group in which radiation damage is most feared. Some physicians have held that ^{131}I therapy should not be given to patients who intend subsequently to have children. In fact, there is at present little if any evidence to support this contention, as discussed above. Chapman[44] studied 110 women treated with ^{131}I who subsequently became pregnant and were delivered of 150 children. There was no evidence of any increase in congenital defects or of accidents of

TABLE 11-8. Gonadal Radiation Dose (in Rads) from Diagnostic Procedures and ^{131}I Therapy

Procedure	Males		Females	
	Median	Range	Median	Range
Barium meal	0.0300	0.005–0.23	0.34	0.06–0.83
Intravenous pyelogram	0.43	0.015–2.09	0.59	0.27–1.16
Retrograde pyelogram	0.58	0.15–2.09	0.52	0.085–1.4
Barium enema	0.3	0.095–1.59	0.87	0.46–1.75
Femur x-ray film	0.92	0.23–1.71	0.24	0.058–0.68
Iodine-131 therapy (5 mCi)	Usually below 1.6		Usually below 1.6	

(Adapted from Robertson and Gorman,[95] with permission.)

pregnancy. Sarkar et al.[96] also found no evidence of excess abnormalities among children who received ^{131}I therapy for cancer. Other studies have confirmed the apparent lack of risk.[42,43] It should be noted that no increase in congenital abnormalities has been detected among the offspring of persons who received much larger radiation doses during atomic bomb explosions.[97]

Often the patient wishes to know about the possibility of carcinogenesis or genetic damage. These questions must be fully but delicately handled. It is not logical to treat a patient of childbearing age with ^{131}I and have the patient subsequently live in great fear of bearing children. These problems and considerations must be faced each time a patient is considered for RAI therapy.

Pregnancy

Pregnancy is an absolute contraindication to ^{131}I therapy. The fetus is exposed to considerable radiation from transplacental migration of ^{131}I, as well as from the isotope in the maternal circulatory and excretory systems. In addition, the fetal thyroid collects ^{131}I after the 12th week of gestation and may be destroyed. The increased sensitivity of fetal structures to radiation damage has already been described.

Physicians treating women of childbearing age with ^{131}I should be certain that the patients are not pregnant when given the isotope. Therapy during or immediately after a normal menstrual period or performance of a pregnancy test are appropriate precautions if pregnancy is possible. Women should be advised to avoid pregnancy for at least six months, since it usually takes this long to be certain that retreatment will not be needed.

Treatment of Thyrotoxicosis with Drugs

Drug therapy for thyrotoxicosis was introduced by Plummer when he observed that the administration of iodide ameliorated the symptoms of this disease[98] (Fig. 11-6). Administration of iodide has since been used occasionally as the complete therapeutic program for thyrotoxicosis, and widely as an adjunct in preparing patients for subtotal thyroidectomy. In 1941 the pioneering observations of MacKenzie and MacKenzie[99] and Astwood[100] led to the development of the thiocarbamide drugs, which reliably block the formation of thyroid hormones. It soon became apparent that, in a certain proportion of patients with Graves' disease, use of these drugs could induce a prolonged or permanent remission of the disease even after the medication was discontinued. It is not yet understood why a temporary reduction in the formation of thyroid hormone should result in permanent amelioration of the disease.

The antithyroid drug that was initially introduced for treatment of Graves' disease was thiourea, but this drug proved to have a large number of undesirable toxic effects. Subsequently a number of derivatives and related compounds were introduced that have potent antithyroid activity without the same degree of toxicity. Among these substances are propyl- and methylthiouracil, methimazole, and carbimazole. In addition to this class of compounds, potassium perchlorate has been used in the treatment of thyrotoxicosis, but is infrequently employed for this purpose because of occasional bone marrow depression. This drug prevents the concentration of iodide by the thyroid. β-sympathetic blockers such as propranolol have a place in the treatment of thyrotoxicosis. These drugs alleviate some of the signs and symptoms of the disease but have little or no direct

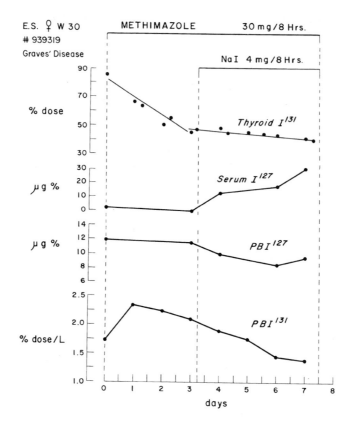

Fig. 11-6. KI in doses over 6 mg/day dramatically inhibits release of hormone from the Graves' thyroid, as shown after treatment in this study starting during day 4. Serum hormone levels (PBI) consequently fall.

effect on the metabolic abnormality itself. They do not uniformly induce a remission of the disease and can be regarded as adjuncts, not as a substitute for more definitive therapy.

Antithyroid drugs inhibit thyroid peroxidase, and PTU (not methimazole) has the further beneficial action of inhibiting T_4 to T_3 conversion in peripheral tissues. A most exciting new idea regarding their action stems from observations that antithyroid therapy is associated with a prompt reduction in circulating antithyroid antibody titers,[101] and anti-receptor antibodies.[77,78,102] Studies by MacGregor and colleagues[103] indicate that antibody reduction also occurs during antithyroid therapy in patients with thyroiditis maintained in a euthyroid state, thus indicating that the effect is not due only to lowering of the FTI in Graves' disease. These authors also found a direct inhibitory effect of PTU and carbimazole on antithyroid antibody synthesis in vitro and postulate that this is the mechanism for diminished

antibody levels.[104] Other data argue against this hypothesis.[105]

Antithyroid drug therapy is also associated with a prompt reduction in the abnormally high levels of activated T lymphocytes in the circulation.[106] Totterman and co-workers have shown this therapy causes a prompt and transient elevation of activated T suppressor lymphocytes in blood.[107] We and others[106,108] have shown that during antithyroid drug treatment the reduced numbers of T suppressor cells present in most thyrotoxic patients return to normal. Antithyroid drugs do not directly inhibit T cell function.[109] All of these data argue that antithyroid drugs exert a powerful beneficial immunosuppressive effect on patients with Graves' disease. While much has been learned about this process, the exact mechanism remains uncertain. Evidence that antithyroid drugs exert their immunosuppressive effect by a direct inhibition of thyroid cell production of hormones has been reviewed recently by Volpe.[109]

Long-Term Antithyroid Drug Therapy with Thiocarbamides

In our practice, many patients with Graves' disease under age 40 to 45 are given a trial of therapy with one of the thiocarbamide drugs. Younger patients, and those with recent onset of disease, small goiters,[110] and mild disease, are especially favorable candidates, since they tend to enter remission most frequently. It is generally found that one-fourth to one-third of these patients who satisfactorily complete a one year course have a long term or permanent remission. The remainder need repeated courses of drug therapy, must be maintained on the drug for years or indefinitely,[111,112] or must be given some other treatment. It appears that the percentage of patients responding has progressively fallen over the past 15 years from about 50 percent to at present 25 to 50 percent.[113,114] This change may reflect an alteration in iodide in our diet,[115] which increased from about 150 μg/day in 1955 to 300 to 600 μg/day. Many physicians do not consider antithyroid drug therapy to be the most efficacious means of treating thyrotoxic patients because of the high recurrence rate. Patients are initially given 100 to 150 mg PTU or 10 to 15 mg methimazole (Tapazole) every eight hours. The initial dosage is varied depending on the severity of the disease, size of the gland, and medical urgency. Antithyroid drugs must usually be given frequently and taken with regularity since the half-life in blood is brief—1.65 hours or less for PTU.[116] Frequent dosage is especially needed when instituting therapy in a severely ill patient. Methimazole has the advantage of a longer therapeutic half-life, and appears to produce fewer reactions when given in low dosage. Propylthiouracil is preferred in patients with very severe hyperthyroidism and in pregnancy.[117,118]

In most thyrotoxic patients, the euthyroid state, as assessed by clinical parameters, and FTI, can be reached within 4 to 6 weeks. If the patient fails to respond, the dosage may be increased. Iodine-131 studies may be performed to determine whether a sufficiently large dose of medication is being employed,[119] but these studies are rarely needed. In general, it is assumed that binding of the ^{131}I should be nearly completely blocked, but the 24-hour ^{131}I thyroid uptake in the patient under therapy may range from 0 percent to 40 percent. This iodide is partly unbound and is usually released rapidly from the gland by administration of 1 g potassium thiocyanate or 400 mg potassium perchlorate. If perchlorate or thiocyanate does not discharge the iodide, it is obvious that binding of iodide is occurring despite the thiocarbamide therapy. The quantity of drug administered may then be increased. In experimental animals, the thiocarbamides block synthesis of iodothyronines more readily than they block formation of MIT and DIT. This observation suggests that a complete block in organification of iodide may not be necessary to produce euthyroidism. The patient's thyroid might accumulate and organify iodide and form iodotyrosines, but be unable to synthesize the iodothyronines. Clinical observations to prove this point are not available.

An RIA for PTU has been developed but has not proven useful in monitoring therapy.[120] Doses of 300 mg PTU produced serum levels of about 7.1 μg/ml, and serum levels of PTU correlated directly with decreases in serum T_3 levels.

It is theoretically possible to give therapeutic doses of methimazole by rectal administration if the oral route is unavailable.[121]

Long-Term Therapeutic Program

After the initial period of high-dose therapy, the amount of drug administered daily is gradually reduced to a level that maintains the patient in a euthyroid condition, as assessed by clinical evaluation and serial observations of serum T_4, FTI, or T_3. These tests should appropriately reflect the metabolic status of the patient. Measurement of TSH level is useful when the FTI falls, to make sure that the patient has not been overtreated, but, as noted previously, TSH may remain suppressed for many weeks after thyrotoxicosis is alleviated. Serum T_3 levels can also be monitored and are occasionally still elevated when the T_4 level is in the normal range. Obviously the RAIU test is not helpful. During the course of treatment, the thyroid gland usually remains the same in size or becomes smaller. If the gland enlarges, the patient has probably become hypothyroid with TSH elevation; this condition should be ascertained by careful clinical and laboratory evaluation. If the patient does become hypothyroid, the dose of antithyroid drug should be reduced. Decrease in size of the thyroid under therapy is a favorable prognostic sign, and more often than not means that the patient will remain euthyroid after the antithyroid drugs have been discontinued. The dose is gradually reduced as the patient reaches euthyroidism, and often one-half or one-third of the initial dose is sufficient to maintain control. The interval between doses—typically six to eight hours initially—can be extended, and patients can often be maintained on twice- or once-a-day therapy.[122] Alternatively, antithyroid drugs can be maintained at a higher dose, and thyroxine can be added to produce euthyroidism. Occasionally ingestion of large amounts of iodide interferes with antithyroid drug therapy.

The appropriate duration of antithyroid drug therapy is uncertain, but usually it is maintained for one year. Treatment for six months has been effective in some clinics but is not general practice.[123] Longer treatment—such as one to three years—does gradually increase the percentage of responders,[124] but this increase must be balanced against the added inconvenience to the patient.[125,126] At least one study suggests that treatment with large doses of antithyroid drugs may increase the remission rate, perhaps because of an immunosuppressive action.[125]

After the patient has taken the antithyroid drugs for a year, the medication is gradually withdrawn over one to two months, and the patient is observed at intervals thereafter. Most of those who will ultimately have an exacerbation of the disease do so within three to six months; others may not develop recurrent hyperthyroidism for several years.[127] Some patients may have a recurrence after discontinuing the drug that lasts for a short time, and then a remission without further therapy.[128] An earlier report that administration of iodide increases the relapse rate after drug therapy is withdrawn has not been confirmed.[129] Hashizume and co-workers recently reported that administration of T_4 to suppress TSH for a year after stopping antithyroid drugs produced a very high remission rate[130] (Fig. 11-7). Similar results were found when T_4 treatment was given after a course of antithyroid drugs during pregnancy.[131] These studies have engendered much interest because of the uniquely high remission rate obtained by the continuation of thyroxine treatment to suppress TSH for a year or more after the usual course of antithyroid drug therapy. Possibly such treatment is beneficial since it inhibits the release of thyroid antigens. While the method can easily be adopted for practice, further studies are needed to ascertain whether the results are generally observed or are, for some reason, peculiar to this study group.

The probability of prolonged remission correlates with reduction in gland size, disappearance of thyroid-stimulating antibodies from serum,[132,133] return of T_3 suppressibility, decrease in serum TG, and a haplotype other than HLA-DR3.[130,134] However, none of these markers predict recovery or continued disease with an accuracy rate above 60 to 70 percent. Long after apparent clinical remission, many patients show continued abnormal thyroid function, including partial failure of T_3 suppression, or absent or excessive TRH responses.[127–140] These findings probably indicate the tenuous balance controlling immune responses in these patients.

The special problems associated with antithyroid drug therapy in pregnant women and in children are reviewed in Chapter 14.

Lactating women taking PTU have PTU levels of up to 7.7 μg/ml in blood, but in milk the level is much lower, about 0.7 μg/ml.[141] Only 1 to 2 mg PTU could be transferred to the baby daily through nursing; this amount is inconsequential except for the possibility of reactions to the drug.

It has long been known that some patients with Graves' disease eventually develop spontaneous hypothyroidism.[68] Reports have shown that most patients who become euthyroid after antithyroid drug therapy, if followed long enough, also develop evidence of diminished thyroid function.[69] In a prospective study, Lamberg et al.[139] found that the annual incidence in these patients of subclinical hypothyroidism was 2.5 percent, and of overt hypothyroidism 0.6 percent.

Toxic Reactions to Antithyroid Drugs

The use of antithyroid drugs may be accompanied by toxic reactions, depending on the drug and dose, in 3 to 12 percent of patients.[117,118,142–146] Most of these reactions probably represent drug allergies.[147–148] Chevalley et al., in a study of 180 patients given methimazole,[143] found an incidence of toxicity of 4.3 percent, broken down as follows:

Total reactions	4.3%
Pruritus	2.2%
Granulocytopenia	1.6%
Urticaria	0.5%

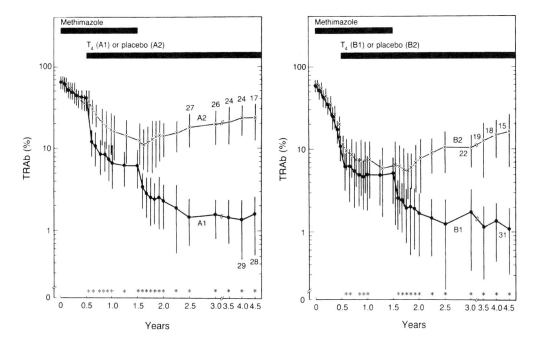

Fig. 11-7. Addition of 1.8 μg/kg T$_4$ for a year or more following ATD treatment is reported to suppress TBII, delay recovery of TSH to normal, and decrease recurrences. This figure shows the effect of added T$_4$ keeping TRAb low over four years in two groups of patients. (From Hashizume et al,[131] with permission.)

The incidence of agranulocytosis in a large series of patients was 0.4 percent.[149] It occurs most frequently in older patients and those given large amounts of the drug (20 to 30 mg every eight hours).[117] Reactions tend to be most frequent in the first few months of therapy but can occur at any time, with small doses of drug, and in patients of all ages.[117] The most common reactions are fever and a morbilliform or erythematous rash with pruritus. Reactions similar to those of serum sickness, with migratory arthralgias, jaundice, lymphadenopathy, polyserositis, and episodes resembling systemic lupus erythematosus have also been observed.[147] Neutropenia and agranulocytosis are the most serious complications. These reactions appear to be due to sensitization to the drugs, as determined by lymphocyte reactivity in vitro to the drugs.[148] Fortunately, even these problems almost always subside when the drug is withdrawn. Aplastic anemia with marrow hypoplasia has been reported (perhaps 10 cases), again with spontaneous recovery in 2 to 5 weeks in 70 percent, but fatal outcome in 3 patients.[149]

Toxic hepatitis (primarily with propylthiouracil) and cholestatic jaundice (primarily with methimazole) are fortunately uncommon.[144] Toxic hepatitis can be severe or fatal, but the incidence of serious liver complications is so low that routine monitoring of function tests has not been advised.[150,151] Diffuse interstitial pneumonitis has also been produced by propylthiouracil.[152]

Methimazole may be the drug least likely to cause a toxic reaction, but there is little difference between it and PTU. When the antithyroid drugs are prescribed, the patient should be apprised of the possibility of reactions, and should be told to report phenomena such as a sore throat, fever, or rash to the physician and to discontinue the drug until the cause of the symptoms has been evaluated. These symptoms may herald a serious reaction.

It is probably wise to see patients receiving the thiocarbamides at least monthly during the initiation of therapy and every two to three months during the entire program. Neutropenia can develop gradually but often comes on so suddenly that a routine white cell count offers only partial protection. A white cell count must be taken whenever there is any suggestion of a reaction, and especially if the patient reports malaise or a sore throat. A white cell count taken at each visit will detect the gradually developing neutropenia that may occur. While many physicians do not routinely monitor these levels, the value of monitoring is suggested by the study of Tajiri et al.[144] Fifty-five of 15,398 patients treated with antithyroid drugs developed agranulocytosis, and 4/5 of these were detected by routine WBC at office visits. Low total leukocyte counts are common in Graves' disease because of relative neutropenia, and for this reason a baseline WBC and differential should be performed before starting anti-thyroid drugs. Total polymorphonuclear counts below 2,000 cells/mm^3, however, should be carefully monitored; below 1,200 cells/mm^3 it is unsafe to continue using the drugs.

If a patient taking a thiocarbamide develops a mild rash, it is permissible to provide an antihistamine and continue using the drug to see whether the reaction subsides spontaneously, as it commonly does. If the reaction is more severe or if neutropenia occurs, another drug should be tried or the medication withdrawn altogether. Usually a switch is made to another thiocarbamide, because cross-reactions do not necessarily occur between members of this drug family. Alternatively, the program of therapy may be changed to the use of RAI, which may be given after the patient has stopped taking the antithyroid drug for 48 to 74 hours, or the patient may be prepared for surgery by the administration of iodides and propranolol.

In the event of severe neutropenia or agranulocytosis, the patient should be monitored closely, given antibiotics if infection develops, and possibly adrenal steroids. There is no consensus on the use of glucocorticoids, since they have not been shown to definitely shorten the period to recovery. However, administration of recombinant human granulocyte colony stimulating factor (75 μg/day given IM) does appear to hasten neutrophile recovery in patients who start with neutrophile counts greater than 0.1 $\times$ 10^9/L.[153] Care must be taken to ensure against exposure to infectious agents, and some physicians prefer not to hospitalize their patients for this reason. If the patient is hospitalized, he or she should be placed in a special-care room with full bacteriologic precautions.

As noted above, thiocarbamides can also cause liver damage ranging from elevation of enzymes,

through jaundice, to fatal hepatic necrosis. Any sign of liver damage must be carefully monitored, and progress of abnormalities in liver function tests demand cessation of the drug.[147,151]

Neutropenia From Propylthiouracil

B.Z., an 18-year-old man, developed symptoms of hyperthyroidism at age 17. He also had a history of diabetes mellitus for six years, requiring insulin twice daily. The insulin requirement had recently increased. His personal physician noted symptoms of hyperthyroidism and thyroid enlargement, and referred him for evaluation. The BP was 140/75 and the pulse rate 110. There was no ophthalmopathy. The thyroid was symmetrically enlarged to about 40 g in weight; there was no nodularity or lymphadenopathy. The heart was hyperactive. There was mild injection of the conjunctiva. The FTI was elevated (13.7) and the TGHA test result was positive at 1/1280. The patient was given PTU, 150 mg every eight hours, and improved clinically, although after one month on therapy the FTI was still 13.5. The patient left for college and did not follow instructions to see a physician at the institution.

He continued to take PTU and returned 10 months later with symptoms of hypothyroidism, including fatigue, weight gain, and a puffy appearance. The skin was dry and cool. The thyroid now weighed 80 g. The T$_4$ level was 0.5 μg/dl, FTI 0.4, and TSH level 117 μU/ml. He had a hemoglobin level of 13 g% and a hematocrit of 37 percent. The white cell count was 2,000 mm^3 with 10 percent polys, 79 percent lymphs, 10 percent monocytes, and 2 percent bands. The platelet count was 189,000/mm^3. Medication was discontinued. He had no evidence of infection. There was no fever or chills and no throat irritation. One day later, the white cell count was 2,200/mm^3 with 1 percent polys. Two days later, it was 2,800/mm^3 with 19 percent polys, and after four days it reached 3,100/mm^3 with 8 percent polys. The thyroid became smaller. After seven days the white cell count was 4,600/mm^3 and the polys were 25 percent. The total neutrophil count was 1,150/mm^3.

One month later, on physical examination there was a 35-g goiter and no evidence of hypothyroidism. The FTI was 10.5, and the T$_4$ level was 8.8 μg/dl. The white cell count was normal.

This young man had severe complications of PTU therapy during a prolonged period of unsupervised care. He developed hypothyroidism and thyroid enlargement, and at the same time a severe neutropenia. With withdrawal of antithyroid medication, the white cell count returned promptly to normal, as did the FTI. There has been no evidence of recurrent hyperthyroidism.

Potassium Perchlorate and Lithium

Potassium perchlorate was introduced into clinical use after it was demonstrated that several monovalent anions, including nitrates, have an antithyroid action. Perchlorate was the only member of the group that appeared to have sufficient potency to be useful. This drug, in doses of 200 to 400 mg every six hours, competitively blocks iodide transport by the thyroid. Accordingly, therapeutic doses of potassium iodide will overcome its effect. Institution and control of therapy with perchlorate are similar to those discussed for the thiocarbamides. Toxic reactions to this agent occur in about 4 percent of cases[154] and usually consist of gastric distress, skin rash, fever, lymphadenopathy, or neutropenia; they usually disappear when the drug is discontinued. The reaction rate is higher when doses of more than 1 g/d are given.[154] Nonfatal cases of neutropenia or agranulocytosis have been reported, and four cases of fatal aplastic anemia have been associated with the use of this drug.[155] Because of toxic reactions, perchlorate is not used at present for routine therapy. It has found a role in therapy of thyrotoxicosis induced by amiodarone.[156] Apparently blocking of iodide uptake is an effective antithyroid therapy in the presence of large body stores of iodide, while in this situation, methimazole and propylthiouracil are not effective alone.

Lithium ion inhibits release of T_4 and T_3 from the thyroid and has been used in the treatment of thyrotoxicosis, but is most effective when used with a thiocarbamide drug. It does not have a well-established place in the treatment of Graves' disease.[156,157] It has possible value in augmenting the retention of ^{131}I[158] and in preparing patients allergic to the usual antithyroid drugs or iodide for surgery, although propranolol is generally used for the latter problem.

Iodine

Plummer originally observed that the administration of iodide to thyrotoxic patients resulted in an amelioration of their symptoms. This reaction is associated with a decreased rate of release of thyroid hormone from the gland and with a gradual increase in the quantity of stored hormone. The effect of iodide on thyroid hormone release and concentration in blood is apparent in Figure 11-5. The mechanism of action is not yet fully understood. Therapeutic quantities of iodide also have an effect on hormone synthesis through inhibition of organification of iodide. Iodide has similar but less intense effects on the normal thyroid gland, apparently because of the adaptive mechanisms described in Chapter 5.

Administration of large amounts of iodide to laboratory animals or humans blocks the synthesis of thyroid hormone and results in an accumulation of trapped inorganic iodide in the thyroid gland (the Wolff-Chaikoff effect, see Ch. 2). The thyrotoxic gland is especially sensitive to this action of iodide. Raising the plasma iodide concentration to a level above 5 μg/dl results in a complete temporary inhibition of iodide organification by the thyrotoxic gland. In normal persons elevation of the inorganic ^{127}I level results, up to a point, in a progressive increase of accumulation of iodide in the gland. When the plasma concentration is above 20 μg/dl, organification is also inhibited in the normal gland.[159] The sensitivity of the thyrotoxic gland, in comparison with that of the euthyroid gland, may be due to an increased ability to concentrate iodide in the thyroid, and its failure to "adapt" by decreasing the iodide concentrating mechanism.

When iodine is to be used therapeutically in Graves' disease, one usually prescribes a saturated solution of potassium iodide (which contains about 50 mg iodide per drop) or Lugol's solution (which contains about 8.3 mg iodide per drop). Thompson and co-workers[160] found that 6 mg of I$^-$ or KI produces a maximum response. This fact was reemphasized by Friend, who pointed out that the habit of prescribing 5 drops of Lugol's or SSKI three times daily is unnecessary.[161] Two drops of Lugol's solution or 1 drop of a saturated solution of potassium iodide two times daily is more than sufficient.

The therapeutic response to iodide begins within two to seven days and is faster than can be obtained by any other methods of medical treatment. Only 3 percent of patients so treated fail to respond.[162] Men, older persons, and those with nodular goiter are in the group less likely to have a response to iodide.[163]

Although almost all patients initially respond to iodide, about one-third respond partially and remain toxic, and another one-third initially respond but relapse after about six weeks.[164] The use of iodide as definitive therapy for thyrotoxicosis has been discarded in favor of the modalities previously described. Iodides are sometimes given after ^{131}I therapy to control hyperthyroidism, and are usually given as part of treatment before thyroidectomy.

Use of Drugs in Adjunctive Therapy for Graves' Disease

Propranolol

Propranolol, a potent β-adrenergic blocking agent, has won a prominent position in the treatment of thyrotoxicosis. Although it alleviates many of the signs and symptoms, it has little effect on the fundamental disease process.[165,166] Palpitations, excessive sweating, and nervousness improve, and tremor and tachycardia are controlled. Many patients feel much improved, but others are depressed by the drug and prefer not to take it. Improvement in myocardial efficiency and reduction in the exaggerated myocardial oxygen consumption have been demonstrated.[167] Propranolol lowers oxygen consumption[168] and reverses the nitrogen wasting of thyrotoxicosis, although it does not inhibit excess urinary calcium and hydroxyproline loss.[124] Propranolol is useful in symptomatic treatment while physician and patient are awaiting the improvement from antithyroid drug or ^{131}I therapy.[169] Some patients appear to respond to this drug alone after six months or so of therapy.[168,170] It has been useful in neonatal thyrotoxicosis[171] and in thyroid storm.[172] The drug must be used cautiously when there is evidence of heart failure, but often control of tachycardia permits improved circulation. Some surgical groups routinely prepare patients for thyroidectomy with propranolol for 20 to 40 days and add potassium iodide during the last week.[173] The BMR and thyroid hormone level remain elevated at the time of operation, but the patient experiences no problems. We prefer conventional preoperative preparation with thio-carbamides, with or without iodide, and would use propranolol as an adjunct, or if the patient is allergic to the usual drugs.

Propranolol is usually given orally as 20 to 40 mg every four to six hours, but up to 200 mg every six hours may be needed. In emergency management of thyroid storm (see also Ch. 12) or tachycardia, it may be given intravenously (1 to 3 mg, rarely up to 6 mg) over 3 to 10 minutes and repeated every four to six hours under electrocardiographic control. Atropine (0.5 to 1.0 mg) is the appropriate antidote if severe brachycardia is produced.

Reserpine and Guanethidine

Drugs such as reserpine[174] and guanethidine[175] that deplete tissue catecholamines were used extensively in the past as adjuncts in the therapy for thyrotoxicosis, but fell into disuse as the value of β-sympathetic blockage with propranolol became recognized.

Glucocorticoids, Ipodate, and Other Treatments

As described elsewhere, potassium iodide acts promptly to inhibit thyroid hormone secretion from the Graves' disease thyroid gland. PTU, propranolol, glucocorticoids,[176] amiodarone, and sodium ipodate (Oragrafin Sodium) inhibit peripheral T_4 to T_3 conversion, and glucocorticoids may have a more prolonged suppressive effect on thyrotoxicosis.[177] Orally administered resins bind T_4 in the intestine and prevent recirculation.[178] All of these agents have been used for control of thyrotoxicosis.[179,180] Combined dexamethasone, potassium iodide, and PTU can lower the serum T_3 level to normal in 24 hours, which is useful in severe thyrotoxicosis.[181] Prednisone has been reported to induce remission of Graves' disease, but at the expense of causing Cushing's syndrome.[182] Ipodate (0.5 to 1 g orally per day) acts to inhibit hormone release because of its iodine content, in addition to its action on T_4 to T_3 conversion. This dose of ipodate given to patients with Graves' disease reduced the serum T_3 level by 58 percent and the T_4 level by 20 percent within 24 hours, and the effect persisted for three weeks.[183,184] This dose of ipodate was more effective than 600 mg of PTU, which decreased the T_3 level by only 23 percent during the first 24 hours, whereas the T_4 level did not drop. Ipodate may prove to be a useful adjunct in the early therapy of hyperthyroidism, but will increase total body and thyroidal iodine. However, when the drug is stopped, the RAIU in Graves' patients usually returns to pretreatment levels within a week.[184] Because it is the most effective agent available in preventing conversion of T_4 to T_3, it has a useful role in managing thyroid storm (Ch. 12).

Surgical Treatment

Subtotal thyroidectomy is an established and effective form of therapy for Graves' disease, providing the patient has been suitably prepared for surgery. In competent hands, the risk of hypoparathyroidism or recurrent nerve damage is under 1 percent, and the discomfort and transient disability attendant upon surgery may be a reasonable price to pay for the rapid relief from this unpleasant disease. In some clinics it is the therapy of choice for most young male adults, especially if a trial of antithyroid drugs has failed. With other effective methods available, it is necessary for the physician and the patient to decide on the form of therapy most suitable for the case at hand. Because of the potential but unproved risks of ^{131}I therapy, it is not always possible to make an entirely rational choice; the fears and prejudices of the physician and the patient will often enter into the decision.

Surgery is clearly indicated in certain patients. Among these are (1) patients who have not responded to prolonged antithyroid drug therapy, or who develop toxic reactions to the drug and for whatever reason are unsuitable for ^{131}I therapy; (2) patients with huge glands, which frequently do not regress adequately after ^{131}I therapy; and (3) patients with thyroid nodules that raise a suspicion of carcinoma. The rate of appearance of progressive ophthalmopathy has been reported to be about the same after treatment with ^{131}I as with surgery,[79] (Table 11-10) but other data indicate that exophthalmos may be exacerbated by RAI therapy.[80] Thus, in the presence of serious eye signs, treatment with antithyroid drugs followed by surgery is one alternative to consider.

More enthusiastic surgeons have in the past recommended surgery for all children as the initial approach, claiming that there is less interference with normal growth and development than with prolonged antithyroid drug treatment.[185] Therapy for childhood thyrotoxicosis is discussed further below.

TABLE 11-9. Approximate Daily Dose of PTU

Surface Area (m^2)	Weight (lbs)*	Approximate Daily Dose (mg)
0.1	5	15
0.2	10	30
0.5	30	75
0.75	60	110
1.0	90	150
1.25	110	190
1.5	140	225
2.0	200	300

* Metrically minded physicians can divide weight by 2 to approximate kilograms.

TABLE 11-10. Incidence of Post-treatment Exophthalmos among Patients Who Did Not Have Clinical Evidence of Infiltrative Ophthalmopathy Pretreatment

Treatment Group	Number of Cases	Percent of Group Developing Exophthalmos Post-treatment
Medical	104	6.7
Surgical	83	7.1
[131]I	144	4.9

The rate of patient rehabilitation is probably quickest with surgery. Although the source of hormone is directly and immediately removed by surgery, the patient usually must undergo one to three months of preparation before operation. The total time from diagnosis through operative convalescence is thus three to four months. Antithyroid drugs, in contrast, provide at best only 30 to 40 percent permanent control after one year of therapy. Iodine-131 can assuredly induce prompt remission. Low-dose protocols, as noted, are plagued by a need for medical management and retreatment over one to three years before all patients are euthyroid. Treatment with higher doses provides more certain remission at the expense of hypothyroidism.

There are several strong contraindications to surgery, including previous thyroid surgery, severe coincident heart or lung disease, the lack of a well-qualified surgeon, and pregnancy in the third trimester, since anesthesia and surgery may induce premature labor. The presence of high levels of antithyroid antibodies may be considered a relative contraindication to surgery, since autoimmunity predisposes to postoperative hypothyroidism.

Preparation for Surgery

Antithyroid drugs of the thiocarbamide group are employed to induce a euthyroid state before subtotal thyroidectomy when surgery is the desired form of treatment. Two approaches are used. PTU or methimazole may be administered until the patient becomes euthyroid. After this state has been reached, and while the patient is maintained on full doses of thiocarbamides, Lugol's solution or a saturated solution of potassium iodide is administered for 7 to 10 days. This therapy induces an involution of the gland and decreases its vascularity, a factor surgeons find helpful in the subsequent thyroidectomy. The iodide should be given only while the patient is under the effect of full doses of the antithyroid drug; otherwise, the iodide may permit an exacerbation of the thyrotoxicosis.

Alternative patients may be prepared by combined treatment with antithyroid drugs and thyroxine. It is not obvious that one method is superior to the other.

Pre-treatment should have the patient in optimal condition for surgical thyroidectomy. By this time the patient has gained weight, the nutritional status has been improved, and the cardiovascular manifestations of the disease are under control. At the time of surgery, the anesthesia is well tolerated without the risk of hypersensitivity to sympathoadrenal discharge characteristic of the thyrotoxic subject. The surgeon finds that the gland is relatively avascular. Convalescence is customarily smooth. The stormy febrile course characteristic of the poorly prepared patient is rarely seen.

Reactions to the thiocarbamide drugs occasionally occur during preparation for surgery. If the problem is a minor rash or low-grade fever, the drug is continued, or a change is made to a different thiocarbamide. More severe reactions (severe fever or rash, leukopenia, jaundice, or serum sickness) continuing after a change to another thiocarbamide necessitate a change to another form of therapy, but no entirely satisfactory alternative is available. One course is to administer iodide and propranolol and proceed to surgery. In some patients, it is best to proceed directly to ^{131}I therapy if difficulties arise in the preparation with antithyroid drugs.

Propranolol has been used alone or in combination with potassium iodide[186] in preparation for surgery, and favorable results have generally been reported.[187,189] This procedure is doubtless safe in the hands of a medical team familiar and experienced with this protocol and willing to monitor the patient carefully to ensure adequate dosage. It is safe to use in young patients with mild disease, but we are reluctant to advise it as a standard protocol. We use propranolol as an adjunct, or combined with potassium iodide as the sole therapy only when complications with antithyroid drugs preclude their use and surgery is strongly preferred to treatment with [131]I.

Techniques and Complications

The standard operation is a one-stage subtotal thyroidectomy. The surgical technique is discussed in Chapter 21. Permanent cure of the hyperthyroidism is produced in 90 to 98 percent of patients treated this way. The amount of tissue left behind is about 4 to 10 grams, but this amount is variable. Taylor and Painter[190] found that the average volume of this remnant in 43 patients achieving a remission was about 8 ml, and Sugino et al recommended leaving 6 grams of tissue.[191] The toxic state recurred in only two patients in their series, and in these twice the amount of tissue mentioned above was left. There seemed to be no relation between the original size of the thyroid and the size of the remnant necessary to maintain normal metabolism.

Although surgery of the thyroid has reached a high degree of perfection, it is not without problems even in excellent hands. The complication rates at present are low.[192] Among 254 patients operated on at three Nashville hospitals in the decade before 1970, there was no mortality, only minor wound problems, a 1.9 percent incidence of permanent hypoparathyroidism, and a 4.2 percent recurrence rate.[193] Hypoparathyroidism is the major undesirable chronic complication. Surgical therapy at the Mayo Clinic has in recent years[194] been associated with a 75 percent rate of hypothyroidism but only a 1 percent recurrence rate, as an effort was made to remove more tissue and prevent recurrences. There is typically an inverse relationship between these two results of surgery. In the recent experience of the University of Chicago Clinics, the euthyroid state has been achieved by surgery in 82 percent; 6 percent became hypothyroid, and the recurrence rate was 12 percent.[195] Recurrence rates are higher in patients with progressive exophthalmos or positive assays for TSAb.[196] Geographic differences in iodine ingestion have been related to the outcome. In Iceland, with a high iodine intake, postoperative hypothyroidism is less frequent, but recurrence is more common than in iodine-deficient Scotland.[197]

Death rates are now approaching the vanishing point.[198] Of the nonfatal complications, permanent hypoparathyroidism is the most serious, and requires lifelong medical supervision and treatment. Experienced surgeons have an incidence under 1 percent. Unfortunately, the general experience is near 3 percent. Davis et al.[199] observed that patients who had previously undergone subtotal thyroidectomy had an average serum calcium concentration below that of normal persons, and also developed hypocalcemia when deprived of calcium. Many had vague neuromuscular symptoms suggestive of hypoparathyroidism. Twenty-four percent of the patients in this report were presumed to have partial hypoparathyroidism and were improved by calcium therapy. This experience seems exceptional.

Unilateral vocal cord paralysis rarely causes more than some hoarseness and a weakened voice, but bilateral injury leads to permanent voice damage even after corrective surgery. Bilateral recurrent nerve injury may be associated with severe respiratory impairment when an acute inflammatory process supervenes and may be life-threatening. Fortunately, it is now extremely rare after subtotal thyroidectomy. Damage to the superior external laryngeal nerve during surgery (see Ch. 21) may alter the quality of the voice and the ability to shout without causing hoarseness. One may speculate whether declining skills in the techniques of subtotal thyroidectomy, attendant upon a dramatic fall in the use of this procedure, may lead to an increase in the hazards of the procedure.

Hypothyroidism, whether occurring after surgery or ^{131}I therapy, can be readily controlled. Transient hypothyroidism is common, with recovery in one to six months. Long-term studies indicate permanent hypothyroidism of 6 to 40 percent.[198,200] The presence of autoimmunity to thyroid antigens predisposes to the development of myxedema after subtotal thyroidectomy for thyrotoxicosis. A positive test for antibodies to the microsomal/TPO antigen was found by Buchanan et al.[201] to correlate with an increased incidence of postoperative hypothyroidism. The incidence of hypothyroidism is certainly of importance in weighing the virtues of ^{131}I and surgical therapy. The ability of surgical therapy to produce a euthyroid state in the majority of patients over long-term follow-up gives it one advantage over RAI therapy, but this must be weighed against the risk of hypoparathyroidism and recurrent nerve damage.

Course after Surgery

In the immediate postoperative period, patients should be followed closely. They should ideally have a special duty nurse during the first 24 hours, and a tracheotomy set and calcium chloride or gluconate for infusion should be at the bedside. During this period, undetected hemorrhage can lead to asphyxiation. Transient hypocalcemia is common, resulting from trauma to the parathyroid glands and their blood supply and also possibly to rapid uptake of calcium by the bones, which have been depleted of calcium by the thyrotoxicosis.[202] Oral or intravenous calcium supplementation suffices in most instances to control the symptoms. The calcium may be given slowly intravenously as calcium gluconate or calcium chloride in a dose ranging from 0.5 to 1.0 g every 4 to 8 hours, as indicated by clinical observation and determination of Ca^{2+}.

Some surgeons give their patients replacement thyroid hormone for an indefinite period after the operation in an attempt to avoid transient hypothyroidism and to remove any stimulus to regeneration of the gland. It is not obvious that this is either necessary or efficacious. In 80 to 85 percent of patients, the residual gland is able to form enough hormone to prevent even transient clinical hypothyroidism. Serum hormone levels should be determined every two to four months until it is clear that the patient does not need replacement.

Probably the thyroid remnant is not normal. It has a rapid ^{131}I turnover rate and a small pool of stored organic iodine. Suppressibility by T_3 administration returns within a few months of operation in some patients. TSAb tend to disappear from the blood in the ensuing 3 to 12 months.[203,205] After subtotal thyroidectomy, thyrotoxicosis recurs in 5 to 10 percent of patients, often many years after the original episode.

Long-Term Follow-Up

Finally, adequate follow-up must be carried out after any kind of treatment of Graves' disease. Recurrence is always possible, either early or late, and there is always the threat that the ophthalmopathic problems may worsen when all else in the progress of the patient seems favorable. A surprisingly large proportion of patients who have had subtotal thyroidectomy for Graves' disease and who are clinically euthyroid can be shown to have an abnormal TRH response (excessive or depressed), and up to a third have elevated serum TSH levels.[205,206] Some of them are undoubtedly mildly hypothyroid, whereas others are euthyroid but require the stimulation of TSH to maintain this state. A measurement of the serum

TSH level is a useful procedure for patients several months after surgery in guiding further management. Over subsequent years the residual thyroid fails in more patients, due either to reduced blood supply, fibrosis from trauma, or continuing autoimmune thyroiditis. After 10 years, and depending on the extent of the original surgery, 20 to 40 percent are hypothyroid. This continuing thyroid failure is also seen after antithyroid drug therapy with ^{131}I and represents the natural evolution of Graves' disease.

Special Considerations in the Treatment of Thyrotoxicosis in Children

Thyrotoxicosis may occur in any age group but is unusual in the first five years of life. The same remarkable preponderance of the disease in females over males is observed in children as in the adult population, and the signs and symptoms of the disease are similar in most respects. Behavioral symptoms frequently predominate in children and produce difficulty in school or problems in relationships within the family. Thyrotoxic children are tall for their age, probably as an effect of the disease. These children are restored to a normal height/age ratio after successful therapy for the thyrotoxicosis. Bone age is also often advanced.[207]

No more is known about the cause of the disease in children than in adults. Diagnosis rests upon eliciting a typical history and signs and upon the standard laboratory test results. Normal values for children are not the same as for adults during the first weeks of life, and these differences, as noted in Chapter 10, should be taken into account.

Therapy

In some clinics, RAI is used in the treatment of thyrotoxicosis in children. In one report, 73 children and adolescents were so treated. Hypothyroidism developed in 43. Subsequent growth and development were normal.[208] In another group of 23 treated with ^{131}I, there were 4 recurrences, at least 5 became hypothyroid, and one was found to have a papillary thyroid cancer 20 months after the second dose.[209] Safa et al.[40] reviewed 87 children treated over 24 years and found no adverse effects except the well-known occurrence of hypothyroidism. Hamburger has examined therapy in 262 children ages 3 to 18 and concludes ^{131}I therapy to be the best initial treatment.[42] Nevertheless, many physicians remain con-

cerned about the risks of carcinogenesis. This problem was more fully discussed earlier in this chapter. Others believe that the risks of surgery and problems with antithyroid drug administration outweigh the potential but so far unproven risk of ^{131}I therapy.

Although ^{131}I therapy is gaining acceptance, the most common choice for therapy is between antithyroid drugs and subtotal thyroidectomy. Proponents of antithyroid drug therapy believe that there is a greater tendency for remission of thyrotoxicosis in children compared to adults and that antithyroid drug therapy avoids the psychic and physical problems caused by surgery in this age group. With drugs the need for surgery (or ^{131}I) can be delayed almost indefinitely until conditions become favorable.

As arguments against surgery, one must consider the morbidity and possible, although rare, mortality. Surgery means a permanent scar, and the recurrence rate is much higher (up to 15 percent) than that observed in adults.[210] If the recurrence rate is kept acceptably low by performing near-total thyroidectomies, there is always an attendant rise in the incidence of permanent hypothyroidism (over 50 percent in some series), and greater potential for damage to the recurrent laryngeal nerves and parathyroid glands. Damage to the parathyroids necessitates a complicated medical program that may be permanent, and is one of the major reasons for opposing routine surgical therapy in this disease. Bacon and Lowrey[211] reported that, in a series of 33 children treated surgically, only one had hypothyroidism, one had permanent hypoparathyroidism, and one had permanent vocal cord paralysis. The low incidence of hypothyroidism in this series is remarkable, but we may note the significant incidence of other serious complications. Others have pointed out the high relapse rate with all forms of therapy in the pediatric age group.[209]

The main argument favoring surgery is that it may correct the thyrotoxicosis with surety and speed, and result in less disruption of normal life and development than is associated with long-term administration of antithyroid drugs and the attendant constant medical supervision. Often children are unable to maintain the careful dosage schedule needed for control of the disease.

Antithyroid drug therapy is the preferable initial therapy in children. Favorable indications for its use are mild thyrotoxicosis, a small goiter, recent onset of disease, and especially the presence of some obvious emotional problem that seems to be related to precipitation of the disease. Antithyroid drug administration necessitates much supervision by the physician and the parents, the permanent remission rate will be 50 percent or less,[210] and there is always the possibility of a reaction to the medication.

There is no consensus on secondary treatment. Some physicians favor surgery if the patient and parents seem incapable of following a regimen requiring frequent administration of medicine for a prolonged period or drug reactions occur. A factor that must be remembered in selecting the appropriate course of therapy is the experience of the available surgeon. Lack of experience contributes to a high rate of recurrence, permanent hypothyroidism, or permanent hypoparathyroidism. Other physicians believe the possible but unproven risks of ^{131}I are more than outweighed by the known risks of operation, and ^{131}I treatment is increasingly accepted for patients over age 15.

If antithyroid drugs are chosen as primary therapy, the patient is initially given a course of treatment for one or two years, according to the dosage schedule shown in Table 11-9. The dosage of PTU needed is usually 120 to 175 mg/m^2 body surface area daily divided into three equal doses every eight hours. Methimazole can be used in place of PTU; approximately one-tenth as much, in milligrams, is required. During therapy the dosage can usually be gradually reduced. Many patients will be satisfactorily controlled by once-a-day treatment.

The program is similar to that employed in adult thyrotoxicosis. It is sensible to see the child once each month, and at that time to make sure that the program is being followed and progress made. Any evidence of depression of the bone marrow should prompt a change to an alternative drug or a different form of treatment, as discussed below.

At the end of one or two years the medication is withdrawn. If thyrotoxicosis recurs, a second course of treatment lasting for one year or more may be given. A decrease in the size of the goiter during therapy is good evidence that a remission has been achieved. Progressive enlargement of the gland during therapy implies that hypothyroidism has been produced. This enlargement can be controlled by reduction in the dose of antithyroid drug or by administration of replacement thyroid hormone.

There is no adequate rule for deciding when medical therapy has failed. After courses of antithyroid

drug therapy totaling two to four years and attainment of age 15, if the patient still has not entered a permanent remission it is probably best to proceed with surgical or ^{131}I treatment.

Occasionally a drug reaction develops while the condition is being controlled with an antithyroid drug. A change to another thiocarbamide may be satisfactory, but patients should be followed carefully. If a reaction is seen again, or if severe neutropenia occurs, it is usually best to stop antithyroid drug therapy and (1) give potassium iodide and an agent such as propranolol and to proceed with surgery, or (2) to give [131]I. RAI therapy will be necessary if surgery is contraindicated by uncontrollable thyrotoxicosis, for whatever reason, or with prior thyroidectomy. If surgery is elected, the patient should be prepared with an antithyroid drug such as PTU in a dosage and duration sufficient to produce a euthyroid state, and then should be given iodide for seven days before surgery. Lugol's solution, or a saturated solution of potassium iodide, 1 or 2 drops twice daily, is sufficient to induce involution of the gland.

Intrauterine and Neonatal Thyrotoxicosis

Thyrotoxicosis in utero is a rare but recognized syndrome occurring in pregnant women with very high TSAb in serum, due to transplacental passage of antibodies, or can develop in the neonate. It is possible to screen for this risk by assaying TSAb in serum of pregnant women with known current or prior Graves' disease. Intra-uterine thyrotoxicosis causes fetal tachycardia, failure to grow, acceleration of bone age, premature closure of sutures, and occasionally fetal death. Multiple sequential pregnancies with this problem have been recorded. Clinical diagnosis is obviously inexact. Fetal blood sampling is feasible in appropriate cases. Antithyroid drugs can be given, but control of the dosage is uncertain.[212] One approach is to monitor heart rate, and possibly to follow fetal blood hormone levels. Plasmapheresis to reduce maternal TSAb has been recommended, but few facts are available. Thyrotoxicosis in pregnancy is discussed in Chapter 14.

Thyrotoxicosis is rare in the newborn infant and is usually associated with past or present maternal hyperthyroidism.[213] Neonatal hypermetabolism usually arises from transplacental passage of TSAb. Frequently the infant is not recognized as thyrotoxic at birth, but develops symptoms of restlessness, tachycardia, poor feeding, occasionally excessive hunger, excessive weight loss, and possibly fever and diarrhea a few days after birth. The fetus converts T_4 to T_3 poorly in utero, but switches to normal T_4 to T_3 deiodination at birth. This phenomenon may normally provide a measure of protection in utero that is lost at birth, allowing the development of thyrotoxicosis in a few days. The syndrome may persist for two to five weeks, until the effects of the maternal antibodies have disappeared. The patient may be treated with propranolol, antithyroid drugs given according to the schedule above, and iodide. The antithyroid drug can be given parenterally if necessary in saline solution after sterilization by filtration through a Millipore filter. Newborn infants with thyrotoxicosis are frequently extremely ill, and ancillary therapy, including sedation, cooling, fluids in large amounts, electrolyte replacement, and oxygen, are probably as important in management as specific therapy for the thyrotoxicosis. Propranolol is used to control the tachycardia. Because of the increased metabolism of such infants, attention to fluid balance and adequacy of nutrition are important.

The patient usually survives the thyrotoxicosis, and the disease is typically self-limiting, with the euthyroid state being established in one or two months. Antithyroid medication can be gradually withdrawn at this time.

Graves' disease can also occur in the newborn because the same disturbance that is causing the disorder in the mother is also occurring independently in the child. Hollingsworth et al.[214] have described their experience in such patients. The mothers did not necessarily have active disease during pregnancy. Graves' disease persisted in these patients from birth far beyond the time during which TSH-RSAb of maternal origin could persist. Advanced bone age was one feature of the disorder. Behavioral disturbances were later found in some of these children at a time when they were euthyroid.

General Therapeutic Relationship of the Patient and Physician

The foregoing discussion explains several methods for specifically decreasing thyroid hormone formation. They are, in a sense, both unphysiologic and traumatic to the patient. As a good physician realizes in any problem, but especially in Graves' disease, attention to the whole patient is mandatory.

During the initial and subsequent interviews, the physician caring for a patient with Graves' disease must determine the nature of any psychic and physical stresses. Frequently major emotional problems come to light after the patient recognizes the sincere interest of the physician. Typically the problem involves interpersonal relationships and often is one of matrimonial friction. The upset may be deep-seated and may involve difficult adjustments by the patient, but characteristically it is related to identifiable factors in the environment. In other words, the problem is not an endogenous emotional reaction but a difficult adjustment to real external problems. On the other hand, one must be aware that the emotional lability of the thyrotoxic patient may be a trial for those with whom he or she must live, as well as for the patient. Thus thyrotoxicosis itself may create interpersonal problems. From whatever cause they arise, these problems are dealt with insofar as possible by the wise physician.

We have been unimpressed by the benefits of formal psychiatric care for the average thyrotoxic patient, but are certain that sympathetic discussion by the physician, possibly together with assistance in environmental manipulation, is an important part of the general attack on Graves' disease. In other cases, personal problems may play a less important etiologic role but may still strongly affect therapy by interfering with rest or by causing economic hardship.

In addition to providing assistance in solving personal problems, two other general therapeutic measures are important. The first is rest. The patient with Graves' disease should have time away from normal duties to help in reestablishing his or her psychic and physiologic equilibria. Patients can and do recover with appropriate therapy while continuing to work, but more rapid and certain progress is made if a period away from the usual occupation can be provided. Often a mild sedative or tranquilizer is helpful.

Another important general measure is attention to nutrition. Patients with Graves' disease are nutritionally depleted in proportion to the duration and severity of their illness. Until metabolism is restored to normal, and for some time afterward, the caloric and protein requirements of the patient may be well above normal. Specific vitamin deficiencies may exist, and multivitamin supplementation is indicated. The intake of calcium should be above normal.

SUMMARY

This chapter has dealt with the diagnosis and treatment of Graves' disease. Diagnosis of the classic form is easy and depends on the recognition of the cardinal features of the disease and confirmation by such tests as TSH and FTI.

The differential diagnosis includes other types of thyrotoxicosis, such as that occurring in a nodular gland, accompanying certain tumors of the thyroid, or thyrotoxicosis factitia, and nontoxic goiter in a patient with symptoms that imitate those of thyrotoxicosis. Types of hypermetabolism not of thyroid origin must also enter the differential diagnosis. Examples are certain cases of pheochromocytoma, polycythemia, lymphoma, and the leukemias. Pulmonary disease, infection, parkinsonism, pregnancy, or nephritis may stimulate certain features of thyrotoxicosis.

Treatment of Graves' disease cannot yet be aimed at the cause because it is still unknown. One seeks to control thyrotoxicosis when that seems to be the major indication, or the ophthalmopathy when that aspect of the disease appears to be more urgent.

The available forms of treatment, including surgery, drugs, and ^{131}I therapy, are reviewed. There is a difference of opinion as to which of these modalities is best, but to a large degree guidelines governing choice of therapy can be drawn.

Antithyroid drugs are widely used for treatment on a long-term basis. About one-third of the patients undergoing long-term antithyroid therapy achieve permanent euthyroidism. Drugs are the preferred initial therapy in children and young adults.

Subtotal thyroidectomy is a satisfactory form of therapy, if an excellent surgeon is available, but is used infrequently by many thyroidologists. The combined use of antithyroid drugs and iodine makes it possible to prepare patients adequately before surgery, and operative mortality is approaching the vanishing point. Many young adults, especially males, are treated by surgery if antithyroid drug treatment fails.

Currently, most endocrinologists consider RAI to be the best treatment, and consider the associated hypothyroidism to be a minor problem. Evidence to date after well over four decades of experience indicates that the risk of late carcinogenesis must be near zero. The authors advise this therapy in most patients over age 40, and believe that it is not con-traindicated above the age of about 15. Dosage is calculated on the basis of ^{131}I uptake and gland size. Most patients are cured by one treatment. The principal side effect is the occurrence of hypothyroidism. This complication occurs with a fairly constant frequency for many years after therapy and may be an inevitable complication in many patients if cure of the disease is to be achieved; many therapists accept this as an anticipated outcome of treatment.

Thyrotoxicosis in children is best handled initially by antithyroid drug therapy. If this therapy does not result in a cure, surgery may be performed. Treatment with ^{131}I is increasingly accepted as an alternative form of treatment.

Neonatal thyrotoxicosis is a rarity and usually subsides with or without therapy. Iodide, antithyroid drugs, and propranolol are required for several weeks.

The physician applying any of these forms of therapy to the control of thyrotoxicosis should also pay heed to the patient's emotional needs, as well as to his or her requirements for rest, nutrition, and specific antithyroid medication.

REFERENCES

1. Wayne EJ: The diagnosis of thyrotoxicosis. Br Med J 1,1, 1954
2. Morley JE, Shafer RB, Elson MK et al: Amphetamine-induced hyperthyroxinemia. Ann Intern Med 93:707, 1980
3. Brown ME, Refetoff S: Transient elevation of serum thyroid Hormone concentration after initiation of replacement therapy in myxedema. Ann Intern Med 92:491, 1980
4. Kaptein EM, Macintyre SS, Weiner JM et al: Free thyroxine estimates in nonthyroidal illness: comparison of eight methods. J Clin Endocrinol Metab 52:1073, 1981
5. Engler D, Donaldson EB, Stockigt JR, Taft P: Hyperthyroidism without triiodothyronine excess: an effect of severe nonthyroidal illness. J Clin Endocrinol Metab 46:77, 1978
6. Mayfield RK, Sagel J, Colwell JA: Thyrotoxicosis without elevated serum triiodothyronine levels during diabetic ketoacidosis. Arch Inter Med 140:408, 1980
7. Sobrinho LG, Limbert ES, Santos MA: Thyroxine toxicosis in patient with iodine-induced thyrotoxicosis. J Clin Endocrinol Metab 45:25, 1977
8. Sterling K, Refetoff S, Selenkow HA: T$_3$ thyrotoxico-

sis due to elevated serum triiodothyronine levels. JAMA 213:571, 1970

9. Hollander CS, Nihei N, Burhay SZ et al: Clinical and laboratory observations in cases of triiodothyronine toxicosis confirmed by radioimmunoassay. Lancet 1: 609, 1972

10. Hollander CS, Mitsuma T, Shenkman L et al: T_3 toxicosis in an iodine-deficient area. Lancet 2:1276, 1972

11. Hollander CS, Mitsuma T, Kastin AJ et al: Hypertiiodothyroninemia as a premonitory manifestation of thyrotoxicosis. Lancet 2:731, 1971

12. Burrow GN: Thyroid dysfunction in the recently pregnant: postpartum thyroiditis. Thyroid 4:363, 1994

13. Ormston BJ, Alexander L, Evered DC et al: Thyrotropin response to thyrotropin-releasing hormone in ophthalmic Graves' disease; correlation with other aspects of thyroid function, thyroid suppressibility, and activity of eye signs. Clin Endocrinol 2:369, 1973

14 Franco PS, Hershman JM, Haigler ED, Pittman JA: Response to thyrotropin-releasing hormone compared with thyroid suppression tests in euthyroid Graves' disease. Metabolism 22:1357, 1973

15. Clifton-Bligh P, Silverstein GE, Burke G: Unresponsiveness to thyrotropin-releasing hormone (TRH) in treated Graves' hyperthyroidism and in euthyroid Graves' disease. J Clin Endocrinol Metab 38:531, 1974

16. Bolk JH, Bussemaker JK, Elte JWF et al: Thyroid stimulating immunoglobulins do not cause non-autonomous, autonomous, or toxic multinodular goiters. Lancet 2:61, 1979

17. Namba H, Ross JL, Goodman D, Fagin JA: Solitary polyclonal autonomous thyroid nodule: a rare cause of childhood hyperthyroidism. J Clin Endocrinol Metab 72:1108, 1991

18. Shimaoka K, Van Herle AJ, Dindogru A: Thyrotoxicosis secondary to involvement of the thyroid with malignant lymphoma. J Clin Endocrinol Metab 43: 64, 1976

19. Spanheimer RG, Bar RS, Hayford JC: Hyperthyroidism caused by inappropriate thyrotropin hypersecretion. Studies in patients with selective pituitary resistance to thyroid hormone. Arch Intern Med 142: 1283, 1982

20. Emerson CH, Utiger RD: Hyperthyroidism and excessive thyrotropin secretion. N Engl J Med 287:328, 1972

21. Gershengron ML: Thytropin-induced hyperthyroidism caused by selective pituitary resistance to thyroid hormone. A new syndrome of "inappropriate secretion of TSH." J Clin Invest 56:271, 1975

22. Woolf PD, Daly R: Thyrotoxicosis with painless thyroiditis. Am J Med 60:73, 1976

23. Gluck FB, Nusynowitz ML, Plymate S: Chronic lymphocytic thyroiditis, thyrotoxicosis, and low radioactive iodine uptake. N Engl J Med 293:624, 1975

24. Ginsberg J, Walfish PG: Post-partum transient thyrotoxicosis with painless thyroiditis. Lancet 1:1125, 1977

25. Amino N, Yabu Y, Miyai K et al: Differentiation of thyrotoxicosis induced by thyroid destruction from Graves' disease. Lancet 1:344, 1978

26. Inada M, Nishikawa M, Naito K et al: Reversible changes of the histological abnormalities of the thyroid in patients with painless thyroiditis. J Clin Endocrinol Metab 52:431, 1981

27. Yabu Y, Amino N, Mori H et al: Postpartum recurrence of hyperthyroidism and changes of thyroid-stimulating immunoglobulins in Graves' disease. J Clin Endocrinol Metab 51:1454 1980

28. Amino N, Miyai K, Azukizawa M et al: Differentiation of thyrotoxicosis induced by thyroid destruction from Graves' disease. Lancet 2:344, 1978

29. Shigemasa C, Ueta Y, Mitani Y et al: Chronic thyroiditis with painful tender thyroid enlargement and transient thyrotoxicosis. J Clin Endocrinol Metab 70: 385, 1990

30. Cave WT Jr, Dunn JT: Choriocarcinoma with hyperthyroidism: probable identity ot the thyrotropin with human chroionic gonadotropin. Ann Intern Med 85: 60, 1976

31. Nagataki S, Mizuno M, Sakamoto S et al: Thyroid function in molar pregnancy. J Clin Endocrinol Metab 44:254, 1977

32. Amir SM, Uchimura H, Ingbar SH: Interactions of bovine thyrotropin and preparations of human chorionic gonadotropin with bovine thyroid membranes. J Clin Endocrinol Metab 45:280, 1977

33. Miyai K, Tanizawa O, Yamamoto T et al: Pituitary-thyroid function in trophoblastic disease. J Clin Endocrinol Metab 42:254, 1976

34. Lahey FH: Apathetic thyroidism. Ann Surg 93:1026, 1931

35. Apathetic thyrotoxicosis. Editorial. Lancet 2:809, 1970

36. Philip JR, Harrison MT, Ridley EF, Crooks J: Treatment of thyrotoxicosis with ionizing radiation. Lancet 2:1307, 1968

37. Glinoer D, Hesch D, LaGasse R, Laurberg P: The management of hyperthyroidism due to Graves' disease in Europe in 1986. Results of an international survey. Presented at the 15th Annual Meeting of the European Thyroid Association; June–July, 1986; Stockholm.

38. Solomon B, Glinoer D, LaGasse R, Wartofsky L: Current trends in the management of Graves' disease. J Clin Endocrinol Metab 70:1518, 1990

39. Dobyns BM, Sheline GE, Workman JB et al: Malignant and benign neoplasms of the thyroid in patients treated for hyperthyroidism: a report of the Cooperative Thyrotoxicosis Therapy Follow-up Study. J Clin Endocrinol Metabl 37:976, 1974

40. Safa AM, Schumacher P, Rodriguez-Antunez A: Long-term follow-up results in children and adolescents treated with radioactive iodine (131-iodine). N Engl J Med 292:167, 1975

41. Holm LE, Dahlqvist I, Israelsson A, Lundell GM: Malignant thyroid tumors after 131-iodine therapy. N Engl J Med 303:188, 1980

42. Hamburger JI: Management of hyperthyroidism in children and adolescents. J Clin Endocrinol Metab 60:1019, 1985

43. Freitas JE, Swanson DP, Gross MD, Sisson JS: Iodine-131: optimal therapy for hyperthyroidism in children and adolescents? et al: Nucl Med 20:847, 1979

44. Hayek A, Chapman E, Crawford E, Crawford JD: Long-term results of treatment of thyrotoxicosis in children and adolescents with radioactive iodine. N Engl J Med 283:949, 1970

45. Chapman EM: History of the discovery of early use of radioactive iodine. J Amer Med Assn 250:2042, 1983

46. Chapman EM, Maloof F: The use of radioactive iodine in the diagnosis and treatment of hyperthyroidism: ten years' experience. Medicine 34:261, 1955

47. Blahd W, Hays MT: Graves' disease in the male. A review of 241 cases treated with an individual-calculated dose of sodium iodide [131]I. Arch Intern Med 129:33, 1972

48. Hagen F, Ouelette RP, Chapman EM: Comparison of high and low dosage levels of ^{131}I in the treatment of thyrotoxicosis. N Engl J Med 277:559, 1967

49. Cevallos JL, Hagen GA, Maloof F, Chapman EM: Low-dosage ^{131}I therapy of thyrotoxicosis (diffuse goiters). N Engl J Med 290:141, 1974

50. Ross DS, Daniels GH, De Stafano P et al: Use of adjunctive potassium iodide after radioactive iodine (^{131}I) treatment of Graves' hyperthyroidism. J Clin Endocrinol Metab 57:250, 1983

51. Reinwein D, Schaps D, Berger H et al: Hypothreoserisyiko nach franktionierter Radiojodtherapie. Dtsch Med Wochenschr 98:1789,1973

52. Rapoport B, Caplan R, DeGroot L: Low-dose sodium iodide ^{131}I therapy in Graves' disease. et al: JAMA 224:1610, 1973

53. Roudebush Cp, Hoye KE, De Groot LJ: Compensated low-dose ^{131}I therapy of Graves disease. Ann Intern med 87:441, 1977

54. Sridama V, McCormick M, Kaplan EL et al: Long-term follow-up study of compensated low-dose ^{131}I therapy for Graves' disease. N Engl J Med 311:426, 1984

55. Glennon JA, Gordon ES, Sawin CT: Hypothyroidism after low-dose I[131] treatment of hyperthyroidism. Ann Intern Med 76:721, 1972

56. Saito S, Sakurada Y, Yamamoto M et al: Long-term results of radioiodine ^{131}I therapy in 331 patient with Graves' disease. Tokyo J Exp Med 132:1 1980

57. DeGroot LJ, Mangklabruks A, McCormick M: Comparison of RA ^{131}I treatment protocols for Graves' disease. J Endocrinol Invest 13:111, 1990

58. Wise PH, Burnet RD, Ahmad A, Harding PE: Intentional radioiodine ablation in Graves' disease. Lancet 2:1231, 1975

59. Marcocci C, Gianchecchi D, Masini I et al: A reappraisal of the role of methimazole and other factors on the efficacy and outcome of radioiodine therapy of Graves' hyperthyroidism. J Endocrinol Invest 13: 513, 1990

60. Greig WR, Gillespie FC, Thomson JA, McGirr EM: Iodine-125 treatment for thyrotoxicosis. Lancet 1: 755, 1969

61. Radioiodine treatment of thyrotoxicosis. Editorial. Lancet 1:23, 1972

62. Bremmer WF, Greig WR, McDougall IR: Results of treating 297 thyrotoxic patients with [131]I. Lancet 2: 281, 1973

63. Benua RS, Dobyns BM; Isolated compounds in the serum, disappearance of radioactive iodine from the thyroid, and clinical response in patients treated with radioactive iodine. J Clin Endocrinol Metab 15:118, 1955

64. Stansbury JB, Janssen MA: The iodinated albumin-like component of the plasma of thyrotoxic patients. J Clin Endocrinol Metab 22:978, 1962

65. Goldsmith RE: Radioisotope therapy for Graves' disease. Mayo Clin Proc 47:953, 1972

66. Slingerland WD, Hershman JM, Dell E, Burrows B: Thyrotropin and PBI in radioiodine-treated hyperthyroid patients. J Clin Endocrinol Metab 35:912, 1972

67. Gordin A, Wagar G, Herberg CA: Serum thyrotropin and response to thyrotrophin-releasing hormone in patients who are euthyroid after radioiodine treatment for hyperthyroidism. Acta med Scand 194:335, 1973

68. Baldwin WW: Graves' disease succeeded by atrophy. Lancet 1:145, 1895

69. Wood LC, Ingbar SH: Hypothyroidism as a late sequela in patients with Graves' disease treated with antithyroid drugs. J Clin Invest 64:1429, 1979

70. Creutzig H, Kallfelz I, Haindl J et al: Thyroid storm and iodine-131 treatment. Lancet 2:145, 1976

71. Hayek A: Thyroid storm following radioiodine for thyrotoxicosis. J Pediatrics 93:978, 1978

72. Lamberg BA, Hernberg CA, Wahlberg P, Hakkila R:

Treatment of toxic nodular goiter with radioactive iodine. Acta Med Scand 165:245, 1959

73. McDermott MT, Kidd GS, Dodson LE Jr, Hofeldt FD: Radioiodine-induced thyroid storm. Case report and literature review. Amer J Med 75:353, 1983

74. Townsend JD: Hypoparathyroidism following radioactive iodine therapy for intractable angina pectoris. Ann Intern Med 55:662, 1961

75. Gilbert-Dreyfus MZ, GAli P: Cataract due to tetany following radioactive iodine therapy. Sem Hop Paris 34:1301, 1958

76. Fulop M: Hypoparathyroidism after ^{131}I therapy. Ann Intern Med 75:808, 1971

77. Fenzi G, Hashizume K, Roudebush C, DeGroot LJ: Changes in thyroid-stimulating immunoglobulins during antithyroid therapy. J Clin Endocrinol Metab 48:572, 1979

78. Teng CS, Yeung RTT, Khoo RKK, Alagaratnam TT: A prospective study of the changes in thyrotropin-binding inhibitory immunoglobulins in Graves' disease treated by subtotal thyroidectomy of radioactive iodine. J Clin Endocrinol Metab 50:1005, 1980

79. Sridama V, DeGroot LJ: Treatment of Graves' disease and the course of ophthalmopathy. Amer J Med 87:70, 1989

80. Tallstedt L, Lundell G, Torring O et al: Occurrence of ophthalmopathy after treatment for Graves' disease. N Engl J Med 326:1733, 1992

81. Gamstedt A, Wadman B, Karlsson A: methimazole, but not betamethasone, prevents ^{131}I treatment-induced rises in thyrotropin receptor autoantibodies in hyperthyroid Graves' disease. J Clin Endocrinol Metab 62:773, 1986

82. Bartalena L, Marcocci C, Bogazzi F et al: Use of corticosteroids to prevent progression of Graves' ophthalmopathy after radioiodine therapy for hyperthyroidism N Engl J med 321:1349, 1989

83. DeGroot LJ, Paloyan E: Thyroid carcinoma and radiation. A Chicago endemic. J Amer Med Assn 225:487, 1973

84. Clark DW: Association of irradiation with cancer of the thyroid in children and adolescents. JAMA 159:1007, 1955

85. Simpson CL, Hempelmann LH, Fuller LM: Neoplasia in children treated with x-rays in infancy for thymic enlargement. Radiology 64:840, 1955

86. Doniach I: The effect of radioactive iodine alone and in combination with methylthiouracil upon tumor production in the rat's thyroid gland. Br J Cancer 7:181, 1953

87. Sampson RJ, Key CR, Buncher CR, Iijuma S: Thyroid carcinoma in Hiroshima and Nagasaki. JAMA 209:65, 1969

88. Conard RA, Dobyns BM, Sutow W: Thyroid neopla-

sia as late effect of exposure to radioactive iodine in fallout. JAMA 214:316, 1970

89. Saenger EL, Seltzer RA, Sterling TD, Kereiakes JG: Carcinogenic effects of the ^{131}I compared with x-irradiation. A review. Health Phys 9:1371, 1963

90. Pochin EE: Leukemia following radioiodine treatment of thyrotoxicosis. Br Med J 2:1545, 1960

91. Saenger EL, Thoma GE, Tompkins EA: Incidence of leukemia following treatment of hyperthyroidism. JAMA 205:855, 1968

92. Advisory Committee on the Biologic Effects of Ionizing Radiation, National Research Council. Biologic effects of ionizing radiation, v: The health effects of exposure to low levels of ionizing radiation. National Academic Press, Washington, DC, 1990

93. Russell WL, Kelly EM: Mutation frequencies in male mice and the estimation of genetic hazards of radiation in men. Proc Natl Acad Sci USA 79:542, 1982

94. Webster EW, Merrill OE; Radiation hazards: II. Measurements of gonadal dose in radiographic examination. N Engl J Med 257:811, 1957

95. Robertson J, Gorman CA: Gonadal radiation dose and its genetic significance in radioiodine therapy of hyperthyroidism. J Nucl med 17:826, 1976

96. Sarkar SD, Bierwaltes WH, Gill SP, Cowley BJ: Subsequent fertility and birth histories of children and adolescents treated with ^{131}I for thyroid cancer. J Nucl Med 17:460, 1976

97. Hollingsworth JW: Delayed radiation effects in survivors of the atomic bombings: a summary of the findings of the Atomic Bomb Casualty Commission, 1947–1959. N Engl J Med 263:481, 1960

99. MacKenzie CG, Mackenzie JB: Effect of sulfonamides and thiourea on the thyroid gland and basal metabolism. Endocrinology 32:185, 1943

100. Astwood EB: Treatment of hyperthyroidism with thiourea and thiouracil. JAMA 122 , 1943

101. Marcocci C, Chiovato L, Mariotti S, Pinchera A: Changes of circulating thyroid autoantibody levels during and after therapy with methimazole in patients with Graves' disease. J Endocrinol Invest 5:13, 1982

102. Pinchera A, Liberti P, Martino E et al: Effects of antithyroid therapy on the long-acting thyroid stimulator and the antithyroglobulin antibodies. J Clin Endocrinol Metab 29:231, 1969

103. MacGregor AM, Ibbertson HK, Smith BR, Hall R: Carbimazole and autoantibody synthesis in Hashimoto's thyroiditis. Br J Med 281:968, 1980

104. McGregor AM, Petersen MM, McLachlan SM et al: Carbimazole and the autoimmune response in Graves' disease. N Engl J Med 303:302, 1980

105. Hallengren B, Forsgren A, Melander A: Effects of antithyroid drugs on lymphocyte function in vitro. J Clin Endocrinol Metab 51:298, 1980

106. Ludgate ME, McGregor AM, Weetman AP et al: Analysis of T cell subsets in Graves' disease: alterations associated with carbimazole. Br Med J 288:526, 1984

107. Totterman TH, Karlsson FA, Bengtsson M, Mendel-Hartvig IB: Induction of circulating activated suppressor-like T cells by methimazole therapy for Graves' disease. N Engl J Med 316:15, 1987

108. Sridama V, Pacini F, DeGroot LJ: Decreased suppressor T lymphocytes in autoimmune thyroid diseases detected by monoclonal antibodies. J Clin Endocrinol Metab 54:316, 1982

109. Volpe R: Evidence that the immunosuppressive effects of antithyroid drugs are mediated through actions on the thyroid cell, modulating thyrocyte-immunocyte signaling: a review. Thyroid 4:217, 1994

110. Laurberg P, Hansen PEB, Iversen E et al: Goiter size and outcome of medical treatment of Graves' disease. Acta Endocrinol 111:39, 1986

111. Shizume K, Irie M, Nagataki S et al: Long-term result of antithyroid drug therapy for Graves' disease: follow-up after more than 5 years. Endocrinol Jpn 17:327, 1970

112. Shizume K: Long-term antithyroid drug therapy for intractable cases of Graves' disease. Endocrinol Jpn 25:377, 1978

113. Wartofsky L: Low remission after therapy for Graves' disease. Possible relation of dietary iodine with antithyroid therapy results. JAMA 226:1083, 1973

114. Hedley AJ, Young RE, Jones SJ et al: Antithyroid drugs in the treatment of hyperthyroidism of Graves' disease: long-term follow-up of 434 patients. Clin Endocrinol 31:209, 1989

115. Alexander WD, Harden RM, Koutras DA, Wayne E: Influence of iodine intake after treatment with antithyroid drugs. Lancet 2:866, 1965

116. McMurray JF Jr, Gilliland PF, Ratliff CR, Bourland PD: Pharmacodynamics of propylthiouracil in normal and hyperthyroid subjects after a single oral dose. J Clin Endocrinol Metab 41:362, 1975

117. Cooper DS: Which antithyroid drug? Amer J Med 80:1165, 1986

118. Cooper DS, Goldminz D, Levin AA et al: Agranulocytosis associated with antithyroid drugs. Ann Int Med 98:26, 1983

119. Barnes V, Bledsoe T: A simple test for selecting the thioamide schedule in thyrotoxicosis. J Clin Endocrinol Metab 35:250, 1972

120. Cooper DS, Saxe VC, Meskell M et al: Acute effects of propylthiouracil (PTU) on thyroidal iodide organification and peripheral iodothyronine deiodination: correlation with serum PTU levels measured by radioimmunoassay. J Clin Endocrinol Metab 54:101, 1982

121. Nabil N, Miner DJ, Amatruda JM: Methimazole: an alternative route of administration. J Clin Endocrinol Metab 54:180, 1982

122. Greer MA, Meihoff WC, Studer H: Treatment of hyperthyroidism with a single daily dose of propylthiouracil. N Engl J Med 272:887, 1965

123. Greer MA, Kammer H, Bouma DJ: Short-term antithyroid drug therapy for the thyrotoxicosis of Graves' disease. N Engl J Med 297:173, 1977

124. Allannic H, Fauchet R, Orgiazzi J et al: Antithyroid drugs and Graves' disease: a prospective randomized evaluation of the efficacy of treatment duration. J Clin Endocrinol Metab 70:675, 1990

125. Romaldini JH, Bromberg N, Werner RS et al: Comparison of high and low dosage regimens of antithyroid drugs. J Clin Endocrinol Metab 57:563, 1983

126. Yamamoto M, Totsuka Y, Kojima I et al: Outcome of patients with Graves' disease after long-term medical treatment guided by triiodothyronine (T_3) suppression test. Clin Endocrinol 19:467, 1983

127. Solomon DH, Beck JC, Vanderlaan WP, Astwood EB: Prognosis of hyperthyroidism treated by antithyroid drugs. JAMA 152:201, 1953

128. McLarty DG, Alexander WD, McHarden R, Robertson JWK: Self-limiting episodes of recurrent thyrotoxicosis. Lancet 1:6, 1971

129. Thalassinos NC, Fraser TR: Effect of potassium iodide on relapse rate of thyrotoxicosis treated with antithyroid drugs. Lancet 2:183, 1971

130. Hashizume K, Ichikawa K, Sakurai A et al: Administration of thyroxine in treated Graves' disease. Effects on the level of antibodies to thyroid-stimulating hormone receptors and on the risk of recurrence of hyperthyroidism. N Engl J Med 324:947, 1991

131. Hashizume K, Ichikawa K, Nishii Y et al: Effect of administration of thyroxine on the risk of postpartum recurrence of hyperthyroid Graves' disease. J Clin Endocrinol Metab 75:6, 1992

132. Zakarija M, McKenzie JM, Banovac K: Clinical significance of assay of thyroid-stimulating antibody in Graves' disease. Ann Intern Med 93:28, 1980

133. Werner RS, Romaldini JH, Farah CS et al: Serum thyroid-stimulating antibody, thyroglobulin levels, and thyroid suppressibility measurement as predictors of the outcome of combined methimazole and triiodothyronine therapy in Graves' disease. Thyroid 1:293, 1991

134. Allannic H, Fauchet R, Lorcy Y et al: A prospective study of the relationship between relapse of hyperthyroid Graves' disease after antithyroid drugs and HLA haplotype. J Clin Endocrinol Metab 57:719, 1983

135. Farid NR (ed): HLA in Endocrine and Metabolic Disorders. p. 357. Academic Press, New York, 1981

136. Schleusener H, Schwander J, Fischer C et al: Prospective multicenter study on the prediction of relapse after antithyroid drug treatment in patients with Graves' disease. Acta Endocrinologica (Copenh) 120:689, 1989

137. Irvine WJ, Gray RS, Toft AD et al: Spectrum of thyroid function in patients remaining in remission after antithyroid drug therapy for thyrotoxicosis. Lancet 1:179, 1977

138. Buerklin EM, Schimmel M, Utiger RD: Pituitary-thyroid regulation in euthyroid patients with Graves' disease previously treated with antithyroid drugs. J Clin Endocrinol Metab 43:419, 1976

139. Lamberg BA, Salmi J, Wagar G, Makinen T: Spontaneous hypothyroidism after antithyroid treatment of hyperthyroid Graves' disease. J Endocrinol Invest 4:399, 1981

140. Hirota Y, Tamai H, Hayashi Y et al: Thyroid function and histology in forty-five patients with hyperthyroid Graves' disease in clinical remission more than ten years after thionamide drug treatment. J Clin Endocrinol Metab 62:165, 1986

141. Kampmann JP, Johansen K, Hansen JM, Helwig J: Propylthiouracil in human milk: revision of a dogma. Lancet 1:736, 1980

142. Wiberg JJ, Nuttall FQ: Methimazole toxicity from high doses. Ann Intern Med 77:414, 1972

143. Chevalley J, McGavack TH, Kenigsberg S, Pearson S: A four-year study of the treatment of hyperthyroidism with methimazole. J Clin Endocrinol Metab 14:948, 1954

144. Tajiri J, Noguchi S, Murakami T, Murakami N: Antithyroid drug-induced agranulocytosis. The usefulness of routine white blood cell count monitoring. Arch Intern Med 150:621, 1990

145. Tamai H, Takaichi Y, Morita T et al: Methimazole-induced agranulocytosis in Japanese patients with Graves' disease. Clin Endocrinol 30:525, 1989

146. Amrhein JA, Kenny F, Ross D: Granulocytopenia, lupus-like syndrome, and other complications of propylthiouracil therapy. J Pediatr 76:54, 1970

147. Pacini F, Sridama V, Refetoff S: Multiple complications of propylthiouracil treatment: granulocytopenia, eosinophilia, skin reaction, and hepatitis with lymphocyte sensitization. J Endocrinol Invest 5:403, 1982

148. Wall JR, Fang SL, Kuroki T et al: In vitro immunoreactivity to propylthiouracil, methimazole, and carbimazole in patients with Graves' disease: a possible cause of antithyroid drug-induced agranulocytosis. J Clin Endocrinol Metab 58:868, 1984

149. Biswas N, Ahn Y-H, Goldman JM, Schwartz JM: Case report: aplastic anemia associated with antithyroid drugs. Am J Med Sci 301:190, 1991

150. Cooper DS: Antithyroid drugs. N Engl J Med 311:1353, 1984

151. Weiss M, Hassin D, Bank H: Propylthiouracil-induced hepatic damage. Arch Intern Med 140:1184, 1980

152. Miyazono K, Okazaki T, Uchida S et al: Propylthiouracil-induced diffuse interstitial pneumonitis. Arch Intern Med 144:1764, 1984

153. Tamai H, Mukuta T, Matsubayashi S et al: Treatment of methimazole-induced agranulocytosis using recombinant human granulocyte colony-stimulating factor (rhG-CSF). J Clin Endocrinol Metab 77:1356, 1993

154. Godley AF, Stanbury JB: Preliminary experience in the treatment of hyperthyroidism with potassium perchlorate. J Clin Endocrinol Metab 14:70, 1954

155. Krevans JR, Asper SP Jr, Rienhoff WF Jr: Fatal aplastic anemia following use of potassium perchlorate in thyrotoxicosis. JAMA 181:162, 1962

156. Georges JL, Normand JP, Lenormand ME, Schwob J: Life-threatening thyrotoxicosis induced by amiodarone in patients with benign heart disease. Eur Heart J 13:129, 1992

157. Lazarus JH, Addison GM, Richards AR, Owen GM: Treatment of thyrotoxicosis with lithium carbonate. Lancet 2:1160, 1974

158. Turner JG, Brownlie BEW, Rogers TGH: Lithium as an adjunct to radioiodine therapy for thyrotoxicosis. Lancet 1:614, 1976

159. Reinwein D, Klein E: Der Einfluss des anorganischen Blutjodes auf den Jodumstaz der menschlichen Schilddruse. Acta Endocrinol 35:485, 1960

160. Thompson WO, Thorp EG, Thompson PK, Cohen AC: The range of effective iodine dosage in exophthalmic goiter. II. The effect on basal metabolism of the daily administration of one-half drop of compound solution of iodine. Arch Intern Med 45:420, 1930

161. Friend DG: Iodide therapy and the importance of quantitating the dose. N Engl J Med 263:1358, 1960

162. Lerman J: Iodine response and other factors in their relation to mortality in thyrotoxicosis. N Engl J Med 217:1041, 1937

163. Nofal MM, Beierwaltes WH, Patno ME: Treatment of hyperthyroidism with sodium iodide [131]I. JAMA 197:605, 1966

164. Emerson CH, Anderson AJ, Howard WJ, Utiger RD: Serum thyroxine and triiodothyronine concentrations during iodide treatment of hyperthyroidism. J Clin Endocrinol Metab 40:33, 1975

165. Shanks RG, Hadden DR, Lowe DC et al: Controlled trial of propranolol in thyrotoxicosis. Lancet 2:1969

166. Mazzaferri EL, Reynolds JC, Young RL et al: Propranolol as primary therapy for thyrotoxicosis. Arch Intern Med 136:50, 1976

167. Wiener L, Stout BD, Cox JW: Influence of β-sympathetic blockade with propranolol on the hemodynamics of hyperthyroidism. Am J Med 46:227, 1969

168. Saunders J, Hall SEH, Crowther A, Sonksen PH: The effect of propranolol on thyroid hormones and oxygen consumption in thyrotoxicosis. Clin Endocrinol 9:67, 1978

169. Hadden DR, Montgomery DAD, Shanks RG, Weaver JA: Propranolol and iodine-131 in the management of thyrotoxicosis. Lancet 2:852, 1968

170. Pimstone N, Marine N, Pimstone B: Beta-adrenergic blockade in thyrotoxic myopathy. Lancet 2:1219, 1968

171. Smith CS, Howard NJ: Propranolol in treatment of neonatal thyrotoxicosis. J Pediatr 83:1046, 1973

172. Rosenberg I: Thyroid storm. N Engl J Med 283:1052, 1970

173. Bewsher PD, Pegg CAS, Steward DJ et al: Propranolol in the surgical management of thyrotoxicosis. Ann Surg 180:787, 1974

174. Moncke C: Treatment of thyrotoxicosis with reserpine. Med Monatsschr Pharm 50:1742, 1955

175. Lee WY, Bronsky D, Waldenstein SS: Studies of the thyroid and sympathetic nervous system interrelationships: effect of guanethidine on manifestations of hyperthyroidism. J Clin Endocrinol Metab 22:879, 1962

176. DeGroot LJ, Hoye K: Dexamethasone suppression of serum T_3 and T_4. J Clin Endocrinol Metab 4:976, 1976

177. Williams DE, Chopra IJ, Orgiazzi J, Solomon DH: Acute effects of corticosteroids on thyroid activity in Graves' disease. J Clin Endocrinol Metab 41:354, 1975

178. Witztum JL, Jacobs LS, Schonfeld G: Thyroid hormone and thyrotropin levels in patients placed on colestipol hydrochloride. J Clin Endocrinol Metab 46:838, 1978

179. Boehm TM, Burman KD, Barnes S, Wartofsky L: Lithium and iodine combination therapy for thyrotoxicosis. Acta Endocrinol 94:174, 1980

180. Sharp B, Reed AW, Tamagna EI et al: Treatment of hyperthyroidism with sodium ipodate (oragraffin) in addition to propylthiouracil and propranolol. J Clin Endocrinol Metab 53:622, 1981

181. Croxson MS, Hall TD, Nicoloff JT: Combination drug therapy for treatment of hyperthyroid Graves' disease. J Clin Endocrinol Metab 45:623, 1977

182. Werner SC, Platman SR: Remission of hyperthyroidism (Graves' disease) and altered pattern of serum-thyroxine binding induced by prednisone. Lancet 2:752, 1965

183. Wu S-Y-, Shyh T-P, Chopra IJ et al: Comparison of sodium ipodate (Oragrafin) and propylthiouracil in early treatment of hyperthyroidism. J Clin Endocrinol Metab 54:630, 1982

184. Shen D-C, Wu S-Y, Chopra IJ et al: Long-term treatment of Graves' hyperthyroidism with sodium ipodate. J Clin Endocrinol Metab 61:723, 1985

185. Arnold MB, Talbot NB, Cope O: Concerning the choice of therapy for childhood hyperthyroidism. Pediatrics 21:47, 1958

186. Feek CM, Stewart J, Sawers A et al: Combination of potassium iodide and propranolol in preparation of patients with Graves' disease for thyroid surgery. N Engl J Med 302:883, 1980

187. Bewsher BD, Pegg CAS, Stewart DJ et al: Propranolol in the surgical management of thyrotoxicosis. Ann Surg 180:787, 1974

188. Toft AD, Irvine WJ, Campbell RWF: Assessment by continuous cardiac monitoring of minimum duration of preoperative propranolol treatment in thyrotoxic patients. Clin Endocrinol 5:195, 1976

189. Toft AD, Irvine WJ, Sinclair I et al: Thyroid function after surgical treatment of thyrotoxicosis. N Engl J Med 298:643, 1978

190. Taylor GW, Painter NS: Size of the thyroid remnant in partial thyroidectomy for toxic goiter. Lancet 1:287, 1962

191. Sugino K, Mimura T, Toshima K et al: Follow-up evaluation of patients with Graves' disease treated by subtotal thyroidectomy and risk factor analysis for postoperative thyroid dysfunction. J Endocrinol Invest 16:195, 1993

192. Colcock BP, King ML: The mortality and morbidity of thyroid surgery. Surg Gynecol Obstet 114:131, 1962

193. Sawyers JL, Martin CE, Byrd BF Jr, Rosenfield L: Thyroidectomy for hyperthyroidism. Ann Surg 175:939, 1972

194. Farnell MB, van Heerden JA, McConahey WM et al: Hypothyroidism after thyroidectomy for Graves' disease. Amer J Surg 142:535, 1981

195. Klementschitsch P, Shen K-L, Kaplan EL: Reemergence of thyroidectomy as treatment for Graves' disease. Surg Clin North Am 59:35, 1979

196. Winsa B, Rastad J, Akerstrom G et al: Retrospective evaluation of the effect of subtotal and total thyroidectomy in the treatment of Graves' disease with and without endocrine ophthalmopathy (thesis). The University of Upsala, Upsala, Sweden, 1993

197. Thjodleifsson B, Hedley AJ, Donald D et al: Outcome of subtotal thyroidectomy for thyrotoxicosis in Iceland and Northeast Scotland. Clin Endocrinol 7:367, 1977

198. Beahrs OH, Sakulsky SB: Surgical thyroidectomy in the management of exophthalmic goiter. Arch Surg 96:511, 1968

199. Davis RH, Fourman P, Smith JWG: Prevalence of parathyroid insufficiency after thyroidectomy. Lancet 2:1432, 1961

200. Green M, Wilson GM: Thyrotoxicosis treated by surgery or iodine-131. With special reference to development of hypothyroidism. Br Med J 1:1005, 1964

201. Buchanan WW, Koutras DA, Crooks J et al: The clinical significance of the complement-fixation test in thyrotoxicosis. J Endocrinol 24:115, 1962

202. Michie W, Duncan T, Hamer-Hodges DW et al: Mechanism of hypocalcemia after thyroidectomy for thyrotoxicosis. Lancet 1:508, 1971

203. Hardisty CA, Talbot CH, Munro DS: The effect of partial thyroidectomy for Graves' disease on serum long-acting thyroid stimulator protector (LATS-P). Clin Endocrinol 14:181, 1981

204. Bech K, Feldt-Rasmussen U, Bliddal H et al: The acute changes in thyroid-stimulating immunoglobulins, thyroglobulin, and thyroglobulin antibodies following subtotal thyroidectomy. Clin Endocrinol 16:235, 1982

205. Fukino O, Tamai H, Fujii S et al: A study of thyroid function after subtotal thyroidectomy for Graves' disease: particularly on TRH tests, T_3 suppression tests, and antithyroid antibodies in euthyroid patients. Acta Endocrinol 103:28, 1983

206. Hedley AJ, Hall R, Amos J et al: Serum-thyrotropin levels after subtotal thyroidectomy for Graves' disease. Lancet 1:455, 1971

207. Hung W, Wilkins L, Blizzard R: Medical therapy of thyrotoxicosis in children. Pediatrics 30:17, 1962

208. Starr P, Jaffe HL, Oettinger L Jr: Late results of ^{131}I treatment of hyperthyroidism in seventy-three children and adosescents. J Nucl Med 5:81, 1964

209. Kogut MD, Kaplan SA, Collipp PJ et al: Treatment of hyperthyroidism in children. N Engl J Med 272:217, 1965

210. Hayles AB, Kennedy RLJ, Beahrs OH, Woolner LB: Exophthalmic goiter in children. J Clin Endocrinol Metab 19:138, 1959

211. Bacon GE, Lowrey GH: Experience with surgical treatment of thyrotoxicosis in children. J Pediatr 67:1, 1965

212. Cheek JH, Rezvani I, Goodner D, Hopper B: Prenatal treatment of thyrotoxicosis to prevent intrauterine growth retardation. Obstet Gynecol 60:122, 1982

213. Jarett SN, Seniour B, Braudo JL, Heymann S: Neonatal thyrotoxicosis. Pediatrics 24:65, 1959

214. Hollingsworth DR, Mabry CC, Eckerd JM: Hereditary aspects of Graves' disease in infancy and childhood. J Pediatr 81:446, 1972

Complications of Graves' Disease

12

THYROID STORM

Thyroid storm is a sudden, life-threatening exacerbation of thyrotoxicosis. In its simplest form, the manifestations are due solely to the actions of excess thyroid hormone. In recent years, this form of thyroid storm has become rare, largely because of earlier diagnoses, better pre- and postoperative medical management, and, possibly, improved nutrition. Acute exacerbations of the symptoms of thyrotoxicosis induced by intercurrent illness, especially infection, are still, however, seen occasionally. Whether or not these episodes should be considered examples of thyroid storm is a question of semantics, but they are indeed life-threatening, and constitute a major therapeutic challenge. In the past, thyroid storm most frequently followed surgery, but today it is usually a complication of an untreated or poorly treated disease.

Clinical Pattern

The classic findings in thyroid storm suggest a sudden and severe exacerbation of hyperthyroidism. There is fever, rapid tachycardia, tremor, nausea

and vomiting, diarrhea, dehydration, and delirium or coma. Fever is perhaps the most characteristic feature; the temperature may rise above 105.8°F (41°C). Occasionally, patients have a true toxic psychosis or a marked deterioration in previously abnormal behavior. Sometimes thyroid crisis takes a strikingly different form, known as *apathetic storm*. This condition is characterized by extreme weakness, emotional apathy, and, sometimes, confusion. The wild delirium and agitation of the classic victim of thyroid storm are missing, and fever, if present, does not rise so high.

Signs and symptoms of decompensation in various organ systems may be present. Delirium is one example. Congestive heart failure may occur, with edema, congestive hepatomegaly, and respiratory distress. Extreme tachycardia or atrial fibrillation is common. Liver damage and jaundice may occur from congestive heart failure or possibly from a direct action of thyroid hormone on the liver coupled with malnutrition (Ch. 10). Fever and vomiting may produce dehydration and prerenal azotemia. Abdominal pain may be a prominent feature. The temperature may

459

rise alarmingly, perhaps because the usual thermal controls have broken down in a manner similar to that occurring in heat stroke. Frequently the clinical picture is clouded by a secondary infection such as pneumonia, a viral infection, or infection of the upper respiratory tract. Death may be caused by cardiac arrythmia, congestive heart failure, hyperthermia, or other unidentified factors.

Storm is typically associated with Graves' disease, but it has also been reported in patients with toxic nodular goiter.[1] In the past, death was the final outcome of storm with awesome regularity.[2] In an unusually large series reported in 1969, three-fourths of the patients with thyroid storm died.[3] These patients typically were nutritionally depleted, had severe thyrotoxicosis, and had coincident serious disease, such as cardiac decompensation. In other series the mortality has been 30 to 75 percent.[1,4] Unfortunately, death from untreated, extremely severe thyrotoxicosis still occurs; we know of two such cases occurring in Chicago within the past decade.

Incidence

In Nelson and Becker's series, reported in 1969,[3] there were 21 cases of storm among 2,329 thyrotoxic admissions. Reports from other clinics, which included all cases manifesting febrile reactions of 38.3°C or more in the postoperative period, set the incidence of storm as high as 10 percent of patients operated on.[4] Few patients are now seen who fit the classic pattern of storm, but patients are occasionally encountered with marked accentuation of the symptoms of thyrotoxicosis in conjunction with infection. Most reports in the published studies of recent years have been accounts of single cases. At present, the incidence of thyroid storm is very low.

Cause

Classically, thyroid storm would begin a few hours after a thyroidectomy had been performed on a patient who was prepared for surgery by potassium iodide alone. Many such patients were not euthyroid and would not be considered appropriately prepared for surgery by today's standards. Exacerbations of thyrotoxicosis are still seen in patients taken too soon to surgery but are unusual in the antithyroid drug-controlled patient. Thyroid storm occasionally occurs in patients operated on for some other illness while severely thyrotoxic. Severe exacerbations of thyrotoxicosis are seen rarely following ^{131}I therapy; some of these may merit the term *storm.*[5]

As reported by Nelson and Becker,[3] thyroid storm appears most commonly following infection, which seems to induce a diastrous escape from control of the thyrotoxicosis. Pneumonia, upper respiratory tract infection, enteric infections, or any other infection can produce an acute exacerbation of the symptoms of thyrotoxicosis. The pathophysiology is incompletely understood.[6] A finding of possible significance is an elevated free T_4 in patients with thyroid storm while total T_4 levels were similar as compared with patients with uncomplicated thyrotoxicosis.[7] These data suggest that precipitated events like infection may decrease serum binding of T_4 resulting in increase in free T_4 that may play a role in the precipitation of the storm.

The decreased incidence of thyroid storm can be largely attributed to the improved methods of diagnosis and therapy available today. In most cases, thyrotoxicosis is recognized before extreme debilitation occurs and is treated by measures of predictable therapeutic value. Patients are routinely made euthyroid before surgery. Under present-day therapy, using thiocarbamides, the glands have only minimal amounts of stored hormone, in contrast to the iodized gland surgeons faced three decades ago. Postoperative storm, once the most frequent kind of storm, has now been virtually eliminated.

Diagnosis

The diagnosis of thyroid storm is made entirely on clinical grounds and involves the usual diagnostic measures for thyrotoxicosis. There are no distinctive laboratory abnormalities. Total and free T_4 and, if possible, total T_3 should be measured. T_3 may rarely be normal because of coexisting nonthyroidal illness.[8] Electrolytes, blood urea nitrogen (BUN), blood sugar, liver function tests, and plasma cortisol should be monitored. The diagnosis of thyroid storm is incomplete until a search for the cause of the crisis, especially infection, has been made.

Therapy

A thyroid storm is a major medical emergency. Continuous attention is required, and optimal nursing care is of central importance (Table 12-1).

If there is any possibility that drugs given orally

TABLE 12-1. Treatment of Thyroid Storm

Supportive
    Rest
    Mild sedation
    Fluid and electrolyte replacement
    Nutritional support and vitamins as needed
    Oxygen therapy
Nonspecific therapy as indicated
    Antibiotics
    Digitalization
    Cooling
Specific therapy
    Propranolol (20 to 200 mg orally every 6 hours, or 1
       to 3 mg intravenously every 4 to 6 hours)
    Antithyroid drugs (150 to 300 mg PTU every 6 hours)
    potassium iodide (after first dose antithyroid drugs)
       (2 drops of SSKI every 6 hours or 0.1 g
    potassium iodide every 12 hours)
    Dexamethasone (2 mg every 6 hours)
Possibly useful therapy
    Ipodate (Oragrafin) or iopanoic acid (Telepaque)
    Plasmapheresis or exchange
    Oral T_4 and T_3 binding resins
    Dialysis

will not be appropriately resorbed, e.g., due to stomach distention, vomiting, diarrhea, or severe heart failure, they should be administered intravenously. An antithyroid drug should be given if the patient has not been under prior treatment. PTU, 150 to 300 mg every 6 hours, should be given, if possible, in preference to methimazole, since PTU prevents peripheral conversion of T_4 to T_3. Since peripheral formation of T_3 is a major source of the hormone, PTU more rapidly reduces the circulating level of T_3 and thus aids recovery. Methimazole (15 to 30 mg every 6 hours) can be given orally or, if necessary, the pure compound can be made up in a 10 mg/ml solution for parenteral administration. Methimazole is also absorbed when given rectally in a suppository.[9] An hour after thiocarbamide has been given, iodide should be administered. A dosage of 100 mg twice daily is more than sufficient. Unless congestive heart failure contraindicates it, propranolol should be given at once, orally or parenterally in large doses, depending on the patient's clinical status. Permanent correction of the thyrotoxicosis by either radioactive iodide or immediate surgery should be deferred. Other supporting measures should be fully exploited. These include the use of sedation, oxygen, treatment for tachycardia or congestive heart failure, rehydration, multivitamins, occasionally sup-

portive transfusions, and cooling the patient to bring the temperature down to a reasonable level. An antibiotic may be given on the presumption of infection while the results of culture are awaited.

The adrenal gland may be limited in its ability to augment steroid production during thyrotoxicosis.[10] If there is any suspicion of hypoadrenalism, hydrocortisone (100 to 300 mg/d) or its equivalent should be given. The dose can be rapidly reduced when the acute process subsides. Pharmacologic doses of steroids (2 mg dexamethasone every 6 hours) acutely depress serum T_3 levels in normal subjects and in Graves' disease patients by reducing T_4 to T_3 conversion. This effect of steroids is beneficial in thyroid storm and supports the routine use of corticosteroids.

Other drugs have been useful in ameliorating some of the more dangerous features of thyrotoxic crisis. Reserpine[11] and guanethidine,[12,13] used in the past, have been replaced by propranolol. Propranolol may not reverse the metabolic insults of thyrotoxicosis but does dramatically suppress tachycardia, restlessness, and other symptoms.[14,15]

Rehydration, repletion of electrolytes, treatment of coincident disease such as infection, and specific agents (antithyroid drugs, iodine, propranolol, and corticosteroids) usually produce a marked improvement within 24 hours. A variety of additional approaches have been reported, but indications for their use are not well defined. For example, oral gallbladder contrast agents such as ipodate and iopanoic acid in doses of 1 to 2 g, which inhibit peripheral T_4 to T_3 conversion, may be of value.[16] Peritoneal dialysis can remove circulating thyroid hormone, as can plasmapheresis, but at the expense of serum protein loss. Orally administered ion-exchange resin[17] (20 to 30g/day as Colestipol-HCl) can trap hormone in the intestine and prevent recirculation. These last treatments will rarely be needed.

The antithyroid treatment should be continued until euthyroidism is achieved, at which point a final decision regarding antithyroid drugs, surgery, or ^{131}I therapy can be made.

OPHTHALMOPATHY IN GRAVES' DISEASE

Recently, Graves' ophthalmopathy has been extensively reviewed.[18,18a] Two types of manifestations may occur in Graves' ophthalmopathy: (1) functional

TABLE 12-2. Classification of the Ocular Changes in Graves' Disease[1]

Classes	Grades	Ocular Symptoms and Signs
0–6	0, a, b, c	No signs or symptoms.
1		Only signs, no symptoms (signs limited to upper lid retraction and stare, with or without lid lag and proptosis). Proptosis associated with class 1 only (specify difference of 3 mm or more, grade 0 included).
	0	Absent (20 mm or less—normal)
	a	Minimal (21–23 mm)
	b	Moderate (24–27 mm)
	c	Marked (28 mm or more)
2		Soft tissue involvement (symptoms of excessive lacrimation, sandy sensation, retrobulbar discomfort, and photophobia, but not diplopia); objective signs as follows:
	0	Absent
	a	Minimal (edema of conjunctivae and lids, conjunctival injection, and fullness of lids, often with orbital fat extrusion, palpable lacrimal glands, or swollen extraocular muscle palpable laterally beneath lower lids)
	b	Moderate (above plus chemosis, lagophthalmos, lid fullness)
	c	Marked
3		Proptosis associated with classes 2 to 6 only (specify if inequality of 3 mm or more between eyes, or if progression of 3 mm or more under observation).
	0	Absent (20 mm or less)
	a	Minimal (21–23 mm)
	b	Moderate (24–27)
	c	Marked (28 mm or more)
4		Extraocular muscle involvement (usually with diplopia)
	0	Absent
	a	Minimal (limitation of motion, evident at extremes of gaze in one or more directions)
	b	Moderate (evident restriction of motion without fixation of position)
	c	Marked (fixation of position of a globe or globes)
5		Corneal involvement (primarily due to lagophthalmos)
	0	Absent
	a	Minimal (stippling of cornea)
	b	Moderate (ulceration)
	c	Marked (clouding, necrosis, perforation)
6		Sight loss (due to optic nerve involvement)
	0	Absent
	a	Minimal (disc pallor or choking, or visual field defect; vision 20/20 to 20/60)
	b	Moderate (disc pallor or choking, visual field defect; 20/70 to 20/200)
	c	Marked (blindness, i.e., failure to perceive light; vision less than 20/200)

[1] Note that in addition to classification by type of involvement, there is also a grading according to severity.

abnormalities due to hyperactivity of the sympathetic nervous system, produced by the thyrotoxicosis, and (2) infiltrative lesions involving the contents of the orbit. The infiltrative type has a far more serious prognosis. A classification of eye sign findings formerly used is given in Table 12-2. Recently, criticism has been voiced regarding this NOSPECS mnemonic. Critics argue that although NOSPECS is "an ingenious, catchy memory aid for medical students who have forgotten how to examine a Graves' eye,"

it is insufficient since its emphasis on the mean status of the eye makes it impossible to evaluate components separately. In other words, the NOSPECS index may not always reflect important improvements or deteriorations in individual components of the eye. For this reason it was proposed that data should be handled separately and not combined in an index.[19] Others, on the basis of these observations, proposed a modification of NOSPECS.[20] In order to assess treatment of active inflammatory

TABLE 12-3. Proposed Classification System to Assess Disease Activity in Graves' Ophthalmopathy

Pain
    Painful, oppressive feeling on or behind the globe
    Pain on attempted up, side, or down gaze
Redness
    Redness of the eyelids
    Diffuse redness of the conjunctiva
Swelling
    Chemosis
    Edema of the eyelid(s)
    Increase of proptosis of 2 mm or more during a period between 1 and 3 months
Impaired function
    Decrease in visual acuity of 1 or more lines on the Snellen chart (using a pinhole) during a period between 1 and 3 months
    Decrease of eye movements in any direction equal to or more than 5 degrees during a period of time between 1 and 3 months

One point is given for each sign present. The sum of these points defines the activity score.
(From Mourits et al.,[21] with permission.)

ophthalmopathy, to predict therapeutic outcome, and to select patients for surgical or nonsurgical treatment, they introduced the clinical activity score (CAS)[21] (Table 12-3). This system was shown to have a high predictive value for therapeutic outcome of immunosuppressive treatment of infiltrative ophthalmopathy.[22] Further trials, however, are necessary to more precisely evaluate it.

Noninfiltrative Ophthalmopathy

Almost all patients with active thyrotoxicosis have an abnormality that is detectable on careful examination of the eyes. This abnormality may be only a widening of the palpabral fissure, a lag of the globe on upward gaze, or a lag of the upper lid on downward gaze, producing an increase in the visible segment of the sclerae and a bright-eyed or pop-eyed appearance. These abnormalities cause the eyes to appear exophthalmic, but measurement may show that there is no proptosis. Similar changes may be produced by administration of thyroid hormone or by local action of sympathetic stimuli on Müller's superior palpebral muscle, causing spasm and retraction of the upper lid.[23] This variety of ophthalmopathy is valuable diagnostically, and although it may have some undesirable cosmetic effect, it poses no hazard to ocular function. These findings are corrected by control of the thyrotoxicosis, no matter which therapeutic route is followed. Lid lag should be noted, is fairly common in normal subjects.

Infiltrative Ophthalmopathy

Infiltrative ophthalmopathy is a characteristic and unique feature of Graves' disease. It may coexist with the noninfiltrative ophthalmopathy described above, but it is a separate disorder.

The signs and symptoms are produced by the following related abnormalities.

Edema of the Orbital Contents

The lids and periorbital tissues are irritated, injected, and characteristically swollen and puffy. The lids may be erythematous. The swollen lids usually feel firm and do not pit. There is chemosis, an edema of the scleral conjunctiva. Edematous conjunctiva may even protrude beyond the palpebral fissure. Excessive lacrimation and photophobia may be associated with this condition. The lacrimal gland may be almost totally destroyed by the infiltrative lesion. Nevertheless, epiphora is typical. Eye pain, irritation, and "grittiness" of the eyes are common complaints.

Protrusion of the Globe

It is unusual for the anterior border of the cornea to protrude normally more than 18 mm beyond the lateral margin of the orbit. If measurements with the Leudde or Hertel exophthalmometer show that the globe is 2 or 3 mm beyond this limit, then true proptosis is present (normal limits may be race-dependent). Often the globes cannot be easily displaced backward by digital pressure. When this displacement is attempted, the examiner senses that the retrobulbar tissue is firm and unyielding. Associated with this condition, and responsible for exophthalmos, is an increase in the volume of orbital contents including fatty tissue and muscles. The lacrimal gland may be enlarged and palpable, sometimes even visible. Prolapse of the globe beyond the orbital fissure in extreme proptosis may permit a startling closure of the lids behind the globe.

The patient or friends usually note these abnormalities as an increased prominence of the eyes or a staring or wild expression. Occasionally there is a severe pain behind the eyes. Exophthalmos causes the exposed conjunctivae to be more readily irritated by noxious agents. If the lids fail to close over the cornea completely while the patient sleeps, development of ulceration is a hazard.

Infiltration of the Extraocular Muscles

The muscles become infiltrated, inflamed, and enlarged. Inflammation of the muscles gives rise to an important and characteristic sign that is helpful in differentiating the ophthalmopathy of Graves' disease from other causes of exophthalmos. The insertion of the swollen lateral rectus is often visible as a beefy red area at the inner and outer canthus when the patient turns the eye laterally or medially. Normally the muscle insertion is barely visible and is pale pink. In tumors or other retrobulbar lesions, this change in muscle insertion is not seen. The muscle enlargement can be recognized by ultrasound or, more certainly, by computed tomography (CT) or nuclear magnetic resonance (NMR) scanning. The enlargement is almost pathognomonic of Graves' disease, but can also occur with pseudotumor.

Paralysis, or paresis, of the extraocular muscles occurs. Upward gaze is affected first and most seriously, and loss of convergence is common. Oculomotor paralysis may be severe when exopthalmos is minimal or absent, but the changes are usually more or less parallel. Initially, these changes in ocular muscle function often produce diplopia. As the lesion progresses, a permanent strabismus may develop, with coincident suppression of the visual image in one eye and loss of the diplopia. Oculomotor function is occasionally lost completely.

The initial inflammatory lesion is followed gradually by recovery and fibrosis, and often the scarred and fibrotic muscle causes a fixed strabismus that persists indefinitely unless corrected surgically.

The oculomotor paresis is occasionally seen without significant exophthalmos or edema, and may be difficult to distinguish from myasthenia gravis or from paresis that is part of the neuropathy of diabetes. In such cases, it is wise to test for the presence of myasthenia by injection of 2 to 10 mg edrophonium intravenously. The function of muscles damaged by the ophthalmopathy of Graves' disease is not significantly improved during the test. Myasthenic weakness will be corrected within 1 minute and the benefit will last for several minutes, depending on the dose.

Damage to the Optic Nerve and the Retina

The retina may be injured by venous congestion or hemorrhages. Occasionally, field defects are found. Papilledema may be present, especially in severe involvement of the eye. If the optic nerve is involved, there may be pallor of the optic disc and a decrease in central visual acuity or field cuts, valuable and ominous signs. Blindness may occur without protrusion of the globe. Thus, the ophthalmopathy of Graves' disease may have the clinical features of optic neuritis.

Increased Intraocular Pressure

Increased intraocular pressure occurs in some patients with Graves' ophthalmopathy, especially in those with infiltrative disease. Two clinical studies showed that upon upgaze, an increase in intraocular pressure correlated with severity of infiltrative disease. No increase in intraocular pressure is seen in healthy patients and those with noninfiltrative ophthalmopathy.[24,25]

The clinical picture is altered by subsequent complications. The edematous conjunctivae are easily irritated by wind, smoke, or dust, and frequently become infected. Panophthalmitis is a most feared complication. Corneal ulcers are a serious hazard and may not heal while exophthalmos persists.

Pathology

Graves' ophthalmopathy involves histologic abnormalities in orbital tissues including extraocular muscles, orbital fat, lacrimal glands, and interstitial connective tissue.

On gross inspection extraocular muscles are enlarged, firm, and have a rubbery consistency. Microscopically intense infiltration is seen by mononuclear inflammatory cells such as lymphocytes, plasma cells, macrophages, and mast cells. Interstitial edema is almost invariably present. The muscle fibers may appear normal under both light and electron microscopy. In end stage ophthalmopathy, fibrosis and infiltration of extraocular muscles is present. Affection of extraocular muscles is usually asymmetrical. The medial and inferior recti are more frequently involved than the superior or lateral recti or the oblique muscles. There is controversy with regard to changes in fat volume in Graves' ophthalmopathy. Recent reports show no significant abnormalities in volume or density of retrobulbar fat in patients with active eye disease in contrast to the marked increase reported earlier. Lacrimal glands often show mild mononuclear infiltration and interstitial edema. Fibrosis, however, does not occur. Orbital tissues characteristically show varying degrees of intercellular edema that has been attributed to increased concentrations of mucopolysaccharides generated by orbital fibroblasts that are stimulated by activated lymphocytes (for review of this material, see ref. 26) (Fig. 12-1).

Cause and Pathogenesis

Despite intensive research, especially in the last two decades, the cause of infiltrative ophthalmopathy is still unknown. It is not simply a manifestation of hyperthyroidism, since feeding toxic amounts of exogenous thyroid hormone reproduces this syndrome in neither animals nor humans. Search for the pathogenesis has been underway for at least 60 years. It is almost of historical importance only to mention factors that were believed to play a role in the production of exophthalmos in the beginning of this era, like TSH and so-called *opthalmotropic factor* (OF). More recently, the cause of OGD has been attributed to immunologic derangement on the basis of autoimmunity. Recent studies show that Graves' hyperthyroidism and ophthalmopathy may share pathogenic mechanisms probably related to cross-reactivity between autoantigens in the thyroid and in retrobulbar tissues. Autoimmune mechanisms lead to accumulation of macrophages, plasma cells, and lymphocytes in extraocular muscles. These lymphocytes may then stimulate fibroblasts to proliferate and to produce glycosaminoglycans leading to infiltrative ophthalmopathy (see below).

Historical Background

When guinea pigs[27] and fish[28] were given crude thyrotropic hormone preparations, changes similar to those seen in human infiltrative ophthalmopathy were elicited. The changes in fatty tissues and muscles were similar, both macroscopically and microscopically.[29–31] Crude TSH fractions that did not possess thyroid-stimulating activity were found to produce similar eye abnormalities in test animals, and the putative factor was called *exophthalmos-producing substance* (EPS).[32,33,34] Similar changes were induced in the guinea pig orbit by a fragment of

TSH containing the intact β subunit coupled with a low-molecular weight fragment of the TSH α-unit.[35] This substance also stimulated ^{35}S-uptake and formation of mucopolysaccharides in Harderian glands of guinea pigs and, finally, bound to retrobulbar tissue.[35–39] Despite these findings it was still considered improbably that TSH or TSH fragments could have any direct relation to Graves' ophthalmopathy. Elevated endogenous TSH levels do not cause exophthalmos, and, furthermore, Graves' ophthalmopathy may occur in hypophysectomized persons. Most importantly, TSH is suppressed in patients with active untreated Graves' disease.

A new impetus in the search for the cause was the finding of an exophthalmos-producing protein in the serum of patients with active ophthalmopathy.[40,41] The presence of this protein, probably a γ globulin,[42] did not correlate well with either exophthalmos during stable periods of the disease or with the degree of hyperthyroidism. It appeared to be distinct from the long-acting thyroid stimulator (LATS) found by Adams and Purves and extensively studied by McKenzie and co-workers (see Ch. 10). In the 70s, attention was focused on the possibility of the involvement of TG in ophthalmopathy. TG and TG-anti TG immune complexes were found to bind to eye muscle membranes with some selectivity.[43] In an in vitro model, evidence was found for immunologically mediated damage produced by killer lymphocytes reacting with surface-bound immune complexes and T-lymphocytes reacting with surface-bound TG.[44] Mullin and co-workers found TG on the surface of normal eye muscle and reported that this material causes T-lymphocytes from patients with Graves' opthalmopathy to develop a delayed-hypersensitivity type of reaction and to secrete migration inhibition factor.[45] Kriss et al.[46] proposed that thyroglobulin from hyperplastic thyroid acini leaks into regional lymphatics and is subsequently transported to cervical lymph nodes. By the formation of antithyroglobulin antibodies, immune complexes and sensitized lymphocytes might reach the orbit. They suggest that thyroglobulin and immune complexes adhere to extraocular muscles and subsequently bind antibodies and antigen-specific sensitized lymphocytes, and cause local tissue injury leading to ophthalmic Graves' disease.[43] This hypothesis, while interesting, has not been supported by subsequent studies and is currently not accepted.[26]

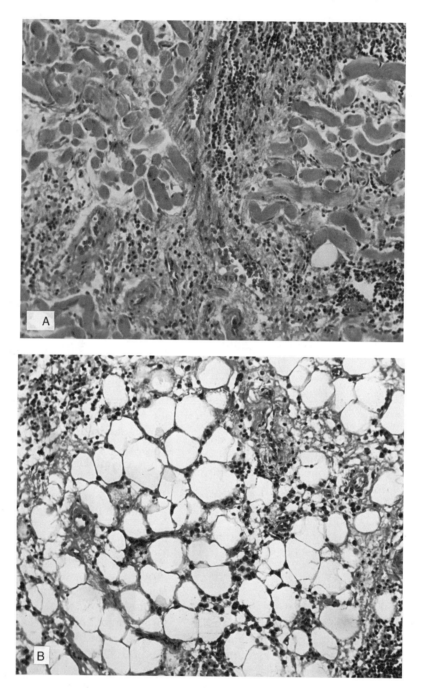

Fig. 12-1. (A) Extraocular muscle from a patient with Graves' disease and infiltrative ophthalmopathy. The lymphocytic infiltration and fibrosis are characteristic findings. (B) Edematous orbital fat and cellular infiltrate. *(Figure continues.)*

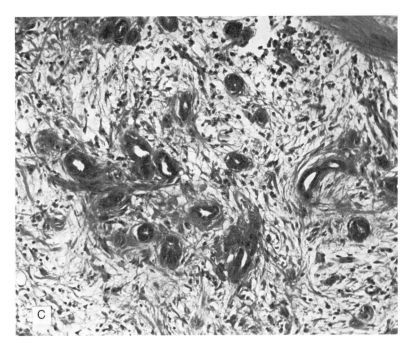

Fig. 12-1 *(Continued)*. (C) Lacrimal gland with mononuclear infiltrate, fibrosis, and an increase in ground substance. (Courtesy of Dr. D. Cogan).

Current Insights

There is little, if any, doubt that the ophthalmopathy of Graves' disease represents an autoimmune disorder. The vast majority of patients with endocrine ophthalmopathy have clear autoimmune thyroid disease. This appears to be the case in almost all patients if careful analysis is performed and patients are closely followed.[26] The specific antigen, however, is still unknown, although intense research is underway. Patients with active Graves' hyperthyroidism and ophthalmopathy almost invariably show circulating thyroidal antibodies such as antithyroglobulin antibodies, antiperoxidase antibodies, and thyroid-stimulating immunoglobulins. About one-third of patients with ophthalmopathy are euthyroid, have thyroid-stimulating immunoglobulins present in their serum, and two-thirds have thyroglobulin or thyroid peroxidase antibodies.[47]

Ophthalmopathy may occur in some patients with typical Hashimoto's thyroiditis. Even patients who appear to be euthyroid and who do not possess serum thyroid peroxidase or antithyroglobulin antibodies, as determined with routine assays, show thyroid-related autoimmunity with more detailed analysis. In 18 patients, for example, cell-mediated

cytotoxicity against fresh thyroid cells, thyroid membrane reactive antibodies, and TSH receptor-binding antibodies were measured.[48] All had positive tests in at least one of the assays. Clinically apparent ophthalmopathy occurs in 25 to 50 percent of patients with hyperthyroid Graves' disease.[49-51] When patients are more closely investigated with orbital ultrasonography, CT scanning, and measurement of intraocular pressure, however, eye abnormalities are found in virtually all cases. All of this evidence suggests a close relationship between ophthalmopathy and autoimmune thyroid disease. Still unexplained, however, is the fact that overt eye disease seldom develops in autoimmune hypothyroidism.[52]

The autoimmune origin of the Graves' disease ophthalmopathy also seems apparent from the histologic changes occurring in extraocular muscles. There is mononuclear cell infiltration, primarily of activated T cells, fewer B cells, and sometimes macrophages and mast cells. Activation of retrobulbar T cells is thought to be caused by the presence of retrobulbar autoantibodies elicited by specific extraocular muscle antigens, but despite intense investigations no definite answers have emerged. The presence of γ globulin that reacts with orbital antigens in the serum of exophthalmic patients has been repeatedly reported.[43] These antibodies were sometimes devoid of any cross-reactivity with thyroid-cell constituents,[53] were not related to serum TSAb activity in patients serum,[54] interacted with several unique eye muscle determinants not present in the skeletal muscle,[55] were found to bind to retro-ocular fibroblasts[56] and apart from binding to retro-ocular muscle, displayed cytotoxic activity.[57] Promising results were reported showing that in a majority of patients with overt ophthalmopathy, immunoglobulins were present that bound to porcine eye muscle membranes. The test in controls and in patients with Graves' hyperthyroidism without overt OGD was negative. Late observations, however, showed that eye-muscle binding antibodies were present in the latter two groups, though at lower levels.[58,59]

Preliminary evidence has been presented of the presence of a 55-kd antigen confined to eye muscle, and that antibodies to this antigen are present in about 50 percent of patients with thyroid-associated eye disease. Recent attention, however, has focused on a 64-kd protein expressed by orbital tissue and by thyroid membranes, and recognized by autoantibodies in serum of patients with thyroid-associated eye disease.[60–61a] Others, however, found sera of normal subjects also react with this 64-kd protein and concluded that this protein was of no pathophysiologic significance.[55,62] Recently a 64-kd antigen was cloned from an eye muscle cDNA library and the mRNA for this gene appeared to be expressed in normal human thyroid and extraocular muscle but not in skeletal muscle. The mRNA for the equivalent gene in the dog, however, was present in the brain, lung, heart, liver, kidney, spleen, and stomach, but not in the thyroid.[63] A recent report[64] showed that a 64-kd antigen derived from human eye muscle reacted positively to 30 percent of sera of patients with ophthalmopathy but also to the same percentage of sera from hyperthyroid Graves' disease patients without ophthalmopathy, and with normal sera. There was significantly more 64 kd antigen reactivity in sera of patients with ophthalmopathy as compared to the normals. Yet when the positive sera of the three patient groups were reacted with a 64-kd antigen derived from other tissues, such as human thyroid, skeletal muscle, brain, and liver, positive reactivity was also found. It was concluded that 64-kd antigen reactivity, though higher in concentration in ophthalmopathy, is frequently encountered in normal sera and

that the found "specificity-crossover" with similar molecular weight transmembrane antigens is likely to be caused by the presence of natural autoantibodies reacting with recurrent autoepitopes. The function of the 64-kd eye muscle antigen in the pathogenesis of Graves' ophthalmopathy was seriously questioned in this investigation. Finally, no evidence that eye muscle membrane or fibroblast antibodies are present in a significant proportion of patients with ophthalmopathy was found, using ELISAs based on antigens derived from porcine eye and skeletal muscle, human eye (membrane and soluble antigen) and skeletal muscle, human thyroid microsomal and TG antigens, and dermal and orbital fibroblasts.[65]

In a search for the same protein, i.e., the thyrotropin receptor (TSH-R) (considered to be the causative autoantigen in Graves' disease), studies were conducted for the expression of TSH-R in retro-orbital tissues. Thus, using polymerase chain reaction (PCR), mRNA for the TSH-R has been identified in cultured retro-ocular fibroblasts and extracts from retro-ocular connective tissues in humans[66,67] as well as laboratory animals,[68] suggesting that the autoantigen causing ophthalmopathy is indeed the same. A later report suggested that ophthalmopathy might be caused by the presence of a genomic point mutation in codon 52 leading to a threonine for proline amino acid shift in the extracellular domain of TSH-R, as found in fibroblasts in two out of 22 patients with severe ophthalmopathy, the other 20 patients having the normal nucleotide sequence corresponding to the full-length extracellular domain of the TSH-R.[69] In a subsequent study from the same group[69a], it was shown that this mutation was associated with Graves' disease, but only in female patients, the prevalence being 15 percent. When ophthalmopathy was present the prevalence was 17 percent, but coexistence of dermopathy and of acropathy raise the prevalence to 40 percent and 60% respectively. In a recent editorial the pathogenic significance of a mutation in autoimmune disease is contested due to the fact that autoantigens have never been shown to be structurally abnormal.[69b] Specific immunological staining of retro-ocular fibroblasts from patients with opthalmopathy was found when using an antiserum against normal human TSH-R.[70] Others, however, using Northern blotting and PCR amplification, could not find mRNA expression of TSH-R in extra-ocular muscle of humans.[71] They did find, however, the presence of a 1.3 kilobase variant of TSH-R containing the first 210 amino acids of the native TSH-R, followed by a unique 22-amino acid tail.[71a] From all these data, it is evident that no firm evidence regarding the specific mechanism of ophthalmopathy is present so far, but most workers in the field believe that immunity to an antigen cross-reacting with TSH-R is probably involved.

Whatever the exact autoimmune mechanism of ophthalmopathy, there seems to be concensus that the primary effector of the autoimmune reaction in the retrobulbar tissue are the fibroblasts of the extra-ocular muscles, stimulated as a result of cytokine release by activated T cells[52,72] (Fig. 12-2). It has been known for a long time that when retrobulbar fibroblasts are stimulated by lymphocytes, they proliferate and produce glycoaminoglycans.[73,74] These substances are hygroscopic and attract water. Accumulation of mucopolysaccharides and the existence of edema and fibrosis are typical endstages of ophthalmopathy in extraocular muscles (Fig. 12-3). Certain cytokines stimulate fibroblasts,[52] including interleukin 1, tumor necrosis factor-α, fibroblast growth factors, platelet-derived growth factor, transforming growth factors-β, lymphotoxin, and fibroblast-activating factors.

There is little, if any, evidence that specific HLA types predispose for ophthalmopathy. Although in patients with Graves' thyrotoxicosis, HLA type DR3 occurs predominantly, this is not so for eye disease, at least in Great Britain.[75,76] In a recent study in Japan, it was found that by using assays of lymphocyte cytotoxicity and restriction fragment length polymorphism, patients with ophthalmopathy showed an increased frequency of HLA DQW3 compared with control subjects. It was concluded, however, that patients with ophthalmopathy form a heterogenous group with respect to HLA type.

Heat shock proteins (HSP) are thought to play a role in modulating immune response, and a strong association between the presence of a particular HSP of 70 kd (HSP-70) and the development of Graves' disease has been reported.[77–79] HSP-70 expression on the surface of retro-ocular fibroblasts and eye muscle cells of patients with ophthalmopathy and the inhibition of expression on these cells during treatment with antithyroid drugs was also found.[80–81a]

Smoking is a predisposing factor for Graves' ophthalmopathy.[82–84] In a recent investigation[85] it was found that smoking increased the risk of Graves' ophthalmopathy about seven times. No relationship was found, however, between the severity of the ophthalmopathy and the number of cigarettes smoked

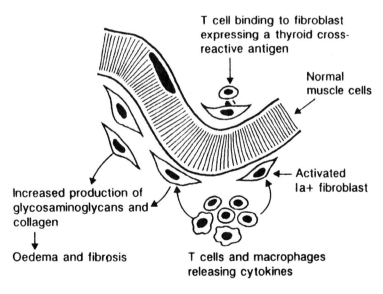

Fig. 12-2. Possible pathogenic mechanisms of Graves' ophthalmopathy. Predominant T-cell infiltration of the retro-ocular muscles may arise from recognition of antigens shared with the thyroid. These T cells, in addition to macrophages, release cytokines (see text) that stimulate fibroblasts, producing edema and fibrosis. (From Feliciello et al,[66] with permission.)

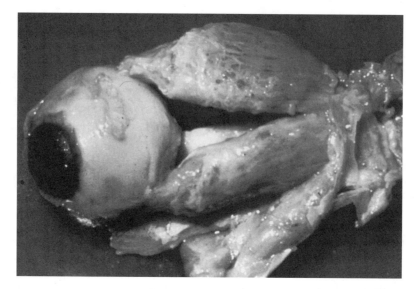

Fig. 12-3. End stage in severe involvement of extraocular muscles in ophthalmopathy (Courtesy of Prof. W. M. Wiersinga, Amsterdam.)

per day or the period of smoking. The relationship to smoking has been explained by the fact that extraocular muscle fibroblasts are stimulated by hypoxia in vitro.[86]

Other predisposing factors for the development of ophthalmopathy or the worsening of eye symptoms may include thyroidectomy[87] or treatment with radioactive iodine for Graves' hyperthyroidism.[88,89] Release of thyroid antigen as a cause of development or aggravation of ophthalmopathy by these forms of treatment may play a role in these phenomena.

Incidence and Course

In 75 percent of patients, ophthalmopathy manifested itself between one year before or one year after appearance of hyperthyroidism.[90,91] Ophthalmopathy, however, may appear long before manifestation of thyrotoxicosis or even decades after hyperthyroidism has been successfully treated. In fact, it may occur in patients who never develop clinical hyperthyroidism. The disease may be unilateral or bilateral, may begin in one eye, or may always be more severe in one eye than in the other. The syndrome usually accompanies hyperthyroidism and is at its worst when the diagnosis is first made. A prospective study[92] of 537 patients with Graves' disease showed that 40 percent had clinical evidence of ophthalmopathy. The data presented by Hamilton et al.[93] suggest a clinical incidence of 30 percent in their series if signs due to noninfiltrative ophthalmopathy are excluded. In about 10 percent of their series, these changes were severe. The prevalence of increased intraocular pressure in 61 percent of such patients shows that infiltrative ophthalmopathy frequently occurs in patients with Graves' disease without clinical evidence for ophthalmic involvement.[94] Yet if more sophisticated techniques are used to detect infiltrative ophthalmopathy, such as ultrasound, virtually all patients with Graves' disease, including those without clinical eyesigns, show signs of extraocular infiltration.[95] Amino and co-workers[96] have reported that measurements of proptosis in Graves' disease fit a normal distribution curve, but the curve is shifted to higher values. This suggests that the complication is not sporadic, but rather that all patients have it to some extent and that we recognize only those with the most severe symptoms.

After therapy for thyrotoxicosis, the infiltrative lesions usually subside or remain stationary. Proptosis is more persistent, tending to remain stationary or to worsen during and after therapy in 92 percent of the patients in Hamilton's series,[93] and in a similar proportion of those reported by Hales and Rundle after a 15-year follow-up period.[97] If hypothyroidism is produced by the therapy, there may be an increase of 1.0 to 1.5 mm in exophthalmos, but this amount decreases if the metabolism returns to normal. In a few patients (perhaps 10 to 20 percent of those with the infiltrative lesion), the disease process gradually increases over a period of time and then remains stationary, with residual abnormalities for many years.

No more than 2 to 5 percent of patients with Graves' disease develop progressive severe exophthalmos. This progression often happens without a clear correlation to the severity the thyrotoxicosis. In some of these patients, the process inexorably progresses to total blindness unless heroic therapeutic measures are taken, and sometimes even then. Although thyrotoxicosis occurs in women about five times more frequently than in men, progressive ophthalmopathy occurs more frequently, and is more severe, in men.[26,98] It is rare in children.

Since exophthalmos usually improves with treatment of thyrotoxicosis,[98a] the patient should be restored to the euthyroid state as soon as possible and kept there. In treating the hyperthyroidism of these patients, it is important that they not be allowed to become hypothyroid later. Hypothyroidism seems to accentuate the signs and symptoms of the ophthalmopathy, possibly by increasing the water content of the tissues.

Insofar as effects on the exophthalmos are concerned, there is no perfect basis for selecting one form of therapy for coincident thyrotoxicosis over another. Some observers advocate antithyroid drug treatment, with an attempt to maintain a minimally toxic state,[99] whereas others believe that antithyroid drug therapy promotes worsening of the eyes.[100] Some reports suggest that surgery exacerbates exophthalmos. Kriss et al.[101] have reported elevations of TSI levels and worsening of the eyes after ^{131}I therapy. Several studies have been published concerning possible effects on development of eye signs after partial thyroidectomy. In a total of five studies[87] comprising 245 patients, no significant worsening or improvement after thyroidectomy was found. The possible effect of the three forms of treatment (medical, RAI, thyroidectomy), on infiltrative ophthalmopathy was recently studied prospectively.[92] No influence of type of treatment on the clinical course of eye signs was found. The authors found that in patients who had no ophthalmopathy before treatment, the occurrence of post-treatment exophthalmos was similar in the surgical, medical, and ^{131}I-treated group (7.1, 6.7, and 4.9 percent, respectively). The incidence and degree of progression of ophthalmopathy in patients who already had exophthalmos before treatment was also not different in the three groups (19.8, 19.2, and 22.7 percent, respectively) as was the improvement of ophthalmopathy (12.7, 14.1, and 12.3 percent, respectively). The most recently published data indicate that ^{131}I therapy is more apt to be followed by worsening of exophthalmos than is surgical treatment. This may occur because of the well-recognized flair of autoimmunity produced by ^{131}I.[102]

A prospective study evaluated the protective effect of prednisone on treatment of radioactive iodine with regard to development of eye signs in patients with only slight or no signs ophthalmopathy. In the group of patients not treated with prednisone, ocular disease worsened in 9 out of 16 patients who had some ophthalmopathy before therapy and did not change in 6 out of 16. In the group of patients treated with prednisone (0.4 to 0.5 mg prednisone/kg bodyweight for 1 month with subsequent tapering and withdrawal after 3 months), ophthalmopathy improved in 11 out of 21 patients and did not change in 10 out of 21. Eye signs did not develop after radio-iodine treatment in ophthalmopathy-negative patients in either group.[87,88] The authors conclude that in patients with Graves' hyperthyroidism and mild to moderate ophthalmopathy, treatment with radioactive iodine should be performed under protection with systemic glucocorticoids. It should be noted, however, that no data have been published about any protective effect of glucocorticoids on possible worsening of eye signs after thyroidectomy. The authors of this volume feel that routine glucocorticoid administration to patients treated with radioactive iodine or by thyroidectomy is currently inadvisable if eye signs are mild. Further studies should be awaited since the extent that the protective effect of glucocorticoids outweighs their side-effects is unknown.

In general, the hyperthyroidism of patients with mild or moderate eye signs should be treated by whatever means seems most appropriate. If, after treatment, eye signs deteriorate despite carefully maintained euthyroidism, administration of a short course of glucocorticoids should be considered.

Diagnosis

The ophthalmopathy of Graves' disease must be differentiated from other conditions that cause oculomotor weakness, proptosis, and congestive phenomena of the orbit and periorbital tissues. If bilateral exopthalmos occurs in patients with thyrotoxicosis, there is little difficulty in diagnosis and the physician need not undertake a rigorous exclusion of other diseases. The same holds true when the exophthalmos follows clinical thyrotoxicosis. Patients who have not been thyrotoxic, however, but who develop exophthalmos—especially if it is unilateral—pose a more difficult problem.[103] A search must be made for orbital or intracranial tumors. Evidence of bone erosion suggests a tumor, although erosion of the orbital roof due to Graves' ophthalmopathy has been seen. Evidence of encroachment upon the optic nerve should be sought. Quadrantic defects are seen in infiltrative ophthalmopathy, but are rare. Occasionally, allergic reactions may produce puffiness of the lids and injection and edema of the conjunctative and sclerae, but not exophthalmos.

Conditions that may be confused with Graves' ophthalmopathy include pseudotumor of the orbit, infiltrative leukemia of the orbit, trichinosis, fibrous dysplasia of bone, retrobulbar hemangiomas, ophthalmic vein thrombosis, cavernous sinus thrombosis, sphenoid ridge meningiomas, retrobulbar hemorrhage, and any other involvement of the orbit by malignancy (Table 12-4).

If the clinical diagnosis is not obvious, circumstantial evidence may be obtained by laboratory examinations. It is useful to determine thyroid-stimulating or thyrotropin-displacing antibodies and antithyroglobin and peroxidase antibodies. A positive result does not certify the cause of exophthalmos but does prove that autoimmune thyroid disease is present. TSH, T_4, FTI, and T_3 levels should be measured. Results will vary from the values typical of hyperthyroidism to the levels suggestive of hypothyroidism. The RAIU may not be suppressed by the administration T_3. The suppression test result, if abnormal, provides an excellent differentiation between patients with Graves' disease and exophthalmos and patients whose thyroid is normal. But a normal response does not rule out the possibility of Graves' exophthalmos. The TRH test result can provide much the same information and is preferred to the T_3 suppression test. Failure of response is typical of active Graves' disease and correlates fairly well with the T_3 suppression test result. Measurement of basal TSH in a sensitive assay probably provides effectively the same information. Currently, we place greatest reliance on the presence of an abnormal CT scan

TABLE 12-4. Conditions That May Be Associated with Exophthalmos

Graves' ophthalmopathy
Pseudo-orbital tumor or cyst of the orbit
Primary orbital tumor including glioma
Metastatic tumors
Lymphomas
Developmental abnormalities of the orbit
Paget's disease
Fibrous dysplasia of bones
Meningioma
Lacrimal tumors
Nasopharyngeal carcinoma
Orbital hematomas secondary to trauma
Subarachnoid hemorrhage
Subdural hematoma
Carotid-cavernous sinus fistular
Carotid aneurysm
Cavernous sinus thrombosis
Nasal sinus emphysema
Granulomatous disease
Cellulitis
Histiocytosis
Pituitary adenoma
Cushing's disease
Acromegaly
Cirrhosis
Arteritis
Trichinosis

showing muscle enlargement (Fig. 12-4). NMR scanning of the orbit may equal or surpass orbital CT scanning.[104–107] Pseudotumor causing a density about the optic nerve is the most frequent problem in the differential diagnosis. Orbital sonography canbe helpful if skillfully done,[108,109] and occasionally angiograms or venograms are required. When iodine containing x-ray contrast are administered, thyrotoxicosis or thyroid autonomy should be ruled out first. The major problem is differentiation of unilateral exophthalmos from a tumor requiring surgery. Time often provides the answer, with the development of other signs of Graves' disease, growth of a lesion on CT scan, or shrinkage on steroids.

The clinical diagnosis of unilateral exophthalmos of Graves' disease may be impossible. Very rarely there may be recourse to exploration of the orbit. Biopsy may then show the microscopic changes in the tissues described above.

It is most important that the degree of exophthalmos, limitations of ocular mobility, visual acuity, and visual fields be determined during the initial evalua-

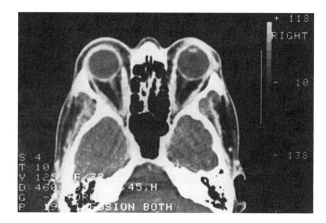

Fig. 12-4. CT scan of the orbital contents in a patient with severe active exophthalmos. The characteristic enlargement of the extraocular muscles is clearly evident, as is the proptosis. Normally the muscles are thin, although visible, and appear to be 2 or 3 mm in diameter.

tion and repeatedly during the course of treatment if the exophthalmos requires active therapy.

Pseudotumor

In a significant number of patients, unilateral exophthalmos and sometimes loss of visual acuity occur without any evidence of Graves' disease and with a posterior orbital density on CT scans being the only laboratory finding. These patients may have *pseudo tumor*, a designation of dubious value. Pseudotumor is said to be a chronic inflammatory process that can be related to some systemic disease or granulomatous process or may be idiopathic. It has been treated with iodide and x-rays, and currently is treated with glucocorticosteroids. The process may be unilateral or bilateral. It can cause muscle thickening[108-111] and visual loss. The authors believe, without certain proof, that many cases of pseudotumor are examples of Graves' ophthalmopathy.

Therapy

Therapeutic possibilities include local measures to combat inflammation, glucocorticoids, plasmapheresis and immune suppressants, orbital radiation, decompressive surgery, and thyroid ablation.

Moderate infiltrative ophthalmopathy is best treated by reassuring the patient and controlling the thyrotoxicosis. It may be helpful to elevate the head of the bed at night, to decrease salt intake, to use

shielded glasses whenever the eyes may be exposed to irritation, and to use protective drops, such as 0.5 percent methylcellulose, or a protective ointment at night. Deeply tinted glasses may help combat photophobia on bright days. A 0.5 percent solution of hydrocortisone may prove beneficial when used as eyedrops three times daily in combatting some of the local irritative phenomena. This therapy is not without danger, however, and should be used briefly since steroid hormones may diminish normal resistance to the herpes simplex virus and may increase intraocular pressure. If there is difficulty in closing the eyelids during sleep, it is necessary to keep them closed with a piece of cellulose tape. (This can be a problem if the tape is dislodged, the eyes open, and the cornea is injured.) Diplopia can sometimes be corrected by prism lenses or be handled temporarily by using an eyepatch or by occluding one lens of the patient's glasses. The majority of patients respond to this program with a gradual improvement as the thyrotoxicosis becomes controlled.

When the ophthalmopathy is severe or progressive, an active approach is required. Diuretic therapy and rigid salt restriction may be helpful. The more active therapeutic modalities most used are administration of glucocorticoids, mostly prednisone in moderate to high doses as a single regimen, x-ray irradiation of the orbit (preferably in combination with glucocorticoids), and surgical decompression of the orbit.

Although in the acute situation administration of prednisone relieves symptoms in most cases, relapse occurs in many patients after glucocorticoids have been withdrawn.[112,113] When prednisone is used in the acute situation, large doses may be required.[114] We usually begin with 40 mg prednisone daily in divided doses and continue until a response is obtained. If vision worsens or no response is obtained, doses of 60 to 200 mg/day may be justified for a short period, and may be helpful when lower doses are ineffective. As soon as the threat to vision is reversed, the dose of prednisone is gradually reduced over 4 to 12 weeks, is switched to an every-other-day program, and is finally reduced to a 5 to 10 mg maintenance dose or discontinued. Antacids, medication to reduce acid secretion, salt restriction, and diuretics may be needed, and one must be prepared to contend with all the usual problems, including weight gain, hypertension, infection, ulcers, diabetes, and osteoporosis.

If steroid therapy does not control the problem—visual acuity is still lower than normal and further deterioration is suspected—then surgical orbital decompression must be considered (see below). An alternative is to institute x-ray irradiation. Two thousand rads are delivered to the orbit with care to avoid the lens. Significant benefit is obtained in a third of patients over 1 to 6 months and another third have some improvement. Side effects, such as retinal damage or flair of exophthalmos, are very unusual.

There is no consensus about which method of treatment should be a first choice in situations in which acute intervention is not necessary. The selection of the procedure, e.g., surgical decompression or x-ray irradiation, is also, of course, dependent on the particular situation. Some of us feel that x-ray irradiation should be a first choice since surgical decompression can be done later if results of irradiation are disappointing. Others, however, feel that surgical treatment is favoured over irradiation, especially in young patients. The different aspects of both treatment modalities are discussed below.

If keratitis is the main problem, eyelid surgery[115] should, if necessary, be performed in combination with radiation therapy or surgical decompression.

Other Medical Therapies

Some patients have been treated with azothioprine or cyclophosphamide with varied results.[116,117] Plasmapheresis, combined with either steroids or immunosuppressants,[118] has also been highly touted for acute exophthalmos, but published experience is limited[119] and our own experience has not been encouraging. Cyclophosphamide, 50 to 100 mg/day for 2.5 months, was reported to give complete or partial clearing of exophthalmos in 28 patients in two studies,[117] but a recent controlled trial showed it to be ineffective.[120] Furthermore, most physicians are afraid of the long-term carcinogenic properties of immunosuppressant drugs other than steroids. Results of a controlled trial on the effects of cyclosporin and prednisone in ophthalmic Graves' disease revealed that cyclosporin is inferior to prednisone as a single drug, but the combined administration of both drugs may be of benefit to patients who do not react favorably to either drug alone.[113] In a recent preliminary report it has been suggested that daily subcutaneous administration of octreotide may benefit patients with active eye disease,[121] but this is not yet proved.

The development of corneal ulceration warrants the most prompt and careful attention in conjunction with an ophthalmologist. Local therapy with antibiotics may be helpful. Local application of cortisone is contraindicated. Emergency suturing of the lids together may be required to protect the cornea. Yet this often fails to help, and the sutures frequently become infected, leaving scarred lids. Scleral implants in the lower lids may protect the cornea. Decompression of the orbits by one of the techniques described below is frequently the only successful method for healing the ulcer.

Surgical Procedures

Orbital decompression is not a treatment intended to influence the basic process; it merely aims at enlarging the intraorbital space to relieve retrobulbar pressure. There are several approaches: the lateral (Fig. 12-5A), the superior (Fig. 12-5B), and the inferior (Fig. 12-5C). In the lateral approach, the lateral orbital wall is removed leaving the lateral orbital rim intact. In the superior approach the superior and lateral wall are removed by means of frontal craniotomy. In the inferior approach, the inferior and medial walls are removed. The approach is usually transantrally, but sometimes the transorbital route is used. The lateral and superior approach are used less often than the inferior approach by the transantral route. When serious proptosis is present, three walls (lateral, inferior, and medial) may be removed. In such cases a reduction of proptosis between 6 and 10 mm may be achieved. In rare cases a four-wall decompression may be indicated, resulting in a reduction of proptoses between 10 to 17 mm.[122] Recently results were reported of transantral orbital decompression in 428 patients with severe ophthalmopathy after a mean follow-up of 8.7 years (in most instances, two walls were probably removed). Optic neuropathy was present in 51 percent of patients and improved or remained unaltered in 89 percent. Scotomas improved or resolved in 91 percent, papilledama in 94 percent, and keratitis in 92 percent of eyes. Mean reduction in proptosis was 4.7 mm. Postoperative diplopia, however, developed in 64 percent of patients and 300 patients needed strabismus surgery. Worsening of any eye signs due to the operation occurred in 10 percent or less of patients.[123] Surgical procedures related to

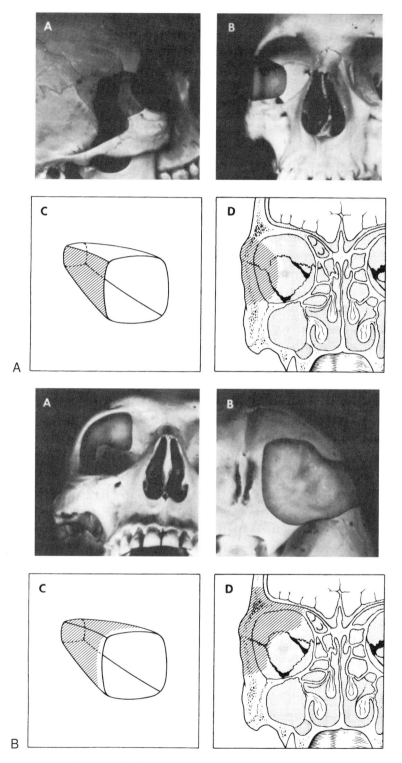

Fig. 12-5. Different approaches in orbital decompression. (A) lateral approach, (B) superior approach, (C) inferior approach. (From Gorman et al,[124] with permission.) *(Figure continues.)*

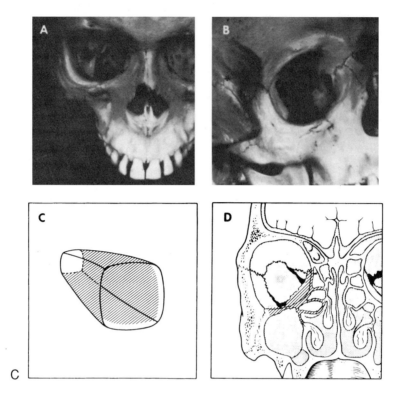

Fig. 12-5. *(Continued).*

eyelid malpositions may also be of benefit. Eyelid surgery is sometimes necessary to prevent keratitis that may result from ocular exposure, particularly when lagophthalmos is present. It may also be necessary to correct disturbing cosmetic upper or lower eyelid retraction (for further reading on surgical treatment, see ref. 124). Operation on the extraocular muscles to restore binocular vision is often helpful.

Orbital X-Ray Treatment

In the series of Gedda and Lindgren,[125] published four decades ago, the roentgen fields often included the posterior parts of the orbit and the pituitaries, and the authors believed that this procedure contributed to the beneficial effect. Three patients were treated only with radiation to the orbit, with success in two instances. Other authors later reported radiation directed to the orbits alone, with good results. Horst and co-workers[126] treated 112 patients with malignant exophthalmos. They used pituitary radiation (1 Gy/d to a total of 10 to 25 Gy), or retrobulbar x-ray (0.3 to 0.4 Gy/d to a total of 3 to 10 Gy), or a combination. In all patients treated within 2 years of the onset of the condition there was a decrease in the intensity of the symptoms, although "neurogenic" symptoms, such as a decreased ocular motility, were not affected. Horst found that the acute inflammatory changes of infiltrative ophthalmopathy and many of the attendant symptoms subsided within a few days.

Interest in orbital irradiation has undergone a revival. Supervoltage irradiation from a linear accelerator with a well-collimated field has been used to deliver approximately 20 Gy to the retro-orbital space in divided doses.[127] Great care is taken to protect the lens. Fifteen out of 23 patients showed improvement and none worsened,[127] and 35 percent improved in the report of Teng et al.[128] Kriss et al.[50] report on a large series of 80 patients treated by radiotherapy alone. An excellent or good result was obtained in 67 percent of cases. On analysis it appeared that improvement was seen in 95 percent for soft tissue involvement, 60 percent for both proptosis and extraocular muscle involvement, 50 percent for cornea lesions, and 85 percent for loss of visual acuity. The same group[129] recently reported on two treatment modalities delivering either 20 Gy per 2 weeks or 30 Gy per 3 weeks to the orbits in a total series of 311 patients. Before therapy, more than 90 percent of patients had soft tissue and eye muscle involvement, 65 to 75 percent had proptosis, and about 50 percent had some degree of sight loss. Both treatment modalities gave the same results, i.e., objective and symptomatic improvement was noted for all parameters assessed, but there was marked individual variability. The best responses were noted for soft tissue infiltration, corneal involvement, and sight loss. Factors that were related to less favorable outcome included male gender, advanced age, need for concurrent therapy for hyperthyroidism, and absent history of hyperthyroidism. No complications were seen and no significant differences in outcome were observed between the two dosage schedules. Pinchera et al. used cobalt units for supervoltage orbital radiotherapy instead of a linear accelerator.[130] After the first irradiation session, they treated the patients with methylprednisolon, 70 and 80 mg per day for the first 3 weeks, and progressively reduced the dose for 5 to 6 months. Others also administered prednisone (15 to 30 mg daily) during irradiation and for a short period thereafter. In a group of 11 treated patients the mean decrease of proptosis was 5.0 mm. Because of the short duration of prednisone administration (less than 3 months), side-effects were acceptable.[112]

Thyroid Ablation

Ablation of thyroid tissue by surgery or ^{131}I therapy to destroy the source of antigens has been recommended by Bauer and Catz,[132] but studies by others[133,134] indicate it is not predictably successful. A role for thyroid ablation remains possible, however, and is currently being studied by some clinics. One author of this text (L. D.) believes that early ablation of thyroid tissue favors progressive resolution of the problem. A recent report claims successful use of this treatment.[131]

Choice of Treatment

The choice among the several therapies available for the control of severe progressive infiltrative exophthalmos (Table 12-5) cannot yet be made with certainty. If local measures, diuresis, and rest are inadequate, our preferred first line of attack is administration of x-rays to the retrobulbar tissues. In a randomized double-blind trial of 3 months predni-

TABLE 12-5. Treatment of Exophthalmos

Local nonspecific
    Head elevation at night
    Dark glasses, side shields
    Ointment-petrolatum, methylcellulose, antibiotic
Protective surgery
    Lid surgery
Therapeutic
    Glucocorticoids
    Radiotherapy
    Surgical decompression
Experimental
    Plasmapheresis
    Antimetabolite treatment
    Thyroid ablation
    Octreotide treatment
Late
    Muscle insertion correction
    Lid surgery
    Removal of redundant eyelid skin

sone versus 20 Gy radiotherapy in patients with moderately severe ophthalmopathy equal results were obtained but side-effects were more frequent and severe with the prednisone.[135] Some physicians prefer to combine treatment with a short course of glucocorticoids. If this therapy does not halt exophthalmos, or if progression of the disease forces further intervention, operative decompression of the orbit should probably be instituted. Use of plasmapheresis or immunosuppressant drugs must be considered experimental. Three recent preliminary reports suggest that disease activity may be assessed using noninvasive techniques. Using ultrasonography, eye muscle reflectivity was lowered in patients with active extraocular orbitopathy and who responded to prednisone treatment, whereas reflectivity was normal in nonresponders.[136] In patients with ophthalmopathy, retrobulbar uptake of labeled octreotide was visualized by isotopic scanning and correlated with activity of eye disease.[137] Signal intensity ratio of orbital connective tissue and extraocular muscle in NMR imaging was significantly greater in responders to prednisone than in nonresponders, and may help to select patients for immunosuppressive therapy.[137a] Further investigations should establish the merits of these techniques in specifically selecting those patients who will respond to immunosuppressive therapy.

Infiltrative ophthalmopathy often becomes stationary and symptoms either progress no further or subside, but an unacceptable cosmetic problem or diplopia may continue to bother the patient. We have not hesitated at times to advise an orbital decompression as an interim procedure. The surgical risk is low when the operation is performed by an experienced surgeon, and the results are often gratifying. Knitting together the lateral quarter of the eyelids may strikingly improve the appearance of a patient with proptosis and a wide palpebral fissure, and scleral implants can help cover the cornea. If established diplopia cannot be helped by prisms or a ground glass, then extraocular muscle balance may be restored, under propitious circumstances, by any of several operative procedures on the muscles. This procedure should be done when the inflammation of the eye has subsided. Many patients find that scleral implants or surgical procedures that remove redundant skin or orbital fat, or both combined, vastly improve the appearance of their eyes.

LOCALIZED MYXEDEMA AND THYROID ACROPACHY

Localized pretibial myxedema often develops along with infiltrative ophthalmopathy. This lesion is a firm localized thickening, usually over the lateral aspect of the lower leg just above the ankle. Patches may be 0.5 to 6.0 cm in the greatest dimensions, or much more, and are elevated, firm, and nonpitting. In rare cases, the infiltrations may be so extensive that they become confluent, giving the leg below the knee a swollen, beefy appearance, and the skin a brawny, porcine texture (Figs. 12-6 and 12-7). The infiltrates are usually bilateral. The color ranges from pink to russet to salmon. The surface over the lesion is usually shiny, but may be scaly and is frequently puckered, like the surface of an orange, or is thrown into fine irregular folds. The lesions on the ankles sometimes take the form of heaped-up masses that interfere with the wearing of shoes. Similar lesions may exist on the dorsum of the feet and the dorsum of the phalanges. In very rare instances, they appear on the abdominal wall and the face. This lesion is almost always associated with infiltrative exophthalmos. Occasionally there is associated clubbing of the fingers and osteoarthropathy, including periosteal new bone formation.[138] These two phenomena constitute thyroid acropachy.[139] Thyroid acropachy differs from hypertrophic pulmonary osteosarthropathy in several respects. The lesions affect mainly the distal portion of the bones. The soft tissue reaction associated with periosteal new bone

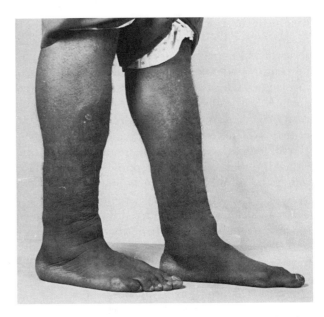

Fig. 12-6. A case of severe pretibial myxedema showing the coarsened, nodular, infiltrated, pigmented lesions on the lower extremities.

formation is firm, pale, and of normal temperature, rather than warm and erythematous, as in the lesion associated with pulmonary disease. Some minor evidence of pretibial myxedema is seen in 5 to 10 percent of patients with Graves' disease. Cosmetically significant lesions occur in 1 to 2 percent, and severe cases are even less frequent.

Apart from their unsightly appearance, the lesions of localized pretibial myxedema usually cause no symptoms. At times they may be somewhat painful, or, more frequently, the source of much itching. If severe, the lesions can be quite troublesome, since stasis changes may occur and it may be impossible to wear ordinary shoes. Studies with quantitative lymphoscintigraphy and fluorescence microlymphography showed functional and structural changes in dermal lymphatics caused by glycoaminoglycan (GAG) deposition and leading to lymphatic compression.[140] Nerve entrapment by the lesion has been reported and was cured by local steroid therapy.[141]

Histologically, the localized pretibial myxedema of Graves' disease is similar to that of hypothyroidism, but the infiltration of GAG is deeper in the skin[142] and is present in higher concentration, appearing more dense in tissue sections. Glycosaminoglycans are the polysaccharide chains in proteogly-

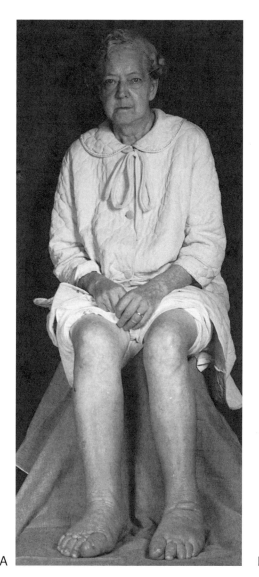

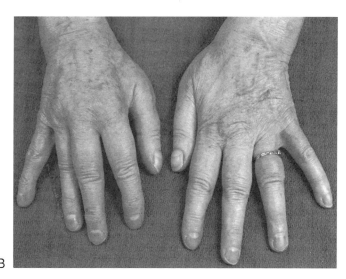

Fig. 12-7. (A) Massive infiltrative, localized myxedema in a female patient with Graves' disease and progressive exophthalmos. The lesions have become confluent over the lower extremities. (B) In the same patient, localized myxedema, involving the phalanges, is evident.

cans and are made up of disaccharide repeating units containing a derivative of an aminosugar, either glucosamine or galactosamine. Hyaluronate, chondroitin sulfate, keratin sulfate, heparin sulfate, dermatin sulfate, and heparin are the major glycosaminoglycans. Proteoglycans are very large polyanions that bind water and cations and thereby form the extracellular medium, or ground substance, of connective tissue. In localized myxedema, collagen appears to be fragmented due to infiltration of GAG

and edema formation. The principal abnormality in pretibial myxedema is the marked increase in GAG concentration in the skin. This may be six- to sixteen times normal.[143,144] Whereas in normal skin approximately 5 percent of the acid mucopolysaccharides is hyaluronic acid, in pretibial myxedema this amount increases to 90 percent. Coupled with the manyfold increase in total GAG, this increase indicates an enormous deposition of hyaluronic acid. Several reports[145–147] on the ultrastructure of pretibial myxedema describe an organized network of microfibrils with knobs within the widened interfibrous spaces. The knobs were supposed to contain glycoprotein and this material was also found in the coating of collagen bundles and on the surface of fibroblasts. These studies suggest that, as in ophthalmic Graves' disease, the fibroblasts may play a central role in the pathogenesis of localized myxedema. Also, immunoglobulins may locally stimulate skin fibroblasts to produce GAGs. It has been known for a long time that patients with localized myxedema have positive LATS and LATS-P assay results, and the levels are often enormously elevated. In some patients, high LATS levels and the pretibial myxedema disappear spontaneously and concurrently. No direct association with LATS or LATS-P, however, has been recorded. There have been several failed attempts to find tissue-bound LATS IgG[148,149] or complement in the lesions. Fibroblasts from control pretibial tissues were found to increase synthesis of hyaluronic acid when exposed to sera of patients with Graves' hyperthyroidism while fibroblasts from pretibial myxedema were stimulated by both normal and Graves' patients' sera.[150]

Cheung and co-workers reported that a non-IgG dialyzable peptide from serum of patients with pretibial myxedema stimulated fibroblast production of hyaluronic acid,[151] especially by fibroblasts from the area of the lesions. Shishiba et al[144] found in in vitro studies that skin fibroblasts of both normals and of skin affected by pretibial myxedema produced GAGs. The rate of synthesis of patients' skin, however, was increased. Synthesis was not affected by normal or patients' serum. Since proteoglycan accumulation is only seen in patients' skin, these authors suspect that impaired clearance of mucopolysaccharides play a causative role in pretibial myxedema. The situation becomes even more confusing when one analyzes the results of a study[152] in which whole serum and the serum immunoglobulin fraction of 20 patients with dermopathy was tested on its activity to alter synthesis of GAGs in rat FRTL cells and in fibroblasts from pretibial skin and from other origins. It was found that serum and IgG fractions stimulated GAG formation in FRTL cells, but not in fibroblasts of any origin, whereas sera and IgG fractions of patients with Graves' disease without dermopathy did not stimulate GAG formation in FRTL cells. It has also been recently reported that thyroid hormone excess stimulates proteoglycan synthesis in normal human skin fibroblasts.[153] Finally, recent attention has been focused on the possible role of heat shock proteins (HSPs) in the development of pretibial myxedema. HSP may have an immunologic role in intracellular antigen processing and presentation of cell membrane-anchored antigens to the immune system. Using fibroblasts from retro-ocular space and pretibial skin from sites affected by Graves' manifestations, it was found that HSPs are differently expressed as compared to tissue taken from unaffected localizations.[154] HSP 72 reactivity in fibroblasts, when exposed to various cytokines and to heat stress, was exclusively detected in those taken from affected tissues, and HSP 70 expression was significantly greater in fibroblasts from these tissues as compared to those from uninvolved tissues. The same group further reported that HSP 72 expression is attenuated both by oxygen radical scavengers and by the antithyroid drugs propylthiouracil and methimazole.[81] The authors suggested that the beneficial effect of these antithyroid drugs on the clinical course of Graves' disease and its extra-thyroidal manifestation may be related to their oxygen free radical scavenging properties.

Summarizing the literature on the pathogenesis of localized myxedema, there is still much confusion and no clearcut answers at present. Despite this, it seems warranted to predict that, as in ophthalmic Graves' disease, in pretibial myxedema mucopolysaccharide synthesis is increased by local fibroblasts stimulated by autoimmune processes. What is not known at present is the primary event leading to these autoimmune processes. Also, in acropachy increased GAG deposits are found.[155] There is thus evidence that the three best known extra-thyroidal manifestations of Graves' disease, i.e., ophthalmopathy, dermatopathy, and acropachy, are pathogenetically related in that mucopolysaccharide synthesis and deposition is probably increased by stimulation of local fibroblasts by autoimmune processes of which the mechanism is not clear. These facts corroborate the clinical observation that these three manifestations frequently occur in the same patient, either simultaneously or separately. The immune reactivity may be related to TSH-R since these manifestations are so closely tied to Graves' disease.

Therapy other than reassurance is usually unnecessary. It is unclear whether treatment of the thyrotoxicosis somehow favors decreased autoimmunity, and thus indirectly favors resolution of pretibial myxedema. The process usually gradually increases in intensity for a period of months or years and then stabilizes or slowly regresses. Local injections of hyaluronidase, T_4, T_3, and adrenocorticosteroids have been given with variable success. Occlusive dressings with fluocinolone or clobetasol propionate have produced gratifying improvement in some patients.[156,157] These dressings may cause temporary regression but don't seem to permanently affect the course of the condition. If necessary, repeated treatments are advised until a spontaneous clinical remission occurs.[158] The effect of hyaluronidase, which persists for 2 to 3 days, is due to removal of the GAGs from the skin. Administration of thyroid hormone has been reported to reduce localized myxedema, but in our experience it has no action comparable to that observed in generalized myxedema due to a deficiency of thyroid hormone.

Plasmapheresis, combined with immunosuppressive therapy, has been reported to be useful.[118] In a patient studied at the University of Chicago Clinics, plasmapheresis had only a temporary and minor effect, although LATS levels were greatly reduced.

CLINICAL ABNORMALITIES OF THE HEART

The biochemical actions of thyroid hormone on the heart have been described in Chapter 10.

Thyrotoxicosis increases the demands on the heart. Cardiac output is much increased on the basis of increased stroke volume and rapid heart rate.[159] It is possible that the metabolic efficiency of heart muscle is decreased. Irritability of the heart is increased.

Mitral valve prolapse is reported to have been present in 43 percent of a series of thyrotoxic patients, whereas it was present in only 18 percent of the control group.[160] This incidence may be due to increased adenergic tone, autoimmunity, or the augmented cardiac output associated with thyroxicosis. Most patients with thyrotoxicosis are adults. Many, especially those with toxic nodular goiter, are in the 50- to 70-years age group, which has a relatively high incidence of organic heart disease anyway. Thus, it is not surprising that cardiac abnormalities are prominent among the symptoms of thyrotoxicosis.

Myocardial infarction may occur in association with thyrotoxicosis.[161] Its relative incidence has been debated in the literature,[162] and we cannot state whether infarction does indeed occur less frequently than in normal patients. Thyrotoxicosis occurs most frequently in middle-aged women, a group having a low incidence of coronary occlusion.

Frequent premature beats and paroxysmal tachycardia sometimes appear in thyrotoxic patients and may disturb the patient. Atrial fibrillation occurs in thyrotoxicosis with or without previous heart disease. It may be episodic or may become fixed during the period of hyperthyroidism. Attempts to correct this arrythmia in patients with persistent atrial fibrillation are usually unsuccessful while they are thyrotoxic. Once they have become euthyroid, the fibrillation may revert spontaneously or may be converted medically[163] or by electroconversion. About two-thirds of patients undergo spontaneous reversion to sinus rhythm after receiving therapy for thyrotoxicosis, usually within a month. If fibrillation persists after the patient has been euthyroid for four months, spontaneous conversion is unlikely to occur.[164] It is always wise to evaluate thyroid function in clinically euthyroid patients with atrial arrhythmias with or without heart disease since in about 20 percent of patients TSH tests and/or FT_4 point to an overactive thyroid and in 50 percent of these patients normal sinus rhythm resumes after treatment with antithyroid drugs.[165] Since embolization occurs in the patients as in others with AF, anticoagulation medication is advised.

Congestive heart failure is a frequent complication in those patients with thyrotoxicosis who already have organic heart disease. In fact, in the older age group, the cardiac symptoms may so dominate the clinical picture that the thyrotoxicosis may be overlooked.[166] Careful attention should be given to this possibility in all patients with resistant congestive heart failure, especially if a goiter is found. Congestive heart failure may occur in patients who have no detectable preexisting organic heart disease.[167,168] It is not always possible to tell how much underlying heart disease is present in a patient with thyrotoxicosis who also has a disorder of rhythm, a cardiac murmur, or congestive heart failure, for all of these conditions may be encountered in thyrotoxicosis alone. Frequently, one sees findings make a gratifying return to normal when the thyrotoxicosis has been corrected.

Angina is worsened if already present, or may be induced de novo.[169] Sometimes this condition occurs in young women with no known heart disease.[170] Evidence of myocardial lactate production when the heart is paced at an accelerated rate,[171] and normal arteries on angiography after episodes of angina or infarction,[172] have suggested that the changes in thyrotoxicosis are due to an imbalance between O_2 demand and supply rather than arterial obstruction. This possibility is corroborated by the finding that coronary artery spasm of an otherwise normal vessel may occur during thyrotoxicosis.[169,173] Histologic examination of the thyrotoxic heart shows only aspecific abnormalities such as necrosis of isolated heart cells, small areas of fibrosis, and roundcell infiltration.[174,175]

We believe that in a few patients permanent enlargement of the heart may be a legacy of thyrotoxicosis, and others are of the same opinion.[176] These patients have hearts that are larger than normal on radiographic examination, and give no clue to the cause other than a history of Graves' disease. Such patients are exceptions to the rule that the cardiac changes found in Graves' disease are reversible. It has become evident that even in the mildest forms of thyrotoxicosis subtle cardiac abnormalities may be present. Thus, in patients with so-called "subclinical" thyrotoxicosis, i.e., suppressed TSH and normal serum free T_4 and T_3 due to multinodular goiter or TSH-suppressive T_4 treatment, mean basal 24-hour heart rate is increased, there is an augmented risk of atrial premature beats and atrial fibrillation, and left ventricular function and wall thickness are increased.[177–179a]

The treatment of heart disease in the presence of thyrotoxicosis is the same as when thyrotoxicosis is absent, but may be more difficult. Rest, salt restriction, diuretic therapy, digitalization, and administration of afterload reducers like angiotensin converting enzyme (ACE) inhibitors are in order. Larger than normal doses of digoxin are required, but there is probably no alteration in the ratio of toxic to therapeutic dosage. Atrial fibrillation may be controlled by digoxin, propranolol, or both. Electroconversion is usually successful only after thyrotoxicosis has been resolved for a few months.

Hyperthyroidism should be controlled as expeditiously as possible. Congestive heart failure is a contraindication to operation. Most patients with thyrotoxicosis and significant heart disease are now treated with RAI. This treatment may be preceded by a 3- to 6-month course of antithyroid drug therapy to deplete their glands of stored thyroid hormone, a program that lessens any chance of an exacerbation of the heart disease caused by a release of hormone from the gland. Fortunately, this complication is rare, but it does occur.[180] Administration of ^{131}I followed by antithyroid drugs, and potassium iodide or ipodate that also inhibit T_4 to T_3 conversion, may be used in severely ill patients in whom a prompt response is needed. This method is described in Chapter 11. Surgical treatment is possible in patients with thyrocardiac disease, as was reported many years ago.[181] If the thyrotoxicosis is controlled before operation, the patient usually tolerates this procedure well.

Propranolol has been used successfully in the control of tachycardia, and also in patients with congestive heart failure if tachycardia appeared to be adding substantially to the problem. In these instances, possible depression of myocardial contractility by the drug was outweighed by the benefit derived from controlling the rate. In such circumstances, one must proceed with caution, and digoxin should often be added.

SUMMARY

In this chapter, some of the important and characteristic complications of Graves' disease have been considered. When these complications occur, particular therapeutic problems arise and must be dealt with.

Thyroid storm, fortunately, is becoming rare. Formerly a complication frequently appearing after surgery on the incompletely prepared patient, it is now usually seen in patients with severe thyrotoxicosis who have neglected therapy or who have an added medical problem, such as an acute infection. Storm may be looked upon as a sudden and violent exacerbation of the signs and symptoms of thyrotoxicosis. Clinically, it is characterized by fever, extreme tachycardia, varied disorders of heart rhythm, and nervous hyperirritability rapidly progressing to exhaustion and often to coma. Mortality is high. A special form of thyroid storm, no less serious, is characterized by apathy and muscle weakness.

The treatment of thyroid storm should include use of antithyroid drugs and iodide, and also general supportive measures such as cooling, oxygen, transfusions, repletion of electrolytes, nutritional repletion, antibiotics if indicated, sedation, and adrenal corticoids. Control of many of the aspects of thyroid storm, especially tachycardia, may be achieved by the use of propranolol.

The infiltrative ophthalmopathy of Graves' disease usually occurs during a period of thyrotoxicosis, but may appear when there is no thyrotoxicosis or even when there is hypothyroidism. Its primary cause is unknown. There is, however, evidence that autoimmune mechanisms in the retro-ocular muscles stimulate fibroblasts to produce glycoaminoglycans (GAGs), leading to water retention and edema and ultimately fibrosis. The primary event responsible for retro-ocular autoimmune reactions is not known and reports are confusing. Ophthalmic Graves' disease presents a therapeutic problem, sometimes of stupendous proportions. If simple local measures fail to halt the progress of the ophthalmopathy, glucocorticoids, surgical decompression of the orbits, or radiotherapy to the orbit may be required.

The curious deposits of a material rich in glycoaminoglycans in the skin of the lower legs and sometimes over the phalanges are discussed in some detail. This material is seen only in patients with Graves' disease and usually coincides with infiltrative ophthalmopathy. Its appearance has no direct relationship to the level of thyroid function.

Cardiac insufficiency in the course of toxic goiter is looked upon as the effect, in most instances at least, of thyrotoxicosis on an already diseased heart. There may be younger patients who sustain permanent heart damage from severe thyrotoxicosis, and long-continued thyrotoxicosis in older age groups may be the only definable etiologic factor in congestive heart failure. The chief indication for treatment in cardiac insufficiency occurring in thyrotoxicosis is to abolish the thyrotoxicosis, but the usual cardiotonic, diuretic, and sometimes vasodilatory measures should be employed as well.

REFERENCES

1. Menendez CE, Rivlin RS: Thyrotoxic crisis and myxoedema coma. Med Clin North Amer 57:1463, 1973
2. Lahey FH: The crisis of exophthalmic goiter. N Engl J Med 199:255, 1928
3. Nelson NC, Becker WF: Thyroid crisis: diagnosis and treatment. Ann Surg 170:263, 1969
4. Mackin JF, Canary JJ, Pittman CS: Thyroid storm and its management. N Engl J Med 291:1396, 1974
5. McDermott MT, Kidd GS, Dodson LE, Hofeldt FD: Radioiodine-induced thyroid storm. Am J Med 75:353, 1983
6. Rosenberg I: Thyroid storm. N Engl J Med 283:1052, 1970
7. Brooks MH, Waldstein SS: Free thyroxine concentrations in thyroid storm. Ann Int Med 93:694, 1980
8. Birkhauser M, Busset R, Burer TH, Burger A: Diagnosis of hyperthyroidism when serum thyroxine alone is raised. Lancet 2:53, 1977
9. Nabil N, Miner DJ, Amatruda JM: Methimazole: an alternative route of administration. J Clin Endocrinol Metab 54:180, 1982
10. Felber J-P, Reddy WJ, Selenkow HA, Thorn GW: Adrenocortical response of the 48-hour ACTH test in myxedema and hyperthyroidism. J Clin Endocrinol Metab 19:895, 1959
11. Canary JJ, Schaaf M, Duffy BJ Jr, Kyle LH: Effects of oral and intramuscular administration of reserpine in thyrotoxicosis. N Engl J Med 257:435, 1957
12. Gaffney TE, Braunwald E, Kahler RL: Effects of guanethidine on triiodothyronine-induced hyperthyroidism in man. N Engl J Med 265:16, 1961
13. Lee WY, Bronsky D, Waldstein SS: Studies on the thyroid and sympathetic nervous system interrelationships, II: effects of guanethidine on manifestations of hyperthyroidism. J Clin Endocrinol Metab 22:879, 1962
14. Abrams JJ, Sandler J: Propranolol for thyroid storm. N Engl J Med 296:1120, 1977
15. Hellmann T, Kelly KL, Mason WD: Propranolol for thyroid storm. N Engl J Med 297:671, 1977
16. Robuschi G, Manfredi A, Salvi M et al: Effect of sodium ipodate and iodide on free T_4 and free T_3 concentrations in patients with Graves' disease. J Endocrinol Invest 9:287, 1986
17. Witztum JI, Jacobs LS, Schonfeld G: Thyroid hormone and thyrotropin levels in patients placed on colestipol hydrochloride. J Clin Endocrinol Metab 46:838, 1978
18. Burch HB, Wartofsky L: Graves' ophthalmopathy: current concepts regarding pathogenesis and management. Endocr Rev 14:747, 1993
18a.Weetman AP, McGregor AM: Autoimmune thyroid disease: further developments in our understanding. Endocr Rev 15:788, 1997
19. Gorman CA: Clever is not enough: NOSPECS is form in search of function. Thyroid 1:353, 1991
20. Wiersinga WM, Prummel MF, Mourits MP et al: Classification of eye signs of Graves' disease. Thyroid 1:357, 1991
21. Mourits MP, Koornneef L, Wiersinga WM et al: Clinical criteria for the assessment of disease activity in Graves' ophthalmopathy: a novel approach. Brit J Ophthalmopathy 73:639, 1989
22. Mourits MP, Prummel MF, Koornneef L et al: Prospective evaluation of the clinical activity score as predictor of therapeutic outcome after immunosuppressive treatment in Graves' ophthalmopathy, abstracted. Thyroid, suppl. 1, 1:S9, 1991

23. Lee WY, Marimoto PK, Bronski D, Waldstein SS: Studies of thyroid and sympathetic nervous system interrelationships, I: the blepharoptosis of myxedema. J Clin Endocrinol Metab 21:1402, 1961

24. Fishman DR, Benes SC: Upgaze intraocular pressure changes and strabysmus in Graves' ophthalmopathy. J Clin Neurol Ophthalmol 11:162, 1991

25. Spierer A, Eisenstein Z: The role of increased intraocular pressure on upgaze in the assessment of Graves' ophthalmopathy. Ophthalmology 98:1491, 1991

26. Jacobson DH, Gorman CA: Endocrine ophthalmopathy: current ideas concerning etiology, pathogenesis, and treatment. Endocrine Rev 5:200, 1984

27. Loeb L, Friedman H: Exophthalmos produced by injections of acid extract of anterior pituitary gland of cattle. Proc Soc Exp Biol Med 29:648, 1932

28. Albert A: The experimental production of exophthalmos in fundulus by means of anterior pituitary extracts. Endocrinology 37:389, 1945

29. Smelser GK: Water and fat content of orbital tissues of guinea pigs with experimental exophthalmos produced by extracts of anterior pituitary glands. Am J Physiol 140:308, 1943

30. Dobyns BM: Studies on exophthalmos produced by thyrotropic hormone: changes induced in various tissues and organs (including orbit) by thyrotropic hormone and their relationship to exophthalmos. Surg Gynaecol Obstet 82:609, 1946

31. Sisson JC, Miles M: Acid mucopolysaccharide alterations in experimental exophthalmos. Endocrinology 37:931, 1973

32. Dobyns MM, Steelman SL: The thyroid-stimulating hormone of the anterior pituitary is distinct from the exophthalmos-producing substance. Endocrinology 52:705, 1953

33. Smelser GK, Ozanies V: Further studies on nature of exophthalmos-producing principles in pituitary extract. Am J Ophthalmol 39:146, 1955

34. Brunish R: The production of experimental exophthalmos. Endocrinology 62:437, 1958

35. Kohn LD, Winand RJ: Structure of an exophthalmos-producing factor derived from thyrotropin by partial pepsin digestion. J Biol Chem 250:6503, 1975

36. Andrews AD, Dunn JT: Effects of TSH on the chemical composition of orbital tissue in guinea pigs. Endocrinology 93:527, 1973

37. Winand RJ, Kohn LD: The binding of (^{3}H)-thyrotropin and an ^{3}H-labeled exophthalmogenic factor by plasma membranes of retro-orbital tissue. Proc Natl Acad Sci USA 69:1711, 1972

38. Bolonkin D, Tate RL, Luber JJ, Kohn LD: Experimental exophthalmos. J Biol Chem 250:6516, 1975

39. Kohn LD, Winand R: Relationship of thyrotropin to exophthalmos-producing substance. J Biol Chem 246:6570, 1971

40. Dobyns BM, Wright A, Wilson L: Assay of the exophthalmos-producing substance in the serum of patients with progressive exophthalmos. J Clin Endocrinol Metab 21:648, 1961

41. Der Kinderen PJ, Houstra-Lanz M, Schwarz F: Exophthalmos-producing substance in human serum. J Clin Endocrinol Metab 20:712, 1960

42. Winand R: Isolement d'un facteur exophtalmiant serique associe aux gamma G globulines. p. 309. In: Rapports de la XLieme Reunion des Endocrinologistes de Langue Français. Masson, Paris.

43. Konishi J, Herman MM, Kriss JP: Binding of thyroglobulin and thyroglobulin-antithyroglobulin immune complex to extraocular muscle membrane. Endocrinology 95:434, 1974

44. Kriss JP, Mehdi SQ: Cell-mediated lysis of lipid vesicles containing eye muscle protein: implication regarding pathogenesis of Graves' ophthalmopathy. Proc Natl Acad Sci USA 76:2003, 1979

45. Mullin BR, Levinson RE, Friedman A et al: Delayed hypersensitivity in Graves' disease and exophthalmos: identification of thyroglobulin in normal human orbital muscle. Endocrinology 100:351, 1977

46. Kriss JP, Konishi J, Herman MM: Studies on the pathogenesis on Graves' ophthalmopathy (with some related observations regarding therapy). Rec Progr Horm Res 31:533, 1975

47. Bech K: Thyroid antibodies in endocrine ophthalmopathy: a review. Acta Endocrinologica, suppl. 2: 117, 1989

48. Salvi M, Zhang Z-G, Haigert D et al: Patients with endocrine ophthalmopathy not associated with overt thyroid disease have multiple thyroid immunologic abnormalities. J Clin Endocrinol Metab 70:89, 1990

49. Mullin BR: Dysthyroid exophthalmos. p. 1077. In: Garner A, Clintworth GK (eds): Pathobiology of Ocular Disease: A Dynamic Approach, Pt B. Marcel Dekker, New York, 1982

50. Kriss JP, McDougall IR, Donaldson SS: Graves's ophthalmopathy. p. 104. In: Krieger DT, Bardin CW (eds): Current Therapy in Endocrinology. Marcel Decker, Philadelphia, 1983

51. Day RM: Extraocular muscle problems associated with Graves' disease: clinical evaluation and diagnosis. Ophthalmology 86:2051, 1979

52. Weetman AP: Thyroid-associated eye disease: pathophysiology. Lancet 338:252, 1991

53. Kendall-Taylor P, Etkinson S, Holcombe M: Aspecific IgG in Graves' ophthalmopathy and its relation to retro-orbital and thyroid autoimmunity. Brit Med J 288:1183, 1984

54. Rotella CM, Zonefrati R, Toccafondi R et al: Ability of monoclonal antibodies to the thyrotropin receptor to increase collagen synthesis in human fibroblasts: an assay which appears to measure exophthalmogenic immunoglobulins in Graves' sera. J Clin Endocrinol Metab 62:357, 1986

55. Ahmann A, Baker JR, Waitman AP et al: Antibodies to porcine eye muscle in patients with Graves' ophthalmopathy: identification of serum immunoglobulins directed against unique determinants by immunoblotting and enzyme-linked immunosorbent assay. J Clin Endocrinol Metab 64:454, 1987

56. Bahn RS, Gorman CA, Woloschak GE et al: Human retro-ocular fibroblasts *in vitro*: a model for the study of Graves' ophthalmopathy. J Clin Endocrinol Metab 65:665, 1987

57. Hiromatsu Y, Fukazawa H, Guinard F et al: A thyroid cytotoxic antibody that cross-reacts with an eye muscle cell surface antigen may be the cause of thyroid-associated ophthalmopathy. J Clin Endocrinol 67:565, 1988

58. Atkinson S, Holcomb M, Kendall-Taylor P: Ophthalmic immunoglobulin in patients with Graves' ophthalmopathy. Lancet 2:374, 1984

59. Perros P, Kendall-Taylor P: Antibodies to orbital tissues in thyroid-associated ophthalmopathy. Acta Endocrinologica 126:137, 1992

60. Salvi M, Miller A, Wall JR: Human orbital tissue and thyroid membranes express a 74-kDa protein which is recognized by autoantibodies in the serum of patients with thyroid associated ophthalmopathy. FEBS Lett 232:135, 1988

61. Boucher A, Zang ZG, Bernard N et al: Immunoprecipitation of eye muscle cell membrane antigens and two-dimension gel electrophoresis confirm the importance of a 64-kd eye muscle antigen in thyroid-associated ophthalmopathy. p. 357. In Gordon A, Gross J, Hennemann G (eds): Progress in Thyroid Research. A. Balkema, Rotterdam, 1991

61a. Wall JR, Hayes M, Scalise D et al: Native gel electrophoresis and isoelectric focusing of a 64-kilodalton eye muscle protein shows that it is an important target for serum autoantibodies in patients with thyroid-associated ophthalmopathy and not expressed in other skeletal muscle. J Clin Endocrinol Metab 80;1226, 1995

62. Weightman D, Kendall-Taylor P: Cross-reaction of eye muscle antibodies with thyroid tissue in thyroid-associated ophthalmopathy. J Endocrinol 122:201, 1989

63. Dong R, Ludgate M, Vassart G: Cloning and sequencing of a novel 64-kDa autoantigen recognized by patients with autoimmune thyroid disease. J Clin Endocrinol Metab 72:1375, 1991

64. Kendler DL, Rootman J, Huber GK, Davies TF: A 64-kDa membrane antigen is a recurrent epitope for natural autoantibodies in patients with Graves' thyroid and ophthalmic disease. Clin Endocrinol 35:539, 1991

65. Tandon N, Yan SL, Arnold K et al: Immunoglobulin class and subclass distribution of eye muscle and fibroblast antibodies in patients with thyroid-associated ophthalmopathy. Clin Endocrinol 40:629, 1994

66. Feliciello A, Porcellini A, Ciullo I et al: Expression of thyrotropin-receptor mRNA in healthy and Graves' disease retro-orbital tissue. Lancet 342:337, 1993

67. Heufelder AE, Dutton CM, Bahn RS: Detection of TSH receptor RNA in cultured retro-ocular fibroblasts from patients with Graves' ophthalmopathy and pretibial myxedema. Thyroid 3:297, 1993

68. Endo T, Ikeda M, Ohmori M et al: Single subunit structure of the human thyrotropin receptor. Biochem Biophys Res Commun 187:887, 1992

69. Bahn RS, Dutton CM, Heufelder AE, Sarkar G: A genomic point mutation in the extracellular domain of the thyrotropin receptor in patients with Graves' ophthalmopathy. J Clin Endocrinol Metab 78:256, 1994

69a. Cuddihy RM, Dutton CM, Bahn RS: A polymorphism in the extracellular domain of the thyrotropin receptor is highly associated with autoimmune thyroid disease in females. Thyroid 5:89,1995

69b. Davies TF: Editorial, the thyrotropin receptors spread themselves around. J Clin Endocrinol Metab 79:1232, 1994

70. Burch HB, Sellitti D, Barnes SG et al: Thyrotropin receptor antisera for the detection of immunoreactive protein species in retroocular fibroblasts obtained from patients with Graves' ophthalmopathy. J Clin Endocrinol Metab 78:1384, 1994

71. Paschke R, Elisei R, Vassart G, Ludgate M: Lack of evidence supporting the presence of mRNA of the thyrotropin receptor in extra-ocular muscle. J Endocrinol Invest 16:329, 1993

71a. Paschke R, Metcalfe A, Alcalde L et al: Presence of nonfunctional thyrotropin receptor variant transcripts in retroocular and other tissues. J Clin Endocrinol Metab 79:1234, 1994

72. McLachlan SM, Prummel MF, Rapoport B: Cell-mediated or humoral immunity in Graves' ophthalmopathy? Profiles of T-cell cytokines amplified by polymerase chain reaction from orbital tissue. J Clin Endocrinol Metab 78:1070, 1994

73. Sisson JC: Mechanisms by which retrobulbar fibroblasts are stimulated by lymphocytes: role of cyclic nucleotide. Proc Soc Exp Biol Med 154:386, 1977

74. Sisson JC, Kothary P, Kirchick H: The effects of lymphocytes, sera, and long-acting thyroid stimulator

from patients with Graves' disease on retrobulbar fibroblasts. J Clin Endocrinol Metab 37:17, 1973

75. Weightman AP, So AK, Warner CA et al: Immunogenetic markers in Graves' ophthalmopathy. Clin Endocrinol 28:619, 1988

76. Kendall-Taylor P, Stephenson A, Stratton A et al: Differentiation of autoimmune ophthalmopathy from Graves' hyperthyroidism by analysis of genetic markers. Clin Endocrinol 28:601, 1988

77. Ratanachaiyavong S, Demaine AG, Campbell RD, McGregor AM: Heat shock protein 70 (HSP70) and complement C4 genotypes in patients with hyperthyroid Graves' disease. Clin Exp Immunol 84:48, 1991

78. Heufelder AE, Goellner JR, Wenzel BE, Bahn RS: Immunohistochemical detection and localization of a 72-kilodalton heat shock protein in autoimmune thyroid disease. J Clin Endocrinol Metab 74:724, 1992

79. Tanaka K, Hiromatsu Y, Sato M et al: Localization of the heat shock protein in orbital tissue from patients with Graves' ophthalmopathy using in situ hybridization. Life Sc 54:355, 1994

80. Heufelder AE, Wenzel BE, Bahn RS: Cell surface localization of a 72-kilodalton heat shock protein in retro-ocular fibroblasts from patients with Graves' ophthalmopathy. J Clin Endocrinol Metab 74:732, 1992

81. Heufelder AE, Wenzel BE, Bahn RS: Methimazole and propylthiouracil inhibit the oxygen free radical-induced expression of a 72-kilodalton heat shock protein in Graves' retroocular fibroblasts. J Clin Endocrinol Metab 74:737, 1992

81a. Hiromatsu Y, Tanaka K, Ishisaka N et al: Human histocompatibility leucocyte antigen-DR and heat shock protein-70 expression in eye muscle tissue in thyroid-associated ophthalmopathy. J Clin Endocrinol Metab 80:685, 1995

82. Hagg E, Asplund K: Is endocrine ophthalmopathy related to smoking? Brit Med J 295:634, 1987

83. Bartalena L, Martino E, Marcocci C et al: More on smoking habits and Graves' ophthalmopathy. J Endocrinol Invest 12:733, 1983

84. Shine B, Fells P, Edwards OM, Waitman AP: Association between Graves' ophthalmopathy and smoking. Lancet 335:1261, 1990

85. Prummel MF, Wiersinga WM: Smoking and risk for Graves' disease. JAMA 269:479, 1993

86. Metcalfe RH, Weetman AP: Stimulation of extraocular muscle fibroblasts by cytokines and hypoxia: possible role in thyroid-associated ophthalmopathy. Clin Endocrinol 40:67, 1994

87. Marcocci C, Bartalena L, Bogazzi F et al: Relationship between Graves' ophthalmopathy and type of treatment in Graves' hyperthyroidism. Thyroid 2:171, 1992

88. Bartalena L, Marcocci C, Bogazzi F et al: Use of corticoids to prevent progression of Graves' ophthalmopathy after radioiodine therapy for hyperthyroidism. N Engl J Med 321:1349, 1989

89. Tallstedt L, Lundell G, Torring O et al: Occurrence of ophthalmopathy after treatment for Graves' hyperthyroidism. N Engl J Med 326:1733, 1992

90. Wiersinga WM, Smit T, van der Gaag R, Koorneef L: Temporal relationship between onset of Graves' ophthalmopathy and onset of thyroidal Graves' disease. J Endocrinol Invest 11:615, 1988

91. Marcocci C, Bartalena L, Bogazzi F et al: Studies on the occurrence of ophthalmopathy in Graves' disease. Acta Endocrinol (Copenh) 120:473, 1989

92. Sridama V, DeGroot L: Treatment of Graves' disease and the course of ophthalmopathy. Am J Med 87:70, 1989

93. Hamilton HE, Schultz RD, DeGowin EL: The endocrine eye lesion in hyperthyroidism. Arch Intern Med 105:675, 1960

94. Gamblin GT, Harper DG, Galentine P et al: Prevalence of increased intra-ocular pressure in Graves' disease: evidence of frequent subclinical ophthalmopathy. N Engl J Med 308:420, 1983

95. Werner SC, Coleman DJ, Franzen LA: Ultrasonographic evidence of consistent orbital involvement in Graves' disease. N Engl J Med 290:1447, 1974

96. Amino N, Yuasa T, Yaba Y et al: Exophthalmos in autoimmune thyroid disease. J Clin Endocrinol Metab 51:1232, 1980

97. Hales IB, Rundle FF: Ocular changes in Graves' disease. Q J Med 29:113, 1960

98. Perros P, Cromble AL, Matthews JNS, Kendall-Taylor P: Age and gender influence the severity of thyroid-associated ophthalmopathy: a study of 101 patients attending a combined thyroid-eye clinic. Clin Endocrinol 38:367, 1993

98a. Perros P, Crombie AL, Kendall-Taylor P: Natural history of thyroid associated ophthalmopathy. Clin Endocrinol 42:45, 1995

99. Aranow H, Day RM: Management of thyrotoxicosis in patients with ophthalmopathy: antithyroid regimen primarily by ocular manifestations. J Clin Endocrinol Metab 25:1, 1965

100. Gwinup G, Elias AN, Ascher MS: Effect on exophthalmos of various methods of treatment of Graves' disease. JAMA 247:2135, 1982

101. Kriss JP, Pleshakov V, Rosenblum AL et al: Studies on the pathogenesis of the ophthalmopathy of Graves' disease. J Clin Endocrinol Metab 27:582, 1967

102. Kung AWC, Yau CC, Cheng A: The incidence of ophthalmopathy after radioiodine therapy for Graves' disease: prognostic factors and the role of methimazole. J Clin Endocrinol Metab 79:542, 1994

103. Choudhury AR: Pathogenesis of unilateral proptosis. Acta Ophthalmologica 55:273, 1977

104. Bydder GM, Steiner RE, Young IR et al: Clinical NMR scanning of the brain: 140 cases. Am J Nucl Res 3:459, 1982

105. Markl AF, Hilberts TH, Mann K: Graves' ophthalmopathy: standardized evaluation of computed tomography examinations and magnetic resonance imaging. Dev Ophthalm 20:38, 1989

106. Forbs G: Computerized imaging evaluation: CT and NMR scanning and computed volume measurement. p. 173. In Gorman CA, Waller RR, Dyer JA (eds): The Eye and Orbit in Thyroid Disease. Raven Press, New York, 1984

107. Hiromatsu Y, Kojima K, Ishiska N et al: Role of magnetic resonance imaging in thyroid-associated ophthalmopathy: its predictive value for therapeutic outcome of immunosuppressive therapy. Thyroid 2: 299, 1992

108. Dallow RL, Momose KJ, Weber AL, Wray SH: Comparison of ultrasonography, computerized tomography (EMI scan), and radiographic techniques in evaluation of exophthalmos. Trans Am Acad Ophthalmol Ontolaryngol 81:305, 1976

109. Ossoinig KC: Ultrasonic diagnosis of Graves' ophthalmopathy. p. 185. In Gorman CA, Waller RR, Dyer JA (eds): The Eye and Orbit in Thyroid Disease. Raven Press, New York, 1984

110. Gorman CA: The presentation and management of endocrine ophthalmopathy. J Clin Endocrinol Metab 7:67, 1978

111. Grove A Jr: Evaluation of exophthalmos. N Engl J Med 292:1005, 1975

112. Ouwerkerk BM, Wijngaarde R, Hennemann G et al: Radiotherapy of severe ophthalmic Graves' disease. J Endocrinol Invest 8:241, 1985

113. Prummel MF, Mourits MP, Berghout A et al: Prednisone and cyclosporin in the treatment of severe Graves' ophthalmopathy. N Engl J Med 321:1353, 1989

114. Ivy HK: Medical approach to ophthalmopathy of Graves' disease. Mayo Clin Proc 47:980, 1972

115. Waller RR, Samples JR, Yeatts RP: Eyelid malpositions in Graves' ophtlmopathy. p. 263. In Gorman CA, Waller RR, Dyer JA (eds): The Eye and Orbit in Thyroid Disease. Raven Press, New York, 1984

116. Burrow GN, Mitchell MS, Howard RO, Morrow LB: Immunosuppressive therapy for the eye changes of Graves' disease. J Clin Endocrinol 31:307, 1970

117. Bigos ST, Nisula BC, Daniels GH et al: Cyclophosphamide in the management of advanced Graves' ophthalmopathy. Ann Intern Med 90:921, 1979

118. Dandona P, Marshall NJ, Bidey SP et al: Successful treatment of exophthalmos and pretibial myxedema with plasmapheresis. Br Med J 1:374, 1979

119. Kelly W, Longson D, Smithard D et al: An evaluation of plasma exchange for Graves' ophthalmopathy. Clin Endocrinol 18:485, 1983

120. Perros P, Weightman DR, Crombie AL, Kendall-Taylor P: Azathioprine in the treatment of thyroid-associated ophthalmopathy. Acta Endocrinol 122:8, 1990

121. Chang TC, Kao SCS, Huang KM: Octreotide and Graves' ophthalmopathy and pretibial myxedema. Brit Med J 304:158, 1992

122. Kennerdell J: The selection of patients for orbital decompression. Thyroid 2, suppl. 1:S12, 1992

123. Garrity J, Faturechi V, Bergstrahl E et al: Results of transantral orbital decompression in 428 patients with severe Graves' ophthalmopathy. Am J Ophthalmol 116:533, 1993

124. Gorman CA, Waller RR, Dyer JA. (eds): The Eye and Orbit in Thyroid Disease. p. 221. Raven Press, New York, 1984

125. Gedda O, Lindgren M: Pituitary and orbital röntgentherapy in the hyperophthalmopathic type of Graves' disease. Acta Radiologica (Stockh) 42:211, 1954

126. Horst W, Sautter H, Ullerich K: Radiojoddiagnostik und Strahlentherapie der endokrinen Ophthalmopathie. Dtsch Med Wochenschr 85:730, 1960

127. Donaldson SS, Bagshaw MA, Kriss JP: Supervoltage orbital therapy for Graves' ophthalmopathy. J Clin Endocrinol Metab 37:276, 1973

128. Teng CS, Crombie AL, Hall R, Ross W: An evaluation of supervoltage orbital irradiation for Graves' ophthalmopathy. Clin Endocrinol 13:545, 1980

129. Peterson IA, Kriss JP, McDougall IR, Donaldson SS: Prognostic factors in the radiotherapy of Graves' ophthalmopathy. Int J Radiat Oncol Biol Phys 19: 259, 1990

130. Bartalena L, Marcocci C, Chiovato L et al: Orbital cobalt irradiation combined with systemic corticoids for Graves' ophthalmopathy: comparison with systemic corticosteroids alone. J Clin Endocrinol Metab 56:1139, 1983

131. DeGroot LJ, Gorman CA, Pinchera A et al: Therapeutic controversies: radiation and Graves' ophthalmopathy. J Clin Endocrinol Metab 80;339, 1995

132. Bauer FK, Catz B: Radioactive iodine therapy for progressive malignant exophthalmos. Acta Endocrinol 51:15, 1966

133. Werner SC, Feind CR, Aida M: Graves' disease and total thyroidectomy: progression of severe eye changes and decrease in serum long-acting thyroid stimulator after operation. N Engl J Med 276:132, 1967

134. Volpe R, Desbarats ML, Schonbaum E et al: The effect of radioablation of the thyroid gland in Graves' disease with high levels of long-acting thyroid stimulator (LATS). Am J Med 46:217, 1969

135. Prummel MF, Mourits MP, Berghout A et al: Randomized double-blind trial of prednisone versus radiotherapy in Graves' ophthalmopathy. Lancet 342: 949, 1993

136. Prummel MF, Suttorp-Schulten MSA, Wiersinga WM et al: A new ultrasonographic method to detect disease activity and predict response to immunosuppressive treatment in Graves' ophthalmopathy. Ophthalmology 100:556, 1993

137. Postema PTE, Krenning EP, Wijngaarde R et al: [111In-DTPA-D-Phe1] octreotide scintigraphy in thyroidal and orbital Graves' disease: a parameter for disease activity. J Clin Endocrinol Metab 79:1845, 1994

137a. Utech CI, Khatibnia U, Winter PF, Wulle KG: MR T2 relaxation time for the assessment of retrobulbar inflammation in Graves' ophthalmopathy. Thyroid 5;185, 1995

138. Diamond MT: The syndrome of exophthalmos, hypertrophic osteoarthropathy, and localized myxedema: a review of the literature and report of a case. Ann Intern Med 50:206, 1959

139. Gimlette TMD: Thyroid acropachy. Lancet 1:22, 1960

140. Bull RH, Coburn PR, Mortimer PS: Pretibial myxoedema: a manifestation of lymphoedema? Lancet 341:403, 1993

141. Siegler M, Refetoff S: Pretibial myxedema: a reversible cause of foot drop due to entrapment of the peroneal nerve. N Engl J Med 294:1383, 1976

142. Gabrilove JL, Alvarez AS, Churg J: Generalized and localized (pretibial) myxedema: effect of thyroid analogues and adrenal glucocorticoids. J Clin Endocrinol Metab 30:825, 1960

143. Sisson JC: Hyaluronic acid in localized myxedema. J Clin Endocrinol Metab 28:433, 1968

144. Shishiba Y, Tanaka T, Ozowa Y et al: Chemical characterization of high buoyant density proteoglycan accumulated in the affected skin of pretibial myxedema of Graves' disease. Endocronol Jpn 33:395, 1986

145. Korting GW, Nürenberger F, Müller G: Zur ultrastruktur der Bindegewebszellen beim Myxoedema zircumscriptum praetibiale. Arch Clin Exp Dermatol 229:381, 1967

146. Konrad K, Brenner W, Hamberger H: Ultrastructural and immunological findings in Graves' disease with pretibial myxedema. J Cutan Pathol 7:99, 1980

147. Ishii M, Nakagawa K, Hamada T: An ultrastructural study of pretibial myxedema utilizing improved ruthenium red stain. J Cutan Pathol 11:125, 1984

148. Diederichsen J, Heydenreich G, Nielsen OS: Long-acting thyroid stimulator (LATS) and immunofluorescent studies in patients with pretibial myxoedema. Dan Med Bull 20:188, 1973

149. Schermer DR, Roenigk HH Jr, Schumacher OP et al: Relationship of long-acting thyroid stimulator to pretibial myxedema. Arch Dermatol 102:62, 1970

150. Hanke CW, Bergfeld WF, Guirguis MN, Lewis LJ: Hyaluronic acid synthesis in fibroblasts of pretibial myxedema. Cleve Clin Q 50:129, 1983

151. Cheung HS, Nicoloff JT, Kamiel MB et al: Stimulation of fibroblast biosynthetic activity by serum of patients with pretibial myxedema. J Invest Dermatol 71:12, 1978

152. Tao T-W, Leu S-L, Kriss JP: Biologic activity of autoantibodies associated with Graves' dermopathy. J Clin Endocrinol Metab 69:90, 1989

153. Shishiba Y, Takeuchi Y, Yokoi N et al: Thyroid hormone excess stimulates the synthesis of proteoglycan in human skin fibroblasts in culture. Acta Endocrinol 123:541, 1990

154. Heufelder AE, Wenzel BE, Gorman CA, Bahn RS: Detection, cellular localization, and modulation of heat shock proteins in cultured fibroblasts from patients with extra-thyroidal manifestations of Graves' disease. J Clin Endocrinol Metab 73:739, 1991

155. Smith TJ, Bahn RS, Gorman CA: Connective tissue, glycosaminoglycans, and diseases of the thyroid. Endocrine Rev 10:366, 1989

156. Kriss J, Pleshakov V, Rosenblum A, Sharp G: Therapy with occlusive dressings of pretibial myxedema with fluocinolone acetonide. J Clin Endocrinol Metab 27:595, 1967

157. Volden G: Successful treatment of chronic skin disease with clobetasol propionate and a hydrocolloid occlusive dressing. Acta Derm Venorol 72:69, 1992

158. Kriss JP: Pathogenesis and treatment of pretibial myxedema. Endocrinol Metab Clin N Am 16:409, 1987

159. Merillon JP, Passa P, Chastre J et al: Left ventricular function and hyperthyroidism. Brit Heart J 46:137, 1982

160. Channick BJ, Adlin EV, Marks AD et al: Hyperthyroidism and mitral-valve prolapse. N Engl J Med 305:497, 1981

161. Burstein J, Lamberg B-A, Erämaa E: Myocardial infarction in thyrotoxicosis. Acta Med Scand 166:379, 1960

162. Littman DS, Jeffers WA, Rose E: The infrequency of myocardial infarction in patients with thyrotoxicosis. Am J Med Sci 233:10, 1957

163. Sandler G, Wilson GM: Thyrotoxic heart disease. Q J Med 28:347, 1959

164. Nakazawa HK, Sakurai K, Hamada N et al: Management of atrial fibrillation in the post-thyrotoxic state. Am J Med 72:903, 1982

165. Rohmer V, Hocq R, Galland F et al: Hyperthyreoidie fruste révélée par un trouble du rythme auriculaire. Press Med 13:145, 1984

166. Summers VK, Surtees SJ: Thyrotoxicosis and heart disease. Acta Med Scand 169:661, 1961

167. Ikram H: The nature and prognosis of thyrotoxic heart disease. Q J Med 54:19, 1985

168. Toft P, Botker HE: Congestive heart failure in thyrotoxicosis. Int J Card 18:444, 1988

169. Featherstone HJ, Stewart DK: Angina in thyrotoxicosis: thyroid-related coronary artery spasm. Arch Int Med 143:554, 1983

170. Proskey MD, Saksina T, Towne WD: Myocardial infarction associated with thyrotoxicosis. Chest 72:109, 1977

171. Resenkov L, Falicov R: Thyrotoxicosis and lactate-producing angina pectoris with normal coronary arteries. Br Heart J 39:1051, 1977

172. Kotler N, Kyriakos M, Bouchard J, Warbasse JR: Myocardial infarction associated with thyrotoxicosis. Arch Intern Med 132:723, 1973

173. Wei JY, Genecin A, Greene HL, Achuff SC: Coronary spasm with ventricular fibrillation during thyrotoxicosis: response to attaining euthyroid state. Am J Card 43:335, 1979

174. Saphiro O: Myocarditis: a general review with an analysis of 240 cases. Arch pathol 33:88, 1942

175. Sachs RN, Vinio M, Modigliani E et al: Absence de lesions histologics ultra-structurales du myocarde dans l'insufficence cardiac the l'hyperthyreoidie. Ann Med Intern (Paris) 137:375, 1980

176. Symons C, Richardson PJ, Wood JB: Unusual presentation of thyrocardiac disease. Lancet II:1163, 1971

177. Ladenson PW: Thyrotoxicosis and the heart: something old and something new. Editorial. J Clin Endocrinol Metab 77:332, 1993

178. Biondi B, Fazio S, Carella C et al: Cardiac effects of long-term thyrotropin-suppressive therapy with levothyroxine. J Clin Endocrinol Metab 77:334, 1993

179. Sawin LT, Geller A, Wolf PhA et al: Low serum thyrotropin concentrations as a risk factor for atrial fibrillation in older persons. N Engl J Med 331:1249, 1994

179a.Fazio S, Biondi B, Carella C et al: Diastolic dysfunction in patients on thyroid-stimulating hormone suppressive therapy with levothyroxine: beneficial effect of β-blockade. J Clin Endocrinol Metab 80:2222, 1995

180. Lamberg B-A, Hernberg CA, Whalberg P, Hakkila R: Treatment of toxic nodular goiter with radioactive iodine. Acta Med Scand 165:245, 1959

181. Likoff WB, Lavine SA: Thyrotoxicosis as a sole cause of heart failure. Am J Med Sci 206:425, 1943

Thyrotoxicosis of Other Etiologies

13

Thyrotoxicosis is defined as the situation in which increased levels of thyroid hormone in the serum lead to biochemical and/or clinical signs of excess thyroid hormone at the tissue level. In other words, the mere presence of increased levels of total and free thyroid hormone is not sufficient for the diagnosis of thyrotoxicosis. For instance, in resistance to thyroid hormone, increased thyroid hormone levels occur even when euthyroidism or sometimes even hypothyroidism is present (see Ch. 16). Increased serum levels of thyroid hormone may result from overproduction of thyroid hormone or leakage of stored iodothyronines due to thyroid gland damage but may also be caused by unintentional or deliberate overingestion of thyroid hormone. A very common cause of thyrotoxicosis is Graves' disease (described in Ch. 12). In this chapter we describe a variety of other causes of the syndrome.

TOXIC ADENOMA

A toxic adenoma of the thyroid is an autonomously functioning thyroid nodule that produces supraphysiologic amounts of thyroid hormone leading to increased serum levels of triiodothyronine (T_3) and/or thyroxine (T_4) and suppression of serum thyroid-stimulating hormone (TSH). The normal thyroid tissue that surrounds the nodule is often atrophic when autonomy is long-standing.

Pathogenesis

Studer et al.[1,2] distinguishes two types of nodular goiter from the pathogenic point of view (i.e., a single nodule in the otherwise normal thyroid and a multinodular enlarged thyroid gland). A single nodule consists either of a true adenoma of monoclonal origin,[3–5] or is of the polyclonal type. Most single nodules are not true adenomas but of polyclonal origin.[6] Although monoclonal at the molecular level, the majority is histomorphologically heterogenous, probably by mechanisms that create phenotypic heterogeneity of growth and morphologic potential.[7] At the genetic level two types of autonomously functioning adenomas have recently been described. Lyons et al.[8] described a somatic mutation in the gene for the α-polypeptide of the G protein (Gsa) resulting in inhibition of GTPase activity and activation of adenylate cyclase in a autonomously functioning thyroid adenoma. O'Sullivan et al.[9] screened Gsa in thyroid adenomas for specific point mutations at codons 201 and 227 and identified such adenylate-activating mutations in 5 out of 13 autonomously functioning adenomas but in none of 16 nonfunctioning adenomas. In an experimental model, transgenic mice expressing the Gsα-subunit gene mutant at codon 201, expressed hyperfunctioning thyroid adenomas.[9a] Gsα expression in thyroid adenomas has recently been discussed in an editorial.[9b] Parma et al.[10] described another type of somatic mutation leading to hyperfunctioning thyroid adenomas. These mutations are present in the carboxy-terminal portion of the third cytoplasmic loop of the thyrotropin receptor (TSH-R) and involve codons 619 and 623; they were identified in 3 out of 11 hyperfunctioning adenomas. The mutant receptors confer constitutive activation of adenylate cyclase when tested by transfection in COS cells. Later, other mutations were reported at codons 631-632-633, located in the sixth transmembrane domain of the TSH-R.[11,12] Parma et al.[12a] completely sequenced exon number 10 of the TSH-R gene in toxic adenomas of eleven patients. Several mutations transfected into LDS. Cells showed not only adenylate cyclase activation, but also constitutive stimulation of the inositol phosphate-diacyglyserol cascade. They conclude that activating mutations of TSH-R constitute a major cause of toxic adenomas. Similarly Russo et al.[12b] screened 37 patients with autonomously functioning thyroid adenomas for mutations in exon 10. They found a mutation in codon 623 in 3 patients. In addition, 9 mutations were found when exon 0 and 9 of the Gsα gene were screened.

Note that the prefix *toxic* defines the adenoma from the *functional* point of view, that is, clinically and scintigraphically a single nodule in combination with biochemical changes and clinical signs of thyroid hormone overproduction. Before the availability of sensitive diagnostic tests, particularly the sensitive TSH assay, it was often necessary to establish the diagnosis of a toxic nodule by administering T_3 or T_4. Uptake in the nodule of radioactive iodine (RAI) or pertechnitate would not be suppressed by this maneuver. In addition, administration of exogenous TSH could cause uptake of isotope in the surrounding, previously suppressed thyroid tissue. Nowadays the presence of elevated serum free T_4 and T_3 levels, and suppressed serum TSH in combination with radionucleide uptake only in the nodule on scintiscan (Fig. 13-1), is sufficient for the diagnosis. Hyperfunc-

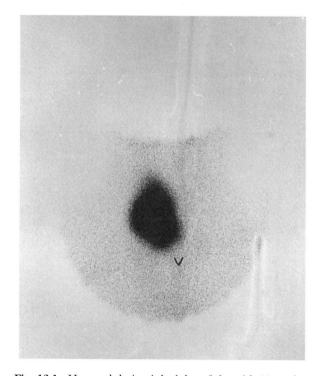

Fig. 13-1. Hot nodule in right lobe of thyroid. Note that uptake of radioactivity in the contralateral lobe is suppressed.

tion of a remnant of thyroid tissue—for instance, after thyroidectomy or after thyroiditis—is not excluded by these tests but is rare. To discriminate between these two possibilities, the presence of a thyroidectomy scar, careful history taking, and measurement of circulating thyroid autoantibodies may be helpful.

The functional development of a toxic adenoma of the thyroid is from a "warm" nodule to a "hot" nodule to a "toxic" nodule. A warm nodule is defined as a nodule that cannot scintigraphically be distinguished from the normal surrounding thyroidal tissue, whereas a hot nodule has more activity than the surrounding tissue. A nodule that is hot on scintiscan may not actually overproduce hormone, in which case serum TSH is still in the normal range and extranodular thyroid tissue is visible on the thyroid scan. The difference between a hot and a toxic nodule is that in the latter TSH is suppressed and there is typically no activity visible on the scan outside the nodule. It is unusual that an autonomously functioning thyroid nodule is toxic when the diameter is less than 3 cm.[13,14]

Epidemiology

Approximately 1 in 10 to 1 in 20 solitary nodules present with hyperthyroidism but this incidence may vary from country to country, being more common in Europe than in the United States.[13,15] The problem is five times more common in women than men. In a group of 349 patients with autonomous functioning thyroid nodules (AFTN), Hamburger found 18 percent to be toxic. The proportion of hyperthyroidism in AFTN was 33 percent in males, but only 17 percent in females.[13] Forty-eight percent of euthyroid subjects were 40 years or older, 57 percent were toxic, whereas this was the case only in 13 percent of patients younger than 60 years. Two hundred thirteen patients had nodules up to 2.5 cm in diameter; of these, only 1.9 percent were toxic, and all of these had a nodule with a diameter of 2.5 cm. In the remaining 136 patients with larger nodules, 42.6 percent were toxic. Of the 266 patients who were younger than 40 years, only 19.5 percent had nodules 3 cm in diameter or larger, whereas in the older patients this figure was 45.9 percent. These data underline the fact that larger AFTN occur in the older age group and that at the time of presentation, nodules less than 2.5 cm in diameter are rarely toxic.

The frequency of toxic adenoma in patients referred for thyrotoxicosis may vary considerably in different geographic areas. Percentages between 1.5 and 44.5 have been reported (Table 13-1). In Europe a female-to-male ratio of 5:1 was reported for toxic autonomous nodules.[16]

Natural History

Autonomously functioning nodules may stay the same, grow, degenerate, or become gradually toxic. In one series, 10 percent of patients became toxic within 6 years. Toxicity may develop independently of age but is much more common in nodules over 3 cm in diameter (up to 20 percent).[13] Using sonography in patients with AFTN, it was found that the critical volume at which hyperthyroidism occurs was 16 ml.[17] Table 13-2 shows changes in nodule size as observed in 159 patients followed from 1 to 15 years.[13] An increase in size was seen in only 10 percent. Four percent decreased in size. Loss of function was seen in four patients because of degeneration. Eight percent developed overt thyrotoxicosis in a mean follow-up period of three to five years. Three percent developed borderline hyperthyroidism (Table 13-3).

Pathology

On macroscopic examination, a solitary toxic nodule is surrounded by normal thyroid tissue that is functionally suppressed. Microscopically one would expect, on the basis of current ideas about pathogenesis, to see the picture of a true adenoma with uniform thyroid follicles without characteristics of malignancy. Studer et al.[1,2] found overwhelming evidence that hot nodules in so-called multinodular goiter appear occasionally to be "monoclonal" in function but usually are composed of heterogenous follicles of different sizes and different capacity to take up radioactive iodine (Fig. 13-2). Although such heterogeneity has been identified in multinodular goiters, it is apparent that also in isolated toxic adenoma multifunctional follicles appear to be present, as opposed to the monotonous picture seen in the less frequent monoclonal adenoma (Fig. 13-3). In addition, old hemorrhage, sometimes reflected by calcification, may be present in toxic adenomas. It has also been shown that on microscopic examination of a thyroid with a single toxic adenoma, autonomously functioning micronodules are often seen in

TABLE 13-1. Frequency of Toxic Adenoma in Various Countries

Location	Period	No. of Thyrotoxic Patients	Percent of Toxic Adenomas
Europe			
Austria	1966–1968	821	44.5
England	1948	107	3.7
Finland	1969	125	18
France			
Paris	1962	24	11.7
Marseille	1964	537	
Montpellier	1965–1967	240	24
Germany	1965	350	19.7
Greece	1968	686	9.5
Italy	1968	1,121	11.4
Switzerland	1967	—	33
General survey	1986	924	27.9[c]
North America			
Cleveland	1962	2,846[a]	1.6
New York	1944	2,431[b]	1.5
Rochester	1912	1,627	23.9
Rochester	1954–1965	215	15.8
Southfield MI	1961–1979	—	2
Australia			
Tasmania	1973[d]	88	17

[a] Graves' disease plus toxic adenomas.
[b] Thyrotoxicosis submitted to surgery.
[c] Patients under 50 years of age.
[d] Six years after bread iodination.
(From Orgiazzi,[81] with permission.)

TABLE 13-2. Correlation of Change in Nodule Size and Duration of Follow-up for Nontoxic AFTN Patients

Change in Nodule Size	Duration of Follow-up (yr)				
	1–2	3–4	5–6	7–15	Total
↑1 cm or more and became toxic	4	0	0	0	4
↑1 cm or more, euthyroid	3	1	0	5	9
↑1 cm or more, euthyroid, degeneration	1	0	1	0	2
No change	60	37	14	11	122
No change, degeneration	3	1	0	0	4
No change, toxic	5	2	3	0	10
↓1 cm or more	1	1	3	1	6
↑1 cm, transient toxicity, then ↓1 cm	2[a]	0	0	0	2
Total	79	42	21	17	159

↑, Nodule increased in size; ↓, nodule decreased in size.
[a] One additional patient presented with acute nodular enlargement and T_3 toxicosis, both of which subsided spontaneously.
(From Hamburder,[13] with permission.)

TABLE 13-3. Results of Follow-up of Untreated Patients with Nontoxic AFTN

Author	Country	Year	No. of Patients	Duration of Follow-up (yr) Range	Mean	Hyperthyroid	Borderline Hyperthyroid
McCormack	U.S.	1967	14	2.5–8.5	4.8	1	0
Silverstein	U.S.	1967	9	2–7	4	0	0
Miller	U.S.	1968	15	1–7	3	0	2
Burman	U.S.	1974	48	⅓–11.3	2	0	0
Blum	U.S.	1975	13	?		4	0
Hamburger	U.S.	1975	51	1–12	3.3	0	0
Hamburger	U.S.	Current	159	1–15	3.5	14	6
Lobo	Brazil	1965	5	½–3		1	1
Wiener	Netherlands	1979	58	1–11.8	4	6	1

(From Hamburger,[13] with permission.)

the extranodular tissue. This finding agrees with the thesis of Studer et al.[1,2] that the true adenoma is one end of a large spectrum of thyroid nodules growing from single follicular cells or tiny cell families, each replicating with an individual growth rate, whereas the grossly abnormal multinodular goiter is situated at the other end of the scale. Presumably the mutation in Gs or thyrotropic receptor (TSH-R) proteins described above are more apt to be present in solitary hyperfunctioning adenomas surrounded by normal tissue.

Clinical Presentation

Patients with toxic adenomas present with a lump in the neck, usually at least 3 cm in diameter, with/or without symptoms compatible with thyrotoxicosis. The symptoms of thyrotoxicosis do not differ from those other causes of thyrotoxicosis except that characteristics of Graves' disease, such as ophthalmic disease, pretibial myxedema, and acropachy, are not present. If so, coincidental occurrence of the two diseases may be present.[18] This coincidence is very rare.

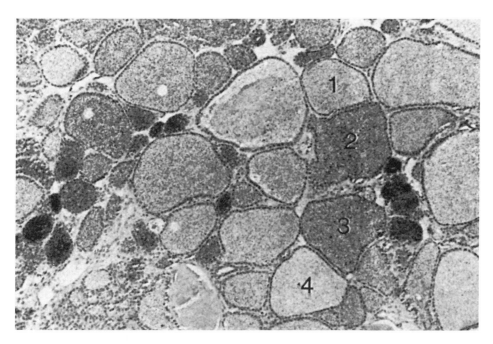

Fig. 13-2. Autoradiograph of a hot nodule illustrating areas with different capacity of uptake of radioactive iodine. (From Studer,[1] with permission.)

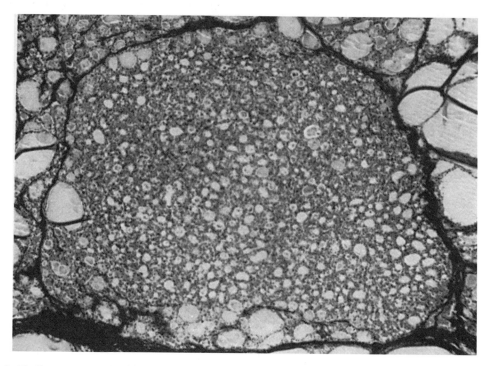

Fig. 13-3. Uniform nature of cells in a nodule formed by proliferation of only one or a few clones of epithelial cells. (From Studer,[2] with permission.)

Patients with toxic adenoma tend to be older than those with Graves' disease, and onset of thyrotoxicosis is generally slow. Many patients are aware of having a lump in the neck for some years, obviously having been nontoxic for a longer time. Nodules hardly ever are of such size that mechanical symptoms, other than a slight discomfort during swallowing, are present. Patients sometimes visit their doctor with cosmetic reasons as the primary complaint.

Laboratory Diagnosis

When clinical symptoms of thyrotoxicosis are evident and a single nodule within the thyroid area is clearly felt with little surrounding tissue on either side, it is theoretically sufficient to establish the diagnosis of a toxic nodule by the finding of a suppressed serum TSH value. However, to ascertain the severity of thyroid overactivity, measurement of a serum (free) T_4 and (when normal) of serum (free) T_3 is of great help and importance. As palpation of the thyroid area may give equivocal results, even where performed by experienced clinicians, it is wise to obtain a thyroid scan using either technetium 99m pertechnetate or iodine 123. The scan of a toxic nodule will show prominent uptake in the nodule with little or no uptake in surrounding thyroid tissue and will show appreciably less uptake in the surrounding tissue in the case of a hot nodule. As TcO_4 is not organified in thyroid tissue (in contrast to radioactive iodine), discrepancies are occasionally seen (Fig. 13-4). Rare nodules may be hot with TcO_4 but cold on scanning with radioactive iodine. In these situations the nodule should be considered to be cold and therefore potentially malignant. Therefore, if a nodule shows prominent activity with technetium, the scan should be repeated using ^{123}I.[19] This is not necessary, however, if TSH is suppressed, which indicates hyperthyroidism.

The presence of carcinoma in a toxic or hot nodule is rare. Horst et al.[16] found no thyroid malignancy in a study of 306 patients with AFTN. Sandler et al.[20] reviewed the literature on occurrence of carcinoma in a solitary hyperfunctioning nodule. They also concluded that the incidence of malignancy in a hot thyroid nodule is exceedingly low. Isolated cases of carcinoma development in a hot nodule have, however, been reported.[21,22] A recent study from the United States[23] reports the occurrence of

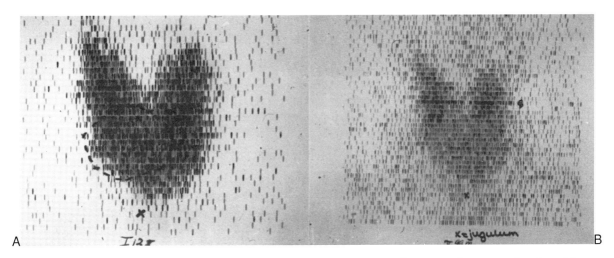

Fig. 13-4. Nodule in isthmus of the thyroid that is **(A)** "hot" on the sodium pertechnetate technetium 99m scan and **(B)** "cold" on the iodine 131 scan (right).

three carcinomas in 30 consecutive patients operated on for solitary hot nodules. Some authors suggest that occurrence of carcinoma in AFTN may be more than coincidental.[24] It is, however, generally felt that the presence of autonomous function is a reassuring characteristic with regard to the possible presence of thyroid carcinoma.

In a thyrotoxic patient with a solitary hot thyroid nodule in which the surrounding tissue is devoid of substantial uptake, the possibility of the presence of Graves' disease in remnant thyroid tissue (e.g., after previous thyroidectomy or in thyroid dysgenesis) is remote. The ultimate proof that surrounding tissue is suppressed but present can only be obtained after administration of TSH and subsequent scanning of the thyroid. However, this is virtually never required to establish the diagnosis. Ultrasound will often reveal a small contralateral thyroid lobe, as well as the dominant nodule, but again adds little to the evaluation. It is of little use to perform fine-needle aspiration in patients with toxic nodules because cytopathologic differentiation between adenoma and thyroid carcinoma is difficult, if not impossible. This will lead to a high proportion of false-positive cytologic diagnoses of follicular carcinoma.

When a hot nodule is present but there is still uptake of isotope in surrounding tissue and serum TSH is within normal limits, autonomous function of the nodule can be proven by administration of T_3 (4 × 25 μg T_3 per day for 10 days). After this, a repeat thyroid scan should show that the surrounding tissue is inactive because of suppressed serum TSH. However, this procedure has no practical consequences and is therefore unnecessary in clinical practice.

Treatment

As discussed in the previous section, the occurrence of malignancy in a hot or toxic nodule is rare. No active treatment is necessary for a hot nodule. The majority of patients remain euthyroid. Clinical observation and serum TSH measurements at intervals of 6 to 12 months are usually sufficient. Anecdotal observations indicate that sometimes, probably due to a hemorrhage in the adenoma, the nodule spontaneously resolves, or the nodule becomes cold on scan. Those nodules that grow and/or lead to overt thyrotoxicosis should be treated since thyrotoxicosis is generally permanent.

Long-term treatment of a toxic nodule with antithyroid drugs is useless, as relapse will almost invariably occur after discontinuation of medication. Three definitive forms of treatment are available: nodulectomy, treatment with radioactive iodine, and ethanol injection. There are advantages and disadvantages to the three approaches. The advantages of nodulectomy are rapid and permanent control of hyperthyroidism with a very low operative complication rate. Usually the patient is treated preoperatively by antithyroid drugs or, if mild thyrotoxicosis is present, by β-blocking agents. The incidence of hypothyroidism after operation is low, but surprisingly not zero. Thus, in a series of 60 patients operated on for autonomously functioning thyroid nodules, 4 (6.6 percent) became hypothyroid after operation. Two of these patients had received either therapeutic doses of ^{131}I or long-term treatment with antithyroid drugs.[25] In another series of patients, also treated surgically by unilateral lobectomy for toxic adenoma, 5 out of 35 became hypothyroid, though in 3 it was only temporary. It is difficult to see how patients become permanently hypothyroid even after hemilobectomy. No information is available, however, about the presence of circulating thyroid autoantibodies and macroscopic status of the contralateral lobe in these cases.[15] Generally it is believed that long-term suppression of the thyroid gland does not lead to permanent inactivation after suppression is relieved (Fig. 13-5). It seems more likely that coexistence of thyroid disease is the culprit. The disadvantages of surgery are the risks of general surgery and the expense as well as the residual scar.

Administration of ^{131}I is also a successful mode of treatment for patients with toxic adenoma (Fig. 13-6). The prevalence of hypothyroidism after treatment with radioactive iodine is reported to be absent or low in most publications. Ratcliffe et al.[26] report no hypothyroidism in 48 patients at 6 months after therapy. Also, at the same time after therapy, Ross et al.[27] report no hypothyroidism in 45 treated patients. However, when the observation period after treatment is longer, hypothyroidism may be documented. In one report[28] 23 patients were followed 4 to 16.5 years after treatment. Eight patients (36 percent) had become hypothyroid. The incidence of hypothyroidism was not related to nodule size, the level of thyroid function at therapy, or the total dose of ^{131}I administered. In 54 percent of patients, nodules were still palpable. In a similar study[29] 126 patients with hot nodules showed an incidence of hypothyroidism of 4.8 percent 10 years after ^{131}I treatment. Here also no relationship was found between the development of hypothyroidism, the size of the nodule, and the total amount of administered radioactivity. Hypothyroidism occurred in 9.7 percent of patients with a euthyroid hot nodule given ^{131}I, and in only 1.5 percent of patients with a toxic adenoma. When antithyroglobulin and/or antithyroid microsomal antibodies were present, the prevalence after 10 years was 18.0 percent versus 1.4 percent in antibody negative patients. From these

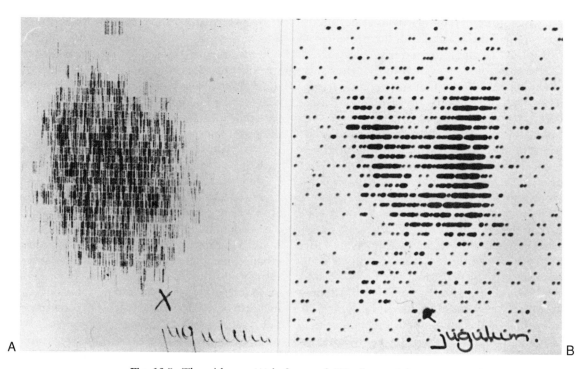

Fig. 13-5. Thyroid scan **(A)** before and **(B)** after nodulectomy.

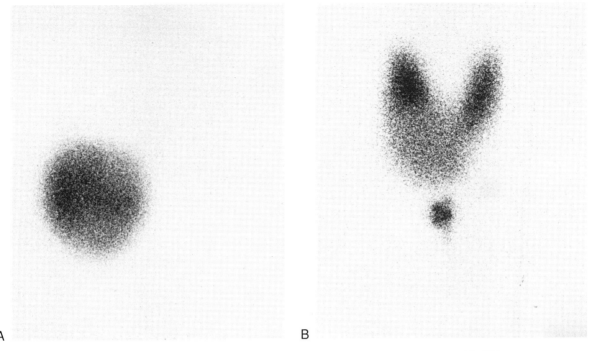

Fig. 13-6. Thyroid with toxic nodule (**A**) before and (**B**) after treatment with [131]I.

results it seems that longer follow-up periods may uncover hypothyroidism, and the prevalence of this may be related to the presence of thyroid autoantibodies and not so much to the size of the thyroid nodule and the ^{131}I dose administered. One possible method of inducing hypothyroidism occurs when patients are rendered euthyroid by treatment with antithyroid drugs before radioactive iodine. In this situation the TSH rises, and suppressed normal thyroid tissue resumes uptake of radioactive iodine and therefore is damaged by the isotope. Some authors administer T_3 for several days, prior to ^{131}I treatment, to be sure that the normal surrounding thyroid tissue is suppressed. It is also possible that high doses of ^{131}I in the nodule provide enough radiation to the surrounding tissue to seriously damage its function. The dose of radioactive iodine administered to patients with toxic nodules differs widely. Between 740 and 2,220 MBq may be administered, depending on the size and the percentage ^{131}I uptake of the nodule. [131]I doses in this range give thousands of rads to the normal tissue surrounding the nodule.

In our opinion, both treatment modalities will cure hot or toxic nodules. Both procedures are safe, but after operation less hypothyroidism may occur. We prefer ^{131}I treatment in general, except when the nodule is large (i.e., diameter 6 cm or more) or when patients are young, in which case operation is advised.

A recent development in the treatment of AFTN, used as an alternative to surgery or ^{131}I treatment, is percutaneous ethanol injection into the nodule under sonographic guidance.[30,31] The preliminary results seem promising. Euthyroidism is achieved in 80 to 85 percent of patients within 3 to 6 months after treatment. Usually injections are repeated three to eight times at weekly intervals. The treatment is generally well tolerated with few side effects.

Prognosis

The prognosis for the autonomous hot nodule is that most patients remain euthyroid and, as stated, clinical observation is sufficient. Whatever treatment is chosen in the case of a toxic nodule—surgery or radioactive iodine—most patients become and remain euthyroid after treatment. The long-term results after ethanol injection are not known yet. Long-term treatment with antithyroid drugs is not indicated. After treatment with ^{131}I and/or surgery, serum TSH measurements at yearly intervals are necessary to detect those patients, especially with circulating thyroid autoantibodies, that will eventually develop hypothyroidism. The occurrence of malignancy in an autonomous or toxic nodule is very rare, but the enlargement of a nodule after ^{131}I would raise this possibility.

TOXIC MULTINODULAR GOITER

Hyperthyroidism may occur in the multinodular thyroid gland, which is discussed in Chapter 17.

DE QUERVAIN'S (ACUTE OR SUBACUTE) THYROIDITIS

De Quervain's acute or subacute thyroiditis leads to temporary thyrotoxicosis in approximately half of the patients due to discharge of stored hormone from the thyroid gland. This disease is discussed in Chapter 19.

SILENT OR PAINLESS THYROIDITIS PRODUCING THYROTOXICOSIS

Although the terms *silent thyroiditis* and *painless thyroiditis* are most commonly used, other names have been given to this syndrome: hyperthyroiditis,[32] spontaneously resolving lymphocytic thyroiditis,[33] transient painless thyroiditis,[34] painless thyroiditis with transient hyperthyroidism,[35] painless subacute thyroiditis,[36] occult subacute thyroiditis,[37] atypical thyroiditis,[38] and transient thyrotoxicosis with lymphocytic thyroiditis.[39]

Incidence

The incidence of painless thyroiditis varies with time and with geography. A retrospective survey conducted in Wisconsin[34] from 1963 through 1977 showed that silent thyroiditis was not found until 1969 and was uncommon up to 1973. The frequency then increased so that silent hyperthyroidism was responsible for about 20 percent of all cases of thyrotoxicosis in this geographic area in the 1980s. In the 1980s a Japanese study[40] found an incidence of 10 percent, but in New York of only 2.4 percent.[41] Schneeberg[42] reported data obtained from a ran-

dom poll indicating silent thyroiditis was uncommon in Argentina, Europe, and the east and west coasts of the United States, but occurred more frequently around the Great Lakes and in Canada. Affected patients are mostly between 30 and 60 years and the female-to-male ratio is about 1.5:1. Our personal experience has been that the disease—apart from pregnancy—is currently rarely recognized.

Etiology

Although the disease was earlier argued to be a mild form of subacute (De Quervain's) thyroiditis, there is now overwhelming evidence that it should be categorized as a lymphocytic thyroiditis.[34,40] Its association with other autoimmune diseases supports the concept that this form of thyroiditis is an autoimmune disease.[43] No significant association has been found with viral infection. There is a significant association with human leukocyte antigen (HLA) genotype DR3. Postpartum thyroiditis (see below) is considered to be identical to silent thyroiditis from the phenomenologic point of view.[44] Here an association is found with HLA types DR3 and DR5.[45]

Pathology

Histologic examination reveals follicles to be disrupted and infiltrated predominantly by lymphocytes and by plasma cells. The infiltration is diffuse and/or focal, sometimes with the formation of lymphoid follicles. The follicular cells have a variable appearance. They can be cuboidal or columnar when stimulated by TSH. Some of the hypertrophied follicular cells have an oxyphilic cytoplasm and are therefore termed *Hürthle* or *Askanazy* cells. Thyroid tissue obtained during the hypothyroid or early recovery phase may show regenerating follicles with little colloid. At times persistent mild lymphocytic thyroiditis is seen, but the tissue may also return to normal in others. Extensive fibrosis may be present. Occasionally multinucleated giant cells, so characteristic of subacute thyroiditis, are observed. The histologic picture of postpartum thyroiditis is identical.

Clinical Presentation

A review[35] compiled the reported clinical manifestations between 1971 and 1980 of 112 patients with 122 episodes of silent thyroiditis. Sixty-eight were

TABLE 13-4. Presenting Symptoms in 52 Episodes of Hyperthyroidism

	No. of Patients
1. Nervousness	23
2. Weight loss	17
3. Palpitations	15
4. Heat intolerance	13
5. Fatigue/malaise	11
6. Hyperdefecation	9
7. Irritability	5
8. Headache	4
9. Insomnia	3
10. Increased appetite	3
11. Angina	2
12. Tremor	2
13. Weakness	2
14. Goiter/neck mass	2
15. Syncope	1
16. Myalgias/arthralgias	1

(From Wolff,[35] with permission.)

female, their mean $\pm$ SD age was 32.4 $\pm$ 18.5 years; the males' were 24.9 $\pm$ 8.2 years. In none of the 122 episodes of silent thyroiditis was thyroidal pain present. Recurrences were uncommon. Table 13-4 summarizes the presenting symptoms in 52 episodes of thyrotoxicosis. These symptoms are similar to those found from other causes of thyrotoxicosis and were mild to severe. The duration of the thyrotoxic phase was variable but for the most part lasted less than 1 year. Mean duration was 3.6 $\pm$ 2.0 (SD) months (range 1 to 12.5 months). Symptoms began 2.5 $\pm$ 2.2 months preceding the initial evaluation. This period is shorter than is usually seen with Graves' disease and certainly than that seen in multinodular toxic goiter. Exophthalmus and pretibial myxedema were absent, although symptoms such as lid lag due to increased sympathetic tone were present. In one patient the consistency of the thyroid was reported to be soft, but most authors described the gland as firm. Forty-three percent of patients had thyroid enlargement, which was generally symmetric, and enlargement was in most instances mild. Nodularity of the thyroid was uncommon. The clinical course of the disease often follows four sequential stages (Fig. 13-7): thyrotoxicosis, euthyroidism, hypothyroidism, and euthyroidism. Fifty-seven out of 112 patients became euthyroid and did not develop clinical hypothyroidism. After a brief period of euthyroidism, transient biochemical hypothyroidism developed in 17 patients. In 32 patients clinical hypothyroidism was present. This was temporary in 24 patients but 8 required thyroid hormone substitution.[35]

Laboratory Findings

During the first phase of the disease, discharge of hormone from the inflamed thyroid results in increases in serum T_4, T_3, and a decrease in serum TSH. At that time there is no uptake of radioactive iodine in the thyroid (Fig. 13-7). When the diagnosis of thyrotoxicosis factitia is suspected, estimation of serum thyroglobulin levels is useful. During ingestion of T_4, little or no thyroglobulin (TG) is present, whereas serum TG levels are elevated in silent thyroiditis. In 17 out of 71 patients with silent thyroiditis, moderate elevations of antithyroglobulin antibodies were also revealed by the tanned red cell hemagglutination assay.[35] Antimicrosomal antibodies were examined in 53 patients using the complement fixation test or by microsomal fluorescence. Using the former technique, 22 patients had positive antibodies, and by the latter 4 out of 7 were positive.[35] The recently developed radioimmunoassay (RIA) for human antithyroglobulin antibodies has greater sensitivity. In a small series of seven patients with silent thyroiditis, all were positive using this RIA.[46] Indicators of inflammation were not useful. The white blood cell count is generally normal. In 53 episodes, 34 had elevated erythrocyte sedimentation rate (ESR), but it was greater than 40 mm/hr in only 8.[35] This contrasts to the typical marked elevation of ESR in patients with subacute granulomatous thyroiditis and helps to differentiate the two conditions. During the acute phase, urinary iodine excretion is high-normal to elevated; after resolution of the thyroiditis, it is reduced to one-third of its original value.[33] As the first phase progresses, T_4 and T_3 levels decline into the euthyroid range (second phase) and reach subnormal levels in the hypothyroid range (third phase) in 40 percent of patients (Fig. 13-7). The erythrocyte sedimentation rate, if elevated, decreases gradually while TG levels decrease as well. After the third phase, patients gradually enter the euthyroid phase, heralded by an increase in thyroid hormone levels and resumption of thyroidal radioactive iodine. Uptake may temporarily rebound above normal before returning to normal values. Serum TSH starts to elevate at the end of the hypothyroid phase. The hypothyroid phase may last several

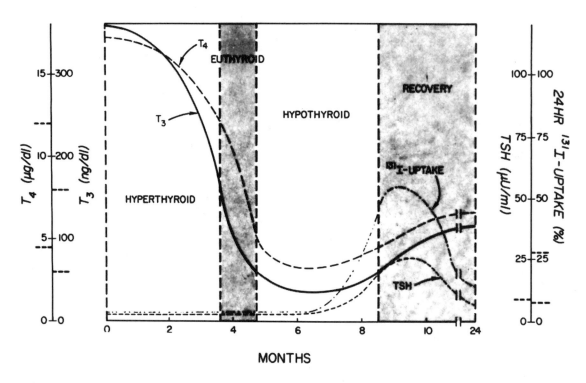

Fig. 13-7. Schematic representation of the four phases of silent thyroiditis. (From Wolff,[35] with permission.)

months. In 26 episodes, patients became euthyroid 6½ months after the onset of the hyperthyroid symptoms. Thyrotropin levels may increase during the recovery phase and can remain elevated for many months. The delayed increase of TSH (i.e., at the end of the hypothyroid phase) is due to TSH suppression during the thyrotoxic phase. This phenomenon is also usually seen after withdrawal of thyroid hormone in patients treated with supraphysiologic doses. The delay time ranges between 2 and 5 weeks.[47] Permanent hypothyroidism occurs in about 7 percent of patients with silent thyroiditis, but "cured" patients may ultimately become permanently hypothyroid (see following section).

Treatment

As thyrotoxicosis in silent thyroiditis is usually mild, treatment to relieve toxic symptoms is usually not necessary. If needed, β-adrenergic blocking agents can be administered. It is not useful to give antithyroid drugs because thyrotoxicosis is not the result of increased thyroid hormone synthesis but of discharge of thyroid hormone from the thyroid

gland due to the inflammatory process. The effect of propylthiouracil or iopanoic acid to block peripheral T_4 to T_3 conversion may be of some clinical benefit. If more serious thyrotoxicosis is present, administration of anti-inflammatory drugs may be of benefit. In this case prednisone can be administered in dosages ranging between 40 and 60 mg/d, which usually rapidly decreases the inflammation.[48] After 1 to 2 weeks the dose can be tapered by 7.5 to 10 mg/wk. In the case of relapsing thyroiditis it is rarely necessary to perform a subtotal thyroidectomy.[40] As an alternative, "thyroidectomy" may be induced by administration of radioactive iodine during a remission. After the thyrotoxic phase, many patients become temporarily hypothyroid (see Clinical Presentation). Often no thyroid substitution is necessary during this period. If it is, the dose should not completely compensate for the hypothyroidism, since a slight TSH elevation will facilitate thyroid recovery. Only a small proportion of patients remain permanently hypothyroid. In these patients, full substitution with L-thyroxine is necessary to keep serum TSH within the normal range. Patients apparently fully recovered from silent thyroiditis may ultimately develop thyroid failure. In a series of 54 patients, Nikolai et al.[49] reported that in about half of patients permanent hypothyroidism ensued. This is in contrast to subacute thyroiditis, which is followed in almost all patients by permanent recovery. Therefore patients with painless thyroiditis should be followed thereafter at yearly intervals with appropriate testing.

POSTPARTUM THYROIDITIS

As mentioned, postpartum thyroiditis is considered to be similar if not identical to silent (painless) thyroiditis.[35] This condition is discussed in Chapter 14.

HASHIMOTO'S THYROIDITIS

Occasionally Hashimoto's thyroiditis is accompanied by mild symptoms of thyrotoxicosis, especially in the early phases of the disease. This condition is discussed in Chapter 8.

THYROTOXICOSIS FACTITIA

Although factitious thyrotoxicosis involves all situations in which usage of (excessive doses) of thyroid hormone leads to symptoms of thyrotoxicosis, the term *factitious* is usually associated with surreptitious ingestion of thyroid hormone in supraphysiologic doses. Patients usually deny taking thyroid hormones in excess. This primarily psychiatric disorder may lead to wrong diagnosis and treatment if physicians are not aware of the phenomenon. Patients are clinically thyrotoxic; however, they do not show eye signs as seen in Graves' disease, except for those related to sympathetic overactivity (lid retraction). Deliberate intake of high doses of thyroid hormone leads to TSH suppression and shrinkage of the thyroid, so that no thyroid tissue is apparent when palpated. Serum TSH and the uptake of ^{123}I or TcO_4^- are suppressed. Thus, factitious thyrotoxicosis is not difficult to differentiate from thyrotoxic Graves' disease, toxic adenoma, or toxic multinodular goiter. In subacute (De Quervain's) thyroiditis, symptoms are typical in that apart from thyrotoxicosis patients may have fever in the initial phase of the disease and the thyroid is very tender. Silent thyroiditis, however, is not so easily distinguished from thyrotoxicosis factitia. In both situations the uptake of radioactive iodine is suppressed, and patients lack eye signs. However, in patients with silent thyroiditis, a palpable, firm, painless thyroid gland is present. Furthermore, patients with silent thyroiditis show high levels of thyroglobulin. In thyrotoxicosis factitia, excessive intake of thyroid hormone leads to suppression of TSH and therefore also to suppression of thyroglobulin leakage from the thyroid gland. Mariotti et al.[50] performed thyroglobulin measurements in six women with thyrotoxicosis factitia. They used a very sensitive TG assay and excluded the presence of TG antibodies, which can interfere with the assay. In all six women, thyroglobulin was undetectable in the serum (lower detection limit 1.25 ng/ml) (Table 13-5).

TABLE 13-5. Results of Thyroid-Function Tests in Patients with Thyrotoxicosis Factitia*

Patient No.	T₄	T₃	T₃ Resin Uptake	TSH	Thyro-globulin	24-Hr Radioiodine Uptake	Thyroid Microsomal Antibody Passive Hemag-glutination	Antithyroglobulin Antibody Passive Hemagglutination	Antithyroglobulin Antibody Radio-Assay
	μg/dl	ng/dl	%	μU/ml	ng/ml	%			
1	>18.0	>450	69.1	>0.6	>1.25	2.0	Negative	Negative	Negative
2	>18.0	410	60.9	>0.6	>1.25	2.0	Negative	Negative	Negative
3	11.5	262	53.6	>0.6	>1.25	3.0	Negative	Negative	Negative
4	>18.0	>450	74.0	>0.6	>1.25	2.0	Negative	Negative	Negative
5	>18.0	>450	72.3	>0.6	>1.25	1.0	Negative	Negative	Negative
6	14.7	ND	63.8	>0.6	>1.25	0.8	Negative	Negative	Negative
Normal	4.6–12.2	100–220	37–59	>0.6–6.0	>1.25–30	28–44	1:100	1:100	Negative

ND = not done.
(From Mariotti,[50] with permission.)

The possibility of this syndrome should be considered, especially when thyrotoxicosis appears to resist treatment or when laboratory data are contradictory. Patients may be persistent in denying the deliberate intake of thyroid hormone and persist in this attitude even after factitious thyrotoxicosis has been unequivocally confirmed. Consultation with a psychiatrist is urgently needed in such patients.

Suppressed radioactive uptake of the thyroid gland in combination with thyrotoxicosis may also exist in patients with hyperfunctioning metastases of follicular thyroid carcinoma. However, in these extremely rare patients, TG levels are almost invariably elevated and radioactive iodine uptake will be detected in metastases with whole-body scanning. Note that the profile of serum thyroid hormones in thyrotoxicosis factitia is determined by the composition of the preparation ingested. Both T_4 and T_3 are elevated in overdosage of L-thyroxine and desiccated thyroid, whereas only T_3 is elevated and T_4 is low or nondetectable when the patient is taking only preparations containing T_3. Treatment of thyrotoxicosis factitia is not difficult with regard to thyrotoxic symptoms, as discontinuation of thyroid hormone ingestion is usually sufficient. In more severe cases treatment with propranolol may be helpful. However, treatment of the psychiatric disorder is more challenging and may fail in the long run.

Thyrotoxicosis induced by excessive thyroid hormone intake that is not the deliberate choice of the patient has been observed in *hamburger thyrotoxicosis* patients. Two epidemics of thyrotoxicosis in the United States were caused by bovine thyroid in hamburger.[51,52] Inclusion of the thyroid in neck muscle trimmings is now prohibited by U.S. Department of Agriculture regulations. Prescription of supranormal amounts of thyroid hormone to suppress serum TSH for medical reasons can be designated as *iatrogenic* (usually subclinical) thyrotoxicosis. TSH suppression is usually given in patients after thyroidectomy for thyroid carcinoma and also to suppress benign thyroid growth in goiter patients. It is discussed further in the relevant chapters (Chs. 17 and 18). Long-term use of excessive amounts of thyroid hormone by patients may enhance osteoporosis and cause cardiac abnormalities, including arrhythmias and heart failure.[53–56b] For these reasons it is important to identify this condition and refer the patient for appropriate treatment.

THYROTOXICOSIS DUE TO PREGNANCY AND TROPHOBLASTIC DISEASE

Due to the intrinsic TSH-like activity of human chorionic gonadotrophin (hCG), many healthy euthyroid pregnant women have reduced serum TSH values. Gestational transient thyrotoxicosis (i.e., increased serum free T_4 and subnormal TSH) is seen in 1.4 percent of pregnant women, mostly when hCG levels are above 70,000 to 80,000 IU/l.[57] Thyrotoxicosis and other thyroid diseases during or after pregnancy are discussed in Chapter 14.

Thyrotoxicosis may be induced by hCG stimulation during molar pregnancy and also by trophoblastic tumors in males and in females. hCG is composed of an α-subunit, identical to the α-subunit in pituitary glycoprotein hormones such as luteinizing hormone (LH), follicle-stimulating hormone (FSH), and TSH, and a β-subunit that is specific for hCG. There is structural homology with the β-subunit of TSH; however, the β-hCG unit is larger in that it is composed of 147 amino acids, whereas that of TSH consists of 110 amino acids and has additional carbohydrate residues on the COOH terminus.

TSH-like Activity of hCG

Weak thyrotropic activity of hCG was found in hCG prepared from a urine sample taken during pregnancy, using a mouse thyrotropin bioassay.[58] In another study[59] hCG was purified from molar tissue and had intrinsic TSH bioactivity in the mouse bioassay, although 4,000 times less than that of human TSH on a molar basis. Despite this weak activity in hydatidiform mole disease, hCG is produced in sufficient amounts to induce hyperthyroidism. In a study of 20 patients[60] with gestational trophoblastic neoplasia, 2 patients were judged to be overtly thyrotoxic, and this was confirmed by elevated serum T_4 levels. These two patients had extremely high serum (3,220,000 IU/L and 6,720,000 IU/L) and urine hCG levels, which correlated closely with TSH-like activity exerted by the serum of these patients in a mouse thyroid bioassay. Patients with moderately (110,000 to 310,000 IU/L) increased serum hCG levels due to trophoblastic neoplasia were euthyroid. In studies using thyroids from different species to test for hCG intrinsic TSH activity, results showed that the mouse thyroid was much more sensitive to stimulation by hCG and that the human thyroid was relatively insensitive.[61] In another study on the activity of hCG on the human thyroid gland,[62] 1.0 IU hCG was found roughly equivalent to 0.27 μIU hTSH. Human luteinizing hormone (hLH) also has intrinsic thyroid-stimulating activity, but higher than hCG. One international unit hLH was found equivalent to 44 μIU hTSH. This lower potency of hCG is caused by its C-terminal extension of the β-subunit that interferes with its binding to the receptor. This extension is lacking in the β-subunit of hLH, its structure being otherwise almost identical to that of hCG.[63] Carboxy peptidase digestion of hCG, cleaving aminoacid residues 142–145 from the β-subunit, dramatically increases its capacity to stimulate adenylate cyclase in human thyroid membranes.[64] A variant of hCG, lacking the C-terminus of the β-subunit due to enzymatic cleavage, has been identified in pregnancy serum and molar tissue.[65] Human chorionic gonadotropin not only stimulated the mouse thyroid but also displaced human TSH from the plasma membrane receptor of follicular cells.[61,62,66] In studies using human thyroid membranes[67] or a cell line transfected with the human TSH receptor,[68]

desialylated forms of hCG exhibited stronger inhibition of TSH-mediated cAMP responses than native hCG. Both TSH binding and TSH-induced adenylate cyclase stimulation were found to be more effectively inhibited by desialylated variants of hCG than by unmodified hCG.[69] From these and other studies[69a] it seems that the biologic effect of hCG is predominantly confined to hCG containing little or no sialic acid. hCG has also been found to increase iodide uptake in cultured Fisher rat thyroid line (FRTL-5) cells and also causes a dose-related increment of adenylate cyclase activity and thymidine uptake.[70,71] Discrepant results regarding TSH-like activity of hHGC when tested in cell systems transported with the human TSH receptor, are not only explained on the basis of different grades of glycosylation of hHGC but also by different expression of the human TSH receptor in the various cell systems.[71a]

Clinical Features of Trophoblastic Disease

In 1955 Tisné and co-workers described a patient with molar pregnancy who had increased thyroidal uptake of radioactive iodine and clinical signs of hy-

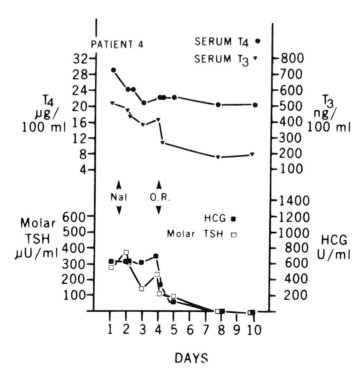

Fig. 13-8. The effect of 1 g of sodium iodide (NaI) and surgical removal of the molar tissue (OR) on the circulating levels of serum T₄, T₃, hCG (immunoassay) and TSH (bioassay) in a patient with hydatidiform mole–induced thyrotoxicosis. (From Higgins,[77] with permission.)

perthyroidism (cited by Hershman and Higgins[72]). Earlier reports[73–76] also described molar pregnancy in combination with hyperthyroidism. In all cases a rapid return to normal thyroid function occurred after removal of the mole. Figure 13-8 shows the effect of removing molar tissue on serum T_4, serum T_3, bioassayable TSH, and hCG (by immunoassay).[77] The patient was pretreated with iodide. After tumor removal serum T_4, T_3, serum TSH, and hCG levels rapidly normalized. From the parallellism of thyroid-stimulating and hCG activity it was concluded that the same molecule, (i.e., hCG) possessed both gonadotrophic and thyrotrophic activity. In another study[72] of two patients with hydatidiform mole with severe hyperthyroidism, the hyperthyroidism rapidly disappeared after removal of the mole. A thyroid stimulator was extracted from the serum of one patient that differed biologically and immunologically from TSH, from hCG found in normal placentas, and from thyroid-stimulating immunoglobulins. The conclusion that the molar thyrotropin differed from normal placenta hCG was based on differences in antigenic properties and molecular size. A recent study showed that hCG extracted from hyatidiform moles contained less sialic acid and was biologically more active than normal pregnancy hCG.[78] Figure 13-9 shows the relationship between bioassayable TSH and serum T_3 values in patients with molar pregnancy. In this study, with the exception of one patient, there is a very high correlation between the two parameters, suggesting a causal relationship between serum thyrotropin activity and thyroid function. A similar correlation between serum hCG levels and thyroid-stimulating activity in both serum and urine was found in two women who had widely metastatic choriocarcinoma and marked hyperthyroidism.[60] In another patient with gestational choriocarcinoma, serum thyroid-stimulating activity correlated precisely with serum T_4, with the β-subunit of human hCG, and with the quantitation of the host tumor burden.[79] The clinical syndrome of hyperthyroidism associated with choriocarcinoma in the male is extremely rare, but several reports have appeared in the literature. Orgiazzi et al.[80] cite four cases from the literature and reported a patient who had choriocarcinoma of the colon associated with gynecomastia and hyperthyroidism. Thyroid-stimulating activity, measured by mouse bioassay, was detected in the serum. Serum thyroid-stimulating activity was partly inactivated by antibovine TSH

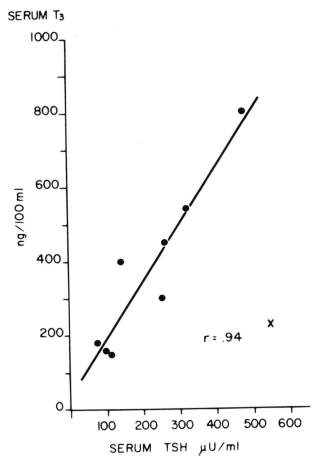

Fig. 13-9. Relationship between T_3 serum levels and bioassayable serum TSH activity in nine patients with hydatidiform mole–induced thyrotoxicosis. The correlation coefficient for eight patients (except x) is 0.94. (From Higgins,[77] with permission.)

antiserum but was completely neutralized by anti-hCG antiserum.

The clinical picture of patients with trophoblastic hyperthyroidism is that of thyrotoxicosis, lacking the characteristic features of Graves' disease, such as ophthalmic disease, pretibial myxedema, and acropatcy. hCG-levels are mostly above 300,000 U/L. The thyrotoxicosis is usually not severe because of its shorter duration.

Therapy

Obviously, removal of the tumor, if feasible, should be carried out as soon as possible. Treatment with antithyroid drugs does not produce euthyroidism rapidly, and patients are therefore also treated preoperatively with oral sodium ipodate, 1 g/d, or saturated potassium iodide, 2 drops every 6 hours, or sodium iodide, 0.1 g IV every 12 hours. Propranolol may be added to the regimen, and additional supportive therapy to replace fluids and electrolytes may be necessary. In patients who are not suitable for surgery because of metastatic disease, antithyroid drug treatment using propylthiouracil or methimazole in combination with chemotherapy is the best treatment available. If hyperthyroidism is so severe that development of thyroid crisis after surgery is possible, antithyroid drug treatment should be combined with iodide and propranolol pretreatment.

IODIDE-INDUCED THYROTOXICOSIS

The earliest report (1821) on thyrotoxicosis induced by administration of iodine is probably that of Coindet (cited by Orgiazzi and Mornex).[81] In 1859 Röser, cited by Hennemann,[82] noted that treating goiter with iodine could result in hyperthyroidism. He used the term *goiter cachexia* for this condition. Later the term *jodbasedow* was applied, although it should be realized that, in many instances, iodide-induced hyperthyroidism does not involve patients with incipient Basedow-Graves' disease. Multinodular goiter may also be rendered thyrotoxic by the administration of stable iodine. In their review on iodide-induced thyrotoxicosis Fradkin and Wolff[83] speculate that a decreased sensitivity to the Wolff-Chaikoff effect under conditions of moderate iodide excess would lead to iodide-induced thyrotoxicosis (IIT). The Wolff-Chaikoff effect (discussed in Ch. 5) involves blockade of iodide organification and hormone synthesis by high intrathyroidal iodide. To date, there is no biochemical or pathologic basis for the hypothetical difference in iodide sensitivity or autoregulation of thyroidal iodide metabolism in IIT. It may even be that the mechanism is heterogeneous in different patients with pre-existing thyroid disorders. IIT may be subdivided into different groups: (1) patients from endemic goiter areas; (2) patients with previous nonendemic goiter; (3) patients with previous or with actual Graves' disease; and (4) patients without apparent previous thyroid

TABLE 13-6. Iodine-containing Compounds

Radiologic contrasts
    Diatrizoate
    Ipanoic acid
    Ipodate
    Iothalamate
    Metrizamide
    Diatrozide
Topical
    Diiodohydroxyquinolone
    Iodine tincture
    Povidone-iodine
    Iodochlorohydroxyquinolone
    Iodoform gauze
Solutions
    Saturated KI
    Lugol
    Iodinated glycerol
    Echothiophate iodide
    Hydriodic acid syrup
    Calcium iodide
Drugs
    Amiodarone
    Expectorants
    Vitamins containing iodine
    Iodochlorohydroxyquinolone
    Diiodohydroxyquinolone
    Potassium iodide
    Food coloring
    Kelp
    Benziodarone
    Isopropamide iodide

disease.[83] Table 13-6 lists sources of iodide in patients with IIT.

One of the best known reports on IIT is that by Connolly et al.[84] They found a steep rise in the incidence of thyrotoxicosis in the late months of 1966 in Tasmania (Australia), which was an area of iodine deficiency with a high prevalence of goiter. It appeared that this increase was due to addition of potassium iodide to bread, a practice that became prevalent in early 1966. The increased incidence occurred predominantly in subjects older than 40 years, in whom a rise in incidence from 50 to a maximum of 130 cases per 100,000 was seen from 1967 to 1968. By 1974 the incidence decreased to about the preepidemic level. It was also evident that most thyrotoxic patients had nodular goiter, and few patients had Graves' disease. Later it was recognized that there was a pre-epidemic increase in incidence of thyrotoxicosis caused by the use of iodofor disinfectants on dairy farms.[85] Figure 13-10 depicts the

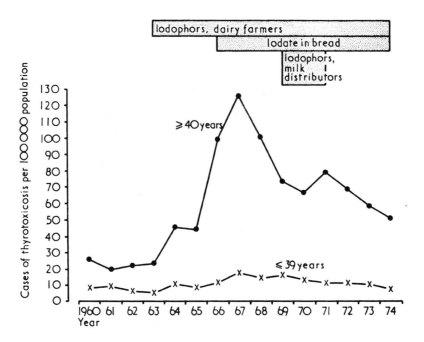

Fig. 13-10. Incidence of iodine-induced thyrotoxicosis in Northern Tasmania from 1960 to 1974 in persons 39 years and younger and 40 years and older. (From Connolly,[84] with permission.)

age-specific incidence of thyrotoxicosis in this area between 1960 and 1974. It can be seen that despite the continued increase in the iodide supply the prevalence of IIT decreased after its peak around 1967 or 1968. It was argued that this increase in thyrotoxicosis, starting from 1964 in this area of relative iodine deficiency with a high prevalence of goiter, was due to autonomy in the nodular goiters. IIT has also been reported after use of iodinated drugs, x-ray contrast agents, iodochloroxyquinoline, iodine-containing contrast agents, desinfectants, and drugs.[83,86,87a] Rarely a thyrotoxic storm is precipitated. Subjects with long-standing goiter are especially susceptible to IIT. A pre-existing thyroid disorder has been present in at least 20 percent of patients. Spontaneous reversal to euthyroidism may occur after a mean period of 6 months in 50 patients. Return to euthyroidism may be preceded by subclinical hypothyroidism.[88] In recent years non-ionic contrast media have been developed. However, use of these agents did not prevent development of IIT in elder subjects.[89] Evidence from human and animal studies indicates that chronic excess iodine intake may modulate thyroid autoimmunity and lead to thyrotoxicosis in genetically susceptible individuals.

Although studies report IIT in subjects without (apparent) pre-existing thyroid disorder, it is still doubtful that iodide on its own merit induces thyroid autoimmunity.[90] A necrotic effect of iodide excess has been demonstrated in vivo in various animal species and also in human thyroid follicles in vitro.[91] Other common sources of iodine causing IIT are iodine-containing drugs, vitamin pills, expectorants, and kelp.

In recent years the antiarhythmic drug amiodarone has been widely used. Because of its high iodine content (37.2 percent), it has caused IIT in many patients from all parts of the world. Its basic molecular structure has some similarities to that of iodothyronines, and amiodarone may also interfere with thyroid hormone transport into cells and with pathways of intracellular thyroid hormone metabolism. In particular it interferes with $5'$-monodeiodination of thyroid hormones, thus leading to a decrease of T_3, both intra- and extracellularly derived from T_4, which subsequently induces tissue hypothyroidism. An exceptional case of myxedema coma leading to death, despite intervention with T_4 and T_3, occurred in a patient after long-term amiodarone therapy.[92] In this patient T_4 administration did not increase serum T_3, evidently because of inhibition of the 5'-deiodinase in T_3-producing tissues. The fact that this patient did not positively react to T_3 administration was explained by interference of nuclear T_3 binding by amiodarone. In a study of 467 patients chronically treated with amiodarone, hypothyroidism developed in 28 patients (6 percent). In 10 out of 19 patients with underlying thyroid disease, thyroid autoantibodies were present, but these were absent in all patients without underlying thyroid abnormalities.

Amiodarone has also caused *hyperthyroidism* in many patients.[83] It is being used in many cardiac patients, particularly in France. Reported incidences of IIT due to amiodarone vary between 0.003 and 11.5 percent. In the largest series of patients, amiodarone-induced IIT occurred in 30 out of 1,448 patients.[83] Estimation of serum total or free T_4 in patients using amiodarone is not specific because these parameters may be elevated in both hyperthyroid and euthyroid patients receiving amiodarone. The latter is explained by a decrease in T_4 metabolic clearance by amiodarone inhibition of T_4 transport into tissues and of subsequent T_4 deiodination. This results in high T_4 plasma values. If, however, the serum TSH is suppressed (and serum T_3 is elevated as well), the patient is thyrotoxic. Amiodarone has recently been reported to cause follicular disruption with iodothyronine release in a manner similar to granulomatous or transient lymphocytic thyroiditis.[93] The effect is mainly due to a direct action of the drug, but the excess iodide released from the drug may contribute to the toxic reaction.[94,94a] Release of iodothyronines from disrupted follicular cells may add to IIT caused by the iodine content of amiodarone.

Amiodarone-associated IIT is a serious problem in many instances because of the coexisting heart disease of these patients; treatment may often be difficult. Administration of a combination of methimazole and potassium perchlorate has been reported to be effective.[95,96] Perchlorate was used in a dosage of 1 g/d for up to 40 days in combination with 40 mg methimazole. After discontinuation of perchlorate, methimazole was continued if the patient continued to use amiodarone. Patients became euthyroid after 2 to 5 weeks despite continued use of amiodarone. Because potassium perchlorate is a drug that potentially causes aplastic anemia, its use should be limited to those patients who cannot be controlled by methimazole alone. However, in cases of amiodarone-induced hyperthyroidism, amiodarone should if possible be discontinued. In a few patients this is not possible, and in a subgroup of these patients temporary use of perchlorate may be necessary. During its use, careful hematologic examinations should be regularly performed. Patients with previous IIT due to amiodarone are at risk to develop hypothyroidism when given excessive iodine.[97]

X-ray contrast agents also cause IIT. They contain 30 to 50 percent of iodine, and many grams are used for roentgenologic visualization of organs. Those patients who have multinodular goiter or who live in countries where iodine intake is low, for instance in parts of Germany and Italy,[98] are especially at risk. Clinicians should be aware that IIT often develops several weeks after administration of x-ray contrast agents. Follow-up of such patients after x-ray procedures is therefore advisable, and in some cases prophylactic administration of methimazole may be necessary. Considering the wide use of x-ray contrast agents (for instance in 1970 an estimated four million persons received x-ray contrast agents in the United States[99]), the probability of inducing IIT by these substances must be low. However, the incidence of IIT may be inversely related to the iodine intake of the area, which is relatively high in the United States.

HYPERTHYROIDISM DUE TO INAPPROPRIATE TSH SECRETION

Normal or even elevated serum TSH in combination with a clinically hyperthyroid patient showing increased serum thyroid hormone levels may be seen in the presence of a TSH-secreting pituitary tumor or due to selective partial pituitary resistance to thyroid hormone.

Selective Tissue Resistance of the Pituitary to Thyroid Hormone

This syndrome (described in Ch. 16) is probably part of the continuous spectrum of the syndromes of thyroid hormone resistance in which the resistance is predominant at the pituitary level. Since the pituitary is partially resistant to thyroid hormone, the *set-point* of the pituitary (i.e., the specific TSH:thyroid hormone ratio needed to ensure normal thyroid gland activation) is set at a higher level of thyroid hormone concentration. As the other body tissues appear more sensitive to thyroid hormones, the clinical picture of thyrotoxicosis is present, although without eye symptoms and other characteristics specific for Graves' disease. This syndrome may be inherited in an autosomal-dominant mode and has been described in a number of patients.[100–102] In this syndrome, since no pituitary tumor is present, the ratio of TSH α-subunits to total TSH is less than 1, whereas in the case of a TSH-producing pituitary tumor (see below) this ratio is usually above 1.

Hyperthyroidism Due to a TSH-producing Pituitary Tumor

Hyperthyroidism due to a TSH-secreting pituitary tumor is rare. In 1978 Tolis et al.[103] reviewed the literature and found that 10 to 20 patients with this condition had been reported. In 1983 another review found 17 women and 16 men with hyperthyroidism due to a TSH-producing pituitary tumor.[104]

The criteria required to confirm this entity are the following: The patient is clinically thyrotoxic while serum levels of free T_4 and/or free T_3 are elevated and serum TSH concentration is normal or increased. Visualization of the pituitary by magnetic resonance imaging (MRI) shows a pituitary tumor. The concentration of TSH α-subunits in blood is above normal, as is the ratio of TSH-α/TSH.

In recent years several more cases have been reported.[105] In a study of nine patients it was found that the mean delay to a correct diagnosis was 6.2 years.[106] Seven of these patients were wrongly treated with either thionamides, radioactive iodine, or even by thyroidectomy prior to the final diagnosis for presumed primary hyperthyroidism. Although in principle this thyrotoxicosis is not accompanied by eye signs, unilateral exophthalmos may ensue from a thyrotropin-secreting pituitary tumor due to invasion of one orbit.[107]

When the diagnosis is established, the pituitary tumor should be treated. Treatment usually consists of surgery plus external radiation. However, this approach is not always successful.[107] During follow-up of 3.5 to 6 years a relapse was seen in four of five patients undergoing surgery and receiving postoperative irradiation. Another report[108] described a relapse in all four similarly treated patients. When the tumor is a macroadenoma, its behavior tends to be aggressive. The prognosis is better in patients with microadenomas.[106] Smallridge and Smith reported

better results with macroadenomas.[104] All patients had large adenomas. Eight out of 9 were cured by surgery plus external radiation, whereas 8 of 16 were cured by surgery alone and 1 out of 4 by radiation alone. Normalization of the elevated biologic to immunologic ratio of serum TSH after operation points to successful treatment of the adenoma.[106] From these results a combination therapy consisting of surgery and irradiation seems imperative, at least in TSH-producing macroadenomas.

Administration of dopamine agonists or of somatostatin analogs have recently been effective in TSH-secreting pituitary tumors.[109–113]

CONGENITAL HYPERTHYROIDISM

Autosomal dominantly inherited nonautoimmune hyperthyroidism has recently been described in two kindreds. The condition was caused by germline mutations, Val 509 Ala and Cys 672 Tyr, respectively, involving the third and seventh transmembrane segment of the thyrotropin receptor. A third mutation, Phe 631 Leu, was described in a similar patient with congenital hyperthyroidism,[114] which was not found in his parents' DNA and thus represented a neomutation.[115] When mutant receptor gene constructs were transfected into COS cells, constitutive cAMP accumulation was observed.[114,115] Results from future studies will teach us how frequently this type hyperthyroidism occurs. It is noteworthy that the mutation in the latter patient was also found in two patients with toxic adenomas (see the section on toxic adenoma, above), except that these were somatic mutations.

THYROTOXICOSIS DUE TO METASTATIC THYROID CARCINOMA

In rare situations metastatic follicular carcinoma may cause thyrotoxicosis. According to Ehrenheim et al.,[116] Leiter et al. was the first to describe, in 1946, thyrotoxicosis due to functioning metastases in a patient with adenocarcinoma of the thyroid. Ehrenheim and co-workers reported 20 similar cases. The age and sex distribution in such patient groups is no different from that of other patients with follicular carcinoma but without thyrotoxicosis. About 85 percent of patients are older than 40 years and the female to male ratio is 3:1. The clinical picture of thyrotoxicosis is similar to the general symptoms of other causes of thyrotoxicosis. There is generally poor efficiency of iodine uptake and thyroid hormone synthesis, and excessive hormone production is due to the large mass of metastatic tissue.[117] The inefficient thyroid hormone synthesis is at least partly due to relative iodine deficiency in tumor tissue and the presence of abnormal thyroglobulin.[118] Other deficiencies and abnormalities may, however, be present in the complicated process of thyroid hormone synthesis in carcinomatous tissue. For instance, there is evidence that expression of the TSH receptor in carcinomatous thyroid tissue may be absent or low.[119] In many cases, clinical symptoms are caused by T_3 toxicosis with suppressed serum TSH and normal, sometimes even low, serum T_4.[117,118,120] Uptake of radioactive iodine in metastatic tissue may be low in the absence of normal thyroid tissue and is often absent when the thyroid gland is still present. The metastatic pattern of this type of adenocarcinoma is as is usually found in thyroid adenocarcinoma patients, that is predominantly in bone, lung, and mediastinum.

Treatment of metastatic functioning thyroid carcinoma consists of RAI administration. The usual dose ranges from 3,700 to 7,400 MBq (100 to 200 mCi). Exacerbation of thyrotoxicosis, even precipitating thyroid storm, has been reported.[121] For this reason RAI therapy of a functioning metastatic thyroid carcinoma should be administered with caution and only after adequate preparation of the elderly patient with cardiovascular disease. If normal thyroid tissue is still present, it is often advantageous to irradicate this tissue either by surgery or by radioactive iodine to ensure more efficient uptake of therapeutic doses of RAI in the metastatic tissue. The combination of Graves' disease and follicular carcinoma may not be a coincidence,[122–124] as recent knowledge suggests an association between Graves' disease and thyroid carcinoma, possibly because of long-standing thyroid stimulation by immunoglobulins.[125] Although it has been postulated that thyroid carcinoma in patients with Graves' disease behaves more aggressively,[126] this has recently been denied.[127]

STRUMA OVARII

Struma ovarii is a rare tumor that occurs in a teratoma or dermoid in the ovarium. It is often admixed with a carcinoid tumor,[128] and has been reported to occur in association with multiple endocrine neoplasia type IIA.[129] Ovarian strumal carcinoid tumors have been found to synthesize different peptide hormones, including calcitonin, adrenocorticotropic hormone (ACTH), somatotropin release inhibiting factor, neuron-specific enolase, chromogranin, synaptophysin, serotonin, and other peptides.[128–130] Struma ovarii is unilaterally localized in about 90 percent of patients, and about 80 percent are benign.[131] Pardo-Mindan and Vazquez[132] reviewed the world literature through 1983 on malignant struma ovarii and found only 17 cases; they added one of their own. As differentiation between carcinoid and struma tissue is sometimes difficult, electron microscopic studies in combination with specific immunochemistry is sometimes necessary.

Struma ovarii seldom causes hyperthyroidism. In thyrotoxicosis due to struma ovarii, RAI uptake by the thyroid gland is low in the presence of elevated serum thyroid hormones and suppressed TSH. RAI uptake over the ovarian tumor confirms the diagnosis. Although one would suspect that in thyrotoxic cases due to struma ovarii the thyroid gland would be reduced in size, the thyroid in several reports was enlarged.[131,133] Treatment of struma ovarii, either with euthyroidism or thyrotoxicosis, should be effected by removing the ovarian tumor. In the case of coexistent thyrotoxicosis, the patient should receive antithyroid drugs before surgery, sometimes in combination with β-blocking agents. Because of the coexisting teratoma, it is sometimes difficult to determine if the thyroid tissue in the tumor is benign or malignant. Patients with thyrotoxic struma ovarii should not receive radioiodine because the tumor may be malignant, which cannot be determined on clinical grounds, and because of the effects of radiation on the other elements of the teratoma are unknown.

SUMMARY

Thyrotoxicosis arises from several etiologies other than Graves' disease. Toxic adenomas are characterized by a single hyperactive nodule in the thyroid leading to clinical and biochemical thyrotoxicosis. Most adenomas are of polyclonal origin. Monoclonal adenomas may originate from somatic mutations in the gene of the Gs protein or the gene of the thyrotropin receptor. On a thyroid scan only the hot nodule is visible. The frequency of toxic nodules varies by geographic region. The frequency of toxic adenoma in patients with hyperthyroidism ranges from 1.5 to 44.5 percent, as reported by different surveys. The possibility of developing thyrotoxicosis in a patient with a hot nodule with a diameter of 3 cm or larger is 20 percent within 6 years. This risk is substantially less for smaller nodules. Also, older patients with a hot nodule are more likely to become toxic as compared to younger patients. Definitive treatment consists of surgical removal of the nodule, administration of ^{131}I, or ethanol injection. The likelihood of malignancy in a toxic nodule is very low.

Thyrotoxicosis due to painless thyroiditis was uncommon until 1973, but the reported incidence has increased since then. This is an autoimmune thyroiditis due to lymphocytic infiltration of the thyroid and is identical to postpartum thyroiditis. About half of the patients pass through four classic phases consisting of thyrotoxicosis, euthyroidism, hypothyroidism, and back to euthyroidism. The other half of the patients do not become hypothyroid or a small minority remains hypothyroid. Biochemically characteristic is the fact that RAI uptake is absent in the thyrotoxic phase, and TG levels are high. Clinical thyrotoxicosis is mild, and treatment with β-blocking agents is often sufficient. Sometimes addition of prednisone is necessary. Relapses may be seen. Although complete recovery is the rule, these patients are at high risk of developing hypothyroidism in later years. Permanent follow-up is therefore necessary.

Thyrotoxicosis factitia (thyrotoxicosis due to surreptitious ingestion of thyroid hormone) is primarily a psychiatric disorder. The diagnosis is straightforward if it is suspected. Patients usually deny ingesting thyroid hormone tablets. Characteristically, thyroid uptake of RAI is low or absent, and thyroglobulin is not detectable in the serum. Furthermore, the thyroid is usually small or absent on palpation. Treatment of the psychiatric disorder is difficult. Another form of excessive thyroid hormone intake is the so-called hamburger thyrotoxicosis. Subjects become thyrotoxic and show characteristic serum abnormalities due to inclusion of thyroid in ground beef made by a meat processor.

Thyrotoxicosis may be seen in association with elevated serum hCG activity in 1 to 2 percent of normal pregnant women. hCG has low intrinsic thyroid-stimulating activity, and hCG acts on the human thyroid cell through the TSH receptor. Desialylation of hCG renders it more biologically active. In hydatidiform mole disease, however, high levels are found in patients' serum, and when values are above 300,000 U/l, thyrotoxicosis is likely. Surgical removal of the mole renders the patient euthyroid.

Administration of moderate or high doses of iodine may induce thyrotoxicosis in patients with or without apparent pre-existing thyroid disease. Iodine may be derived from iodine solutions, radiographic contrast agents, and medications. A notorious iodine-containing agent is the antiarrhythmic drug amiodarone. Due to its structure it may block pathways of thyroid hormone metabolism and action, leading to hypothyroidism, but it can also cause hyperthyroidism due to its iodine content. Amiodarone may also disrupt thyroid follicles, resulting in thyrotoxicosis due to release of stored iodothyronines.

Inappropriate TSH secretion by a TSH-secreting pituitary tumor may cause hyperthyroidism. Treatment of the pituitary tumor will lead to euthyroidism. The prognosis is better in patients with microadenoma. Treatment consists of surgery with postoperative external irradiation. Administration of dopamine antagonists or somatostatin analogs has been shown to be successful as well.

Inherited toxic thyroid hyperplasia is a nonautoimmune type of hyperthyroidism caused by germline point mutations in the thyrotropin receptor.

Rarely, follicular carcinoma metastases may result in thyrotoxicosis with suppressed activity of the thyroid gland. Treatment of the metastases with radioactive iodine will ameliorate thyrotoxicosis. Struma ovarii, in itself a rare tumor occurring in a teratoma or dermoid in the ovarium, rarely causes hyperthyroidism. Most patients with struma ovarii are clinically and biochemically euthyroid. Treatment consists of surgically removing the tumor.

Other causes of thyrotoxicosis, such as multinodular goiter, (sub)acute thyroiditis of De Quervain, postpartum thyroiditis, Hashimoto's thyroiditis, and partial selective pituitary resistance to thyroid hormone, are considered elsewhere in this volume.

REFERENCES

1. Studer H, Gerber H, Peter HJ: Multinodular goiter. In DeGroot LJ (ed): Endocrinology. Vol 1, p. 722. WB Saunders, Philadelphia, 1989

2. Studer H, Ramelli F: Simple goiter and its variants: Euthyroid and hyperthyroid multinodular goiters. Endocr Rev 3:40, 1982

3. Ferriman D, Hennebry TM, Tassopoulos CN: True thyroid adenoma. Q J Med 41:127, 1972

4. Meissner WA, Warren S: Tumours of the thyroid gland. In Firminger HI (ed): Atlas of tumour pathology. 2nd series, Fasscicle 4, Washington DC, Armed Forces Institute of Pathology, 1969

5. Williams ED: Hyperplasia and neoplasia in endocrine glands. In Williams ED (ed): Current Concepts. p. 3. Praeger Publishers, London, 1982

6. Ramelli F, Studer H, Bruggisser D: Pathogenesis of thyroid nodules in multinodular goiter. Am J Pathol 109:215, 1982

7. Aeschimann S, Kopp PA, Kimura ET: Morphological and functional polymorphism within thyroid nodules. J Clin Endocrinol 77:846, 1993

8. Lyons J, Landis CA, Harsh G et al: Two G protein oncogenes in human endocrine tumors. Science 249: 655, 1990

9. O'Sullivan C, Barton CM, Staddon SL et al: Activating point mutations of the GSP oncogene in human thyroid adenomas. Molec Carcinogen 4:345, 1992

9a. Oncogenic potential of guanine nucleotide stimulatory factor α subunit in thyroid glands of transgenic mice. Proc Natl Acad Sci USA 91:10488, 1994

10. Parma J, Duprez L, Van Sande J et al: Somatic mutations in the thyrotropin gene cause hyperfunctioning thyroid adenomas. Nature 365:649, 1993

11. Porcelli A, Cinillo I, Laviola L et al: Novel mutations of thyrotropin receptor gene in thyroid hyperfunctioning adenomas. J Clin Endocrinol Metab 79:657, 1994

12. Paschke R, Tonacchera M, Van Sande J, Parma J, Vassart G: Identification and functional characterization of two new somatic mutations causing constitutive activation of the thyrotropin receptor in hyperfunctioning autonomous adenomas of the thyroid. J Clin Endocrinol Metab 79:1785, 1994

12a. Parma J, Van Sande J, Swillens S et al: Somatic mutations causing constitutive activity of the thyrotropin receptor are the major cause of hyperfunctioning thyrotropin adenomas: identification of additional mutations activating both the cyclic adenosine 3,'5'-monophosphate and inositol phosphate − Ca2 + cascades. Molec Endocrinol 9:725, 1995

12b. Russ D, Arturi F, Wicker R et al: Genetic alterations in thyroid hyperfunctioning adenomas. J Clin Endocrinol Metab 80:1347, 1995

13. Hamburger JI: Evolution of toxicity in solitary nontoxic autonomously functioning thyroid nodules. J Clin Endocrinol Metab 50:1089, 1980

14. Thomas CG, Croom RD: Current management of the patient with autonomously functioning nodular goiter. Surg Clin North Am 67:315, 1987

15. Bransom CJ, Talbot CH, Henry L, Elemenoglou J: Solitary toxic adenoma of the thyroid gland. Br J Surg 66:590, 1979

16. Horst W, Rösler H, Schneider C, Labhart A: 306 Cases of toxic adenoma: clinical aspects, findings in radioiodine diagnostics, radiochromatography and histology; results of I^{131} and surgical treatment. J Nucl Med 8:515, 1967

17. Emrich D, Erlenmaier U, Pohl M, Luig H: Determination of the autonomously functioning volume of the thyroid. Eur J Nucl Med 20:410, 1993

18. McKenzie JM, Zakarija M: Hyperthyroidism. In DeGroot LJ (ed): Endocrinology. Vol 1, p. 646. WB Saunders, Philadelphia, 1989

19. Barth JD, Bakker WH, Hennemann G: Discrepancies between iodine and technetium thyroid scintigraphy. JAMA 240:463, 1978

20. Sandler MP, Fellmeth B, Salhany KE, Patton JA: Thyroid carcinoma masquerading as a solitary benign hyperfunctioning nodule. Clin Nucl Med 13: 410, 1988

21. Becker FO, Economou PG, Schwartz TB: The occurrence of carcinoma in "hot" thyroid nodules: report of two cases. Ann Intern Med 58:877, 1963

22. Fujimoto Y, Oka A, Nagataki S: Occurrence of papillary carcinoma in hyperfunctioning thyroid nodule: report of a case. Endocrinol Jpn 19:371, 1972

23. Smyth M, McHenry C, Jarosz H et al: Carcinoma of the thyroid in patients with autonomous nodules. Am J Surg 54:448, 1988

24. Hamburger JI: Solitary autonomously functioning thyroid lesions: diagnosis, clinical features and pathogenetic considerations. Am J Med 58:740, 1975

25. Eyre-Brooke IA, Talbot CH: The treatment of autonomous functioning thyroid nodules. Br J Surg 69: 577, 1982

26. Ratcliffe GE, Cooke S, Fogelman I, Maisey MN: Radioiodine treatment of solitary functioning thyroid nodules. Br J Radiol 59:385, 1986

27. Ross DS, Ridgway EC, Daniels GH: Successful treatment of solitary toxic nodules with relatively low-dose I^{131} with low prevalence of hypothyroidism. Ann Intern Med 101:488, 1984

28. Goldstein R, Hart IR: Follow-up of solitary autonomous thyroid nodules treated with I^{131}. N Engl J Med 309:1473, 1983

29. Mariotti S, Martino E, Francesconi M et al: Serum thyroid auto-antibodies as a risk factor for development of hypothyroidism after radioactive iodine therapy for single thyroid "hot" nodule. Acta Endocrinol (Copenh.) 113:500, 1986

30. Monzani F, Goletti O, Caraccio N et al: Percutaneous

ethanol injection treatment of autonomous thyroid adenoma: hormonal and clinical evaluation. Clin Endocrinol 36:491, 1992

31. Papini E, Panunzi C, Pacella CM et al: Percutaneous ultrasound-guided ethanol injection: a new treatment of toxic autonomously functioning thyroid nodules? J Clin Endocrinol Metab 76:411, 1993

32. Jackson IMD: Hyperthyroiditis, a diagnostic pitfall. N Engl J Med 293:661, 1975

33. Nicolai TF, Brusso J, Kettrick MA et al: Lymphocytic thyroiditis with spontaneously resolving hyperthyroidism (silent thyroiditis). Arch Intern Med 140: 478, 1980

34. Wolff PD, Daly R: Thyrotoxicosis with painless thyroiditis. Am J Med 60:73, 1977

35. Wolff PD: Transient painless thyroiditis with hyperthyroidism: a variant of lymphocytic thyroiditis? Endocr Rev 1:411, 1980

36. Gegick CG, Harring WB: Painless subacute thyroiditis: a report of two cases. NC Med J 38:387, 1977

37. Hamburger JI: Occult subacute thyroiditis-diagnostic challenge. Mich Med 70:1125, 1971

38. Morrison J, Caplan RH: Typical and atypical ("silent") subacute thyroiditis in a wife and husband. Arch Intern Med 138:45, 1978

39. Gorman CA, Duick DS, Woolner LB, Wahner HW: Transient hyperthyroidism in patients with lymphocytic thyroiditis. Mayo Clinic Proc 53:359, 1978

40. Tokuda Y, Kasagi K, Lida Y et al: Sonography of subacute thyroiditis: changes in the findings during the course of the disease. J Clin Ultrasound 18:21, 1990

41. Vitug AC, Goldman JM: Thyrotoxic silent thyroiditis: a geographic puzzle. Arch Intern Med 145:2263, 1985

42. Schneeberg NG: Silent thyroiditis. Arch Intern Med 143:2214, 1983

43. Parker M, Klein I, Fishman LM, Levey GS: Silent thyrotoxic thyroiditis in association with chronic adrenocortical insufficiency. Arch Intern Med 140: 1108, 1978

44. Hamburger JI: Are silent thyroiditis and postpartum silent thyroiditis forms of chronic thyroiditis, or different (new) forms of viral thyroiditis? In Hamburger JI, Miller JM (eds): Controversies in Clinical Thyroidology. p. 21. Springer-Verlag, New York, 1981

45. Farid NR, Hawe BS, Walfish PG: Increased frequency of HLA-DR3 and 5 in the syndromes of painless thyroiditis with transient thyrotoxicosis: evidence for an autoimmune etiology. Clin Endocrinol 19:699, 1983

46. Dorfman SG, Cooperman MT, Nelson RL et al: Painless thyroiditis and transient hyperthyroidism without goiter. Ann Intern Med 86:24, 1977

47. Vagenakis AG, Braverman LE, Asisi F et al: Recovery of pituitary thyrotropic function after withdrawal of prolonged thyroid-suppression therapy. N Engl J Med 293:681, 1975

48. Nikolai TF, Coombs GJ, McKenzie AK et al: Treatment of lymphocytic thyroiditis with spontaneously resolving hyperthyroidism (silent thyroiditis). Arch Intern Med 142:2281, 1982

49. Nikolai TF, Coombs GJ, McKenzie AK: Lymphocytic thyroiditis with spontaneously resolving hyperthyroidism and subacute thyroiditis. Long-term follow-up. Arch Intern Med 141:1455, 1981

50. Mariotti S, Martino E, Cuppini C et al: Low serum thyroglobulin as a clue to the diagnosis of thyrotoxicosis factitia. N Engl J Med 307:410, 1982

51. Kinney JS, Hurwitz ES, Fishbein DB et al: Community outbreak of thyrotoxicosis: Epidemiology, immunogenetic characteristics, and long-term outcome. Am J Med 84:10, 1988

52. Hedberg CW, Fishbein DB, Janssen RS et al: An outbreak of thyrotoxicosis caused by the consumption of bovine thyroid gland in ground beef. N Engl J Med 316:993, 1987

53. Baran DT, Braverman LE: Editorial: Thyroid hormones and bone mass. J Clin Endocrinol Metab 72: 1182, 1991

54. Diamond T, Nery L, Hales I: A therapeutic dilemma: Suppressive doses of thyroxine significantly reduce bone mineral measurements in both premenopausal and postmenopausal women with thyroid carcinoma. J Clin Endocrinol Metab 72:1184, 1991

55. Harvey RD, McHardy KC, Reid IW et al: Measurement of bone collagen degradation in hyperthyroidism and during thyroxine replacement therapy using pyridiium cross-links as specific urinary markers. J Clin Endocrinol Metab 72:1189, 1991

56. Tseng KH, Walfish PG, Persaud JA, Gilbert BW: Concurrent aortic and mitral valve echocardiography permits measurement of systolic time intervals as an index of peripheral tissue thyroid functional status. J Clin Endocrinol Metab 79:633, 1989

56a. Biondi B, Fario S, Carella C et al: Cardiac effects of long-term thyrotropin-suppressive therapy with levothyroxine. J Clin Endocrinol Metab 77:334, 1993

56b. Fario S, Biondi B, Carella C et al: Diastolic dysfunction in patients on thyroid-stimulating hormone suppressive therapy with levothyroxine: beneficial effect of β-blockade. J Clin Endocrinol Metab 80:2222, 1995

57. Glinoer D, Lemone M: Goiter and pregnancy: a new insight into an old problem. Thyroid 2:65, 1992

58. Nisula BC, Ketelslegers J-M: Thyroid-stimulating activity and chorionic gonadotropin. J Clin Invest 54: 494, 1974

59. Kenimer JG, Hershman JM, Higgins HP: The thyrotropin in hydatidiform moles is human chorionic gonadotropin J Clin Endocrinol Metab 40:482, 1975

60. Nisula BC, Taliadouros GS: Thyroid function in gestational trophoblastic neoplasia: Evidence that the thyrotropic activity of chorionic gonadotropin mediates the thyrotoxicosis of choriocarcinoma. Am J Obstet Gyn 138:77, 1980

61. Amir SM, Endo K, Osathanondh R, Inbar SH: Divergent responses by human and mouse thyroids to human chorionic gonadotropin in vitro. Molec Cell Endocrinol 39:31, 1985

62. Carayon P, Lefort G, Nisula BC: Interaction of human chorionic gonadotropin and human luteinizing hormone with human thyroid membranes. Endocrinology 106:1907, 1980

63. Yoshimura M, Hershman JM, Pang X-P et al: Activation of the thyrotropin (TSH) receptor by human chorionic gonadotropin and luteinizing hormone in Chinese hamster ovary cells expressing functional human TSH receptors. J Clin Endocrinol Metab 77: 1009, 1993

64. Carayon P, Amir S, Nisula B, Lissitzky S: Effect of carboxypeptidase digestion of the human choriogonadotropin molecule on its thyrotropic activity. Endocrinology 108:1891, 1981

65. Cole LA, Kardana A: Discordant results in human chorionic gonadotropin assays. Clin Chem 38:263, 1992

66. Davies TF, Taliaduros GS, Catt KJ, Nisula BC: Assessment of urinary thyrotropin-competing activity in choriocarcinoma and thyroid disease: further evidence for human chorionic gonadotropin interacting at the thyroid cell membrane. J Clin Endocrinol Metab 49:353, 1979

67. Ouchimoura H, Nagataki S, Ito K et al: Inhibition of the thyroid adenylate cyclase response to thyroid-stimulating immunoglobulin G and asialo-human chorionic gonadotropin. J Clin Endocrinol Metab 55:347, 1982

68. Hoermann R, Broecker M, Grossman M et al: Interaction of human chorionic gonadotropin (hCG) and asialo-hCG with recombinant human thyrotropin receptor. J Clin Endocrinol Metab 78:933, 1994

69. Hoermann R, Amir SM, Ingbar SH: Evidence that partially desialylated variants of human chorionic gonadotropin (hCG) are the factors in crude hCG that inhibit the response to thyrotropin in human thyroid membranes. Endocrinology 123:1535, 1988

69a. Yamanaki K, Sato K, Shizume K et al: Patient thyrotropic activity of human chronic gonadotropin variants in terms of ^{125}I incorporation and *de novo* synthesized thyroid hormone release in human thyroid follicles. J Clin Endocrinol Metab 80:473, 1995

70. Davies TF, Platzer M: hCG-induced TSH receptor activation and growth acceleration in FRTL-5 thyroid cells. Endocrinology 118:2149, 1986

71. Hershman JM, Lee H-Y, Sugawara M et al: Human chorionic gonadotropin stimulates iodide uptake, adenylate cyclase, and deoxyribonucleic acid synthesis in cultured rat thyroid cells. J Clin Endocrinol Metab 67:74, 1988

71a. Variation in the thyrotropic activity of human chorionic gonadotropin in Chinese hamster ovary cells arises from differential expression of the human thyrotropin receptor and microheterogeneity of the hormone. J Clin Endocrinol Metab 80:1605, 1995

72. Hershman JM, Higgins P: Hydatidiform mole—a cause of clinical hyperthyroidism. N Engl J Med 284: 573, 1971

73. Dowling JT, Ingbar SH, Frenkel N: Iodine metabolism in hydatidiform mole and choriocarcinoma. J Clin Endocrinol Metab 20:1, 1960

74. Kock H, Kessel HV, Stolte L, van Leusden H: Thyroid function in molar pregnancy. J Clin Endocr Metab 26:1128, 1966

75. Galton VA: Abnormalities of thyroid hormone economy in patients with hydatidiform mole. Progr Annual meeting of the ATA. p. 35. Washington DC, Oct. 10–12, 1968

76. Mann LI, Lutz M, Schulman H, Romney SL: Hydatidiform mole with hyperthyroidism. Am J Obstet Gynecol 98:1151, 1967

77. Higgins HP, Hershman JM, Kenimer JG et al: The thyrotoxicosis of hydatiform mole. Ann Intern Med 83:307, 1975

78. Yoshimura M, Pekary AE, Pang X-P et al: Thyrotrophic activity of basic isoelectric forms of human chorionic gonadotropin in extracted from hydatiform mole tissues. J Clin Endocrinol Metab 78:862, 1994

79. Anderson NR, Lokich JJ, McDermott WV Jr et al: Gestational choriocarcinoma and thyrotoxicosis. Cancer 44:304, 1979

80. Orgiazzi JJ, Rousset B, Cosentino C et al: Plasma thyrotropic activity in a man with choriocarcinoma. J Clin Endocrinol Metab 39:653, 1974

81. Orgiazzi JJ, Mornex R: Hyperthyroidism. In Greer MA (ed): The Thyroid Gland. p. 442. Raven Press, New York, 1990

82. Hennemann G: Historical aspects about the development of our knowledge of morbus Basedow. J Endocrinol Invest 14:617, 1991

83. Fradkin JE, Wolff J: Iodide-induced thyrotoxicosis. Medicine 62:1, 1983

84. Connolly RJ, Vidor GI, Stewart JC: Increase in thyrotoxicosis in endemic goiter area after iodination of bread. Lancet 1:500, 1970

85. Stewart JC, Vidor GI: Thyrotoxicosis induced by iodine contamination of food—a common unrecognized condition? Br Med J 1:372, 1976

86. Leger AF, Laurent M-F, Savoie J-C: Surcharge iodée pathologie thyreoïdienne iatrogène. Ann Endocrinol 42:446, 1981

87. Herrmann J, Krüskemper HL: Gefardung von Patienten mit latenter und manifester Hyperthyreose durch jodhaltige Röntgenkontrastmittel und Medikamente. Deutsche Medizin Wochenschr 103:1437, 1978

87a. Breadmore R, McKenzie AM, Arkles LB, Hicks RJ: Hyperthyroidism after radiographic contrast in a patient with separate cervical and intrathoracic multinodular goiters. Clin Nucl Med 20:413, 1995

88. Leger AF et al: Iodine-induced thyrotoxicosis: analysis of eighty-five consecutive cases. Eur J Clin Invest 14:449, 1984

89. Martin FIR, Tress BW, Colman P, Deam DR: Iodine-induced hyperthyroidism due to nonionic contrast radiography in the elderly. Am J Med 95:78, 1933

90. Mariotti S, Pinchera A: Role of the immune system in the control of thyroid function. In Greer MA (ed): The Thyroid Gland. p. 147. Raven Press, New York, 1990

91. Many M-C, Mestdagh C, van den Hove M-F, Denef JF: In vitro study of acute toxic effects of high iodide dosis in human thyroid follicles. Endocrinology 131:621, 1992

92. Mazson PD, Williams ML, Cantley LK et al: Myxedema coma during long-term amiodarone therapy. Am J Med 77:751, 1984

93. Brennan MD, Klee GG, Carney JA: Pathogenesis of amiodarone-associated thyrotoxicosis (AAT). Thyroid 1, suppl. 1:S-1, 1991

94. Chiovato L, Martino E, Tonacchera M et al: Studies on the *in vitro* cytotoxic effect of amiodarone. Endocrinology 134:2277, 1994

94a. Brennan MD, Erickson DZ, Carney JA, Bahn RS: Nongoitrous (type I) amiodarone-associated thyrotoxicosis: evidence of follicular disruption *in vitro* and *in vivo*. Thyroid 5:177, 1995

95. Martino E, Aghini-Lombardi F, Mariotti S et al: Treatment of amiodarone-associated thyrotoxicosis by simultaneous administration of potassium perchlorate and methimazole. J Endocrinol Invest 5:201, 1986

96. Reichert LJ, de Rooy HA: Treatment of amiodarone induced hyperthyroidism with potassium perchlorate and methimazole during amiodarone treatment. Br Med J 298:1547, 1989

97. Roti E et al: Iodine-induced subclinical hypothyroidism in euthyroid subjects with a previous episode of amiodarone-induced thyrotoxicosis. J Clin Endocrinol Metab 75:1273, 1992

98. Martino E, Aghini-Lombardi F, Mariotti S et al: Amiodarone: a common source of iodine-induced thyrotoxicosis. Horm Res 26:158, 1987

99. U.S. Department of Health, Education and Welfare. Food and Drug Administration: Population exposure to X-rays U.S. 1970 D.H.E.W. Publication (F.D.A.) 73-8047. p. 92. U.S. Department of Health, Education and Welfare, Rockville, Maryland, 1973

100. Emerson CH, Utiger RD: Hyperthyroidism and excessive thyrotropin secretion. N Engl J Med 287:328, 1972

101. Gershengorn MC, Weintraub BD: Thyrotropin-induced hyperthyroidism caused by selective pituitary resistance to thyroid hormone. J Clin Invest 56:633, 1975

102. Rösler A, Litvin Y, Hage C et al: Familial hyperthyroidism due to inappropriate thyrotropin secretion successfully treated with triiodothyronine. J Clin Endocrinol Metab 54:76, 1982

103. Tolis G, Bird C, Bertrand G et al: Pituitary hyperthyroidism. Am J Med 64:177, 1978

104. Smallridge RC, Smith CE: Hyperthyroidism due to thyrotropin-secreting pituitary tumors. Diagnostic and therapeutic considerations. Arch Intern Med 143:503, 1983

105. Kiso Y, Yoshida K, Kaise K et al: A case of thyrotropin (TSH)-secreting tumor complicated by periodic paralysis. Jap J Med 92:399, 1990

106. Gesundheit N, Petrick PA, Nissim M et al: Thyrotropin-secreting pituitary adenomas: Clinical and biochemical heterogeneity. Case reports and follow-up of 9 patients. Ann Intern Med 111:827, 1989

107. Yovos JG, Falko JM, O-Dorisio TM et al: Thyrotoxicosis and a thyrotropin-secreting pituitary tumor causing unilateral exophthalmos. J Clin Endocrinol Metab 53:338, 1981

108. Hill SA, Falko JM, Wilson CB, Hunt WE: Thyrotrophin-producing pituitary adenomas. J Neurol Surg 57:515, 1982

109. Benoit R et al: Hyperthyroidism due to a pituitary TSH secreting tumour with amenorrhoea-galactorrhoea. Clin Endocrinol 12:11, 1980

110. Lamberg BA et al: Hyperthyroidism and acromegaly caused by a pituitary TSH- and GH-secreting tumour. Acta Endocrinol (Copenh) 103:7, 1983

111. Chanson P: Les adenomes hypofysaire thyreotrope. Aspect clinique, evolution et traitement. Presse-Med 16:1644, 1987

112. Polak M et al: A human TSH-secreting adenoma: endocrine, biochemical and morphological studies. Evidence of somatostatin receptors by using quantitative autoradiography. Clinical and biological improvement by SMS 201-995 treatment. Acta Endocrinol (Copenh) 1224:479, 1991

113. Chanson Ph, Weintraub BD, Harris AG: Octreotide therapy for thyroid-stimulating hormone secreting pituitary adenomas. Ann Intern Med 119:236, 1993

114. Duprez L, Parma J, Van Sande J et al: Germline mutations in the thyrotropin receptor gene cause non-autoimmune autosomal dominant hyperthyroidism. Nat Genet 7:396, 1994

115. Kopp P, Van Sande J, Parma J et al: Brief report: Congenital hyperthyroidism caused by a mutation in the thyrotropin receptor gene. N Engl J Med 332:150, 1995

116. Ehrenheim C, Heintz P, Schober O et al: Jodinduzierte T_3-Hyperthyreose beim metastasierenden follikularen Schilddrüsen Karzinom. Nuklear Medizin 25:201, 1986

117. Paul SJ, Sisson JC: Thyrotoxicosis caused by thyroid cancer. Endocrinol Metab Clin North Am 19:593, 1990

118. Nakashima T, Enue K, Shiro-osu A et al: Predominant T_3 synthesis in the metastatic thyroid carcinoma in a patient with T_3-toxicosis. Metabolism 30:327, 1981

119. Verschueren CP, Rutteman GR, Vos JH et al: Thyrotrophin receptors in normal and neoplastic (primary and metastatic) canine thyroid tissue. J Endocrinol 132:461, 1992

120. Sung LC, Cavalieri RR: T_3 toxicosis due to metastatic thyroid carcinoma. J Clin Endocrinol Metab 36:215, 1973

121. Cerletty JM, Listwan WJ: Hyperthyroidism due to functioning metastatic thyroid carcinoma. Precipitation of thyroid storm with therapeutic radioactive iodine. JAMA 242:269, 1979

122. Grayzel EF, Bennett B: Graves' disease, follicular thyroid carcinoma and functioning pulmonary metastases. Cancer 43:1885, 1979

123. Kasagi K, Takeichi R, Miyamoto S et al: Metastatic thyroid cancer presenting as thyrotoxicosis: Report of three cases. Clin Endocrinol 40:429, 1994

124. Steffensen FH, Aunsholt NAA: Hyperthyroidism associated with metastatic thyroid carcinoma. Clin Endocrinol 41:685, 1994

125. Mazzaferri EL: Editorial. Thyroid cancer and Graves' disease. J Clin Endocrinol Metab 70:826, 1990

126. Belfiore A, Charofalo MR, Giuffrida D et al: Increased aggressiveness of thyroid cancer in patients with Graves' disease. J Clin Endocrinol Metab 70:830, 1990

127. Hales IB, McElduff A, Crummer P et al: Does Graves' disease or thyrotoxicosis affect the prognosis of thyroid cancer. J Clin Endocrinol Metab 75:886, 1992

128. Tamsen A, Mazur MT: Ovarian strumal carcinoid in association with multiple endocrine neoplasia, type IIA. Arch Pathol Lab Med 116:200, 1992

129. Sakura H, Fujii T, Okamoto K: A study of human calcitonin in an ovarian carcinoid and ovarian cancers. Exp Clin Endocrinol 97:91, 1991

130. Ozerwenka KF, Schon HJ, Bock P: Immunochemical and ultrastructural studies of an ovarian strumal carcinoid. Wien Klin Wochenschr 102:687, 1990

131. Kempers RD, Dockerty MB, Hoffman DL et al: Struma ovarii-ascitic, hyperthyroid and asymptomatic syndromes. Ann Intern Med 72:883, 1970

132. Pardo-Mindan FJ, Vazquez JJ: Malignant struma ovarii. Light and electron microscopic study. Cancer 51:337, 1983

133. Smith FG: Pathology and physiology of struma ovarii. Arch Surg 53:603, 1946

Thyroid Dysfunction in the Pregnant Patient

14

Pregnancy significantly affects thyroid function, particularly the course of thyroid disease in patients with pre-existing autoimmune thyroid dysfunction. Since autoimmune thyroid disease is especially common in women and has significant prevalence during the childbearing period, it is important to understand both the expected changes in thyroid function tests in normal pregnancy and how this condition can affect pre-existing thyroiditis, hypothyroidism, and Graves' disease in these women. In this chapter the normal changes in thyroid function are discussed in relation to both iodine-sufficient and iodine-deficient patients. In addition, those aspects of the diagnosis and treatment that must be kept in mind in the care of pregnant patients with thyroid disease will be emphasized. In the past decade a profusion of new information regarding the effects of normal pregnancy on thyroid function have clarified many aspects of the interaction of the gestational processes and the normal thyroid system.

THYROID FUNCTION IN NORMAL PREGNANCY

Table 14-1 summarizes the changes occurring during normal pregnancy that relate to thyroid function or thyroid function testing. Early in pregnancy there is an increase in renal blood flow and glomerular filtration, which leads to an increase in iodide clearance from the plasma.[1–5] This results in decreased plasma iodide and an increased requirement for iodide in the diet.[1] This increase is over and above changes due to an increase in thyroxine production rate, which also may occur. In iodine-sufficient patients this increased iodide excretion has little impact in terms of thyroid function. However, in geographic areas where iodine supply is borderline or low, significant changes occur.[2,3,6] While 24-hour radioiodine (RAI) uptake determinations are not now performed during pregnancy, past stud-

TABLE 14-1. Effects of Pregnancy on Thyroid Physiology

Physiologic Change	Thyroid-related Consequences
Increased renal I⁻ clearance	Increased 24-hr RAIU
Decreased plasma I⁻ and placental I⁻ transport to the fetus	In I⁻-deficient women, decreased T_4, increased TSH, and goiter
Increased O_2 consumption by fetoplacental unit, gravid uterus and mother	Increased BMR
First-trimester increase in hCG	Increased free T_4 and T_3 Decreased basal TSH
Increased serum TBG	Increased total T_4 and T_3
Increased plasma volume	Increased T_4 and T_3 pool size
Inner-ring deiodination of T_4 and T_3 by placenta	Accelerated rates of T_4 and T_3 degradation and production

ies have shown this value is increased.[7] In addition, there is a further increment in iodine requirement due to the transplacental transport of iodide that is required for iodothyronine synthesis by the fetal thyroid, which becomes functional by the end of the first trimester. The increase in iodine requirement is illustrated especially well in studies by Glinoer and co-workers that document modest thyroid enlargement during pregnancy in areas of borderline iodine adequacy.[2,3,8,9] In normal pregnancy in iodine-sufficient areas there appears to be little, if any, increase in the size of the thyroid gland.[10,11] This indicates that, while there is thyroid stimulation by human chorionic gonadotropin (hCG), this modest change does not normally result in anatomic changes, at least as assessed by physical examination and ultrasound studies.[11–14]

Oxygen Consumption

Oxygen consumption increases during pregnancy; this can be attributed to the metabolic requirements of the fetus, the placenta, the gravid uterus, and increased maternal cardiac output. This increase is reflected in the increased basal metabolic rate, although this test is rarely used to assess thyroid function in practice.

Human Chorionic Gonadotropin

Human chorionic gonadotropin is comprised of two subunits, termed α- and β-chains. The α subunit is shared with three other pituitary glycoprotein hormones, thyroid-stimulating hormone (TSH), luteinizing hormone (LH), and follicle-stimulating hormone (FSH). The structural similarity between the β subunit of hCG and of TSH and in in vitro bioassays indicates that hCG has intrinsic thyroid-stimulating activity.[14–16] While early studies using tissue extracts of hydatidiform mole or choriocarcinoma suggested that there was a second non-hCG placental thyrotropin (and there is still some disagreement about this[17,18]), current evidence suggests that hCG is the thyroid stimulator of early pregnancy (Table 14-2).[15,16,19,20] A very small but definite increase in free thyroxine occurs during the first trimester of normal pregnancy (Fig. 14-1).[21,22] Especially noteworthy is the fact that the modest increase in free thyroxine (T_4) and free triiodothyronine (T_3) are disproportionate to the increases in total T_4 and T_3, which are a consequence of the estrogen-induced increase in serum thyroxine-binding globulin (TBG) (discussed below). The parallelism between the levels of circulating hCG, the increases in free T_4 and T_3, and the suppression of TSH during normal pregnancy are quite compelling.[19,23–27] This finding has been further supported by studies in which the thyroid-stimulating activity of sera from first-trimester pregnancies was abolished by immunoprecipitation of hCG with anti-hCG antibody.[19,28] This treatment lowered the thyroid cell–stimulating activity (measured in a rat thyroid FRTL-5 cell assay) from pretreatment values of 200 to 400 percent of normal to negligible levels. Further evidence supporting a pathophysiologic role of hCG in stimulating the human thyroid is found in studies of patients with hydatidiform mole and choriocarcinoma (see Chapter 13). In these conditions clinical and biochemical manifestations of hyperthyroidism often occur.[29,30] As expected, this thyroid stimulation is relieved rapidly

TABLE 14-2. Evidence Favoring hCG as the Endogenous Thyroid Stimulator in Early Pregnancy

1. Maternal thyroid status parallels serum hCG during normal pregnancy.
2. Thyroid-stimulating activity of pregnant serum detected in vitro is absorbed by anti-hCG antibody.
3. TSH is suppressed and free T_4 and hCG elevated in many patients with hyperemesis gravidarum.
4. Most patients with molar pregnancy and choriocarcinoma have biochemical hyperthyroidism.

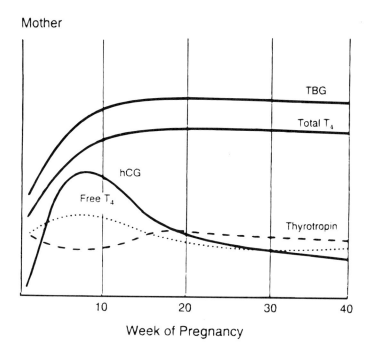

Mother

Week of Pregnancy

Fig. 14-1. Relative changes in parameters of maternal thyroid function during gestation. The trends and relative magnitude of changes in serum thyroxine-binding globulin (TBG), thyrotropin, total and free T_4, and T_3 are shown. (From Burrow et al,[13] with permission.)

after appropriate surgical therapy. Thus, in molar pregnancy, serum TSH is suppressed, as it is in patients with hyperthyroidism due to Graves' disease, and this has been confirmed.[31] Fig. 14-1 summarizes the inverse relationship between serum hCG concentrations and serum TSH in normal pregnancy. TSH levels decrease during the first trimester to reach a nadir at the time of peak hCG concentrations at weeks 10 to 12. TSH may even be reduced below the normal range in a small fraction of otherwise euthyroid pregnant women at this time.[9,32,33]

Hyperemesis Gravidarum

Patients with hyperemesis gravidarum may have increases in free T_4 and free T_3.[34–40] This, together with the generalized illness associated with this syndrome, may make differentiation of this condition from Graves' disease difficult. Some studies have indicated that in patients with hyperemesis, hCG may be higher than in unaffected women.[41] This may be associated with an exaggerated stimulation of the thyroid in the first trimester. One report indicated that 66 percent of patients with hyperemesis have biochemical hyperthyroidism (increased free thy-

roxine index and or suppressed TSH) and that the more seriously ill of these subjects also had an elevation in the serum free T_3 index.[36,37] Thus, the increase in the free T_4 in hyperemesis may be attributed to hCG-induced thyroid stimulation. This may even extend to an elevation in serum free T_3, despite the fact that these patients are often nutritionally compromised and would be expected to have a suppressed T_3 due to impairment of T_4 to T_3 conversion. In many patients, appropriate fluid replacement will resolve the clinical symptoms and, as gestation proceeds and hCG levels fall, normal thyroid function will resume.[42] In patients with more severe illness antithyroid drug therapy is needed as described below. In a few patients, hyperemesis is a symptom of coexistent hyperthyroidism due to Graves' disease.[38,43] In such patients, appropriate treatment for hyperthyroidism is required. While true hyperthyroidism is a rare cause of hyperemesis, it remains one of the differential diagnostic considerations in this syndrome (see below). Others have observed that there may be an even more subtle form of hyperthyroidism associated with morning sickness.[41] The severity of morning sickness correlated with the levels of free T_4 and hCG, suggesting again that hyperemesis reflects the extreme of the spectrum of the physiologic changes that occur in normal pregnancy. One tempting hypothesis to connect the two is that higher hCG levels cause increased estrogen secretion as well as mild hyperthyroidism and that this explains the coexistence of nausea and vomiting on the one hand and mild hyperthyroidism on the other.

Changes in Circulating Thyroid Hormone–Binding Proteins

The increase in total serum T_4 and T_3 during pregnancy is due to an increase in the serum thyroxine-binding globulin (TBG). This change appears early in pregnancy, TBG having doubled by the end of the first trimester. Figure 14-1 shows the impact of this change on circulating thyroid hormones. Pregnancy is also associated with an increase in several other serum glycoproteins, including cortisol-binding globulin, clotting factors I, VII, and IX, and sex hormone–binding globulin (SHBG). The cause of the increased serum TBG may be multifactorial. Early studies showed an increase in TBG synthesis in primary cultures of hepatocytes from rhesus monkeys treated with estradiol.[44] This indicates that estrogen may increase the hepatic synthesis of this protein during pregnancy. However, the lack of increase of TBG and SHBG by estrogen in HEP-G2 cells raised the possibility that other factors might be operative in the pregnant individual.

A recent reevaluation of this issue[45] indicates that estrogen-induced alterations in the glycosylation pattern of TBG increase circulating TBG (as well as the other serum glycoproteins) by reducing their plasma clearance (see also Chaps. 3 and 5). There is an increase in the fraction of more heavily sialylated and therefore more negatively charged fractions of TBG in the sera of pregnant or estrogen-treated individuals. Since this increase in sialic acid content of TBG inhibits the uptake of these proteins by the asialoglycoprotein receptors on hepatocytes, the more heavily sialylated proteins from pregnant sera have a longer plasma half-life.[46] This alteration in sialylation is not found in the TBG isolated from patients with a congenital elevation in TBG, the latter due to a true overproduction of the protein.[47] Thus, in addition to whatever stimulatory effects estrogen might have on TBG synthesis, a major contri-

bution to the increased TBG concentration in the sera of pregnant women is the reduced clearance of the more highly glycosylated proteins. This explanation is attractive, since it would also account for the increases in the concentration of other circulating glycoproteins in hyperestrogenemic states. To date, there are no data demonstrating that the enzyme or enzymes responsible for sialylation are increased by estrogen. Nonetheless the evidence supporting this possibility is quite compelling. Delivery leads to a rapid reversal of this process, and serum TBG concentrations return to normal within 4 to 6 weeks. With that, serum T_4 and T_3 also return to normal. Perhaps the increase in TBG-bound T_4 and T_3 subserves the function of redistributing thyroid hormones to the placenta.[48] In addition to two to threefold increases in serum TBG, modest decreases in both serum transthyretin (TTR) and serum albumin are also found in pregnancy.[49] The physiologic impact of these changes, if any, is not known.

Increased Plasma Volume

The increased plasma concentration of TBG, together with the increased plasma volume, results in a severalfold increase in the total T_4 pool during pregnancy. While the changes in TBG are most dramatic during the first trimester, the increase in plasma volume continues up until the time of delivery. Thus, if the free T_4 concentration is to remain normal, T_4 production rate must increase or the degradation rate must decrease to allow the additional T_4 to accumulate. One would predict that in a situation where T_4 input was constant, there would be an iterative increment in T_4 as TBG increased due to the reduced availability of T_4 to degradative enzymes. The evidence that levothyroxine requirements are enhanced during pregnancy in hypothyroid women (see below) suggests that not only is T_4 degradation decreased during early pregnancy but also that increased T_4 production must also occur throughout gestation.[50–52]

Placental Metabolism of Thyroid Hormones

The placenta contains high concentrations of the type 3 or inner-ring (5) iodothyronine deiodinase.[53–55] The inner-ring deiodination of T_4 catalyzed by this enzyme is the source of the high concentrations of reverse T_3 present in amniotic fluid.

These parallel maternal serum T_4 concentrations.[56-59] This enzyme may function to reduce the concentration of T_3 and T_4 in the fetal circulation, and the latter is quite low up to the time of parturition. Fetal tissue T_3 levels can, however, reach adult levels due to the action of the type 2 deiodinase[13] (see Ch. 15). The type 3 deiodinase may also provide a source of iodide for the fetus via iodothyronine deiodination. However, despite the presence of placental type 3 deiodinase under circumstances in which fetal T_4 production is reduced or maternal free T_4 is markedly increased, transplacental T_4 passage (at least) does occur and fetal serum T_4 levels are about one-third of normal.[60] Thyroxine is also detectable in amniotic fluid before onset of fetal thyroid function.[61] Thus, the placental barrier to maternal iodothyronines, at least in the third trimester, is modest.[13]

Thyroxine Production Rate

The only direct measurements of T_4 turnover rates in pregnancy were performed approximately 25 years ago by Dowling et al.[62] In eight pregnant subjects, four in the first half and four in the second half of gestation, T_4 turnover rates were estimated not to be significantly different from those of nonpregnant women. However, the considerations raised above and summarized in Table 14-1 argue that T_4 production rates are enhanced during pregnancy. Evidence supporting this concept has been developed from analyses of the effects of pregnancy on levothyroxine replacement in patients with primary hypothyroidism. Nine of 12 women with primary hypothyroidism and receiving stable doses of levothyroxine experienced a significant increase in TSH during gestation that required an increase in thyroxine.[50] The three patients who did not require an increase were receiving slightly excessive replacement doses prior to gestation. If the increased levothyroxine dose was maintained into the postpartum period, there was a subsequent increase in free T_4 and a decrease in TSH (Fig. 14-2). These results indicated there was an increase in T_4 requirements beginning early in gestation that persisted until the time of delivery. An alternative explanation is that the absorption of levothyroxine was reduced throughout gestation. This seems unlikely but cannot be unequivocally eliminated. In a subsequent study, thyroxine replacement was evaluated in two groups of hypothyroid patients during pregnancy; one group had Hashimoto's disease and the second thyroid ablation for either Graves' disease or thyroid cancer.[51] A 45 percent increase in levothyroxine requirements during gestation occurred in patients with thyroid ablation and a 25 percent increase in those with Hashimoto's disease. This indicates that patients with some residual thyroid function were able to compensate for the increased requirement, whereas those without thyroid tissue could not. From the point of view of maternal thyroid function during pregnancy, these results suggest there is about a 50 percent increase in T_4 production during gestation.

Thyroid Function Studies in Normal Pregnancy

Total and Free Serum T_4 and T_3

The increase in TBG during gestation causes an increase in total serum thyroid hormones. To estimate the free hormone concentration a thyroid-hormone-binding ratio (THBR), free T_4 index, or direct free T_4 measurement must be obtained.[5,22,23,33,63] The reduction in the free fraction of T_3 is approximately equal to that of T_4. Thus the standard approach for these determinations employing tracer T_3 can be used. However, it is important to recognize that as the free fraction is reduced, the resin T_3 uptake (and similar assessments of the free fraction) asymptotically approach a fixed lower limit. This is not linearly related to the increase in unoccupied TBG binding sites. Thus, the decrease in the THBR does not usually match the 50 percent decrease in the T_4 and T_3 free fractions estimated directly and in some sera, the free T_4 index or estimate will be slightly elevated relative to the true free T_4 or T_3.

Direct measurements of free T_4 using older T_4 analog technologies often resulted in a decreased free T_4 estimate in pregnant euthyroid subjects. This has been attributed to the physiologic decrease in albumin that occurs in pregnancy, which in turn reduces the binding of labeled T_4 analog making more available for binding to the antibody. A specific normal range for pregnant patients must be employed when using such methods. On the other hand, those techniques in which a direct assay of thyroid hormones is performed in an ultrafiltrate or dialysate should provide accurate estimates of the free hormone concentrations. The development of the sensi-

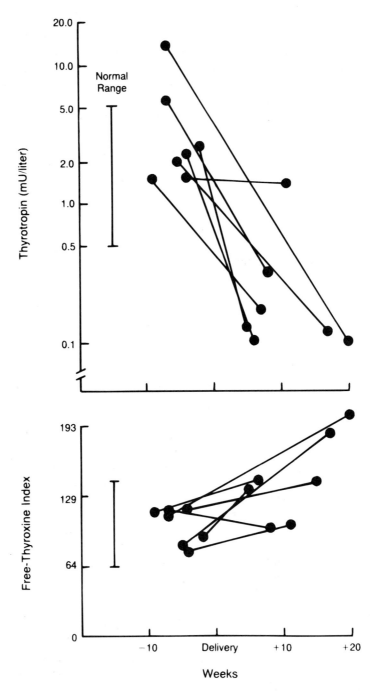

Fig. 14-2. Individual serum free-thyroxine indexes and thyrotropin concentrations during the third trimester and post partum in women with hypothyroidism. Results are shown for seven patients whose measurements were made within 10 weeks before and 20 weeks after delivery. Each patient is represented by a single line. The normal ranges for serum thyrotropin and the free thyroxine index are indicated by the vertical bars. (From Mandel et al,[50] with permission.)

tive TSH assay, which is now used to confirm the diagnosis of thyrotoxicosis, has obviated the technical difficulties in the rapid and accurate assessment of the free T_4 and T_3 during pregnancy.

Serum TSH

As noted, serum TSH concentrations may be modestly subnormal (0.2 to 0.5 mU/L) during the first trimester in a small fraction of "euthyroid" pregnant women.[2,4,9,31,33] Therefore, such a result should not automatically lead to a diagnosis of pathologic hyperthyroidism. This tendency may be exacerbated in patients with hyperemesis gravidarum. During the second and third trimester, serum TSH returns to the normal range of 0.5 to 5.0 mU/L.

Other Tests

Because isotopic tracers are no longer administered during pregnancy, altered iodine kinetics in the pregnant patient are not a source of confusion. In evaluating the clinical status during gestation, it should be recalled that many physical findings suggestive of hyperthyroidism are normally present, including increased pulse pressure, tachycardia, heat intolerance, and decreased peripheral vascular resistance.

AUTOIMMUNE THYROID DISEASE AND PREGNANCY

Effects of Pregnancy on Immune Function

The alterations in the maternal immune system that permit the successful implantation of the fetal allograft have not been definitively identified. However, the factors leading to this tolerance seem likely to be partially responsible for the generalized improvement in autoimmune thyroid disease that is so characteristic of the pregnant state. Table 14-3

TABLE 14-3. Effects of Pregnancy on Lymphocyte Subsets in Patients with and Without Thyroid Autoantibodies

1. Decreased CD4$^+$ and increased CD8$^+$ T cells in all patients.
2. Increase in CD29$^+$/CD45RA$^+$ ratio (suppressor-inducer T cell function) postpartum in all patients.
3. Decrease in TPO$^-$ and TgAb during pregnancy and a marked increase postpartum.

summarizes the effects of pregnancy on lymphocyte subsets in patients with and without thyroid autoantibodies.[64–68] The precise mechanism by which thyroid autoantibodies, as well as those directed against other tissues, are suppressed during pregnancy and exacerbated thereafter remains obscure. Presumably the rapid reduction in "immune suppressor proteins" following delivery leads to the reestablishment and exacerbation of these conditions. The postpartum exacerbation of autoimmune thyroid disease is one of the most striking examples of this phenomenon. This pattern is especially well illustrated in patients with untreated Hashimoto's disease, asymptomatic patients with positive thyroid antibodies who develop postpartum thyroiditis often with hyperthyroidism, and in those with Graves' disease.[69–79] A report suggesting that women who are thyroid-autoantibody-positive in the first trimester miscarry twice as often as women who are thyroid-antibody-negative raises the possibility that the presence of autoantibodies may be a marker for less readily recognized but more generalized autoimmune dysfunction.[66,80,81] There is, however, no evidence that thyroid autoantibodies per se play a causative role in spontaneous abortion.[80]

The prevalence of elevated thyroid autoantibodies in the pregnant population is surprisingly high—18.7 percent of 500 women in one study.[80] The high prevalence in this study may be a consequence of the increased sensitivity of the ELISA assays used in assessing the presence of autoantibodies as well as the fact that there may be some enhancement of autoimmunity in the first trimester of pregnancy. The prevalence of autoantibodies during the first trimester in patients with type I diabetes is even higher than this—approximately 20 to 25 percent.[67,82] The high prevalence of positive autoantibodies and the observation that biochemical postpartum thyroid disease occurs in a significant fraction of those individuals with positive antibodies has led some to recommend that all pregnant patients be screened for the presence of thyroid peroxidase (TPO) antibodies during the first trimester of pregnancy.[66] It is likely that hypo- or hyperthyroidism will be found to be common in the antibody-positive group when systematic follow-up studies of thyroid function are performed during the postpartum period. Table 14-4 summarizes the types of autoimmune thyroid disease that can be expected in the pregnant and postpartum population. These are

TABLE 14-4. Autoimmune Thyroid Disease During Pregnancy and the Postpartum Period

Primary hypothyroidism
    Thyroid destruction (Hashimoto's disease)
    Circulating TSH-receptor-blocking antibody
Asymptomatic (euthyroid) autoimmune thyroid disease
Postpartum thyroid disease (PPTD)
    Hyperthyroidism
    Hypothyroidism
    Combinations
Graves' disease
    Pre-existing
    Gestational exacerbation and remission
    Postpartum exacerbation

discussed in greater detail below. Postpartum thyroiditis is also reviewed in Chapters 8 and 13.

PRIMARY HYPOTHYROIDISM

Prevalence

Primary hypothyroidism is usually caused by autoimmune thyroiditis or radioiodine or surgical treatment of Graves' disease (see Ch. 9). Roughly 1 to 2 percent of patients who become pregnant are already receiving levothyroxine therapy for hypothyroidism due to one or another of these conditions. A recent study evaluated the prevalence of elevated serum TSH concentrations (greater than 6 μU/ml) in 2,000 serum samples that had been obtained for α-fetoprotein screening from pregnant women at 15 to 18 weeks' gestation.[83] TSH concentrations greater than 6 μU/ml were found in 49 women, or 2.5 percent of the unselected pregnant population (Table 14-5). Serum thyroid hormone concentrations and anti-TPO antibodies were compared by assaying these abnormal samples and those with normal TSH results just before and after those in the series. Of the 49 specimens with TSH elevation, 6 were found to have subnormal free T_4 values. The remaining 43

had an elevated TSH with serum T_4 results still in the normal range. Fifty-eight percent of the patients with an elevated TSH were positive for anti-TPO antibodies, as opposed to only 11 percent of the controls. The design of this study did not permit the investigators to determine whether the individuals with an elevated TSH had recognized thyroid disease or were taking inadequate levothyroxine or excessive antithyroid drugs. The prevalence of subnormal serum T_4 results of 0.3% in this study presumably represents the lower limit of the estimate of hypothyroidism in the pregnant population, since adequately treated hypothyroid patients would not be recognized.

A much rarer cause of hypothyroidism during pregnancy is that associated with the presence of TSH receptor blocking antibody.[74,84-87] In such patients, hypothyroidism is caused by interference in TSH–TSH receptor interaction. The significance of this problem during pregnancy is that blocking antibody may be transmitted to the fetus and cause intrauterine or transient neonatal hypothyroidism. While this is an unusual cause of congenital hypothyroidism, it has been confirmed in several instances.[86,87]

Pregnancy Outcome

The reported increase of spontaneous abortions in women with circulating antithyroid antibodies has been mentioned previously. This is not a consequence of associated hypothyroidism, and it is not clear what, if any, causal relationship there is between the two observations. There are only a few reports of the outcome of pregnancy in patients with untreated hypothyroidism.[88-90] One suggests that there were no significant consequences that could be directly attributed to the hypothyroidism.[88] In a second study, hypothyroidism was present but was also associated with a number of other problems, including anemia, hypertension, and nutritional inadequacy.[89] While in the latter series, significant ma-

TABLE 14-5. Prevalence of Elevated TSH in 200 Consecutive Women at 15 to 18 Weeks' Gestation

	n	Median mU/L	Free T_4 pmol/L	TPO Antibody (% pos)
Total screened	2000	2.1	—	—
Elevated TSH (>6 mU/L)	40	10	11.5 ± 0.44	58
Controls	99	2.3	13.4 ± 0.28	11

ternal complications including preeclampsia and placenta abruptio occurred, it is difficult to know which were the most important causative factors.

In congenital hypothyroidism due to athyreosis, maternal T_4 is the only source of fetal thyroid hormone. Thus, in mothers with untreated hypothyroidism, damage to the central nervous system development of the athyreotic fetus may be greater in the absence of placentally transported thyroxine.[91] A similar problem might occur in the infant with an intact thyroid if untreated maternal hypothyroidism is due to blocking antibodies. A comparison of children of mothers with hypothyroidism during the first trimester with their siblings did not suggest any difference in intellectual development, although the numbers were small.[90]

Diagnosis

The diagnosis of primary hypothyroidism during pregnancy can be readily established by measuring the free T_4 index and TSH. It should be recalled that total serum T_4 should be increased approximately 4 to 5 μg/dl (50 to 60 nmol/L) in the pregnant patient, whereas free T_4 is in the normal range (Fig. 14-1). The symptoms of hypothyroidism are similar to those in the nonpregnant individual. However, they may be difficult to separate from symptoms such as the fatigue associated with normal pregnancy. A high index of suspicion is necessary, and any patient with positive TPO or TG antibodies should also have a serum TSH determination to screen for this condition.

Therapeutic Considerations

The newly diagnosed hypothyroid patient should receive a full replacement dose of levothyroxine immediately, assuming there are no abnormalities in

TABLE 14-7. Serum Free T_4 and TSH Concentrations Before and During Pregnancy in Women with Previous Thyroid Ablation Taking Constant T_4 Doses

	Before Mean ± SD	During
T_4 dose (μg/day)	112 ± 27	112 ± 27
T_4 dose (μg/kg/day)	1.77 ± 0.48	1.66 ± 0.42[a]
Serum free T_4 (pmol/L)	21 ± 7	11 ± 4
Serum TSH (mU/L)	1.4 ± 1.4	14 ± 15[a]

[a] $P < 0.001$.
(From Kaplan.[51])

cardiac function. For maintenance, recent results suggest that patients with thyroid failure due to Hashimoto's disease should receive approximately 1.9 μg levothyroxine/kg ideal body weight (Table 14-6). Patients with a history of thyroid ablation should receive somewhat more, approximately 2.3 μg/kg/d (or roughly 1 μg/lb). To normalize the T_4 pool rapidly, therapy may be initiated by giving 3 days of a levothyroxine dose, which is three times the estimated daily replacement. This will allow more rapid normalization of the plasma T_4 and a more rapid return to the euthyroid state.

As mentioned earlier in this chapter, there is compelling evidence that in patients with pre-existing hypothyroidism, levothyroxine requirements will increase during gestation (Table 14-7). This change has been observed within 4 weeks of implantation.[51] If the pregnancy is planned, the patient should have thyroid function tests soon after the missed period. If serum TSH is not increased at that time, the test should be repeated at 8 weeks' and 6 months' gestation, since the increase in requirements may not be-

TABLE 14-6. Doses of Thyroxine Required for Normal Serum TSH Concentration Before and During Pregnancy in Patients with Primary Hypothyroidism

	Patients with Hashimoto's Disease (n = 15)		Patient's with Thyroid Ablation (n = 18)	
	Before	During	Before	During
T_4 dose (μg/day)	111 ± 25	139 ± 52	114 ± 33	166 ± 64[a]
T_4 dose (μg/kg/day)	1.7 ± 0.6	1.9 ± 0.9	1.8 ± 0.5	2.3 ± 0.8[a]
Serum TSH (mU/L)	2.0 ± 1.8	1.8 ± 1.1	1.5 ± 1.3	1.9 ± 1.1

[a] $P < 0.01$.

come apparent until later. At the time of delivery, the levothyroxine dose should be reduced to its pregestational level and the TSH concentration reassayed 6 to 8 weeks later (Fig. 14-2).[50,92]

As mentioned, there has been suspicion that the intellectual development of infants born to hypothyroxinemic mothers may be impaired, although more recent reassessments of this issue are reassuring.[90,91] Nonetheless, common sense dictates that levothyroxine replacement should be designed to duplicate normal physiology and that patients with hypothyroidism should be monitored by serum TSH measurements with sufficient regularity to permit achievement of this goal.[93]

THYROTOXICOSIS

One of the most difficult challenges for the endocrinologist is the management of Graves' disease in the pregnant patient. It has been estimated that approximately 1 in 500 pregnancies is complicated by hyperthyroidism due to Graves' disease, thus representing one of the most common endocrine disorders during gestation. Since the most common cause of hyperthyroidism in the pregnant patient is Graves' disease, this section will focus primarily on that disorder. However, other conditions such as toxic nodules or multinodular goiter may also occur. These are rarely severe enough to require definitive therapy during gestation and thus can be managed expectantly.

Clinical Indications

The historic clues and physical findings of hyperthyroidism in the pregnant patient are the same as occur in the nonpregnant patient. What makes it difficult to recognize these findings as symptoms of elevated thyroid hormone levels is the similarity to the symptoms of normal pregnancy to those of thyrotoxicosis (see Tables 14-1 and 14-8). Fatigue, palpitations, anxiety, heat intolerance, and diaphoresis are all symptoms that can be found in the pregnant female without thyrotoxicosis. In general, the patient with complicating thyrotoxicosis has more severe symptoms or notes that the symptoms of this pregnancy are somewhat different from those of her earlier experiences. In the evaluation of patients in whom the presence of thyrotoxicosis is an issue, the clinician should pay special attention to a prior his-

TABLE 14-8. Symptoms and Signs Suggesting the Presence of Hyperthyroidism in a Pregnant Patient

1. Prior history of hyperthyroidism or autoimmune thyroid disease in the patient or her family.
2. Presence of typical symptoms of hyperthyroidism, including weight loss (or failure to gain weight), palpitations, proximal muscle weakness, emotional lability, or pruritus.
3. Symptoms suggesting Graves' disease, such as ophthalmopathy or pretibial myxedema
4. Accentuation of normal symptoms of pregnancy, such as heat intolerance, diaphoresis, and fatigue.
5. Pulse rate >100 and widened pulse pressure.
6. Eye signs of Graves' disease, pretibial myxedema, or onycholysis.
7. Thyroid enlargement, especially in iodine-sufficient geographic areas.
8. Thyroid nodule (>3 cm) or multinodular goiter.

tory of thyrotoxicosis or autoimmune thyroid disease in the patient, her relatives, or children. However, since Graves' disease may appear for the first time in the first trimester, a negative family or personal history does not eliminate this possibility. A useful historical point is that instead of the customary weight gain, patients report weight loss, usually with an increased appetite. However, nausea or emesis occur during normal pregnancies or patients may have hyperemesis gravidarum leading to weight loss and raise the possibility of hyperthyroidism. Additional historical factors suggesting the presence of excess thyroid hormone are excessive palpitations, proximal muscle weakness, and emotional lability. The presence of Graves' ophthalmopathy or pretibial myxedema (Ch. 12) should further alert the physician to the diagnosis of hyperthyroid Graves' disease as the cause of the thyrotoxicosis. In general, patients are not aware of thyroid enlargement. If it occurs, it is likely that the hyperthyroidism will be of moderate or severe degree. Occasionally pruritus is a symptom of hyperthyroidism in the younger patient and may be an early manifestation of hyperthyroidism during pregnancy.

On physical examination, the pulse rate is almost universally elevated. However, tachycardia may be a part of the normal response to pregnancy and, as with other manifestations of hypermetabolism, the thyrotoxicosis only exacerbates this tendency. If the pulse rate is greater than 100 and there is no respiratory variation or bradycardia during a Valsalva maneuver, one should suspect that thyrotoxicosis is present. As occurs during thyrotoxicosis in the non-pregnant individual, the systolic pressure is increased and the diastolic pressure reduced due to a decrease in peripheral vascular resistance. However, the latter is again characteristic of pregnancy and thus this represents only a relative criteria. Eye signs and pretibial myxedema are especially helpful, though these may be mild. Thyroid enlargement is highly suggestive of thyroid pathology when iodine intake is sufficient. Thyroid enlargement may occur as a physiologic response to the thyroid stimulation, particularly in the first trimester of pregnancy in those areas of the world where iodine is deficient or borderline, such as Belgium, parts of Italy, Germany, Scandinavia, and portions of the United Kingdom and South America.[2,8,11,12] The presence of a thyroid nodule or multinodular goiter, while rare, should also lead to an evaluation of thyroid status. Lastly, onycholysis is virtually limited to the young hyperthyroid female, and its presence on the fourth and fifth fingers should lead to a search for this diagnosis. In many situations, it will be the obstetrician who makes the diagnosis of hyperthyroidism based on lack of weight gain and excessive tachycardia or goiter. In such patients, thyroid function tests will often have already been performed and the diagnosis established prior to the first visit to the endocrinologist.

Laboratory Diagnosis

The immunometric TSH has simplified the diagnosis of thyrotoxicosis during pregnancy (see Chs. 4 and 6). Virtually all patients with significant clinical symptoms will have a serum TSH less than 0.1 mU/L and will at the same time show elevations in the serum free T_4 and free T_3 estimates (Table 14-9).

TABLE 14-9. Laboratory Confirmation of Hyperthyroidism During Pregnancy

1. Increased free T_4 and T_3 index or free T_4 and T_3. The total T_4 and T_3 are increased above normal range for pregnancy. The resin T_3 uptake or THBR is not reduced as it normally is when TBG is elevated.
2. Serum TSH <0.1 except in the presence of markedly elevated hCG values or severe hyperemesis gravidum or in rare patients with TSH-induced hyperthyroidism.
3. The presence of TPO antibodies or TSH receptor antibodies points to autoimmune thyroid disease as the cause of the hyperthyroidism.

If second- or third-generation TSH assays are not available, then the combination of clinical symptoms and serum free T_4 estimates should generally allow the diagnosis to be established. A serum T_4 above the elevated normal range for pregnancy (approximately 9 to 18 μg T_4/dl, 120 to 240 nmol/L), with a resin T_3 uptake or THBR value that is not reduced (as it should be in normal pregnancy), should confirm the diagnosis. As mentioned, in the first trimester the serum TSH may be less than 0.5 mU/L in 10 to 20 percent of euthyroid individuals.[2,4,9,16,31,33] Therefore, it is the degree of TSH suppression during the first trimester that must be considered in making the diagnosis. Screening of pregnant patients for antibodies against thyroid antigens is now performed with increasing frequency. Since many patients with Graves' disease will have TPO antibodies, their presence should alert the clinician to the possibility that autoimmune thyroid disease is the cause of the symptoms associated with hyperthyroidism.

If the abnormalities in the thyroid function tests are only borderline, it is not likely that significant clinical thyrotoxicosis is present. Since the principle of treatment of the pregnant patient with hyperthyroidism is to avoid antithyroid drugs whenever possible, treatment is not indicated in such circumstances. This fact is sometimes lost sight of in the enthusiasm to establish a definitive diagnosis.

Etiology

Graves' disease is the cause of over 95 percent of thyrotoxicosis during pregnancy (Table 14-10). The hyperthyroidism of hyperemesis gravidarum tends to be transient and usually not so severe and is associated with less marked abnormalities in thyroid function tests.[31] Differentiation from Graves' disease may be impossible in the absence of eye signs or positive thyroid-stimulating antibodies (TSAb) or thyroid-binding inhibitory immunoglobulins (TBII) assay.

TABLE 14-10. Differential Diagnosis of Thyrotoxicosis in Pregnancy

1. Graves' disease
2. Hyperemesis gravidarum
3. Molar pregnancy or choriocarcinoma
4. Subacute thyroiditis
5. Toxic nodule(s)
6. Exogenous thyrotoxicosis

Painless thyroiditis is a common cause of hyperthyroidism in the postpartum period but is quite rare during gestation. Molar pregnancy and choriocarcinoma, both associated with marked elevations in hCG, may be accompanied by thyrotoxicosis due to thyroid stimulation. However, the relative size of the uterus for gestational age, the marked elevation in hCG levels, and abdominal ultrasound will allow an accurate diagnosis even though there may be slight thyroid enlargement. In general, the symptoms of hyperthyroidism in these two conditions are much milder than occur in Graves' disease, presumably due to the shorter duration of the hyperthyroidism. Multinodular goiter and toxic nodules may lead to hyperthyroidism in pregnancy as in other patients. However, it should be recalled that since the use of radioisotopes is precluded during pregnancy, the size and configuration of the thyroid must be ascertained by palpation or by ultrasound. Solitary functioning thyroid nodules must be of significant size, more than 3 to 4 cm in diameter, before they can produce quantities of thyroid hormone sufficient to cause thyrotoxicosis. Such nodules are generally associated with a suppressed TSH and a smaller contralateral lobe.

While not common, the possibility of exogenous thyrotoxicosis must always be kept in mind. This condition should be suspected when hyperthyroidism coexists with a small thyroid gland. Further evidence that exogenous thyroid hormone administration is a possibility can be achieved by measuring serum TG, which will be low, and determination of the T_3:T_4 molar ratio, which will also be low relative to that in the typical Graves' patient (T_3/T_4 in Graves' disease is 0.02 to 0.03, in normal subjects, 0.01 to 0.02[94]).

Treatment

Graves' Disease

The treatment of Graves' disease during pregnancy has been discussed extensively over the past 30 years and reviewed recently.[95] The design of appropriate therapy for this condition requires an understanding of the previously mentioned effects of pregnancy on the natural history of Graves' disease. In a study of 35 pregnant Japanese patients with Graves' disease there was a transient increase in the free T_4 index at 10 to 15 weeks in about half the patients, with a restoration to normal values during the second and third trimesters.[96] In the 2 to 4 months following delivery, 32 of 35 patients developed hyperthyroidism. A number of investigators have demonstrated a decrease in the concentration of thyroid-stimulating antibodies as pregnancy continues.[74,75,78,97] The cause of this improvement has not been specifically identified; however, there is a clear decrease in the helper T lymphocytes during pregnancy, which reflects the generalized ameliorative effects of pregnancy on autoimmune diseases (Table 14-3). Amino and co-workers, as well as others, have described similar changes in patients with Hashimoto's thyroiditis in whom TPO antibody titers decrease during pregnancy only to rise to high levels again in the postpartum period.[69-71] Further knowledge of the specific immunopathology of the Graves' patient will be required before more specific explanations can be found for this clinical phenomenon. However, the *first* principle is that the hyperthyroidism will usually become less severe as pregnancy continues.

While there are few studies on the course of pregnancy in patients with untreated Graves' disease, several reports have identified a number of consequences such as preeclampsia, fetal malformations, premature delivery, and low-birth-weight infants.[95] In most of these studies, the general medical care of these patients was suboptimal, and it is not clear which of the potentially causative factors leading to the suboptimal fetal outcome was more important. Nonetheless, recent studies of over 200 pregnancies (summarized in Table 14-11) indicate that there is no adverse impact of adequately treated Graves' disease on pregnancy.[98] The treatment goal in these studies was to keep the patients at a high euthyroid or mildly hyperthyroid level of thyroid function throughout pregnancy using as low a dose of antithyroid drugs as possible. This is the *second* general prin-

TABLE 14-11. Fetal Outcome in 230 Consecutive Pregnancies in 172 Japanese Women with Graves' Disease

Normal distribution of birth weight.
No increase in obstetrical complications.
16.5% incidence of neonatal thyroid dysfunction.
No increase in the prevalence of fetal anomalies.
No instances of aplasia cutis (91 women received methimazole, 20 received propylthiouracil).

ciple for successful therapy of the pregnant hyperthyroid patient.

The *third* consideration is that *all* antithyroid drugs cross the placenta and in most cases will affect fetal thyroid function.[54,99–101] The thiourea drugs, propylthiouracil (PTU) and methimazole (MMI), have been compared with respect to their use in the pregnant patient. Propylthiouracil is more water soluble and is therefore less well transferred from the maternal to the fetal circulation, as well as from the maternal circulation into breast milk.[99,101–104] This has led to the recommendation that during pregnancy PTU should be used in preference to MMI unless specific attempts are being made to suppress thyroid function in the fetus. However, MMI is used commonly in during pregnancy in Japan and carbimazole (which is metabolized to MMI) in the United Kingdom. Specific comparisons of the effectiveness and complications of PTU and MMI in the same pregnant patient have not been reported.

Some years ago a prospective study was performed on the effects of maternal propylthiouracil therapy on thyroid function in the newborn.[105] Patients received frequent adjustments of PTU during pregnancy to achieve the lowest dose compatible with the mildly hyperthyroid state. This resulted in a range of PTU doses from 100 to 200 mg in these 11 patients during the third trimester. Some received supplemental T_4 or T_4/T_3 combinations, as was the practice in some clinics during that time. No mother developed a TSH elevation. These results indicate that the goal of not overtreating these patients was met. On the other hand, in the neonates, T_4 concentrations in cord serum and at 1 day of age were subnormal. Serum TSH concentrations peaked at day 1 at a level of approximately 45 mU/L in the infants of PTU-treated mothers, whereas in normal infants, the mean day one TSH is approximately 20 mU/ml. However, by 3 days of age, TSH and T_4 values were normal. (See Fig. 15-5 in Ch. 15) Even using these modest doses of PTU, there was clear evidence of newborn thyroid dysfunction, albeit of a modest degree.

The effect of 400 mg PTU on fetal thyroid function was dramatically exemplified in one patient who was the impetus for the prospective study. This infant had respiratory distress, APGAR scores of 1 and 2, a cord serum T_4 value of 4.4, and TSH greater than 480 (see Table 15-3 in Ch. 15). There was no history of iodide exposure. The causal relationship

between maternal PTU and neonatal hypothyroidism in this patient was reflected in the rapid increase of T_3 and T_4 to normal levels by day 4, concomitant with a dramatic reduction in serum TSH to near normal without exogenous levothyroxine. A similar but much larger experience showed that there was a correlation between the level of the maternal free T_4 and that of the neonate during antithyroid drug therapy. If maternal T_4 was maintained elevated or in the upper one-third of the normal range, only 1 of the 19 infants had a decreased free T_4. Of the 24 mothers in whom the free T_4 was reduced to levels lower than this, 15 had infants with a reduced free T_4.[106]

Table 14-12 summarizes further data correlating the impact of antithyroid drug therapy with neonatal thyroid function in another group of pregnant Japanese patients.[98] Four of nine infants of mothers receiving more than 1,000 antithyroid drug tablets (~3.7/d) during gestation were hypothyroid or had an elevated TSH, whereas only 7 of 55 receiving 100 to 499 tablets were so affected. Hypothyroidism and elevated TSH were not found in any infants of 134 mothers with Graves' disease who had received 1 to 100 tablets. Thus, one can attribute the hypothyroidism or elevated TSH results to the therapy rather than to the presence of autoimmune thyroid disease.

Thus, the moderate to severely hyperthyroid pregnant patient presents the major therapeutic dilemma. The antithyroid drug doses required to regulate the thyroid function of the mother may be too high for the fetus. Since both the TSH-receptor antibody and the antithyroid drug can cross the placenta, but thyroid hormone passes in only limited amounts, there is no simple way to resolve this issue. One cannot easily avoid the hypothyroidism of the fetus, but one can eliminate the requirement for antithyroid drug during pregnancy by prior treatment of the mother. This has led many experts to conclude that patients with more severe Graves' disease should be treated definitively prior to becoming pregnant. There are no risk-benefit analyses of either approach.

These data also raise the question of whether the clinical syndrome of Graves' disease might differ in the Japanese and North American populations. None of the 11 patients whose data are presented in Fig. 15-5 had particularly severe Graves' disease by North American standards, and none of the neonates developed hyperthyroidism. In fact, the preva-

**TABLE 14-12. Relationship Between Antithyroid Drug Dose
and Neonatal Thyroid Dysfunction**

Dose[a]	n (%)	Hyperthyroid n (%)	Hypothyroid n (%)	Elevated TSH n (%)
≥1000	9 (4)	4 (44)	1 (11)	3 (33)
500–1000	30 (13)	6 (20)	5 (17)	4 (13)
100–499	55 (24)	2 (4)	1 (2)	6 (11)
1–99	17 (7)	0	0	0
0 and T4[b]	119 (52)	1 (1)	0	0

[a] Total dose as tablets of PTU (50 mg) or MMI (5 mg) during pregnancy.
[b] No antithyroid drug (110) or thyroxine therapy (9).

lence of neonatal hyperthyroidism in the United States is estimated to be only 1 percent.[75] The figure derived from the Japanese patients listed in Table 14-12 is five times this (13/230)—an unexplained difference.

Iodide alone is not traditionally used in pregnant patients because of the potential for causing iodide-induced goiter and possible hypothyroidism in the fetus. Therefore, while iodide (2 qtts saturated solution of potassium iodide [SSKI] bid ~ 200 mg total I⁻/day) can be safely used for 5 to 10 days in the preoperative preparation of pregnant patients for thyroid surgery, chronic therapy at these levels is not recommended. However, small amounts of iodide (6 to 20 mg) have been given to women with moderate Graves' disease without causing fetal goiter.[107] This treatment reduced serum T_4 in all patients, although the serum free T_4 remained above normal in more than half. None of the 35 infants of these mothers had a subnormal free T_4 and only one an elevated TSH. While no comment was made about the presence of neonatal goiter, presumably it did not occur, since the TSH levels in cord sera were not elevated. A possible explanation for the lack of complications of iodide therapy in this group may be that these occur only in other patients receiving concomitant thiourea drugs or in the fetuses of mothers receiving iodide for nonthyroid disease who do not have maternal thyroid-stimulating immunoglobulin to maintain thyroid function. It should also be noted that the doses used (6 to 40 mg iodide/d) are low compared to that supplied by the 5 qtts SSKI per day. The content of iodide in SSKI is about 35 mg per drop. While further experience with this approach is necessary for confirmation, these results suggest that *modest* quantities of maternal iodide may not be as deleterious to fetal thyroid function as was once thought.

There is little experience with other nonthiourea antithyroid drugs such as lithium during pregnancy.

In an attempt to alter the tendency of Graves' disease to relapse in the postpartum period, one group has administered 100 μg of levothyroxine/d to a group of pregnant patients who had a remission of Graves' disease during therapy with MMI during the first portion of pregnancy.[108] This strategy was based on earlier results from this group suggesting that TSH suppressive levothyroxine therapy could ameliorate the tendency for relapse of Graves' disease after cessation of antithyroid drug therapy (see Ch. 11). The rate of increase of TSH receptor antibodies was more rapid in patients who had not received T_4 than in those who had. Furthermore, postpartum recurrence of hyperthyroidism in the first year after delivery was only 5 percent in the levothyroxine-treated group but was 32 percent in the controls. This approach could have considerable importance in the treatment of patients who become euthyroid during pregnancy. Since it is a relatively new strategy, there is need for further study before the conclusions can be assumed to be generally applicable.

Table 14-13 summarizes the important aspects of the treatment of patients with Graves' disease. These recommendations are based on the considerations already discussed, with particular emphasis on the natural history of the condition. The main principle of therapy is to administer the lowest dose of antithyroid drug feasible for regulating the clinical symptomatology of the patient. Thus, mild degrees of thyrotoxicosis can be tolerated as long as the pregnancy is progressing satisfactorily. Such patients should be followed closely with the obstetrician with careful monitoring of weight gain and fetal heart rate. A typical starting dose of antithyroid drug might be 50 to 100 mg PTU twice daily. We prefer PTU to

TABLE 14-13. Treatment Guidelines for Graves' Disease During Pregnancy

1. Monitor pulse, weight gain, thyroid size, free T_4 and T_3 indices, and TSH at monthly intervals.
2. Use the lowest doses of antithyroid drug that will maintain the patient in a mildly hyperthyroid state but not higher than ~300 mg PTU (20 mg methimazole).
3. Communicate regularly with the obstetrician, especially with respect to fetal pulse and growth.
4. One should not attempt to normalize serum TSH. Serum TSH concentrations between 0.1 and 0.4 mU/L are generally appropriate, but lower levels are acceptable if the patient is clinically satisfactory.
5. Propylthiouracil is usually preferable to methimazole due to the higher transplacental transport and potency of the latter drug.
6. While even as little as 100–200 mg of PTU/day may affect fetal thyroid function, dosages of as high as 300 mg PTU (~20 mg methimazole) have been employed. Iodides should not be used during pregnancy except to prepare patient for surgery.
7. Indications for surgery are:
   a. Requirements for high doses of PTU (>300 mg) or MMI (>20 mg) with inadequate control of clinical hyperthyroidism.
   b. Poor compliance with resulting clinical hyperthyroidism.
   c. The appearance of fetal hypothyroidism (retarded bone age, bradycardia) at antithyroid drug doses required for control of the mother.
8. Usually the dose of antithyroid drug can be adjusted downward after the first trimester and often discontinued during the third.
9. Antithyroid drugs will often need to be reinstituted or increased after delivery.

methimazole for two reasons. First, while the evidence linking aplasia cutis to maternal methimazole is not conclusive, it is also not sufficient to rule out a causal role.[95] This condition, an absence of skin and its accessory structures—usually over the scalp, has not been reported in mothers treated with PTU. Second, one tablet of PTU (50 mg) is less potent than 5 mg of methimazole or carbimazole. Monitoring antithyroid drug requirements at monthly intervals is necessary because it is often possible to reduce the PTU dose after the hyperthyroidism is controlled. The choice of the maximal safe antithyroid drug dose for pregnancy is somewhat arbitrary, since results vary with the individual maternal-fetal thyroid pairs. Limits as low as 150 mg or as high as 400 mg have been suggested. If, for one of various reasons stated in Table 14-13, it appears that surgery is required, the administration of 1 or 2 drops of SSKI

twice a day may facilitate patient preparation. Following surgery, levothyroxine therapy should be instituted at a dose of about 2.2 μg/kg, typical for that required in the hypothyroid pregnant patient.

Neonatal Thyroid Function and Graves' Disease

As indicated, neonatal hyperthyroidism is extremely uncommon—approximately 1 percent of pregnancies in patients with Graves' disease in North America.[4,75] There is a rough relationship between the level of TSH-receptor antibody and the risk of neonatal Graves' disease in that higher levels of maternal antibody are more likely to be transmitted to the fetus. Since there is no internationally recognized standard for TSAb, this relationship is imprecise, and an absolute antibody "titer" at which neonatal hyperthyroidism is more likely to occur cannot be defined. On the other hand, experienced laboratories may be able to be much more precise in this prediction.[109] Neonatal Graves' disease may occur in patients whose TSAb titer is barely elevated and not in infants where it has been quite elevated, presumably in the latter case due to the coexistence of blocking antibodies. Patients who have had previous surgical or radioiodine therapy for Graves' disease and are receiving levothyroxine may still have significant quantities of TSH receptor antibody.[74,78,97] Therefore, while it is difficult to argue that all individuals with a history of (or the presence of) Graves' disease should have TSH receptor antibody determinations during pregnancy, those with clinical signs generally associated with higher titers, such as moderate to severe ophthalmopathy, pretibial myxedema, large goiter, or high antithyroid drug requirement (or a history thereof), should be considered at high risk. In such individuals, assessment of TSH receptor antibody titer may provide some general guidance, especially if the laboratory can provide documentation of the correlation between a given assay result and the severity of Graves' disease. The best estimate is the bioassay in the patient with an intact thyroid, as reflected in the size of the thyroid and the antithyroid drug dose requirement. Mothers with a history of bearing infants with neonatal Graves' are at extremely high risk of repeated episodes.[75]

On the other hand, the most helpful and specific observations are those that indicate fetal hyperthyroidism. These include fetal tachycardia (> 160 bpm), advanced bone age, a small-for-gestational-age fetus, and on occasion fetal goiter.[75] If persistent fetal tachycardia is present it is reasonable to institute antithyroid drug therapy (200 to 400 mg propylthiouracil or 20 mg methimazole) to the mother and to supplement this with levothyroxine. This approach has been used prospectively in a few instances, but it is difficult to monitor.[110] Cordocentesis can be used to obtain fetal blood samples for diagnosis or for monitoring therapy, but this procedure is associated with complications and/or fetal loss in as many as 1 percent of procedures.[111] We have had success in monitoring the PTU dose to the fetus by giving sufficient antithyroid drug to the mother to maintain the fetal heart rate at about 160.

More often, neonatal Graves' disease will be diagnosed at or shortly following delivery after the maternal antithyroid drugs have been cleared from the neonatal thyroid and serum. Signs of hyperthyroidism in the neonate are congestive heart failure, goiter, proptosis, jaundice, hyperirritability, failure to thrive, and tachycardia. Once considered, the diagnosis is easily made. Cord serum T_4 and TSH determinations should be performed in all deliveries of patients with a history or the presence of Graves' disease.

Treatment should be implemented in collaboration with the neonatologist and should include iodide, antithyroid drugs, glucocorticoids, and digoxin with β-adrenergic blocking agents (depending on cardiovascular status). In some patients, particularly those in whom both TSH receptor blocking and stimulating antibodies are present, neonatal hyperthyroidism may be delayed in onset.[97] This circumstance can also confound the results of thyroid-stimulating and thyrotropin receptor–blocking antibody tests in the diagnosis of maternal Graves' disease. Thus, the pediatrician should be alerted by the endocrinologist to obtain a serum T_4 if any symptoms suggesting the presence of hyperthyroidism appear during the first 6 weeks of life, even if the cord serum assay results are normal, but especially if cord serum TSH concentration is suppressed.

Graves' Disease in Lactating Mothers

Both PTU and MMI are secreted in human milk, although PTU may be less so.[102–104] In one study performed to evaluate effects of 15 mg of carbimazole or 150 mg of PTU on the infants of nursing mothers, there was no evidence of neonatal hypothyroidism as evidenced by elevated TSH or reduced T_4 over the first 21 days of life.[112] Even with carbimazole or MMI, only small quantities of drug enter the milk. On the other hand, to be weighed against this is the necessity for periodic monitoring of the infant's thyroid function when antithyroid drugs are being administered to the mother. Furthermore, there is a remote possibility that the allergic reactions associated with antithyroid drugs, such as agranulocytosis or rash, will occur in the infant. While these would be rare, they should be kept in mind when evaluating the febrile infant or the presence of a rash.

For these reasons, most endocrinologists advise against concomitant antithyroid drug therapy and nursing. This consideration should influence the decision regarding definitive therapy in those individuals requiring high doses of antithyroid drugs who are contemplating pregnancy and wanting to breastfeed. In most circumstances, the safest course of action for the fetus and newborn is definitive treatment of the mother surgically or with ^{131}I prior to pregnancy. If ^{131}I is employed as the treatment, an arbitrary time period—about 6 months—should be allowed to elapse between the ^{131}I therapy and pregnancy to minimize the possibility of transient radiation-induced changes in the ovum.

Treatment of Other Causes of Hyperthyroidism

The hyperthyroidism of hyperemesis gravidarum is mild and often not clinically significant.[34,36] The major problems are restitution of fluids and therapy for nausea. In the patient in whom Graves' disease and hyperemesis cannot be differentiated, even using receptor antibody measurements, and in whom hyperemesis continues and symptomatology is significant, a therapeutic trial of antithyroid drugs is indicated.[34,38] The hyperthyroidism of hydatidiform mole or choriocarcinoma is generally mild to moderate, and patients can be prepared for surgery with iodide, antithyroid drugs, or even β-adrenergic receptor antagonists alone. The condition is self-limited and ends after removal of the tumor producing the thyroid-stimulating hCG.[113]

The treatment of hyperthyroidism due to single or multiple thyroid nodules depends on the degree of hyperthyroidism. If this is mild, therapy can be withheld until after pregnancy, at which time radioiodine can be used if the physical size of the nodule is not causing significant obstruction. On the other hand, if more severe hyperthyroidism is present, one must choose between using antithyroid drugs until the end of pregnancy and surgery during pregnancy. The major clinical problem in using antithyroid drugs for hyperthyroidism due to an autonomous nodule (or nodules) is that there is no transplacental passage of thyroid-stimulating antibody to protect the infant against the maternal antithyroid drug. While this makes thiourea agents potentially a riskier approach to therapy of nodular hyperthyroidism than of Graves' disease, the risk is more theoretical than real. Most young patients with hyperthyroidism due to autonomous nodules have a mild form of hyperthyroidism and should not require large doses of antithyroid drug.

NODULAR THYROID DISEASE

A thyroid nodule or a dominant nodule in a multinodular gland may be recognized for the first time in the pregnant patient.[114,115] If this occurs prior to the third trimester and the patient is not hyperthyroid, a fine-needle aspiration should be performed (see Ch. 18). If a clear-cut diagnosis of malignancy is made (usually only with papillary, medullary, or anaplastic carcinoma) appropriate thyroid surgery should be performed as indicated by diagnosis. If a diagnosis of follicular neoplasm or a suspicious result is obtained, surgery can be postponed until after delivery so that appropriate radioisotope studies can be performed to eliminate a diagnosis of autonomously functioning (benign) thyroid nodules. There is no evidence that the natural history of any form of thyroid cancer is altered by pregnancy.[114–118]

SUMMARY

Thyroid dysfunction occurs in 1 to 2 percent of pregnant patients. Despite the low prevalence of the coexistence of the two conditions, the concerns are much broader for two reasons. First, the physiologic changes of pregnancy simulate those of hyperthyroidism and, second, the treatment of the pregnant patient with thyroid dysfunction has implications for fetal and neonatal health and development. With respect to the physiologic changes of pregnancy, in addition to pregnancy-induced increases in metabolic rate, blood flow, heart rate, and cardiac output,

various subjective sensations such as fatigue and heat intolerance may suggest the possibility of coexistent thyrotoxicosis. Furthermore, the estrogen-induced increase in thyroxine-binding globulin increases serum T_4, which can potentially be confused with a true elevation in free T_4. Other changes that impact the hypothalamic pituitary thyroid system are the potential stimulation of thyroid function by hCG and the accelerated metabolism of thyroxine, presumably due to the placental fetal inner ring deiodinase.

With respect to diagnosis, the increasing dependence of the endocrinologist on the quantitation of serum thyrotropin as an indirect reflection of thyroid status has simplified the laboratory assessment of the pregnant patient with possible thyroid dysfunction. Increases in serum TSH generally mean subnormal thyroid hormone production rates, whereas a TSH less than 0.1 mU/L generally implies excess thyroid hormone supply of either endogenous or exogenous origin. With respect to hypothyroidism, it is important to recognize that requirements for exogenous levothyroxine increase 50 percent on average during pregnancy. This should be taken into account in the management of these patients. Appropriate diagnostic studies should be performed to titer the patients levothyroxine dose during gestation and reduce it thereafter. With respect to thyrotoxicosis, the commonest cause of this condition in the pregnant patient is Graves' disease. Since radioiodine is absolutely contraindicated during pregnancy, most patients are treated with antithyroid drugs during the course of gestation. It is critical for the clinician to recognize that the natural history of Graves' disease is altered during pregnancy, with a tendency for an exacerbation in the first trimester, an amelioration of the condition during the second and third trimesters, and a typical reexacerbation in the postpartum period. These changes are thought to be a consequence of the normal suppression of immune function during gestation, although the specific cause has not been elucidated. This natural history must be kept in mind when treating the Graves' disease patient since all antithyroid drugs pass the placenta and can, to a greater or less extent, impair thyroid function of the fetus. This is not a sufficiently severe factor to cause a clinical problem in the mildly hyperthyroid patient; however, in patients with more severe forms of Graves' disease the dose of antithyroid drugs required to control the patient's hyperthyroid manifestations may be in excess of the amounts that can be tolerated in terms of fetal thyroid function. While a specific upper limit of dosage has not been defined (and in fact may very significantly between patients or pregnancies), most authorities agree that requiring quantities of propylthiouracil in excess of 300 mg or methimazole in excess of 20 mg per day would significantly risk impairing fetal thyroid function, which would in turn lead to fetal goiter, possible hypothyroidism, and respiratory difficulty in the newborn. Accordingly, such patients are usually treated by surgery in the second trimester. While such a need is not common, it should be recognized as a suitable approach. In addition, to achieve the lowest dose of antithyroid drugs, the clinical symptomatology and progress of the pregnancy should be used as end points rather than an attempt to normalize the serum TSH. Because of the risks of administering high doses of antithyroid drugs during pregnancy, many authorities prefer to treat such patient with radioactive iodine or surgery prior to the onset of pregnancy to avoid these risks.

Neonatal hyperthyroidism is due to the transplacental transfer of maternal antibody. In the United States this occurs in only 1 to 2 percent of pregnancies in patients with Graves' disease; however, it may be higher in other countries, for example, Japan. The diagnosis of neonatal hyperthyroidism is usually made on the basis of fetal tachycardia, accelerated bone age, and intrauterine growth retardation. It may occur in patients with active Graves' disease or in patients who have had definitive treatment by surgery or radioactive iodine. The condition can be treated by surgery or radioactive iodine. The condition can be treated by administering antithyroid drugs to the mother, although monitoring the precise dose is difficult and is usually done indirectly by monitoring fetal pulse. The proper management of the pregnant patient with Graves' disease is thus one of the most challenging in clinical endocrinology.

Thyroid nodules in euthyroid pregnant patients should be aspirated for diagnosis. If malignancy is present, surgery should be performed; timing depends on the nature of the lesion and the time of parturition. Pregnancy itself does not adversely affect the natural history of thyroid carcinoma.

REFERENCES

1. Dworkin HJ, Jacquez JA, Beierwaltes WH: Relationship of iodine ingestion to iodine excretion in pregnancy. J Clin Endocrinol Metab 26:1329, 1966

2. Glinoer D, De Nayer P, Bourdoux P et al: Regulation of maternal thyroid during pregnancy. J Clin Endocrinol Metab 71:276, 1990

3. Glinoer D, Delange F, Laboureur I, De Nayer PH: Maternal and neonatal thyroid function at birth in an area of marginally low iodine intake. J Clin Endocrinol Metab 75:800, 1992

4. Burrow GN: Thyroid function and hyperfunction during gestation. Endocr Rev 14:194, 1993

5. Burrow GN: Thyroid status in normal pregnancy. J Clin Endocrinol Metab 71:274, 1990

6. Bauch K, Meng W, Ulrich FE et al: Thyroid status during pregnancy and post partum in regions of iodine deficiency and endemic goiter. Endocrinol Exp 20:67, 1986

7. Halnan KE: The radioiodine uptake of the human thyroid in pregnancy. Clin Sci 17:281, 1958

8. Crooks J, Tulloch MI, Turnbull AC et al: Comparative incidence of goitre in pregnancy in Iceland and Scotland. Lancet 2:625, 1969

9. Glinoer D, De Nayer P, Robyn C et al: Serum levels of intact human chorionic gonadotropin (HCG) and its free alpha and beta subunits, in relation to maternal thyroid stimulation during normal pregnancy. J Endocrinol Invest 16:881, 1993

10. Levy RP, Newman DM, Rejali LS, Barford DA: The myth of goiter in pregnancy. Am J Obstet Gynecol 137:701, 1980

11. Nelson M, Wickus GG, Caplan RH, Beguin EA: Thyroid gland size in pregnancy: an ultrasound and clinical study. J Reproduct Med 32:888, 1987

12. Glinoer D, Leome M: Goiter and pregnancy: a new insight into an old problem. Thyroid 2:65, 1992

13. Burrow GN, Fisher DA, Larsen PR: Mechanisms of disease: Maternal and fetal thyroid function. N Engl J Med 331:1072, 1994

14. Hershman JM: Role of human chorionic gonadotropin as a thyroid stimulator. J Clin Endocrinol Metab 74:258, 1992

15. Hershman JM, Lee HY, Sugawara M et al: Human chorionic gonadotropin stimulates iodide uptake, adenylate cyclase, and deoxribonucleic acid synthesis in cultured rat thyroid cells. J Clin Endocrinol Metab 67:74, 1988

16. Pekonen F, Alfthan H, Stenman UH, Ylikorkala O: Human chorionic gonadotropin (hCG) and thyroid function in early human pregnancy: Circadian variation and evidence for intrinsic thyrotropic activity of hCG. J Clin Endocrinol Metab 66:853, 1988

17. Harada A, Hershman JM, Reed AW et al: Comparison of thyroid stimulators and thyroid hormone concentrations in the sera of pregnant women. J Clin Endocrinol Metab 48:793, 1979

18. Kennedy RL, Cohn DM, Price A et al: Human chori-

onic gonadotropin may not be responsible for thyroid-stimulating activity in normal pregnancy serum. J Clin Endocrinol Metab 74:260, 1992

19. Kimura M, Amino N, Tamaki H et al: Physiologic thyroid activation in normal early pregnancy is induced by circulating hCG. Obstet Gynecol 75:775, 1990

20. Ballabio M, Poshyachinda M, Ekins RP: Pregnancy-induced changes in thyroid function: Role of human chorionic gonadotropin as putative regulator of maternal thyroid. J Clin Endocrinol Metab 73:824, 1991

21. Guillaume J, Schussler GC, Goldman J: Components of the total serum thyroid hormone concentrations during pregnancy: high free thyroxine and blunted thyrotropin (TSH) response to TSH-releasing hormone in the first trimester. J Clin Endocrinol Metab 60:678, 1985

22. Weeke J, Dybkjaer L, Granlie K et al: A longitudinal study of serum TSH, and total and free iodothyronines during normal pregnancy. Acta Endocrinol 101:531, 1982

23. Chan BY, Swaminathan R: Serum thyrotropin concentration measured by sensitive assays in normal pregnancy. Br J Obstet Gynecol 95:1332, 1988

24. Yamamoto T, Amino N, Tanizawa O et al: Longitudinal study of serum thyroid hormones, chorionic gonadotrophin and thyrotropin during and after normal pregnancy. Clin Endocrinol 10:459, 1979

25. Ylikorkala O, Kivinen S, Reinila MI: Serial prolactin and thyrotropin responses to thyrotropin-releasing hormone throughout normal human pregnancy. J Clin Endocrinol Metab 48:288, 1979

26. Yoshikawa N, Nishikawa M, Horimoto M et al: Thyroid-stimulating activity in sera of normal pregnant women. J Clin Endocrinol Metab 69:891, 1989

27. Pacchirotti A, Martino E, Bartalena L et al: Serum thyrotropin by ultrasensitive immunoradiometric assay and serum free thyroid hormones in pregnancy. J Endocrinol Invest 9:185, 1986

28. Pekonen F, Alfthan H, Stenman UH, Ylikorkala O: Human chorionic gonadotropin (hCG) and thyroid function in early human pregnancy: Circadian variation and evidence for intrinsic thyrotropic activity of hCG. J Clin Endocrinol Metab 66:853, 1988

29. Norman RJ, Green-Thompson RW, Jialal I et al: Hyperthyroidism in gestational trophoblastic neoplasia. Clin Endocrinol 15:395, 1981

30. Nagataki S, Mizuno M, Sakamoto S et al: Thyroid function in molar pregnancy. J Clin Endocrinol Metab 44:254, 1977

31. Berghout A, Endert E, Wiersinga WM, Touber JL: The application of an immunoradiometric assay of plasma thyrotropin (TSH-IRMA) in molar pregnancy. J Endocrinol Invest 11:15, 1988

32. Gow SM, Kellett HA, Seth J et al: Limitations of new thyroid function tests in pregnancy. Clin Chim Acta 152, 1985

33. Gow SM, Kellett HA, Seth J et al: Limitations of new thyroid function tests in pregnancy. Clin Chim Acta 152:325, 1985

34. Kirshon B, Lee W, Cotton DB: Prompt resolution of hyperthyroidism and hyperemesis gravidarum after delivery. Obstet Gynecol 71:1032, 1988

35. Bober SA, McGill AC, Tunbridge WMG: Thyroid function in hyperemesis gravidarum. Acta Endocrinol 111:404, 1986

36. Goodwin TM, Montoro M, Mestman JH: Transient hyperthyroidism and hyperemesis gravidarum: clinical aspects. Am J Obstet Gynecol 167:648, 1992

37. Goodwin TM, Montoro M, Mestman JH et al: The role of chorionic gonadotropin in transient hypothyroidism of hyperemesis gravidarum. J Clin Endocrinol Metab 75:1333, 1992

38. Lao TT, Chin KH, Chang AMZ: The outcome of hyperemetic pregnancies complicated by transient hyperthyroidism. Aust NZ J Obstet Gynaecol 27:99, 1987

39. Wilson R, McKillop JH, MacLean M et al: Thyroid function tests are rarely abnormal in patients with severe hyperemesis gravidarum. Clin Endocrinol 37:331, 1992

40. Dozeman R, Kaiser FE, Cass O, Pries J: Hyperthyroidism appearing as hyperemesis gravidarum. Arch Intern Med 143:2202, 1983

41. Mori M, Amino N, Tamaki H et al: Morning sickness and thyroid function in normal pregnancy. Obstet Gynecol 72:355, 1988

42. Kirshon B, Wesley L, Cotton DB: Prompt resolution of hyperthyroidism and hyperemesis gravidarum after delivery. Obstet Gynecol 71:1032, 1988

43. Bouillon R, Naesens M, Van Assche FA et al: Thyroid function in patients with hyperemesis gravidarum. Am J Obstet Gynecol 143:922, 1982

44. Glinoer D, McGuire RA, Dubois A et al: Thyroxine-binding globulin metabolism in rhesus monkeys: Effects of hyper- and hypothyroidism. Endocrinology 104:175, 1979

45. Ain KB, Mori Y, Refetoff S: Reduced clearance rate of thyroxine-binding globulin (TBG) with increased sialylation: a mechanism for estrogen-induced elevation of serum TBG concentration. J Clin Endocrinol Metab 65:689, 1987

46. Ain KB, Refetoff S: Relationship of oligosaccharide modification to the cause of serum thyroxine-binding globulin excess. J Clin Endocrinol Metab 66:1037, 1988

47. Refetoff S: Inherited thyroxine-binding globulin abnormalities in man. Endocr Rev 10:275, 1989

48. Ekins R, Edwards P, Newman B: The role of binding-proteins in hormone delivery (appendix). In Albertini A, Elkins RP (eds): Free Hormones in Blood. p. 3. Amsterdam, Elsevier Biomedical, 1982

49. Bartalena L: Recent achievements in studies on thyroid hormone–binding proteins. Endocr Rev 11:47, 1990

50. Mandel SJ, Larsen PR, Seely EW et al: Increased need for thyroxine during pregnancy in women with primary hypothyroidism. N Engl J Med 323:91, 1990

51. Kaplan MM: Monitoring thyroxine treatment during pregnancy. Thyroid 2:147, 1992

52. Larsen PR: Monitoring thyroxine treatment during pregnancy. Thyroid 2:153, 1992

53. Roti E, Fang SL, Green K et al: Human placenta is an active site of thyroxine and 3,3′,5-triiodothyronine tyrosyl ring deiodination. J Clin Endocrinol Metab 53:498, 1981

54. Roti E, Gnudi A, Braverman LE: The placental transport, synthesis and metabolism of hormones and drugs which affect thyroid function. Endocr Rev 4: 131, 1983

55. Hidal JT, Kaplan MM: Characteristics of thyroxine 5′-deiodination in cultured human placental cells: regulation by iodothyronines. J Clin Invest 76:947, 1985

56. Burman KD, Read J, Dimond RC et al: Measurements of 3,3′,5′-triiodothyronine (reverse T_3), 3,3′-L-diiodothyronine, T_3, and T_4 in human amniotic fluid and in cord and maternal serum. J Clin Endocrinol Metab 43:1351, 1976

57. El-Zaheri MM, Vagenakis AG, Hinerfeld L et al: Maternal thyroid function is the major determinant of amniotic fluid 3,3′,5′-triiodothyronine in the rat. J Clin Invest 67:1126, 1981

58. Landau H, Sack J, Frucht H et al: Amniotic fluid 3,3′,5′-triiodothyronine in the detection of congenital hypothyroidism. J Clin Endocrinol Metab 50:799, 1980

59. Meinhold H, Dudenhausen JW, Wenzel KW, Saling E: Amniotic fluid concentrations of 3,3′,3′-tri-iodthyronine (reverse T_3), 3,3′-di-iodothyronine, 3,5,3′-tri-iodothyronine (T_3) and thyroxine (T_4) in normal and complicated pregnancy. Clin Endocrinol 10: 355, 1979

60. Vulsma T, Gons MH, DeVijlder JMM: Maternal fetal transfer of thyroxine in congenital hypothyroidism due to a total organification defect of thyroid dysgenesis. N Engl J Med 321:13, 1989

61. Contempre B, Jauniaux E, Calvo R: Detection of thyroid hormones in human embryonic cavities during the first trimester of pregnancy. J Clin Endocrinol Metab 77:1719, 1993

62. Dowling JT, Appleton WG, Nicoloff JT: Thyroxine turnover during human pregnancy. J Clin Endocrinol Metab 27:1749, 1964

63. Osathanondh R, Tulchinsky D, Chopra IJ: Total and free thyroxine and triiodothyronine in normal and complicated pregnancy. J Clin Endocrinol Metab 42: 98, 1976

64. Sridama V, Pagini F, Yang SL et al: Decreased level of helper T cells: a possible cause of immunodeficiency in pregnancy. N Engl J Med 307:352, 1982

65. Simeone A, Acampora D, Arcioni L et al: Sequential activation of HOX2 homeobox genes by retinoic acid in human embryonal carcinoma cells. Nature 346: 763, 1990

66. Stagnaro-Green A, Roman SH, Cobin RH et al: A prospective study of lymphocyte-initiated immunosuppression in normal pregnancy: evidence of a T-cell etiology for postpartum thyroid dysfunction. J Clin Endocrinol Metab 74:645, 1992

67. Bech K, Hoier-Madsen M, Feldt-Rasmussen U et al: Thyroid function and autoimmune manifestations in insulin-dependent diabetes mellitus during and after pregnancy. Acta Endocrinol 124:534, 1991

68. DeGroot LJ, Quintans J: The causes of autoimmune thyroid disease. Endocr Rev 10:537, 1989

69. Amino N, Miyai K, Onishi T et al: Transient hypothyroidism after delivery in autoimmune thyroiditis. J Clin Endocrinol Metab 42:296, 1976

70. Amino N, Miyai K, Kuro R et al: Transient postpartum hypothyroidism: fourteen cases with autoimmune thyroiditis. Ann Intern Med 87:155, 1977

71. Amino N, Mori H, Iwatani Y et al: High prevalence of transient post-partum thyrotoxicosis and hypothyroidism. N Engl J Med 306:849, 1982

72. Jansson R, Bernander S, Karlsson A et al: Autoimmune thyroid dysfunction in the postpartum period. J Clin Endocrinol Metab 58:681, 1984

73. Bech K, Hertel J, Rasmussen NG et al: Effect of maternal thyroid autoantibodies and post-partum thyroiditis on the fetus and neonate. Acta Endocrinol 125:146, 1991

74. McKenzie JM, Zakarija M: The clinical use of thyrotropin receptor antibody measurements. J Clin Endocrinol Metab 69:1093, 1989

75. McKenzie JM, Zakarija M: Fetal and neonatal hyperthyroidism due to maternal TSH receptor antibodies. Thyroid 2:155, 1992

76. Roti E, Emerson CH: Postpartum thyroiditis. J Clin Endocrinol Metab 74:3, 1992

77. Rasmussen NG, Hornnes PJ, Hoier-Madsen M et al: Thyroid size and function in healthy pregnant women with thyroid autoantibodies: Relation to development of postpartum thyroiditis. Acta Endocrinol 123:395, 1990

78. Zakarija M, McKenzie JM: Pregnancy-associated changes in the thyroid-stimulating antibody of Graves' disease and the relationship to neonatal hyperthyroidism. J Clin Endocrinol Metab 57:1036, 1983

79. Jansson R, Totterman TH, Sallstrom J, Dahlberg PA: Intrathyroidal and circulating lymphocyte subsets in different stages of autoimmune postpartum thyroiditis. J Clin Endocrinol Metab 58:942, 1984

80. Stagnaro-Green A, Roman SH, Cobin RH et al: Detection of at-risk pregnancy by means of highly sensitive assays for thyroid autoantibodies. JAMA 264:1422, 1990

81. Glinoer D, Soto MF, Bourdoux P et al: Pregnancy in patients with mild thyroid abnormalities: Maternal and neonatal repercussions. J Clin Endocrinol Metab 73:421, 1991

82. Gerstein HC: Incidence of postpartum thyroid dysfunction in patients with type I diabetes mellitus. Ann Intern Med 118:419, 1993

83. Klein RZ, Haddow JE, Faix JD et al: Prevalence of thyroid deficiency in pregnant women. Clin Endocrinol 35:41, 1991

84. Ginsberg J, Walfish PG, Rafter DJ et al: Thyrotrophin blocking antibodies in the sera of mothers with congenitally hypothyroid infants. Clin Endocrinol 25:189, 1986

85. Bogner U, Grüters A, Sigle B et al: Cytotoxic antibodies in congenital hypothyroidism. J Clin Endocrinol Metab 68:671, 1989

86. Tamaki H, Amino N, Aozasa M et al: Effective method for prediction of transient hypothyroidism in neonates born to mothers with chronic thyroiditis. Am J perinatol 6:296, 1989

87. Brown RS, Keating P, Mitchell E: Maternal thyroid-blocking immunoglobulins in congenital hypothyroidism. J Clin Endocrinol Metab 70:1341, 1990

88. Montoro M, Collea JV, Frasier SD, Mestman JH: Successful outcome of pregnancy in women with hypothyroidism. Ann Intern Med 94:31, 1981

89. Davis LE, Leveno KJ, Cunningham FG: Hypothyroidism complicating pregnancy. Obstet Gynecol 72:108, 1988

90. Liu H, Momotani N, Noh JY et al: Maternal hypothyroidism during early pregnancy and intellectual development of progeny. Arch Intern Med 154:785, 1994

91. Man EB, Brown JF, Serunian SA: Maternal hypothyroxinemia: Psychoneurological deficits of progeny. Ann Clin Lab Ser 21:227, 1991

92. Mandel SJ, Brent GA, Larsen PR: Levothyroxine therapy in patients with thyroid disease. Ann Intern Med 119:492-502, 1993

93. Larsen PR: Maternal thyroxine and congenital hypothyroidism. N Engl J Med 321:44, 1989

94. Abuid J, Larsen PR: Triiodothyronine and thyroxine in hyperthyroidism. J Clin Invest 54:201, 1974

95. Mandel SJ, Brent GA, Larsen PR: Review of antithyroid drug use during pregnancy and report of a case of aplasia cutis. Thyroid 4:129, 1994

96. Amino N, Tanizawa O, Mori H et al: Aggravation of thyrotoxicosis in early pregnancy and after delivery in Graves' disease. J Clin Endocrinol Metab 55:108, 1982

97. Zakarija M, Garcia A, McKenzie JM: Studies on multiple thyroid cell membrane-directed antibodies in Graves' disease. J Clin Invest 76:1885, 1985

98. Mitsuda N, Tamaki H, Amino N et al: Risk factors for developmental disorders in infants born to women with Graves' disease. Obstet Gynecol 80:359, 1992

99. Marchant B, Brownlie BEW, Hart DM et al: The placental transfer of propylthiouracil, methimazole and carbamizole. J Clin Endocrinol Metab 45:1187, 1977

100. Skellern GG, Knight BI, Otter M: The pharmacokinetics of methimazole in pregnant patients after oral administration of carbamizole. Br J Clin Pharmacol 9:145, 1980

101. Gardner DF, Cruikshank DP, Hays PM, Cooper DS: Pharmacology of propylthiouracil (PTU) in pregnant hyperthyroid women: Correlation of maternal PTU concentrations with cord serum thyroid function tests. J Clin Endocrinol Metab 62:217, 1986

102. Low LCK, Lang J, Alexander WD: Excretion of carbimazole and propylthiouracil in breast milk. Lancet 2:1011, 1979

103. Kampmann JP, Johansen K, Hansen JM, Helweg J: Propylthiouracil in human milk. Lancet 1:736, 1980

104. Tegler L, Lindstrom B: Antithyroid drugs in milk. Lancet 2:591, 1980

105. Cheron RG, Kaplan MM, Larsen PR et al: Neonatal thyroid function after propylthiouracil therapy for maternal Graves' disease. N Engl J Med 304:525, 1981

106. Momotani N, Noh J, Oyanagi H et al: Antithyroid drug therapy for Graves' disease during pregnancy: optimal regimen for fetal thyroid status. N Engl J Med 315:24, 1986

107. Momotani N, Hisaoka T, Noh J et al: Effects of iodine on thyroid status of fetus versus mother in treatment of Graves' disease complicated by pregnancy. J Clin Endocrinol Metab 75:738, 1992

108. Hashizume K, Ichikawa K, Nishii Y et al: Effect of administration of thyroxine on the risk of postpartum recurrence of hyperthyroid Graves' disease. J Clin Endocrinol Metab 75:6, 1992

109. Tamaki H, Amino N, Aozasa M et al: Universal predictive criteria for neonatal overt thyroxicosis requiring treatment. Am J Perinatol 5:152, 1988

110. Burrow GN: The management of thyrotoxicosis in pregnancy. N Engl J Med 313:562, 1985

111. Thorpe-Beeston JG, Nicolaides KH, Felton CV et al: Maturation of the secretion of thyroid hormone and thyroid-stimulating hormone in the fetus. N Engl J Med 324:532, 1991

112. Lamberg BA, Ikonen E, Osterlund K et al: Antithyroid treatment of maternal hyperthyroidism during lactation. Clin Endocrinol 21:81, 1984

113. Forsbach G, Contreras J, de Hoyos R, Martinez-Campos A: Neuroendocrine regulation of anterior pituitary function in patients during and after molar pregnancy. Acta Endocrinol 116:373, 1987

114. Rosen IB, Walfish PG, Nikore V: Pregnancy and surgical thyroid disease. Surgery 98:1135, 1985

115. Hamburger JI: Thyroid nodules in pregnancy. Thyroid 2:165, 1992

116. Asteris GT, DeGroot LJ: Thyroid cancer: Relationship to radiation exposure and to pregnancy. J Reproduct Med 4:209, 1976

117. Rosen IB, Walfish PG: Pregnancy as a predisposing factor in thyroid neoplasia. Arch Surg 121:1287, 1986

118. Hod M, Sharony R, Friedman S, Ovadia J: Pregnancy and thyroid carcinoma: a review of incidence, course and prognosis. Obstet Gynecol Survey 44:774, 1989

Ontogenesis of Thyroid Function, Thyroid Hormone and Brain Development, Diagnosis and Treatment of Congenital Hypothyroidism

15

Hypothyroidism that begins during adult life does not have any particularly ominous significance. Appropriate therapy completely restores the patient to normal. If hypothyroidism occurs before birth or during infancy, the developing brain and the skeleton may be permanently damaged, especially if the disorder is long unrecognized, and subsequent therapy may not correct these changes. Hypothyroidism that begins during childhood or adolescence is comparable to adult hypothyroidism but, if it begins early and is of long duration, treatment may not completely correct certain of the attendant abnormalities.

If hypothyroidism due to a lack of functionally competent thyroid is present before birth or appears in the first few postnatal months, it may produce the type of physical and mental retardation that is discussed here in some detail. This disorder is known as *sporadic congenital hypothyroidism* and occurs in about 1 in every 4,000 live births. When the state of hypothyroidism is quite complete and prolonged, the term *cretin* may be applied. Cretinism is a term originally used in endemic goiter regions and applied to members of a class of defective persons with a characteristic habitus and facies, often short stature, and mental retardation, frequently with deaf-mutism and pyramidal tract signs. Perhaps this term should not be applied to patients with congenital hypothyroidism in nonendemic regions. This does not imply that there is a fundamental difference between the two types of patients, but rather that the more severe signs and symptoms usually found in the endemic cretin may be the result of the hypothyroid state of both mother and fetus during gestation, whereas this combination is found only rarely in the background of the sporadic congenitally hypothyroid patient. While the term congenital hypothyroidism is perhaps more appropriate for the patients considered in this chapter, *sporadic cretinism* is deeply rooted in traditional parlance. The subject of endemic cretinism is discussed in greater detail in Chapter 20. A description of the inherited defects in thyroid hormone biosynthesis, which may also lead to sporadic cretinism, are discussed in detail in Chapter 16.

ONTOGENESIS OF THYROID FUNCTION IN THE FETUS AND INFANT

Fetal Thyroid Physiology

Thyroid hormones are detectable in fetal serum by 12 weeks of gestational age with both thyroxine (T_4) and triiodothyronine (T_3) being measurable.[1–5] However, at this early stage it is not certain what fraction of these hormones are contributed by the fetus versus the mother through transplacental transfer. Four aspects of thyroid physiology in the fetus need to be considered. These are the development of the fetal thyroid, the maturation of the hypothalamic-pituitary system, the potential contributions of maternal thyroid function and, lastly, the

pathways of thyroid hormone activation and inactivation in the various fetal tissues.

Maturation of the Fetal Thyroid

Embryogenesis of the human thyroid is largely complete by 10 to 12 weeks' gestation, and tiny follicle precursors can be seen. In the 10 to 11-week fetus, iodine binding can be identified and thyroglobulin detected in follicular spaces.[2,5–8] Thyroid hormones continue to increase gradually over the entire period of gestation, as does serum thyroxine-binding globulin (TBG) (Fig. 15-1). While thyroglobulin can be identified in the fetal thyroid as early as the fifth week, and is certainly present in follicular spaces by 10 to 11 weeks, maturation of thyroglobulin secretion takes much longer, and it is not known when circulating thyroglobulin first appears in the fetal serum. By the time of gestational age 27 to 28 weeks, however, thyroglobulin levels average approximately 100 ng/ml, much higher than in the adult, and they remain approximately stable until the time of birth.[9] Thyroglobulin is undetectable in the serum of athyreotic infants, indicating the absence of any transplacental passage of this large protein.[10]

Based on samples obtained by cordocentesis, TBG

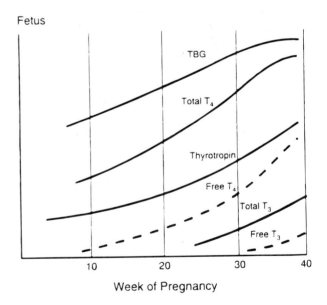

Fig. 15-1. Relative changes in parameters of fetal thyroid function during gestation. The trends and relative magnitude of changes in serum thyroxine-binding globulin (TBG), thyrotropin, total and free T_4, and T_3 are shown. (From Burrow et al.,[5] with permission.)

is present at levels of 100 nmol/L at gestational age 12 weeks and progressively increases up to the time of birth, reaching concentrations of 400 to 500 nmol/L.[3,4] The serum TBG concentrations are higher in the infant then in adult humans (~300 nmol/L) as a consequence of placental estrogen effects on the fetal liver. In addition to the increase in total T_4 however, there is also a progressive increase of free T_4 concentrations between 18 and 36 weeks' gestation, indicating a maturation of the hypothalamic-pituitary thyroid axis.

The Hypothalamic-Pituitary Axis

Thyroid-stimulating hormone (TSH) is detectable at levels of 3 to 4 mU/L at gestational age 12 weeks and increases moderately over the last two trimesters to levels of 6 to 8 mU/L at the time of delivery.[4] The maturation of the negative feedback control of thyroid hormone synthesis occurs by approximately midgestation, and elevated serum TSH concentrations have been noted in infants as early as 28 weeks. The administration of 700 μg of thyroxine into the amniotic fluid 24 hours before cesarean section elevates fetal T_4 and reduces cord serum TSH.[11] In addition, the neonatal surge in TSH (see below) is suppressed by such treatment, indicating that the hypothalamic-pituitary feedback is intact. Similar inferences can be made from observations that TSH is reduced in the cord serum of infants with neonatal thyrotoxicosis due to the transplacental passage of thyroid-stimulating antibodies from mothers with Graves' disease.

As mentioned, iodide-concentrating capacity can be detected in the thyroid of the 10- to 11-week fetus. Unlike the case for the adult thyroid, the fetus does not reduce iodide trapping in response to excess iodide. The latter capacity does not appear until 36 to 40 weeks' gestation. This is clinically relevant in that the exposure of the premature infant to large quantities of iodide in the form of antiseptics can impair thyroid hormone synthesis through the Wolff-Chaikoff effect and lead to transient elevations in serum TSH and reductions in serum T_4.[12,13] Similar events may occur after iodide exposure following amniofetography.

Maturation of Peripheral Thyroid Hormone Activation and Inactivation Processes

As discussed in Chapter 3, there are three iodothyronine deiodinases involved in the activation and inactivation of thyroid hormone. All three are coordi-

nately regulated during gestation. Figure 15-2 is a diagram of the complex pattern of interactions between the maternal circulation, the placenta, amniotic fluid, and the fetus. The selenoenzyme type 1 iodothyronine deiodinase, which in adult life catalyzes the bulk of T_4 to T_3 conversion but which also catalyzes thyroid hormone inactivation via removal of the inner-ring iodine from T_4 and T_3, is low throughout gestation. As a consequence, circulating T_3 concentrations in the fetus are quite low and at birth are on the order of 50 to 60 ng/dl (~1 nmol/L).[14] The type 2 deiodinase, which converts T_4 to T_3, is detectable by midgestation, as is the type 3 or inner-ring deiodinase. The latter two enzymes are especially important in defining the level of T_3 in the brain and pituitary.[15] These activities have been found to be critically important in defending the rat fetus against the effects of fetal hypothyroidism pro-

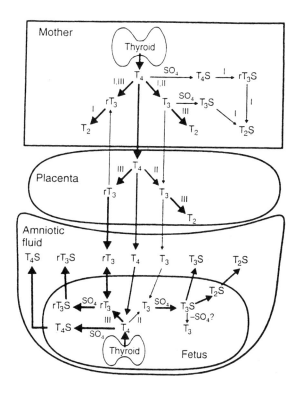

Fig. 15-2. Interrelationships of maternal, placental, and fetal thyroid hormone metabolism. I, II, and III refer to type 1, type 2, and type 3 iodothyronine deiodinases. SO_4 indicates a sulfation pathway; T_2, 3,3'-diiodothyronine; T_2S, 3,3'-diiodothyronine sulfate. (From Burrow et al.,[5] with permission.)

viding the maternal T_4 levels are maintained at normal concentrations.[16] While it is generally appreciated that type 2 deiodinase is the source of most of the T_3 in the adult central nervous system,[17] this situation is even more critical in the fetus as a consequence of the extremely low concentrations of circulating T_3.

As indicated in Figure 15-2, transplacental passage of T_4 does occur and is potentially of critical importance in the athyreotic fetus.[18] However, the physiologic interrelationships between the various deiodinases in the fetus and placenta[19–21] seem designed to maintain circulating T_3 concentrations at a reduced level.[5] On the other hand, since brain maturation requires active thyroid hormone, specific mechanisms have evolved for maintaining T_3 concentrations in that tissue so that normal development can proceed. The physiologic rationale for the maintenance of reduced circulating T_3 concentrations throughout fetal life is still unknown. Despite the low levels of circulating T_3, brain T_3 levels are 60 to 80 percent of those of the adult by fetal age 20 to 26 weeks.[8,22]

As would be predicted from the fact that the type 1 deiodinase activity in the fetus is low, the concentrations of the specific substrates metabolized by this deiodinase, namely reverse T_3 and the sulfate conjugates of T_4, reverse T_3, T_3, and $3'T_2$ (Fig. 15-3), are markedly elevated in the fetal circulation and to a considerable extent in amniotic fluid.[23–27] This oc-

curs because the type 3 (inner-ring) deiodinase has a very low capacity for their deiodination.[28]

Type 2 deiodinase has been detected in brain, brown adipose tissue, and pituitary by midgestation in rats and sheep.[29] If such animals are made hypothyroid or iodine-deficient, type 2 deiodinase activities increase while types 1 and 3 deiodinases are reduced.[30,31] These coordinate adjustments maintain T_3 concentrations in tissues such as the brain, where type 2 and type 3 deiodinases are highly expressed.[16]

Contributions of the Maternal Thyroid to Fetal Thyroid Economy

Interest in the role of maternal T_4 in the fetal thyroid economy has been reawakened in recent years with the recognition that in infants with the congenital absence of thyroid peroxidase (hence, the complete inability to synthesize T_4), T_4 is present in cord serum at concentrations between 25 and 50 percent of normal.[18] Similar results are obtained in retrospective studies of cord serum in infants with sporadic congenital athyreosis.[18] This T_4 disappears rapidly from the newborn circulation with a half-life of approximately 3 to 4 days. Thus, as discussed further in the section on congenital hypothyroidism, the transplacental passage of maternal T_4 may explain the relatively normal clinical appearance at birth of over 90 percent of infants with congenital hypothyroidism. This may also explain the fact that it has been possible, at least in certain screening programs, to prevent the development of mental retardation by early institution of adequate levothyroxine therapy. This can be achieved despite the clear requirement for thyroid hormone in CNS development reflected in the mental retardation and neurologic abnormalities of infants in endemic goiter areas who presumably fail to get adequate maternal, as well as fetal, T_4.

The critical role of maternal T_4 as a source of T_3 in the fetal central nervous system has been particularly well studied in the rat. In a series of careful studies, Morreale de Escobar et al. have demonstrated that in the iodine-deficient or chemically thyroidectomized fetal rat, the concentration of T_3 in the CNS can be maintained at normal levels by the transplacental passage of maternal T_4.[16,32–35] It seems likely that when fetal thyroid function is normal, the net flux of T_4 from mother to fetus may be relatively limited.[36]

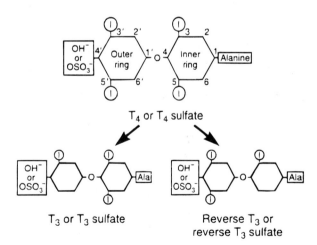

Fig. 15-3. Structures of thyroxine (T_4), triiodothyronine (T_3) and reverse triiodothyronine (rT_3). Sulfation at the 4' hydroxyl position produces the sulfate conjugates of T_4, T_3, and rT_3. (From Burrow et al.,[5] with permission.)

TABLE 15-1. Average Iodothyronine Concentrations in Human Maternal and Fetal Serum and in Amniotic Fluid[a]

	Maternal Serum (Midgestation)	Amniotic Fluid		Fetal Serum	
		20 Weeks	Term	20 Weeks	Term
T_4	160,000	3,220	7,370	40,000	140,000
T_3	3,100	132	101	200	750
T_2	43	112	119		211
rT_3	370	2,000	1,060	3,800	4,160
T_4-sulfate	21	322	—		245
T_3-sulfate	40	90	—	92	164
rT_3-sulfate	52	1,176	—		684

[a] Results recorded in pmol/L; values developed from reference 5.

However, the presence of a high concentration gradient between the euthyroxinemic mother and hypothyroxinemic fetus permits significant bulk transfer of T_4 to the fetal circulation. This can occur both at the level of the placental maternal capillary interface and via uptake of thyroid hormone from the amniotic fluid through the immature epidermis. T_4 uptake by the fetus can also occur via fetal ingestion of amniotic fluid, thus permitting the intestinal absorption of significant quantities of the T_4 therein (Table 15-1). Instillation of T_4 into the amniotic cavity causes significant increases in fetal serum T_4 and suppression of TSH in the term fetus.[11] This approach has been advocated as a method of delivery of T_4 to an athyreotic infant, e.g., following inadvertent radioiodine administration during pregnancy.[37]

Table 15-1 shows the pattern of maternal, amniotic fluid, and fetal iodothyronine concentrations in the human.[5] While the T_4 concentrations in amniotic fluid appear modest, the fraction of T_4 free in amniotic fluid is approximately tenfold higher than that of serum, and thus the free T_4 concentration in amniotic fluid is approximately equal to that in fetal serum at 20 weeks' gestation.

It has been shown on numerous occasions in both animals and humans that maternal amniotic fluid iodothyronine concentrations reflect those in the maternal circulation.[27] Despite significant transplacental transfer of thyroid hormones in the human and rat, little transplacental T_4 passage occurs in sheep.[38] This difference in placental permeability may be due to the fact that the sheep placenta contains components of both maternal and fetal origin, whereas humans and rats have hemochorial placentas consisting of exclusively fetal tissue.

Placental Permeability to Maternal TRH and TSH

When thyrotropin-releasing hormone (TRH) is given to mothers during the second or third trimester, serum TSH rises in the fetal circulation.[19] This has been demonstrated as early as 25 weeks' gestation in humans. Thus, the fetal thyrotroph responds to TRH as early as 25 weeks' gestation and, in fact, the fetal TSH increment after TRH administration was greater than was the paired-maternal response. This can be explained either on the basis of enhanced TSH release or impaired TSH degradation, perhaps due to immaturity of the hepatic glycoprotein metabolic clearance system. Maternal TSH does not cross the placenta.

In summary, these results illustrate that human prenatal thyroid physiology is the consequence of a complicated series of interactions between the pituitary-hypothalamic thyroid axis and various pathways for activation and inactivation of thyroid hormones. Maternal thyroid function can play a critical role in the fetus. Accordingly, maintaining normal T_4 concentrations during gestation is of greater importance to the fetus than has been recognized previously. The potential for T_4 transfer from amniotic fluid to the fetus provides a pathway by which levothyroxine can be administered to fetus in the rare circumstances where this is indicated.

Thyroid Function in the Full-term Neonate and Infant and During Childhood

The Neonate

Marked changes occur in thyroid physiology at the time of birth in the full-term newborn (Fig. 15-4). One of the most dramatic changes is an abrupt rise

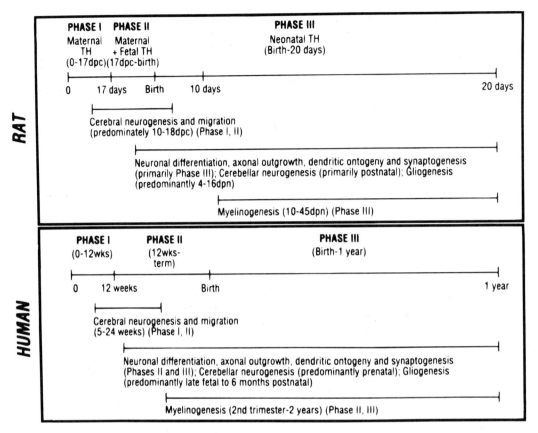

Fig. 15-4. Brain neurologic development relative to thyroid function in the rat and human. TH, Thyroid hormones; dpc, days postconception; dpn, days postnatal. (From Porterfield and Hendrich,[57] with permission.)

in the serum TSH, which occurs within 30 minutes of delivery. Peak TSH concentrations in the full-term infant can reach 60 to 70 mU/L.[39] This causes a marked stimulation of the thyroid and an increase in the concentrations of both serum T_4 and T_3.[40,41] These consist of an approximate doubling of the serum T_4 and an increase of three- to fourfold in the concentration of serum T_3 within 24 hours (Fig. 15-4). Studies in experimental animals suggest that the increase in TSH is a consequence of the relative hypothermia of the ambient extrauterine environment.[2] However, while a significant portion of the marked increase in T_3 from its low basal levels in cord serum can be explained by the abrupt increase in TSH, there is also an apparent increase in the type 1 deiodinase activity at the time of delivery.[42,43] Thus, serum T_3 concentrations rise to levels typical of those expected in adults. As a consequence, the elevated concentrations of the other substrates of

type 1 deiodinase, reverse T_3, and T_3 sulfate, decrease relatively rapidly during the newborn period.[23] Type 2 deiodinase has also been identified in human brown adipose tissue, and the acute increase in T_3 in this tissue at birth is required for optimal uncoupling protein synthesis and thermogenesis.[44,45]

Infants and Children

Following the acute perturbations of the neonatal period there is a slow and progressive decrease in the concentrations of T_4, T_3, and TSH during infancy and childhood.[2,46] The most important aspect of thyroid physiology in the infant and child, however, is the markedly higher T_4 turnover in this age group relative to that in the adult. In infants, T_4 production rates are estimated to be on the order of 5 to 6 μg/kg/d, decreasing slowly over the first few years of life to about 2 to 3 μg/kg/d at ages 3 to 9 years.[2,47] This is to be contrasted with the production rate of T_4 in the adult, which is about 1.5 μg/kg/day. Serum thyroglobulin levels also fall over the first year of life, reaching concentrations typical of adults by about 6 months of age.[10] The size of the infant thyroid gland increases quite slowly. The thyroid gland of the newborn weighs approximately 1 g and increases about 1 g/year until age 15, when it achieves its adult size of about 15 to 20 g. In general, the size of the thyroid lobe is comparable to that of the terminal phalanx of the infant or child's thumb.

Thyroid Function in the Premature and Small-for-Gestational-Age Infant

Premature Infants

Thyroid function in the premature infant reflects that which is found in comparable gestational age infants in utero. Thus, depending on the gestational age, there are variable degrees of immaturity of the hypothalamic-pituitary thyroid axis. The smaller the infant, the lower the serum T_4 and TSH.[48,49] As infants approach full-term status, the level of TSH increases to that characteristic of full-term infants. Studies of very small preterm infants (400 to 1,500 g) in the New England screening program have shown mean serum T_4 concentrations ranging from as low as 5.7 μg/dl (70 nmol/L) to 8.0 μg/dl (105 nmol/L) in the 1.2- to 1.5-kg infants. Despite the reduced total T_4, TSH is less than 40 mU/L in most, although the prevalence of TSH levels greater than 40 mU/l varies from 3 to 7 percent, as opposed to less than 1 percent in preterm infants of greater than 2 kg birth weight. In addition to reduced serum T_4 and TSH at delivery, the serum reverse T_3 and T_3 tend to reflect the immaturity of the type 1 deiodinase system. Serum reverse T_3 tends to stay higher, and serum T_3 reduced for a longer period in the premature infant.

However, the situation is further complicated by the appearance of transient elevations in TSH, suggesting transient hypothyroidism in some premature or small-for-gestational-age (SGA) infants. In some geographic areas, this can be explained on the basis of iodine deficiency. Thus, it is more likely to occur in countries with modest iodine deficiency, such as Belgium, than in North America, where iodine deficiency does not exist.[50] In addition, since the capacity of the immature thyroid to adapt to exogenous iodide is reduced, there is an increase in sensitivity to the thyroid suppressive effects of excess iodide, the Wolff-Chaikoff effect. Various antiseptics containing iodine used in the preterm nursery are readily absorbed by the immature epidermis, which may contribute to the problem of impaired thyroid function in this age group.[51,52]

To some extent the increase in TSH seen in the preterm infants at several weeks of age may reflect the elevated TSH observed in adults who are recovering from severe illness.[53] Such individuals may develop transient TSH elevations that are associated with still reduced serum T_4 and T_3 concentrations. These have been interpreted as reflecting a "reawakening" of the illness-induced suppression of the hypothalamic-pituitary axis (see Ch. 4 and 5). As the infant recovers from prematurity-associated illnesses such as respiratory distress syndrome (RDS), a recovery of the illness-induced suppression of the hypothalamic-pituitary thyroid axis would also occur. While most of the infants with an elevated TSH do eventually have normal thyroid function, there is concern that the incidence of true permanent congenital hypothyroidism may be higher in this population than in full-term infants.[54] It is still not clear whether such infants should be given levothyroxine. If they are not, appropriate follow-up studies should be done to screen premature infants for hypothyroidism after discharge from the hospital. It is important to recall that the hypothalamic-pituitary axis of the immature infant is only relatively insensitive in that even premature infants who have true primary hypothyroidism, such as that due to maternal antithyroid drug administration, will have the expected elevations in TSH.

Somewhat surprisingly, given the relative immaturity of the thyroid gland, serum TG concentrations may be higher in the premature than in the full-term infant. For example, median serum TG concentrations of 102 μg/L were observed in 45 premature infants, as opposed to levels of 73 ng in the full-term infant.[55] This could be explained on the basis of impaired clearance of this glycoprotein from the circulation by the immature liver. However, because of the attenuated TSH burst at the time of birth, the serum TG concentrations tend not to rise as greatly in the postpartum period in the premature as in the full-term infant.

Small-for-Gestational-Age Infant

SGA infants have significantly higher TSH and lower total and free T_4 values than do infants of normal weight.[56] This can be related to the severity of the malnutrition in these infants, presumably in part due to fetal hypoxemia and acidemia. This may reflect impaired placental perfusion and chronic starvation. This pattern of reduced T_4 and elevated TSH differs from the response to starvation in older individuals and healthy adults in whom TSH is reduced. The explanation for the relatively higher TSH in such infants is not known.

THYROID HORMONES AND CENTRAL NERVOUS SYSTEM DEVELOPMENT

It is well known that adequate thyroid hormone is required for normal central nervous system development. However, despite numerous studies, specific thyroid hormone–dependent rate-limiting steps required for CNS maturation have not as yet been identified. Rather, the impairment of intellectual function in the untreated, congenitally hypothyroid infant is most likely due to modest deficits or in even just a modest delay in the occurrence of certain events critical for the normal maturation process.

The best studied model for thyroid hormone–related events in central nervous system development is the rat. Many of the concepts developed from this animal model appear to be applicable to the human. However, a major advantage of the rat as an experimental model is that at the time of birth the rat central nervous system is relatively immature compared with the human full-term infant. Therefore, events that take place in the latter third of gestation in the human can be studied in the rat over the first 2 to 3 weeks of life. To compare the two species, however, it must be recognized that the differences in the timing of these critical steps in brain maturation need to be correlated with the timing of the development of thyroid function in the two species.

Chronologic Correlations of Thyroid and CNS Development in Humans and Experimental Animals

Fig. 15-4 depicts the various phases of fetal and neonatal thyroid hormone physiology and the correlations in the rat and human of those events with the critical stages of central nervous system maturation.[57] The development of the human thyroid and studies of circulating thyroid hormones at various stages have already been discussed. The major difference between the rat and human in this process is the relatively long period of intrauterine life of the rat, during which the maternal thyroid is the only source of fetal hormone available to the fetus. Thyroid function in the rat fetus does not begin until approximately 4 days prior to birth. Thus, in the rat a substantial portion of cerebral neurogenesis and migration takes place during the time when thyroid-hormone dependent processes would be markedly influenced by maternal thyroid status. In addition, most of neuronal differentiation and synaptogenesis in the human has been initiated just at the end of the first trimester and myelinogenesis is well underway at the time of birth, this does not occur until much later in the rat. It is thus apparent that the impact of congenital hypothyroidism will be different in the two species, since the human fetus is dependent for a much longer period on its intrinsic thyroid function than is the rat. Given this, it is all the more surprising that in a large percentage of infants with congenital hypothyroidism, the initiation of levothyroxine therapy by age 3 to 4 weeks can normalize CNS function, whereas if treatment is delayed, an estimated 3 to 5 IQ points are lost for each month of uncorrected hypothyroxinemia.[47] The relative contributions of the maternal versus fetal thyroid to human fetal T_4 production in normal pairs are still not known. The data previously alluded to, namely that in the human fetus unable to synthesize thyroid hormone, a serum T_4 level of approximately 33 to 50 percent of normal is present at delivery, indicates that maternal thyroid function can at least partially compensate for fetal athyreosis.[18,58]

While it is not possible to determine precisely when thyroid hormone–dependent central nervous system developmental processes begin, there is a critical period in neurogenesis after which reversal of hypothyroidism cannot normalize brain function. In the rat, this period extends from approximately 18 to 19 gestational days up until age 3 weeks.[57,59] In the human, studies of infants with congenital hypothyroidism show that normal or near-normal intellectual development can be achieved in most if adequate and sustained levothyroxine replacement is instituted within a few weeks of birth.[60,61] However, not all authorities agree with this assessment.[62-64] For example, Tillotson et al. reported that in the United Kingdom program, 55 percent of all infants with more severe disease, defined as a plasma T_4 ~<43 mol/L (3.3 μg/dl) at diagnosis, had an IQ at age 5 years that was 10 points lower than those with higher values, regardless of the quality of treatment in the first year.[63] The reason or reasons for these differences are not apparent from the data available. One factor may be the experience of the New England Program, which showed significant level of poor compliance, particularly in the adolescent age group. This, perhaps combined with recommendations for levothyroxine replacement that we now recognize to have been suboptimal in the early phases of screening programs, are potential explanations for a failure to achieve normal intellectual function in the most severely affected infants.[61] However, it is clear that early diagnosis and treatment have improved the intellectual function of children with congenital hypothyroidism in all programs.

Thus, the model of congenital hypothyroidism in the human neonate argues either that early events in human central nervous system development are not thyroid hormone–dependent or require such minimal levels that maternal thyroid hormone is adequate to supply these needs. Is it possible to differentiate between these two possibilities? The studies of individuals with endemic goiter provide an excellent model for recognizing which specific processes in human central nervous system development require thyroid hormone. Individuals living in areas of severe iodine deficiency have impairment of both maternal and fetal thyroid function. Thus, CNS abnormalities observed in these individuals are those that can be assumed to be a consequence of both fetal and maternal thyroid hormone deficiency.

This subject, that is the origins of the significant neurologic impairment of endemic cretinism in hypothyroidism, has been reviewed by many authorities in recent years.[65-69] It is discussed at greater length in Chapter 20, and the reader should review this chapter for more details. Endemic cretinism provides a critically important clinical model for elucidating the thyroid hormone–dependent events in the human central nervous system. A specific neurologic syndrome has been described. The major features of this syndrome are mental disability, deafmutism, pyramidal tract disturbance, extrapyramidal dysfunction with a spastic diplegia or quadriplegia, and a characteristic gait disorder. This differen-

tiation has been particularly well described in studies in China and Indonesia by Boyages and Halpern.[69] The most common manifestation of pyramidal dysfunction is hyperreflexia of the patellar (but not Achilles) reflexes. Extrapyramidal features of neurologic endemic cretinism include rigidity, dystonic posturing, and other lesions indicating a disorder of the basal ganglia. Supporting these observations have been recent magnetic resonance imaging (MRI) studies demonstrating abnormalities in the corpus striatum and substantia nigra in three adult Chinese endemic cretins.[70] The clinical features suggest the abnormalities typical of cerebral palsy. Delong has attributed the timing of damage to these systems to about 14 weeks' gestation with persistence through to the third trimester. An impairment of thyroid hormone–dependent events in the second trimester can also explain the abnormalities in the cochlea (developing during the 10th to 18th weeks), the impairment of cerebrocortical function (developing during the 14th to 18th weeks), and abnormalities in the basal ganglia (12th to 18th weeks).[57,66,69] It has been demonstrated by Pharaoh et al. that iodized oil will prevent the development of the neurologic manifestation of cretinism, providing it is given before the second trimester of pregnancy.[71]

None of the neurologic features of severe endemic cretinism have been identified in infants with sporadic congenital hypothyroidism. Even infants who displayed clinical manifestations of hypothyroidism at birth, presumably indicating a severe deficiency of endogenous thyroid function and a failure of maternal T_4 to compensate for this, do not have evidence of extrapyramidal or pyramidal disease, nor do they usually have impaired hearing.[61,62,72] This would appear to provide unequivocal evidence that the neurologic damage sustained by infants with endemic cretinism is prevented by maternal T_4 in infants with congenital athyroetic hypothyroidism.

Given the potential importance of the transplacental passage of maternal T_4, it is notable that a study comparing siblings has shown that maternal hypothyroxinemia in early pregnancy due to primary hypothyroidism is not associated with impaired intellectual development of the progeny.[73] This disagrees with the conclusions of earlier reports,[74] and more extensive studies are required to confirm it. If this observation is borne out in future studies, one would conclude that a combined impairment of both fetal and maternal thyroid function is required for the complete clinical syndrome of thyroid-related impaired CNS development to appear. This situation would occur only rarely outside areas of endemic iodine deficiency.[50,75-79] There is evidence from experimental studies that maternal hypothyroidism can alter brain biochemistry in adult progeny.[80]

Ontogenesis of α and β Thyroid Hormone Receptors in the Central Nervous System of Humans and Experimental Animals

The developmental effects of thyroid hormone occur through interaction of T_3 with its nuclear receptor.[81] Accordingly, considerable attention has been given to the study of ontogenesis of T_3 receptors in the central nervous system, since such data are critically important for assessing the timing and localization of thyroid hormone–dependent processes. Little information is available for the human fetus. Specific nuclear T_3 binding proteins have been identified in human fetal brain by 10 weeks' gestation, and during the period between 10 and 18 weeks there is an increase in the level of these receptors.[22,82] This is subsequent to the appearance of fetal thyroid hormone in the circulation (Fig. 15-1).[3,4,6] Specific radioimmunoassay techniques have demonstrated a high degree of saturation of the receptors with T_3.[8,22]

In the rat, T_3-binding nuclear proteins in the cerebral cortex have been identified by day 13 of fetal life, and these increase progressively to the time of birth.[83-87] At that time, the nuclear T_3 binding capacity is about half that of the adult. Similarly, studies using specific antisera directed against the $\beta 1$ isoform of the T_3 receptor have shown a marked increase in this protein during the late gestational period, presumably in neurons.[84] In the case of the brain, this is associated with a marked increase in the mRNA encoding this species. A number of investigators have compared the levels of mRNA encoding, the $\alpha 1$, $\alpha 2$, $\beta 1$, and $\beta 2$ mRNAs in the central nervous system.[85,88-90] As discussed in Chapter 3, the $\alpha 1$, $\beta 1$, and $\beta 2$ receptors are the biologically active isoforms. However, the $\beta 2$ form of the receptor is of special interest with respect to central nervous system development, since it appears to be localized to specific structures, including the pituitary, paraventricular nuclei, arcuate and ventromedial nuclei of hypothalamus, as well as the median eminence.[91]

This relatively specific CNS β receptor isoform has also been identified in the basal ganglia by day 19 of rat gestation. Given the fact that hypothyroid neonatal rodents develop deafness and cochlear dysfunction, the detection of $\beta 1$ and $\beta 2$ mRNA in the portions of the embryonic ear giving rise to the cochlea at 12.5 days of fetal life is quite intriguing.[86,92] The $\beta 2$ isoform has been identified in the chick's retinal outer nuclear layer early in embryogenesis, though this decreases at later times in development.[90] This is especially important since thyroid hormone has a marked influence on the development of the amphibian eye. It is of interest that while the $\alpha 1$ and $\alpha 2$ mRNA isoforms are dominant in the central nervous system, they do not undergo developmental changes. Since these are present prior to the increase in the $\beta 1$ mRNA, it has been speculated that in the central nervous system, as in the tadpole in general, T_3-induced induction of $\beta 1$ thyroid hormone receptor may occur by its interaction with the $\alpha 1$ receptor protein in this tissue.[88,93-95]

While T_3 receptors have been identified in both neurons and glia, their highest concentration is in neurons.[96-99] In the rat, the neuronal nuclei express TR$\beta 1$, whereas only c-erb-A$\alpha 2$ protein was detected in astroglial nuclei.[98] As is discussed below, specific thyroid hormone–dependent processes have been identified in both neurons and glia. Thyroid hormone nuclear receptors appear during the time of neuroblast proliferation and, at least as judged by studies in the rat, increase markedly as this animal enters phase 3 of central nervous system development (Fig. 15-4). This is a logical pattern of development and implicates thyroid hormone receptors in these effects. Furthermore, while the quantities of mRNA encoding the $\alpha 1$ and $\alpha 2$ isoforms of the thyroid hormone receptor are much higher than those of TR $\beta 1$, developmental changes appear to be most specifically associated with increases in TR$\beta 1$ (and perhaps $\beta 2$) mRNAs, suggesting that these receptors may be the critical inducers of thyroid hormone effects. Changes in the $\beta 1$ isoform have been especially well demonstrated by immunofluorescent studies in the cerebellar Purkinje cells, which develop relatively later in neonatal life than do cerebrocortical cells. These correlate well with specific effects of T_3-directed transcription of certain Purkinje cell genes.[84,100] Studies of the TR mRNAs during differentiation suggest the possibility that the $\alpha 1$ thyroid hormone receptor could play a role in the differentiation process once neuroblast development has occurred.

Overview of Effects of Hypothyroidism on the Central Nervous System of Various Species

In humans, the association between congenital hypothyroidism or endemic cretinism and mental retardation has been recognized for centuries. A clinical manifestation of this abnormality is the impairment of intelligence as measured by IQ tests. This syndrome presumably occurs due to hypothyroidism in the postnatal period, since it can be prevented or ameliorated by appropriate treatment of infants with congenital athyreosis. The pyramidal and extrapyramidal signs found in endemic cretins are irreversible and presumably result from damage sustained during the second and third trimesters of fetal life.

There are few data in humans regarding the pathologic concomitants of the functional abnormalities of the hypothyroid central nervous system. Some information regarding the anatomic defects is being generated by application of advanced radiologic techniques to the evaluation of adult human endemic cretins. The radiologic studies mentioned earlier have demonstrated a remarkably normal appearance of the brain with the exception of gliotic lesions of the globus pallidus and substantia nigra. In the few histopathologic studies that have been performed, the brain has been found to be small, with poor development of cerebral and cerebellar cortex, basal ganglia, and thalamus.[66,101] Abnormalities have been identified in the hippocampus that show hypoplasia of pyramidal and granular cells, suggesting that hippocampal defects could be an explanation for the dementia of the endemic cretin, though whether such effects are produced during intrauterine life or during the neonatal period is not clear. EEG studies in endemic cretins have demonstrated characteristic slowing of the α rhythm and other signs suggesting diffuse cerebral dysfunction.[102–104]

Extensive morphologic, biochemical, molecular biologic, and functional studies have been carried out in rats and, more recently, in mouse models of congenital hypothyroidism. Taken together, the results point to the diffuseness of abnormalities in brain development in hypothyroidism, which affect most of the structures and functions examined to a greater or lesser degree. Interpretation of some of the earlier cross-sectional studies on biochemical changes induced by hypothyroidism was confounded by the fact that the absence of thyroid hormone appears to delay, rather than eliminate, the appearance of certain specific morphologic features or gene products.[105,106] Such delays, however, could obviously have critical functional importance in an organ with the complexity of the central nervous system.

In addition, thyroid hormone–dependent effects have been identified in the adult as well as the developing rodent.[107,108] This indicates that thyroid hormone–dependent effects in the CNS continue throughout life. Such effects can explain the clinical alterations in mental processes that occur in the individual with acquired hypo- or hyperthyroidism

A thorough evaluation of this literature is beyond the scope of this text, and the reader is referred to the reviews cited earlier for a more complete discussion. However, several generalizations and specific examples can be provided to illustrate the types of abnormalities observed over many years of study of this problem. A number of years ago, Eayrs and colleagues demonstrated that a functional learning disability can be induced in rats by making them hypothyroid and that a functional learning disability can be induced in rats by making them hypothyroid and that the earlier in neonatal life hypothyroidism was produced, the greater the disability.[109] More recent studies have taken advantage of the congenitally hypothyroid (hyt/hyt) mouse.[110,111] Due to a defect in the TSH receptor signal transduction process, these animals develop hypothyroidism in utero and demonstrate many manifestations of the specific effects of hypothyroxinemia.[112,113] Affected mice show retarded eye opening and ear raising and reduced bone growth and body weight. From a functional point of view, they demonstrate delayed reflex behavior and abnormal motor function. Studies of optic nerves in this model have shown impaired axonal flow of specific proteins involved in synaptic function, as well as fewer microtubules and neurofilaments.[114,115]

Morphologic studies of cortical neurons in the hypothyroid adult rat provide an example of the postnatal effects of thyroid hormone deficiency.[107,108] The numbers of spines along the apical shaft of pyramidal cells are markedly reduced in hypothyroid rats, and effects on pyramidal neurons could be demonstrated at all ages. It is possible to reverse or prevent these effects if T_4 is given within a few days of thyroidectomy. Partial reversal could be obtained if treatment were instituted at a later time. Legrand performed similar studies of Purkinje cells in the cerebellar cortex many years ago.[116] These showed striking abnormalities of the granular cell layer with disorganized and reduced numbers of dendrites, impairment of Purkinje cell migration to deeper layers of the cerebral cortex, and impaired or absent synapses in certain cells of the cerebellar cortex.

Studies of the effects of hypothyroidism on cerebellar development have been extended to the molecular biologic level. Pups made hypothyroid in utero and continuously treated with methimazole showed delayed expression of mRNAs encoding for calbindin, the myoinositol, 1,4,5 triphosphate receptor, and a specific Purkinje cell protein, PCP 2. Myelin basic protein mRNA expression was also reduced.[117,118] This protein is present in the oligodendroglia and is critical for axonal myelination. T_3 injection reversed these changes.

Microtubular polymerization has been shown to be impaired in the brain of congenitally hypothyroid rats. This has been attributed to abnormalities in the microtubular associated tau protein.[105,119] In addition, the appearance of the dendrite-specific protein MAP_2 is delayed in the cerebellum in congenitally hypothyroid rats. Furthermore, the migration of the protein into the dendrites did not occur.[120] Interestingly, the level of mRNA for the MAP_2 protein is not affected by hypothyroidism, indicating that hypothyroidism may also affect translational events critical for brain development.

Further studies of both neonatal hypothyroidism and hypothyroidism induced in adult rats have shown abnormalities in specific neuronal gene expression. One such gene, RC3, encodes a neuronal-specific protein of unknown function. It appears to be similar to neurogranin, which is a protein kinase substrate thought to be involved in long-term potentiation mechanisms.[121,122] RC3 expression is reduced in adult rats made hypothyroid on day 40 with effects demonstrable in cerebral cortex and striatum. This effect could be prevented by thyroxine administration. On the other hand, other studies have shown that a specific oligodendroglial protein, myelin-associated glycoprotein (Mag), is reduced at the level of mRNA in hypothyroid rats but no effects on alteration of Mag gene transcription rates were observed.[123] This indicates that hypothyroidism can also influence mRNA stability.

Inherited Thyroid Hormone Resistance and Brain Development

An extensive discussion of thyroid hormone resistance syndromes is presented in Chapter 16.[124] However, this is an important model from the point of view of the effects of thyroid hormone on the central nervous system. In the autosomal-dominant form of the disorder, attention deficit hyperactivity disorder has been identified in 70 percent of affected children, as opposed to only 20 percent of their unaffected siblings.[125] This gives a relative risk ratio of about 15-fold for the development of this syndrome in such patients. The relationship between this βTR receptor disorder and neuropsychiatric manifestations was particularly impressive given the similar genetic and environmental background of the individual families. The authors attributed this abnormality to a lack of expression of thyroid hormone effects, but it could also relate to the supranormal levels of thyroid hormone present in these individuals. However, attention deficit disorder is not common in hyperthyroid children as it is in these individuals.

Unfortunately, little is known of the specific functional or anatomic abnormalities leading to this syndrome. Recent studies have reported decreased hearing in some thyroid hormone–resistant patients,[126] and the original patient of Refetoff who has no functional β receptor is deaf but has no labyrinthine dysfunction.[127] This is quite intriguing given the evidence of early appearance of TR $\beta 1$ and $\beta 2$ mRNAs in the embryonic cochlear tissue of the rat fetus.[86,92] It would point to hearing loss as a marker for early fetal hypothyroidism in humans as it is in rats.[59]

In summary, it is clear that thyroid hormone–dependent effects in the central nervous system are produced by a variety of mechanisms in both neurons and glia. While certain areas of the brain appear to be more susceptible to hypothyroidism than do others, particularly in the developing human central nervous system, the abnormality is more likely to be generalized rather than due to a disruption in a specific rate-limiting step. It is characterized by delays and concomitant disorganization in intercellular communication rather than in absolute deficiencies in function.[128–130] On the one hand, it is surprising that cerebrocortical function can be as well maintained as it is in the presence of these diffuse abnormalities. On the other hand, the generality of the process and the critical nature of the chronology of CNS development make identification of specific defects very difficult to unravel.

SPORADIC CONGENITAL HYPOTHYROIDISM

Causes and Prevalence

Our knowledge of the cause and prevalence of congenital hypothyroidism has expanded geometrically in the last two decades. This great increase is a consequence of programs for screening newborn infants for congenital hypothyroidism that have been instituted in most industrialized countries. Such programs have been so effective that by 1982 some 25 million infants had been screened worldwide, and now seven to nine million newborns are currently evaluated. This screening is now expanding throughout Europe, Asia, and Oceania, and into regional areas of China and South America. A prevalence of hypothyroidism of 1 in 3,800 to 1 in 4,000 newborns is found in Europe and North America. The incidence of hypothyroidism in Japan is somewhat lower, about 1 in 5,500 and in the African-American population in North America the prevalence of congenital hypothyroidism is 1 in 32,000. Thyroid ectopy and agenesis are the causes of approximately 60 and 25 percent of the cases of permanent hypothyroidism, respectively.[47,131–133] The remainder of patients with permanent hypothyroidism include those with inborn errors in thyroid hormone synthesis and thyroid hormone resistance (see Ch. 16) and infants with hypothalamic pituitary hypothyroidism (Table 15-2).

Cost-Benefit Analysis

Before discussing the pathophysiology of congenital hypothyroidism, it is appropriate to comment on the cost-benefit ratio of programs that have led to the identification and treatment of over 20,000 infants with this condition. Fortunately, at the time when the question of such testing was raised, screening programs were already in place in many coun-

TABLE 15-2. Causes of Congenital Hypothyroidism

Thyroid dysgenesis including agenesis, hypoplasia, or ectopia
Thyroid dyshormonogenesis including TSH resistance
Hypothalamic or pituitary hypothyroidism
Maternal antithyroid drug ingestion; iodides, thiourea derivatives, [131]I
Maternal autoimmunity
Immaturity
    Transient hypothyroxinemia
    Transient hyperthyrotropinemia
Iodide exposure
    Amniofetography
    Neonatal povidone or other antiseptics containing iodine

tries for heritable diseases such as phenylketonuria. Thus, in the most thorough analysis of one typical program in the northwestern United States, the total cost in 1977 for screening one infant for phenylketonuria, galactosemia, maple syrup urine disease, homocystinuria, tyrosinemia, and congenital hypothyroidism was $1.71.[132] The costs attributable to the hypothyroidism alone were estimated to be one-third of the total cost of this program, or approximately $0.60. In 1977, the U.S. General Accounting Office estimated that the average untreated hypothyroid child would incur total institutional medical care costs of $330,000 throughout life. It has been estimated that only 1 in 10 such infants would require institutionalization, but even taking this figure, the cost-benefit ratio ($330,000 divided by $27,000, the cost of discovering 10 such infants in 45,000 normal children) is greater than 10. This ratio does not include the loss of tax income to the state and federal governments that would result from impaired intellectual capacity in the untreated, but noninstitutionalized, person. Such an accounting also does not place a monetary value on the anguish to the family and patient as a consequence of untreated congenital hypothyroidism. Congenital hypothyroidism screening is a prime example of the social and economic benefits of preventive medicine to the individual and to the community.

Screening Strategies

Full-term Infants

Initial strategies in the Quebec program and in the northeast and northwest United States employed primary screening using estimated concentration of serum T_4 in a dried blood spot obtained from infants 2 to 3 days of age. In the initial phases of the Quebec model program, the lowest few percent of the population were located and repeat tests performed.[131] However, because of the difficult logistics involved in the follow-up program and consequent high cost, this and many other programs subsequently adopted a two-tiered strategy consisting of a T_4 estimate on all samples obtained at 2 to 3 days of age followed by a TSH estimation in those samples in which serum T_4 concentrations were less than 6 to 7 μg/dl (80 nmol/L). Other programs, particularly those used in western Europe, have employed a TSH measurement as the screening strategy.[134,135] A TSH greater than 40 mU/L leads to an evaluation of the infant for congenital hypothyroidism, whereas a level between 15 and 40 mU/L leads to a T_4 measurement in the same sample and a follow-up T_4/TSH in a second blood spot. There are fewer causes of false-positive elevations in serum TSH than of falsely low serum T_4 concentrations. On the other hand, a TSH screening program will generally not identify the 3 to 4 percent of the infant population with hypothyroidism due to hypothalamic or pituitary causes. Also, geographic areas in which dietary iodine is limited, such as Belgium, will have a relatively higher frequency of infants with transient TSH elevation, especially in the premature population.[50]

In the United States, many mother-infant pairs are now discharged within 24 hours of delivery. Obtaining reliable samples requires taking them within that period. This has increased the number of false-positive results by TSH screening, since it takes several days for the neonatal TSH surge to dissipate completely (Fig. 15-5).[39,136] Thus, in California, the early discharge program increased the ratio of false to true positives by TSH assay from 2.5:1 to 5:1.[134] While this could be reduced by increasing the upper

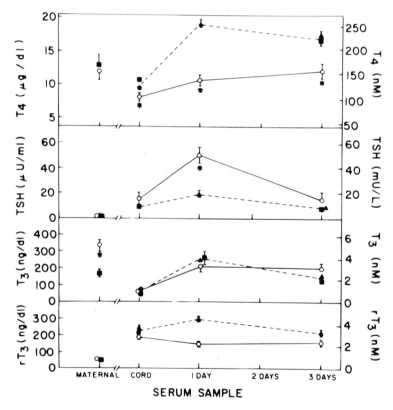

Fig. 15-5. Effects of PTU treatment on maternal and neonatal serum thyroid hormone and TSH concentrations. Bars indicate the standard error of the mean (SEM). Where bars are absent, the SEM is smaller than the symbol. Open circles denote PTU-treated mothers and infants, and solid symbols, control values from several sources. An asterisk indicates a significant difference from normal (p<0.05). T_4 denotes thyroxine, T_3 triiodothyronine, and rT_3 reverse triiodothyronine. (From Cheron et al.,[136] with permission.)

limits of normal for TSH, the possibility of missing infants with slowly rising TSH values is significant. This observation was confirmed in an Oregon study showing that when a second screen at 4 to 6 weeks was performed, an additional 19 infants previously thought to be normal were found to have congenital hypothyroidism.[133] The missed group constituted 10 percent of the total with congenital hypothyroidism. By retrospective analysis of the blood spots obtained from the undiagnosed infants, the causes of the false-negative results were characterized. Of the 19 infants, 14 had had a low serum T_4 at the time of the initial screen, but the TSH was not elevated. Another 20 percent of the group had a normal serum T_4, but an elevated TSH that had not been measured since the T_4 estimate was above the cut-off point for TSH testing. A worrisome aspect of these results is the fact that a significant fraction of this missed population has had a delayed rise in serum TSH. The reason for this is not understood at this time. It justifies the policy of all screening programs to emphasize to pediatricians and parents alike that signs suggesting the possibility of congenital hypothyroidism should not be ignored merely because the infant has "passed" the neonatal hypothyroidism screening test.[47] In addition to the physiologic causes for missed cases, there are a number of reports that emphasize the possibility for human error in failing to identify affected infants. This can occur due to poor communication, lack of receipt of requested specimens, and the failure to test an infant who is transferred between hospitals during the neonatal period.[137,138]

Very-Low-Birth-Weight Infants

The New England program has called attention to the problem that has arisen in testing very-low-birth-weight infants, a subject already alluded to in the discussion of prematurity.[56,139] It is in this population that the possibility of a low initial T_4, and a several-month delay in TSH elevation, is especially common. This program reported nine infants with birth weights between 400 and 1,300 g in whom clearly subnormal T_4 levels were associated with serum TSH values less than 20 mU/L. By age 30 to 45 days, TSH in most had risen to the high levels typical of congenital hypothyroidism. However, in a few infants, a TSH elevation did not occur until almost 2 months of age. The authors concluded that a high index of suspicion must be maintained for the very-low-birth-weight infant with a subnormal serum T_4 concentration. Unfortunately, there is a significant tendency for serum T_4 concentrations to be subnormal in this population due to illness, immaturity of hepatic protein synthesis, and of the hypothalamic pituitary axis. This will be more of a problem in a program that depends on TSH assay as the initial screening test. Such programs may need to give specific attention to this issue in the very-low-birth-weight population. A consensus on whether or not premature infants with transient hypothyroidism should be treated has not been achieved. A decision to institute treatment with levothyroxine must be made on a case-by-case basis. If treatment is instituted, it should be with doses of 10 to 15 $\mu g/kg$ levothyroxine, but the infants should be followed carefully to allow the recognition as to whether or not endogenous thyroid function has resumed.

Etiology

Table 15-2 lists the potential causes of congenital hypothyroidism.[2,131,132,140–143] In North America about 60 percent of infants were found to have aplastic or hypoplastic glands and another 28 percent to have functioning thyroid tissue in an ectopic location.[2] In Europe, thyroid agenesis was found in 40 percent and ectopic thyroid location in 60 percent.[140] Whether this difference in the prevalence of thyroid ectopy and agenesis in Europe and North America is real or apparent cannot be determined as yet, since many infants did not have thyroid scans before the onset of treatment. The ectopic thyroid glands are usually lingual or sublingual in location. Thyroid dysgenesis is about twice as common in girls as in boys. The reason for failure of both biochemical and clinical evidence of hypothyroidism to appear is that thyroid hormone deficiency is less severe in patients with ectopic thyroid tissue than in those with no demonstrable tissue. No association of sporadic congenital hypothyroidism with potential environmental or ingested toxins or drugs has been made. This lack of association, of course, does not apply to hypothyroidism appearing endemically where iodine deficiency or thiocyanate ingestion have been found to be causative factors. Familial cases of sporadic congenital hypothyroidism have been described, but this pattern is the exception rather than the rule.

The next most common cause of congenital hypothyroidism is dyshormonogenesis due to defects in one or another of the steps involved in thyroid hormone synthesis. These defects are discussed in Chapter 16.

Two children with apparent inherited resistance of the thyroid to TSH have been described.[142,143] One infant had an elevated serum TSH concentration, and the TSH was both immunologically and biologically normal.[143] There was a history of consanguinity, and the patient was severely retarded. There was no response of the thyroid to exogenous bovine TSH, suggesting that there was a defect in response to all forms of TSH. A similar possibility has been proposed for the hypothyroidism in familial pseudohypoparathyroidism, and a genetic defect in the *Gs* protein linking the TSH receptor with adenylate cyclase has been identified in such families.[144]

Hypothalamic or pituitary hypothyroidism is distinctly less common than primary hypothyroidism. In the screening programs of North America, this rare condition accounts for less than 5 percent of patients. Various types of abnormalities have been described.[145,146] They include an apparent defect in TRH production, isolated TSH deficiency (familial), familial panhypopituitarism, and congenital absence of the pituitary gland. In addition, genetic defects in the TSH gene, such as the CAGYC mutation in the TSH β subunit gene[147,148] and mutations in the gene encoding Pit-1, which can cause not only TSH deficiency but also deficiencies of growth hormone and prolactin, though not of luteinizing hormone (LH) and FSH.[76,149,150]

There is some disagreement as to whether or not maternal autoimmunity can play a role in the genesis of congenital hypothyroidism. Several infants with transient hypothyroidism due to maternal TSH receptor blocking antibodies have been reported, but this is quite rare.[77,79,151] There is no relationship between circulating maternal anti-TPO antibodies and the appearance of congenital hypothyroidism.[77] On the other hand, evidence of antibody-dependent, cell-mediated cytotoxicity was reported in 61 patients with congenital hypothyroidism and in 46 of their mothers.[78] The presence of cell-mediated toxicity was much higher in infants with athyreosis and ectopic thyroid than it was in individuals with a normal thyroid gland. Such antibodies could conceiva-

bly play a role in the induction of thyroid cell destruction in utero, although it is still not clear how frequently this mechanism plays a role in the sporadic form of the disease.

Other causes of transient hypothyroidism include maternal or fetal iodine exposure. This is particularly problematic in the premature infant, in whom adaptation to a high plasma iodide does not readily occur.[51,52] Iodide can enter the fetal circulation either from medications or dietary ingestion. Iodine deficiency can also impair neonatal thyroid function.

The most common cause of transient neonatal hypothyroidism is that due to neonatal administration of antithyroid drugs during pregnancy.[136,152] Figure 15-5 shows results of a prospective study analyzing this issue in 11 mothers receiving 200 mg of propylthiouracil (PTU) or less per day. Despite the relatively modest dose of PTU, well within the allowable dose according to current guidelines, there was clear-cut impairment of thyroid function in the newborn infants as evidenced by a lower neonatal T_4 surge and higher TSH at 3 days of age. The impaired thyroid function in these infants was biochemical, not clinical, and transient. The results show conclusively, however, that even low daily doses of PTU impact fetal thyroid function. Furthermore, as with iodide ingestion, respiratory obstruction due to thyroid enlargement can be significant. This fact is illustrated by the following case report.[136]

A 20-year-old woman with Graves' disease was treated with 400 mg PTU daily throughout her pregnancy. No iodide was given. With cesarean delivery for cephalopelvic disproportion and polyhydramnios, a 2,700-g boy was born. The infant was apneic, with a pulse of 80, had 1- and 5-minute Apgar scores of 1 and 2, respectively, and required assisted ventilation for 20 minutes. The thyroid was enlarged bilaterally, each lobe measuring 3.5 × 2 cm. Respiratory distress required 40 to 50 percent oxygen for 5 days. The infant was placed in the prone position to avoid tracheal compression. Table 15-3 shows results of sequential laboratory studies. They demonstrate the rapid spontaneous recovery of thyroid function after elimination of maternal antithyroid drug.

Pathology

The structural changes of untreated congenital hypothyroidism may include an imposing array of developmental retardations, among which are the

TABLE 15-3. Serum Thyroid Hormone and TSH Concentrations in an Infant whose Mother Received 400 mg/day PTU

Sample	T_4 (μg/dl)	T_3 (ng/dl)	TSH (μU/ml)	rT_3 (ng/dl)
Mother[a]	9.0	196	2.8	—
Cord	4.4	75	>480	176
1 day	3.5	250	>480	40
2 days	8.3	300	126	—
3 days	9.5	250	33	—
4 days	10.0	180	12.5	—
5 days	10.5	178	9.0	—
6 days	10.8	210	9.0	—
14 days	10.7	196	—	70

[a] At the time of delivery.
(From Cheron et al.,[136] wtih permission.)

delayed appearance of epiphyseal union, epiphyseal dysgenesis, delayed dentition, and hypoplasia of the brain. In addition, one may find the characteristic changes of adult hypothyroidism. Among the changes in the central nervous system are low brain weight, nerve cell loss, and delayed myelinization.[101] It must be admitted, however, that the number of patients carefully studied from the pathologic point of view is small. There has been no pathologic study of the ear of these patients. Hearing is usually normal, in contrast to the endemic cretin. A significant finding is hypertrophy of the anterior pituitary and accompanying enlargement of the sella with prolonged hypothyroidism. This condition has been reported by many writers, beginning with Niepce in 1841,[153,154] and coincides well with the remarkably elevated plasma TSH concentration often found in these patients (~<400mU/L).

Clinical Features

The most important clinical observation in infants with congenital or neonatal hypothyroidism identified by the screening programs is that they are usually asymptomatic. Thus, a report of an abnormal thyroid screening test result in an apparently normal infant is quite consistent with the diagnosis of congenital hypothyroidism. This point is well illustrated by the list in Table 15-4 and is similar to the results of several authors.[146,155,156] It is safe to say that no abnormal symptom or sign is found in more than about one-third of infants with congenital hypothyroidism, and no clinical feature can be said to be pathognomonic.

As untreated infants grow older, the clinical features of hypothyroidism described in the prescreening era appear or become more obvious. Failure of linear growth, listless feeding, constipation, hoarse cry, somnolence, and noisy respiration are commonly observed. Such infants may have a puffy face, eyelids, and hands, a thickened or protruding tongue due to myxedema, pallor or mottled cool skin, umbilical hernia, bradycardia, and a hoarse cry, with a slow response to noxious stimuli. The thyroid gland is usually not palpable. The posterior fontanel may remain open even at 4 to 8 weeks. The clinical picture should be kept in mind because the screening programs are not 100 percent effective, and hypothyroidism may appear in the first months of life even when screening test results have been normal.

Diagnosis

The confirmatory diagnosis of congenital hypothyroidism is relatively straightforward when the condition is associated with primary thyroid disease. In such patients, the serum T_4 is reduced, the free T_4 index is low, and serum TSH is elevated, often to remarkably high levels (>200 mU/L). The older the infant at the time T_4 is measured, the greater will be the difference between the serum T_4 in affected infants and the result in normal infants of the same age. This is due to the rapid clearance of maternal T_4 from the circulation. As discussed in Chapter 6 and elsewhere, measurement of the serum T_3 concentration is not of additional value in establishing the diagnosis of primary hypothyroidism, since it may be within the normal range even in infants with marked TSH elevation.[155]

If causes of transient hypothyroidism such as maternal drug ingestion, maternal or fetal iodide exposure, and prematurity-related hypothyroidism can be ruled out, then a presumptive diagnosis of congenital hypothyroidism can be made. In some infants it may be necessary to wait several days to establish a clear diagnosis before instituting further diagnostic evaluation. However, a longer delay is contraindicated, and when serious consideration is being given to the diagnosis, time is of the essence.[47,61,135,157] A serum thyroglobulin (TG) measurement may be of use in confirming the diagnosis of athyreosis, since in that condition it is universally reduced or undetectable.[10] Serum TG concentrations vary considerably in individuals with ectopic

TABLE 15-4. Symptoms and Signs of Congenital Hypothyroidism in Infants Diagnosed by a Screening Program

Symptoms	No. of Infants	Signs	No. of Infants
Constipation	9/22	Temperature <36°	1/12
Lethargy	7/22	Large anterior fontanel	4/18
Prolonged jaundice	6/21	Large posterior fontanel	2/17
Poor feeding	5/22	Macroglossia	4/21
		Goiter	0/21
		Umbilical hernia	6/21
		Hypotonia	7/21
		Slow relaxation of deep tendon reflexes	3/21

(Modified from LaFranchi et al.,[146] with permission.)

thyroid gland but are generally elevated in individuals with goitrous hypothyroidism. The combination of a low total T_4 and TSH in the normal range should lead to an evaluation for reduced TBG, which has been estimated to be present in approximately 1 in 7,500 individuals.[158] This diagnosis is established by measuring the free T_4 index or assay of TBG and calculation of the T_4/TBG ratio (see Ch. 6). Computed tomography (CT) or MRI is useful in characterizing the possibility of hypothalamic pituitary anomalies, and the administration of 7 μg/kg TRH will confirm that TSH is, in fact, absent. When central hypothyroidism is present, it is also necessary to evaluate the infant for adrenocorticotropic hormone (ACTH) and growth hormone (GH) deficiency. A family history of similar diseases will raise the possibility of a genetic abnormality in pituitary-dependent function.

Infants with apparent primary hypothyroidism should have either an iodine or technetium 99m pertechnetate (TcO4) scan if this is available, but treatment should not be delayed to perform this study. In infants with primary hypothyroidism, the serum TSH will remain elevated for days to weeks after levothyroxine therapy begins, thus permitting recognition of any functioning tissue. If the thyroid gland is in an abnormal location, the scan will establish the diagnosis of thyroid ectopy. While the absence of uptake in the normal thyroid and the lack of palpable tissue in this area suggest athyreosis, infants with transient causes of hypothyroidism (e.g., excess iodide, TSH receptor-blocking antibody) can also have low uptakes. Ultrasound evaluation of the neck may permit a definitive identification of thyroid tissue. An x-ray of the knee and foot to assess bone age is a useful index of the duration and severity of the intrauterine hypothyroidism.

There is generally little difficulty in discriminating between infants with congenital hypothyroidism and those with Down's syndrome alone (in which the incidence of congenital hypothyroidism is increased) or other inborn errors such as of the mucopolysaccharidoses.

Treatment

Recognition of the critical role played by serum T_4 as a source of cerebrocortical T_3 (see above and Ch. 3) has led to the consensus that the serum T_4 concentrations should be normalized as rapidly as possible in infants with congenital hypothyroidism. With a half-life of 3.6 days, maternal T_4 is rapidly cleared from the infant's circulation (based on data from the Dutch study.[18,58]) Early guidelines suggested a dose of between 8 and 10 μg/kg/d would be appropriate for initial treatment.[131] However, on such a regimen, as long as 4 to 6 weeks may be required before the serum T_4 reaches the desirable level of 10 to 16 μg/dl (130 to 260 nmol/L). It is conceivable that this delay could explain the slightly subnormal intellectual outcome in infants treated using these initial guidelines.[60,62–64,159–163] The current recommendation is to use a levothyroxine dose of 10 to 15 μg/kg/day.[47,135] This can be achieved by giving about 50 μg levothyroxine per day to a full-term infant. Using this approach, follow-up studies in 15 infants showed that at 1 year of age, the height, bone age, and head circumference were all normal, and no evidence was found for craniosynostosis in any infant.[157] Both serum free T_4 index and TSH should be monitored.

As the infant grows, the total levothyroxine dose does not change substantially. It should decrease very gradually from the initial level of 10 to 15 μg/

kg in the newborn to approximately 1.5 μg/kg in the adult. Thus, a typical daily dose of levothyroxine for an infant is 50 μg, whereas that for an adult female is about 88 to 125 μg. This reflects the marked reduction in T_4 production/kg body weight with increasing age.[5]

The treatment of infants with central hypothyroidism should follow the same guidelines with respect to levothyroxine replacement as those for infants with primary thyroid dysfunction. The serum free T_4 index is the critical parameter to monitor in these infants. It will also be necessary to evaluate such infants for other pituitary hormone deficiencies and replace these as necessary, depending on the type of central abnormality.

In addition to recommending rapid normalization of the serum T_4 concentration, the experience of the New England program suggests that close attention must be maintained to ensure that compliance with the medication schedule is achieved. These investigators noted that at all ages, a significant number of individuals received inadequate therapy as reflected in serum T_4 concentrations less than 8 μg/dl (103 nmol/L) and elevated TSH levels.[61,137] In the first 1 to 2 years of life, it may not be possible to normalize the serum TSH concentration even though serum free T_4 concentrations are elevated. This has been attributed to a reduced sensitivity of the hypothalamic-pituitary axis to feedback inhibition by thyroid hormone due to fetal hypothyroidism. The axis usually achieves normal sensitivity by 1 year of age.[6,135] If TSH is elevated, increasing the total serum T_4 concentration to 10 to 16 μg/dl (130 to 206 nmol/L) will reduce it to less than 20 mU/L in over 80 percent of infants.[61] In the residual 20 percent, providing levothyroxine at doses adequate to maintain T_4 at or above 12 μg/dl (155 nmol/L) should reduce the serum TSH to less than 20 mU/L in all infants.[47] Modest TSH elevations, up to 20 mU/L, are acceptable during the first year of treatment if the serum free T_4 index or free T_4 are maintained slightly above the upper limits of normal.

Continuous monitoring of these patients is essential. There is a correlation between success in cognitive test scores and adequacy of treatment even in adolescent children.[61] For example, at age 14 years, 16 of the 36 children tested had serum TSH values greater than 15 mU/L and serum T_4 concentrations less than 6.6 μg/dl (85 nmol/L). Attention to compliance, education of the parents, and random testing with finger-stick TSH specimens resulted in a considerable improvement in compliance. Such improvements were associated with higher cognitive test results, and with an increase of IQ from 106 to 112. While it is not clear that these two events are causally related, it calls attention to the fact that with levothyroxine, as with any chronically administered medication, compliance is difficult to sustain without constant monitoring.

Prognosis for Psychoneurologic Development

Follow-up data are still being collected on this issue, since the oldest patients under treatment are only now reaching 20 years of age. There is general agreement that the prognosis for the development of normal intelligence is markedly improved by early recognition and treatment of congenital hypothyroidism. All groups who have studied this matter in depth have found normalization or near normalization of intelligence when compared with the population as a whole or when compared with siblings within the same family. However, all groups have identified certain patients who have not achieved normal intelligence. In the Quebec program, infants with severe hypothyroidism at birth, as reflected in a serum T_4 less than 2 μg/dl (<30 nmol/L) and markedly retarded bone age as assessed by the ossification center in the knee, often did not achieve a developmental quotient of 90.[62,160,161] No other factors that could be evaluated could account for these differences, although the monitoring of compliance in the early phases of this program, as in most others, was not as systematic as it has been in more recent years. Accordingly, these authors concluded that infants with severe biochemical hypothyroidism and physical evidence of delayed bone maturation at birth have sustained irreversible impairment of intellectual function. On the other hand, the New England program has reported that in the 15- to 17-year age group, the only factor identified that influenced IQ was inadequate treatment in the first year of life, as defined by two or more serum T_4 results less than 8 μg/dl (103 nmol/L).[58,61] They also reported that IQ was positively correlated with mean serum T_4 concentration in the first year. Noncompliance has been documented by this program in earlier years, and the studies already alluded to indicated that this was a problem in as many as 50 percent of the patients during adolescence. An improvement in compliance in the teenage years was associated an improved performance on intelligence testing, although some potential for an improved performance due to enhanced test taking skills cannot be completely eliminated. The conclusion of the New England group is that the IQ results are normally distributed in infants who received early and adequate treatment and in whom compliance was maintained.

Reports from other programs, while not as old as those in these two series, are similar; namely, most children will develop normally.[162,164] Nonetheless, there are exceptions. The evidence from the United Kingdom that severely affected children show an average 10 point lower IQ than less affected patients is quite convincing.[63,64] However, the entire group was treated with lower doses of levothyroxine and with less rigorous monitoring than would be recommended under current guidelines. Whether changes in these aspects of treatment will prevent or reverse the dysfunction in the more severely affected individuals in the U.K. program remains to be seen.

It would seem likely that all programs will experience the same difficulties with patient compliance. One would expect that, on average, an infant with more severe thyroid impairment would sustain greater postnatal damage if compliance is not adequately maintained than would one with a less severe thyroid malfunction. Thus, the two factors that have been shown to be important in this issue, severity of deficit and adequacy of compliance, are not independent. The importance of the early normalization of serum T_4 in enhancing the childhood intelligence quotient has also been emphasized by the Toronto group.[159,165] They noted an approximately 4 to 5 point higher IQ in infants receiving an initial levothyroxine dose of 8 to 10 μg/kg, as opposed to those receiving 7 to 9 μg/kg/d. They also observed a 5 to 10 point lower IQ in infants in whom treatment was delayed beyond age 4 weeks and who had a delayed bone age at birth. Based on these data, Fisher has estimated that untreated congenitally hypothyroid infants with severe hypothyroidism could lose approximately 3 to 5 IQ points per month in the first year of life.[47]

The New England Collaborative has recommended the following guidelines for monitoring treatment in patients with congenital hypothyroidism: that serum T_4 and TSH be measured monthly, as well as 2 weeks after any change in levothyroxine dose during the first 2 years of life.[61] This should be done using filter paper heel-stick samples. The monitoring should then be continued at 3- to 4-month intervals from early childhood through adolescence. Based on this experience, the serum T_4 concentrations should reach 10 μg/dl (130 nmol/L) within 2 weeks of the start of treatment and be maintained between 10 and 15 μg/dl (130 to 190 nmol/L) over the first year of life. In 80 to 90 percent of infants this will be associated with a reduction in TSH to less than 15 mU/L. After the first year of life, sufficient levothyroxine should be given to normalize the TSH. Similar recommendations have been made by others.[47,135,166]

In conclusion, congenital hypothyroidism screening programs are remarkably successful in identifying affected infants. The major challenges at this time are how to institute treatment rapidly with levothyroxine doses adequate to raise and maintain the serum T_4 concentrations consistently at appropriate levels throughout infancy and childhood.

SUMMARY

Thyroid gland function develops early in the human fetus with establishment of a functional thyroid gland by 10 to 12 weeks' gestation. Circulating thyroid hormones continue to increase gradually thereafter. For reasons not yet understood, the fetus has low levels of the outer-ring type 1 deiodinase and high levels of type 3 (inner-ring deiodinase) in immature skin as well as in the placenta. This results in extremely low serum T_3 concentrations until delivery. Despite this, significant quantities of nuclear T_3 are present in the central nervous system, even in the first trimester, as a consequence of the action of type 2 deiodinase on the circulating T_4. At birth, serum reverse T_3 is high, serum T_3 is low, and serum free T_4 is similar to that in the maternal serum. TSH increases abruptly at delivery with a consequent rise in serum T_3 and T_4. Type 1 deiodinase increases as well, and a pattern of circulating T_4, T_3, and reverse T_3 concentrations similar to those found in the adult is rapidly established. The stimulus for the acute release of TSH in the neonate is presumably the rapid decrease in environmental temperature. Premature infants exhibit hypothalamic-pituitary thyroid function typical of their gestational age, namely, relatively normal free T_4, but reduced T_3 and a blunted TSH response at delivery. Premature infants are prone to develop hypothalamic-pituitary hypothyroidism as a consequence of respiratory distress syndrome.

Under normal circumstances there is probably little transfer of maternal thyroid hormone to the fetus after the first trimester. However, if fetal thyroid function is impaired, transfer of maternal hormone from the amniotic fluid and placental circulations occurs so that serum T_4 concentrations in the athyreotic newborn are between 25 and 50 percent of normal. Thus, maternal hormone can support normal development of the central nervous system.

Thyroid hormone is required for many steps in the development of the central nervous system and for normal bone maturation. The central nervous system is particularly sensitive to thyroid hormone deprivation, and its development is severely impaired when both maternal and fetal thyroid function are compromised. This rarely occurs except in areas of endemic iodine deficiency. The clinical picture of severe combined maternal and fetal iodine deficiency is manifested in the endemic cretin by extrapyramidal dysfunction, strabismus, deafness, and mental retardation. While the anatomic abnormalities in the brain of patients with endemic cretinism are few, the functional disorders reflect the abnormal development of those areas of the central nervous system that are most sensitive to a lack of thyroid hormone. Features of endemic cretinism are rarely seen in patients with sporadic congenital hypothyroidism, presumably due to an adequate supply of maternal thyroid hormone.

Congenital hypothyroidism occurs in about 1 in 4,000 births. The cause is generally thyroid dysgenesis with absent, hypoplastic, or ectopic thyroid tissue present. Thyroid dyshormonogenesis, hypothalamic-pituitary hypothyroidism, and transient hypothyroidism due to either iodine supplementation, antithyroid drug therapy to the mother or, rarely, maternal or transplacental passage of maternal antithyroid antibody should also be considered. Newborn screening for this condition is performed by measuring T_4 and or TSH in dried blood spots obtained by heel puncture shortly after birth. In many screening programs an initial quantitation of spot T_4 is made with a TSH assay performed on the lowest 5 to 10 percent of the population. All studies have shown that the intellectual development of infants

treated within the first month of life with adequate amounts of levothyroxine have improved intellectual development. There is still some disagreement as to whether the development of severely affected hypothyroid infants can be completely normalized even with early treatment. Some programs seem to have been able to achieve this, while others have not. Possible explanations for this discrepancy are that there is poor compliance or levothyroxine misadministration or that the initial doses of levothyroxine recommended for treatment were too low to normalize serum T_4 concentrations rapidly enough. The current recommendations are that 10 to 15 mg/kg of levothyroxine be administered per day and that frequent monitoring of serum T_4 and TSH by heel or finger-stick specimens be maintained throughout infancy and adolescence. Serum T_4 concentrations should be 130 to 206 nmol/L (10 to 16 mg/dl). This will generally be associated with serum TSH values that are less than 15 mU/L but that normalize after age 1 year.

REFERENCES

1. Fisher DA, Dussault JH, Sack J, Chopra IJ: Ontogenesis of hypothalamic-pituitary thyroid function and metabolism in man, sheep, and rat. Recent Prog Horm Res 33:59, 1977
2. Fisher DA, Klein AH: Thyroid development and disorders of thyroid function in the newborn. N Engl J Med 304:702, 1981
3. Thorpe-Beeston JG, Nicolaides KH, McGregor AM: Fetal thyroid function. Thyroid 2:207, 1992
4. Thorpe-Beeston JG, Nicolaides KH, Felton CV et al: Maturation of the secretion of thyroid hormone and thyroid-stimulating hormone in the fetus. N Engl J Med 324:532, 1991
5. Burrow GN, Fisher DA, Larsen PR: Mechanisms of disease: maternal and fetal thyroid function. N Engl J Med 331:1072, 1994
6. Bellabio M, Nicolini U, Jowett T et al: Maturation of thyroid function in normal human fetuses. Clin Endocrinol 31:565, 1989
7. Contempre B, Jauniaux E, Calvo R: Detection of thyroid hormones in human embryonic cavities during the first trimester of pregnancy. J Clin Endocrinol Metab 77:1719, 1993
8. Costa A, Arisio R, Benedetto C et al: Thyroid hormones in tissues from human embryos and fetuses. J Endocrinol Invest 14:550, 1991
9. Gitlin D, Biasucci A: Ontogenesis of immunoreac-

tion thyroglobulin in the human conceptus. J Clin Endocrinol Metab 29:849, 1969

10. Heinze HJ, Shulman DI, Diamond FB Jr, Bercu BB: Spectrum of serum thyroglobulin elevation in congenital thyroid disorders. Thyroid 3:37, 1993

11. Klein AH, Hobel CJ, Sack J, Fisher DA: Effect of intraamniotic fluid thyroxine injection on fetal serum and amniotic fluid iodothyronine concentrations. J Clin Endocrinol Metab 47:1034, 1978

12. Wolff J: Iodide goiter and the pharmacologic effects of excess iodide. Am J Med 47:101, 1969

13. Delange F, Dodion J, Wolter R et al: Transient hypothyroidism in the newborn infant. J Pediatr 92:974, 1978

14. Montalvo JN, Wahner HW, Mayberry WE, Lum RK: Serum triiodothyronine, total thyroxine, and thyroxine-to-triiodothyronine ratios in paired maternal-cord sera and at one week and one month of age. Pediatr Res 7:706, 1973

15. Larsen PR, Silva JE, Kaplan MM: Relationships between circulating and intracellular thyroid hormones: physiological and clinical implications. Endocr Rev 2:87, 1981

16. Calvo R, Obregon MJ, Ruiz de Ona C et al: Congenital hypothyroidism as studied in rats: crucial role of maternal thyroxine (T_4), but not of 3,5,3' triiodothyronine (T_3) in the protection of the fetal brain. J Clin Invest 86:889, 1990

17. Crantz FR, Silva JE, Larsen PR: Analysis of the sources and quantity of 3,5,3'-triiodothyronine specifically bound to nuclear receptors in rat cerebral cortex and cerebellum. Endocrinology 110:367, 1982

18. Vulsma T, Gons MH, DeVijlder JMM: Maternal fetal transfer of thyroxine in congenital hypothyroidism due to a total organification defect of thyroid dysgenesis. N Engl J Med 321:13, 1989

19. Roti E, Gnudi A, Braverman LE: The placental transport, synthesis and metabolism of hormones and drugs which affect thyroid function. Endocr Rev 4: 131, 1983

20. Roti E, Fang SL, Green K et al: Human placenta is an active site of thyroxine and 3,3',5-triiodothyronine tyrosyl ring deiodination. J Clin Endocrinol Metab 53:498, 1981

21. Ruiz de Ona C, Morreale de Escobar G, Calvo R et al: Thyroid hormone and 5'-deiodinase in the rat fetus late in gestation: effects of maternal hypothyroidism. Endocrinology 128:422, 1991

22. Ferreiro B, Bernal J, Goodyer CG, Branchard CL: Estimation of nuclear thyroid receptor saturation in human fetal brain and lung during early gestation. J Clin Endocrinol Metab 67:853, 1988

23. Chopra IJ, Wu SY, Chua Teco GN, Santini F: A radio-immunoassay for measurement of 3,5,3'-triiodothyronine sulfate; studies in thyroidal and non-thyroidal disease, pregnancy and neonatal life. J Clin Endocrinol Metab 75:189, 1992

24. Sharifi J, St. Gernain DL: The cDNA for the type I iodothyronine 5'-deiodinase encodes an enzyme manifesting both high K_m and low K_m activity. J Biol Chem 267:12539, 1992

25. Wu SY, Huang WS, Polk D et al: Identification of thyroxine sulfate (T_4S) in human serum and amniotic fluid by a novel T_4S radioimmunoassay. Thyroid 2:101, 1992

26. Polk DH, Reviczky A, Wu SY et al: Metabolism of sulfoconjugated thyroid hormone derivatives in developing sheep. Am J Physiol 266:E892, 1994

27. Meinhold H, Dudenhausen JW, Wenzel KW, Saling E: Amniotic fluid concentrations of 3,3',3'-tri-iodthyronine (reverse T_3), 3,3'-di-iodothyronine, 3,5,3'-tri-iodothyronine (T_3) and thyroxine (T_4) in normal and complicated pregnancy. Clin Endocrinol 10: 355, 1979

28. Santini F, Hurd RE, Chopra IJ: A study of metabolism of deaminated and sulfoconjugated iodothyronines by rat placental iodothyronine 5-monodeiodinase. Endocrinology 131:1689, 1992

29. Kaplan MM, Yakoski KA: Maturational patterns of iodothyronine phenolic and tyrosyl ring deiodinase activities in rat cerebrum, cerebellum, and hypothalamus. J Clin Invest 67:1204, 1980

30. Silva JE, Larsen PR: Comparison of iodothyronine 5'-deiodinase and other thyroid-hormone-dependent enzyme activities in the cerbral cortex and hypothyroid neonatal rat. J Clin Invest 70:1110, 1982

31. Silva JE, Matthews PS: Production rates and turnover of triiodothyronine in rat-developing cerebral cortex and cerebellum: responses to hypothyroidism. J Clin Invest 74:1035, 1984

32. Obregon MJ, Mallol J, Pastor RM et al: L-thyroxine and 3,5,3'-triiodothyronine in rat embryos before onset of fetal thyroid function. Endocrinology 114: 305, 1984

33. Morreale de Escobar G, Obregon MJ, Ruiz de Ona C, Escobar del Rey F: Transfer of thyroxine from the mother to the rat fetus near term: effects on brain 3,5,3'-triiodothyronine deficiency. Endocrinology 122:1521, 1988

34. Calvo R, Obregon MJ, Escobar del Rey F, Morreale de Escobar G: The rat placenta and the transfer of thyroid hormones from the mother to the fetus: effects of maternal thyroid status. Endocrinology 131: 357, 1992

35. Morreale de Escobar G, Calvo R, Obregon MJ, Escobar del Rey F: Contribution of maternal thyroxine

to fetal thyroxine pools in normal rats near term. Endocrinology 126:2765, 1990

36. Fisher DA, Lehman H, Lackey C: Placental transport of thyroxine. J Clin Endocrinol 24:393, 1964

37. Davidson KM, Richards DS, Schatz DA, Fisher DA: Successful in utero treatment of fetal goiter and hypothyroidism. N Engl J Med 324:543, 1991

38. Polk DH, Wu SY, Wright C et al: Ontogeny of thyroid hormone effect on tissue 5' monodeiodinase activity in fetal sheep. Am J Physiol 17:E337, 1988

39. Fisher DA, Odell WD: Acute release of thyrotropin in the newborn. J Clin Invest 48:1670, 1969

40. Abuid J, Klein AH, Foley Jr TP, Larsen PR: Total and free triiodothyronine and thyroxine in early infancy. J Clin Endocrinol Metab 39:263, 1974

41. Abuid J, Stinson DA, Larsen PR: Serum triiodothyronine and thyroxine in the neonate and the acute increases in these hormones following delivery. J Clin Invest 52:1195, 1973

42. Wu S-Y, Klein AH, Chopra IJ, Fisher DA: Alterations in tissue thyroxine 5'-monodeiodinating activity in the perinatal period. Endocrinology 103:235, 1978

43. Harris ARC, Fang S-L, Prosky J et al: Decreased outer ring monodeiodination of thyroxine and reverse triiodothyronine in the fetal and neonatal rat. Endocrinology 103:2216, 1978

44. Bianco AC, Kieffer JD, Silva JE: Adenosine 3' 5'-monophosphate and thyroid hormone control of uncoupling protein messenger ribonucleic acid in freshly dispersed brown adipocytes. Endocrinology 130:2625, 1992

45. Houstek J, Vizek K, Stanislav P, Kopecky J, et al: Type II iodothyronine 5'-deiodinase and uncoupling protein in brown adipose tissue of human newborns. J Clin Endocrinol Metab 77:382, 1993

46. AvRuskin TW, Tang SC, Shenkman L et al: Serum triiodothyronine concentrations in infancy, childhood, adolescence, and pediatric thyroid disorders. J Clin Endocrinol Metab 37:235, 1973

47. Fisher DA: Clinical Review 19; Management of congenital hypothyroidism. J Clin Endocrinol Metab 72:523, 1991

48. Klein AH, Foley B, Kenny FM, Fisher DA: Thyroid hormone and thyrotropin responses to parturition in premature infants with and without the respiratory distress syndrome. Pediatrics 63:380, 1979

49. Hadeed A, Asay LD, Klein AH, Fisher DA: Significance of transient postnatal hypothyroxinemia in premature infants with and without respiratory distress syndrome. Pediatrics 68:4. 494-498. 1981

50. Glinoer D, Delange F, Laboureur I, De Nayer PH: Maternal and neonatal thyroid function at birth in an area of marginally low iodine intake. J Clin Endocrinol Metab 75:800, 1992

51. Mitchell ML, Larsen PR: Screening for congenital hypothyroidism in New England using the T$_4$-TSH strategy. In Burrow GN, Dussault JH (eds): Neonatal Thyroid Screening p 105. New York, Raven Press, 1980

52. Miyai K, Amino N, Nishi K et al: Transient infantile hyperthyrotropinaemia: Report of a case. Arch Dis Child 54:965, 1979

53. Guillaume J, Schussler GC, Goldman J: Components of the total serum thyroid hormone concentrations during pregnancy: High free thyroxine and blunted thyrotropin (TSH) response to TSH-releasing hormone in the first trimester. J Clin Endocrinol Metab 60:678, 1985

54. Mitchell ML, Potischman N, Larsen PR, Klein RZ: Screening very-low-birthweight infants for congenital: hypothyroidism. p. 95. In Naruse H, Irie M (eds) Neonatal Screening. Excerpta Medica, Amsterdam, 1983

55. Pezzino V, Filetti S, Belfiore A et al: Serum thyroglobulin levels in the newborn. J Clin Endocrinol 52: 364, 1981

56. Thorpe-Beeston JG, Nicolaides KH, Snijders RJ et al: Thyroid function in small for gestational age fetuses. Obstet Gynecol 77:701, 1991

57. Porterfield SP, Hendrich CE: The role of thyroid hormones in prenatal and neonatal neurological development—current perspectives. Endocr Rev 14: 94, 1993

58. Larsen PR: Maternal thyroxine and congenital hypothyroidism. N Engl J Med 321:44, 1989

59. Hebert R, Langlois JM, Dussault JH: Permanent defects in rat peripheral auditory function following perinatal hypothyroidism: determination of a critical period. Dev Brain Res 23:161, 1985

60. Heyerdahl S, Kase BF, Lie SO: Intellectual development in children with congenital hypothyroidism in relation to recommended thyroxine treatment. J Pediatr 118:850, 1991

61. New England Congenital Hypothyroid Collaborative: Correlation of cognitive test scores and adequacy of treatment in adolescents with congenital hypothyroidism. J Pediatr 124:383, 1994

62. Glouieux J, Dussault J, Van Vliet G: Intellectual development at age 12 years of children with congenital hypothyroidism diagnosed by neonatal screening. J Pediatr 121:581, 1992

63. Tillotson SL, Fuggle PW, Smith I et al: Relations between biochemical severity and intelligence in early treated congenital hypothyroidism: a threshold effect. Br Med J 309:440, 1994

64. Fuggle PW, Grant DB, Smith I, Murphy G: Intelligence, motor skills, and behavior at 5 years in early-treated congenital hypothyroidism. Eur J Pediatr 150:570, 1991

65. Dunn JT: Iodine supplementation and the prevention of cretinism. Ann NY Acad Sci 678:158, 1993

66. Halpern JP, Boyages SC, Maberly GF: The neurology of endemic cretinism. a study of two endemias. Brain 114:825, 1991

67. Xue-Yi C, Xin-Min J, Zhi-Hong D et al: Timing of vulnerability of the brain to iodine deficiency in endemic cretinism. N Engl J Med 331:1739, 1994

68. Boyages SC: Clinical review of 49: Iodine deficiency disorders. J Clin Endocrinol Metab 77:587, 1993

69. Boyages SC, Halpern JP: Endemic cretinism: toward a unifying hypothesis. Thyroid 3:59, 1993

70. Ma T, Lian ZC, Qi SP et al: Magnetic resonance imaging of brain and the neuromotor disorder in endemic cretinism. Ann Neurol 34:91, 1993

71. Pharoah POD, Connolly KJ, Ekins RP, Harding AG: Maternal thyroid hormone levels in pregnancy and the subsequent cognitive and motor performance of the children. Clin Endocrinol 21:265, 1984

72. New England Congenital Hypothyroidism Collaborative: Effects of neonatal screening for hypothyroidism; prevention of mental retardation by treatment before clinical manifestations. Lancet 2:1095, 1981

73. Liu H, Momotani N, Noh JY et al: Maternal hypothyroidism during early pregnancy and intellectual development of progeny. Arch Intern Med 154:785, 1994

74. Man EB, Brown JF, Serunian SA: Maternal hypothyroxinemia: Psychoneurological deficits of progeny. Ann Clin Lab Ser 21:227, 1991

75. Chanoine JP, Safran M, Farwell AP et al: Selenium deficiency and type II 5′-deiodinase regulation in the euthyroid and hypothyroid rat: evidence of a direct effect of thyroxine. Endocrinology 130:479, 1992

76. Pfäffle RW, DiMattia GE, Parks JS et al: Mutation of the POU-specific domain of Pit-1 and hypopituitarism without pituitary hypoplasia. Science 257:1118, 1992

77. Brown RS, Keating P, Mitchell E: Maternal thyroid-blocking immunoglobulins in congenital hypothyroidism. J Clin Endocrinol Metab 70:1341, 1990

78. Bogner U, Grüters A, Sigle B et al: Cytotoxic antibodies in congenital hypothyroidism. J Clin Endocrinol Metab 68:671, 1989

79. Ginsberg J, Walfish PG, Rafter DJ et al: Thyrotrophin blocking antibodies in the sera of mothers with congenitally hypothyroid infants. Clin Endocrinol 25:189, 1986

80. Hadjzadeh M, Sinha AK, Pickard MR, Ekins RP: Effect of maternal hypothyroxinemia in the rat on brain biochemistry in adult progeny. J Endocrinol 124:387, 1990

81. Brent GA: The molecular basis of thyroid hormone action. N Engl J Med 331:847, 1994

82. Bernal J, Pekonen F: Ontogenesis of the nuclear 3,5,3′-triiodothyronine receptor in the human fetal brain. Endocrinology 114:677, 1984

83. Rodd C, Schwartz HL, Strait KA, Oppenheimer JH: Ontogeny of hepatic nuclear triiodothyronine receptor isoforms in the rat. Endocrinology 131:2559, 1992

84. Strait KA, Schwartz HL, Perez-Castillo A, Oppenheimer JH: Relationship of c-erbA mRNA content in tissue triiodothyronine nuclear binding capacity and function in developing and adult rats. J Biol Chem 265:10514, 1990

85. Bradley DJ, Towle HC, Young III WS: Spatial and temporal expression of α- and β-thyroid hormone receptors mRNAs, including the $\beta2$-subtype, in the developing mammalian central nervous system. J Neurosci 12:2288, 1992

86. Bradley DJ, Towle HC, Young WS III: α and β thyroid hormone receptor (TR) gene expression during auditory neurogenesis: Evidence for TR isoform-specific transcriptional regulation in vivo. Proc Natl Acad Sci USA 91:439, 1994

87. Mellstrom B, Naranjo JR, Santos A et al: Independent expression of the alpha and beta c-erbA genes in developing rat brain. Molec Endocrinol 5:1339, 1991

88. Yaoita Y, Brown DD: Correlation of thyroid hormone receptor gene expression with amphibian metamorphosis. Gene Dev 4:1917, 1990

89. Forrest D, Hallbook F, Persson H, Vennstrom B: Distinct functions for thyroid hormone receptors α and β in brain development indicated by differential expression of receptor genes. EMBO J 10:269, 1991

90. Sjösberg M, Vennström B, Forrest D: Thyroid hormone receptors in chick retinal development: differential expression of mRNAs for α and N-terminal variant β receptors. Development 114:39, 1992

91. Cook CB, Kakucska I, Lechan RM, Koenig RJ: Expression of thyroid hormone receptor $\beta2$ in rat hypothalamus. Endocrinology 130:1077, 1992

92. Van Middlesworth L, Norris CH: Audiogenic seizures and cochlear damage in rats after perinatal antithyroid treatment. Endocrinology 106:1686, 1980

93. Baker BS, Tata JR: Accumulation of proto-oncogene c-erbA related transcripts during *Xenopus* development: association with early acquisition of response to thyroid hormone and estrogen. EMBO J 9:879, 1990

94. Yaoita Y, Shi YB, Brown DD: *Xenopus laevis* α and β thyroid hormone receptors. Proc Natl Acad Sci USA 87:7090, 1990

95. Banker DE, Bigler J, Eisenman RN: The thyroid hormone receptor gene (c-*erb*Aα) is expressed in ad-

vance of thyroid gland maturation during the early embryonic development of *Xenopus laevis*. Molec Cell Biol 11:5079, 1991

96. Leonard JL, Larsen PR: Thyroid hormone metabolism in primary cultures of fetal rat brain cells. Brain Res 327:1, 1985

97. Kolodny JM, Leonard JL, Larsen PR, Silva JE: Studies of nuclear 3,5,3′-triiodothyronine binding in primary cultures of rat brain. Endocrinology 117:1848, 1985

98. Leonard JL, Farwell AP, Yen PM et al: Differential expression of thyroid hormone receptor isoforms in neurons and astroglial cells. Endocrinology 135:548, 1994

99. Castiglia D, Cestelli A, Di Liegro C et al: Accumulation of different c-erbA transcripts during rat brain development and in cortical neurons cultured in a synthetic medium. Cell Molec Neurobiol 12:259, 1992

100. Strait KA, Zou L, Oppenheimer JH: β1 isoform-specific regulation of a triiodothyronine-induced gene during cerebellar development. Molec Endocrinol 6:1874, 1992

101. Rosman NP: The neuropathology of congenital hypothyroidism. In Stanbury JB, Kroc RL (eds): Human Development and the Thyroid Gland: Relation to Endemic Cretinism. Plenum Press, New York, 1972

102. D'Avignon M, Melin KA: The electroencephalogram in congenital hypothyreosis. Acta Paediatr Scand 38:37, 1949

103. Gupta SP, Gupta PC, Kumar V, Ahuja MMS: Electroencephalic changes in hypothyroidism. Indian J Med 60:1101, 1972

104. Nickel SN, Frame B: Neurologic manifestations of myxedema. Neurology 8:511, 1958

105. Nunez J: Effects of thyroid hormones during brain differentiation. Molec Cell Endocrinol 37:125, 1984

106. Patel AJ, Hunt A, Meier E: Effects of undernutrition and thyroid state on the ontogenic changes of D1, D2 and D3 brain specific proteins in rat cerebellum. J Neurochem 44:1581, 1985

107. Sanchez-Toscano F, Escobar del Rey F, Morreale de Escobar G, Ruiz-Marcos A: Measurement of the effects of hypothyroidism on the number and distribution of spines along the apical shaft of pyramidal neurons of the rat cerebral cortex. Brain Res 126:547, 1977

108. Ruiz-Marcos A, Sanchez-Toscano F, Escobar del Rey F, Morreale de Escobar G: Severe hypothyroidism and the maturation of the rat cerebral cortex. Brain Res 162:315, 1979

109. Eayrs JT, Taylor SH: The effect of thyroid deficiency induced by methyl thiouracil on the maturation of the central nervous system. J Anat 85:350, 1951

110. Adams PM, Stein SA, Palnitkar M et al: Evaluation and characterization of the hypothyroid hyt/hyt mouse. I. Somatic and behavioral studies. Neuroendocrinology 49:138, 1989

111. Anthony A, Adams PM, Stein SA: The effects of congenital hypothyroidism using the hyt/hyt mouse on locomotor activity and learned behavior. Horm Behav 27:418, 1993

112. Stein SA, Shanklin DR, Krulich L et al: Evaluation and characterization of the hyt/hyt hypothyroid mouse. II. Abnormalities of TSH and the thyroid gland. Neuroendocrinology 49:509, 1989

113. Stein SA, Zakarija M, McKenzie JM et al: The site of the molecular defect in the thyroid gland of the hyt/hyt mouse: Abnormalities in the TSH receptor-G protein complex. Thyroid 1:257, 1991

114. Stein SA, Kirkpatrick LL, Shanklin DR et al: Hypothyroidism reduces the rate of slow component A (SCa) axonal transport and the amount of transported tubulin in the hyt/hyt mouse optic nerve. J Neurosci Res 28:121, 1991

115. Stein SA, McIntire DD, Kirkpatrick LL et al: Hypothyroidism selectively reduces the rate and amount of transport for specific SCb proteins in the hyt/hyt mouse optic nerve. J Neurosci Res 30:28, 1991

116. Legrand J: Variations as a function of age, of the response of the cerebellum to morphogenetic action of the thyroid in rats. Microscopy Morphol Exp 56:291, 1967

117. Munoz A, Rodriguez-Pena A, Perez-Castillo A et al: Effects of neonatal hypothyroidism on rat brain gene expression. Molec Endocrinol 5:273, 1991

118. Munoz A, Wrighton C, Seliger B et al: Thyroid hormone receptor/c-erbA: Control of commitment and differentiation in the neuronal/chromaffin progenitor line PC12. J Cell Biol 121:423, 1993

119. Nunez J, Couchie D, Aniello F, Bridoux AM: Thyroid hormone effects on neuronal differentiation during brain development. Acta Med Austriaca 19 Suppl 1:36, 1992

120. Silva JE, Rudas P: Effect of congenital hypothyroidism on microtubule-associated protein-2 expression in the cerebellum of the rat. Endocrinology 126:1276, 1990

121. Iniguez MA, Rodriguez-Pena A, Ibarrola N et al: Adult rat brain is sensitive to thyroid hormone. Regulation of RC3/neurogranin mRNA. J Clin Invest 90:554, 1992

122. Iniguez MA, Rodriguez-Pena A, Ibarrola N et al: Thyroid hormone regulation of RC3, a brain-specific gene encoding a protein kinase-C substrate. Endocrinology 133:467, 1993

123. Rodriguez-Pena A, Ibarrola N, Iniguez MA et al: Neonatal hypothyroidism affects the timely expres-

sion of myelin-associated glycoprotein in the rat brain. J Clin Invest 91:812, 1993

124. Weiss RE, Refetoff S: Thyroid hormone resistance. Ann Rev Med 43:363, 1992

125. Hauser PH, Zametkin AJ, Martinez P et al: Attention deficit-hyperactivity disorder in people with generalized resistance to thyroid hormone. N Engl J Med 328:997, 1993

126. Mixson AJ, Parrilla R, Ransom SC et al: Correlations of language abnormalities with localization of mutations in the β-thyroid hormone receptor in 13 kindreds with generalized resistance to thyroid hormone: identification of four new mutations. J Clin Endocrinol Metab 75:1039, 1992

127. Refetoff S, Weiss RE, Usala SJ: The syndromes of resistance to thyroid hormone. Endocr Rev 14:348, 1993

128. Barres BA, Lazar MA, Raff MC: A novel role for thyroid hormone, glucocorticoids and retinoic acid in timing oligodendrocyte development. Development 120:1097, 1994

129. Garcia-Fernandez LF, Iniguez MA, Rodriguez-Pena A et al: Brain-specific prostaglandin D2 synthetase mRNA is dependent on thyroid hormone during rat brain development. Biochem Biophys Res Comm 196:396, 1993

130. Ruiz de Elvira MC, Sinha AK, Pickard M et al: Effect of maternal hypothyroxinemia during fetal life on the calmodulin-regulated phosphatase activity in the brain of the adult progeny in the rat. J Endocrinol 121:331, 1989

131. Fisher DA, Dussault JH, Foley TP Jr et al: Screening for congenital hypothyroidism: Results of screening one million North American infants. J Pediatr 94:700, 1979

132. LaFranchi SH, Murphey WH, Foley TP Jr et al: Neonatal hypothyroidism detected by the Northwest Regional Screening Program. Pediatrics 63:180, 1979

133. La Franchi S, Hanna CE, Krainz PL et al: Screening for congenital hypothyroidism with specimen collection at two time periods: results of northwest regional screening program. Pediatrics 76:734, 1985

134. Fisher DA: Screening for congenital hypothyroidism. Trends Endocrinol Metab 2:129, 1991

135. American Academy of Pediatrics, American Thyroid Association: Newborn screening for congenital hypothyroidism: Recommended guidelines. Thyroid 3:257, 1993

136. Cheron RG, Kaplan MM, Larsen PR et al: Neonatal thyroid function after propylthiouracil therapy for maternal Graves' disease. N Engl J Med 304:525, 1981

137. Mitchell ML, Larsen PR, Levy HL et al: Screening for congenital hypothyroidism. Results in the new-born populations of New England. JAMA 239:2348, 1978

138. Mitchell ML, Bapat V, Larsen PR et al: Pitfalls in screening for neonatal hypothyroidism. Pediatrics 70:16, 1982

139. Dussalt JH, Letarte J, Guyda H, Laberge C: Thyroid function in neonatal hypothyroidism. J Pediatr 89:550, 1976

140. Newborn Committee of the European Thyroid Association: Neonatal screening for congenital hypothyroidism in Europe. Acta Endocrinol suppl 223:1, 1979

141. Robertson EF, Olfield R, Wilkins A et al: Screening of newborn infants for hypothyroidism. Med J Aust 1:593, 1979

142. Stanbury JB, Rocmans P, Buhler UK, Ochi Y: Congenital hypothyroidism with impaired thyroid response to thyrotropin. N Engl J Med 279:1132, 1968

143. Codaccioni JL, Carayon P, Michael-Bechet M et al: Congenital hypothyroidism associated with thyrotropinunresponsiveness and thyroid cell membrane alterations. J Clin Endocrinol Metab 50:932, 1980

144. Mallet E, Carayon P, Amr S et al: Coupling defect of thyrotropin receptor and adenylate cyclase in a pseudohypoparathyroid patient. J Clin Endocrinol Metab 54:1028, 1982

145. Miyai K, Azukizawa M, Onishi T et al: Familial isolated thyrotropin deficiency. p. 345. In James VHT (ed): Endocrinology. Excerpta Medica, Amsterdam 1976

146. LaFranchi SH: Hypothyroidism. Pediatr Clin North Am 26:33, 1979

147. Hayashizaki Y, Hiraoka Y, Endo Y, Matsubara K: Thyroid-stimulating hormone (TSH) deficiency caused by a single base substitution in the CAGYC region of the β-subunit. EMBO J 8:2291, 1989

148. Hayashizaki Y, Hiraoka Y, Tatsumi K: Deoxyribonucleic acid analyses of five families with familial inherited thyroid stimulating hormone deficiency. J Clin Endocrinol Metab 71:792, 1990

149. Tatsumi K, Miyai K, Notomi T et al: Cretinism with combined hormone deficiency caused by a mutation in the PIT1 gene. Nat Genet 1:56, 1992

150. Radovick S, Nations M, Du Y et al: A mutation in the POU-homeodomain of Pit-1 responsible for combined pituitary hormone deficiency. Science 257:1115, 1992

151. Goldsmith RE, McAdams AJ, Larsen PR et al: Familial autoimmune thyroiditis: maternal-fetal relationship and the role of generalized autoimmunity. J Clin Endocrinol Metab 37:265, 1973

152. Burrow GN: The management of thyrotoxicosis in pregnancy. N Engl J Med 313:562, 1985

153. Konig MP: Di knogenitale hypothyreose und der

endermische Kretinismus. New York. Springer Publishers Inc. 1968

154. Niepce B: Traite du goitre et du cretonisme, suivi de la statistique des goitreux et des cretins dans le bassin de l'Isere en Savoie. dans les departements de l'Isere. des Hautes-Alps et des Basses-Alpes. Paris, JB Ballier, 1851

155. Klein AH, Foley TP Jr, Larsen PR et al: Neonatal thyroid function in congenital hypothyroidism. J Pediatr 89:545, 1976

156. Letarte J, Guyda H, Dussault JH: Clinical biochemical and radiological features of neonatal hypothyroid infants. p. 225. In Burrow GN, Dussault JH (eds): Neonatal Thyroid Screening. Raven Press, New York, 1980

157. Fisher DA, Foley BL: Early treatment of congenital hypothyroidism. Pediatrics 83:785, 1989

158. Refetoff S: Inherited thyroxine-binding globulin abnormalities in man. Endocr Rev 10:275, 1989

159. Rovet J, Ehrlich R, Sorbara D: Intellectual outcome in children with fetal hypothyroidism. J Pediatr 110:700, 1987

160. Glorieux J, Dussault JH, Morissette J et al: Follow-up at ages 5 and 7 years on mental development in children with hypothyroidism detected by Quebec screening program. J Pediatr 107:913, 1986

161. Glorieux J, Desjardins M, Letarte M et al: Useful parameters to predict the eventual outcome of hypothyroid children. Pediatr Res 24:6, 1988

162. Ilicki A, Larsson A, Mortensson W: Neonatal skeletal maturation in congenital hypothyroidism and its prognostic value for psychomotor development at 3 years in patients treated early. Horm Res 33:260, 1990

163. Rochiccioli P, Roge B, Alexandre F, Tauber MT: School achievement in children with hypothyroidism detected at birth and search for predictive factors. Horm Res 38:236, 1992

164. Ilicki A, Larsson A: Psychological development at 7 years of age in children with congenital hypothyroidism. Timing and dosage of initial treatment. Acta Paediatr 80:199, 1991

165. Rovet JF, Sorbara DL Ehlrich RM: The intellectual and behavioral characteristics of children with congenital hypothyroidism identified by neonatal screening in Ontario: the Toronto prospective study. p. 281. In Carter TB, Willey AM (eds): Genetic Disease Screening and Management. Alan R Liss, New York, 1986

166. Germak JA, Foley THP: Longitudinal assessment of L-thyroxine therapy for congenital hypothyroidism. J Pediatr 117:211, 1990

Genetic Defects of Thyroid Hormone Supply, Transport, and Action

16

DEFECTS OF THYROID HORMONE SYNTHESIS

The conditions of patients with the inherited thyroid disorders described herein are reviewed in detail elsewhere.[1-3] Included are patients whose conditions are related biochemically, but in whom the tendency toward hypothyroidism has been overcome by compensatory growth and function of the thyroid. In others with familial thyroid diseases the size of the thyroid gland cannot increase. In spite of the similarity of these cases, the conditions fall into several categories, each representing an abnormality at a separate step in thyroid hormone synthesis. These metabolic disorders are inborn errors of metabolism. We also include here a group of hypothyroid patients with thyroid glands that are insensitive to thyroid-stimulating hormone (TSH), who secrete insufficient amounts of TSH or defective

TSH due to abnormalities in the TSH-β gene. Emphasis is placed on disorders that provide insight into the nature of the disease process. Each appears to occur because of the genetic absence of a single enzyme or protein. For most we have information on the biochemical mechanisms involved, and they are inherited according to classic Mendelian rules. The disorders are rare, but their significance extends far beyond their numbers because the study of these conditions has provided valuable information about thyroid gland function. Furthermore, it is possible for heterozygotes in the same abnormality to present with only goiter but not with the retarded development that often characterizes the homozygous patient with the full defect. This appealing concept has often proved difficult to substantiate.

Patients may be grouped as shown in Table 16-1. Each of these categories is reviewed, and the

**TABLE 16-1. Disorders of Thyroid
Hormone Supply**

Defective hormone synthesis
    Iodide trapping (transport) defect
    Iodide organification defect
        Without familial deafness
        With familial deafness (Pendred's syndrome)
    Iodothyrosine dehalogenase defect
    Defective iodothyronine and TG synthesis
        Iodotyrosyl coupling defect
        Defective TG synthesis
        Plasma iodoprotein defect
Defective TSH response or supply[a]
    TSH unresponsiveness
    Defective TSH synthesis
    TRH deficiency
    Defective TSH-β subunit synthesis
    Defective synthesis of Pit-1

[a] Not characterized by goiter.

procedures necessary for diagnosis are indicated in the following sections. The normal pathways of iodine transport are described in Chapter 2.

Iodide Transport Defect

The first step in the synthesis of the thyroid hormones is the transport of iodide from the blood into the thyroid gland.[4] Saito et al. have studied in some detail a patient with iodide transport defect.[5]

A 32-year-old man was admitted for study to the Jichi Medical School in Tochigi, Japan, because of goiter. His early development had been moderately delayed, and although he had learned to read and write, his school performance was poor. A goiter had appeared at age 15. The diagnosis of schizophrenia was made, as well as hypothyroidism, for which he was treated intermittently with thyroid hormone. A left hemithyroidectomy was performed at age 17.

At the time of the study his height was only 144.8 cm and weight 64.5 kg. His face was puffy. The right thyroid lobe was an elastic soft mass with a hard nodule. Serum level of T_3 was 39 ng/dl; T_4, 1 μg/dl, and TSH, 217 μU/ml. The RAIU was less than 1 percent at 24 hours. The result of kinetic analysis was consistent with an absence of a significant pool of iodine in the gland. Biopsy of the thyroid gland disclosed intense hyperplasia. When the patient was given iodide, the euthyroid state was quickly established.

Interpretation

The interpretation of the findings in this patient is that an essential component of the iodide transport system was defective. The salivary gland, the gastric mucosa, the mammary glands, the lacrimal glands, and the choroid plexus share a common iodide transport system with the thyroid. Since iodide transport is an energy-requiring system and may involve a specific transport protein, absence of this protein or synthesis of a defective molecule are distinct possibilities. Whatever the defect, it must be fairly specific to iodide transport and related anions, since other transport processes are intact. Indeed, Saito et al. found that in this patient the thyroid microsome peroxidase activity was higher than normal, and the ouabain-sensitive Na^+-K^+-ATPase activity was normal. Although the ATPase activity is required for iodide transport, the defect must have been elsewhere, perhaps in the iodide carrier protein.[6] Apart from iodide transport, the thyroid cells seemed to be functioning normally.

To date, 35 patients with the iodide transport defect have been described. The most recent case was detected through neonatal screening[7] the first[8] became euthyroid and a practicing attorney 20 years after this hypothyroidism was corrected with daily administration of iodide. He was a member of a consanguinous family. Most persons with this defect are hypothyroid when not treated. Some have been permanently retarded, others not. The inheritance pattern appears to be autosomal recessive.[9,10]

It is interesting that some thyroid nodules fail to transport iodide, and consequently appear "cold" on thyroid scan. These nodules may be acquired analogs of the transport defect, but the precise defect remains to be determined.

Papadopoulos et al.[11] reported studies on a 9-year-old Greek boy with goiter and growth and mental retardation, who had a partial defect of iodide transport. The patient was below the third percentile in height, had a bone age of 5 years, and an intelligence quotient of 65. The mean ratio of iodide in the saliva to that in the plasma of 17.2, far lower than the 84.3 in the authors' normal subjects. The serum thyroxine (T_4) iodine concentration was 0.5 μg/dl. Tissue slices prepared from the surgically excised thyroid gland achieved an iodide concentration ratio against the incubating medium of only 1.7, as compared to a normal value of 7.1 in their laboratory. Two siblings with mental retardation from a consanguinous family in Brazil have been reported.[12] Iodide transport into the thyroid was demonstrable but was much reduced.

An interesting point at issue in cases described in

the preceding paragraph is mental retardation with a partial iodide transport defect. In contrast, some patients with a complete transport defect have not been permanently retarded. A possible reason for this discrepancy is the very low dietary iodide in the patients from Brazil and Greece. In the patient of Papadopoulos et al.[11] the daily urinary excretion was only 16 μg. The thyroid clearance of iodide was 4.5 ml/min (normal 8 to 40 ml/min), and the absolute iodine uptake by the thyroid was 0.7 μg/hr (normal, 0.5 to 6.0 μg/hr). The Brazilian siblings also lived in a region that was poor in iodine. Since the disease can be corrected by administration of large doses of iodide[16] and since those patients without developmental retardation resided in regions of iodine abundance, it seems reasonable to conclude that the clinical features in some patients are the result of more severe hormone deprivation due to limitation on thyroid hormone synthesis imposed by the small amount of iodide available in the diet.

Diagnosis and Treatment

Diagnosis of defective iodide transport should rest primarily on a demonstration that iodide transport into a palpable thyroid is limited or absent in spite of TSH stimulation. Other causes of low radioactive iodine uptake (RAIU) should be excluded. In addition, limited or absent iodide transport by the salivary glands should be demonstrated. This is most easily established by determining the ratio of iodine 125 or iodine 123 in saliva versus that in serum 1 to 2 hours after administration of a small oral tracer dose of the isotope. Usually it will exceed 10:1. Finding a low iodine content of the thyroid is also helpful. Based on the information from three cases, it might be suggested that partial defect in thyroid transport would manifest as hypothyroidism and goiter in areas of limited iodide in the diet. Demonstration that administration of therapeutic doses of iodide restored hormone synthesis to normal would be a strong point in favor but not pathognomonic of this disorder. Although these patients may be successfully treated by administering a few milligrams to several grams of iodine daily[17] (depending on the severity of the defect), it is wiser to treat them with standard replacement dosis of L-thyroxine.

Disorders of Iodide Organification

Iodide that is trapped in the thyroid gland must be oxidized to iodine before it can displace hydrogen and bind to the 3 position of tyrosyl residues present in peptide linkage in thyroglobulin (TG) (see Ch. 2). An impairment in this step of thyroid hormonegenesis was the first metabolic defect in familial goiter to be defined.[18–20] Several cretins with this disorder have been studied. Four were siblings from a family of seven children of consanguinous parents. The three oldest children were normal and without thyroid disease. Growth and development of the affected children were reported to be normal during the first months of life but thereafter they became retarded. Thyroid hormone was given only intermittently.

These patients were dwarfed and grossly retarded mentally (Fig. 16-1). Their thyroid glands were enlarged, nodular, and firm, and bruits and thrills were present. The thyroid hormone concentrations in serum were very low.

When iodine 131 was given, the labeled iodine in the gland reached a plateau in less than 2 hours. At this juncture, oral administration of 1 g potassium thiocyanate or perchlorate caused an immediate and striking fall in the labeled iodine accumulated in the gland. At the end of 2 hours the counts had fallen to 25 percent of the preperchlorate level (see Fig. 16-2). Histologically, the gland showed intense hy-

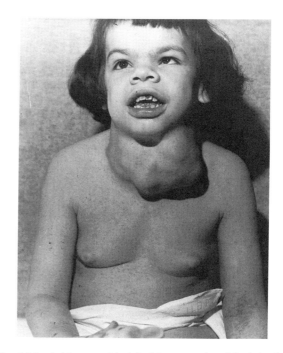

Fig. 16-1. A 16-year-old girl with a complete block in the organification of iodine. There is gross retardation in stature and intellect. Note the huge nodular thyroid mass.

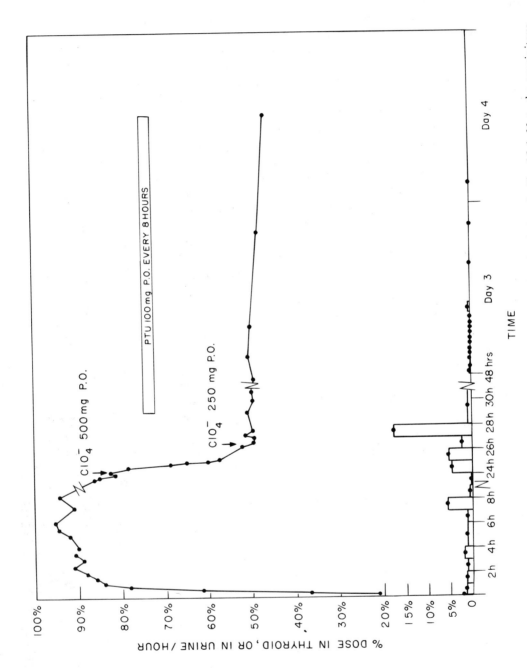

Fig. 16-2. Uptake and retention of ^{131}I by the thyroid of a grandniece of the patient in Fig. 16-1. Note the precipitous discharge of iodide on administration of perchlorate. This patient had a moderate-sized goiter and some retardation of growth but was normal intellectually. PTU was given to observe the turnover of the iodine remaining in the gland. There was little metabolic activity of this component.

perplasia, cystic degeneration, and fibrosis. The concentration of iodine in the thyroid gland was very low.

The observations strongly suggested that these patients harbored a defect in iodine organification, and further studies confirmed this hypothesis. The kinetics of iodine metabolism indicated that the rate of disappearance of labeled iodine from the gland and its excretion in the urine were consistent with free exchange of all the iodine between the gland and the perfusing blood.[19] Chemical analysis of biopsy specimens obtained after administration of ^{131}I indicated that the only labeled iodine in the gland was inorganic.

Identical twin girls, grandnieces of these cretins, had normal intelligence, retarded statural growth, and enlarged thyroids that discharged iodide precipitously with administration of perchlorate[20] They are presumed to be compound heterozygotes for the abnormal gene of their great-aunts and great-uncles and for another gene that impairs thyroid peroxidase activity inherited from their father.

Precipitous discharge of labeled iodine from the thyroid gland after administration of thiocyanate or perchlorate has become generally accepted as the central criterion for impaired iodide organification. If discharge of more than 10 percent of the labeled iodide from the thyroid occurs when 1 g $KC10_4$ is given orally 2 hours after administration of a tracer, then one may assume that defective organification exists.[21,22] Such discharge is usually not detectable in the normal person. At least two problems may arise with this test. Impaired absorption of the administered thiocyanate or perchlorate may obscure the results. A more important problem is that of obtaining statistically significant counting rates over the thyroid gland against a high background of radioisotope in the blood at 2 hours, especially in glands that do not have a high uptake. Also, rapid turnover of RAI by a small thyroid gland may cause a drop in the level of labeled iodine measured over the thyroid gland after administration of the blocking anion. This latter difficulty may be resolved by serial measurement of labeled protein-bound iodine (PBI) in the plasma. If the fall in counts over the thyroid gland is due to this problem, one should observe a high level of labeled PBI. Still another unresolved problem is the time thiocyanate or perchlorate should be given after the RAI. If the defect in organification is partial, the longer one waits after

administering the RAI, the less likely is there to be a significant demonstrable pool of dischargeable thyroidal iodide.

Haddad and Sidbury[23] were the first to demonstrate an absence of peroxidase activity in the thyroid of a patient with familial goiter, hypothyroidism, and virtually complete thiocyanate discharge of thyroidal iodide. Further observations by a number of investigators have led to the conclusion that there may be at least five types of organification defects, and that heterogeneity may exist within each type. This categorization is based on functional changes in thyroid peroxidase (TPO) activity. Presumably all are due to mutations that alter the structure of the molecule, cause it to be unstable, or prevent synthesis, but this has been proven only for a few of the cases with clinically evident TPO deficiency.

1. Absent, inactive, or abnormal thyroid peroxidase. Peroxidase activity is not demonstrable in thyroid tissue from these patients under any circumstances, including enzyme solubilization and addition of the prosthetic group, hematin. Candidates for this category have been described by Pommier et al.,[24] Medeiros-Neto et al.,[25] and others.[26–29] Evidently, this defect may be either complete or incomplete. Recently two patients have been described with a mutation in the coding sequence of the human TPO gene. One is a boy with an iodide organification defect, and no TPO activity in resected thyroid tissue. A four base pair (bp) insertion in the eighth exon of the TPO gene was identified, and it was shown that the patient was homozygous for this frameshift mutation.[30] The other patient with a total iodide organification defect and congenital hypothyroidism and without TPO activity or messenger RNA in the thyroid gland had a homozygous mutation in exon 2 of the TPO gene. Sequence analysis showed a 20-bp duplication, 47 bp downstream of the ATG start codon. The duplication results in a frameshift and a termination signal in exon 3 compatible with complete absence of TPO. Both parents of the patient were heterozygous for the same duplication.[31]

2. Peroxidase apoenzyme-prosthetic group defect. Peroxidase activity may be restored in gland preparations if hematin is added to the reacting system. This defect was first described by Niepomniszcze et al.[32,33]

3. Inhibition or abnormal intracellular location of peroxidase. In thyroid specimens from some patients the peroxidase activity can be restored by solubilization with digitonin, whereas in others the predominant activity has abnormal sedimentation characteristics.[34-36] Recently defective peroxydase activity was described in two cats with congenital hypothyroidism. It appeared that activity was decreased because this peroxidase was not membrane bound.[37]

4. Deficiency in H_2O_2 production. One patient has been described with a presumed defect in the synthesis of flavine adenine dinucleotide, a cofactor in H_2O_2 production.[38] In another patient with defective H_2O_2 generation, organification could be restored by adding a source of H_2O_2 to the incubation mixture of isolated thyroid tissue. The defect in the H_2O_2 generating system in this patient was not elucidated.[39]

5. Receptor abnormality. Peroxidase is normally present but fails to generate organic iodine because of a presumed defect in binding to or absence of TG, its acceptor. Several patients who appear to have this defect have been described.[40,41]

Interpretation

From the foregoing, it may be appreciated that the organification defect encompasses a constellation of disorders that almost surely have a diverse genetic background. The common denominator is evidence of reduced peroxidase activity, as indicated by release of iodide from the gland after administration of thiocyanate or perchlorate.

Another group of patients with a related disorder have Pendred syndrome.[42-44] These patients are either euthyroid or mildly hypothyroid, have sensorineural deafness, usually have a normal IQ, and have a partial defect in iodide organification, as indicated by the result of the perchlorate discharge test.[45,46] The precise defect in the Pendred syndrome has not been identified. There is no evidence of fetal hypothyroidism in these patients. In this regard, it is interesting to note that sensorineural deafness is common in iodine-deficient endemic cretinism, where there is clear evidence of fetal retardation, and not in sporadic cretinism.

The origin of deafness in Pendred's syndrome is now known. Individuals with Pendred's syndrome have a characteristically deformed ear—a "Mondini cochlea"—which can be recognized by computed tomography (CAT) scans. It seems probable that the thyroid and cochlear abnormalities represent pleomorphic effects of a heritable genetic defect.[47,48] Changes have been induced in the inner ear of developing chicks by injecting PTU into the yolk sac[49] and in neonatal rats by administering PTU to their mothers.[50] In rats, abnormalities were found especially in the organ of Corti, particularly in the tectorial membrane. The membrane was thickened, displaced, and at times split. The hair cells were often small, irregular, and reduced in number. Development was much retarded. Since the changes can be reversed by simultaneous injection of T_4, normal thyroid function is necessary for the development of the middle ear in the chick.

Several publications have dealt with the inheritance pattern of the Pendred syndrome and some of its clinical features.[51-53] Although in most instances the pattern is that of an autosomal-recessive trait with tight concordance between goiter and deafness, there are reports of dissociation within kindreds of deafness and goiter.[54-56] In some instances, there are patients who are only partially deaf, and in some the deafness is much more severe in one ear than in the other. Most but not all[55] of these patients are euthyroid, but an exaggerated response to thyrotropin-releasing hormone (TRH) suggests a tendency toward hypothyroidism.[56] TG, iodoalbumin, and an insoluble iodoprotein have been identified in the thyroid glands of patients with this syndrome.[57,58] Cave and Dunn have described heterogeneity in the TG from a patient with Pendred's syndrome.[59] TG from thyroid tissue from two siblings with Pendred's syndrome showed low hormone and iodine content, but could easily be iodinated in vitro. Reverse transcription of mRNA and amplification of specific regions encoding the most important hormonogenic sites of TG revealed a normal complementary DNA sequence corresponding to the first hundred amino acids in TG's N-terminus. However, variants of mRNA corresponding to the TG C-terminus were detected. As some of the variants also occur in other human thyroids, further studies are needed to relate these alterations to defective hormone synthesis and goiter.[59a]

Diagnosis and Treatment

In vivo diagnosis of the peroxidase defect depends on the demonstration of a large pool of readily exchangeable iodide in the thyroid gland. This demonstration is most conveniently done by administering a tracer dose of RAI, measuring its accumulation within the gland over the next 2 hours, and then demonstrating that a significant fraction of it can be discharged from the gland within a few minutes after oral administration of 1 g thiocyanate or perchlorate. Severe forms of peroxidase defect can give rise to growth and mental retardation as well as goiter. If retardation is mild or absent and if the patient has nerve deafness, the diagnosis of Pendred's syndrome can be presumed.

Biochemical studies of peroxidase function are required to differentiate the various causes of organification defect. These studies include measurement of thyroid peroxidase activity using different substrates, the effect of added hematin on enzyme activity, studies on the H_2O_2 supply in the gland, and the presence of normal TG substrate. For patients with hypothyroidism and/or goiter, supplementation with T_4 is indicated. When large goiters are present that do not shrink with T_4 therapy, thyroidectomy is sometimes indicated.

Iodotyrosine Dehalogenase Defect

In the normal thyroid gland, TG undergoes proteolytic degradation, which causes the release of monoiodothyrosine (MIT) and diiodotyrosine (DIT), in addition to iodothyronines. The latter are deiodinated by a dehalogenase present in the thyroid gland, and the iodide released is reused in the synthesis of thyroid hormone.[60] Related dehalogenases are also present in liver and other tissues.[61,62]

A number of cretins with goiter have been described who are unable to deiodinate iodotyrosines.[63-67] Some of them appeared in closely inbred families, and at least one has had a number of relatives with thyroid defect but without hypothyroidism or developmental retardation.[65] This group of patients was first clinically described by Hutschison and McGirr, who reported 12 patients from the Royal Hospital for Sick Children and the Royal Infirmary in Glasgow.[64,68] Four of these patients were siblings and were from the same kindred. They were, for the most part, from intinerant tinker stock, an isolated group of people living a nomadic existence in Argyllshire and the Isle of Selay. The tinker cretins were all goitrous. The thyroidal uptake of ^{131}I was high, and the maximal value was quickly reached. Most of the glands lost a large fraction of the accumulated labeled iodine within a few hours after maximal uptake.

The first demonstration of the dehalogenase defect was made in a patient who was studied by Stanbury, Querido, and colleagues.[65-66] P.J., a 27-year-old man, had been found to have a goiter at birth. Thyroid hormone was given for many years but was discontinued 4 years before investigation, during which time the goiter increased relentlessly in size. The serum PBI was 0.5 $\mu g/$dl. His parents were not consanguinous and were normal, as was his older brother. A younger brother also had goiter at birth and was physically and mentally retarded.

RAI accumulated rapidly in the thyroid, but after the first hour the labeled iodine began to leave the thyroid gland and to appear in the blood as a component that was only partially precipitable with trichloracetic acid. The serum contained large amounts of monoiodotyrosine (MIT) and diiodotyrosine (DIT), as well as other components that proved to be metabolites and conjugates of these two amino acids. These substances are normally encountered only in trace amounts, or not at all, outside the thyroid.

It was postulated that the reason for the metabolic anomaly was an absence of dehalogenase in the thyroid gland and in all other tissues of the body. Indeed, labeled DIT administered intravenously was almost completely recovered in the urine. When thyroid tissue became available at the time of surgery, no deiodinating ability was observed, whereas normal thyroid tissue and that from nodular goiter rapidly deiodinated MIT and DIT. Other investigators, especially McGirr and his coworkers, also found an identical metabolic defect in their patients.[68]

The patients who were originally characterized as lacking deiodinase activity were found to have this defect not only in the thyroid gland but also in other tissues, as evidenced by the fact that intravenously administered labeled iodotyrosines were not deiodinated, indicating complete enzyme deficiency. Impaired deiodination of intravenously administered labeled DIT by some family members was interpreted as evidence that they were heterozygotes for the same defect; others have made similar observations.[69-71]

Later, families have been described with partial deficiency of dehalogenase activity.[72,73] Patients have also been described in whom deficiency of deiodinase activity was restricted to the thyroid gland[74]; others have had no deiodination in any tissue except for the thyroid.[75] Lissitzky et al.[76] also described a patient who had no deiodinating activity and who in addition had a large amount of iodinated albumin in the thyroid gland. In contrast, other patients who have been similarly studied have had no iodoalbumin detected in the thyroid gland or in blood.[77] Some patients with this disorder had an associated neurologic syndrome resembling Werdnig-Hoffmann's paralysis.[78]

Interpretation

These patients are unable to deiodinate iodotyrosines due to inherited absence of tissue deiodinase activity. In this defect, as in the iodide transport defect described above, the disorder is not usually confined to the thyroid but is also present in other tissues. Since the reaction is highly important to thyroid hormone biosynthesis, the defect manifests as impaired thyroid function.

Continued loss of hormone precursors from the gland and from the body depletes the iodine stores and sets up a vicious cycle of thyroid hyperplasia, followed by increased synthesis and secretion of hormone precursors, increasing iodide loss, and further hyperplasia. Thus, it should be possible to restore hormone synthesis and put the gland at rest by supplying iodide in a large excess. The initial demonstration of the validity of this hypothesis by Choufoer et al.[66] has been confirmed. The iodide concentration in blood appears to govern the rate of hormone synthesis in these patients. Harden et al.[79] found that hormone synthesis proceeded normally when serum iodide concentration was 1.0 μg/dl. This was attained by increasing the intake of iodide to 612 μg/d. Lissitzky et al.[80] found that the administration of 1.25 mg iodide daily restored thyroid function to normal. In the United States, where iodine is used in the bread-making industry and in other products that introduce it into the food chain, many persons receive nearly this amount of iodine or even more. Under such conditions the disorder is not expected to become clinically evident.

Diagnosis and Treatment

The laboratory diagnosis is not difficult. Chromatography of a sample of urine taken within the first 12 hours after administration of RAI will show, in addition to inorganic RAI, some in the positions of MIT and DIT and their metabolic products. If a sample of serum is taken within 24 hours of the administration of RAI and extracted with acid butanol, chromatography of the extract will disclose iodinated tyrosines, their conjugates and metabolic products. Definitive proof of dehalogenase defect may be obtained by demonstrating that more than 50 percent

of the intravenously administered DIT appears unchanged in the urine.

No clinical features clearly distinguish this disorder from others with hypothyroidism and goiter, though one clinical laboratory feature seems to be characteristic of many of these patients. Their early RAI uptake is high, followed by rapid disappearance of the labeled iodine from the thyroid gland. Thus, the RAIU at 1 or 2 hours may be more than 50 percent, with low or normal values at 24 hours. When hypothyroidism and/or goiter is present, T_4 therapy is indicated. While administration of large doses of iodide may prevent hypothyroidism, its administration in subjects with hyperplastic glands can cause transient thyrotoxicosis.

Disorders of Iodothyronine and Thyroglobulin

A number of patients with familial goiter have been characterized as having impaired coupling of iodotyrosyl residues to form triiodothyronine (T_3) and T_4 (coupling defect), impaired synthesis of TG (TG synthesis defect), or the presence of abnormal iodinated peptide in the peripheral blood for no apparent reason (plasma iodopeptide defect). Evidence that these are distinct disorders is not strong. Patients are described under these rubrics in the following paragraphs, and interpretation of the findings is offered.

Iodotyrosyl Coupling Defect

T_4 and T_3 are formed in the thyroid gland by coupling of two molecules of iodotyrosyl precursors. (This process is described in detail in Ch. 2.) This coupling depends on the integrity of the iodide organification processes in the gland and probably on the intact structure of the TG molecule.

Iodotyrosyl Coupling Defect

Two sisters (M.D. and L.D.) had large goiters, hypothyroidism, and retarded mental and physical development.[81] There were at least three consanguinous marriages among the progenitors of these patients. RAIU by the thyroid gland was extremely rapid and reached nearly 100 percent. When PTU was given to block iodide organification, iodine was discharged from the gland, but was not in hormonal form, since the thyroid hormone levels in the blood were low. Furthermore, when methimazole was given several days after a tracer of ^{131}I, the specific activity of the iodine in the urine rose to 17 percent per milligram, yet the specific activity of ^{131}I in the gland was only 2.9 percent per milligram. Thus, the iodide discharged from the gland during methimazole administration was derived from a small pool of labeled iodine of high specific activity. Evidently this iodine pool was in the process of recycling rapidly within the thyroid gland. In addition, analysis of thyroid tissue from one of these subjects 4 days after the administration of ^{131}I disclosed a large quantity of MIT and DIT but only trace amounts of stable T_4 and no labeled T_4. The gland was very hyperplastic. Several patients who showed the same clinical and laboratory findings[81,83] have been described.

Patients assigned to this group do not make enough iodothyronines from the abundant stores of iodotyrosyl precursors in the thyroid gland. Patients with iodide deficiency and some with nodular goiter also have large amounts of iodotyrosyl residues relative to the small amounts of iodothyronines, but the mechanisms responsible for these findings may be different. If the defect is indeed that of iodotyrosyl coupling, it could be attributed to a deficiency in the activity of the iodine organification process, lack of a hypothetical coupling enzyme, an error in the structure of the protein substrate impairing coupling, or other, not yet identified abnormality. Very recently a coupling defect was described in a patient whose parents are first cousins. When thyroid tissue of this patient was analyzed, TG was not properly sialylated due to deficient sialyltransferase activity. There was no deficiency in glucosamine, galactose, or manose content. It was concluded that the presence of severely hyposialylated TG is linked to the defective iodotyrosine coupling with a possibly abnormal migration of TG into the follicular lumen.[84]

The diagnosis of coupling defect has followed the finding of hypothyroidism and a hyperplastic overactive thyroid gland, absence of other defects in hormonogenesis, and an abnormally high ratio of iodotyrosines to iodothyronines in thyroid specimen. Demonstration of a small pool of recycling iodine of high specific activity in the thyroid glands has strengthened the interpretation concerning the nature of the disorder, but this finding is not in itself diagnostic because it has also been observed in certain patients with severe iodide deficiency in an endemic goiter area and in other unrelated thyroid disease. Treatment consists of T_4 administration for goiter and/or hypothyroidism.

Abnormal, Diminished, or Absent TG Synthesis

TG is a large glycoprotein of complex structure. It is thus expected that errors in TG synthesis and structure exist and might be detected by physical and chemical means. An error in primary structure might alter the conformation of the molecule in such a way that its physical properties would be altered and iodination or coupling would be impeded. Alternatively, the gland might form little or no TG or might process it abnormally. Sometimes the predominant iodoprotein found in the thyroid gland is iodinated albumin. It has been suggested that this "thyralbumin" is synthesized in the follicular cell. However, recently it has been shown that albumin is bloodborne and not synthesized locally.[85]

In the many reports of abnormalities of TG, it is impossible to determine from the evidence whether the defect is in a primary DNA error for TG that leads to diminished, absent, or abnormal structure, to an error in mRNA leading to impaired transcription, to an error in translation or to one in the processing or transport of the molecule to the recovery of hormone formed within its matrix, or even to some subtle change in structure that impedes hormone synthesis. An attempt for a rational classification appears in Table 16-2.

The results of a number of studies have been consistent with impaired or absent TG synthesis.[86–97] Defective synthesis of TG was reported in a patient

TABLE 16-2. Tentative Classification of Reported Instances of TG Abnormalities[a]

1. Defective DNA code for TG
   Humans[86–99]
   Sheep[100–105]
   Cattle[106–112]
   Goat[113–120]
   Rat (tumor)[124,122]
   Mice[123–125]
2. Abnormal mRNA processing[116,117]
3. Abnormal translation[93]
4. Abnormal intracellular processing
   Abnormal transport, segregation, or exocytosis[92,126,127]
   Abnormal glycosylation[128]
5. Abnormal TG mobilization (unestablished)

[a] It should be understood that allocation of cases to the categories is usually based on limited information, and assignment is accordingly tentative. Also, each category is doubtless heterogeneous. Furthermore, it is probable that abnormalities allocated under 2 to 5 may be secondary to the defects in the DNA code for TG.

born to consanguineous marriage from a family without goiter, indicating autosomal-recessive inheritance.[96] This was caused by a mutation involving cytosine to thymine transition creating a stop codon at position 1510 of the protein. Translation of the mutated transcript would generate a severely truncated polypeptide of 1509 amino acids. However, in a minor proportion of normal transcripts, position 1510 is removed by alternative splicing. Thus a minor transcript encoding for a TG protein missing only 57 residues escapes early termination. Thyroid hormone synthesis in this patient is thus expected to operate on two protein precursors. Ieiry et al.[99] studied a 33-year-old female whose parents were first cousins and who is the fifth of six siblings. Three, including the patient, had voluminous goiters. She was only 132 cm tall, and her mental age was that of a 13-year-old child. Tests of thyroid function were as follows: T_4, 1.0 μg/dl (normal range 5.0 to 13.0 μg/dl): free T_4, 0.2 ng/dl (0.8 to 2.4 ng/dl): T_3, 1.8 ng/dl (1.0 to 2.0 ng/ml): PBI 8.7 μg/dl (4.0 to 8.0 μg/dl): TSH, 57 mU/ml (<9 mU/ml); and RAIU, 60

percent before and 55 percent after perchlorate administration. The thyroid gland removed after surgery weighted 350 g. Normal thyroid peroxidase and coupling activity were reported. It appeared that defective TG was synthesized due to aberrant splicing caused by a point mutation at the acceptor splice site of intron 3, which produced a deletion of exon 4 from the major TG transcript. Since exon 4 encodes the tyrosine residue involved in thyroid hormone formation, its deletion explains the hypothyroid status of the patient despite a relatively minor alteration of the TG molecule (see Fig. 16-3).

An iodoprotein resistant to trypsin and others with abnormal solubility have been reported. Other iodinated species found in the thyroid glands of congenital goiter have been subunits of TG or proteins with abnormal carbohydrate residues. These findings suggest the possibility of TG molecules with abnormal amino acid sequences.

Similar observations have been made in animals. Falconer et al.,[100–103] Rac et al.,[104] and Dolling and Good[105] have studied merino sheep that appear to

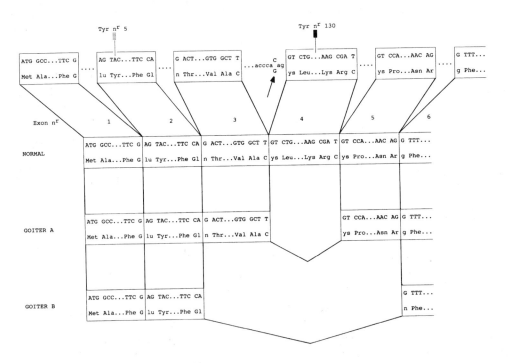

Fig. 16-3. Organization of genomic and cDNA thyroglobulin sequence. Schematic representation of the genomic organization of the 5'region (6 first exons) of the thyroglobulin gene, together with the normal and goitrous (A,B) cDNA sequences. The arrow points to the mutation (C-G). Tyrosine no. 5 (the major hormonogenic acceptor residue), and tyrosine no. 130 (putative donor residue) are highlighted. (From Ieiri et al.,[99] with permission.)

have impaired synthesis of TG. Falconer et al. detected a small amount of immunoprecipitable TG-like iodoprotein in the hyperplastic glands. Two abnormal TG polypeptides were found in the thyroid glands of South African cattle with congenital goiter, with autosomal-recessive defect of TG synthesis. In vitro translation of TG mRNA produced one polypeptide with a molecular weight of 250,000 and another with a molecular weight of 75,000. Both polypeptides were immunoprecipitated by a purified TG antibody. Northern blot analysis revealed a mRNA of slightly reduced size (30 S) as compared to that in normal bovine thyroid tissue (33 S). Furthermore, a 10-to 15-fold decrease in relative concentration of TG mRNA was observed.[109,110] The thyroid glands of a well-studied strain of goats from the Netherlands produce only a trace amounts of TG.[113–120] The goitrous thyroid glands do not contain the normal 19S TG but have small amounts of 7S TG. The total TG mRNA concentration is only 2.5 to 10 percent the normal level. It is polyadenylated and of normal size, but in contrast to normal TG mRNA, it cannot be translated into 19S Tg or other distinct translation products. The TG gene of normal and goitrous goats has been cloned,[119] and sequence analysis of the 3′ end of the abnormal TG genes, as compared to that of the normal gene, has revealed one transition mutation 3′ to the reading frame in a stem-loupe structure region of the last exon near the poly(A) addition site. Analysis of the promotor site and the first five exons has revealed only one difference between the normal and goitrous TG genes, i.e., a Ser-Leu transition in exon 5. Also an insertion was found in the fifth intron of the abnormal gene. A strain of mice with inherited congenital colloid-deficient goiter and hypothyroidism (cog/cog) has been described. The cog mutation is linked to the thyroid TG gene, but no gross deletion of the gene or quantative abnormalities of TG mRNA have been observed. Apart from the presence of a 12S and 19S TG subunit, the majority of iodoproteins in the goiter are in the smaller area of 3-8S.[123–125]

Can criteria be established for the diagnosis of TG synthesis defects? Evidence favoring such a diagnosis would be the demonstration of a thyroid gland protein that is immunologically related to TG but with other properties that are abnormal. A number of methods are available for testing the properties of proteins in thyroid extracts and their relationship to normal TG. If the protein has the mobility of 19 S TG on polyacrylamide gel electrophoresis and is immunoprecipitable with TG antibody, then it is safe to assume that it is authentic TG. Additional proof is the demonstration of precipitation between 1.7 and 1.9 M phosphate buffer (salting out), a 19 S sedimentation constant (with a slight band at 27 S) on analytic centrifugation, appropriate elution from Sephadex or similar columns, and a clean peak at 19 S after sucrose density sedimentation. If an immunoprecipitable iodoprotein fails to meet other criteria, then the possibility of synthesis of an abnormal TG may be entertained. Abnormalities in TG mRNA with regard to its size and abundance may be detected using hybridization with TG cDNA (Northern blotting). Analysis of abnormalities at the gene level may be done using restriction fragment length analysis and sequencing the DNA region suspected to be abnormal.

It is much more difficult to establish a limitation in the rate of synthesis of a normally structured TG molecule. Evidence favoring such a deduction might be the presence of a heavily iodinated TG of normal structure and properties but in greatly reduced concentration and quantity. The conclusion that a patient has a complete inability to synthesize TG or its subunits might follow the finding of only nonthyroglobulin-related iodinated protein in the thyroid gland in the absence of other well-defined defects in thyroid cell function.

Plasma Iodoprotein Defect

Based on current knowledge this is not a tenable diagnosis. A soluble iodoprotein with properties similar to those of an iodinated albumin may comprise as much as 4 percent of the iodine in the normal thyroid gland. Under normal circumstances, only small amounts of iodoproteins escape into the blood. Of the 10 to 15 percent of serum iodine present as iodinated (covalently linked) protein a greater portion is formed during peripheral metabolism of thyroid hormones. Under certain circumstances, increased amounts of iodinated proteins are found circulating in blood. These proteins contain iodinated amino acids in peptide linkage, and MIT is their main iodinated constituent.

Patients with hypothyroidism and goiter have been described whose sera contain an abnormal amount of nonhormonal iodine in peptide linkage. In these patients, 60 to 70 percent of the serum iodine is butanol extractable, but the remaining fraction is not extractable. This component is an iodoprotein that can be hydrolyzed by proteolytic enzymes to yield MIT and DIT and, at times, a little T_4.

Iodinated peptides have been detected in peripheral blood in several disorders of the thyroid. For example, an iodinated albuminlike protein constitutes a large fraction of the precipitable iodine in blood of patients with Hashimoto's disease and Graves' disease and has been found in certain patients with endemic goiter, sporadic goiter, multinodular goiter, and thyroid carcinoma.[3] Strong evidence suggests that when the thyroid gland becomes hyperplastic, plasma albumin circulating through the thyroid gland penetrates the thyroid cells, where it serves as a substrate for iodination when normal TG is in short supply.[85] This is also the case in congenital goiters due to a defect in TG synthesis. Thus, the presence of an iodinated albuminlike component in the blood does not in itself indicate the presence of inborn error of the thyroid hormone synthese, but may only be indicative of thyroid hyperplasia. On the other hand, not all patients with hyperplastic thyroid glands have an iodinated peptide in the blood.

Interpretation

In contrast to defects in iodide transport, iodide organification, and iodothyrosine dehalogenation, which can clearly be discriminated, it is very difficult to precisely define the three categories of abnormalities mentioned under disorders of iodothyronine and TG synthesis.

Is a separate designation of iodotyrosyl coupling defect tenable? In order to establish this diagnosis as a separate entity, it is necessary to show that TG of normal structure is formed in amounts adequate to act as substrate for iodination, and that its MIT and DIT content is normal in amount and ratio, but that for such an amount and ratio the iodothyronine concentration is low, and low for reasons other than rapid turnover or iodide deficiency. In addition, at the present level of understanding, it would probably be necessary to show that TG prepared from such a patient is normal insofar as it can form iodothyronine in vivo at a normal rate in the presence of a thyroid peroxidase–catalyzed iodinating system or during reaction with I_2. Such criteria have not yet been rigorously met for any patient. In our own patients with a coupling defect, the findings still do not exclude the possibility of complete or nearly complete absence of TG synthesis as the primary defect.

From another point of view, if a patient synthesized a TG of abnormal structure that impeded coupling, such condition could be designated either as coupling defect or as defective TG synthesis. Perhaps the term *coupling defect* should be reserved for those instances in which thyroid gland extract would fail to support iodothyronine synthesis using a normal TG as substrate.

As has been stated earlier, the classification of abnormalities in TG synthesis is arbitrary in many instances due to incomplete analysis of the abnormalities. Also attention must be directed to abnormalities that are secondary to undetected events. For instance, reported increasing turnover of TG mRNA[117] is probably secondary to abnormal TG mRNA on the basis of a coding defect in the TG gene.[119] Also, abnormalities in glycosylation of TG may be secondary to a defect in transport of TG from the endoplasmatic reticulum and Golgi apparatus to the follicular lumen.[126] The latter may be the consequence of abnormalities in TG structure gene or to abnormal mRNA processing.

Patients with disorders of iodothyronine and TG synthesis, whatever the cause, are best treated with L-thyroxine. If a goiter causing discomfort or cosmetic problems does not regress under thyroid hormone replacement, thyroidectomy should be considered.

TSH Unresponsiveness

Thyrotropin stimulates most if not all functions of the thyroid follicular cell including cell division TG synthesis and hormone formation. Lack of TSH is expected to result in thyroid gland failure. The same finding might also arise if the thyroid gland failed to respond normally to TSH. The following case report concerns a patient whose thyroid gland appeared not to respond to TSH.

Thyroid Unresponsiveness to TSH

An 8-year-old boy appeared normal at birth but developed slowly[129] (Fig. 16-4). The diagnosis of hypothyroidism was first made at 2 years of age. Desiccated thyroid (15 to 60 mg/day) was given until age 8. His IQ at age 7 was 50. The parents were first cousins once removed. They had three normal children and one other who had mental and growth retardation.

The patient was 110 cm in height (below the third percentile) and weighed 19.3 kg. He could feed and dress himself and to say a few intelligible words. His

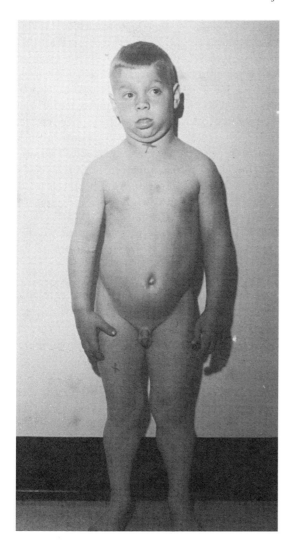

Fig. 16-4. An 8-year-old boy with a thyroid that failed to respond to TSH. There was severe physical and intellectual retardation.

bone age was 3.5 years and face was typically cretinoid. Hearing was normal. The thyroid gland was not enlarged. Reflex relaxation time was strikingly slow. Excretion of [127]I in the urine was normal.

PBI concentration was 1.0 μg/dl and RAIU was 27 percent. Administration of perchlorate induced a discharge of 22 percent of the iodide trapped by the thyroid gland in 30 minutes. There was no response to the administered bovine TSH in terms of either increase in thyroidal ^{131}I uptake or net rate of loss of iodine from the gland.

Thyroxine binding globulin (TBG) capacity was slightly low, but thyroxine-binding prealbumin (TBPA) capacity and resin T_3 uptake (rT_3U) were normal. TSH

measured by the McKenzie bioassay showed activity of 393 ± 65 percent of control at 2 hours and 340 ± 34 percent at 8 hours. The concentration of serum TSH by RIA was 145 μU/ml (normal, 1.5 to 20).

The metabolism of glucose in slices of thyroid issue obtained at biopsy was not stimulated by TSH, whereas control slices were briskly stimulated. No TG could be demonstrated in the gland.

The microscopic picture of the thyroid gland was unusual. There was a diffuse increase in the stroma. Some follicles had cells that were very flat and involuted or even atrophic. Others, often adjacent to the inactive ones, were lined with hypertropied large cuboidal cells typical of reactive hyperplasia. Another feature was the frequency of atypical nuclear forms, which were often bizarre in shape and hyperchromatic.

A remarkably similar patient was studied by Codaccioni et al.[130] Uptake of ^{131}I by the thyroid gland was stimulated by intravenously administered dibutyryl cAMP, and membranes prepared from a biopsy specimen bound TSH normally. These membranes appeared to be abnormal on electron microscopy, showing extensive increases in the width and surface of the basal plasma membrane and lamina. Adenyl cyclase activity was stimulated by fluoride but not by TSH in these membrancs. Thus, the error appeared to be in the coupling of the TSH receptors to cAMP stimulation. Patients who had similar or identical disorders have been studied by Medeiros-Neto et al., (personal communication, 1980) Job et al.,[131] Aarseth et al.,[132] Leger et al.,[133] and Takamatsu.[134] A point mutation in the gene of the TSH receptor (TSH-R) has been identified in a strain of *hyt/hyt* hypothyroid mice that also fails to respond to TSH.[135] This mutation resulted in a leucine for proline substitution at amino acid position 556 in the fourth transmembrane domain of the receptor. COS cells transfected with this mutant showed no TSH binding and response to TSH stimulation.[136] Further studies showed that plasma membrane targeting of this mutant was intact but that binding of TSH was eliminated. These findings suggest interactions between the transmembrane and extracellular domains of the TSH-R.[136a] Recently three sisters were described who were euthyroid and had normal serum thyroid hormone levels but elevated TSH concentrations between 40 and 60 mU/L.[137] All three had mutations in both alleles of the TSH-R gene, one inherited from each parent. In the paternal allele, thymine at position 599 was replaced by adenine, resulting in replacement of isoleucine by asparagine at position 167. In the maternal allele, cytocine at position 583 was replaced by guanine, leading to replacement of proline by alanine at position 162. Both mutations are located in exon 6, which encodes the midportion of the extracellular domain of the TSH-R.

As compared to the TSH response in COS cells transfected with the wild-type TSH-R, cells transfected with the maternal mutant showed about 10 times less responsiveness to TSH, whereas cells transfected with the paternal mutant showed almost no TSH-inducible activity. Cotransfection of the wild-type TSH-R which each of the mutant TSH receptors, in order to simulate the heterozygous state of the parents, resulted in almost equal response activity as compared to cells expressing the wild-type TSH-R. However, cells transfected with equal amounts of mutant maternal and paternal receptors in order to simulate the compound heterozygous state of the three daughters responded with 20 times less activity to TSH. The mechanism that enables the subjects to maintain high TSH levels to ensure normal thyroid hormone levels is a matter of speculation but may be related to resetting of the sensitivity of the thyrotroph for the TSH-suppressive effect of thyroid hormone. Resistance to TSH occurs frequently in patients with pseudohypoparathyroidism but is due to mutations in the G protein.[138]

Interpretation

Most of the reported patients with TSH unresponsiveness had severe clinical hypothyroidism.[131–135] In spite of this, the avidity of the thyroid gland for iodine was normal. The TSH level in the blood was high, and there was much cellular hypertrohpy in the biopsy specimen, but there was no goiter. No evidence of a protein resembling thyroglobulin could be found.

Many of the abnormalities indicated a failure of the thyroid gland to respond adequately to TSH. There was a high concentration of TSH in the blood without hypertrophy of the gland or increased thyroidal ^{131}I uptake, and administration of TSH caused no change in glandular function. Thus, the epithelial cells appeared to be unable to respond to TSH in three ways that are specific to the hormone-gland interaction: cell division, synthesis of the organ-specific protein, TG, and stimulation of glucose oxidation. Failure to respond to TSH, but a response to dcAMP, suggests a problem in coupling of the receptor–TSH complex to activation of adenyl cyclase and synthesis of cAMP.

While the defect in these patients has not been localized, Refetoff et al.[137] recently described three sisters in whom a mutation in both alleles of the TSH-R gene, one inherited from each parent, was the cause of the TSH unresponsiveness. In transfection studies in COS cells, both mutants had less but different activity, apparently related to the location of the mutation. These siblings were, contrary to the previously reported patients, clinically euthyroid and had normal thyroid hormone serum levels but high serum TSH concentrations. The fact that the other patients were clinically hypothyroid might be related to different mutations in the TSH-R gene or to the fact that the abnormality is located somewhere else in the TSH-R—cAMP activating complex.

Diagnosis

Identification of a patient with TSH unresponsiveness should depend upon the demonstration of a reduced gland function and a failure to respond to the administration TSH. Obviously unresponsiveness to the high levels of endogenous TSH may theoretically also be due to a defective TSH of lesser biologic activity (see below). In addition, the presence of a thyroid in normal position should be confirmed. If possible, thyroid biopsy should disclose absence of TG and hypoplastic epithelial cells. Additional studies of TSH binding to thyroid cell plasma membranes and observations on the function of the adenyl cyclase system from such patients might prove particularly revealing. Sequencing of the genes of the TSH-receptor and the G proteins provide a method to establish the cause of the defect by noninvasive means.

Congenital Pituitary Failure

Inherited defects of synthesis or secretion of TRH have not yet been described, although isolated cases of TRH deficiency with hypothyroidism have been reported.[139,140] It may be the cause of secondary amenorrhea, and normal menstruation resumes after treatment with thyroid hormone.[141,142] The diagnosis may be presumed if the pituitary gland of a hypothyroid patient with low serum TSH levels responds to administration of TRH with a rise in serum TSH concentration.

Isolated TSH deficiency should be considered when central hypothyroidism is present, whereas other pituitary functions are normal.[143] Serum TSH levels are low as measured by a sensitive immunoradiometric assay (IRMA).[144] Characteristically, the concentration of pituitary glycoprotein α subunit significantly increases in serum after TRH administration, whereas serum free TSH-β subunit remains undetectable. From this observation abnormalities in the TSH-β gene were presumed to be present.[144] This was subsequently confirmed in patients with congenital isolated TSH deficiency combined with cretinism and growth retardation. They appeared to have a single base substitution in the codon for the 29th amino acid of the TSH-β subunit gene. The alteration is in the center of the CAGYC sequence of amino acids conserved among all known glycoprotein hormone β subunits. In these patients the TSH deficiency was an autosomal-β recessive disease.[145] So far three families have been described with this single base substitution, while in two other families with defective TSH-β subunit synthesis, the genetic defect has not been located yet.[146] Of interest is the fact that normal prolactin release in response to TRH is normal.[147] Recently patients have been detected who are hypothyroid because of mutations in the Pit-1 gene. This gene is essential for the development of cells secreting growth hormone (GH), prolactin (PRL), and TSH. These patients have hypoplastic pituitary glands and multiple pituitary hormone failures.[148–149b]

Patients with these syndromes should be treated with thyroid hormone replacement therapy as soon as diagnosis is made.

Congenital Hyperthyroidism

Autosomal dominantly inherited nonautoimmune hyperthyroidism is caused by a germlike mutation of the thyrotropin receptor gene leading to constitutive thyroid activation and is discussed in Chapter 13.

General Interpretations

One may anticipate with considerable confidence that in the course of time other metabolic abnormalities that interfere with the synthesis of the thyroid hormones will be described and characterized. The defects described are probably each genetically heterogeneous.

The number of patients described are so few that inheritance patterns often cannot be assigned with certainty. Observations are consistent with point mutations and autosomal-recessive inheritance for the full defect. Consanguinity has been the rule. There are, nevertheless, instances consistent with dominant inheritance. The finding of goiter without hypothyroidism in family members of some patients has suggested that the disorders are expressed in the heterozygote as thyroid enlargement. For example, a minimal but detectable dehalogenase deficiency was demonstrated in goitrous but otherwise normal family members of patients with the full defect. Routine screening programs for neonatal hypothyroidism in the United States, Canada, Europe, and Japan are identifying approximately 1 child in 4,000 with congenital hypothyroidism, and of these approximately one-third have some form of defect of thyroid hormone synthesis rather than a congenital absence of the gland.[150] Further studies of these patients should permit better definition of inheritance patterns.

The wide spectrum of clinical manifestations is worth noting. Many of the patients are severely hypothyroid and developmentally retarded, but as many are normal and have thyroid glands that have grown to a size and activity that permits the patient to be euthyroid or nearly so. Two of these groups illustrate the interaction of the genetic endowment with the environment in the production of disease. In both the dehalogenase defect and in the iodide transport defect, ingestion of sufficient iodide caused the manifestations of the disease to vanish. In order for the disease to appear, not only is the specific constitution necessary, but the environment must be appropriate as well.

The role of these metabolic defects in the production of neoplastic change in the thyroid gland must be mentioned. The thyroids of patients with familial goiter and cretinism tend to be intensely hyperplastic. In one of the author's patients and several others reported in the literature,[151] all the criteria of malignant change have been found. It is interesting to note in this regard that Wollman has developed several lines of experimental tumors in rats that appear to have metabolic defects similar or identical to those that have been described among the various patients with familial goiter and hypothyroidism.[152]

Treatment

Satisfactory treatment of familial goiter depends on the degree to which irreversible changes have occurred in the skeleton and central nervous system. Remarkable shrinkage of the goiter may be expected from treatment with L-thyroxine in usual maintenance doses, providing the changes of degeneration, cyst formation, and fibrous replacement have not taken place. The goiter will invariably recur if medication is discontinued. In some instances, as in the transport and dehalogenase defects, potassium iodide supplementation may be entirely effective.

Care should be exercised in treating familial goiter medically in view of the tendency of some of these goiters to undergo malignant changes.[153] In general, it is prudent to remove a nodule that fails to shrink after a few months of replacement therapy, especially if it continues to grow. Unfortunately, many well-established goiters eventually require surgery. We have encountered a complication of surgery, tracheomalacia, in one of these patients. Interestingly, symptoms developed only several years after a large goiter was removed.

Often, unless hormone replacement therapy is begun during the first few weeks of life, there is considerable risk of permanent retardation of intellectual development or skeletal growth. These patients can be identified by the neonatal hypothyroid screening programs. Determination of plasma TG concentrations may be helpful in distinguishing infants with absent thyroid glands from those with thyroid glands that are ectopic or have TG that is abnormal but immunologicaly identifiable.[154] If hypothyroidism is confirmed by serum analysis, we advise that the patient not be tested further, but rather treated at once because of the risk of damage to the growing nervous system. Testing to establish the cause of hypothyroidism can be delayed until the child is 4 or 5 years old, when it is safe to withdraw the hormone for a few weeks and to proceed with a thorough investigation. There are reasons to suspect that in some instances damage may have occurred in utero, so that hormone therapy will not fully reverse developmental arrest or mental retardation. L-thyroxine should be given in sufficient amount based on measurement of serum TSH and free T_4, since often attempts to normalized TSH may cause thyrotoxicosis.

Management of the patient with fully developed goiter, hypothyroidism, and permanent growth and mental retardation is unsatisfactory. Unacceptable aggressiveness or other undesirable behavior may be the result of excessive thyroid medication. The dosage is best adjusted to keep the patient active and comfortable without arousing unwanted side effects. Patients with Pendred's syndrome usually synthesize an adequate or nearly adequate amount of hormone to develop normally. They require thyroid hormone treatment only to prevent goiter formation, to which they are genetically predisposed. Patients whose thyroids fail to respond to TSH or those with pituitary failure should be treated with thyroid hormone.

Summary

Patients with familial goiter and hypothyroidism have been classified into several categories according to fairly well-defined inborn errors of thyroid hormone synthesis. The defect in each group prevents the secretion of normal amounts of thyroid hormone.

Patients with the iodide accumulation defect are unable to maintain a sufficient concentration of iodide in the gland. This defect is also found in the salivary gland an the gastric mucosa. Presumably it arises either because of a defect in the supply of energy that is necessary for the thyroidal iodide transport system or because of an abnormality of a membrane receptor or intracellular carrier.

The iodide organification defect is characterized by an expanded pool of readily exchangeable iodide in the thyroid gland and impaired formation of iodotyrosyl residues. It includes several distinct defects. In one, iodide perioxidase activity is lacking. This type is heterogeneous in that hematin will restore peroxidase activity in some and not in others. In some the defect is complete, whereas in others there is goiter but not hypothyroidism. Another type of disorder with deficient iodide organification is Pendred's syndrome. Peroxidase activity is present, and the nature of the defect is not known.

Patients with the iodotyrosine dehalogenase defect lack the deiodinase of MIT and DIT.

Groups of patients have been described who are said to have defective coupling of thyroid hormone precursors into hormones, or who have impaired synthesis of TG, or who secrete abnormal iodopeptides into the blood. These defects have not been adequately defined, and the patients may all have abnormalities in TG synthesis.

Patients have also been described in whom mutations in the coding region of the TSH β gene leads to a defective TSH, which is usually not secreted and consequently leads to thyroid failure. Recently patients have been reported with deficiencies in TSH, prolactin, and growth hormone due to a mutation in the gene that is essential for development of the pituitary cells secreting these peptides. Other patients have been reported whose thyroid glands fail to respond to thyrotropin, and mutations in the gene for the TSH receptor have been detected.

Treatment of these abnormalities consists of administration of thyroid hormone in an amount to restore euthyroidism.

DEFECTS OF THYROID HORMONE TRANSPORT IN SERUM

Abnormalities in thyroid hormone transport serum proteins do not alter the metabolic state and do not cause thyroid disease. However, they do produce alterations in thyroid hormone concentration in serum and, when unrecognized, have led to inappropriate treatment. When the abnormality is the consequence of altered synthesis, secretion, or stability of the variant serum protein, the free thyroid hormone level estimated by any of the clinically available techniques remains within the range of normal. In contrast, when the defect results in an alteration of the affinity of the variant protein for the hormone, estimates of the free thyroid hormone level give erroneous results, and it is thus prudent to measure the free hormone concentration by more direct methods, such as equilibrium dialysis or ultrafiltration.

The existence of inherited defects of thyroid hormone transport in serum was first recognized in 1959 with the report of TBG excess.[155] Genetic variants for each of the three major thyroid hormone transport proteins have been since described, and in recent years the molecular basis of a number of these defects has been identified.[156] Clinically, these defects manifest as either euthyroid hyperthyroxinemia or hypothyroxinemia. Associated abnormalities such as thyrotoxicosis, goiter, and familial hyperlipidemia are usually coincidental.[157] However, individuals with thyroid disorders are more likely to undergo thyroid testing leading to the fortuitous detection of a thyroid hormone transport defect.

Thyroxine Binding Globulin Defects

Familial TBG abnormalities are inherited as X chromosome–linked traits,[158,159] which is compatible with the location of the TBG gene on the long arm of the X chromosome (Xq21q22).[160] This mode of inheritance also suggests that the defects involve the TBG gene proper, rather than the rate of TBG disposal, as previously postulated.[158] The normal, common type TBG (TBG-C) has a high affinity for iodothyronines (affinity constants: $10^{-10}M^{-1}$ for T_4 and 10^{-1} for T_3) and binds 75 percent of the total T_4 and T_3 circulating in blood. Thus, among the inherited abnormalities of thyroid hormone transport proteins, those involving the TBG molecule have the potential to produce the most profound alterations of thyroid hormone concentration in serum.

Clinically TBG defects are classified according to the level of TBG in serum of affected hemizygotes (XY males or XO females) that express only the mutant allele: complete TBG deficiency (TBG-CD), partial TBG deficiency (TBG-PD), and TBG excess (TBG-E). In families with TBG-CD, affected males have no detectable TBG, and carrier females (mothers or daughters) have on the average half the normal TBG concentration. In families with partially TBG deficient males, the mean TBG concentration in heterozygous females is usually above half the normal. Serum TBG concentration in males with TBG-E is three-to five-fold the normal mean and that in the corresponding carrier females is slightly higher than half that of the affected males. These observations indicate an equal contribution of cells expressing the normal and mutant TBG genes.

Inherited TBG defects can be further characterized by the level of denatured TBG (dnTBG) in serum and the physicochemical properties of the molecule. The latter can be easily determined without the need of purification. These properties are (1) immunologic identity; (2) isoelectric focusing (IEF) pattern; (3) rate of inactivation when exposed to various temperatures and pH; and (4) affinity for the ligands T_4 and T_3. More precise identification of TBG defects requires sequencing of the TBG gene.

Complete TBG Deficiency
   M.I.P., a phenotypic female, was 13 years old when first seen because of retarded growth, amenorrhea, and absence of secondary sexual traits. She was the first sibling of a second marriage for both parents. The family included a younger brother and four older half-siblings, two maternal and two paternal. The propositus was born to her 30-year-old mother after a full-term, uncomplicated pregnancy. Infancy and early childhood development were normal until 4 years of age, when it

became apparent that she was shorter than her peers. She was 12 years of age when a low PBI of 2.2 μg/dl (normal range 4.0 to 8.0) was noted, and treatment with 120 mg of desiccated thyroid (equivalent to 200 μg L-T4) daily was initiated. Since, during the ensuing 6 months, no change in her growth rate occurred and because PBI remained unchanged (2.0 μg/dl), the dose of desiccated thyroid was increased to 180 mg/day. This produced restlessness, perturbed sleep, and deteriorating school performance necessitating discontinuation of thyroid hormone treatment. No family history of thyroid disease or short stature was elicited, and the parents denied consanguinity.

On physical examination, the patient appeared younger than her chronologic age, was short (137 cm), and showed no signs of sexual development. She had a webbed neck, low nuchal hairline, bilateral eyelid ptosis, shield-shaped chest, increased carrying angle, and short fourth metacarpals and metatarsals. The thyroid gland was normal in size and consistency.

Buccal smear was negative for Barr bodies, and karyotyping revealed 45 chromosomes consistent with XO Turner's syndrome. No chromosomal abnormalities were found in lymphocytes from the mother and father. Bone age was 12 years and x-ray of the scull showed a mild degree of hyperteliorism. PBI and butanol-extractable iodine (BEI) were low at 2.0 and 1.8 μg/dl, respectively. Resin T_3 uptake was high at 59.9 percent (normal range 25 to 35 percent) indicating reduced TBG-binding capacity. A 24-hour thyroidal radioiodide uptake was normal at 29 percent, BMR was +20 percent (normal range −10 to +20), and TG autoantibodies were not present. Serum cortisol was normal, as were the responses to ACTH and metyrapone. Basal growth hormone concentration was normal at 8.0 ng/ml, which rose to 32 ng/ml following insulin hypoglycemia.

Studies were carried out in all first-degree relatives, and the propositus was treated cyclically with diethylstilbesterol, which produced withdrawal uterine bleeding and gradual breast development, accompanied by the appearance of scant pubic and axillary hair.

Five family members, in addition to the propositus, had thyroid function test abnormalities. Two were males and three females. The two males (maternal grandfather and maternal half-brother) and the propositus had the lowest PBI levels and undetectable T_4 binding to serum TBG. In contrast, the three females (mother, maternal aunt, and maternal half-sister) had a lesser reduction of their PBI and T_4-binding capacity to TBG approximately one-half the normal mean value. The two sons of the affected grandfather (maternal uncles to the propositus) had normal PBI and T_4 binding to TBG. No interference with T_4 binding to

TBG or other serum protein abnormalities were found in affected members of the family. In vivo T_4 kinetic studies revealed a rapid extrathyroidal turnover rate but normal daily secretion and degradation, compatible with their eumetabolic state.

Interpretation

The incidental identification of thyroid test abnormalities in the propositus is typical for most subjects with TBG deficiency as well as TBG excess. So is, in many, the initial unnecessary treatment. The inherited nature of the defect is suspected by exclusion of factors known to cause acquired TBG abnormalities (see Ch. 3 and 5) and should be confirmed by the presence of similar abnormalities in members of the family. The absence of male-to-male transmission and the carrier state of all female offspring of the affected males is a typical pattern of X chromosome-linked inheritance. This is further supported by the complete TBG deficiency in individuals having a single X chromosome (males and the XO female) and only partial TBG deficiency in carrier XX females.

Sixteen TBG variants have been so far identified, in 12 the precise genetic defect has been determined by gene sequencing. Their primary structure, some of their physical and chemical properties, and the resulting serum T_4 concentrations are summarized in Fig 16-5 and 16-6.

Complete TBG Deficiency

Complete TBG deficiency (TBG-CD) is defined as undetectable TBG in serum of affected hemizygous subjects or a value lesser than 0.03 percent the normal mean, the current limits of detection being 5 ng/dl.[161] The prevalence is approximately 1:15,000 newborn males. Three TBG variants having this phenotype have been characterized at the gene level. Two, TBG-CD6[162] and TBG-CDJ,[163] have a single nucleotide insertion and deletion, respectively, resulting in a frameshift and premature termination of translation (Fig. 16-4). While this finding explains the complete lack of TBG in serum, this is not the case with the mutation in TBG-CD5, which involves the replacement of a single amino acid (Leu-227–Pro)[161]) (Fig. 16-4 and see below). TBG-CDJ has been so far identified only in Japanese patients, but its allele frequency in the population remains unknown.[164,165]

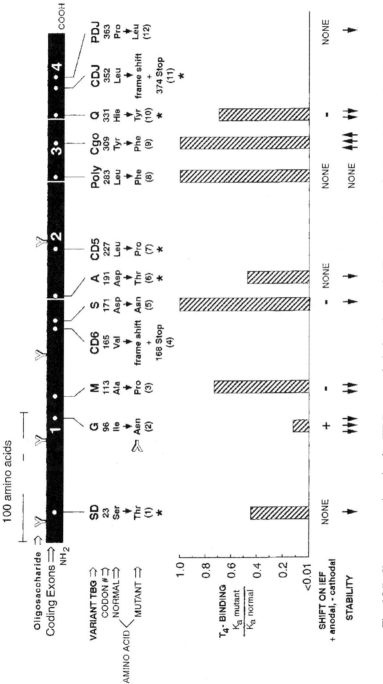

Fig. 16-5. Known mutations in the TBG gene, their location and effect on the properties of the molecule. The TBG variants are -SD, San Diego; -G, Gary; -M, Montreal, -CD6, complete deficiency 6; -S, slow; -A, Aborigine; -CD5, complete deficiency 5; -Cgo, Chicago; -Poly, polymorphic; -Q, Quebec; -CDJ, complete deficiency Japan; and -PDJ, partial deficiency Japan. Asterisks indicate the coexistence of TBG-Poly. (From Hayashi and Refetoff,[156] with permission.)

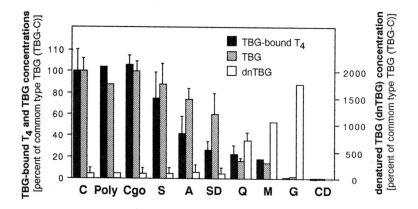

Fig. 16-6. Serum T_4 bound to TBG and the concentration of TBG and denatured TBG (dnTBG) in hemizygous subjects expressing different TBG variants. Results, shown as mean ± SD, were normalized by expressing them as percentage of those for TBG-C. For abbreviations used in the nomenclature of the TBG variants, see legend to Fig. 16-4. (Adapted from Janssen et al.,[168] with permission.)

Partial TBG Deficiency

Partial TBG deficiency (TBG-PD) is the most common form of inherited TBG deficiency, having a prevalence of 1:4,000 newborn. Identification of heterozygous females by serum TBG measurement may be difficult because levels often overlap the normal range. Six different mutations, producing a variable degree of reduction of TBG concentration in serum, have been identified (TBG-A, TBG-G, TBG-SD, TBG-M, TBG-Q, and TBG-PDJ) (Fig. 16-4). In addition, some of these variants are unstable or have lower binding affinity for T_4 and T_3, and some exhibit an abnormal migration pattern on IEF electrophoresis (Fig. 16-4). Variants with decreased affinity for T_4 and T_3 have a disproportionate reduction in hormone concentration relative to the corresponding serum TBG level; estimations of the free hormone levels by any of the index methods give erroneous results[166,167] (Fig. 16-5).[168] One of these variants, TBG-A, is found with high frequency in Australian aborigines (allele frequency of 51 percent).[169]

TBG Excess

TBG excess (TBG-E) has a lower prevalence than TBG deficiency, with values obtained from neonatal screening programs from 1:6,000 to 1:40,000.[170,171] Considering that some newborn may have noninherited, transient TBG excess, a conservative overall estimate of inherited TBG-E would be 1:25,000.[172]

The molecular basis of TBG excess has remained elusive. The molecule has properties identical to TBG-C. Thus, it is not surprising that complete sequencing of the coding regions derived from a subject with inherited TBG-E failed to show any defects.[173]

TBG Variants with Unaltered TBG Concentrations in Serum

Six TBG variants have been identified that present with normal or clinically insignificant alterations in their concentration in serum. Four occur with high frequency in some population groups and thus can be considered polymorphic. TBG-Poly (Fig. 16-4), with no alterations of its physical or biologic properties, has been detected in 16 and 20 percent of the French Canadian and Japanese populations, respectively.[161,165] TBG-S exhibits a slower mobility on polyacrylamide gel electrophoresis and cathodal shift on IEF, owing to the loss of a negative change due to the replacement of the normal Asp-171 by Asn[174] (Fig. 16-4). It has an allele frequency of 5 to 16 percent in black populations of African origin and 2 to 10 percent in Pacific Islanders. The molecular structure of two other polymorphic TBG variants has not been identified. TBG-F has an allele frequency of 3.2 percent in Eskimos residing on the Kodiak and St. Lawrence islands. It has a slight anodal (fast) mobility on IEF.[175] TBG-C1 has been recently identified in subjects inhabiting two Mali villages.[176] It has a small cathodal shift on IEF and an allele frequency of 5.1 percent. TBG-Cgo, resistant to high temperatures,[177] has normal affinity for T_4 and T_3. Its molecular basis has been recently identified.[178] Structure modeling suggests that the replacement of the normal Tyr-309 by Phe (Fig. 16-4) ties one of the α-helices to the molecule, thus stabilizing its tertiary structure. A new variant TBG, TBG-Houston (TBG-H), has been also recently identified.[179] It has normal electrophoretic and physical properties and is present in normal concentration in serum. However, due to relatively marked reduction in thyroid hormone-binding affinity, subjects present with serum T_4 and T_3 levels almost as low as those found in subjects with complete TBG deficiency. Although the structural defect of this TBG variant has not been identified, the mutation is likely to involve a crucial site in the ligand-binding domain of the molecule.

Biologic Consequences of Mutations in the TBG Gene

Researchers have investigated the mechanisms whereby structural abnormalities of the TBG molecule produce the variant phenotypes by expressing some of these molecules in living cells. Contrary to previous speculation, intracellular retention and degradation of the defective TBG molecules, rather than increased extracellular degradation due to in-

stability, is responsible for their presence in low concentrations in serum.[180–183] Of note is the full intracellular retention of TBG-CD5 despite synthesis in normal quantities. A single amino acid substitution in TBG-CD5 is sufficient to alter its tertiary structure and thus prevent export. The same finding in the case of TBG-CDJ has been traced to its retention within the endoplasmic reticulum. Furthermore, the increased amount of GRP78 mRNA in cells transfected with TBG-PDJ suggests that association of this TBG variant with the GRP78 molecular chaperon is responsible for its impaired secretion.[183]

Transthyretin Defects

Sequencing of the transthyretin (TTR) gene, formerly known as thyroxine-binding prealbumin (TBPA) on chromosome 18 (18q11.2-q12.1), has uncovered mutations that produce variant TTR molecules with or without alterations in the binding affinity for iodothyronines.[156] Only those known to affect iodothyronine binding are listed in Table 16-3. Some of the TTR variants are responsible for the dominantly inherited *familial amyloidotic polyneuropaty (FAP)*, which causes, multiple organ failure and death in early adulthood.[194] Because TTR has a relatively lower affinity for T_4 (100-fold less than that of TBG), it plays a minor role in thyroid hormone

TABLE 16-3. TTR Variants with Altered Affinity for T_4 and Potentially an Effect on Tests of Thyroid Function in Serum

Affinity for T_4 Mutant/Normal		TTR Concentration	Codon Number	Amino Acid (Normal → Variant)	References
Homo[a]	Hetero[a]				
Decreased[b]					
<0.1	0.17–0.41	N	30	Val → Met	184, 185
	0.54		58	Leu → His	185
	0.45		77	Ser → Tyr	185
	0.19–0.46	N	84	Ile → Ser	184, 185
~1.0	0.44		122	Val → Ile	185
Increased					
	3.5†	N	6	Gly → Ser	185, 187, 188
	3.2–3.9	N	109	Ala → Thr	185, 189
	1–2.1	↑ or N	119	Thr → Met	190, 191, 192, 193

[a] HOMO, homozygous; HETERO, heterozygous.
[b] Probably overestimated since the subjects harboring this TTR variant have normal serum TT$_4$ concentrations. Variant TTR tested and shown not to have altered affinity to T_4 are Ala-60, (heter)[184,185]

N, normal; ↑, increased.

Endonucleases useful in the identification of TTR variants: Msp I −ve for Ser-6 in exon 2 associated PHA; Fnu 4H −ve for Thr-109 and Nco I +ve for Met-119, both in exon 4.

transport in blood. Accordingly, changes in the TTR concentration in serum and variant TTRs with reduced affinity for T_4 have little effect on the concentration of serum T_4.[184,195] Only variant TTRs with increased affinity for iodothyronines produce significant elevation in serum T_4 and rT_3 concentrations and account for 2 percent of subjects with euthyroid hyperthyroxinemia.[191]

A family with elevated total T_4 concentration that was predominantly bound to TTR was first described in 1982.[196] The inheritance was autosomal dominant, and affected members were clinically euthyroid with normal free T_4 levels measured by equilibrium dialysis. The variant TTR has a single nucleotide substitution replacing the normal Ala-109 with a Thr that increases its affinity for T_4, rT_3, and 3,3′,5,5′-tetraiodothyroacetic acid (TETRAC).[189] Crystallographic analysis of this variant TTR revealed an alteration in the size of the T_4-binding pocket.[197]

A more common defect found in subjects with *pre-albumin-associated hyperthyroxinemia (PHA)* is a point mutation in exon 4 of the TTR gene replacing the normal Thr-119 with Met.[191] First described in a single individual with normal serum total and free T_4 levels,[190] the majority of subsequently identified heterozygous subjects harboring the TTR Met-119 had an increase in the fraction of T_4 and rT_3 associated with TTR, but only few had serum T_4 levels above the upper limit of normal. Furthermore, their hyperthyroxinemia appears to be transient, usually in association with nonthyroidal illness.[191] The variant TTRs associated with PHA are not amyloidogenic.

Albumin Defects

Another form of dominantly inherited euthyroid hyperthyroxinemia, later to be linked to the albumin gene on chromosome 4 (4q11–q13), was first described in 1979.[198,199] Known as *familial dysalbuminemic hyperthyroxinemia (FDH)*,[200] it is the most common cause of inherited increase in total T_4 in serum in the Caucasian population. In a study of 430 subjects suspected of having euthyroid hyperthyroxinemia, 12 percent were proven to have FDH.[191] The prevalence varies from 0.01 to 1.8 percent, depending on ethnic origin, with the highest prevalence in Hispanics.[201–204] No FDH has been reported in subjects of African or Asian origin. The euthyroid status of subjects with FDH has been confirmed by normal

TSH response to TRH, normal free T_4 concentration measured by equilibrium dialysis using appropriate buffer systems, normal T_4 production rate, and normal serum sex hormone–binding globulin concentration.[198,200,205,206] Nevertheless, the falsely elevated free T_4 value, when estimated by standard clinical laboratory techniques, has often resulted in inappropriate thyroid gland ablative or drug therapy.[207–209]

FDH is suspected when serum total T_4 concentration is increased without proportional elevation in total T_3 level and nonsuppressed serum TSH. Half of affected subjects have also rT_3 values above the normal range.[210] Since the same combination of test results is found in subjects with the Thr-109 TTR variant, the diagnosis of FDH should be confirmed by the demonstration that an increased proportion of the total serum T_4 migrates with ALB on nondenaturing electrophoresis or precipitates with anti-ALB serum.

A tight linkage between FDH and the ALB gene (logarithm of the odds ratio [LOD] score 5.25) was found in a large Swiss Amish family using two polymorphic markers.[210] This was followed by the identification of a missense mutation in codon 218 of the ALB gene replacing the normal Arg with His.[211,212] Furthermore, the same mutation was present in all subjects with FDH from 11 unrelated families. Its association with a Sac I+ polymorphism suggests a founder effect and is compatible with ethnic predilection of FDH.[212] The coexistence of FDH and a TTR variant with increased affinity for T_4 in the same individual[186,188] and FDH with TBG-PD in another[213] has been reported. In both instances these individuals were the product of parents each heterozygous for one of the two defects.

DEFECTS OF THYROID HORMONE ACTION

During the last 5 years considerable knowledge has been gained concerning the molecular events that mediate thyroid hormone action at the intracellular level. The interplay of thyroid hormone receptors (TRs), auxiliary nuclear transcription factors (TRAPs), and thyroid hormone response elements (TREs), their multiplicity and in-tissue specificity are beginning to explain the diversity as well as the complexity of thyroid hormone action (see Ch. 3). When tissue sensitivity to thyroid hormone appears to be reduced because increased serum free hormone does not suppress TSH and is not accompanied by stigmata indicative of thyrotoxicosis, a defect in thyroid hormone action is usually considered. This can, theoretically, be due to reduced hormone transfer into cells, faulty metabolism of T_4 required for hormone activation, or a true defect of hormone action resulting from abnormalities in the steps involving its expression. The term resistance to thyroid hormone encompasses inherited defects at the site of hormone action, the cell nucleus.

Resistance to Thyroid Hormone

Resistance to thyroid hormone (RTH) is a clinically heterogeneous syndrome characterized by reduced responses of target tissues to a supply of thyroid hormone that under normal circumstances would be excessive. RTH was originally described in 1967.[214] It involved a 6-year-old girl who sustained injuries in a car accident. Radiologic evaluation disclosed stippling of all major secondary ossification centers. She was also deaf, mute, and her thyroid gland was slightly enlarged. Since these findings are usually encountered in individuals deficient in thyroid hormone during infancy and early childhood, measurement of her PBI in serum was obtained, which at the time was the routine test for the estimation of thyroid hormone content. Surprisingly, the value was high and in agreement with the absence of other signs and symptoms of thyroid hormone deprivation. However, the high PBI value also was not in agreement with the lack of manifestations commonly associated with thyroid hormone excess. These unusual features led to further studies in the key subject and two of her siblings, who exhibited the same abnormalities of bones, thyroid gland, and PBI, as well as in three normal siblings and consanguineous parents. The results were rather unexpected. The children had not only normal metabolism, but we failed to demonstrate the presence of any of the known inborn errors of thyroid hormone synthesis. Data suggested that the disorder was due to partial failure of body tissues to recognize thyroid hormone, later termed the *syndrome of generalized resistance to thyroid hormone* (GRTH). The crucial experiments that removed any doubt that the defect was at the level of target tissues were the demonstration that the T_3 of the affected subjects and its precursor,

T_4, were the natural and active L-isomers and that administration of large doses of these thyroid hormones were required to observe an effect in the same individuals.[215]

A subject with RTH

J.F. the proband, was 3 years old when delayed verbal expression and hyperactivity led to the diagnosis of attention deficit hyperactivity disorder (ADHD). Treatment with methylphenidate failed to produce beneficial effects. At 5.5 years of age, thyroid gland enlargement and elevated serum T_4 and T_3 levels were interpreted as indictive of thyrotoxicosis. Treatment with propylthioracil also did not result in symptomatic improvement. As a matter of fact, normalization of the thyroid hormone levels in blood slowed his growth rate and substantially augmented the size of his goiter as a consequence of a striking increase in in serum TSH concentration to 175 μU/ml.

Although no family history of thyroid disease could be elicited, the father had also had delayed speech development, hyperactivity, and learning disability. However, he did graduate from high school, proceeded to obtain a master's degree, and became the principal of an elementary school.

On physical examination, 2 months without any therapy, revealed a child of poor attention span and immature speech. Other than sinus tachycardia and a diffuse thyroid gland enlargement (35 g estimated weight), there were no other physical stigmata of thyrotoxicosis or hypothyroidism. His height and weight were at the 75th percentile for his chronologic age of 6.5 years.

Total concentrations of T_4 and T_3 in serum were high at 24.7 μg/dl (normal range 5 to 12) and 369 ng/dl (normal range 90 to 210), respectively. TBG concentration was normal and the FT_{4I} was 25.1 (normal range 6.0 to 10.5), with a normal serum TSH concentration of 2.3 μU/ml that increased to 23.5 μU/ml 30 minutes following the intravenous administration of TRH. While he showed expressive deficit (verbal IQ of 85 percent), his performance IQ was 120 percent.

The responses to the administration of graded doses of L-T3 were examined in the proband and his father, who showed at base line the same thyroid test abnormalities. Doses of L-T3 that achieved highly elevated serum levels of T_3 (from 600 to 1,000 ng/dl) and that completely suppress serum TSH and its response to TRH in normal individuals, had only a partial suppressive effect in the proband and his father. Furthermore, attenuated or paradoxic effects of L-T_3 on peripheral tissues were also observed. These included changes in serum cholesterol, sex hormone–binding globulin, and ferritin. Also there was no significant increase in the sleeping heart rate and basal metabolic rate. Most revealing was the failure of supraphysiologic doses of L-T$_4$ to increase the excretion of urea nitrogen. As a matter of fact, the reduction in this measurement suggested an anabolic rather than a catabolic effect of this large amount of thyroid hormone.

Reduced responses of L-T$_3$ in skin fibroblasts from these subjects, grown in tissue culture, established the intracellular nature of their defect; these same fibroblasts served to later identify their inherited defect in the TRβ gene.[216]

Interpretation

A characteristic of RTH is the paucity of clinical manifestations. In all subjects so far identified, the defect has been only partial, probably because a complete insensitivity to thyroid hormone would be incompatible with life. This conclusion is based on the observation that the consequences of untreated hypothyroidism in athyreotic neonates are more devastating than those of untreated subjects resistant to thyroid hormone. Usually the syndrome of resistance to thyroid hormone is first suspected when serum thyroid hormone levels are found to be elevated in association with nonsuppressed TSH and in the absence of intercurrent illness, drugs, or alterations of thyroid hormone–binding serum proteins. More importantly, full replacement doses of thyroid hormone fail to produce the expected degree of suppression on the secretion of TSH and/or induce the appropriate responses in peripheral tissues.

Classification

Until very recently, RTH has been subclassified into various forms; these are based on clinical observations owing to the paucity of specific tests for determining hormone responsiveness at the level of the different target tissues. The majority of cases appeared to have generalized tissue resistance to thyroid hormone (GRTH), in which the participation of the pituitary thyrotrophs provided a mechanism of partial compensation of the defect through an increase in the synthesis and secretion of thyroid hormone. Isolated pituitary resistance to thyroid hormone (PRTH) was assigned to a few cases with apparent signs of hypermetabolism and a preponderance for sporadic occurrence. Isolated peripheral tissue resistance to thyroid hormone (PTRTH) has been reported in only one individual.[217]

Doubts were later expressed that GRTH and PRTH represent distinct entities because subjects with tachycardia, commonly responsible for assigning the diagnosis or PRTH, had objective evidence for resistance to thyroid hormone in tissues other than the pituitary.[218,29] A recent study showed no significant differences in clinical features or laboratory findings in 312 patients with presumed GRTH compared to 72 with PRTH, pointing to the subjective nature of the subclassification of RTH.[220] This is further supported by the identification of identical mutations in families formerly classified as GRTH and PRTH.[221] Although the First Workshop on Thyroid Hormone Resistance (Cambridge, UK, 1993) recommended that the term RTH be adopted to describe the syndrome, the qualification of "generalized" and "pituitary" was not abolished because its descriptive value was considered to be useful to clinicians.

Prevalence and Inheritance

The prevalence of GRTH is unknown. Since the first report in 1967,[214] more than 450 cases have been identified, 349 of which have been reviewed in detail.[219] Most are familial, with the 13 percent of sporadic cases corresponding to the incidence of do novo mutations (see below). Inheritance is autosomal dominant, with the exception of then key family in which transmission was clearly recessive.[222] Contrary to most thyroid diseases that affect predominantly females, RTH has been found with equal frequency in both genders. The condition has a wide geographic distribution, having been reported in Caucasians, Orientals, and blacks. However, the prevalence may vary among different ethnic groups.

Clinical Features

The majority of untreated subjects maintain a normal metabolic state at the expense of high levels of thyroid hormone. The degree of this compensation of tissue hyposensitivity to the hormone is, however, variable among individuals, as well as in different tissues. As a consequence, clinical and laboratory evidence of thyroid hormone deficiency and excess often coexist. For example, RTH can present with mild to moderate growth retardation and delayed bone maturation, along with hyperactivity and tachycardia. More importantly, the clinical manifestations of RTH are often influenced by the effect of inappropriate treatment intended to normalize the thyroid hormone level but which aggravate further the delay in growth and development.[223]

Goiter has been by far the most common clinical finding (38 percent of cases), which has led to the suspicion of thyroid gland dysfunction has prompted further testing (Fig. 6-1). Next in order of frequency, clinical manifestations leading to the identification of key family cases are hyperactivity or learning disability (10 percent) and developmental delay (8 percent), followed by tachycardia (7 percent). Thus, symptoms and signs in subjects with RTH have suggested both thyrotoxicosis and hypothyroidism. Careful evaluation of subjects with GRTH has shown that almost one-half have some degree of learning disability with or without attention deficit hyperactivity disorder (ADHD).[219,224] One-quarter have intellectual quotients (IQ) lesser than 85 percent, but frank mental retardation (IQ <60) has been found only in 3 percent of cases. Impaired mental function was found to be associated with impaired or delayed growth (<5th percentile) in 20 percent of subjects, through growth retardation alone is rare (4 percent).[219] Despite the high prevalence of ADHD in patients with RTH, the occurrence of RTH in children with ADHD must be very rare, none having been detected in 330 such children studied.[225,226] Furthermore, current data do not support a genetic linkage of RTH with ADHD. Rather the association with low IQ scores may confer a higher likelihood for subjects with RTH to exhibit ADHD symptoms.[227]

Diagnosis

Diagnostic procedures need to be initiated only after persistence of elevated serum T_4 and T_3 concentrations in association with nonsuppressed TSH levels has been confirmed on samples obtained several weeks apart. Normal T_3 levels are typical of FDH (see preceding section). This condition as well as TBG excess or the presence of antibodies to T_3 and T_4 can be excluded by specific tests and by measurement of the free T_4 and T_3 levels.

Because of the occurrence of subclinical thyrotoxicosis, current diagnostic evaluation relies on a number of dynamic tests based on the responses to substances known to either stimulate or suppress TSH. Any of the following results are strongly suggestive of a TSH-producing adenoma: (1) failure of serum TSH to appropriately increase in response to TRH, (2) failure of serum TSH to decrease in response to supraphysiologic doses of thyroid hormone, and (3) an increase of the pituitary glycoprotein α subunit to whole TSH ratio.[228]

Several tests that are altered by thyroid hormone through its effects on peripheral tissues have potential diagnostic value. They are serum sex hormone–binding globulin, ferritin, angiotensin-converting enzyme, cholesterol, triglycerides, carotene and creatine phosphokinase; urine hydroxyproline, carnitine, and magnesium; and measurement of sleeping pulse, basal metabolic rate (BMR), cardiac contractility by echocardiography and deep tendon reflex relaxation time. However, because of considerable overlap of values between hyperthyroid, euthyroid, and hypothyroid subjects, they are useful only if changes in their response to the administration of thyroid hormone are compared to the individual's baseline results (Fig. 16-7).

Genetics

Using the technique of restriction fragment length polymorphism (RFLP), Usala et al.[229] were first to demonstrate linkage between a TR β locus on chromosome 3 and the RTH phenotype. Subsequent studies at the University of Chicago and at the National Institutes of Health have identified distinct point mutations in the TR β gene of two unrelated families with RTH.[216,230] In both families only one of the two TR β alleles was involved, compatible with the apparent dominant mode of inheritance.

Mutations in the TR β gene have now been identified in subjects with RTH belonging to 94 families (Table 16-4). All mutations are located in the TR β gene and involve the functionally relevant areas of the T_3-binding domain (see below). Since only 56 of the mutations identified in 94 families are unique, 38 occur in more than one family. Haplotyping by analysis of satellite DNA has established that in most instances identical mutations among families have occurred independently.[237] Furthermore, the frequency of de novo mutations (those that occurred within the last 50 years) is 13 percent (Table 16-4). The majority of mutations involve a single nucleotide substitution resulting in the replacement of an amino acid and in two cases a truncated receptor protein due to a translation terminator codon. In three instances, a three-base deletion resulted in the

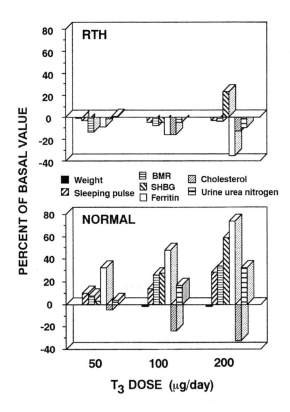

Fig. 16-7. Responses of peripheral tissues to the administration of L-T₃. Each L-T₃ dose level was given for three consecutive days and was administered in six doses every 12 hours. Average responses for each parameter and treatment period are expressed as percent increment (+) or decrement (−) from the corresponding mean basal value. Results of a patient with GRTH are compared to those of a normal relative. Serum levels of T₃ achieved on each dose of L-T₃ were comparable or higher to those of the normal subject, yet the responses in the patient with RTH are clearly attenuated. (Adapted from Sakurai,[216] with permission.)

loss of an amino acid and in three others a frameshift was caused by single nucleotide deletion or insertion and seven-base duplication, respectively. Deletion of all coding regions of the TR β gene has been encountered in only one family (F1) representing the only example of recessive inheritance of RTH. Sixty-nine percent of mutations occur in CG-rich areas (four or more consecutive Cs or Gs) and, in particular, in CpG dinucleotide hot spots (47 percent),[237] which are frequent sites of polymorphism in humans. It is thus not surprising that of the 11 mutations identified in more than one family, 9 occurred in CpG hot

spots, that are also frequently the sites for de novo mutations. Most notable is the C to T transition in codon 338 replacing the normal Arg (CGG) with Trp (TGG), which has been detected in 10 families. Four different amino acid replacements have been identified in codons 345 and 453. Silent mutations (codons 319 and 417) were found in conjunction with missense mutations in two families, F100 and F45, respectively.

No mutations have been so far detected in the TR α gene, which suggests that either its products may play a minor role in TSH regulation or that TR α defects are lethal.

Molecular Basis

With the exception of the family with TR β deletion, all mutations are localized in the T₃-binding domain of the TR β gene, resulting in variable reduction of the affinity of the receptor for T₃ but normal binding to TRE. They are clustered in two mutational "hot" areas spanning codons 310 to 349 and 429 to 460 (Fig. 16-8). Not a single mutation has been so far identified in the "cold" area, though it is not devoid of mutational CpG hot spots. Introduction of artificial mutations in this cold area, according to the hot spot mutational rule, yielded mutant TR β with either normal T₃-binding affinity of impairments of a lesser degree than that of natural mutations with the mildest functional and clinical defect.[238] Thus, natural mutations expected to occur in the cold region of the TR β should fail to manifest as RTH and would escape detection.

The family with deletion of all coding sequences of the TR β but intact TR α exhibited an autosomal-recessive inheritance of RTH. Thus, complete absence of the TR β is compatible with life. Since some effects of thyroid hormone could be demonstrated in these subjects, it is logical to conclude that TR α1, expressed in virtually all tissues, is capable of partially substituting for the function of TR β. In all other families, RTH is inherited in a dominant fashion, and affected individuals harbor mutations in only one of the two TR β alleles. The finding that subjects with deletion of one of the two TR β alleles have no clinical or laboratory abnormalities indicates not only that a single copy of the TR β gene is sufficient for normal function but also that the dominant inheritance of RTH, caused by point mutations in the TR β gene, is not simply due to a reduc-

TABLE 16-4. Mutations in the TR β Gene Associated with RTH, Their Location and Affinity For T_3

Kindred ID[a]	References	Nucleotides		Codons and Amino Acids	Codon Number and Amino Acids	$\dfrac{K_a \text{ Mutant}}{Ka \text{ Normal}}$
[F1]	(222)	deletion	244–1704	All deleted		
T[F109]	(231)	G → A	985	*(C)* GCC → ACC	A234T	0.34
				Ala → **Thr**		
no ID	(232)	G → A	1013	*C*GG → CAG	R243Q	
				Arg → **Gln**		
GP,8[b]	(221, 233)	T → A	1076	GTT → GAT	V264D	<0.01
				Val → **Asp**		
(XV)[F99]	(234)	T → C	1214	ATG → ACG	M310T	
				Met → **Thr**		
[F98]	(personal observation)	T → C	1223	ATG → ACG	M313T	
				Met → **Thr**		
G-H	(236)	G → A	1232	*C*GC → CAC	R316H	0.019
deG(II); 9, 10, 11	(221, 233)			A**R**g → **His**		<0.01
[F120][b]	(227, 236)					0.05
(XVIII)[F89]	(234, 236, 237)	G → A	1234	*(C)* GCT → ACT	A317T	0.16
[F52][b]	(236, 237)			Ala → **Thr**		0.16
E-D[F100][b]	(238)					0.22
Mlo	(personal observation)					0.16
AM	(221)					0.13
PC[b]	(221)					0.13
W.R.[F54]	(241)	C → T	1243	*C*GC → TGC	R320C	0.49
[F88]	(237)			Arg → **Cys**		
CL[F67]	(241)	G → A	1244	*C*GC → CAC	R320H	0.46
[F95]	(236, 237, 241)			Arg → **His**		0.42
PM 7	(221, 233)					0.38
4,5	(233)					
no ID	(221)					
SC	(221)	G → T	1244	*C*GC → CTC	R320L	0.10
GM	(221)			Arg → **Leu**		0.10
ST	(221)	A → G	1247	TAT → TGT	Y321C	0.018
				Tyr → **Cys**		
Mo	(242)	G → A	1249	GAC → A**A**C	D322N	
				Asp → **Asn**		
I-R[F110]	(243)	G → C	1249	GAC → C**A**C	D322H	0.39
				Asp → **His**		
Pt H	(244)	G → C	1275	TTG → TT**C**	L330F	0.01
				Leu → **Phe**		
(VII)F-W)[F14]	(234, 238)	G → A	1279	GGG → AGG	G322R	
				Gly → **Arg**		
BB	(221)	G → A	1280	GGG → GAG	G332E	0.02
				Gly → **Glu**		
So	(242)	G → C	1282	GAA → CAA	E333Q	
				Glu → **Gln**		
no ID	(221)	T → G	1286	ATG → AGG	M334R	
				Met → **Arg**		
S[F66]	(245)	deletion	1295–1297	A**CA** CGG → AGG	T337Δ	0.001
				Thr Arg → Arg		
[F29]	(236)	C → T	1297	*C*GG → TGG	R338W	0.21
[106]	(236)			A**R**g → **Trp**		0.21
F.E.	(246)					0.019

(Continued)

TABLE 16-4. *(Continued)*

Kindred ID[a]	References	Nucleotides		Codons and Amino Acids	Codon Number and Amino Acids	K_a Mutant Ka Normal
K-T[F111][b]	(243)					0.21
JM	(221)					0.10
RM[b]	(221)					0.10
LM	(221)					0.10
2 fam no ID	(221)					
L-F	(247)					0.23
NM	(221)	G → T	1298	CGG → CTG Arg → **Leu**	R338L	0.26
D-C(D)[F56]	(249)	G → C	1305	CAG → CAC Gln → **His**	Q340H	0.46
BK	(221)	G → A	1316	GGG → GAG Gly → **Glu**	G344 E	<0.01
Mf[F44]	(216, 249)	G → C	1318	GGT → CGT Gly → **Arg**	G345R	0.001
[F18]	(250)	G → A	1318	GGT → AGT Gly → **Ser**	G345S	<0.01
G-S[F101][b]	(250)	G → T	1319	GGT → GTT Gly → **Val**	G345V	
(VII)[F17]	(238)	G → A	1319	GGT → GAT Gly → **Asp**	G345D	
N-N[F102]	(234)	G → A	1325	GGG → GAG Gly → **Glu**	G347E	
SS	(238)	G → A	1330	GTG → ATG Val → **Met**	V349M	0.23
MS	(221)	G → A	1571	CGG → CAG Arg → **Gln**	R429Q	0.21
MA	(221)					0.21
no ID	(236, 251)					0.9 (± 0.2)
no ID,2	(221, 233)	deletion		ATG Met	M430Δ	<0.01
[F51]	(234)	T → C	1577	ATA ± ACA Ile → **Thr**	I431T	0.05
LO[b]	(221)					0.01
no ID	(221)	deletion		GGA Gly	G432Δ	<0.01
Pt B[F34]	(252)	A → T	1589	CAT → CTT His → **Leu**	H435L	
Pt C	(252)	T → A	1590	CAT → CAA His → **Gln**	H435Q	
CMa	(221)	C → T	1597	CGC → TGC Arg → **Cys**	R438C	0.30
no ID	(221)					
(XII)Mt[F45]	(234, 236, 253)	G → A	1598	CGC → CAC Arg → **His**	R438H	0.14 (0.25)
[F68]	(254)					
[F114][b]	(255)					0.25
BW	(221)					0.23
CS	(221)					0.23
GS	(221)					0.23
JH	(221)					0.23
O-K[F103]	(238)	A → G	1609	ATG → GTG Met → **Val**	M442V	0.17
K fam [F107]	(256)	A → G	1612	AAG → GAG Lys → **Glu**	K443E	0.09–0.046
DiG[F117]	(242)	G → C	1614	AAG → AAC Lys → **Asn**	K443N	<0.03
[F119]	(257)	T → C	1621	TGC → CGC Cys → **Arg**	C446R	
[F108]	(258)	C → A	1623	TGC → TGA Cys → **Stop**	C446X	
P-V[F104][b]	(238)	insertion	1627	CCC ACA → CCC **CAC** AGA Pro Thr → Pro **His Arg**	448fr shift463	<0.05

TABLE 16-4. *(Continued)*

Kindred ID[a]	References	Nucleotides		Codons and Amino Acids	Codon Number and Amino Acids	$\dfrac{K_a \text{ Mutant}}{K_a \text{ Normal}}$
T-P[F112]	(243)	T → A	1634	CTC → C**A**C Leu → **His**	L450H	0.39
Pt A [F86]	(252)	T → A	1636	TTC → **A**TC Phe → **Ile**	F451I	
no ID	(259)	T → A C → A	1637 1638	TTC → T**AA** Phe → **Stop**	F451X	
BN	(221)	7 base duplication	1638	A CTC TTC **ACT CTT CCC** CCC TTT Leu Phe **Thr Pro** Pro Pro **Phe**	452fr shift463	<0.01
no ID	(260)	3 base deletion	1639–1641	TTC CCC CCT → TTC CCT Phe Pro Pro → Phe Pro	P452Δ	
Q-W[F105] [F85] SH[b] PA	(238) (261) (221) (221)	C → A	1642	CCT → **A**CT Pro → **Thr**	P453T	0.41 0.46 0.20 0.20
(X)[F27] [F94] MC	(234, 262) (262) (221)	C → T	1642	CCT → **T**CT Pro → **Ser**	P453S	0.36
TB	(221)	C → G	1642	CCT → **G**CT Pro → **Ala**	P453A	0.17
A (Mh) [F22]	(230, 234, 263)	C → A	1643	CCT → C**A**T	P453H	0.16
no ID	(221)			Pro → **His**		
XI[F26]	(234)	insertion	1644	CCT **T**TG → CCC TTT GTT Pro Leu → Pro **Phe Val**	454fr shift463	
R-L[F113]	(243)	T → G	1661	TTC → T**G**C Phe → **Cys**	F459C	0.33
MP	(221)	G → A	1663	(C) GAG → **A**AG Glu → **Lys**	E460K	0.25

[a] Numbers preceded by F and in square brackets represent family members according Refetoff et al.[219]

[b] De novo mutations.

tion in the amount of the normal TR β. This finding supports the hypothesis that the mechanism of dominant inheritance of RTH requires the interference of a mutant TR with the function of the normal TR (dominant negative effect).

Early work has postulated three mechanisms to explain the dominant negative effect of a mutant TR (mTR) based on the cotransfection of a mTR β with the normal (wild type) TR (wTR).[264–266] They are (1) competition of mTR with wTR at the level of TRE, (2) heterodimer formation between mTR and TRAP that exhausts a limited amount of cofactor (squelching), and (3) formation of inactive mTR/wTR dimers. It is likely that all three mechanisms are operative, though dimerization appears to play a central role since when prevented by the introduc-

tion of a second mutation, the dominant negative effect of a mTR is abrogated.[267] It remains, however, unclear whether homodimerization of two mTRs[249,268] or heterodimers between a mTR with a cofactor[267,269] play a major role. The dominant negative effect of mTRs is undoubtedly more complex, since preferential formation of the different dimeric forms appears to vary with the substituted amino acid in the mTR[270] and is influenced by other nuclear factors and the structure of the various TREs.

Of interest are the observations made in one subject with homozygous deletion of Thr-337 in the TR β gene belonging to a family with dominantly inherited RTH (F66). This subject manifested the most severe form of RTH with signs of both hypo- and hyperthyroidism despite astronomic levels of thy-

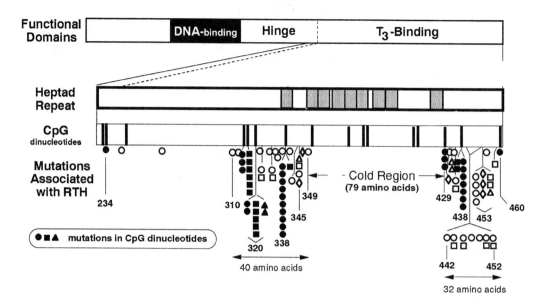

Fig. 16-8. Location of natural mutations in the TR β gene associated with RTH. Schematic representation of the TR β and its functional domains for interaction with TREs (DNA-binding) and hormone (T₃-binding). The latter domain is expanded and the locations of the 56 different mutations detected in 93 unrelated families are indicated by dots. Identical mutations in members of unrelated families are indicated by the same shading pattern of vertically placed dots. Note the "cold region" of 79 amino acids devoid of mutations associated with RTH. Amino acids are numbered consecutively starting at the amino terminus of the molecule.

roid hormone.[245,271] The severe hypothyroidism manifested in bone and brain of this subject is explained by the interference of the double dose mTR with the function of TR α, a situation that does not occur in homozygous subjects with TR β deletion. In contrast, manifestations of thyrotoxicosis in other tissues may be explained by the effect high thyroid levels have on tissues that normally express predominantly TR α1.

The earlier expectation that differences in functional impairment resulting from a particular amino acid substitution in a mutant TR β would explain the variable manifestations of RTH was not borne out. In fact, the in vitro potency of dominant negative activity of mutant TR βs appears to correlate better with the RTH phenotype than the impairment of their T₃ binding.[272] Furthermore, the phenotype of RTH may vary among individuals harboring the same TR β mutation not only among families but also in affected members of the same family.[235,237,241] The most striking example is the mutation R316H, which in family G.H. did not cosegregate with the RTH phenotype.[235] Indeed, only one of three members of this family harboring the TR β

mutation presented symptoms and serum thyroid hormone and TSH abnormalities typical of RTH. This variability in clinical and laboratory manifestations was not observed in affected members of two other families harboring the same mutation.[221,227] While the precise mechanism of intrafamilial heterogeneity in RTH remains unknown, studies in a large family with the R320H TR β mutation suggest that genetic variability of factors other than TR that contribute to the action of thyroid hormone may modulate the phenotype of RTH.[241]

Of interest is a recent study carried out with the TR β mutant R429Q, which has normal affinity for T₃.[236,251] While this mutant TR β mediated a normal transactivation on positive TREs, it exhibited a reduced constitutive activation through a negative TRE and thus a weaker T₃-mediated inhibition. This mutant TR β possesses properties that could impair selectively the action of T₃ on thyrotrophs.

Treatment

No specific treatment is available to fully correct the defect. The ability to identify specific mutations in the TR β provides a mean for prenatal diagnosis and family counseling. In subjects adequately compensated by an increase of the endogenous supply of thyroid hormone, no further treatment is required. In those subjects in whom compensation appears to be incomplete, judicious administration of supraphysiologic doses of the hormone is indicated. Requirements should be determined on an individual basis by assessing tissue responses to incremental doses of the hormone. In children, particular attention must be paid to growth, bone maturation, and mental development. The emergence of a catabolic state is an indication of overtreatment. Adults who have received ablative therapy due to erroneous diagnosis and thus have limited thyroidal reserve also need treatment with thyroid hormone. Suppression of the elevated serum TSH values is an appropriate guide to therapy.

Pituitary Defect in Generating T_3 from T_4

The most convincing evidence for the existence of inherited impairment of the pituitary to generate T_3 from T_4 is contained in a report by Rösler et al.[273] It deals with six women belonging to three generations of the same family with high serum levels of T_4 and T_3, elevated serum TSH concentrations, and increased thyroidal radioiodide uptake. The appropriate response of peripheral tissues to the elevated thyroid hormone levels was documented not only by the clinical symptoms and signs of thyrotoxicosis but also by the unequivocal presence of hypermetabolism with BMR values ranging from +32 to +100 percent. Thus, these individuals fulfill the criteria for PRTH. However, contrary to all other individuals presumed to have PRTH, administration of physiologic doses of L-T_3 but not L-T_4 normalized their serum T_4, T_3, and TSH levels as well as their BMR and induced goiter regression as well as a complete remission of the clinical manifestations of thyroid hormone excess. The apparent paradox of normalization of serum T_3 levels by the administration of L-T_3 was achieved by giving this short-acting hormone in a single daily dose which produced an acute but brief rise in the serum T_3 concentration sufficient to suppress TSH secretion. This, in turn, reduced the excessive synthesis and release of T_4 that, prior to L-T_3 treatment served as a continual source of T_3 generated in peripheral tissues. As suggested by the authors, the etiology of apparent PRTH in this family may be explained by a selective abnormality or deficiency in type II 5'-deiodinase, an enzyme pres-

ent in the pituitary but not in most peripheral tissues (see Ch. 4). However, as about 50 percent of nuclear T_3 in the thyrothroph is derived from intracellular generation from T_4,[273a] selective inhibition of T_4 transport into the pituitary may be an alternative explanation. Decreased transport of T_4 but not of T_3 into the liver has recently been described in an isolated case.[273b] This defect results in increased serum total and free T_4 and low serum T_3, as the liver plays a dominant role in the production of plasma T_3. Two other isolated cases showed the same pattern, i.e. high total and free serum T_4, low serum T_3. Normal serum TSH and normal serum thyroid hormone binding-proteins have been described[273c,d] but no further analysis was conducted in these cases as to the cause of the abnormalities. In one of these patients signs of tissue hypothyroidism were detected, that disappeared upon treatment with physiological doses of L–T_3.[273c]

REFERENCES

1. Dumont JE, Vassart G, Refetoff S: Thyroid disorders. In Scriver CR, Beaudet AL, Sly WS, Valle D (eds): The Metabolic Basis of Inherited Disease II. 6th ed. p. 1843. McGraw-Hill, New York, 1989
2. Lever EG, Medeiros-Neto GA, DeGroot LJ: Inherited disorders of thyroid metabolism. Endocr Rev 4: 213, 1983
3. Ryan M, DeGroot L: Congenital defects in hormone formation and action. In DeGroot, LJ (ed): Endocrinology. p. 784. WB Saunders, Philadelphia, 1989
4. Wolff J: Iodide concentrating mechanism. In Rall JE, Kopin IJ (eds): The Thyroid and Biogenic Amines. Chapter 8. North Holland Publishing Co, Amsterdam, 1972
5. Saito K, Yamamoto K, Yoshida S et al: Goitrous hypothyroidism due to iodide-trapping defect. J Clin Endocrinol Metab 53:1267, 1981
6. Wolff J: Congenital goiter with defective iodide transport. Endocr Rev 4,420, 1983
7. Vulsma T, Rammeloo JA, Gons MH, de Vijlder JJ: The role of serum thyroglobulin concentration and thyroid ultrasound imaging in the detection of iodide transport defects in infants. Acta Endocrinol 124:405, 1991
8. Stanbury JB, Chapman EM: Congenital hypothyroidism with goitre: Absence of an iodide-concentrating mechanism. Lancet 1:1162, 1960
9. Wolff J, Thompson RH, Robbins J: Congenital goitrous cretinism due to absence of iodide-concentrating ability. J Clin Endocrinol 24:699, 1964
10. Gilboa V, Ber A, Lewitis Z, Hasenfratz J: Goitrous

myxedema due to iodide trapping defect. Arch Intern Med 112:212, 1963

11. Papadopoulos SN, Vagenakis AG, Moschos A et al: A case of a partial defect of the iodide trapping mechanism. J Clin Endocrinol 30:302, 1970

12. Medeiros-Neto GA, Bloise W, Uloah-Cintra A: Partial defect of iodide trapping mechanism in two siblings with congenital goiter and hypothyroidism. J Clin Endocrinol Metab 35:370, 1972

13. Toyoshima K, Matsumoto Y, Nishida M, Yabuuchi H: Five cases of absence of iodide concentrating mechanism. Acta Endocrinol 84:527, 1977

14. Pannal PR, Steyn AF, Van Reenen O: Iodide-trapping defect of the thyroid. SA Med J 53:414, 1978

15. Struwe FrE, Seseke G, Kempe H, Hoffman G: Seltene Form der Hypothyreose bei Geschwietern (Jodakkumulationsstörung). Mschr Kinderheilk 117:189, 1969

16. Léger FA, Doumith R, Courpotin C, Helal OB et al: Complete iodide trapping defect in two cases with congenital hypothyroidism: adaptation of thyroid to huge iodide supplementation. Eur J Clin Invest 17:249, 1987

17. Albero R, Cerdan A, Sanchez-Franco F: Congenital hypothyroidism from complete iodide transport defect: long-term evolution with iodide treatment. Postgrad Med J 63:1043, 1987

18. Stanbury JB, Hedge AN: A study of a family of goitrous cretins. J Clin Endocrinol 10:1471, 1950

19. Stanbury JB, Ohela K, Pitt-Rivers R: The metabolism of iodine in 2 goitrous cretins compared with that in 2 patients receiving methimazole. J Clin Endocrinol Metab 15:54, 1955

20. Perez-Cuvit E, Crigler JF Jr, Stanbury JB: Partial and total iodide organification defect in different subships in a kindred. Am J Hum Genet 29:142, 1977

21. Murray IPC, Stewart RDH: An evaluation of the perchlorate discharge test. J Clin Endocrinol Metab 26:1050, 1966

22. Jaffiol C, Baldet L, Khalil R, Mirouze J: Confrontation de deux techniques d'etude du test au thiocyanate de potassium. Application cliniques. Ann Endocrinol 30:447, 1969

23. Haddad HM, Sidbury JB Jr: Defect of the iodinating system in congenital goitrous cretinism: Report of a case with biochemical studies. J Clin Endocrinol Metab 19:1446, 1959

24. Pommier J, Tourniaire J, Rahmoun B et al: Thyroid iodine organification defects: a case with lack of thyroglobulin iodination and a case without any peroxidase activity. J Clin Endocrinol Metab 42:319, 1976

25. Medeiros-Neto GA, Knobel M, Yamamoto K et al: Deficient thyroid peroxidase causing organification

defect and goitrous hypothyroidism. J Endocrinol Invest 2:353, 1979

26. Valenta LJ, Bode H, Vickery A et al: Lack of thyroid peroxidase activity as the cause of congenital goitrous hypothyroidism. J Clin Endocrinol Metab 36:830, 1973

27. Eggo MC, Burrow GN, Alexander NM, Gordon JH: Iodination and the structure of human thyroglobulin. J Clin Endocrinol Metab 51:7, 1980

28. Niepomniszcze H, Degrossi OJ, Scavini LM, Curutchet HP: Familial goiter with partial iodine incorporation block and euthyroidism due to the deficient peroxidase defect. p. 470. In Thyroid Research, 7th International Thyroid Conference Boston, 1976

29. Niepomniszcze H, Castells S, DeGroot LJ et al: Peroxidase defect in congenital goiter with complete organification block. J Clin Endocrinol Metab 36:347, 1973

30. Abramovicz MJ et al: Identification of a mutation in the coding sequence of the human thyroid peroxidase gene causing congenital goiter. J Clin Invest 90:1200, 1992

31. Bikker H, den Hartog MT, Baas F et al: A 20-basepair duplication in the human thyroid peroxidase gene results in a total iodide organification defect and congenital hypothyrodism. J Clin Endocrinol Metab 79:248, 1994

32. Niepomniszcze H, Rosenbloom AL, DeGroot LJ et al: Differentiation of two abnormalities in thyroid peroxidase causing organification defect and goitrous hypothyroidism. Metabolism 24:57, 1975

33. Niepomniszcze H, DeGroot LJ, Hagen GA: Abnormal thyroid peroxidase causing iodide organification. J Clin Endocrinol Metab 34:607, 1972

34. Pommier J, Tourniaire J, Deme D et al: A defective thyroid peroxidase solubilized from a familial goite with iodine organification defect. J Clin Endocrinol Metab 39:69, 1979

35. Medeiros-Neto GA, Nakashima T, Taurog A et al: Congenital goitre and hypothyroidism with impaired iodide organification and high thyroid peroxidase concentration. Clin Endocrinol 11:123, 1979

36. Pommier J, Dominici R, Bougneres P et al: A dialysable inhibitor bound to thyroglobulin and from two goitres with iodine organification defect. J Molec Med 2:169, 1977

37. Sjollema BE, den Hartog MT, de Vijlder JJ et al: Congenital hypothyroidism in two cats due to defective organification: data suggesting loosely anchored thyroperoxidase. Acta Endocrinol 125:435, 1991

38. Kusakabe T: Deficient cytochrome b$_5$ reductase activity in nontoxic goiter with iodide organification defect. Metabolism 24:1103, 1975

39. Niepomniszcze H, Targovnik HM, Gluzman BE,

Curutchet P: Abnormal H_2O_2 supply in the thyroid of a patient with goiter and iodine organification defect. J Clin Endocrinol Metab 65:344, 1987

40. Kusakabe T: Goitrous subject with defective synthesis of diiodotyrosine due to thyroglobulin abnormalities. J Clin Endocrinol Metab 37:317, 1973

41. Niepomniszcze H, Medeiros-Neto GA, Refetoff S et al: Familial goiter with partial iodine organification defect, lack of thyroglobulin and high levels of thyroid peroxidase. Clin Endocrinol 6:27, 1977

42. Pendred V: Deaf mutism and goitre. Lancet 2:532, 1896

43. Fraser GR, Morgans ME, Trotter WR: The syndrome of sporadic goitre and congenital deafness. Q J Med 29:279, 1960

44. Johnsen S: Familial deafness and goitre in persons with a low level of protein bound iodine. Acta Otolaryngol, suppl. 40:168, 1958

45. Burrow GN, Spaulding SW, Alexander NM, Bower BF: Normal peroxidase activity in Pendred's syndrome. J Clin Endocrinol Metab 36:522, 1973

46. Ljunggren JG, Vecchio G: Studies on a patient with congenital deafness, nodular goitre, positive perchlorate test, abnormal biosynthesis of thyroglobulin and a high total concentration of thyroid peroxidase, abstracted. Acta Endocrinol, suppl 138:174, 1969

47. Ryan M, DeGroot LJ: Congenital defects in hormone formation and action. In DeGroot LJ (ed): Endocrinology. p. 782. WB Saunders Co, Philadelphia, 1989

48. Johnsen T, Jurgensen MB, Johnsen S. Mondini cochlea in Pendred's syndrome. Acta Otolaryngol (Stockh) 102:239, 1986

49. Bargman GJ, Gardner LI: Experimental production of otic lesions with antithyroid drugs. In Stanbury JB, Kroc RL (eds): Human Development and the Thyroid Gland. Advances in Experimental Medicine and Biology, vol 30. p. 305. Plenum Press, New York, 1972

50. Deol MS: An experimental approach to the understanding and treatment of hereditary syndromes with congenital deafness and hypothyroidism. J Med Genet 10:235, 1973

51. Vislakhmi S, Khanna KK: Pendred's syndrome. J Indian Med Assoc 53:199, 1969

52. Fraser GR: The genetics of thyroid disease. In Steinberg AG, Bearn AG (eds): Progress in Medical Genetics, vol 6. Chapter 3. Grune & Stratton, New York, 1969

53. Thompson J, Maguire NC, Hurwitz LJ: A family with deafness: goitre, epilepsy and low intelligence segregating independently. Ir J Med Sci 3:427, 1970

54. Papasov G: Untersuchungen uber das Wesen des Pendred-syndroms. Z Gesamte Inn Med 24:766, 1969

55. Safar A, Chaussain J-L, Vassal J et al: Hypothyreoidie precoce majeure, partiellement regressive, dans deux cas de syndrome de Pendred. Arch Fr Pediatr 30:843, 1973

56. Gomez-Pan A, Evered DC, Hall R: Pituitary-thyroid function in Pendred's syndrome. Br Med J 2:152, 1974

57. Medeiros-Neto GA, Nicolau W, Kieffer J, Ulhoa Cintra AB: Thyroidal iodoproteins in Pendred's syndrome. J Clin Endocrinol 28:1205, 1968

58. Milutinovic PS, Stanbury JB, Wicken JV, Jones EW: Thyroid function in a family with the Pendred syndrome. J Clin Endocrinol 20,962, 1969

59. Cave WT Jr, Dunn J: Studies on the thyroidal defect in an atypical form of Pendred's syndrome. J Clin Endocrinol Metab 41:590, 1975

59a. Mason ME, Dunn AD, Wortsman J et al: Thyroids from siblings with Pendred's syndrome contain thyroglobulin messenger ribonucleic acid variants. J Clin Endocrinol Metab 80:407, 1995.

60. Roche J, Michel R, Gorbman A, Lissitzky S: Sur la deshalogenation enzymatique des iodotyrosines par le corps thyroids et sur son role physiologique. II. Biochim Biophys Acta 12:570, 1953

61. Stanbury JB, Morris ML: Deiodination of diiodotyrosine by cell-free systems. J Biol Chem 233:106, 1958

62. Rosenberg IN, Ahn CS: Enzymatic deiodination of diiodotyrosine: possible mediation by reduced flavin nucleotide. Endocrinology 84:727, 1969

63. Stanbury JB, Kassenaar AAH, Meijer JWA: The metabolism of iodotyrosines. I. The fate of mono- and diiodotyrosine in normal subjects and in patients with various diseases. J Clin Endocrinol Metab 16:735, 1956

64. McGirr EM, Hutchison JH: Radioactive iodine studies in non-endemic goitrous cretins. Lancet 1:1117, 1953

65. Stanbury JB, Meijer JWA, Kassenaar AAH: The metabolism of iodotyrosines. II. The metabolism of mono- and diiodotyrosine in certain patients with familial goiter. J Clin Endocrinol Metab 16:848, 1956

66. Choufoer JC, Kassenaar AAH, Querido A: The syndrome of congenital hypothyroidism with defective dehalogenation of iodotyrosines: Further observations and a discussion of the pathophysiology. J Clin Endocrinol Metab 20:983, 1960

67. Querido A, Choufoer JC: Congenital hypothyroidism: Defective dehalogenation of iodotyrosines. p. 134. Proceedings of the 6th Congress of Internal Med, Basle, 1961

68. McGirr EM, Hutchison JH, Clements WE: Sporadic nonendemic goitrous cretinism: Identification and significance of monoiodotyrosine and diiodotyrosine in serum and urine. Lancet 2:906, 1956

69. Codaccioni JL, Rinaldi JP, Bismuth J: The test of overloading of I-diiodotyrosine (DIT) in the screening of iodotyrosine dehalogenase deficiency. Acta Endocrinol 87:95, 1978

70. Niall HD, Wellby ML, Hetzel BS et al: Biochemical and clinical studies in familial goitre caused by an iodotyrosine deiodinase defect. Aust Ann Med 17:89, 1968

71. Murray P, Thomson JA, McGirr EM, Wallace TJ: Absent and defective iodotyrosine deiodination in a family some of whose members are goitrous cretins. Lancet I:183, 1965

72. Larkander O, Larsson L-G, Ottosson J-O: Hereditary goitrous cretinism. Acta Psychiatr Scand, suppl. 22:103, 1971

73. Ismail-Beigi F, Rahimifar M: A variant of iodotyrosine-dehalogenase deficiency. J Clin Endocrinol Metab 44:499, 1977

74. Kusakabe T, Miyake T: Thyroidal deiodination defect in three sisters with simple goiter. J Clin Endocrinol 24:456, 1964

75. Kusakabe T, Miyake T: Defective deiodination of ^{131}I-labeled 1-diiodotyrosine in patients with simple goiter. J Clin Endocrinol Metab 23:132, 1963

76. Lissitzky S, Bismuth J, Codaccioni J-L Cartouzou G: Congenital goiter with iodoalbumin replacing thyroglobulin and defect of deiodination of iodotyrosines. Serum origin of the thyroid iodoalbumin. J Clin Endocrinol 28:1797, 1968

77. Thomson JA, McGirr EM: Defective deiodinase activity and abnormal thyroidal iodoproteins. J Clin Endocrinol 29:1259, 1969

78. Hutchison JG, McGirr EM: Hypothyroidism as an inborn error of metabolism. J Clin Endocrinol Metab 14:869, 1954

79. Harden R McG, Alexander WD, Papadopoulos S et al: The influence of the plasma inorganic iodine concentration on thyroid function in dehalogenase deficiency. Acta Endocrinol 55:361, 1967

80. Lissitzky S, Comar D, Riviere R, Codaccioni J-L: Etude quantitative du metabolisme de l'iode dans un cas d'hypothyroidie avec goitre due a un defaut d'iodotyrosine-deshalogenase. Rev Franc Clin Biol 10:631, 1965

81. Stanbury JB, Riccabona G, Janssen MA: Iodotyrosyl coupling defect in congenital hypothyroidism with goitre. Lancet 1:917, 1963

82. Jacobsen BB: Normal serum T_3 value in one of two siblings with goitrous hypothyroidism and dyshormonogenesis. Dan Med Bull 20:192, 1973

83. Morris JH: Defective coupling of iodotyrosine in familial goiters. Arch Int Med 114:417, 1964

84. Grollman EF, Doi SQ, Weiss P et al: Hyposialylated thyroglobulin in a patient with congenital goiter and hypothyroidism. J Clin Endocrinol Metab 74:43, 1992

85. de Vijlder JJM, Veenboer GJM, van Dijk JE: Thyroid albumen originates from blood. Endocrinology 131:578, 1992

86. Sulton C, Bismuth J, Castay M et al: Hypothyroidié par anomalie congenitale de synthése de la thyroglobuline. Arch Fr Pediatr 31:11, 1974

87. De Luca F, Michel R, Salabe GB, Baschieri L: Cretinismo sporadico congenito con gozzo da alterata struttura della tireoglobulina. Folia Endocrinol 16:141, 1963

88. Torresani J, Lissitzky S: Further studies on abnormal thyroglobulin from congenital goitres likely related to defective thyroglobulin export. In Robbins J, Braverman LE (eds): Advances in Thyroid Research. p. 453. Exerpta Medica, American Elsevier, New York, 1976

89. Wägar G, Lamberg BA, Saarinen P: Congenital goitre with thyroglobulin deficiency. In Robbins J, Braverman LE (eds): Advances in Thyroid Research. p. 463. Exerpta Medica, American Elsevier, New York, 1976

90. Kusakabe T: A goitrous subject with structural abnormality of thyroglobulin. J Clin Endocrinol Metab 35:785, 1972

91. Kusakabe T: A goitrous subject with defective synthesis of diiodotyrosine due to thyroglobulin abnormalities. J Clin Endocrinol Metab 37:317, 1973

92. Silva JE, Santelices R, Kishihara M, Schneider A: Low molecular weight thyroglobulin leading to a goiter in a 12-year-old girl. J Clin Endocrinol Metab 58:526, 1984

93. Medeiros-Neto GA, Knobel M, Bronstein MD et al: Impaired cyclic-AMP response to thyrotropin in congenital hypothyroidism with thyroglobulin deficiency. Acta Endocrinol (Copenhagen) 92:62, 1979

94. Baas F, Bikker H, van Ommen GJ, de Vijlder JJ: Unusual scarcity of restriction site polymorphism in the human thyroglobulin gene. A linkage study suggesting autosomal dominance of a defective thyroglobulin allele. Hum Genet 67:301, 1984

95. Medeiros-Neto GA, Knobel M, Cavaliere H et al: Heriditary congenital goitre with thyroglobulin deficiency causing hypothyroidism. Clin Endocrinol 20:631, 1984

96. Cabrer B, Brocas H, Perez-Castillio A et al: Normal level of thyroglobulin messenger ribonucleic acid in a human congenital goiter with thyroglobulin deficiency. J Clin Endocrinol Metab 63:931, 1986

97. McKenna TJ, Loughlin T, Ohman M et al: Mild familial goitrous hypothyroidism associated with prolongued ^{131}I retention: Possible defect in thyroglobulin synthesis. J Endocrinol Invest 12:229, 1989

98. Targovnik HM, Medeiros-Neto G, Varela V et al: A nonsense mutation causes human hereditary congenital goiter with preferential production of a 171-nucleotide-deleted thyroglobulin ribonucleic acid messenger. J Clin Endocrinol Metab 77:210, 1993

99. Leiri T, Cochaux P, Targovnik H et al: A 3'splice site mutation in the thyroglobulin gene responsible for congenital goiter with hypothyroidism. J Clin Invest 88:1901, 1991

100. Dolling CE, Good BF: Congenital goitre in sheep: Isolation of the iodoproteins which replace thyroglobulin. J Endocrinol 71:179, 1976

101. Falconer IR: Biochemical defect causing congenital goitre in sheep. Nature 205:978, 1965

102. Falconer IR: Studies of the congenitally goitrous sheep. The iodinated compounds of serum and circulating thyroid-stimulating hormone. Biochem J 100:190, 1966

103. Falconer IR: Studies of the congenitally goitrous sheep. Composition and metabolism of goitrous thyroid tissue. Biochem J 100:197, 1966

104. Falconer IR, Roitt I, Scamark RF, Torrigiani G: Studies of the congenitally goitrous sheep. Iodoproteins of the goitre. Biochem J 117:417, 1970

105. Rac R, Hill GN, Pain RW, Mulhearn CJ: Congenital goitre in merino sheep due to an inherited defect in the biosynthesis of thyroid hormone. Vet Sci 9:209, 1968

106. Pammenter MD: The biochemical nature of the primary defect in the genetically determined goitre of Afrikander cattle, thesis. University of Stellenbosch, Stellenbosch, South Africa, September 1978

107. Van Jaarsveld PP, Sena L, Van der Walt B, Van Zijl A: Abnormal iodoproteins in a congenital bovine goitre. In Fellinger K, Höfer R (eds): Further Advances in Thyroid Research. p. 465. G. Gistel & Cie, Vienna, 1971

108. Van Jaarsveld PP, Van der Walt B, Theron CN: Afrikander cattle congenital goiter: Purification and partial identification of the iodoprotein pattern. Endocrinology 91:470, 1972

109. Tassi VP, DiLauro R, van Jaarsveld P, Alvino CG: Two abnormal thyroglobulin-like polypeptides are produced from Afrikander cattle congenital goiter mRNA. J Biol Chem 259:10507, 1984

110. Ricketts MH, Vandenplas S, van der Walt M, van Jaarsveld PP: Afrikaner cattle congenital goiter: size heterogenity: thyroglobulin mRNA. Biochem Biophys Res Commun 126:240, 1985

111. Van Zyl A, Van der Walt B, Van der Walt K, Robbins J: Thyroidal iodoproteins in a congenital goitre. S Afr Med J 43:100, 1969

112. Doi S, Shifrin S, Santisteban P et al: Familial goiter in Bongo antelope (*Tragelaphus eurycerus*). Endocrinology 127:857, 1990

113. Rijnberk A, de Vijlder JJM, van Dijk JE et al: Congenital defect in iodothyronine synthesis. Clinical aspects of iodine metabolism in goats with congenital goitre and hypothyroidism. Br Vet J 133:495, 1977

114. de Vijlder JJM, van Voorthuyzen WF, van Dijk JE et al: Hereditary congenital goiter and thyroglobulin deficiency in a breed of goats. Endocrinology 102:1214, 1978

115. van Voorthuyzen WF, de Vijlder JJM, van dijk JE, Tegelaers WHH: Euthyroidism via iodide supplementation in hereditary congenital goiter with thyroglobulin deficiency. Endocrinology 103:2105, 1978

116. Van Voorthuyzen WF, Dinsart C, Flavell RA et al: Abnormal cellular localization of thyroglobulin mRNA associated with hereditary congenital goiter and thyroglobulin deficiency. Proc Natl Acad Sci USA 75:74, 1978

117. de Vijlder JJM, van Ommen GJB, van Voorthuyzen WF et al: Non-functional thyroglobulin messenger RNA in goats with hereditary congenital goiter. J Molec Appl Genet 1:51, 1981

118. De Vijlder JJM, Sterk A, Kok K, Vass F: Enhanced turnover of thyroglobulin RNA in the thyroid of goitrous goates. In Medeiros-Neto G, Gaitan E (eds): Frontiers in Thyroidology, vol 2. p. 809. Plenum Press, New York, 1986

119. van Ommen GJ, Sterk A, Mercken LO et al: Studies on the structures of the normal and abnormal goat thyroglobulin genes. Biochimie 71:211, 1989

120. Sterk A, van Dijk JE, Veenboer GJM et al: Normal-sized thyroglobulin messenger ribonucleic acid in Dutch goats with a thyroglobulin synthesis defect is translated into a 35,000 molecular weight N-terminal fragment. Endocrinology 124,477, 1989

121. Monaco F, Robbins J: Defective thyroglobulin synthesis in an experimental rat thyroid tumor. J Biol Chem 248:2328, 1973

122. Fukasawa N: Studies on the iodide metabolism and the expression of thyroglobulin and thyroid peroxidase mRNA in the thyroid of BB/W rats. Nippon Naibunni Gakkai Zasshi 67:1178, 1991

123. Basche M, Beamer WG, Schneider AB: Abnormal properties of thyroglobulin in mice with inherited congenital goiter (cog/cog) Endocrinology 124:1822, 1989

124. Adkinson LR, Taylor S, Beamer WG: Mutant gene-induced disorders of structure, function and thyroglobulin synthesis in congenital goiter (coc/coc) in mice. J Endocrinol 162:51, 1990

125. Fogelfeld L, Harel G, Beamer WG, Schneider AB: Low-molecular-weight iodoproteins in the congenital goiters of cog/cog mice. Thyroid 2:329, 1992

126. Lissitzky S, Torresani J, Burrow GN et al: Defective thyroglobulin export as a cause of congenital goitre. Clin Endocrinol 4:363, 1975

127. Ohyama Y, Nosoy T, Kameya T et al: Congenital euthyroid goitre with impaired thyroglobulin transport. Clin Endocrinol 41:129, 1994

128. Monaco F, Andreoli M, Beretta-Anguissola A: Isolation and characterization of soluble and particulate thyroid iodoproteins in human congenital goiter. Horm Res 5:141, 1974

129. Stanbury JB, Rocmans P, Buhler UK, Ochi Y: Congenital hypothyroidism with impaired thyroid response to thyrotropin. N Engl J Med 279:1132, 1968

130. Codaccioni JL, Carayon P, Michel-Bechet M et al: Congenital hypothyroidism associated with thyrotropin unresponsiveness and thyroid cell membrane alterations. J Clin Endocrinol Metab 50:932, 1980

131. Job JC, Canlorbe P, Thomassin N, Vassal J: L'hyperthyroidie infantile a debut precoce avec glande en place, fixation fiable de radio-iode et defaut de response a la thyrostimuline. Ann Endocrinol 30:696, 1979

132. Aarseth HP, Hang E, Raknerud N, Frey HM: TSH unresponsiveness, a case report. Acta Endocrinol 102:358, 1983

133. Leger FA, Thomas G, Helal OB et al: Hypothyréoidie congénitale avec probable anomalie de la récptivite thyréoidienne à l'hormone thyréotrope. Deux observations. Presse Med 13:491, 1984

134. Takamatsu J, Mishikawa M, Horimoto M, Oksawa N: Familial unresponsiveness to thyrotropin by autosomal recessive inheritance. J Clin Endocrinol Metab 77:1569, 1993

135. Bemaer WG, Eicher EM, Maltais LJ, Southard JL: Inherited primary hypothyroidism in mice. Science 212:61, 1981

136. Stein SA, Oates EL, Hall CR et al: Identification of a point mutation in the thyrotropin receptor of the hyt/hyt hypothyroid mouse. Molec Endocrinol 8:129, 1994

136a.Gu W-X, Du G-G, Kopp P et al: The thyrotropin (TSH) receptor transmembrane domain mutation (Pro556-Leu) in the hypothyroid *hyt/hyt* mouse results in plasma membrane targeting but defective TSH binding. Endocrinology 136:3164, 1995

137. Sunthornthepvarakul T, Gottschalk ME, Hayashi Y, Refetoff S: Brief report: resistance to thyrotropin caused by mutations in the thyrotropin-receptor gene. N Engl J Med 332:155, 1995

138. Weinstein LS, Shenker A: G protein mutations in human disease. Clin Biochem 26:333, 1993

139. Pittman JA, Haigler ED, Hershman JM, Pittman CS: Hypothalamic hypothyroidism. N Engl J Med 285:844, 1971

140. Mori M, Shoda Y, Yamada M et al: Central hypothyroidism due to isolated TRH deficiency in a depressive man. J Intern Med 229:285, 1991

141. Kramer MS, Kauschansky A, Gend M: Adolescent secondary amenorrhea: association with hypothalamic hypothyroidism. J Pediatr 94:300, 1979

142. Tanaka Y, Sawa H, Iden M et al: A case of idiopathic hypothalamic hypothyroidism. Jap J Med 20_2, 1981

143. L'Abbé A, Dubray C, Gaillard G et al: Familial growth retardation with isolated thyroid-stimulating hormone deficiency. Clin Pediatr 23:675, 1984

144. Miyai K, Endo Y, Iijima Y et al: Serum free thyrotropin subunit in congenital isolated thyrotropin deficiency. Endocrinol Jap 35:517, 1988

145. Hayashizaki Y, Hiraoka Y, Ando Y, Matsubara K: Thyroid stimulating hormone (TSH) deficiency caused by a single base substitution in the CAGYC region of the beta-subunit. EMBO J 8:2291, 1989 (Published erratum EMBO J 8:3542, 1989)

146. Hayashizaki Y et al: Deoxyribonucleic acid analyses of five families with familial inherited thyroid stimulating hormone deficiency. J Clin Endocrinol Metab 71:792, 1990

147. Böhm TM, Diamond RC, Wartofsky L: Isolated thyrotropin deficiency with thyrotropin releasing hormone induced TSH secretion and thyroidal release. J Clin Endocrinol Metab 43:1041, 1976

148. Radovick S, Nations M, Du Y et al: A mutation in the POU-homeodomaine of Pit-1 responsible for combined pituitary hormone deficiency. Science 257:1115, 1992

149. Pfäffle RW, DiMattia GE, Parks JS et al: Mutation of the POU-specific domain of Pit-1 and hypopituitarism without pituitary hypoplasia. Science 257:1118, 1992

149a.Cohen LE, Wondisford FE, Salvatoni A et al: A "hot spot" in the Pit-1 gene responsible for combined pituitary hormone deficiency: Clinical and molecular correlates. J Clin Endocrinol Metab 80:679, 1995

149b.Irie Y, Tatsumi K-I, Kusuda S et al: Screening for *PIT1* abnormality by PCR direct sequencing method. Thyroid 5:207, 1995

150. Burrow GN, Dussault JH: Neonatal Thyroid Screening Raven Press, New York, 1980

151. Savoie JC, Massin JP, Savoie: Studies on mono- and diiodohistidine. II Congenital goitrous hypothyroidism with thyroglobulin defect and iodohistidine-rich iodoalbumin production. J Clin Invest 52:116, 1973

152. Wollman SH: Production and properties of transplantable tumors of the thyroid gland in the Fisher rat. Recent Progr Horm Res 19:579, 1963

153. Cooper DS, Axelrod L, DeGroot LJ et al: Congenital goiter and the development of metastatic follicular carcinoma with evidence of a leak of nonhormonal iodide: clinical, pathological, kinetic, and biochemical studies and a review of the literature. J Clin Endocrinol Metab 52:294, 1981

154. Scernichow P, Schlumberger M, Pomarede R, Fragu P: Plasma thyroglobulin measurements help determine type of thyroid defect in congenital hypothyroidism. J Clin Endocrinol Metab 56:241, 1983

155. Beierwaltes WH, Robbins J: Familial increase in the thyroxine-binding sites in serum alpha globulin. J Clin Invest 38:1683, 1959

156. Hayashi Y, Refetoff S: Genetic abnormalities of thyroid hormone transport serum proteins. In Weintraube B (ed): Molecular endocrinology: Basic concepts and clinical correlations. p. 371. Raven Press, New York, 1995

157. Refetoff S: Inherited thyroxine-binding globulin (TBG) abnormalities in man. Endocr Rev 10:275, 1989

158. Refetoff S, Robin NI, Alper CA: Study of four new kindreds with inherited thyroxine-binding globulin abnormalities: Possible mutations of a single gene locus. J Clin Invest 51:848, 1972

159. Burr WA, Ramsden DB, Hoffenberg R: Hereditary abnormalities of thyroxine-binding globulin concentration. Q J Med 49:295, 1980

160. Trent JM, Flink IL, Morkin E et al: Localization of the human thyroxine-binding globulin gene to the long arm of the X chromosome (Xq21-22). Am J Hum Genet 41:428, 1987

161. Mori Y, Takeda K, Charbonneau M, Refetoff S: Replacement of Leu[227] by pro in thyroxine-binding globulin (TBG) is associated with complete TBG deficiency in three of eight families with this inherited defect. J Clin Endocrinol Metab 70:804, 1990

162. Li P, Janssen OE, Takeda K et al: Complete thyroxine-binding globulin (TBG) deficiency caused by a single nucleotide deletion in the TBG gene. Metabolism 40:1231, 1991

163. Yamamori I, Mori Y, Seo H et al: Nucleotide deletion resulting in frameshift as a possible cause of complete thyroxine-binding globulin deficiency in six Japanese families. J Clin Endocrinol Metab 73:262, 1991

164. Yamamori I, Mori Y, Miura Y et al: Gene screening of 23 Japanese families with complete thyroxine-binding globulin deficiency: identification of a nucleotide deletion at codon 352 as a common cause. Endocr J 40:563, 1993

165. Takeda K, Iyota KY et al: Gene screening in Japanese families with complete deficiency of thyroxine-binding globulin demonstrates that a nucleotide deletion at codon 352 may be a race specific mutation. Clin Endocrinol 40:221, 1994

166. Sarne DH, Refetoff S, Murata Y et al: Variant thyroxine-binding globulin in serum of Australian Aborigines. A comparison with familial TBG deficiency in Caucasians and American Blacks. J Endocrinol Invest 8:217, 1985

167. Sarne DH, Refetoff S, Nelson JC, Dussault J: A new inherited abnormality of thyroxine-binding globulin (TBG-San Diego) with decreased affinity for thyroxine and triiodothyronine. J Clin Endocrinol Metab 68:114, 1989

168. Janssen OE, Bertenshaw R, Takeda K et al: Molecular basis of inherited thyroxine-binding globulin defects. Trends Endocrinol Metab 3:49, 1992

169. Takeda K, Mori Y, Sobieszczyk S et al: Sequence of the variant thyroxine-binding globulin of Australian Aborigines: Only one of two amino acid replacements is responsible for its altered properties. J Clin Invest 83:1344, 1989

170. Griffiths KD, Virdi NK, Rayner PHW, Green A: Neonatal screening for congenital hypothyroidism by measurement of plasma thyroxine and thyroid stimulating hormone concentrations. Br Med J 291:117, 1985

171. Brown SK, Bellisario R: Measurement of thyroxine-binding globulin (TBG) levels from dried blood spot specimens: Detection of TBG deficiency and TBG excess in infants. In: Carter TP, Wiley AH (eds): Genetic Disease: Screening and Management. p. 373. Alan R. Liss, New York 1986

172. Refetoff S, Charbonneau M, Sarne DH et al: Resistance to thyroid hormones and screening for high thyroxine at birth. In: Research for Congenital Hypothyroidism. p. 165. Plenum, New York, 1989

173. Hayashi Y, Mori Y, Janssen OE et al: Human thyroxine-binding globulin gene: Complete sequence and transcriptional regulation. Molec Endocrinol 7:1049, 1993

174. Waltz MR, Pullman TN, Takeda K et al: Molecular basis for the properties of the thyroxine-binding globulin-slow variant in American Blacks. J Endocrinol Invest 13:343, 1990

175. Kamboh MI, Ferrell RE: A sensitive immunoblotting technique to identify thyroxine-binding globulin protein heterogeneity after isoelectric focusing. Biochem Genet 24:273, 1986

176. Constans J, Ribouchon MT, Gouaillard C et al: A new polymorphism of thyroxin-binding globulin in three African groups (Mali) with endemic nodular goitre. Hum Genet 89:199, 1992

177. Takamatsu J, Refetoff S: Inherited heat stable variant thyroxine-binding globulin (TBG-Chicago). J Clin Endocrinol Metab 63:1140, 1986

178. Janssen OE, Chen B, Büttner C et al: Sequence analysis and in-vitro expression of the heat-resistant variant thyroxine-binding globulin-Chicago. p. 254 The 75th Annual meeting of The Endocrine Society, Las Vegas, Nevada, 1993

179. Janssen OE, Büttner C, Treske B et al: The new variant thyroxine-binding globulin-Huston has reduced

thyroxine-binding affinity but normal concentration in serum. The 76th Annual meeting of The Endocrine Society, Anaheim, California, 1994

180. Janssen OE, Refetoff S: In-vitro expression of thyroxine-binding globulin (TBG) variants: Impaired secretion of TBG[PRO-227] but not TBG[PRO-113]. J Biol Chem 267:13998, 1992

181. Kambe F, Seo H, Mori Y et al: An additional carbohydrate chain in the variant thyroxine-binding globulin-Gary (TBG[Asn-96]) impairs its secretion. Molec Endocrinol 6:443, 1992

182. Miura Y, Kambe F, Yamamori I et al: A truncated thyroxine-binding globulin due to a frameshift mutation is retained within the rough endoplasmic reticulum: a possible mechanism of complete thyroxine-binding globulin deficiency in Japanese. J Clin Endocrinol Metab 78:283, 1994

183. Miura Y, Mori Y, Kambe F et al: Impaired intracellular transport contributes to partial thyroxine-binding globulin (TBG) deficiency in a Japanese family. J Clin Endocrinol Metab 79:740, 1994

184. Refetoff S, Dwulet FE, Benson MD: Reduced affinity for thyroxine in two of three structural thyroxine-binding prealbumin variants associated with familial amyloidotic polyneuropathy. J Clin Endocrinol Metab 63:1432, 1986

185. Rosen HN, Moses AC, Murrell JR et al: Thyroxine interactions with transthyretin: a comparison of 10 naturally occurring human transthyretin variants. J Clin Endocrinol Metab 77:370, 1993

186. Lalloz MR, Byfield PG, Goel KM et al: Hyperthyroxinemia due to the coexistence of two raised affinity thyroxine-binding proteins (albumin and prealbumin) in one family. J Clin Endocrinol Metab 64:346, 1987

187. Akbari MT, Fitch NJ, Farmer M et al: Thyroxine-binding prealbumin gene: a population study. Clin Endocrinol 33:155, 1990

188. Fitch NJS, Akbary MT, Ramsden DB: An inherited non-amyloidogenic transthyretin variant, [Ser[6]]-TTR, with increased thyroxine-binding affinity, characterized by DNA sequencing. J Endocrinol 129:309, 1991

189. Moses C, Rosen HN, Moller DE et al: A point mutation in transthyretin increases affinity for thyroxine and produces euthyroid hyperthyroxinemia. J Clin Invest 86:2025, 1990

190. Harrison HH, Gordon ED, Nichols WC, Benson MD: Biochemical and clinical characterization of prealbumin[CHICAGO]: an apparently benign variant of serum prealbumin (transthyretin) discovered with high-resolution two-dimensional electrophoresis. Am J Med Gen 39:442, 1991

191. Scrimshaw BJ, Fellowes AP, Palmer BN et al: A novel variant of transthyretin (prealbumin), Thr[119] to Met, associated with increased thyroxine binding. Thyroid 2:21, 1992

192. Alves IL, Divino CM, Schussler GC et al: Thyroxine binding in a TTR met 119 kindred. J Clin Endocrinol Metab 76:484, 1993

193. Curtis AL, Scrimshaw BL, Topliss DJ et al: Thyroxine binding by human transthyretin variants: mutations at position 119, but not 54, increase thyroxine binding affinity. J Clin Endocrinol Metab 78:459, 1994

194. Benson MD: Amyloidosis. In Scriver CR, Beaudet AL, Sly WS, Valle D (eds): The Metabolic Basis of Inherited Diseases. Chapter 131. McGraw-Hill, New York, 1994

195. Woeber KA, Ingbar SH: The contribution of thyroxine-binding prealbumin to the binding of thyroxine in human serum, as assessed by immunoadsorption. J Clin Invest 47:1710, 1968

196. Moses AC, Lawlor J, Haddow J, Jackson IMD: Familial euthyroid hyperthyroxinemia resulting from increased thyroxine binding to thyroxine-binding prealbumin. N Engl J Med 306:966, 1982

197. Steinrauf LK, Hamilton JA, Braden BC et al: X-ray crystal structure of the Ala-109 → Thr variant of human transthyretin which produces euthyroid hyperthyroxinemia. J Biol Chem 268:2425, 1993

198. Hennemann G, Krenning EP, Otten M et al: Raised total thyroxine and free thyroxine index but normal free thyroxine. A serum abnormality due to inherited increased affinity of iodothyronines for serum binding protein. Lancet 1:639, 1979

199. Lee WNP, Golden MP, Van Herle AJ et al: Inherited abnormal thyroid hormone-binding protein causing selective increase of total serum thyroxine. J Clin Endocrinol Metab 49:292, 1979

200. Ruiz M, Rajatanavin R, Young RA et al: Familial dysalbuminemic hyperthyroxinemia: a syndrome that can be confused with thyrotoxicosis. N Engl J Med 306:635, 1982

201. DeCosimo DR, Fang SL, Braverman LE: Prevalence of familial dysalbuminemic hyperthyroxinemia in Hispanics. Ann Intern Med 107:780, 1987

202. Jensen IW, Faber J: Familial dysalbuminaemic hyperthyroxinemia: a review. J Royal Soc Med 81:34, 1988

203. Sapin R, Gasser F, Chambron J: Hyperthyroxinémie familiale avec dysalbuminémie: Dépistage sur 21 000 patients a l'occasion d'un bilan thyroïden. Pathol Biol (Paris) 37:785, 1989

204. Arevalo G: Prevalence of familial dysalbuminemic hyperthyroxinemia in serum samples received for thyroid testing. Clin Chem 37:1430, 1991

205. DeNayer P, Malvaux P: Hyperthyroxinemia associ-

ated with high thyroxine binding to albumin in euthyroid subjects. J Endocrinol Invest 5:383, 1982

206. Mendel CM, Cavalieri RR: Thyroxine distribution and metabolism in familial dysalbuminemic hyperthyroxinemia. J Clin Endocrinol Metab 59:499, 1984

207. Fleming SJ, Applegate GF, Beardwell CG: Familial dysalbuminemic hyperthyroxinemia. Postgrad Med J 63:273, 1987

208. Wood DF, Zalin AM, Ratcliffe WA, Sheppard MC: Elevation of free thyroxine measurement in patients with thyrotoxicosis. Q J Med 65:863, 1987

209. Croxson MS, Palmer BN, Holdaway IM et al: Detection of familial dysalbuminaemic hyperthyroxinaemia. Br Med J 290:1099, 1985

210. Weiss RE, Angkeow P, Sunthornthepvarakul T et al: Linkage of albumin (ALB) to familial dysalbuminemic hyperthyroxinemia (FDH) in a large Amish kindred. J Clin Endocrinol Metab 80:116, 1995

211. Petersen CE, Scottolini AG, Cody LR et al: A point mutation in the human serum albumin gene results in familial dysalbuminaemic hyperthyroxinaemia. J Med Genet 31:355, 1994

212. Sunthornthepvarakul T, Angkeow P, Weiss RE et al: A missense mutation in the albumin gene produces familial disalbuminemic hyperthyroxinemia in 8 unrelated families. Biochem Biophys Res Commun 202:781, 1994

213. Langsteger W, Stockigt JR, Docter R et al: Familial disalbuminaemic hyperthyroxinaemia and inherited partial TBG deficiency: first report. Clin Endocrinol 40:751, 1994

214. Refetoff S, DeWind LT, DeGroot LJ: Familial syndrome combining deaf-mutism, stippled epiphyses, goiter, and abnormally high PBI: possible target organ refractoriness to thyroid hormone. J Clin Endocrinol Metab 27:279, 1967

215. Refetoff S, DeGroot LJ, Benard B, DeWind LT: Studies of a sibship with apparent hereditary resistance to the intracellular action of thyroid hormone. Metabolism 21:723, 1972

216. Sakurai A, Takeda K, Ain K et al: Generalized resistance to thyroid hormone associated with a mutation in the ligand-binding domain of the human thyroid hormone receptor β. Proc Natl Acad Sci (USA) 86:8977, 1989

217. Kaplan MM, Swartz SL, Larsen PR: Partial peripheral resistance to thyroid hormone. Am J Med 70:1115, 1981

218. Beck-Peccoz P, Roncoroni R, Mariotti S et al: Sex hormone–binding globulin measurement in patients with inappropriate secretion of thyrotropin (IST): Evidence against selective pituitary thyroid hormone resistance in nonneoplastic IST. J Clin Endocrinol Metab 71:19, 1990

219. Refetoff S, Weiss RE, Usala SJ: The syndromes of resistance to thyroid hormone. Endocr Rev 14:348, 1993

220. Beck-Peccoz P, Chatterjee VKK: The variable clinical phenotype in thyroid hormone resistance syndrome. Thyroid 4:225, 1994

221. Adams M, Matthews C, Collingwood TN et al: Genetic analysis of 29 kindreds with generalized and pituitary resistance to thyroid hormone: Identification of thirteen novel mutations in the thyroid hormone receptor β gene. J Clin Invest 94:506, 1994

222. Takeda K, Sakurai A, DeGroot LJ, Refetoff S: Recessive inheritance of thyroid hormone resistance caused by complete deletion of the protein-coding region of the thyroid hormone receptor-β gene. J Clin Endocrinol Metab 74:49, 1992

223. Refetoff S, Salazar A, Smith TJ, Scherberg NH: The consequences of inappropriate treatment due to failure to recognize the syndrome of pituitary and peripheral tissue resistance to thyroid hormone. Metabolism 32:822, 1983

224. Hauser P, Zametkin AJ, Martinez P et al: Attention deficit-hyperactivity disorder in people with generalized resistance to thyroid hormone. N Engl J Med 328:997, 1993

225. Weiss RE, Stein MA, Trommer B, Refetoff S: Attention-deficit hyperactivity disorder and thyroid function. J Pediatr 123:539, 1993

226. Elia J, Gulotta C, Rose SR et al: Thyroid function and attention-deficit hyperactivity disorder. J Am Acad Child Adolesc Psychiatr 33:169, 1994

227. Weiss RE, Stein MA, Duck SC et al: Low intelligence but not attention deficit hyperactivity disorder is associated with resistance to thyroid hormone caused by mutation R316H in the thyroid hormone receptor β gene. J Clin Endocrinol Metab 78:1525, 1994

228. Beck-Peccoz P, Persani L, Faglia G: Glycoprotein hormone α-subunit in pituitary adenomas. Trends Endocrinol Metab 3:41, 1992

229. Usala SJ, Bale AE, Gesundheit N et al: Tight linkage between the syndrome of generalized thyroid hormone resistance and the human c-erbAβ gene. Molec Endocrinol 2:1217, 1988

230. Usala SJ, Tennyson GE, Bale AE et al: A base mutation of the c-erbAβ thyroid hormone receptor in a kindred with generalized thyroid hormone resistance. Molecular heterogeneity in two other kindreds. J Clin Invest 85:93, 1990

231. Behr M, Loos U: A point mutation (Ala^{229} to Thr) in the hinge domain of the c-erbAβ thyroid hormone receptor in a family with generalized thyroid hormone resistance. Molec Endocrinol 6:1119, 1992

232. Onigata K, Yagi H, Hagashima K, Kuroume T: Point mutation in exon of the c-erbAβ thyroid hormone

receptor gene in a family with generalized thyroid hormone resistance. 98th Meeting of the Japanese Pediatric Society, Yokohama, Japan, 1993

233. Persani L, Asteria C, Tonacchera M et al: Evidence for secretion of thyrotropin with enhanced bioactivity in syndromes of thyroid hormone resistance. J Clin Endocrinol Metab 78:1034, 1994

234. Takeda K, Weiss RE, Refetoff S: Rapid localization of mutations in the thyroid hormone receptor-β gene by denaturing gradient gel electrophoresis in 18 families with thyroid hormone resistance. J Clin Endocrinol Metab 74:712, 1992

235. Geffner ME, Su F, Ross NS et al: An arginine to histidine mutation in codon 311 of the C-erbAβ gene results in a mutant thyroid hormone receptor that does not mediate a dominant negative phenotype. J Clin Invest 91:538, 1993

236. Hayashi Y, Sunthornthepvarakul T, Refetoff S: Mutations of CpG dinucleotides located in the triiodothyronine (T$_3$)-binding domain of the thyroid hormone receptor (TR) β gene that appears to be devoid of natural mutations may not be detected because they are unlikely to produce the clinical phenotype of resistance to thyroid hormone. J Clin Invest 94:607, 1994

237. Weiss RE, Weinberg M, Refetoff S: Identical mutations in unrelated families with generalized resistance to thyroid hormone occur in cytosine-guanine-rich areas of the thyroid hormone receptor beta gene: Analysis of 15 families. J Clin Invest 91:2408, 1993

238. Parrilla R, Mixson AJ, McPherson JA et al: Characterization of seven novel mutations of the c-erbAβ gene in unrelated kindreds with generalized thyroid hormone resistance. Evidence for two "hot spot" regions of the ligand binding domain. J Clin Invest 88:2123, 1991

239. Burman KD, Djuh YY, Nicholson D et al: Generalized thyroid hormone resistance: Identification of an arginine to cystine mutation in codon 315 of the c-erb A beta thyroid hormone receptor. J Endocrinol Invest 15:573, 1992

240. Cugini CD Jr, Leidy JW Jr, Chertow BS et al: An arginine to histidine mutation in codon 315 of the c-erbAβ thyroid hormone receptor in a kindred with generalized resistance to thyroid hormones results in a receptor with significant 3,5,3'-triiodothyronine binding activity. J Clin Endocrinol Metab 74:1164, 1992

241. Weiss RE, Marcocci C, Bruno-Bossio G, Refetoff S: Multiple genetic factors in the heterogeneity of thyroid hormone resistance. J Clin Endocrinol Metab 76:257, 1993

242. Bartolone L, Regalbuto C, Benvenga S et al: Three new mutations of thyroid hormone receptor-β associated with resistance to thyroid hormone. J Clin Endocrinol Metab 78:323, 1994

243. Mixson AJ, Parrilla R, Ransom SC et al: Correlations of language abnormalities with localization of mutations in the β-thyroid hormone receptor in 13 kindreds with generalized resistance to thyroid hormone: Identification of four new mutations. J Clin Endocrinol Metab 75:1039, 1992

244. Usala SJ, Menke JB, Hao EH et al: Mutations in the c-erbA-beta gene in two different patients with selective pituitary resistance to thyroid hormones. 135 Abstract Q335. 74th Annual Meeting of The Endocrine Society, San Antonio, Texas, 1992

245. Usala SJ, Menke JB, Watson TL et al: A homozygous deletion in the c-erbAβ thyroid hormone receptor gene in a patient with generalized thyroid hormone resistance: isolation and characterization of the mutant receptor. Molec Endocrinol 5:327, 1991

246. Sasaki S, Nakamura H, Tagami T et al: Pituitary resistance to thyroid hormone associated with a base mutation in the hormone-binding domain of the human 3,5,3'-triiodothyronine receptor-β. J Clin Endocrinol Metab 76:1254, 1993

247. Mixson AJ, Renault JC, Ransom S et al: Identification of a novel mutation in the gene encoding the β-triiodothyronine receptor in a patient with apparent selective pituitary resistance to thyroid hormone. Clin Endocrinol 38:227, 1993

248. Usala SJ, Menke JB, Watson TL et al: A new point mutation in the 3,5,3'-triiodothyronine-binding domain of the c-erbAβ thyroid hormone receptor is tightly linked to generalized thyroid hormone resistance. J Clin Endocrinol Metab 72:32, 1991

249. Yen PM, Sugawara A, Refetoff S, Chin WW: New insights on the mechanism(s) of the dominant negative effect of mutant thyroid hormone receptor in generalized resistance to thyroid hormone. J Clin Invest 90:1825, 1992

250. Adams M, Nagaya T, Tone Y et al: Functional properties of a novel mutant thyroid hormone receptor in a family with generalized thyroid hormone resistance syndrome. Clin Endocrinol 36:281, 1992

251. Flynn TR, Tollin S, Cohen O et al: Pituitary thyroid hormone resistance caused by a novel mutation in the beta isoform of the thyroid hormone receptor, abstracted. Clin Res 42:208A, 1994

252. Tsukaguchi H, Yoshimasa Y, Fujimoto K et al: An analysis of the thyroid hormone receptor genes in patients with generalized thyroid hormone resistance. Thyroid, 2 Suppl. 1:S-57, 1992

253. Sakurai A, Miyamoto T, Hughes IA, DeGroot LJ: Characterization of a novel mutant human thyroid hormone receptor β in a family with hereditary thyroid hormone resistance. Clin Endocrinol 38:29, 1993

254. Boothroyd CV, Teh BT, Hayward NK et al: Single base mutation in the hormone binding domain of the thyroid hormone receptor β gene in generalized thyroid hormone resistance demonstrated by single stranded conformation polymorphism analysis. Biochem Biophys Res Commun 178:606, 1991

255. Gharib H, Nagaya T, Stelter A et al: Characterization of the c-erbAβ R438H mutant in generalized thyroid hormone resistance. Endocr J 1:193, 1993

256. Sasaki S, Nakamura H, Tagami T et al: A point mutation of the T_3 receptor beta 1 gene in a kindred of generalized resistance to thyroid hormone. Molec Cell Endocrinol 84:159, 1992

257. Weiss RE, Chyna B, Duell PB et al: A point mutation (C446R) in the thyroid hormone receptor-β gene of a family with resistance to thyroid hormone. J Clin Endocrinol Metab 78:1253, 1994

258. Groenhout EG, Dorin RI: Generalized thyroid hormone resistance due to a deletion of the carboxy terminus of the c-erbAβ receptor. Molec Cell Endocrinol 99:81, 1994

259. Nakamura H, Sasaki S, Tagami T et al: Identification and functions of abnormal T_3 receptors in patients with thyroid hormone resistance, (abstract). Thyroid, Suppl. 3:T-3, 1993

260. Nakamura H, Sasaki S, Tagami T et al: Analysis of the T_3 receptor genes in patients with generalized resistance to thyroid hormone and selective pituitary form, abstracted. Thyroid, 2 Suppl. 1:S-36, 1992

261. Shuto Y, Wakabayashi I, Amuro N et al: A point mutation in the 3,5,3'-triiodothyronine-binding domain of thyroid hormone receptor β associated with a family with generalized resistance to thyroid hormone. J Clin Endocrinol Metab 75:213, 1992

262. Refetoff S, Weiss RE, Wing JR et al: Resistance to thyroid hormone in subjects from two unrelated families is associated with a point mutation in the thyroid hormone receptor β gene resulting in the replacement of the normal proline 453 with serine. Thyroid 4:249, 1994

263. Usala SJ, Wondisford FE, Watson TL et al: Thyroid hormone and DNA binding properties of a mutant c-erbAβ receptor associated with generalized thyroid hormone resistance. Biochem Biophys Res Commun 171:575, 1990

264. Sakurai A, Miyamoto T, Refetoff S, DeGroot LJ: Dominant negative transcriptional regulation by a mutant thyroid hormone receptor β in a family with generalized resistance to thyroid hormone. Molec Endocrinol 4:1988, 1990

265. Chatterjee VKK, Nagaya T, Madison LD et al: Thyroid hormone resistance syndrome. Inhibition of normal receptor function by mutant thyroid hormone receptors. J Clin Invest 87:1977, 1991

266. Nagaya T, Madison LD, Jameson JL: Thyroid hormone receptor mutants that cause resistance to thyroid hormone. Evidence for receptor competition for DNA sequences in target genes. J Biol Chem 267: 13014, 1992

267. Nagaya T, Jameson JL: Thyroid hormone receptor dimerization is required for the dominant negative inhibition by mutations that cause thyroid hormone resistance. J Biol Chem 268:15766, 1993

268. Hao E, Menke JB, Smith AM et al: Divergent dimerization properties of mutant β1 thyroid hormone receptors are associated with different dominant negative activities. Molec Endocrinol 8:841, 1994

269. Au-Fliegner M, Helmer E, Casanova J et al: The conserved ninth C-terminal heptad in thyroid hormone and retinoic acid receptors mediates diverse responses by affecting heterodimer but not homodimer formation. Molec Cell Endocrinol 13:5725, 1993

270. Zavacki AM, Harney JW, Brent GA, Larsen PR: Dominant negative inhibition by mutant thyroid hormone receptors is thyroid hormone responce element and receptor isoform specific. Molec Endocrinol 7:1319, 1993

271. Ono S, Schwartz ID, Mueller OT et al: Homozygosity for a "dominant negative" thyroid hormone receptor gene responsible for generalized resistance to thyroid hormone. J Clin Endocrinol Metab 73:990, 1991

272. Nagaya T, Eberhardt NL, Jameson JL: Thyroid hormone resistance syndrome: correlation of dominant negative activity and location of mutations. J Clin Endocrinol Metab 77:982, 990

273. Rösler A, Litvin Y, Hage C et al: Familial hyperthyroidism due to inappropriate thyrotropin secretion successfully treated with triiodothyronine. J Clin Endocrinol Metab 54:76, 1982

273a. Larsen PR, Silva JE, Kaplan MM: Relationships between circulating and intracellular thyroid hormones: physiological and clinical implications. Endocr Rev 2:87, 1981

273b. Hennemann G, Vos AR, de Jong M, Krenning EP, Docter R: Decreased peripheral 3,5,3'-triiodothyronine (T_3) production from thyroxine (T_4): a syndrome of impaired thyroid hormone activation due to transport inhibition of T4- into T3-producing tissues. J Clin Endocrinol Metab 77:1431, 1993

273c. Jansen M, Krenning EP, Dostdÿk W et al: Hyperthyroxinaemia due to decreased peripheral triiodothyronine production. Lancet 2:849, 1982

273d. Kleinhaus N, Faber J, Kahana L, Sneer J, Scheinfeld M: Euthyroid hyperthyroxinaemia due to a generalized 5'-deiodinase defect. J Clin Endocrinol Metab 66:684, 1988

Multinodular Goiter

17

Although the normal thyroid gland is a fairly homogenous structure, nodules often form within it. These nodules may be simply the growth and fusion of localized colloid-filled follicles, or more or less discrete adenomas, or cysts. Nodules larger than 1 cm are detectable by palpation, and careful examination finds them in at least 4 percent of the general population. Nodules less than 1 cm in diameter are not clinically detectable unless located on the surface of the gland, and are much more common. The terms *adenomatous goiter, nontoxic nodular goiter,* and *colloid nodular goiter* are used interchangeably for multinodular goiters.

INCIDENCE

In the past the prevalence of goiter throughout the United States varied considerably, with zones of high frequency in the Midwest and Northwest.[1] These differences in prevalence have diminished sharply in recent years. In Framingham, Massachusetts, a small community where iodide intake is ample, Vander and his colleagues[2] examined 5,000 persons and found that 4 percent had nodular goiters. Of these, one-quarter were thought to be multinodular. In a subsequent study the same authors[3] showed that over 15 years, new nodules appeared in 1.4 percent of the population.

In a study of 2,779 persons in northern England, Tunbridge et al.[4] found obvious goiters in 6.9 percent with a female/male ratio of 13:1. Thyroid nodules were found in 0.8 percent of men and 5.3 percent of women, with an increased frequency in women over 45 years of age. Twenty years later a follow-up survey was performed in 96 percent of the 1877 survivors of the original studied population. A marked reduction was found in goiter frequency that now reached a value of 3 percent.[4a] Routine autopsy surveys usually produce a much higher incidence. In a study of 2,185 routine postmortem examinations in Boston, 8 percent had one or more thyroid nodules at least 1 cm in diameter,[5] but in women over 50 years of age a 15 percent incidence was found, with up to 40 percent in certain groups. Another study of consecutive autopsy cases disclosed that 50 percent of the thyroid glands were nodular (though not necessarily enlarged), although clinically the glands had been considered normal. Three-quarters of these glands were multinodular, and one-quarter contained solitary adenomas.[6] A survey of periadolescent schoolchildren has been performed in four widely separated communities in the United States.[7] The incidence of readily palpable thyroids among these children varied from 4.4 percent in Savannah, Georgia, to 9.8 percent in Tecumseh, Michigan. The iodine supply was ample or more than ample for all groups studied. Most of the goiters were small, and they occurred more often in girls than boys. This rate and pattern of occurrence is typical where iodine supplies are ample; the goiters found presumably have some cause other than iodine deficiency, including autoimmune thyroid disease.

The weight and nodularity of the thyroid increase with age, and by the eighth decade nearly all thyroid glands contain macroscopic nodules. The incidence of clinically detectable goiter is two- to ten times higher in women than in men.[2–5]

CAUSE

A nodular goiter may be the result of any chronic, low-grade, intermittent stimulus to thyroid hyperplasia. Supporting evidence for this view is circumstantial. David Marine first suggested that in response to iodide deficiency, the thyroid first goes through a period of hyperplasia, but eventually—possibly because of iodide repletion or a decreased requirement for thyroid hormone—enters a resting phase characterized by colloid storage and the histologic picture of a colloid goiter. Marine believed that repetition of these two phases of the cycle eventually resulted in the formation of nontoxic multinodular goiter.[8] Taylor's studies of thyroid glands removed at surgery led him to believe that the initial lesion is diffuse hyperplasia, but that discrete nodules develop eventually.[9] By the time the goiter is well developed, serum TSH levels and TSH production rates are usually normal or even suppressed.[10]

Dige-Petersen and Hummer evaluated basal and TRH-stimulated serum TSH levels in 15 patients with diffuse goiter and 47 patients with nodular goiter.[11] They found impairment of TRH-induced TSH release in 27 percent of the patients with nodular goiter, suggesting thyroid autonomy, but in only 1 of the 15 with diffuse goiter. Smeulers et al. studied 22 clinically euthyroid women with multinodular goiter and found that there was an inverse relationship between the increment of TSH after administration of TRH and the size of the thyroid gland (Fig. 17-1). It was also found that, while still within the normal range, the mean serum T_3 concentration of the group with impaired TSH secretion was significantly higher than the normal mean whereas mean value serum T_4 level was not elevated.[12] These results are consistent with the hypothesis that a diffuse goiter may precede the development of nodules;

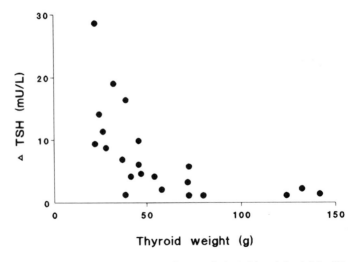

Fig. 17-1. Relationship of ΔTSH (after 400 μg TRH i.v.) and thyroid weight (g) in 22 women with clinically euthyroid multinodular goiter. (From Smeulers et al,[12] with permission.)

TABLE 17-1. Factors That May Be Involved in the Evolution of Multinodular Goiter

Primary factors
  Functional heterogeneity of normal follicular cells, cause unknown, possibly genetic
  Acquisition of new inheritable qualities by replicating epithelial cells
  Subsequent functional and structural abnormalities in growing goiters
Secondary factors (Stimuli to New Follicle Generation)
  TSH (induced by, e.g., iodine deficiency, goitrogens, inborn errors of thyroid hormone synthesis)
  Other thyroid-stimulating factors

(From Studer et al.,[13–15] with permission.)

they are also consistent with the clinical observation that, with time, autonomy with suppression of TSH release may occur even though such goiters were originally TSH dependent. Studer et al. have published comprehensive reviews of recently developed insights into the evolution of multinodular goiter.[13–16] A summary of the major factors discussed by these authors is presented in Table 17-1.

PRIMARY FACTORS

Genetic Heterogeneity of Normal Follicular Cells

In theory the genetic information of all cells in a human must be homogenous, except for x/y gene expression. In practice, however, it appears that through developmental processes the thyroid epithelial cells forming a follicle are functionally polyclonal and possess widely differing qualities regarding the different biochemical steps leading to growth and to thyroid hormone synthesis such as iodine uptake (i.e., transport), thyroglobulin production and iodination, iodothyrosine coupling, endocytosis, and dehalogenation. As a consequence there is some heterogeneity of growth and function within a thyroid and even within a follicle (Fig. 17-2). In a recent study, polyclonal and monoclonal nodules were found to coexist in multinodular glands.[17]

Acquisition of New Inheritable Qualities by Replicating Epithelial Cells

Newly generated cells appear to somehow acquire qualities not present in mother cells. These qualities can subsequently be passed on to further generations of cells. A possible example of this process is the

acquired abnormal growth pattern that is reproduced when a tissue sample is transplanted into a nude mouse.[16] Other examples are acquired variable responsiveness to TSH.[13] These changes may be related to mutations in oncogenes such as ras, or others, which do not produce malignancy, per se, but can alter growth and function.

Subsequent Functional and Structural Abnormalities in Growing Goiters

Follicles of second and later generations are less well formed and compartmentalization of key enzymes may become altered. Intercellular communication may become disrupted. As a consequence, inter- and intrafollicular growth and function may become poorly integrated resulting in further heterogeneity.[13,18]

SECONDARY FACTORS

The secondary factors discussed below stimulate thyroid cell growth and function and, because of differences in cellular responsiveness that are presumed to exist, aggravate the expression of heterogeneity which leads to further growth and focal autonomic function of the thyroid gland. Local necrosis, cyst formation (sometimes with bleeding), and fibrosis may be the anatomic end stage of such processes[13] (see the section *Pathology*, below).

Iodine Deficiency

Stimulation of new follicle growth seems to be necessary for the formation of simple goiter. Many studies indicate that iodine deficiency or impairment of iodine metabolism by the thyroid gland, perhaps due to congenital biochemical defects, may be an important mechanism leading to increases in TSH secretion. Since in experimental animals the level of iodine per se may modulate the response of thyroid cells to TSH, this is an additional mechanism by which relatively small increases in serum TSH level may cause substantial effects on thyroid growth in iodine-deficient areas. Koutras et al.[19] found that the thyroidal iodine clearance of patients in Scotland with nontoxic nodular goiter was, on average, higher than that in normal persons (Fig. 17-3). This seemed to be because the patients weren't getting enough iodine. Similar observations have been made in Belgium and France but not in the United States. When

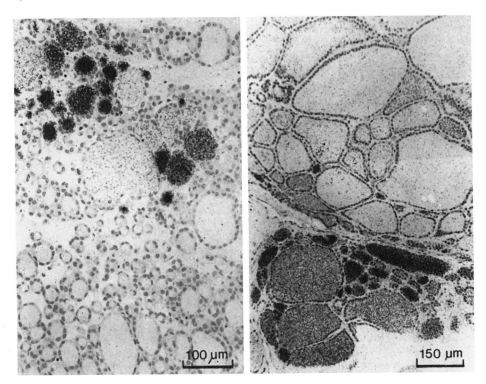

Fig. 17-2. Heterogeneity of morphology and function in a human multinodular goiter. Autoradiographs of two different areas of a typical multinodular euthyroid human goiter excised after administration of radioiodine tracer to the patient. There are enormous differences of size, shape, and function among the individual follicles of the same goiter. Note also that there is no correlation between the size or any other morphologic hallmark of a single follicle and its iodine uptake. (From Studer et al,[15] with permission.)

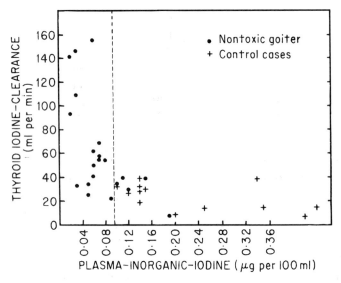

Fig. 17-3. Relationship between nontoxic goiter and thyroidal iodine clearance. (From Koutras et al,[19] with permission.)

data regarding thyroid volume and iodine excretion from several major cities in Western Europe were combined,[20] an inverse relation was found between urinary iodine excretion and thyroid volume (Fig. 17-4). It may also be that physiologic stresses, such as pregnancy, increase the need for iodine and require thyroid hypertrophy to increase an iodine uptake that might otherwise be satisfactory. An elevated renal clearance of iodine occurs during normal pregnancy.[21,22] It has been suggested that in some patients with endemic goiter there are similar increases in renal iodine losses.[23,24] Increased need for thyroxine during pregnancy may also lead to thyroid hypertrophy when iodine intake is limited. Recently it has been shown that iodide need in pregnancy is not only increased by increased iodide loss through the kidneys, but also because of significant transfer of thyroid hormone from the mother to the fetus.[25] Glinoer and co-workers found that thyroid volume increase is predominantly effected by a higher HCG serum concentration during the first trimester of pregnancy, and by a slightly elevated serum TSH level present at delivery, especially in areas of moderate iodine intake.[20]

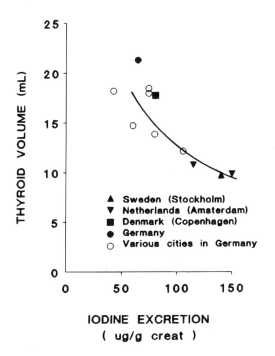

Fig. 17-4. Correlation between thyroid volume and urinary iodine excretion in normal populations from various areas. (From Glinoer and Lemone,[20] with permission.)

The declining prevalence of multinodular goiter in the United States in areas where iodine intake has reached levels of 240 to 700 $\mu g/d$[26] suggests that borderline iodine deficiency played an etiologic role in past decades.

Dietary Goitrogens

Patients occasionally have thyroid enlargement either because of goitrogenic substances in their diet[27] or because of drugs they are taking for other conditions. Peltola[28] has demonstrated this experimentally by feeding rats minute doses of a natural goitrogen over many months. Similar results have been obtained by Langer[29,30] using combinations of the three most prevalent goitrogens contained in cabbage. The explanation for the effect of such substances is that the goitrogen is much more effective at the level of iodothyronine synthesis than at earlier steps in hormone production, such as iodide trapping. Thus, the radioactive iodide uptake (RAIU) may be high, but with a block in hormone synthesis, goiter may be produced. This mechanism remains to be documented in humans, but if present, it would operate most effectively in a situation of borderline iodine supply. As discussed in Chapter 5, the goitrogen KSCN potentiates the effect of severe iodine deficiency in endemic areas of Africa.

Inherited Defects in T_4 Synthesis

An intriguing clue to the cause of nontoxic goiter in some patients is that it is familial. No particular pattern of inheritance has been found, but the condition can often be traced through several generations. Occasionally, other members of the family may have Graves' disease. It may be that patients with nontoxic goiter are heterozygous for genes that in the homozygous state lead to clinically apparent hypothyroidism.

Some investigators have evaluated iodide transport in patients with multinodular goiter and found it to be normal.[31] Parker and Beierwaltes[32] observed that many relatives of patients with defective iodine organification had goiter, but the results of iodine-binding studies were normal in these subjects. Some relatives of patients with the iodotyrosine dehalogenase defect have goiter and are euthyroid. In these cases, it has been possible to demonstrate that relatives have a deficiency in the deiodinating enzyme system, but this deficiency is not severe enough to cause hypothyroidism. Similar results have been reported by McGirr.[33]

Multinodular Goiter Produced by a Congenital Metabolic Defect

The birth and early development of R.S., a 42-year-old clerk, were entirely normal. Although his progress in school was slow, he managed to complete trade school. A goiter was first noted at age 14; because of slowly increasing pressure symptoms, it necessitated a subtotal thyroidectomy 9 years later. The specimen showed hyperplasia and involution. By age 37 a goiter again was present. The patient ultimately sought help because of difficulty in passing a preemployment examination. His mother had a goiter, and one sister died at age 13 at operation for removal of a goiter. Two other siblings were well.

The patient appeared well developed and adequately nourished. The thyroid was four times the normal size, lobulated, and without a bruit or thrill. The patient's intelligence was below average; otherwise, his physical examination was normal. The RAIU was 60 percent at 2 hours and 82 percent at 24 hours. The PBI concentration in serum was 4.6 μg/dl (normal 4 to 8 μg/dl).

A second subtotal thyroidectomy was performed. Slices from the specimen deiodinated MIT and DIT normally. The tissue was fractionated by centrifugation, and 99 percent of labeled iodine was found in the 1,000,000 $\times$ g supernatant fraction. On ultracentrifugation, 51 percent of the protein was present as a 19.4 S component and 49 percent as a 4.3 S component. The latter fraction, which would contain lightweight proteins such as albumin, was much increased over normal values. On enzymatic digestion of the supernatant fraction (presumably containing TG), 40 percent of the ^{131}I, administered before surgery, was DIT; 21 percent, MIT; and 3 percent iodothyronine. Twenty-one percent resisted hydrolysis. Electrophoresis of the supernatant fraction showed that ^{131}I was associated with a visible TG band, and in addition, a protein moving in the position of albumin, present in high concentration. This protein behaved immunologically as albumin. It was estimated that the thyroid contained approximately 5 g/dl of this iodinated albumin or albumin-like protein.

The pathologic diagnosis was multinodular goiter with multiple adenomas. Numerous adenomas of the fetal and embryonal type were interspersed with colloid nodules; this suggested prolonged stimulation of the thyroid gland.

After the second operation, the patient was maintained on thyroid hormone replacement and did well. There was no further recurrence of the goiter.

The appearance of the goiter by age 14, the strong familial tendency to thyroid disease, and the mental retardation all suggest that this patient had a congenital goiter that may have been associated with hypothyroidism early in life. The tendency of the goiter to recur, as well as the histologic pattern of the second surgical specimen, support the interpretation that the goiter grew in response to an abnormality in hormone synthesis. Metabolic compensation was apparently achieved during adult life by means of hypertrophy of the gland. The thyroid appeared to form and release into the serum an abnormal iodoprotein. This iodoprotein was metabolically inactive, and it indicated inefficient use of iodide by the thyroid. Formation of this protein presumably was secondary to some metabolic block in hormone synthesis.

Despite the possibility that inherited defects are involved in patients with multinodular goiter, most examinations for such defects have been negative. Major problems of analysis are the limited ability of tests to identify recessive states and the marked heterogeneity of function that exists within a single gland.[13] For example, Niepomniszcze and co-workers[34] evaluated peroxidase function in 13 patients with nontoxic multinodular goiter. Both "cold" and "warm" nodules were identified by scintiscanning before thyroidectomy. The iodide peroxidase activity of cold nodules was generally reduced, whereas in 10 warm nodules studied, 7 had normal activity and 3 decreased activity. Thus, one may conclude that the cold nodules of these multinodular glands were peroxidase deficient. In the same glands, however, normal activity could be found in other nodules that were active in concentrating RAI. Heterogeneity of iodide organification was confirmed by Peter et al.[35] and summarized by Studer.[36] Later, using autoradiography, two types of cold follicles were found—those that failed to accumulate iodide because of deficient trapping and those that could transport iodide but could not organify it, suggesting failure of apical membrane peroxidase.[37] At this time, it is reasonable to assume that some form of a partial biosynthetic abnormality is the most likely explanation for sporadic multinodular goiter. This assumption appears to be borne out by the recent reports of a family in which goiter was associated with a mutation in thyroglobulin (TG) in the area of a "hormonogenic" thyroxine residue.[38] Molecular endocrinology will probably provide answers to more cases in the future.

Other Thyroid-Stimulating Factors

Recently, Drexhage et al.[39,40] identified another possible stimulus to growth in the sera of patients with simple goiter. Using an assay system in which stimulation of thyroid cell replication was quantitated, evidence of a growth stimulation factor was found in the immunoglobulin fraction of sera from these patients. This substance, thyroid growth immunoglobulin (TGI) was also found in patients with goitrous Graves' disease but not in those with primary myxedema or goiter secondary to inborn defects of thyroid hormone synthesis. This factor was not TSH, nor was it the same thyroid-stimulating immunoglobulin found in patients with nongoitrous Graves' disease. The authors proposed that some patients, particularly those who showed recurrence of goiter after surgery, might have thyroid enlargement as a consequence of yet another form of thyroid autoimmunity. The findings of Drexhage et al. have, however, been challenged.[40a,40b,40c] Some suggest that the effects they found are due to contamination of their immunoglobulin fraction by a common growth factor and that they used as target FRTL5 cells which are not human and not normal.[41]

Other substances that could be involved in stimulating thyroid enlargement are epidermal growth factor (EGF) and insulin-like growth factors (IGF). EGF stimulates the proliferation of thyrocytes from sheep, dogs, pigs, calves, and humans.[42] While stimulating growth, EGF reduces trapping and organification of iodide, TSH receptor binding, and release of thyroglobulin, T_3, and T_4. On the other hand, TSH may modulate EGF binding to thyroid cell membranes, and thyroid hormone may stimulate EGF production and EGF receptor number.[42] In a study on adenomatous tissue, obtained from patients with multinodular goiter, it was found by immunohistochemistry that expression of EGF was increased.[43] IGF-2 interacts with trophic hormones to stimulate cell proliferation and differentiation in a variety of cell types. The interaction between TSH and IGF-2 is synergestic.[44] Increased IGF-1 expression may contribute to goiter formation.[45] A similar synergistic effect as with IGF-2 has recently been reported to exist between IGF-1 and TSH.[46] In these latter studies it was suggested that this synergism on DNA synthesis is mediated by complex interactions including the secretion of one or more autocrine amplification factors. Recently it was found that non-functioning nodules in patients with multinodular goiter contain the same IGF-1 receptors that were present in the normal adjacent extranodular follicles but were expressed in higher concentrations.[47] Acidic fibroblast growth factor stimulates colloid accumulation in thyroids of rats but only in the presence of TSH.[48] Other factors promoting cell growth and differentiation have been identified in the past decade. These include cytokinines, acetylcholine, norepinephrine, prostaglandins, substances of neural origin, such as vasoactive intestinal peptides, and substances of C-cell origin. It is not known, however, to what extent these compounds play a role in the genesis of multinodular goiter. These substances are discussed in Chapter 1.

The hypothesis that the development of thyroid autonomy is due to a gradual increase in the numbers of cells having relatively autonomous thyroid hormone synthesis is supported by data. In patients with nodular goiter, 27 percent exhibited impaired TSH responses to TRH as opposed to only 7 percent of patients with diffuse goiter.[11] Such partial autonomy may appear only with time and could possibly be prevented by TSH-suppressive therapy. The fact that it is possible to induce hyperthyroidism in some patients with multinodular goiters by administering iodide suggests that certain of the nodules in the multinodular gland are autonomous but unable under normal iodine intake to concentrate sufficient quantities of iodide to cause hyperthyroidism.[49] Presumably iodide administration provides sufficient substrate for generation of excessive amounts of hormone, although it does not readily account for the long persistence of the hyperthyroidism in some of those cases.

Thus, there may be several etiologic factors in simple and nodular goiter, and some of these factors may act synergistically. The result is a collection of heterogeneously functioning thyroid follicles, some of which may be autonomous and produce sufficient amounts of thyroid hormone to cause hyperthyroidism.

PATHOLOGY

Although thyroid glands in the early phases of development of multinodular goiters are rarely examined pathologically, such glands generally show areas of hyperplasia with considerable variation in follicle size. The more typical specimen, however, is that of the goiter that has developed a nodular consistency. Such goiters characteristically present a variegated appearance, with the normal homogeneous parenchymal structure deformed by the presence of nodules (Fig. 17-5A, B). The nodules may vary considerably in size (from a few millimeters to several centimeters); in outline (from sharp encapsulation in adenomas to poorly defined margination for ordinary nodules); and in architecture (from the solid follicular adenomas to the gelatinous, colloid-rich nodules or degenerative cystic structures). The graphic term *Puddingstone goiter* has been applied. Frequently the nodules have degenerated and a cyst has formed, with evidence of old or recent hemorrhage, and the cyst wall may have become calcified. Often there is extensive fibrosis, and calcium may

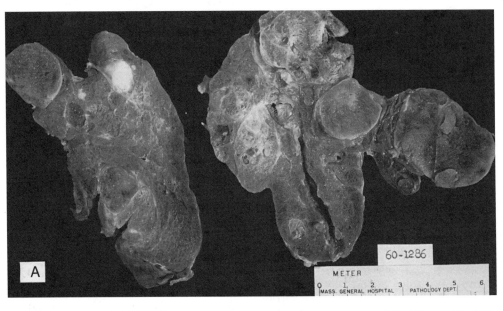

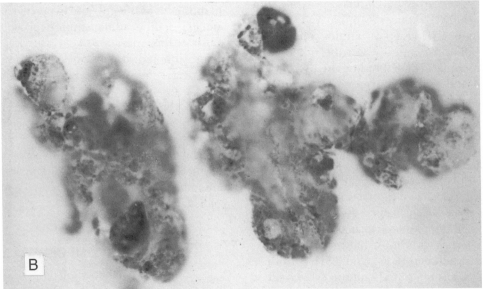

Fig. 17-5. (A) Cross section of multinodular goiter. (B) Gross radioautograph of the thyroid in part A. Observe the variation in ^{131}I uptake in different areas.

also be deposited in these septae. Scattered between the nodules are areas of normal thyroid tissue, and often focal areas of lymphocytic infiltration. Radioautography shows a variegated appearance, with RAI localized sometimes in the adenomas and sometimes in the paranodular tissue. Occasionally, most of the radioactivity is confined to a few nodules that seem to dominate the metabolic activity of the gland.

If careful sections are made of numerous areas, 4 to 17 percent of these glands removed at surgery will be found to harbor microscopic papillary carcinoma.[43,50–52] The variable incidence can probably be attributed to the different criteria used by the pathologists and the basis of selection of the patients for operation by their physicians. These factors are discussed below.

NATURAL HISTORY OF THE DISEASE

Multinodular goiter is probably a lifelong condition that has its inception in adolescence or at puberty. Minimal diffuse enlargement of the thyroid gland is found in many teenage boys and girls, and is almost a physiologic response to the complex structural and hormonal changes occurring at this time. It usually regresses, but occasionally (much more commonly in girls) it persists and undergoes further growth during pregnancy. This course of events has not been documented as well as might be desired in sporadic nodular goiter, but it is the usual evolution in areas where mild endemic goiter is found.

Patients with multinodular goiter seek medical attention for many reasons. Perhaps most commonly, they consult a physician because a lump has been discovered in the neck, or because a growth spurt has been observed in a goiter known to be present for a long time. Sometimes the increase in the goiter's size will cause pressure symptoms, such as difficulty in swallowing, cough, respiratory distress, or the feeling of a lump in the throat. Rarely, an area of particularly asymmetrical enlargement may impinge upon or stretch the recurrent laryngeal nerve. Of course, the most common sequence of events is for the goiter to be discovered accidentally by a physician in the course of an examination for some other condition. An important and frequently overlooked sequence of events is the patient's seeking medical

attention because of cardiac irregularities or congestive heart failure, which proves to be the result of slowly developing thyrotoxicosis. (This scenario is discussed more fully later in this chapter). Frequently the goiter grows gradually for a period of a few to many years, and then becomes stable with little tendency for further growth. It is rare for any noteworthy spontaneous reduction in the size of the thyroid gland to occur, but patients often describe fluctuations in the size of the goiters and the symptoms they give. These are usually subjective occurrences, and more often than not the physician is unable to corroborate the changes that the patient describes. On the other hand, it could be that changes in blood flow through the enlarged gland account for the symptoms.

Occasionally, a sudden increase in the size of the gland is associated with sharp pain and tenderness in one area. This event suggests hemorrhage into a nodular cyst of the goiter, which can be confirmed by ultrasound. Within 3 to 4 days the symptoms subside, and within 2 to 3 weeks the gland may revert to its previous dimensions. In such a situation, acute thyrotoxicosis may develop and subside spontaneously[53,54] (Fig. 17-6).

Rarely, if ever, do the patients become hypothyroid and if they do, the diagnosis is more probably Hashimoto's thyroiditis than nodular goiter. In a study of clinically euthyroid subjects with multinodular goiter, 13 out of 22 had subnormal TSH release after TRH.[12] If the goiter is present for a long time, thyrotoxicosis develops in a large number of patients. In a series collected many years ago at the Mayo Clinic, 60 percent of patients over 60 were thyrotoxic.[55] The average duration of the goiter before the onset of thyrotoxicosis was 17 years; the longer the goiter had been present, the greater was the tendency for thyrotoxicosis to develop. This condition appears to occur because with the passage of time autonomous function of the nodules develops. In a recent study of patients with euthyroid multinodular goiter, thyroid function was autonomous in 64 and normal in 26. After a mean follow-up of 5 (maximum 12 years) 18 patients with autonomous thyroid function became overtly hyperthyroid, and in 6 patients with primarily normal thyroid function autonomy developed.[56] In Figure 17-7, a typical course of thyroid function tests for a patient with multinodular goiter is illustrated, from complete euthyroidism to overt thyrotoxicosis. Occasionally a

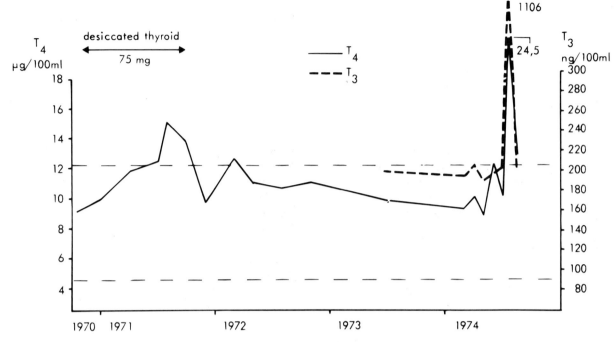

Fig. 17-6. T_4 and T_3 levels in a patient with multinodular goiter. Desiccated thyroid was withdrawn because of thyrotoxic symptoms. Note high T_3 and T_4 peak values in mid-1974 due to acute homorrhage in thyroid nodule. (From Smeulers et al,[53] with permission.)

single discrete nodule in the thyroid gland becomes sufficiently active to cause thyrotoxicosis and to suppress the activity of the rest of the gland (see Ch. 13). If these patients are given thyroid hormone, continued function of nodules can be demonstrated by radioiodine scanning techniques. Thus, these nodules have become independent of pituitary control. When patients with euthyroid multinodular goiter are frequently tested, it appears that in some of them occasional transient increases of serum T_3 and T_4 are seen[57] (Fig. 17-8). The possibility that the abrupt development of hyperthyroidism may follow administration of large amounts of iodine to these patients has already been mentioned.[49]

Occasionally an invasive thyroid cancer develops in a multinodular goiter. This fact brings the discussion to one of the most serious problems relating to multinodular goiter—carcinoma.

THE CARCINOMA PROBLEM

If surgical specimens of multinodular goiters are examined carefully, 4 to 17 percent are found to harbor a carcinoma.[43,50–52] These carcinomas vary widely in size and are typically of the papillary variety. Similar tumors are occasionally found in thyroid glands affected by Hashimoto's thyroiditis and in otherwise normal glands. Stoffer et al.[58] reported that 13 percent of the glands resected in thyroid operations contained papillary adenocarcinoma. In Japan, in routine autopsies of patients who were not suspected of having thyroid disease and who had no known irradiation experience, 17 percent of the patients were found to have small carcinomas when careful serial sections of the thyroid glands were done.[59] If the recently confirmed figures of Stoffer et al.[50] truly represent the prevalence of invasive carcinoma, all multinodular goiters should be resected in order to prevent dissemination of malignant disease. It seems quite unlikely, however, that all lesions that appear to satisfy the criteria for malignant neoplasia are potentially lethal. This view is strongly supported by the final report of the study on the significance of nodular goiter by Vander et al.[3] in Framingham, Massachusetts. For 15 years, they followed all 218 nontoxic thyroid nodules previously detected in a total population of approximately 5,000 persons. None of these lesions showed any

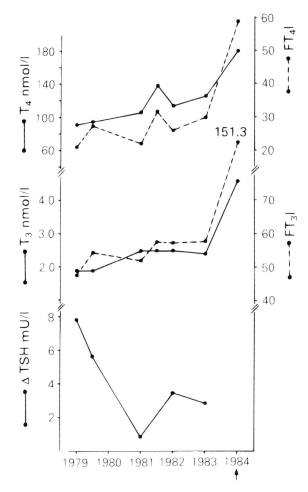

151.3

Fig. 17-7. Course of thyroid function tests, including the increment of TSH in response to TRH in a patient who demonstrated the whole functional cycle from nonautonomy (1979), through autonomy (1981), to overt hyperthyroidism (1984). (From Elte et al,[56] with permission.)

clinical evidence of malignancy at the end of that time.

We believe that there is only minimal risk from carcinoma in multinodular goiter. Sokal[60,61] has presented this position in detail, and we can do no better than to borrow directly from his analysis. The prevalence of clinical nodularity of the thyroid is at least 4 percent, or 40,000 per 1,000,000 population.[2] Use of a much higher figure can be justified by the autopsy studies described above. Despite the high frequency of nodular goiter, only 36 to 60 thyroid tumors appear per 1,000,000 persons each year[62,63] or by analysis of reported statistics on thyroid surgical

specimens.[61] This incidence has not changed during a more recent national cancer survey in the United States that came up with an incidence of 40 per 1,000,000.[63] In his monograph, Riccabona[64] published an overview of the incidence of thyroid cancer in 40 countries, both with and without endemic goiter. The range of incidence varies between 7.5 and 56 per 1,000,000 persons each year. There is no increased goiter rate in endemic goiter areas. The prevalence of significant thyroid carcinoma at routine autopsy is less than 0.1 percent[61,65,66] and persons with this type of tumor are probably examined as frequently as are those with other forms of neoplasia. In the United States, mortality figures for thyroid carcinoma are constant at about 6 per 10^6 population each year. Riccabona also summarizes death rate from thyroid cancer in nonendemic and in endemic countries.[64] For some countries death rates were published at intervals. For Austria this was 16 per 10^6 per year in 1952 and 10 per 10^6 per year in 1983. For Switzerland this was 18 per 10^6 per year in 1952 and 9 per 10^6 per year in 1979. The death rate per year for the United States was 3 per 10^6 in 1979, for Israel, 1 per 10^6 per year in 1952 and for the United Kingdom, 7 per 10^6 in 1963. Death rates from thyroid cancer in endemic goiter areas as published from regions in Austria, Yugoslavia, Finland, and Israel were between 10 and 16 per 10^6 per year between 1980 and 1984.

Lastly, it should be recognized that meticulous examination of autopsy specimens from persons dying of nonthyroid disease may show small (less than 0.5 cm) papillary lesions in 4 to 24 percent of human thyroid glands.[67–69] A recent report of 1,020 sequential autopsies revealed the presence of microscopic papillary carcinoma in 6 percent.[66] Although the prevalence of this type of lesion increases with age, there is no question that such lesions may be present in young persons. The proportion of these lesions that even become clinically apparent is unknown, but their presence in otherwise normal thyroid glands should be kept in mind when evaluating reports of similar prevalences of thyroid carcinoma in multinodular thyroid glands.

If 4 percent of patients with nodular goiter actually have thyroid carcinoma, the prevalence of tumor in the general population would be 1,600 per 1,000,000. It is remarkable that only about 25 of these 1,600 hypothetical tumors become apparent each year, and that only about 10 prove fatal. Thus, there appears to be a gross discrepancy between the

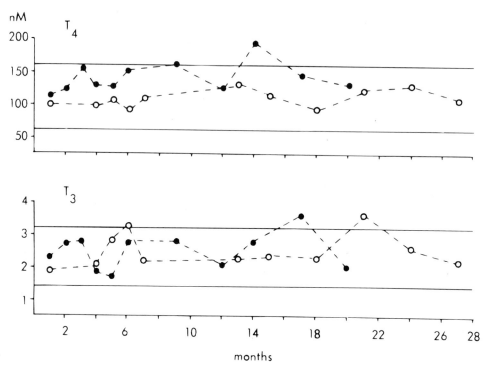

Fig. 17-8. Serum T_4 and T_3 levels during a follow-up of 20 and 27 months in 2 patients (●--● and ○--○), both aged 60 years, with euthyroid multinodular goitre. The continuous lines indicate 95 percent confidence limits of the normal range. (From Smeulers et al,[57] with permission.)

mortality from thyroid carcinoma and its reported frequency in surgical specimens of multinodular goiters. Reasonable arguments, however, can be mustered in an effort to reconcile the information. Perhaps the most important single factor is selection. Persons with nodular goiter who come to operation are not representative of the general population but are patients with clinically significant thyroid disease who have been selected by their physicians for thyroid surgery. One of the factors controlling the selection process is the suspicion of malignant tumor. In fact, the selection process is especially good, as reflected by the high recovery of malignant thyroid tumors in patients operated on with this presumptive diagnosis.[70] A second factor is that the histologic diagnosis of thyroid carcinoma may not correlate well with true invasiveness. It is impossible to prove this thesis, but pathologists agree that the criteria for judging malignancy are variable and that it is exceedingly difficult to predict with any degree of certainty the growth potential of a particular thyroid lesion.

Other arguments may be used to defend a conservative therapeutic posision. In the first place, the tumors that are usually found in multinodular goiters are papillary tumors, and their degree of invasiveness is low. Indeed, the survival rate for intrathyroid papillary carcinoma is only slightly less than that for normal persons of the same age and sex.[71] Furthermore, prophylactic subtotal thyroidectomy is not a guarantee of protection from cancer arising in a nodular goiter, since the process is usually diffuse, and it may be assumed that abnormal tissue is left in the neck after operation. In fact, unless replacement therapy is given, partial thyroidectomy might be expected to induce a tremendous growth stimulus in the remaining gland. A further point is that thyroidectomy, even in the best of hands, carries its own risk and its own morbidity, whose dimensions may be comparable to those of missing a small papillary carcinoma within a multinodular goiter. Obviously this last possibility does not apply when a focus of unusual induration or rapid growth rate is detected clinically.

SIGNS AND SYMPTOMS

Many of the symptoms of multinodular goiter have already been described. They are chiefly due to the presence of an enlarging mass in the neck and its impingement upon the adjacent structures. There may be dysphagia, cough, and hoarseness. Paralysis of a recurrent laryngeal nerve may occur when the nerve is stretched taut across the surface of an expanding goiter, but this event is very unusual. When unilateral vocal cord paralysis is demonstrated, the presumptive diagnosis is cancer. Pressure on the superior sympathetic ganglions and nerves may produce Horner syndrome.

As the gland grows it characteristically enlarges the neck, but frequently the growth occurs in downward, producing a substernal goiter. Sometimes a history given by an older patient that a goiter in the neck has disappeared may mean that it has fallen down into the upper mediastinum, where its upper limits can be felt by careful deep palpation. Hemorrhage into this goiter can produce acute tracheal obstruction. Sometimes substernal goiters are attached only by a fibrous band to the goiter in the neck and extend downward to the arch of the aorta. They have even been observed as deep in the mediastinum as the diaphragm. Occasionally the skilled physician can detect a substernal goiter by percussion, particularly if there is a hint from tracheal deviation, or the presence of a nodular mass in the neck above the manubrial notch.

Symptoms suggesting constriction of the trachea are frequent, and displacement of the trachea is commonly found on physical examination. Radiographic examination is useful in defining the extent of tracheal deviation and compression. Compression is frequently seen but is rarely functionally significant. The authors have expected to find softened tracheal cartilage after the removal of some large goiters, but tracheomalacia has been observed only on the rarest occasions. Dr. George Riccabona has described to us his experience in Innsbruck, where tracheomalacia is still occasionally seen and may pose a serious threat after removal of the huge endemic goiters, especially in elderly patients.

Patients may be remarkably tolerant of nodular goiter even when the enlargement is striking; this is especially true in endemic goiter areas. On the other hand, when the facilities for removal are available, most patients like to be rid of their goiters.

HYPERTHYROIDISM IN THE NODULAR THYROID GLAND

A significant proportion of patients with nodular thyroid glands develop thyrotoxicosis, and this proportion directly correlates to the goiter's duration. Possible explanations for this occurrence were discussed earlier. Typically, the thyrotoxicosis develops so insidiously that the patient is unaware of the symptoms.

The symptoms of thyrotoxicosis are those observed with other causes of thyroid hormone excess, and are discussed in Chapter 10. Emotional lability, heightened neuromuscular activity, altered integument, increased metabolic rate, cardiac irritability and tachycardia, and increased motility of the intestine are seen, as in Graves' disease, but infiltrative ophthalmopathy is absent. Toxic adenomatous goiter was first clearly distinguished from Graves' disease by H. S. Plummer and is sometimes known as *Plummer's disease*.[72]

Certain features are much more prominent than in Graves' disease, perhaps because the disease usually appears first in the fifth through seventh decades.[73] Congestive heart failure occurs, which is often resistant to the usual therapeutic measures. Recurrent or permanent atrial fibrillation, or recurrent episodes of atrial tachycardia, may dominate the picture. In fact, thyrotoxicosis should be carefully excluded in any goitrous adult with congestive heart failure or tachyarrhythmia. Occasionally muscle weakness is so severe that the patient is unable to climb stairs, or even to walk, when few other symptoms or signs of the disease have become manifest. Emotional lability is often unusually prominent in these patients. Depression, crying episodes, emotional fatigue, and irritability may lead one to conclude that the problem is that of an agitated depression. Frequently the symptoms are confusing because they are coincidentally mixed with those of menopause. Although emotional problems may be caused by thyrotoxicosis, the contribution of the thyroid often cannot be defined until the patient has been rendered euthyroid.

Thyrotoxicosis in multinodular goiter can occur for reasons other than nodular autonomy. First, any patient with long-standing diffuse hyperplasia of Graves' disease may develop nodules in the thyroid gland. Second, the normal glandular elements between the nodules may become diffusely hyperplastic, as in any other gland. This condition would be Graves' disease in a multinodular goiter. If the circulating thyroid immunostimulator, typical of Graves' disease, is present in the serum, it would indicate the presence of autoimmune thyroid disease. The presence of another thyroid-stimulating immunoglobulin, i.e. stimulating thyroid growth, as suggested by Drexhage et al.,[39] has been disputed.[40a,40b,40c,41]

Several clinical observations support a fundamental distinction between Graves' disease and Plummer's disease. Frequently the hyperactive tissue in Plummer's disease is confined to one or a few nodules, as demonstrated by isotopic scan. Exophthalmos is not present in toxic nodular goiter, unless there is concomitant Graves' disease, and these patients have a family background of thyrotoxicosis less frequently. Usually they are older, and thyrotoxicosis is milder and often exists for a long time without many symptoms, but responds much less readily to the administration of antithyroid drugs and iodide. Very few patients have recurrent thyrotoxicosis after surgery, and few become hypothyroid. There is a widespread clinical impression that all patients with multinodular goiter will develop thyrotoxicosis if given sufficient time.

Thyrotoxicosis can also develop because a single nodule in the thyroid has become overactive and independent of pituitary control. In as many as 46 percent, this condition may be T_3 thyrotoxicosis.[74] Nodules causing hyperthyroidism are generally 3 cm or more in diameter. The function of the rest of the gland is suppressed due to the lack of circulating TSH.

DIAGNOSIS

A clinical diagnosis of multinodular goiter based on an enlarged multinodular gland in a euthyroid adult is usually accurate. If the nodules are largely confined to one part of the thyroid gland, clinical examination may suggest a solitary nodule. If multiple nodules are not obvious and the gland is diffusely enlarged, the differentiation from other conditions causing goiter, such as Hashimoto's thyroiditis, is more difficult. The FT_4I, FT_3 level, and 24-hour RAIU are normal in most instances. Scanning after administration of RAI or $^{99m}TcO^{4-}$ may delineate areas of decreased or increased concentration of the

isotope in some nodules; this finding suggests a nonuniform rather than a diffuse process. Scanning may also be helpful in demonstrating the boundaries of the goiter when it extends substernally. An objective and very sensitive technique to detect even small nodules is that of high-resolution ultrasonography which can detect lesions with a diameter of a few millimeters. Antibody titers against thyroid proteins usually are absent or low. Needle biopsy may suggest multinodular goiter but does not provide enough information about the overall architecture of the gland for the diagnosis to be made with assurance. Nevertheless, needle biopsy of a prominent nodule is usually performed to reassure physician and patient that a cancer is not present. Needle aspiration of large cysts can occasionally produce gratifying reduction in goiter size, especially after several aspirations.

Radiographic examination of the neck and chest are helpful in defining the extent of the goiter and its distortion of structures in the neck. Tracheal deviation produced by the goiter is compatible with a multinodular rather than a diffuse process. Fluoroscopy during a barium swallow will often be helpful in giving information regarding the degree of esophageal deviation or obstruction. Anterior-posterior and lateral views of the trachea, obtained during inspiration with and without the glottis closed, can be used to identify tracheal compression or tracheomalacia. If tracheomalacia is present, the airway will decrease in width when the patient inspires against the closed glottis. Calcification in the wall of cysts may give some indication of the nature of lesions and the length of time they have been present. Sandy or gritlike calcification suggests the presence of papillary carcinoma of long duration. Rings, coarse flakes, and streaks are typical of benign processes. Ultrasound examination of the thyroid may give added information on the extent of the nodular enlargement of the thyroid gland and may reveal cystic areas or calcification. A CT or MRI scan of the neck may be required in unusual circumstances, although less expensive scanning techniques and physical examination are often sufficient to make a precise diagnosis.

The differential diagnosis includes Hashimoto's thyroiditis, solitary adenomas, and carcinomas. In Hashimoto's thyroiditis the gland is usually diffusely involved and the pyramidal lobe is enlarged. Antibodies against thyroid proteins are present in the serum, and the needle biopsy or aspiration may be diagnostic. The possibility of carcinoma, of course, cannot be settled without histologic proof. Rapid enlargement of the thyroid or the presence of a dominant hard nodule or of lymph nodes is suggestive. The presence of carcinoma in a nodular goiter cannot be absolutely excluded except by excisional biopsy.

The diagnosis of thyrotoxicosis should be considered in all patients with nodular goiter, particularly the elderly. TSH is suppressed to a variable degree depending on thyrotoxicity, and characteristically the plasma hormone concentrations are only moderately elevated. Occasionally T_3 thyrotoxicosis, with normal plasma T_4 levels, occurs. The RAIU may be above normal or borderline, but is an unreliable diagnostic procedure.

The T_3 suppression test was formerly used in defining autonomous hyperfunction in multinodular goiter. Administration of T_3 (50 to 75 μg/d for 1 week) will not depress the RAIU in the thyrotoxic gland. Often multinodular goiters that are not toxic will also fail to suppress.[11,12] The test is considered outdated for routine practice, since the administered T_3, additive to the endogenous hormone supply, may precipitate cardiac difficulties. Until recently the TRH stimulation test was used more safely to gain evidence of thyroid autonomy. As discussed in more detail in Chapter 6, autonomous release of thyroid hormone in amounts equivalent to the daily requirement of the subject or slightly above will lead to suppression of TSH secretion by in the pituitary gland. Reduced or absent TSH responses to TRH[11,12] are extremely common in patients with long-standing multinodular thyroid disease. The availability of more sensitive IRMA-TSH determination has made the use of TRH tests unnecessary since basal TSH generally correlates with the increment of TSH after TRH. Therefore, a subnormal IRMA-TSH level, or a value near the lower normal limit, is suggestive of autonomy of thyroid function or subclinical hyperthyroidism when free hormone levels are in the normal range. If the diagnosis of autonomy is established but hormone levels are only borderline, then a therapeutic trial with PTU or methimazole may be helpful to see if any symptoms or signs that the patient shows are related to thyroid function. If adequate quantities of the antithyroid agent result in reduction of the circulating free thy-

roid hormones and symptomatic improvement, the diagnosis of thyrotoxicosis is established and definitive treatment can be provided.

THERAPY FOR THE NONTOXIC NODULAR GOITER

If the enlargement of the gland is moderate and there are no symptoms, therapy is not required. But if there are symptoms due to pressure, if the patient is disturbed by the appearance of the goiter, if there is growth of one nodule, or if possible toxicity develops, therapy is necessary. Attempts to reduce multinodular goiter by administering suppressive doses of thyroid hormone may be considered, but this is usually ineffective and carries the risk of inducing thyrotoxicosis since autonomy of thyroid function is already present. Although some reports found suppressive therapy in multinodular goiter efficacious, less favorable results have been published as well.[75] Our experience has been less favorable. After treatment for 4 to 6 months with thyroid hormone, perhaps 30 to 50 percent of all multinodular goiters decrease in size, and this is mainly due to regression of the paranodular tissue. It has been said that T_3 may be a more effective agent than T_4, but no convincing evidence has been published to support this view. Therapy must be followed with some care, because of the risk of thyrotoxicosis. These patients may be those who might subsequently develop endogenous thyrotoxicosis.[12] Long-term suppression of TSH to the bottom of normal range, however, may still be of value in helping to prevent further growth of the goiter.

There is a growing trend to administer ^{131}I in euthyroid or hyperthyroid multinodular goiter, to both decrease the size and to treat thyrotoxicosis.[76,77] Although many were somewhat skeptical about reducing the size of large multinodular goiters, results are better than was expected.[76,78–80] A substantial reduction in goiter size after one or more treatment doses, though not always complete, occurs in virtually all patients.[81] Hypothyroidism ensues in a substantial number of patients varying from 25 percent after five years[81,82] to 100 percent after eight years[79] depending on the cumulative ^{131}I dose administered and the sensitivity of the thyroid to [131]I. After administering large doses of ^{131}I, temporary increases of thyroid hormone levels may complicate the clinical situation.[83] In the anticipation of such situations, administration of antithyroid drugs for several weeks before administration of ^{131}I or treatment with β-adrenergic blocking agents after ^{131}I administration should be considered. Multiple small doses of 5 to 10 MCi [131]I (185 to 370 MBq) may also be administered. In doing so, however, the uptake of ^{131}I may be lowered so that chances for a positive result are ultimately reduced.

Explorative surgery should be performed in cases of sudden growth in the goiter, when a hard nodule is present, suspicious enlarged lymph nodes are palpable, or vocal cord paralysis is found. Surgery is also necessary in the presence of bleeding leading to mechanical symptoms or any other disturbing local symptoms causing substantial tracheal compression. Surgery may be needed for large goiters, especially those with serious compression of the trachea, since administration of ^{131}I may lead to edema formation which might cause acute obstruction. In the experience of the authors, this has been prevented by the administration of multiple small doses of [131]I. Recent experience shows that even in large compressive goiters a single treatment with ^{131}I is often sufficient. Hkysmans et al.[83a] treated 19 elderly patients (mean age 66.14 years) with a multinodular goiter with a mean thyroid volume of 269 ml (range 108 to 1002 ml) with a single intravenous dose of ^{131}I, aimed at delivering 3.7 MBq (100 rli) per g thyroid tissue. No exacerbation of compressive symptoms occurred. A mean reduction in thyroid volume of 43 percent was noted after one year. Chemical and objective symptoms of tracheal compression improved dramatically. The authors do not endorse prophylactic surgery to prevent the occurrence of carcinoma.

After surgical removal of a nodular goiter, it is sound practice to give the patient replacement doses of thyroid hormone. This therapy will depress pituitary TSH production and may prevent regeneration of the goiter, but it is doubtful that it will totally prevent regrowth. Although in one report no recurrences were found during thyroid hormone administration,[84] others found no differences between untreated patients and patients treated with thyroid hormone after operation.[85–87] In one of these studies[87] carried out over 9 years, no effect of T_4 treatment of thyroidectomy was seen in 104 patients operated on for nontoxic goiter (recurrence rate 9.5 percent) as compared with 71 untreated patients (recurrence rate 11.3 percent). If regrowth occurs, early

ablative treatment with ^{131}I should be considered to prevent the necessity for future reoperation.

Administration of iodide generally has little or no beneficial therapeutic effect, and in an occasional patient may be followed by a rise in plasma hormone concentration and symptoms of thyrotoxicosis.[49,88] This condition is the *jodbasedow phenomenon*, and is dependent on autonomy of function of some elements of the goiter. Its occurrence is not confined to regions of iodine deficiency and is seen on occasion wherever iodide is administered to patients with well-established multinodular goiter.

THERAPY FOR THE TOXIC NODULAR GOITER

Treatment of toxic nodular goiter with RAI is generally satisfactory and will cause a reversion to euthyroid state. The dose of ^{131}I is calculated on the basis of uptake determinations and gland weight, as discussed in Chapter 11. These glands are relatively resistant to ^{131}I, and for this reason some therapists increase the standard dose by 20 to 50 percent. (This is done as part of the schedule given in Chapter 11 since dose is increased with weight.) It is probable that areas in the thyroid of low functional activity at the time of therapy may become activated after destruction of the hyperfunctioning tissue unless these larger doses of ^{131}I are given. Frequently doses are between 15 and 50 mCi (555 and 1850 MBq). Jensen et al.[78] treated their patients with a mean dose of 37 mCi (1369 MBq) range 6.3 to 150 mCi (233 to 5550 MBq). After one year of follow-up 16 percent of patients were hypothyroid. Hamburger et al.[77] used higher doses, 25 to 200 mCi (925 to 7400 MBq) but they treated many patients with large goiters. Danaci et al.[82] treated multinodular toxic goiters with a fixed dose of 16.6 mCi (614 MBq) [131]I and they reported a cumulative relapse rate of 39 percent at 5 years and a cumulative incidence of hypothyroidism of 24 percent at 5 years.

An increase in the severity of thyrotoxicosis after treatment with ^{131}I has occasionally occurred, presumably because these glands contain a large amount of stored TG that is released by radiation damage. Therapy with ^{131}I usually reduces the gland to a cosmetically satisfactory size, but rarely to normal dimensions. Also, in the case of *toxic* nodular goiters of large size more thyroidologists use ^{131}I as first choice of treatment. Careful pretreatment with antithyroid drugs in these cases is imperative. When using large doses, it is important to consider the radiation dose administered. This can be very large and causes serious local reactions, including damage to the laryngeal or tracheal cartilage, and will typically cause significant local pain and tenderness.

Thyroidectomy is indicated if there is a question of cancer or a serious cosmetic problem. The patient may then be prepared with an antithyroid drug administered until the euthyroid state is achieved. The degree of thyrotoxicosis in this group of patients is usually rather mild. Thus, it is permissible and is common practice to prepare the patient simply by the administration of propranolol and iodide for 1 week. After this time most patients will have had some amelioration of their mild thyrotoxicosis and can be carried through thyroidectomy with little difficulty. Thyroid storm occurs only with the greatest rarity after surgical treatment of toxic nodular goiter. When, after operation, airway patency is significantly compromised because of tracheomalacia, a tracheotomy tube is often inserted and left in place for several weeks until peritracheal scarring has produced a rigid airway. Alternatively, the trachea is sutured to surrounding tissues, or plastic rings are sutured to the outside of the trachea in order to provide support.

Unfortunately, many patients with toxic nodular goiter first come to the attention of the physician because of cardiac symptoms, especially congestive heart failure. This condition poses a particularly knotty therapeutic problem. It is obvious that the patient must be given the best available cardiosupportive and diuretic program, but in addition, it is important to relieve the burden of thyrotoxicosis as expeditiously as possible. Propranolol may be helpful in controlling the symptoms of thyrotoxicosis and in controlling the heart rate. Whether propranolol should be used in the presence of congestive heart failure, however, has been much debated. It should probably be avoided unless tachycardia due to thyrotoxicosis is the principal contributing factor. At times patients with moderately severe thyrotoxicosis and advanced congestive heart failure may present a virtually insoluble therapeutic dilemma. Usually RAI therapy is satisfactory despite slow response in this type of patient. As described in Chapter 12, antithyroid drugs and then iodide can be given beginning one day after ^{131}I therapy in order to speed the return to normal. On the other hand, it is our experience that with rest, maximal attention to cardiac

function, appropriate preparation with a antithyroid drug such as PTU or methimazole, great care with anesthesia, and a skillful surgeon, these patients can be quickly relieved of their thyrotoxicosis by subtotal thyroidectomy. Either form of therapy is satisfactory, but ^{131}I treatment is generally preferred in severely ill patients.

COLLOID OR DIFFUSE GOITER

Colloid goiter is histologically distinct from non-toxic nodular goiter, but it may be closely related etiologically. For this reason, it is discussed here briefly. Colloid goiter occurs occasionally as a diffuse enlargement of the thyroid gland in adolescent girls, and is especially frequent in this age group in endemic goiter areas. It occurs much less frequently in adults. Typically, the goiter is asymptomatic. It occasionally causes dysphagia or dyspnea, but it is rare for a colloid goiter to produce significant compression of the trachea or esophagus. The gland is usually symmetrically enlarged and feels soft or spongy.

On gross inspection the excised gland is reddish-tan or pale tan in color and homogeneous on the cut surface. On histologic section, the parenchyma is seen to be nonnodular and composed of uniform follicles filled with colloid. The follicles may be of normal size, in which case it must be considered that an increase in the number of normal follicles has produced the increased bulk of the gland, or the follicles may be uniformly distended to several times the usual diameter. Fibrosis and lymphocyte infiltration are not prominent.

The cause of the condition is unknown. In the past it has been ascribed to the intermediate phase of the Marine cycle (i.e., between the hyperplastic stage and the multinodular or end stage of the thyroid gland as described above). More recent studies in mice suggest that such goiters can be induced in animals by TSH without a prior hyperplastic phase.[13,89] The stimulus to TSH secretion in these patients may be an increased requirement for thyroid hormone, possibly associated with puberty or pregnancy, a period of decreased iodide intake, or the presence within the thyroid of a biochemical lesion interfering with the normal synthesis of thyroid hormone.

The small colloid goiter of adolescent girls may disappear over 1 to 3 years. On the other hand, it may grow gradually and evolve into the nontoxic multinodular goiter found in adults.

A diagnosis of colloid goiter cannot be made with certainty without histologic confirmation. Thyroid function tests are variable, but the results are frequently normal. Antithyroid antibodies are absent if Hashimoto's thyroiditis is not present. Needle biopsy will confirm the diagnosis but is seldom warranted.

Reassurance that the lesion is not a malignant neoplasm, and that the thyroid is not overactive, is often the only therapy required. If the goiter is large, thyroid hormone may be given in an attempt to decrease its size. If one accepts the theory that the goiter has grown in response to a need for more thyroid hormone, it is logical to expect that exogenous thyroid hormone would cause it to decrease in size. Unfortunately, practice does not always bear out this theory. Only about 70 percent[71] of patients will respond with complete or partial regression of goiter. If there are significant pressure symptoms or if the goiter is a serious cosmetic problem, administration of ^{131}I or surgical resection may be indicated. Subsequent replacement therapy with T_4 will then be necessary.

SUBSTERNAL AND ACQUIRED INTRATHORACIC GOITER

The terms *substernal* and *intrathoracic goiter* include instances in which there is a pronounced downward prolongation of the lower pole or poles of the thyroid gland or a downward growth of a nodule from the lower pole below the level of the manubrial notch. The original development site of the thyroid is presumed to be normal. It is an acquired rather than an embryologic abnormality. Displacement of the thyroid through the thoracic strait changes the situation from one where surgery is simple to one where it is potentially difficult, and the symptoms may change from relatively slight to severe. The term *substernal* may be used for those goiters with the greatest diameter above the level of the sternal notch and *intrathoracic* for those in which it is below this notch. Intrathoracic goiter is by far the most common of the important thyroid anatomic anomalies.

Cause

The downward prolongation of the thyroid is due to growth from the lower pole of either a single nodule or one of several nodules in a nodular goiter. When one remembers the anatomy of the thyroid, it is easy to see why at times the growth may be downward rather than anterior, where it is limited by the pretracheal muscles, or posterior or lateral, where it meets resistance from firm structures. The deeper layer of pretracheal muscles is inserted into the posterior part of the clavicle and sternum, and as the nodule slides up and down with deglutition and other movements of the neck, it is guided behind the bony structures of the cervical ring. For a varying length of time, generally a long period, the mass will descend into and come out of the thorax with perfect ease. After a time, more and more of the mass falls below the superior bony margin. The moment the nodule reaches a size that precludes its moving upward into the neck itself, it becomes a completely intrathoracic goiter and, because of its fixed position, is potentially more dangerous in case of sudden swelling from any cause. The size of the growth within the thorax may increase markedly. A tongue of tissue may extend behind the trachea and esophagus, and the lower level may be below the level of the aortic arch and even descend as far as the diaphragm. Although the lower pole is the usual starting point, it is possible for the growth to start from a lateral lobe and thus add to the difficulties of diagnosis because of the apparent freedom of the lower pole from any connection with the intrathoracic growth.

Substernal and intrathoracic goiters are typically found in older persons. A kyphosis, a stooped posture, and an increased anterior-posterior thoracic diameter no doubt promotes an intrathoracic position of the gland. By having the patient lie supine with a pillow under the shoulders, a large part of the gland may be delivered into the neck, and at surgery it is sometimes surprising how easily a large substernal goiter may be pulled out through the cervical inlet and removed without recourse to splitting of the sternum.

Clinical Picture

The symptoms are most often due to mechanical factors, the result of pressure from the mass on surrounding structures. Thyrotoxicosis may also arise from such a gland. Often the first thing that bothers the patient is an obstruction to breathing when the head is in a particular position or when he or she is asleep and the head is lying at a fixed angle. Patients may give a history of attacks during the day or night during which they fear they will suffocate. Dyspnea may suddenly become severe during a respiratory infection and can lead to respiratory failure unless recognized. Bleeding into a cystic lesion is also a cause of sudden accentuation of obstructive symptoms. An irritative cough or slight hoarseness may occur. Difficulty in swallowing may develop so insidiously that the patient is not aware of the problem until it has assumed considerable proportions. One of our patients was unable to swallow anything but liquids for more than a year preceding admission to the hospital. Patients with large, strategically located masses may show a striking pattern of dilated veins over the upper chest. Very rarely a vena cava superior syndrome may ensue.

Diagnosis

A patient with a substernal goiter may show tracheal deviation or evidence of dilated cervical or facial veins. Venous obstruction may be made apparent by having the patient elevate the arms above the head. If external jugular vein dilatation is seen (Pemberton's sign), a significant obstruction to venous return is present due to the mass in the thoracic inlet. The radiograph will show a substernal tumor and often deviation of the trachea. Radioisotope scanning (with ^{131}I) is of much help in defining the limits as well as in identifying the nature of the mass. CT or MRI imaging may be necessary, especially to distinguish a goiter from a vascular tumor or aneurysm.

Treatment

The small, asymptomatic substernal goiter does not require therapy. If necessary ^{131}I treatment can be applied. When the gland causes symptoms, especially the blocking of the thoracic inlet or respiratory symptoms, ^{131}I treatment may be ineffective and sometimes even dangerous because of the risk of edema resulting in further obstruction. Surgical removal is then necessary. Little need be said of the operative procedure for the most commonly observed substernal glands. These glands do not demand any change in anesthesia or special surgical

treatment. Since their greatest diameter is above the level of the strait, they lift out easily and there is no greater danger of nerve damage than in routine thyroidectomy nor is there any increased risk of postoperative complications.

When the growth is lodged below the bony strait, however, the problem may be more serious. Tracheal intubation ensures the continuity of breathing if it should become necessary to exert pressure against the trachea during the surgical procedure. The blood supply of the mass comes from the regular sources to the thyroid and is carried down into the thorax with the descent of the goiter. Consequently, the procedure is first to control the blood supply from above by tying the upper pole and the lateral vessels, and then to find the line of cleavage that will allow the mass to be separated from the bed in which it lies. Because the tracheal tube insures an adequate supply of air, it is possible, in practically all cases, to deliver the growth with a finger lifting below and traction from above.

SUMMARY

Perhaps the most common of all the disorders of the thyroid gland is multinodular goiter. Even in nonendemic regions it is clinically detected in about 4 percent of all adults over the age of 30. Pathologically it is much more frequent, the percentage of incidence being roughly the same as the age of the group examined. The disease is much more common in women than in men.

Multinodular goiter is thought to be the result of primarily two factors: the genetic heterogenity of follicular cells with regard to function (i.e., thyroid hormone synthesis) and growth; and the acquisition of new qualities that were not present in mother cells and which are inheritable during further replication. These two factors may lead to loss of anatomic and functional integrity of the follicles and of the gland as a whole. This process ultimately leads to goiter formation and is accelerated by stimulatory factors. These stimulatory factors may be TSH, brought about by events such as iodine deficiency, inborn errors of thyroid hormone synthesis, goitrogens, immunogenic growth factors, or local tissue growth-regulating factors. These basic and secondary factors may cause the thyroid to grow and gradually evolve into an organ containing hyperplastic islands of normal glandular elements together with nodules and cysts of varied histologic pattern.

Nodular goiter is most often detected simply as a mass in the neck, but at times an enlarging gland produces pressure symptoms on the trachea or esophagus. Occasionally tenderness and a sudden increase in size herald hemorrhage into a cyst. Thyrotoxicosis develops in a large proportion of these goiters after a few decades. Rare complications are paralysis of the recurrent laryngeal nerve and pressure on the superior sympathetic ganglion, which causes Horner's syndrome.

The diagnosis is based on the physical examination. Serum free T_4 and T_3 are usually normal and thyroid autoantibodies are absent, excluding Hashimoto's thyroiditis. Serum TSH is often low especially in large goiters. Imaging procedures may reveal distortion of the trachea, calcified cysts, or impingement of the goiter on the esophagus.

From 4 to 17 percent of multinodular thyroids removed at operation contain foci that on microscopic examination fulfill the criteria of malignant change. The infrequency of thyroid cancer as a cause of death clearly proves that the vast majority of these lesions are not lethal. One of the reasons for the high incidence of cancer in surgical specimens is that patients with enlarging or otherwise clinically suspicious multinodular goiters are selected for surgery.

If a euthyroid multinodular goiter is small and is producing no symptoms, treatment is not necessary. T_4 given in an effort to shrink the gland or to prevent further growth is often unsuccessful. This therapy is more likely to be effective if begun at an early age while the goiter is still diffuse than in older patients in whom certain nodules may have already become autonomous. If the goiter is unsightly or if it is causing pressure symptoms, treatment with ^{131}I is successful in almost all cases but causes hypothyroidism to varying degrees. Sometimes surgery is necessary. Frequently the patient is given T_4 replacement after treatment in order to prevent regrowth. The efficacy of the treatment, however, is doubtful.

Toxic nodular goiter is usually treated with radioactive iodine (RAI). A gratifying reduction in the size of the goiter and control of the thyrotoxicosis may be expected. Alternatively, surgical removal may be successfully employed, particularly if the gland is large. The term *colloid goiter* is applied to glands composed of uniformly distended follicles appearing as a diffuse enlargement of the thyroid gland. The condition is found almost exclusively in young women. With time and due to a number of primary and secondary factors it may gradually develop into a multinodular goiter which becomes increasingly prominent as the decades pass. Appropriate therapy, if required, is the administration of thyroid hormone.

An intrathoracic goiter is usually an acquired rather than a developmental abnormality. It may originate in embryonic life by a carrying downward into the thorax of the developing thyroid anlage, or in adult life by protrusion of an enlarging thyroid through the superior thoracic inlet into the yielding mediastinal spaces. These lesions may produce pressure symptoms and may also be associated with hyperthyroidism or, rarely, with cancer formation. The appropriate therapy is resection of the goiter through the neck, if possible. Locating the attachment of the intrathoracic goiter to the gland in the neck ordinarily proves the site of origin and provides a method for its easy surgical removal.

REFERENCES

1. Trowbridge FL, Hand KA, Nichaman MZ: Findings relating to goiter and iodine in the Ten-State Nutrition Survey. Am J Clin Nutr 28:712, 1975
2. Vander JB, Gaston EA, Dawber TR: Significance of solitary non-toxic thyroid nodules. Final report of a 15-years study of the incidence of thyroid malignancy. N Engl J Med 251:970, 1954
3. Vander JB, Gaston EA, Dawber TR: The significance of nontoxic thyroid nodules. Ann Int Med 69:537, 1968
4. Tunbridge WGM, Evered DC, Hall R et al: The spectrum of thyroid disease in a community: the Whickham survey. Clin Endocrinol 7:481, 1977
4a.Vanderpump MPJ, Turnbridge WMG, French JM et al: The incidence of thyroid disorders in the community: a twenty-year follow-up of the Wickham survey. Clin Endocrinol 43:55, 1995
5. Schlesinger MJ, Cargill GL, Saxe IH: Studies in nodular goiter I. Incidence of thyroid nodules in routine necropsies in non-goitrous region. JAMA 110:1638, 1938
6. Mortensen JD, Woolner LB, Bennett WA: Gross and microscopic findings in clinically normal thyroid glands. J Clin Endocrinol Metab 15:1270, 1955
7. Trowbridge FL, Matovimovic J, McLaren GD, Michaman MZ: Iodine and goiter in children. Pediatrics 56:82, 1975
8. Marine D: Etiology and prevention of simple goiter. Medicine 3:453, 1924

9. Taylor S: The evolution of nodular goiter. J Clin Endocrinol Metab 13:1232, 1953

10. Beckers C, Cornette C: TSH production rate in nontoxic goiter. J Clin Endocrinol Metab 32:852, 1971

11. Dige-Petersen H, Hummer L: Serum thyrotropin concentrations under basal conditions and after stimulation with thyrotropin-releasing hormone in idiopathic non-toxic goiter. J Clin Endocrinol Metab 44:1115, 1977

12. Smeulers J, Docter R, Visser TJ, Hennemann G: Response to thyrotrophin-releasing hormone and triiodothyronine suppressibility in euthyroid multinodular goitre. Clin Endocrinology 7:389, 1977

13. Studer H, Ramelli F: Simple goiter and its variants: euthyroid and hyperthyroid multinodular goiters. Endocrine Rev 3:40, 1982

14. Studer H, Gerber H, Peter HJ: Multinodular goiter. p. I:722. In DeGroot LJ (ed): Endocrinology. Vol. 1. WB Saunders, Philadelphia, 1989

15. Studer H, Peter HJ, Gerber H: Natural heterogeneity of thyroid cells: the basis for understanding thyroid function and nodular growth. Endocr Rev 10:125, 1989

16. Peter HJ, Gerber H, Studer H, Smeds S: Pathogenesis of heterogeneity in human multinodular goiter. J Clin Invest 76:1992, 1985

17. Kopp P, Kimura ET, Alochimann S et al: Polyclonal and monoclonal thyroid nodules co-exist within human multinodular goiters. J Clin Endocrinol Metab 79:134, 1994

18. Masini-Repiso AM, Cobanillas AM, Bonaventura M, Coleoni AH: Dissociation of thyrotropin-dependent enzyme activities, reduced iodide transport, and preserved iodide organification in nonfunctioning adenoma and multinodular goiter. J Clin Endocrinol Metab 79:39, 1994

19. Koutras DA, Alexander WD, Buchanan WW et al: Stable iodine metabolism in non-toxic goitre. Lancet 2:784, 1960

20. Glinoer D, Lemone M: Goiter and pregnancy: a new insight into an old problem. Thyroid 2:65, 1992

21. Baschieri L, Andreani D, Andreoli M et al: Il ricambio dello iodio in gravidanza. Folia Endocrinol 12:3, 1959

22. Aboul-Khair SA, Crooks J, Turnbull AC, Hytten FE: The physiological changes in thyroid function during pregnancy. Clin Sci 27:195, 1964

23. Cassano C, Baschieri L, Andreani D: Etude de 48 cas de goitre simple avec élévation de la clearance rénale de l'iode. p. 307. In Pitt-Rivers R (ed): Advances in Thyroid Research. Pergamon Press, Oxford, 1961

24. Akerman M, DiPaola R, Tubiana M: Estimation of the absolute thyroid uptake of stable ^{127}I using a simplified method and comparison of the results with two classic methods. J Clin Endocrinol Metab 27:1309, 1967

25. Vulsma T, Gons MH, de Vijlder JJM: Maternal-fetal transfer of thyroxine in congenital hypothyroidism due to a total organification defect or thyroid agenesis. New Engl J Med 321:13, 1989

26. Oddie TH, Fisher DA, McConahey WM, Thompson CS: Iodine intake in the United States: a reassessment. J Clin Endocrinol 30:659, 1970

27. Gaitan E: Goitrogens. Clin Endocrinol Metab 2:683, 1988

28. Peltola P: The role of L-5-vinyl-2-thiooxazolidone in the genesis of endemic goiter in Finland. p. 872. In Cassano C, Andreoli M (eds): Current Topics in Thyroid Research. San Diego, Academic Press, 1965

29. Langer P: Antithyroid action in rats of small doses of some naturally occurring compounds. Endocrinology 79:1117, 1966

30. Langer P, Greer MA. Antithyroid substances and naturally occurring goitrogens. Basel, S. Karger, 1977

31. Harden RM, Alexander WD, Chisholm CJS, Shimmins J: The salivary iodide trap in nontoxic goiter. J Clin Endocrinol Metab 28:117, 1968

32. Parker RH, Beierwaltes WH: Inheritance of defective organification of iodine in familial goitrous cretinism. J Clin Endocrinol Metab 21:21, 1961

33. McGirr EM: Sporadic goiter due to dyshormonogenesis. p. I:133. In Astwood EB (ed): Clinical Endocrinology. Vol. 1. Orlando Grune & Stratton, 1960

34. Niepomniszcze H, Altschuler N, Korob MH, Degrossi OJ: Iodide-peroxidase activity in human thyroid. Studies on non-toxic nodular goiter. Acta Endocrinol 62:192, 1969

35. Peter HJ, Studer H, Forster R, Gerber H: The pathogenesis of "hot" and "cold" follicles in multinodular goiters. J Clin Endocrinol Metab 55:941, 1982

36. Studer H: A fresh look at an old thyroid disease: euthyroid and hyperthyroid nodular goiter. J Endocrinol Invest 5:156, 1982

37. Schürch M, Peter HJ, Gerber H, Studer H: Cold follicles in a multinodular human goiter arise partly from a failing iodide pump and partly from deficient iodine organification. J Clin Endocrinol Metab 71:1224, 1990

38. Ieiri T, Cochaux P, Targovnik HM et al: A 3′ splice-site mutation in the thyroglobulin gene responsible for congenital goiter with hypothyroidism. J Clin Invest 88:1901, 1991

39. Drexhage HA, Bottazzo GF, Doniach D: Evidence for thyroid-growth-stimulating immunoglobulins in some goitrous diseases. Lancet 2:287, 1980

40. Wilders-Truschnig MM, Drexhage HA, Leg G et al: Chromatographically purified immunoglobulin G of endemic and sporadic goiter patients stimulates FRTL5 cell growth in a mitotic arrest assay. J Clin Endocrinol Metab 70:444, 1990

40a. Vitti P, Chiovato L, Tonacchera M et al: Failure to detect thyroid growth promoting activity in immunoglobulin G of patients with endemic goiter. J Clin Endocrinol Metab 78:1020, 1994

40b. Davies R, Lawry J, Bhatia V, Weetman AP: Growth stimulating antibodies in endemic goitre: a reappraisal. Clin Endocrinol 43:189, 1995

40c. Brown RS: Editorial: Immunoglobulins affecting thyroid growth: a continuing controversy. Endocrinology 80:1506, 1995

41. Zakarija M, McKenzie JM: Do thyroid growth-promoting immunoglobulins exist? Editorial. J Clin Endocrinol Metab 70:308, 1990

42. Cheng YL, Birman KD, Schaudies RP et al: Effects of epidermal growth factor on thyroglobulin and adenosine 3',5'-monophosphate production by cultured human thyrocytes. J Clin Endocrinol Metab 69:771, 1989

43. Sugenoya A, Masuda H, Komatzu M et al: Adenomatous goitre: therapeutic strategy, postoperative outcome, and study of epidermal growth factor receptor. Br J Surg 79:404, 1992

44. Maciel RM, Moses AC, Villone G et al: Demonstration of the production and physiological role of insulin-like growth factor II in rat thyroid follicular cells in culture. J Clin Invest 82:1546, 1988

45. Phillips ID, Becks GP, Logan A et al: Altered expression of insulin growth factor-1 (IGF-1) and IGF binding proteins during rat hyperplasia and involution. Growth Factors 10:207, 1994

46. Takahashi S-I, Conti M, Van Wyk JJ: Thyrotropin potentiation of insulin-like growth factor-I dependent deoxyribonucleic acid synthesis in FRTL-5 cells: mediation by an autocrine amplification factor(s). Endocrinology 126:736, 1990

47. Vanelli GB, Barni T, Modigliani U et al: Insulin-like growth factor-I receptors in non-functioning thyroid nodules. J Clin Endocrinol Metab 71:1175, 1990

48. deVito WJ, Chanoine J-P, Alex S et al: Effect of in vivo administration of recombinant acidic fibroblast growth factor on thyroid function in the rat: induction of colloid goiter. Endocrinology 131:729, 1992

49. Vagenakis AG, Wang CA, Burger A et al: Iodide-induced thyrotoxicosis in Boston. N Engl J Med 287:523, 1972

50. Pelizzo MR, Piotto A, Rubello D et al: High prevalence of occult papillary thyroid carcinoma in a surgical series for benign thyroid disease. Tumori 76:255, 1990

51. McCall A, Jarosz H, Lawrence AM, Paloyan E: The incidence of thyroid carcinoma in solitary cold nodules and in multinodular goiters. Surgery 100:1128, 1986

52. Koh KB, Chang KW: Carcinoma in multinodular goiter. Br J Surg 79:266, 1992

53. Smeulers J, Docter R, Visser TJ, Hennemann G: Acute thyrotoxicosis in multinodular goiter. Neth J Med 20:275, 1977

54. Hamburger JI, Taylor CI: Transient thyrotoxicosis associated with acute hemorrhagic infarction of autonomously functioning thyroid nodules. Ann Intern Med 91:406, 1979

55. Plummer HS: The clinical and pathologic relationship of hyperplastic and nonhyperplastic goiters. JAMA 61:650, 1913

56. Elte JW, Bussemaker JK, Haak A: The natural history of euthyroid multinodular goiter. Postgrad Med J 66:186, 1990

57. Smeulers J, Visser TJ, Docter R, Hennemann G: Occasional thyroxine and triiodothyronine hypersecretion in euthyroid multinodular goiter. Neth J Med 23:152, 1980

58. Stoffer RP, Welch JW, Hellwig CA et al: Nodular goiter. Arch Intern Med 106:10, 1960

59. Sampson RJ, Key CR, Buncher CR, Iijima S: Thyroid carcinoma in Hiroshima and Nagasaki. I. Prevalence of thyroid carcinoma at autopsy. JAMA 209:65, 1969

60. Sokal JE: A long term follow-up of non-toxic nodular goiter. Arch Intern Med 99:60, 1957

61. Sokal JE: The incidence of thyroid cancer and the problem of malignancy in nodular goiter. p. I:168. In Astwood EB (ed): Clinical Endocrinology. Grune & Stratton, Orlando 1960

62. Mustacchi P, Cutler SJ: Some observations on the incidence of thyroid cancer in the United States. N Engl J Med 255:889, 1956

63. Butler SJ, Young JL: National Cancer Institute: Third national cancer survey incidence data. p. 775. Washington, DC, Dept. of Health, Education and Welfare (NIH), 1975

64. Riccabona OA: Thyroid cancer: its epidemiology, clinical features and treatment. Springer-Verlag, New York 1987

65. Catler SJ, Scotto J, Devesa SS, Connally RR: Third National Cancer Survey: an overview of available information. J Natl Cancer Inst 53:1565, 1974

66. Lang W, Borrusch H, Bauer L: Occult carcinomas of the thyroid: evaluation of 1,020 sequential autopsies. Am J Clin Pathol 90:72, 1988

67. Fukunaga FH, Lockett LJ: Thyroid carcinoma in the Japanese in Hawaii. Arch Pathol Lab Med 92:6, 1971

68. Sampson RJ, Key CR, Buncher CR, Iijima S: Smallest form of papillary carcinoma of the thyroid. Arch Pathol Lab Med 91:334, 1971

69. Sampson RJ, Woolner LB, Bahn RC, Kurland LT: Occult thyroid carcinoma in Olmsted County, Minnesota: prevalence at autopsy compared with that in Hiroshima and Nagasaki. Jpn Cancer 34:2072, 1974

70. Harvey HK: Diagnosis and management of the thyroid nodule. Otolaryngol Clin N Am 23:303, 1990

71. McConahey WM, Hay ID, Woolner LB et al: Papillary thyroid cancer treated at the Mayo Clinic, 1946 through 1970: initial manifestations, pathologic findings, therapy, and outcome. Mayo Clin Proc 61:978, 1986

72. Plummer HS: The function of the thyroid gland containing adenomatous tissue. Trans Assoc Am Physicians 43:159, 1928

73. Davis PJ, Davis FB: Hyperthyroidism in patients over the age of 60 years. Clinical features in 85 patients. Medicine 53:161, 1974

74. Hamburger JI: Evolution of toxicity in solitary nontoxic autonomously functioning thyroid nodules. J Clin Endocrinol Metab 50:1089, 1980

75. Hennemann G: Non-toxic goitre. Clin Endocrinol Metab 8:167, 1979

76. Hegedüs L, Hansen BM, Knudsen N, Hansen JM: Reduction of size of thyroid with radioactive iodine in multinodular nontoxic goitre. Brit Med J 297:661, 1988

77. Hamburger JI, Hamburger SW: Diagnosis and management of large toxic multinodular goiters. J Nucl Med 26:888, 1985

78. Kay TW, d'Emden MC, Andrews JT, Martin FI: Treatment of non-toxic multinodular goiter with radioactive iodine. Am J Med 84:19, 1988

79. Verelst J, Bonnyns M, Glinoer D: Radioactive therapy in voluminous multinodular non-toxic goitre. Acta Endocrinol (Copenh) 122:417, 1990

80. Guermazi F, Fekih MA, Kraiem A, Mtimet S: Efficacité thérapeutique de l'iode[131] dans l'adenome thyréoidien autonome et le goitre multinodulaire toxique: a propos de 59 cas. Ann Endocrinol (Paris) 52:323, 1991

81. Nygaard B, Hegedüs L, Gervil M et al: Radioiodine treatment of multinodular non-toxic goitre. Br Med J 307:828, 1993

82. Danaci M, Veek CM, Notghi A et al: [131]I radioiodine therapy for hyperthyroidism in patients with Graves' disease, uninodular goiter and multinodular goiter. N Z Med J 101:784, 1988

83. Aach R, Kissane J: Thyroid storm shortly after ^{131}I therapy of a toxic multinodular goiter. Am J Med 52:786, 1972

83a. Hksymans DAKC, Hermus ARMM, Corstens FHM, Barentsa JO, Kloppenborg PWC: Large, compressive goiters treated with radioiodine. Ann Int Med 121:757, 1994

84. Bergfelt G, Risholm L: Postoperative thyroid hormone therapy in nontoxic goitre. Acta Chir Scand 126:531, 1963

85. Hegedüs L, Hansen JM, Veiergang D, Karstrup S: Does prophylactic thyroxine treatment after operation for nontoxic goitre influence thyroid size? Brit Med J 294:801, 1987

86. Berghout A, Wiersinga WM, Drexhage HA et al: The long-term outcome of thyroidectomy for sporadic nontoxic goitre. Clin Endocrinol 31:193, 1989

87. Geerdsen JP, Frölund L: Recurrence of nontoxic goitre with and without postoperative thyroxine medication. Clin Endocrinol 21:529, 1984

88. Ermans AM, Camus M: Modifications of thyroid function induced by chronic administration of iodide in the presence of autonomous thyroid tissue. Acta Endocrinol 70:463, 1972

89. Gerber H, Studer H, Conti A et al: Reaccumulation of thyroglobulin and colloid in rat and mouse thyroid follicles during intense thyrotropin stimulation: a clue to the pathogenesis of colloid goiters. J Clin Invest 68:1338, 1981

Thyroid Neoplasia 18

Thyroid cancer accounts for only 0.4 percent of all cancer deaths and for about 5 deaths per 1 million population in the United States each year. Its clinical importance, however, is out of all proportion to its incidence, because cancers of the thyroid must be differentiated from the much more frequent benign adenomas and multinodular goiters. The latter, depending on the criteria employed, occur in up to 4 percent of the population.

This chapter is concerned with both benign and malignant tumors that develop in the thyroid. In a sense, multinodular goiter can be classified as a thyroid tumor, but because it is probably etiologically distinct from the neoplasms considered here and because of its clinical importance, it is discussed separately in Chapter 17.

Numerous classifications of thyroid tumors have been proposed. The one we currently follow groups the lesions on the basis of histologic findings (Table 18-1). The frequently encountered papillary tumors can be subdivided into the small proportion that have only papillary histologic characteristics and the larger group having in addition follicular elements. There is no agreement that these groups differ functionally, and current terminology treats them as one.

THYROID ADENOMAS AND THE PROBLEM OF THE SOLITARY NODULE

The thyroid adenoma is a benign neoplastic growth contained within a capsule. If the tumor reaches 0.5 to 1.0 cm in diameter, it may be detected by careful physical examination.

The terms *adenoma* and *nodule* are often used interchangeably in the literature. This practice is imprecise because adenoma implies a specific benign new tissue growth with a glandlike cellular structure, whereas a nodule could as well be a cyst, carcinoma, lobule of normal tissue, or other focal lesion different from the normal gland. In the following section, the term *nodule* appears frequently when there is need for a nonspecific term.

Incidence and Prevalence

Solitary adenomas occur without recognized geographic preference. Multinodular goiters contain numerous discrete follicular adenomas,[1] however, and if these tumors are included, a high prevalence of adenomas would be recorded in areas of iodide

TABLE 18-1. Neoplasms of the Thyroid

I. Adenomas (Fig. 18-1)
  A. Follicular
    1. Colloid variant
    2. Embryonal
    3. Fetal
    4. Hürthle cell variant
  B. Papillary (probably malignant)
  C. Teratoma
II. Malignant tumors
  A. Differentiated
    1. Papillary adenocarcinoma
      a. Pure papillary adenocarcinoma
      b. Mixed papillary and follicular carcinoma
    2. Follicular adenocarcinomas (variants: "malignant adenoma," Hürthle cell carcinoma or oxyphil carcinoma, clear-cell carcinoma, insular carcinoma)
  B. Medullary carcinoma
  C. Undifferentiated
    1. Small cell (to be differentiated from lymphoma)
    2. Giant cell
    3. Carcinosarcoma
  D. Miscellaneous
    1. Lymphoma, sarcoma
    2. Squamous cell epidermoid carcinoma
    3. Fibrosarcoma
    4. Mucoepithelial carcinoma
    5. Metastatic tumor

Adapted from Hedinger et al.[12]

deficiency and endemic goiter. Palpable thyroid nodules were found in 4 percent of the population sampled in the Framingham, Massachusetts study.[2] One-quarter were considered multinodular and three-quarters solitary. New nodules appeared with an incidence of about 0.1 percent per year.[3] Tunbridge et al. found nodules in 3.7 percent of women in a large survey in England; the prevalence increased with age.[4] Of all the thyroid glands that on surgical resection prove to contain solitary nodules, 70 to 80 percent are benign adenomas and about 10 to 30 percent are malignant growths.[5–7]

In a 1955 report from the Mayo Clinic on 1,000 consecutive autopsies on individuals with clinically normal thyroid glands, the glands weighed on average 20 g at age 20 and gradually increased to 35 g at age 65.[8] The increase occurred in both men and women and did not seem to be related to place of residence. In 50 percent there was one or more nodules, and in 12 percent there was a solitary nodule. Nodularity was more frequent in women than in men, and the prevalence of thyroid carcinomas was

2.1 percent. Surprisingly, nearly 2 percent of the thyroid glands harbored metastatic malignant tumors (carcinomas or lymphomas) originating elsewhere, but it should be noted that, due to the nature of the series, many may have died of malignant disease. Almost identical data were reported from New Haven.[9] In a study from Brazil of 300 autopsies in a goitrous area, 4.3 percent of the glands harbored an adenoma and 2.3 percent a primary carcinoma, of which half were small or "occult."[10] Thus the prevalence of solitary thyroid nodules, and therefore presumably of adenomas, may be approximately 3 percent if one relies on clinical surveys, or as high as 12 percent if one accepts data derived from autopsy studies. Of clinically detected nodules, 5 to 10 percent are in fact carcinomas.[11]

Pathology

These tumors are divided into embryonal, fetal, follicular, Hürthle, and possibly papillary adenomas on the basis of their characteristic pattern.[12] Examples appear in Figure 18-1. The adenomas usually exhibit a uniform orderly architecture and few mitoses, and show no lymphatic or blood vessel invasion. They are characteristically enveloped by a discrete fibrous capsule or a thin zone of compressed surrounding thyroid tissue.

Whether papillary adenoma is a real entity is debatable; most observers believe that all papillary tumors should be considered as carcinomas. Others consider that some papillary tumors are benign adenomas. It is our impression that papillary tumors are best thought of as carcinomatous, although the degree of invasive potential may be very slight in some instances. The same confusion extends to Hürthle cell adenomas. Many pathologists consider all of these tumors as low-grade carcinomas in view of their frequent late recurrences. For this reason, the nondefinitive term *Hürthle cell tumor* is commonly used. Hürthle cell tumors are found on electron microscopy to be packed with mitochondria, which accounts for this special eosinophilic staining quality.

Nearly half of all single nodules have on gross inspection a gelatinous appearance, are composed of large colloid-filled follicles, and are not completely surrounded by a well-defined fibrous capsule. These nodules are listed as colloid variants of follicular adenomas in our classification. Many pathologists report these as colloid nodules, and suggest that each

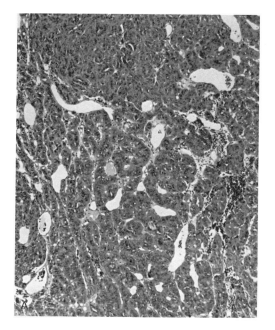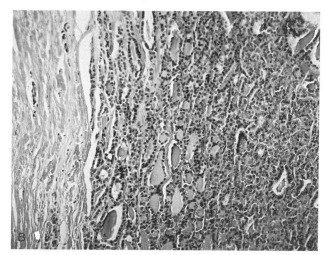

Fig. 18-1. Histologic pattern of benign tumors of the thyroid: (A), Embryonal adenoma. (B), fetal adenoma. Note the sharp margin, capsule, and tiny follicles. (Courtesy of Dr. F. Straus.)

is a focal process perhaps related to multinodular goiter rather than a true adenoma. These tumors are usually not surrounded by a capsule of compressed normal tissue, and often show degeneration of parenchyma, hemosiderosis, and colloid phagocytosis (Fig. 18-2). Recent studies indicate that most adenomas, as well as carcinomas, are truly clonal—derived from one cell—whereas colloid nodules, at least in multinodular goiters, tend to be polyclonal.[13]

Cause

Thyroid adenomas are monoclonal "new growths" that are formed in response to the same sort of stimuli as are carcinomas. Heredity does not appear to play a major role in their appearance. One clue to their origin is that they are four times more frequent in women than in men, although no definitive relation of estrogen to cell growth has been demonstrated. Thyroid radiation, chronic TSH stimulation, and oncogenes believed to be related to the origin of these lesions are discussed below in the section on thyroid cancer.

Course and Symptoms

Thyroid adenomas grow slowly and may remain dormant for years. This is presumably related to the fact that adult thyroid cells normally divide once in eight years.[14] An adenoma may first come to attention because the patient accidentally finds a lump in the neck or because a physician discovers it upon routine examination. Rarely, symptoms such as dysphagia, dysphonia, or stridor may develop, but it is unusual for these tumors to attain sufficient size to cause significant symptoms. Typically, they are entirely asymptomatic. Occasionally there is bleeding into the tumor, causing a sudden increase in size and local pain and tenderness. After bleeding into an adenoma, transient symptoms of thyrotoxicosis may appear with elevated serum T_4 levels, and suppression of thyroidal radioactive iodine uptake (RAIU). Spontaneous regression of adenomas can occur.

Hemorrhage into a Nodule

When M. G., a 47-year-old woman, was first examined, enlargement of the thyroid had been known for at least 6 years. A scan showed a cold nodule in the left lobe. The patient was thought to have a thyroid nodule and to be euthyroid. These was on exam a normal right thyroid lobe, and a 4- × 5-cm soft mass occupying the position of the left lobe. The impression at this time was that she had an adenoma that might be cystic. Antithyroid antibodies were not detectable.

The patient was examined by several observers who palpated the thyroid. One-half hour after leaving the clinic, the patient's neck gradually began to enlarge,

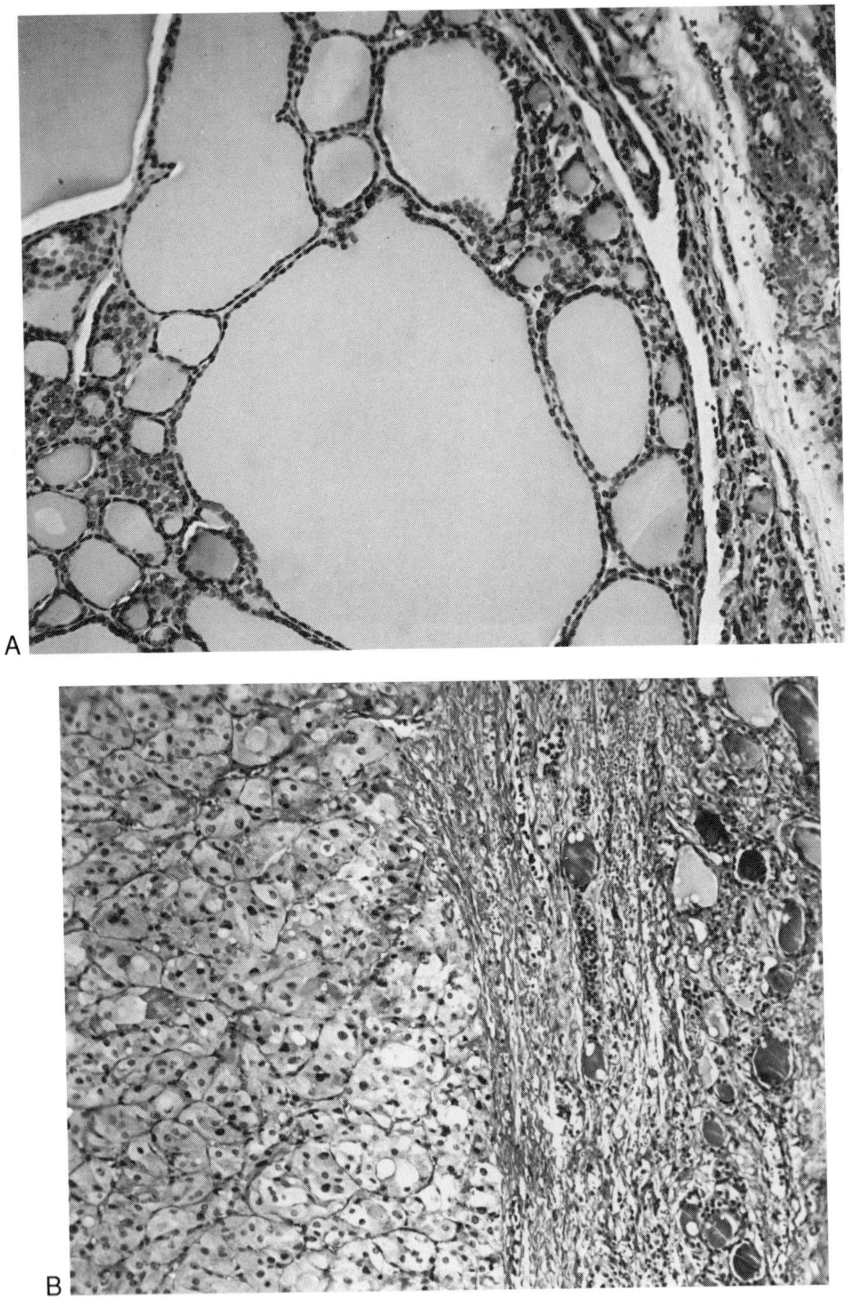

Fig. 18-2. (A) Colloid nodule or adenoma. The macrofollicular pattern and minimal capsule are evident. (B) Hürthle cell adenoma.

and she developed pain in the area of the thyroid and a rasping hoarseness. She had no difficulty in swallowing or breathing. The pain was significant enough to keep her awake that night, and she returned to the hospital the next day.

The patient was very anxious, and there was a 10- ×

12-cm tender fluctuant swelling occupying the area of the thyroid. Inspiratory stridor was present, and there were a few rhonchi in the lungs.

During the subsequent 3 days the pain in the neck gradually diminished, but the size of the mass remained more or less the same. Chest radiographs revealed marked deviation of the trachea to the right. Operation was elected. A greatly enlarged left lobe of the thyroid was found, with hemorrhage into an adenoma. The encapsulated mass measured 6.5 × 5.5 cm and was smooth and cystic. There was a large multiloculated hematoma and considerable necrotic tissue. A left lobectomy was performed. Microscopic examination showed a microfollicular thyroid adenoma with recent hemorrhage and necrosis. The postoperative course was unremarkable. The patient remained well after surgery without further difficulty.

Usually hemorrhage occurs without known provocation, but occasionally is seen after trauma to the neck. In this instance, palpation may have been sufficient to induce bleeding.

Does an adenoma ever develop into a carcinoma? Most pathologists and surgeons believe that thyroid adenomas are benign from the start and that most thyroid carcinomas are likewise malignant from their inception. In animals chronically given ^{131}I and antithyroid drugs, a gradual progression of types of lesions from adenomas to carcinomas is seen. Pathologic examination occasionally gives evidence for conversion of an adenoma to a carcinoma. Transformation of hyperplastic thyroid tissue into invasive cancer occasionally occurs in patients with congenital goitrous hypothyroidism, and cancers are sometimes seen inside an adenoma or in a gland that was known to have harbored a nodule for many years. Occasionally a patient develops metastatic cancer years after resection of an embryonal or Hürthle cell adenoma. All of these points suggest that transformation of an adenoma into a carcinoma occurs occasionally, but it must be an unusual sequence of events.

About 10 percent of thyroid adenomas are functional enough (are "hot" on scan) to produce overt thyrotoxicosis and account for perhaps 2 percent of all thyrotoxic patients. Another 10 percent may be borderline in function and are classified as "hot" (or hyperfunctioning, in comparison to the remainder of the thyroid gland) on isotopic scans. Although hyperfunctioning nodules may remain unchanged for years, some gradually develop into toxic nodules, especially if their diameter exceeds 3 cm.[15] Others undergo spontaneous necrosis with a return of function in the formerly suppressed normal gland. Patients with functioning autonomous nodules may be overtly thyrotoxic; more commonly, however, the nodule functions enough to suppress the remainder of the gland, but not enough to produce clinical hyperthyroidism.[16] In such patients, T_3 levels may be

slightly elevated, serum TSH will be below normal, and the pituitary response to TRH is typically suppressed.[17] If the nodule is resected, the gland resumes normal function, and serum TSH and the TRH response is normalized (see also Ch. 13).

In certain areas such as Switzerland, up to one-third of all thyrotoxic patients have hyperfunctioning adenomas,[18] largely in multinodular glands. Perhaps this situation is generally true in endemic goiter areas.

Biochemical Studies

The biochemical defect responsible for diminished iodine metabolism in the "cold" (i.e., inactive) nodule can result from deletion of specific metabolic processes required for hormone synthesis. Slices of cold nodules incubated in vitro were unable to accumulate iodide against a concentration gradient, although peroxidase and iodide organification activities were present.[19] This finding was consistent with a specific defect of the iodide transport process. Others have also observed this phenomenon and have shown that TSH can bind to the membranes of the cells and activate adenyl cyclase as usual, but that subsequent metabolic steps are not induced.[20] Activity of the sodium-potassium-activated ATPase, thought to be related to iodide transport, is intact, and ATP levels are normal, even though iodide transport is inoperative. Other nodules appear to be cold because they lack peroxidase.[21] These nodules can be "hot" when scanned with $^{99m}TcO_4$ due to active transport of the isotope, but relatively cold on scanning at 24 hours after ^{131}I is given, since iodide binding is poor.[22] The adenyl cyclase system in the plasma membrane of of some hyperfunctioning nodules has been found to be hyper-responsive to TSH in some studies[23] but not in others.[24] All of the foregoing reports suggest that adenoma formation is associated with mutational events that cause loss or dysfunction of normal metabolic activities. It has been suggested that functioning nodules grew because they were unusually responsive to TSH, but this does not appear to be a characteristic finding. However, activating mutations of the TSH receptor have now been shown to be an important cause of toxic adenomas (and hereditary hyperthyroidism) as discussed below.

TABLE 18-2. Differential Diagnosis of the Thyroid Nodule

Adenoma
Cyst
Carcinoma
Multinodular goiter
Hashimoto's thyroiditis
Subacute thyroiditis
Effect of prior operation or ^{131}I therapy
Thyroid hemiagenesis
Metastasis
Parathyroid cyst or adenoma
Thyroglossal cyst
Nonthyroidal lesions
    Inflammatory or neoplastic nodes
    Cystic hygroma
    Aneurysm
    Bronchocele
    Laryngocele

CLINICAL EVALUATION AND MANAGEMENT OF NODULES

Conditions to be considered in the differential diagnosis are listed in Table 18-2. They include adenoma, cyst, multinodular goiter, a prominent area of thyroiditis, an irregular regrowth of tissue if surgery has been performed, thyroid hemiagenesis, and of course, thyroid cancer.

Factors that must be considered in reaching a decision for management include the history of the lesion, age, sex, and family history of the patient, physical characteristics of the gland, local symptoms, and laboratory evaluation. The age of the patient is an important consideration since the ratio of malignant to benign nodules is higher in youth and lower in older age. Male sex carries a similar importance.[25] Nodules are less frequent in men, and a greater proportion are malignant.

Rarely, the family history may be helpful in the decision regarding surgery. Patients with the hereditable multiple endocrine neoplasia syndrome (MEN), type I, may have thyroid adenomas, parathyroid adenomas, islet cell tumors, and adrenal tumors, whereas patients with MEN types II and III, have pheochromocytomas, medullary thyroid carcinomas, hyperparathyroidism, and mucosal neuromas[26-28] (see below). Furthermore, we have observed that 6 percent of our patients with thyroid carcinoma have a history of malignant thyroid neoplasm in other family members, and familial medullary cancer (without MEN) is well known. Familial

thyroid tumors occur in Cowden's disease, Gardner syndrome, and familial polyposis coli (see below).

A most important piece of information regarding a nodule is a history of prior neck irradiation. Any irradiation above 50 rads (50 cGrays) to the thyroid during childhood should be viewed with concern. Exposure to 100 to 700 rads during the first 3 or 4 years of life has been associated with a 1 to 7 percent incidence of thyroid cancer occurring 10 to 30 years later.[29-34] Radiation exposure during adolescence or early adulthood for acne or for other reasons has also been identified as a cause of this disease. Although this association has been known since 1950, patients are still being seen with radiation-related tumors who received x-ray treatment as late as 1959. Radiation therapy for other benign or malignant lesions in the neck is still in use in selected patients; such exposure will thus continue to be a relevant part of the history. Because of the high prevalence (20 to 40 percent) of carcinoma in nodules resected from irradiated glands, the finding of one or more clear-cut nodules in a radiated gland, or a cold area on scan, must be viewed with alarm and requires consideration for removal, as indicated below. In this instance, multiple nodules do not indicate that the lesions are benign. Although ^{131}I therapy is generally considered not to induce thyroid cancers, observation of a nodule in a patient previously treated with ^{131}I must raise the index of suspicion and requires definitive proof of benign nature, or resection.

The history of the neck lump itself is important. Recent onset, growth, hoarseness, pain, nodes in the supraclavicular fossae, symptoms of brachial plexus irritation, and local tenderness all suggest malignancy, but of course do not prove it. The usual cause of sudden swelling and tenderness in a nodule is hemorrhage into a benign lesion. Although the presence of a nodule for many years suggests a benign process, some cancers grow slowly. In our series, the average time from recognition of a nodule to diagnosis of cancer was 3 years. A history of residence in an endemic goiter zone during the first decades of life is also relevant and must raise the possibility of multinodular goiter as the true diagnosis.

The adenoma is typically felt as a discrete lump in an otherwise normal gland, and it moves with the thyroid. Enlarged lymph nodes should be carefully sought, particularly in the area above the isthmus, in the cervical chains, and in the supraclavicular areas. Their presence suggests malignant disease unless a good alternative diagnosis is apparent, such as recent oropharyngeal sepsis or viral infection. Fixation of the nodule to strap muscles or the trachea is alarming. Characteristically a benign thyroid adenoma is part of the thyroid and moves with deglutition, but can be moved in relation to strap muscles and within the gland substance to some extent. Pain, tenderness, or sudden swelling of the nodule usually indicates hemorrhage into the nodule but can also indicate an invasive malignancy. Hoarseness may arise from pressure or by infiltration of a recurrent laryngeal nerve by a neoplasm. Obviously the presence of a firm, fixed lesion, associated with pain, hoarseness, or any one of these features, should signal some degree of alarm. The converse situation, the absence of such characteristics, suggests but does not prove benignity. Fluctuance in the lesion suggest the presence of a cyst that is, usually, benign.

The presence of a diffusely multinodular gland, ascertained on the basis of palpation or scanning, is usually interpreted as a sign of safety. Multinodular goiters coming to surgery have a significant prevalence of carcinoma (4 to 17 percent), but this finding is believed to be due largely to selection of patients for surgery, and not to be typical of multinodular goiter in the general population.[35,36] If there is one area within a multinodular goiter that seems different from the remainder of the gland on the basis of palpation or function, or has demonstrated rapid growth, or if there are two discrete nodules in a gland that is otherwise normal, then one should consider malignant change rather than a benign multinodular goiter.

Occasionally the gland has, in addition to a nodule, the diffuse enlargement and firm consistency of chronic thyroiditis, a palpable pyramidal lobe, and antibody test results that may be positive. These findings strongly suggest thyroiditis but do not disclose the nature of the nodule, which must be evaluated independently. It should be remembered that 14 to 20 percent[34,37] of thyroid cancer specimens contain diffuse or focal thyroiditis. In addition, a positive association of thyroid cancer and Hashimoto's thyroiditis has been reported, but is not proven (see below).

The patient is usually euthyroid, and this impression is supported by normal values for the serum FTI and T_3 levels. Thyrotoxicity produced by an adenoma is discussed below. Low FTI or elevated TSH results should raise the question of thyroiditis. The serum TG concentration may be elevated, as in all other goitrous conditions, and therefore is not a valuable tool in differential diagnosis. The calcitonin

assay is not cost effective in the diagnosis of the usual nodule, but is indicated in the presence of a suggestive family history or of coincident features of the MEN-II syndromes. A chest radiograph should be taken if a normal film has not been reported in the prior 6 months. Soft tissue radiographs of the neck may disclose indentation or deviation of the trachea if the tumor is more than 3 or 4 cm in diameter. Fine, stippled calcifications through the tumor (psammoma bodies) are virtually pathognomonic of papillary cancer. Patchy or "signet ring" calcification occurs in old cysts and degenerating adenomas, and has no such connotation.

The scintiscan received much attention as an aid in the differential diagnosis of thyroid lesions (Ch. 5). The scan may provide evidence for a diagnosis in a multinodular goiter, in Hashimoto's thyroiditis, and rarely in thyroid cancer when functioning cervical metastases are seen. If the scan demonstrates a hyperfunctioning nodule suppressing the remainder of the gland, and the patient is thyrotoxic as demonstrated by an elevated serum FTI or T_3 level, or suppressed sTSH, the chance of malignancy is very low. Tumors that accumulate RAI in a concentration equal to or greater than that of the surrounding normal thyroid tissue, but that do not produce thyrotoxicosis, are also typically benign.[38,39] In fact, some observers insist that functioning nodules cannot be malignant,[39] in spite of reports of malignant change in occasional warm or hot nodules.[39–43] Malignant tumors usually fail to accumulate iodide to a degree equal to that of the normal gland. Most cold nodules, however, turn out to be benign adenomas and cysts, not cancers. The reported incidence of cancer in cold nodules is highly variable; a review of 400 cases found 10 percent to be cancer,[44] and this experience is typical. Tumors smaller than 1 cm in size are below the discriminating power of most of the available scanning devices. Thus, a nodule 1 cm or less in diameter that fails to collect RAI (cold nodule) might not be delineated at all on the scintiscan. Further, many nodules turn out to be neither cold nor hot (preferential isotope accumulation); rather, they accumulate RAI in approximately the same concentration as the surrounding thyroid tissue. Normal tissue in front of or behind the nodule may also accumulate isotope and in this way obscure a deficit in collection within the lesion itself. For all of these reasons, it is our impression that the thyroid scintiscan has value, but except for the clearly toxic nodule, does not form an absolute judgment as to whether a palpable nodule is malignant or benign. Usually pertechnetate scanning provides the same information as RAI scanning, but exceptions occur.

Several alternative techniques have been introduced for scanning, all showing some promise for selection of dangerous lesions. Lesions that are cold on conventional RAI scan but active on selenomethionine scan are said to be usually malignant.[45] Radioactive phosphate has been used in a similar fashion. Radioactive gallium and technetium-labeled bleomycin have also been studied as possible scanning agents, but without notable success. Fluorescent thyroid scanning[46] offers the possibility of quantitating the distribution of ^{127}I in thyroid nodules, but in our clinical experience with the technique, it has not proven to be a more discriminating diagnostic method than conventional radioisotope scanning. ^{201}Thallium is accumulated in thyroid cancer tissue. So far, it has mainly been employed to identify metastatic sites.[47]

Hyperfunctioning Nodule versus Carcinoma

R. B., a 15-year-old girl, was found on routine examination to have thyroid enlargement. Examinations revealed a nodule that gradually enlarged to 4 cm in diameter. The patient was told by her physician that her thyroid was slightly overactive. There was a history of diagnostic dental radiographs but no other head or neck irradiation.

On examination the thyroid was normal except for a soft 4 cm nodule in the left lower pole. There was no bruit and no fixation to the trachea (Fig. 18-3). The right lobe could be palpated and was normal. There were no palpable lymph nodes.

The serum T_3 level was 249 ng/dl and the FTI was 12.2 (normal, 6.0 to 10.5). Antibody test results were negative. TG was 12.2 ng/ml and TSH was 3.4 μU/ml (in a first generation TSH assay). Thyroid needle aspiration showed normal epithelial cells and macrophages. On scintiscan the nodule was clearly functioning and suppressed the remainder of the gland.

Because of concern over growth of the nodule in a young girl, and to treat the hyperthyroidism, the patient underwent a left thyroid lobectomy. The pathologic diagnosis was hyperplastic nodule, a variant of the common colloid nodule and possibly a type of follicular adenoma. She subsequently was placed on thyroxine replacement and has been well to date.

This patient had an 18-g nodule suppressing the normal gland. Most young patients with this problem have benign hyperplastic colloid nodules rather than typical follicular adenomas.

It is now common to perform ultrasound examination of thyroid nodules. Good technique demonstrates nodules of more than 3 mm in size, indicates cystic areas, may demonstrate a capsule around the nodule, and the size of the lobes. It often displays multiple nodules when only one is noted clinically.

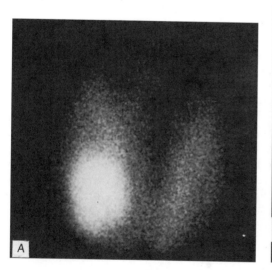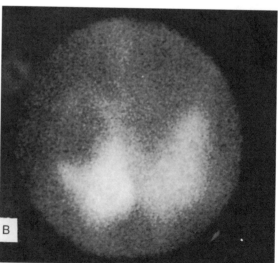

Fig. 18-3. Scintiscans of thyroid nodules. The function of the nodule detected in (A) is typical of a warm but not "toxic" nodule, since residual function is present in the remainder of the thyroid gland. (B) Typical technetium pyrophosphate scan of a "cold" thyroid nodule failing to accumulate isotope. This nodule could be functional on iodide scanning.

The technique is more sensitive than scintiscanning, is noninvasive, involves less time, allows serial exams, and is usually less expensive. From 3 to 20 percent of lesions are found to be totally or partially cystic. Purely cystic lesions are reported to have a lower incidence of malignancy than solid tumors (3 percent versus 10 percent), and diagnosis of a cyst raises the possibility of aspiration therapy.[47] Mixed solid and cystic lesions allegedly have a higher frequency of malignant change than either pure cysts or solid lesions.

Thyroid thermography also has been done and may hold promise, but it is not yet a well-defined procedure.

For many years core needle biopsy of the thyroid was employed successfully in some clinics to provide a histologic diagnosis on which to base therapy.[48] Difficulties in acceptance of the procedure by surgeons, patients, and pathologists prevented its widespread application. As an alternative technique, thin needle aspiration cytologic examination has been widely adopted after favorable reports by Walfish et al.[49] and Gershengorn et al.[50] The procedure is technically simple and acceptable to patients, but requires an experienced operator and collaboration with a skilled cytopathologist (Fig. 18-4). Adequate specimens can be obtained in over 90 percent of patients. False-negative and false-positive diagnoses do of course occur, but are each under 5 percent with experienced hands. Willems and Lowhagen,[6] in reviewing a collected series of nearly 4,000 surgically proven fine needle aspiration studies, found that 11.8 percent were considered to be malignant lesions. False-negative diagnoses of cancer were made in 6.6 to 27.5 percent and false-positive diagnoses in only 0 to 2 percent. Currently the results of FNA are viewed as the gold standard for diagnosis in most cases, and play a crucial role in the selection of patients for operation. Gharib and co-workers recently analyzed data on 10,000 FNAs, and found the procedure to be the preferred first step in diagnosis.[51] Miller et al.[52] compared fine needle aspiration, large needle aspiration, and cutting needle biopsy. They found fine needle aspiration cytologic examination was able to detect almost all carcinomas, but believe that cutting needle biopsy is a useful additional procedure, especially in larger (over 2 to 3 cm) nodules.

In our practice, 5 to 8 percent of aspirates are found diagnostic of malignancy, 10 to 20 percent are considered suspicious but not diagnostic, 2 to 5 percent fail to provide an adequate specimen, and the remainder are considered benign, usually suggestive of a "colloid nodule" or thyroiditis. An inadequate specimen should lead to reaspiration. A positive diagnosis of cancer, of course, leads to surgery. We, as others, tend to operate on patients with suspicious FNA histology, since about 25 percent prove at surgery to be malignant. In the remainder, continued observation and suppressive thyroxine therapy are offered. Patients who are not operated on are seen at 6 or 12 month intervals, and examined for any sign such as pain, growth, hoarseness, or nodes that might indicate a change in the character of the tumor. Patients are usually rebiopsied after 2 to 3 years to document again the benign nature of the lesion.

Most patients are given thyroxine in a dose adjusted to keep TSH in the minimally depressed range—e.g., .3 to .5 μU/ml. It is recognized that the efficacy of this treatment to shrink nodules is poor, but it does appear to reduce the size of 10 to 20 percent of the lesions[53,54] and may prevent further growth. This level of hormone replacement is chosen in the belief that it is unlikely to cause symptoms of hyperthyroidism, such as palpitations, and unlikely to cause osteoporosis, even with prolonged use, while it presumably does reduce growth stimulation to the nodule. It is not appropriate to maintain postmenopausal women on doses of hormone that produce even mild hyperthyroidism for a long period, in view of the potential induction of osteoporosis. Serum TG is usually measured at each visit. Suppression to a normal level by T_4 therapy is a gratifying and reassuring response, and is correlated with nodule shrinkage.[55] Progressive elevation suggests resection should be considered.

While FNA clearly has reduced the initial incidence of surgery in the management of nodules, the long term effect is less clear. Over three years of follow-up, at least 30 percent of our patients, who are believed to have a benign nodule, eventually undergo surgery. This occurs because they, or their physicians, remain concerned about the nodule, or the nodule is painful or grows, or is cosmetically unsatisfactory. But in most cases operation probably occurs because the patient cannot be entirely reassured by the physician that the lesion is safe.

The Value of Surgery

Probably less than one-quarter of the nodules in the population eventually come to surgery, and these represent a highly selected fraction of the total.[3] Of

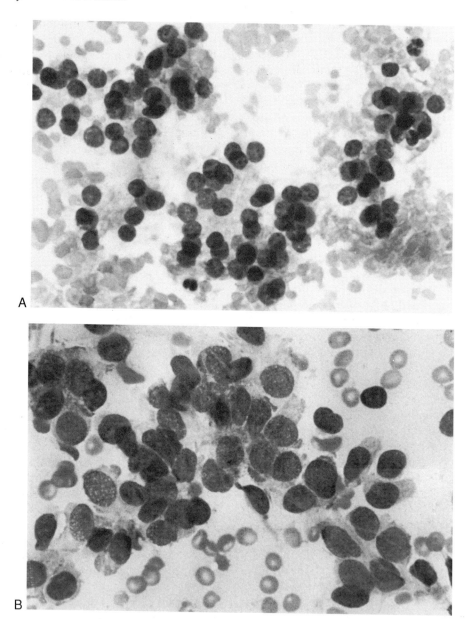

Fig. 18-4. Fine needle aspiration cytology specimens. (A) Epithelial cells in a follicular arrangement suggesting adenoma, but which could be from a follicular carcinoma. (B) Epithelial cells in a papillary formation from a papillary thyroid carcinoma. Nuclear grooves are also apparent. (Courtesy of Dr. M. Bibbo.)

those who are caught in the selection process, including "cocktail party" observation, family physician screening, palpation by the gynecologist, referral to an internist, endocrinologist, or surgeon, and who finally have microscopic examination by a pathologist, a few turn out not to have discrete nodules, but rather to have multinodular goiters in which one region of the gland is especially prominent. In past

years, up to one-half of all nodules clinically regarded as single prove at surgery to reside in multinodular goiters.[3] But with the decreased incidence of multinodular goiter, this is less frequent. The reported incidence of surgically proven thyroid carcinoma in specimens resected because of a clinically defined solitary nodule varies from 10 to 30 percent among different observers.[5–7] In a series of 104 patients at the University of Chicago Clinics operated on for a suspicion of thyroid carcinoma, the diagnosis was established at surgery in 36 percent. Of 64 patients in the group with a clinically single nodule, 33 percent had cancer. Less than 10 percent of the total number had multinodular goiter. Almost identical statistics came from Hoffman et al., who found carcinoma in 29 percent of 202 single nodules.[37] A reminder that the above experience may not be typical comes again from the Framingham study; of 60 nodules resected over a period of 15 years, none was declared malignant by the pathologist. Most probably this finding indicates a peculiarity of this series, which selected an entire population group, rather than patients who came to the physician for care.

What is the prognosis, with or without treatment, for these thyroid malignancies? The majority are papillary or mixed papillary-follicular tumors, with fewer pure follicular and rare solid or anaplastic carcinomas. In general, the death rate due to thyroid carcinoma (4.5 per 10^6 persons per year) is approximately one-tenth the incidence rate of 30 to 60 per million people each year.[56,57] Although it would be comforting to believe that the difference between the incidence and death rates is due to the effectiveness of surgical and medical therapy, it also reflects the remarkable benignity of many of these tumors. Some patients carry them throughout their lives and die from other causes. Although no controlled series is

available, it seems obvious that some carcinomas that occur first as nodules will cause death. About all that can be stated with certainty is that some patients do die from thyroid carcinoma, and that if the surgeon removes a nodule that is really an invasive tumor before it has metastasized, or while it is still under the control of the defense mechanisms of the body, a cure is effected. Quantitating the results of resection of thyroid nodules is virtually impossible. There is even some hope for survival if an anaplastic tumor is observed and resected promptly, since surgery cures 5 to 15 percent of patients with these tumors.[58]

Therapy for Nodules

Toxic nodules are treated by resection or ^{131}I therapy (Table 18-3). Since surgery is safe, removes the lesion, provides histologic diagnosis, avoids leaving a hard nodule in the thyroid gland, and avoids irradiation and possible hypothyroidism, we prefer this approach in most young adults through age 45 to 50.

Toxic nodules may also be treated by administration of single 30- to 60-mCi doses of ^{131}I, and some thyroidologists use this treatment in most persons over age 25. The ease and convenience of ^{131}I, lower expense, avoidance of a scar, and avoidance of hospitalization make it the preferable approach in older

TABLE 18-3. Management of Cold Nodules

History	Physical Examination	Laboratory Tests
Radiation	Size	FTI
Age	Fixation	Antithyroid antibodies
Sex	Cystic nature	TG
Duration	Tenderness	Chest x-ray film
Local symptoms	Adenopathy	Ultrasound scan
Growth	Diffuse/local process	Isotope scan (?)
MEN syndrome	Vocal cord paralysis	X-ray of soft tissues of the neck
Thyrotoxicity	Single versus multiple nodules	Fine needle aspiration
Geographic residence		
Family history		

Management	
Thyrotoxic hot nodules ⟶	Surgery (or ^{131}I therapy)
"Mainly cystic" ⟶	Aspirate for Dx and therapy; reaspirate as needed; T_4 therapy
	Probable cancer → operate
	Inadequate specimen → reaspirate
Other nodules ⟶ Aspiration cytology	Suspicious → operate
	Benign → follow on replacement T_4 therapy

patients and those with coincident serious illness. This therapy usually spares the uninvolved parts of the gland because, at the time, they are inactive. Results are to some extent unpredictable. Smaller doses may be ineffective or must be repeated, and the remainder of the gland receives 1,000 to 8,000 rads, which induces hypothyroidism in up to one-third of cases.[59] Although, in theory, this radiation could induce tumor formation, this has not been reported. Further, the patient receives 30 to 60 rads of whole body irradiation.[60] A nodule is usually left in the gland after treatment,[59] but surgery is avoided.

Autonomous thyroid adenomas are currently being treated by some physicians through repeated percutaneous injection of ethanol under ultrasonic guidance. Volumes of .4 to 2 ml are injected, and patients may receive up to 9 or more treatments at intervals of several days. The response is a gradual return to a euthyroid state and shrinking of the nodule.[61] Leakage of ethanol can cause local pain and tissue damage. A firm or partially cystic nodule usually remains.

Cystic lesions are aspirated and often reaspirated one or more times. Long-term suppression with thyroid hormone may tend to prevent recurrence, although this outcome is uncertain.[53] If, after repeated aspiration, the lesion is still clearly evident, it must be considered a mixed solid/cystic lesion and probably should be resected. Cytologic examination of the aspirated fluid should be done, but the specimens are often not satisfactory for diagnosis.

Some physicians attempt to sclerose cysts by aspirating fluid, and then reinjecting one-half volume of a 10/1 mixture of saline and an injectable form of tetracycline containing 100 mg/ml of the drug. Care must be taken to avoid subcutaneous leakage which is very painful. The technique is not widely used, but is reported to be effective[62] by some (but not all) clinicians.

Sclerotherapy is also possible using ethanol instillation. In a recent report,[63] recurrent cysts were aspirated and one-third volume of ethanol was instilled, and then removed after 5 minutes. Some patients were treated twice. The overall effect was a major reduction in cyst size.

Solid, mixed, functioning, or "cold" nodules constitute the remaining group and indeed the majority of cases. Here major reliance is placed on aspiration cytology. If the results are positive for carcinoma, resection is offered. If no specimen is obtained, reaspiration is performed. If the specimen is suspicious, reaspiration or resection is mandatory. If a benign result is obtained on cytologic examination, the patient is followed while receiving suppressive therapy with thyroid hormone. The dose may consist of .05 to 0.15 mg L-T_4, or equivalent amounts of other preparations. The dose should be enough to largely suppress TSH stimulation, as evidenced by a serum TSH level of .3 to 1 μU/ml, reduction in nodule size, reduction of serum TG, and should not be so high as to produce chemical or clinical hyperthyroidism. Patients receiving thyroxine therapy are followed indefinitely at 6- to 12-month intervals, and future management varies with the patient's course. Adverse factors to be noted include growth, development of local symptoms, or adenopathy. In all patients under age 25, all men, and those with a history of neck irradiation, any change usually constitutes grounds for resection. In women 25 years of age and up, the situation should be carefully reviewed and reaspiration performed. If the changes can be explained in the context of a benign process and the reaspirate is benign, continued careful medical follow-up is acceptable, but operation will often be preferred by the patient or physician. The desired course in follow-up is for a gradual reduction and disappearance of the offending lesion. Although this result occasionally is seen, most often the lump remains the same or a bit smaller and persists year after year.

The most important requirement for surgery is the selection of an experienced surgeon in an institution with an adequate department of pathology. The patient is occasionally pretreated for several weeks with of thyroid hormone to suppress the normal thyroid and thereby better delineate the nodule from the normal gland. The surgeon should be prepared to do a lobectomy if the lesion is benign, or a more extensive operation and appropriate lymph node removal if, from the operative findings and examination of frozen sections, it is malignant. If the lesion is described as a hypercellular follicular adenoma, we feel it is best to do a lobectomy and contralateral subtotal lobectomy. Many of these lesions turn out on final pathology to be malignant, and reoperation is then avoided.

The first operation is the time for definitive surgery. Although a surgeon with limited experience in neck surgery can remove a thyroid nodule, an adequate near-total thyroidectomy and modified radical neck dissection requires experience, if damage to the recurrent laryngeal nerves or induction of hypoparathyrodism is to be avoided. In this day of specialization, patients deserve a surgeon who has more than a casual interest in the field. Indeed, in the absence of such surgical skill, medical therapy may offer significantly fewer problems for certain patients with nodules than those arising out of inadequate surgery.

Lobectomy for benign solitary adenomas is a relatively harmless procedure. The incidence of death, recurrent laryngeal nerve paralysis, or permanent hypoparathyrodism should be zero. It is less of a procedure than is subtotal thyroidectomy for Graves' disease. Only 2 to 3 days are required in the hospital. Postoperative morbidity is slight and transient, and the cosmetic appearance is almost always satisfactory. Complications increase if a carcinoma is discovered, and thyroidectomy and node dissection are required. However, this risk is more than balanced by the benefits,[64] since long-term survival after surgery for intrathyroidal or locally metastatic thyroid carcinoma is almost equal to that of the normal population.

A satisfactory outcome often depends on a pathologist competent in thyroid histopathology. Occasionally the difficulty of interpreting frozen sections will lead to thyroidectomy for a tumor that is ultimately classified as benign. Performance of an occasional unnecessary thyroidectomy is not a serious problem in the hands of a surgeon who has few operative complications. On the other hand, reoperation at a later date for cancer erroneously diagnosed at initial surgery as benign is all too often required, and does not offer the patient the best chance of operative cure and freedom from operative complications.

After operation, some thyroidologists favor treating patients with long-term replacement therapy with thyroid hormone. Although the recurrence of "solitary" nodules is infrequent, replacement therapy is safe, inexpensive, and probably provides some protection. There is no general agreement, however, on this point. We note that thyroxine treatment has been shown to decrease recurrence of nodules in patients operated for thyroid disease induced by childhood irradiation.[65]

Occasionally, when the patient is recuperating from lobectomy for a presumed benign lesion, the permanent tissue sections indicate to the pathologist that the diagnosis is actually carcinoma of the follicular or papillary type. If the lesion is over 1 cm in size, there is a history of irradiation, or the lesion is follicular, completion of the thyroidectomy is advisable, as discussed below.

THYROID CARCINOMA

Incidence and Distribution

The incidence of thyroid cancers is about 36 to 60 new cases per 1 million population each year[57] (Fig. 18-5). The annual mortality from thyroid cancer in 1977 was 4 per million for men and 5 per million for women.[57] The discrepancy between incidence and mortality presumably reflects the good prognosis for most thyroid cancers. Autopsy studies indicate a surprising frequency ranging from 0.01 to over 2.0 percent.[8,9] A survey of consecutive autopsies at Grace-New Haven Hospital found 2.7 percent of thyroids to harbor unsuspected thyroid cancer.[9] Another 2.7 percent had discrete benign adenomas, and nearly half showed nodularity. The high prevalence was attributed to careful examination of the gland, but probably also reflects a highly selected group of older patients dying in a hospital. Most studies suggest that the average prevalence of thyroid car-

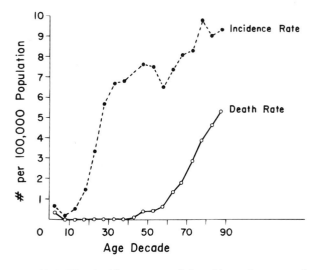

Fig. 18-5. The incidence rate of thyroid carcinoma and death rate from thyroid carcinoma are diagrammed in relation to the experience per 100,000 population in each decade. Sharply increased mortality occurs after age 50. (Data from Young et al.[57])

cinoma at autopsy is about 1 per thousand. In many instances, thyroid cancer is not diagnosed during life or is not the immediate cause of death. Both suggestions are in accord with the rather leisurely growth of the majority of thyroid tumors, especially the frequent small papillary types.

The incidence of thyroid cancer in a well-defined population was studied by Verby et al.[66] They found no certain increase in the past three decades if lesions over 1.5 cm in diameter were tallied; the rate was 17 per 10^6 people per year in the earlier period and 36 per 10^6 in the most recent decade—a difference not statistically significant. However, they also detected an almost equal frequency of tumors under 1.5 cm in size in the most recent decades, making a final total incidence of 60 per 10^6 each year. These data are open to interpretation and may indicate an increasing frequency. Up to 6 percent of thyroid glands in autopsied adults in the United States, and over 20 percent in Japan, also harbor microscopically detectable foci of thyroid carcinoma, which are believed to be of no biologic significance (see *Occult Tumors*, below).

Thyroid tumors are rare in children and increase in frequency in each decade. The variety of tumor is also related to age (see below). Carcinomas are three times as frequent in women as in men. In the past, it was generally believed that thyroid tumors were more frequent in areas of endemic goiter, and reports from Colombia and Austria support this association[67] (see Ch. 11). Surveys conducted in the United States found no relation between usual geographic residence and incidence of thyroid cancer.

Cause

Most, if not all, thyroid adenomas are monoclonal, as, presumably, are carcinomas.[13] Thus the tumor represents the persistent growth of the progeny of one cell which has somehow escaped the mechanisms which maintain normal cell division at about once each 8.5 years.[14]

The process of oncogenesis is conceived to be a series of events induced by genetic and environmental factors which alter growth control. At the phenomenologic level these factors may be considered as "initiators" and "promoters." Initiators include such agents as chemicals and irradiation which induce tumors, and promoters are agents such as phenobarbital, which in rats augments TSH secretion and radi-

cally increases tumor development. In man x-ray treatment is the sole known initiator, and other than elevated TSH, no promoters are known. Compounds such as phenobarbital, dilantin, and PCBs, which are known thyroid tumor promoters in animals through liver microsomal hormone degrading enzyme induction leading to increased thyroid hormone metabolism, do not appear to have a detectable adverse effect in man in doses usually employed.[68]

We now begin, however, to understand oncogenesis at another level.[69] More than 30 "oncogenes" have been recognized in the human genome. These genes, normally silent, can become activated by chromosomal translocations, deletions, or mutations, and then can "transform" normal cells into a condition of uncontrolled growth. Most oncogenes appear to be closely related to normal growth factors, genes that control cell division, or to hormone receptors. In general, these genes, when turned on, promote cell growth and division and depress differentiation. Typically, activation of one such gene may not be enough to produce malignancy, but if accompanied by expression of another oncogene, or if gene mutation or reduplication occurs, the cell may progress toward a malignant potential. Information on expression of oncogenes in human thyroid tissue is rapidly accumulating. Expression of c-myc is stimulated in normal thyroid cells by TSH, and the proto-oncogene is expressed in adenomas and carcinomas. Activating mutations of h-ras at codons 12, 13, and 61, and over expression of h-ras, are found in adenomas and carcinomas, but h-ras mutations are also found in nodular goiter tissue,[70] suggesting that h-ras mutations could be an early event in oncogenesis.[70,71] Other studies, it should be noted, find ras mutations uncommon.[72] Santoro and co-workers[73] have cloned an oncogene which is frequently and specifically expressed in papillary thyroid cancers. This oncogene is found on chromosome 10 (the area of the MEN I gene as well), and involves an intrachromosomal rearrangement of the tyrosine kinase domain of the ret oncogene.

Studies on patients with MEN I and MEN II indicated linkage to chromosomes 11[74] and 10, respectively. Subsequent studies demonstrated that the ret oncogene is present at 10q11.2. Germline mutations have been detected in this oncogene in all patients with MEN I and MEN II, and familial MTC.[75] Somatic mutations are present in up to half of patients with sporadic MTC (personal communication, Dr. Furio Pacini).

Mutations in the proteins involved in the normal TSH-receptor-G protein-adenylyl cyclase-kinase signal transduction pathway also play a role in tumor formation. Activating TSH receptor mutations have been found by Vassart and co-workers[76] to be the cause of most hyperfunctional nodules. Mutations of the stimulatory GTP binding protein α subunit are present in 25 percent of hyperfunctioning thyroid adenomas.[77] TSH-R mutations are, however, unusual in thyroid cancer,[78] excepting hyperfunctional adenomas. TSH-R expression tends to be lost as cancers dedifferentiate, and persistence of expression is associated with a better prognosis.[79]

In addition to positive factors, oncogenesis may frequently involve loss of tumor suppressor genes. This has been proven in hereditary retinoblastoma. These genes appear in some instances to function as dominant factors, and are normally present on both sets (maternal and paternal) of chromosomes. In retinoblastoma the inherited lack of one suppressor (RB) gene does not cause disease, but if a genetic event (deletion, recombination, mutation, etc.) causes failure of expression of the second allele, cancer ensues. The presence of tumor-specific suppressor genes is often detected because of lack of heterozygosity of chromosomal markers associated with deletions of segments of genetic material. Evidence for characteristic chromosomal abnormalities within tumor cells may lead to recognition of a tumor suppressor gene. Deletion of the tumor suppressor genes, P53 and the RB gene, have now been detected in differentiated and undifferentiated thyroid cancer.[80]

Thyroid carcinomas rarely occur as part of several familial syndromes, which may involve hereditable loss of tumor suppressor genes. Cowden's disease is a familial syndrome which includes a variety of hamartomas, multinodular goiter, and carcinomas of several tissues including breast, colon, lung, and thyroid, especially in women.[81] Thyroid carcinoma also co-occurs in patients with familial adenomatous polyposis of the colon.[82] Differentiated thyroid carcinoma is reported to co-occur with chemodactomas of the carotid body, which can be inherited in a familial autosomal dominant form.[83] Thyroid carcinoma is also associated with Gardner syndrome.[84]

In subsequent discussions we note the carcino-genic effects of irradiation and excess TSH secretion, and other related thyroid tumor initiators or promoters. Very likely the mechanism through which these agents work is by altering expression of positively acting oncogenes or tumor-suppressor genes, but specific connections have yet to be made.

Experimental Thyroid Tumor Formation

Thyroid tumors have been induced experimentally in rodents by several procedures having as their common denominator a prolonged increase in pituitary thyrotropin production and thyroid stimulation.

Goitrogenic drugs, if administered to animals for a prolonged period, can induce tumors, as numerous investigators[85] have demonstrated. These tumors are typically papillary adenocarcinomas, and are associated with a diffuse hyperplasia of the thyroid gland. Old rats of some strains appear to develop thyroid cancers spontaneously.[86]

Radiographic irradiation of the thyroid and administration of ^{131}I have both induced carcinomas in the experimental animal.[87] A combination of ^{131}I injury to the thyroid cell and prolonged administration of a goitrogen is especially likely to produce carcinomas, as shown by Doniach.[88]

Cell metabolism is altered by ^{131}I, even when small amounts are administered. In the rat, 5 μCi prevents subsequent response to a goitrogenic drug.[89] With larger doses the colloid is sparse, the follicles are variable in size, and large eosinophilic acinar cells appear. Very large doses of [131]I (several thousand rads) to the rat thyroid radically alter cell metabolism, liberate TG within 1 or 2 weeks, and subsequently reduce the efficiency of hormone synthesis.

[131]I irradiation in rats in doses so low as not to alter hormone biosynthesis immediately inhibits DNA synthesis and cell replication, as shown by a failure to respond to subsequent goitrogenic challenge. The cells also have a shortened life span. Similar inhibition of hyperplasia follows x-irradiation to the thyroid.

Therapeutic doses of ^{131}I to patients also induce atypical nuclei, which may remain for many years.[90] The doses of RAI needed to produce neoplastic change in the thyroid glands of animals closely parallel those given in the treatment of thyrotoxicosis in humans. The morphologic changes are intensified by a goitrogenic stimulus and reduced by thyroid hormone treatment.

The effects of radiation may be twofold. The nuclear morphologic changes may derive from an abnormality in cell division or replication of nucleic acids, which may predispose to carcinomatous change. Also, the damaged cell produces less thyroid hormone, and thereby ultimately comes under intense TSH stimulation, as in experiments with goitrogens. Thus, it seems certain that chronic TSH stimulation in animals is associated with the evolution of a neoplasm, especially if it is combined with radiation damage to the cell nuclei.

Experimental thyroid tumors induced by ^{131}I are initially TSH dependent. At first, they can be transplanted successfully only into thyroidectomized animals that are producing much TSH. After serial passages through several generations, the tumors may become autonomous and will then grow in a normal host. Partial or complete dependence on TSH is also observed in some human papillary and follicular tumors.

Human Radiation Exposure and Thyroid Cancer

Duffy and Fitzgerald[9] first made the important observation that a high proportion of children with thyroid carcinoma had received therapeutic x-irradiation to the upper mediastinum or neck during childhood for control of benign lesions such as enlarged thymus, tonsils, or adenoids. Their finding has been amply confirmed.[30-34,91-93] Winship and Rosvoll[94] studied 562 children with thyroid carcinoma from all parts of the world. Among those for whom adequate historical data were available, 80 percent had a history of prior x-ray treatment. this relationship is not so obvious for carcinomas developing after age 35. Significant x-irradiation to the head, neck, and chest in childhood increases the frequency of thyroid cancer by 100-fold,[95] and the incidence is proportional to the dose, reaching at least 1.7 percent at 500 rads, or 5.5 per million persons per rad each year (Fig. 18-6). Our own data disclose a 7 percent incidence by 30 years after irradiation[34] (Fig. 18-7). The latent period averages 10 to 20 years, but tumors occur even after 20 to 40 years (Fig. 18-8). There appears to be no true threshold, since even doses as low as 9 rads increase the incidence of cancer.[31] There is a direct dose-response relationship through 1,000 rads.[95] Higher doses of

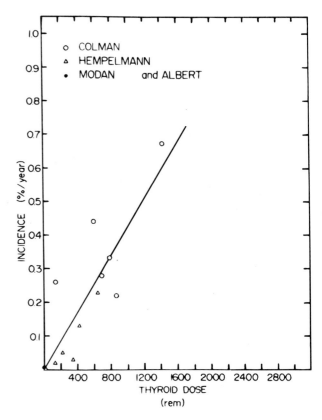

Fig. 18-6. Estimated dose response for thyroid cancer in humans from external irradiation. The incidence of carcinomas each year is plotted against the original thyroid irradiation dose. (From Maxon et al,[95] with permission.)

irradiation also induce tumors, and the true dose-response curve in the range of 1,000 to 5,000 rads in humans is not known. Benign nodules occur with nearly ten times the frequency of cancers. Interestingly, the type of tumor induced is not different from those occurring spontaneously, and there is no relation between dose and latent period. For some reason, women are more prone to develop radiation-induced tumors than men, and both ethnic and familial factors may influence tumor development.[96]

Probably any x-ray exposure of the thyroid has some carcinogenic potential, although the risk may decrease with age. Adults were extensively treated by x-irradiation for Graves' disease from 1930 to 1950. There is reported to be an increased incidence of carcinoma in these patients.[97] A significant incidence of thyroid neoplasia was observed in patients who received x-ray therapy for cervical tuberculous adenitis.[98] These patients were treated at ages up to

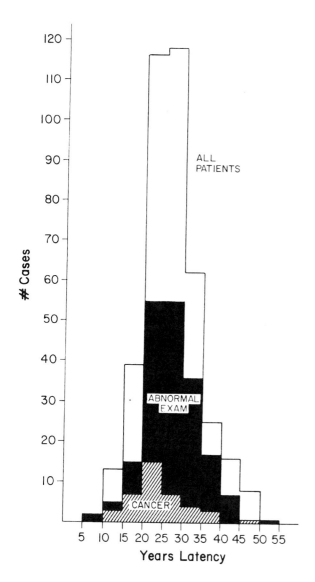

Fig. 18-7. Distribution of patients with a history of irradiation to the head and neck, according to the time after irradiation at which they were examined. The majority of patients were seen 20 to 35 years after irradiation, but the incidence of tumors peaked 5 to 10 years earlier. Tumors continued to occur through 40 years after irradiation, and it is unclear whether there is a finite latency period.

34, received 500 to 1,500 rads, and developed tumors 10 to 27 years after treatment. In a study of survivors of the atomic blasts at Nagasaki and Hiroshima, an increased incidence of thyroid cancer was found among persons who had received large amounts of radiation.[99] Thus, the thyroid of the adult is sensitive to the carcinogenic action of x-rays, although not so sensitive as that of the child. Thyroid nodularity also occurred as a sequela of nuclear fallout in the accident at Rongelap in the Marshall Islands.[100] In those patients, who received 200 to 1,400 rads, the incidence of nodularity is 40 percent, and nearly 6 percent proved to have cancer. Children in Utah exposed to small amounts of fallout from atomic bomb testing[101] have not developed nodules or carcinomas.

Radiation-associated tumors of the thyroid continue to occur, although x-ray treatment of thymic enlargement and tonsillar or adenoid hypertrophy has been discontinued since 1959. A recent analysis of 1787 patients treated with x-ray for Hodgkin's disease found 1.7 percent to have thyroid cancer.[102]

Radiation-associated tumors are generally found among younger patients. They are rarely undifferentiated, but some have been fatal. In a review of x-ray associated thyroid tumors at the University of Chicago Thyroid Clinic,[34] the latent period among children treated predominantly in adolescence for tonsillar enlargement or acne averaged 20 years. It appears that the peak incidence of lesions is at 10 to 25 years after exposure (Fig. 18-8), and it is probable that the occurrence of new cancers decreases over time. Among 100 consecutive patients seen in 1973 and 1974, only because they knew of prior radiation exposure, 15 percent had lesions suggestive of tumor and 7 percent had cancer proven at operation.[33] Favus et al.[103] found a similar incidence of cancer (60 per 1056) in irradiated patients called back for evaluation. Although one case-controlled study suggests a lack of effect of radiation,[104] the evidence, reviewed by Maxon et al,[95] clearly confirms the importance of this problem.

Based on these facts, it has been accepted by most physicians in the field that patients with a history of thyroid irradiation (over 20 rads, and certainly 50 rads) should be located and advised to have an assessment. This evaluation should consist at least of a physical examination and, if any thyroid abnormality is found, a scan or ultrasound. If one or more clear-cut nodules is found, or if one or more clear-cut inactive areas is found by scan, then surgical intervention may be indicated. As noted below, needle aspiration cytology can alter this approach in some cases. Benign adenomas are also found in these glands, with an incidence three times or more than that of cancers. Our own studies show that almost

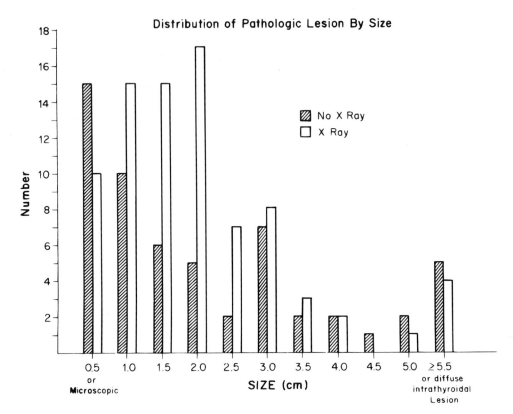

Fig. 18-8. Comparison of the distribution of the size of primary tumors among 100 non-radiation associated thyroid malignancies, and an equal number of radiation-associated tumors. All were differentiated thyroid carcinomas. The distribution of sizes was not statistically different, although the radiation-associated tumors were slightly larger on average in this comparison than the tumors lacking association with prior x-ray treatment.

all clinically detectable cancers are found by careful physical examination, and that scans are of supplementary value and rarely turn up a cancer missed on palpation. Serum TG levels tend to be elevated in irradiated patients, and antithyroid antibodies are more commonly present, but these tests are not of diagnostic value. When excised these glands often show multiple benign as well as malignant nodules as well as areas of fibrosis and hyperplasia[105] (Fig. 18-9).

Thyroid Radiation and Multiple Gland Abnormalities

M. P., a 52-year old woman, was first seen with a history of irradiation for acne during her teens. She subsequently developed telangiectasia of the skin of her face. The month before the examination, she had observed a lump on the right side of the neck. Examination disclosed a 1-cm nodule in the right lobe of the thyroid and some irregularity of the left lobe. Thyroid scintiscan showed a cold nodule of the lower pole of the

right lobe. Ultrasound examination of the right lobe identified a partially cystic nodule and a small cystic structure of the left. The FTI was slightly elevated at 10.9. RAIU was above normal. Thyroid antibodies were not present. Thyroid needle aspiration showed cells indicative of malignancy.

Routine blood tests disclosed alkaline phosphatase of 107 units (normal, 25 to 100 units), calcium 10.9 and 11.5 mg/dl (normal, 8.5 to 10.2 mg/dl), and phosphate 2.7 ng/dl. Repeated assay of FTI again demonstrated an elevated value of 15 (normal = 6 to 10.5). The level of parathyroid hormone was 0.65 ng/ml (with a coincident calcium level of 11.5 mg/dl), values indicative of primary hyperparathyroidism.

The patient was treated with potassium iodide for 1 week and admitted for exploratory surgery. A right upper parathyroid adenoma weighing 908 mg was found. The adenoma showed areas of cystic degeneration and fibrosis. The thyroid gland was multinodular and was suspicious on frozen section for follicular carcinoma. There was extensive fibrosis around and adher-

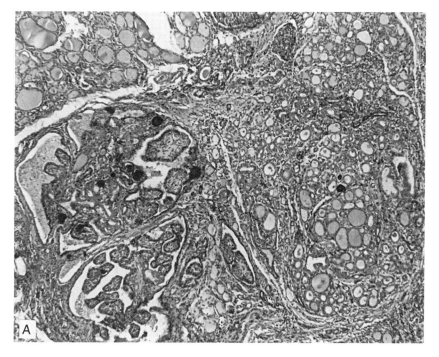

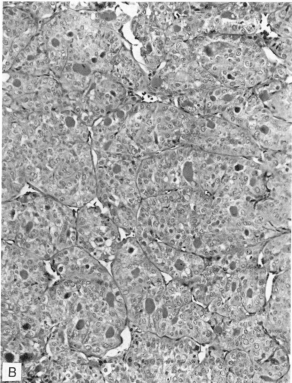

Fig. 18-9. Histologic pattern of malignant tumors of the thyroid. (A) Papillary carcinoma. Note the tall cells and the fibrovascular core of the papillae. (B) Follicular adenocarcinoma showing fair preservation of architecture, and vesicular nuclei. *(Figure continues.)*

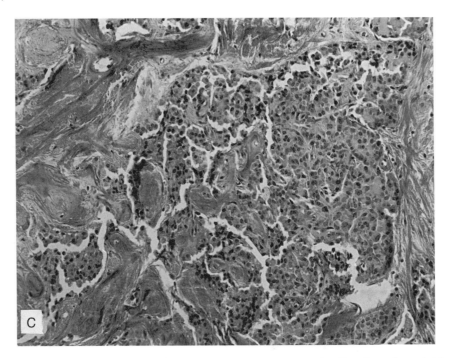

Fig. 18-9. *(Continued).* (C) Medullary carcinoma, with sheets of large cells, fibrosis and amyloid visible with Congo red staining. (Courtesy of Dr. F. Straus.)

ent to the thyroid gland. A near-total thyroidectomy was performed. The gland weighed 17 g. Multiple nodules in the gland measured 1 to 18 mm in diameter. An 18-mm nodule in the right lobe was identified as follicular carcinoma. There were, in addition, multiple follicular adenomas and multiple Hürthle cell tumors, focal hyperplasia, and colloid nodules in the right and left lobe.

Postoperatively the patient received thyroid hormone. When seen 1 month after surgery, her calcium level was 9.4 mg/dl, phosphorus 3.5 mg/dl, and parathyroid hormone 0.28 ng/ml (normal). The FTI was 9.2 while taking 0.15 mg L-T_4.

This patient developed a cystic parathyroid adenoma with hyperparathyroidism, multiple adenomas of the thyroid, follicular carcinoma, and multiple functioning adenomas that produced thyrotoxicosis. All of these tumors occurred concurrently in a gland showing changes typical of prior radiation exposure.

Development of Thyroid Carcinoma, After X-Ray Therapy, While Receiving Thyroid Hormone

At age 10, D. C., a 19-year-old woman, had respiratory distress and was found to have a superior-anterior mediastinal mass. There was left cervical lymphadenopathy and bilateral supraclavicular lymphadenopathy. Biopsy revealed Hodgkin's disease of the nodular scle-

rosing variety. The result of staging laparotomy was negative. She was treated with 4,000 rads to a neck mantle field.

One year later the results of thyroid function tests were normal, but two years after x-ray treatment the FTI was 4.1 and the TSH level was 24 μU/ml. Thyroid hormone replacement therapy was begun, and the patient was carefully monitored over subsequent years with periodic FTI and TSH determinations. Six years after irradiation a 2-cm nodule was noted in the left lobe of the thyroid. This nodule was found to be cold on ^{123}I scan. Fine needle aspiration revealed cells suggestive of malignancy.

At surgery a papillary adenocarcinoma with capsular and vascular invasion was found, and a near-total thyroidectomy was performed. Postoperatively residual thyroid tissue was ablated by administration of 30 mCi ^{131}I. The skeletal survey findings were negative; chest and bone radiographs were normal. She has remained free of evidence of thyroid carcinoma or Hodgkin's disease in the subsequent three years.

This history demonstrates the occurrence of thyroid carcinoma, in a gland heavily irradiated during therapy for Hodgkin's disease, while the patient was taking adequate replacement doses of thyroid hormone. Possibly the period of x-ray induced hypothyroidism played a

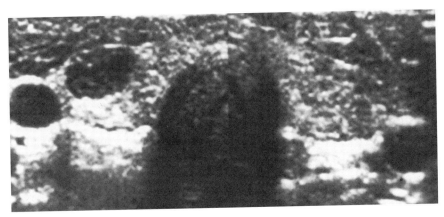

Fig. 18-10. Ultrasonographic examination by transverse image of the thyroid containing a solid nodule in the right lobe and a homogeneous appearance of the left lobe. The structure peripheral to the nodule is the internal jugular vein.

role in tumor induction. The tumor developed within 6 years of the radiation therapy. Fortunately, the tumor was not metastatic and has presumably been eradicated by surgery and RAI ablation of residual tissue.

In our series, postradiation carcinomas averaged 1.7 cm in size (Fig. 18-10), and 14 percent were below 0.5 cm. The size distribution was similar to that of non-x-ray-associated tumors. They were more frequently multicentric than those in nonirradiated glands and as aggressive, or more so, in behavior than tumors arising without known irradiation.[106] The tumors are mainly papillary or follicular, but an occasional anaplastic cancer is also found. In examining patients, it should be remembered that benign and malignant salivary gland neoplasms, neuromas, parathyroid adenomas,[107] laryngeal cancer, skin malignancies, and breast cancer also occur with undue frequency in this group of patients.

Lack of Association of [131]I Treatment and Thyroid Carcinoma

Iodine-131 treatment induces abnormalities in the thyroid gland that persist for many years.[108] Giant nuclei, increased mitotic activity, hyperchromatic nuclei, and other abnormalities appear. It seems reasonable that these nuclear changes could lead to carcinomatous degeneration. Chromosomal damage in circulating lymphocytes has also been reported after ^{131}I administration.[109] Patients have developed thyroid nodules or tumors after ^{131}I therapy for Graves' disease; it has been suggested, but not proved, that the highest incidence has been among those treated during childhood. Two of the lesions found in ^{131}I-treated children may actually have been carcinomas, but there has been debate[110] among the various pathologists who examined the specimens. Several reports of isolated instances of cancer after ^{131}I treatment of adults for Graves' disease have appeared, but the large United States Public Health Service cooperative study failed to show an increased risk in this group.[111–113] Studies by Holm et al.[113] have again failed to show an increase in cancer incidence among persons given ^{131}I either for diagnosis or for therapy for thyrotoxicosis. These patients were adults, and usually in the 40 to 60-year-age group. Also, very large radiation doses may be less carcinogenic than small ones, and in half or more of these patients, the thyroid has been totally destroyed. Lastly, the follow-up time averages 8 to 13 years, which may be too soon to see radiation-induced neoplasia. Thus the evidence is reassuring but the question cannot be considered closed.

Thyroid Hyperplasia and Cancer

Chronic stimulation of the thyroid with TSH probably can lead to carcinogenesis in humans, as it can in animals. There are several reports of intensely hyperplastic congenital goiters, untreated for long periods, in which carcinomas have finally developed.[114–118] Fortunately, most patients with congenital goiter are recognized and treated with replacement thyroid hormone at some time during early childhood, so that chronic TSH stimulation does not occur.

Relation of Cancer to Other Thyroid Disease

The relationship of thyroid tumors to other thyroid disease is still debated. In the preceding section we discussed whether carcinomas arise from adenomas, occurring either singly or as a component of a multinodular gland. While this must happen rarely, it is not the ordinary course of events. In support of this view one may note, for example, that, whereas adenomas are rarely if ever papillary, approximately 60 percent of all thyroid carcinomas are papillary. If carcinomas arise from adenomas, one might expect that the majority would be follicular rather than papillary, and this is not the case. Also, although carcinomas, largely of the papillary type, occur in nontoxic nodular goiters with a reported frequency of 4 to 17 percent of cases, the age of diagnosis of papillary carcinomas does not follow that for nontoxic goiter.[119] papillary carcinomas occur in children and adolescents, and reach their highest frequency during the middle decades of life. Multinodular goiter, by contrast, is infrequent in childhood, but increases with each decade. The high frequency of carcinomas detected in nodular goiter appears to reflect the efficiency of selection of patients for operation on the basis of suspicious clinical findings in the gland.

Parathyroid adenomas occur in a small percentage of patients with thyroid cancer. The converse relationship may also exist; 2 to 11 percent of patients with parathyroid adenomas also have thyroid cancer.[120–122] An important reason for this association is the induction of both tumors by x-ray exposure.

An increased incidence of cancer in Hashimoto's thyroiditis has been reported, but our clinical experience does not suggest an important relationship between this relatively common disease and thyroid cancer. Certainly the diseases can coexist in the same gland. Further, focal thyroiditis may occur as an immunologic response to thyroid cancer.

Neoplasia and Graves' Disease

Many reports on Graves' disease stress a normal or low coincidence of cancer. In contrast, one report gives an association of 9 percent.[122] In our recent review, 4 of 50 patients with thyroid cancer had coincident Graves' disease.[34] Belfiore et al found the risk of thyroid cancer in Graves' disease to be increased 2 to 3 fold.[123] Valenta and co-workers[124] reported that patients with thyroid cancer may have a LATS-like substance in the blood. A TSH-like component that cross-reacted with bovine TSH was also found in cancer patients and was not suppressed by thyroid hormone.[125] This phenomenon was explained on the basis of antibovine TSH antibodies present in these sera, induced by prior testing or treatment with bovine TSH.[126] TSAb can stimulate thyroid cancers when Graves' disease coexists, however, so the idea that TSAb might induce malignant change is tenable, if not proven. It is also possible, but unproven, that continued stimulation of a tumor may make it behave in a more aggressive manner.[123,127] Patients with Graves' disease and thyroid cancer who underwent total thyroidectomy and ^{131}I ablation fared as well in follow-up as did patients without Graves' disease.

Hereditable Tumors

Genetic factors clearly play a role in some cancers. Individuals with familial adenomatous polyposis of the colon have an increased frequency of thyroid tumors. Also, patients with Cowden's disease and Gardner syndrome have associated thyroid tumors.

Panza et al.[128] found a strong association between histocompatibility antigen HLA-Dr1 and the occurrence of papillary and follicular cancer in Italy. This observation needs confirmation, and it is surprising in view of the usual sporadic rather than familial occurrence of these tumors. We found an association between HLA-Dr7 and differentiated thyroid cancer in patients not exposed to x-ray.[129] Others have found no association with HLA-DR genes.[130] Medullary thyroid cancers are associated in inherited syndromes with bilateral pheochromocytomas, parathyroid hyperplasia, neurofibromas, and mucosal neuromas. The associated gene deletions are noted above.

"Occult" Carcinomas

Tiny carcinomas, usually papillary and often sclerotic, have been found in 5.7 percent of thyroids of adults coming to autopsy in the United States.[131] This prevalence is noted only when the thyroid is sectioned completely at 1 to 2 mm intervals and every abnormality is studied. The tumors have a mean diameter of 2 mm, and almost all are under 5 mm. The prevalence is best known in adults[132] and may be lower in young people. Since, in some glands, collections of psammoma bodies also exist in tiny scarred areas, it is hypothesized that such lesions may spontaneously regress. Because of their small size, they are detectable only at surgical or pathologic examination of the gland.

These observations, now widely accepted, have provoked much discussion. Certainly most of these tiny tumors cannot be biologically significant, considering the low incidence of clinically recognized cancer. Most of the lesions are probably missed during routine surgical or autopsy pathologic studies. Their cause is unknown. They may be a variant of the occult sclerosing carcinomas described by Hazard, but the latter tumors are usually larger, have a predominant sclerotic component, and clearly do metastasize. It has been suggested that such lesions are in fact the cancers found after thyroid irradiation, but they probably can explain only a small proportion of radiation-associated tumors. Most of these lesions would go undetected in a standard surgical pathologic examination, and the great majority of radiation-associated lesions are larger. In our own series, the radiation-associated lesions were on average 1.7 cm in diameter and only 14 percent were under 0.5 cm. Whether such "minimal"[131] cancers are in fact the occasional precursors of clinically evident cancers is a moot point. It is clear that they are at present an important pathologic—but not clinical—entity.

Although there are a few leads, the total information available does not provide anything approaching an understanding of the causes of thyroid tumors. Certainly long-term stimulation of the thyroid by thyrotropin and injury to the gland by radiation are two important contributing factors. Whether they act on abnormal substrate, such as a genetically susceptible cell, or require the concomitant action of a virus or other factors is entirely unknown. It seems probable that numerous causes are involved, since the age incidence of tumors such as papillary carcinoma differs radically from that of others such as the small-cell malignant carcinoma of the thyroid, which occurs primarily in elderly people.

Neoplastic cell growth may normally be controlled by immunologic defense mechanisms. Some thyroid tumors appear to have lost the normal thyroid antigen reacting with the "cytotoxic factor" antibody found in the sera of patients with Hashimoto's disease,[133] but this loss is probably a response, not a cause, of the malignant process. A defect in immune surveillance is believed to be involved in the unhampered proliferation of all neoplastic cell clones, and

may exist in thyroid cancer, although no data are available to support this claim.

Pathology

Pathologists are agreed that there are peculiar difficulties in the classification and diagnosis of malignant tumors of the thyroid. The histologic changes required for diagnosis of carcinoma include absence of a true capsule, invasion of surrounding normal tissue, invasion of blood and lymph channels, loss of normal follicular architectural arrangements, and cellular abnormalities such as an increase in the ratio of nucleus to cytoplasm, enlarged vesicular nuclei, nuclear folding, increased mitoses, and hyperchromasia of the nucleus. Recently, aneuploidy of nuclear DNA content has been added to this list. Obviously the presence of distant metastases is the most certain criterion. Most students of the disease agree that the ordinary criteria of malignancy have little prognostic value in thyroid tumors, except perhaps in the wildly growing anaplastic tumors. It may be noted, however, that pathologists at the Mayo Clinic believe a histologic typing by their criteria provides significant information on prognosis.

Examples of the histologic patterns of several of these tumors are given in Figure 18-11. The papillary adenocarcinoma typically shows tumor cells around a fibrovascular core and, not infrequently, areas of follicular differentiation. Papillary lesions tend to be infiltrative, and encapsulation is rare. Lymphocytic "reactions" are prominent. The cell nuclei have a ground-glass or "cat's eye" appearance and intracellular inclusions are common. Vascular invasion is rare. Psammoma bodies are often abundant. Multiple intraglandular foci are frequent, especially in children. Areas of lymphocyte infiltration, and even extensive lymphocytic thyroiditis, are common, especially in papillary tumors. Many tumors look much like follicular cancers, but have the characteristic nuclei of papillary cancers. These constitute the "follicular variant" of papillary cancer, and behave more or less as do other papillary cancers.

Follicular adenocarcinomas vary from those with a definite follicular pattern to those with solid sheets of cells. The lesions are more frequently encapsulated, but capsular and blood vessel invasions are typical. The nuclei are normo- or hyper chromated, or may be quite vesicular. One variant, the so-called malignant adenoma, appears to be nearly benign and can be identified as malignant only by the dem-

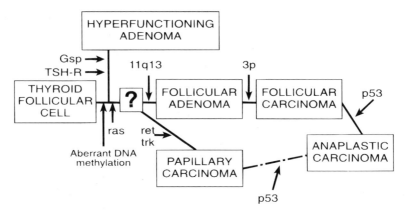

Fig. 18-11. Genetic defects in thyroid neoplasms. Information is based on the relative prevalence of genetic lesions in the various phenotypes, suggesting that a sequence of mutations affecting oncogenes or tumor suppressor genes can determine thyroid tumor histology and behavior. (Courtesy of Dr. J. A. Fagin.)

onstration of invasion of vessels or capsule, or because of the presence of distant metastases, which may also be composed of normal-appearing thyroid tissue. Hürthle cell carcinomas usually grow as solid sheets of large eosinophilic granular cells with much cytoplasm, and less often with a follicular pattern.

Medullary tumors have an ominous histologic pattern, with solid masses of cells with large vesicular nuclei.[134] There may be considerable associated fibrosis, and deposits of amyloid are a helpful diagnostic point. At the time of initial histologic examination, the pathologist should recognize these tumors as entities distinct from the undifferentiated cancers, for the medullary carcinomas have a much better prognosis.

In the undifferentiated group of small-cell tumors, giant-cell tumors, and carcinosarcomas, or in the miscellaneous group, the histologic pattern has little resemblance to the original thyroid structure.

The general experience of pathologists has been that, in the absence of irradiation, the substrate in which thyroid tumor forms is usually normal thyroid tissue or displays the changes of multinodular goiter or adenoma in approximately the proportion found in any sampling of the general population. This finding was obtained both by Sloan in the Presbyterian Hospital and in the Mayo Clinic studies.[135] There is a slightly increased frequency of association with benign adenomas and with Hashimoto's thyroiditis.[136] Lymphosarcomas are associated with Hashimoto's thyroiditis, and there is considerable evidence that lymphosarcoma actually evolves from a gland with thyroiditis.[137]

Multicentricity is a common feature of thyroid cancer, especially papillary cancer. Innumerable separate foci are sometimes found. Estimates of multicentricity range from 20 to 80 percent.[138,139] Whether this phenomenon represents truly multicentric sites of origin or intrathyroidal dissemination is not clear. This multifocality is thought to be one cause of recurrences in patients treated by subtotal rather than total thyroidectomy.

Both papillary and follicular tumors may appear as small (less than 1.5-cm) tumors surrounded by a densely fibrotic reaction. Although it is frequently said that these "occult" (because they may be found incidentally at operation) tumors are benign, the original report by Hazard[140] and subsequent studies show that cervical lymph node metastases occur.[141]

Occasionally pathologic examination suggests conversion of differentiated papillary or follicular cancers into anaplastic forms or conversion of an adenoma into a carcinoma.

An interesting aspect of thyroid tumor pathology is the frequency of metastatic tumors to the thyroid—5 percent in the data of Silverberg and Vidone[142] for unselected autopsies and 24 percent for patients dying of metastatic malignant disease.

Course of the Disease: Characteristics of the Various Types of Neoplasia

The tumor may be discovered accidentally by the patient or physician as a lump in the neck. It may appear as a gradually enlarging, painful mass with associated symptoms of hoarseness, dysphagia or dysphonia, or there may be difficulty in breathing. Occasionally a patient arrives with metastatic nodules in the neck, pulmonary symptoms from metastases, or a pathologic fracture of the spine or hip. Usually there are no symptoms of hyper- or hypothyroidism, but in rare instances the tumor can produce enough hormone to cause hyperthyroidism[143,144] (see Ch. 13).

Upon examination of the neck, carcinoma of the thyroid characteristically appears as an asymmetrical lump in the gland. If it is still within the confines of the gland, it will move with the gland when the patient swallows and may be moveable within the gland. If it invaded the trachea or neighboring structures, it may be fixed; this is a useful sign. Lymph nodes containing metastases may be found in the supraclavicular triangles, in the carotid chain, along the thyroid isthmus, and rarely in the axillary nodes. A sentinel or "Delphic" node above the isthmus may be present. Although carcinoma of the thyroid is typically firm or hard, rapidly growing lesions may sometimes be soft or even fluctuant. We have seen multiple lesions undergo necrosis and discharge through sinuses that developed in the skin of the neck.

Patients with thyroid cancer are also prone to develop other cancers, the risk being about double the average. Among these cancers is an excess incidence of leukemia, perhaps related to ^{131}I therapy.[145–147]

Age at diagnosis has an important bearing on the patient's subsequent course. The adverse effect of age on the prognosis increases gradually with each decade.[148] For practical assessment purposes, it is clear that patients diagnosed before age 45 have a much better prognosis than those detected later.[149] Age is also directly related to the incidence of undifferentiated tumors and to overall mortality.[148] Pregnancy does not seem to worsen the course of established or previously treated thyroid cancer.[150] Overall, women have a better prognosis than men with cancer.[151] Other characteristics of the tumor, including (as would be expected) extraglandular extension, gross invasion of the tumor capsule, and increasing size also carry a worsened prognosis.[151]

Papillary Carcinoma

Papillary carcinoma has a peak incidence in the third and fourth decades[152] (Fig. 18-12). It occurs three times more frequently in women than in men, and accounts for 60 to 70 percent of all thyroid cancers in adults and about 70 percent of those found in children. The disease tends to remain localized in the thyroid gland and in time metastasizes locally to the cervical or upper mediastinal nodes. The lesions are multicentric in 20 percent or more of patients, especially in children. Using rigid pathologic criteria, perhaps two-thirds of predominantly papillary thyroid cancers are found to have follicular elements. The natural history of these tumors is similar to that of pure papillary lesions. The metastases may conform to either histologic pattern. At present, the mixed tumors are lumped together with all other papillary cancers.

This tumor tends to be indolent and may exist for decades without killing the host. In a Mayo Clinic series of papillary tumors that were detected because of lymph node metastasis or found incidentally dur-

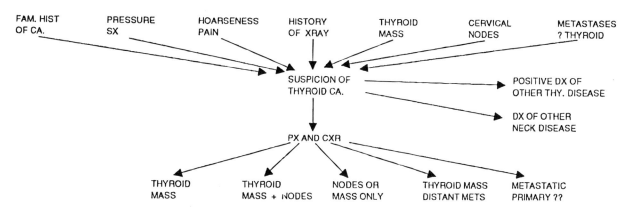

Fig. 18-12. Triage of patients who have symptoms that may be suggestive of thyroid carcinoma, indicating the categorization recognized clinically at the end of the initial examination.

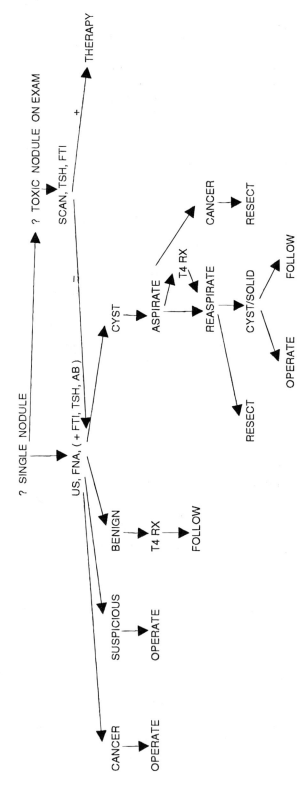

Fig. 18-13. Diagnostic sequence and therapeutic decisions in managing a patient with an apparent single nodule of the thyroid.

ing surgery of the thyroid gland, all the patients were unaffected by the tumors over several decades.[153]

The frequent occurrence of occult or minimal, incidentally found thyroid cancers, usually papillary and under 0.5 cm in size, is described above. The term occult has been used in a variety of ways, however, including reference to tumors with malignant nodes but no obvious primary, or in reference to any tumor under 1.5 cm in diameter. Mayo Clinic reports of papillary tumors under 1.5 cm in diameter, treated with conservative subtotal thyroidectomy and node dissection, have stressed their nonlethal nature, but a 1980 follow-up report on 820 patients treated by this group notes that 6 patients eventually died after spread of tumor from such "occult" primaries.[154] Patients with appropriately treated Clinical Class I or II lesions have 96 to 100 percent survival even after 15 to 30 years. Survival lowers to 87 percent for Class III and 35 percent for Class IV lesions at 15 years.

While the disease may be aggressive in children, it is distinctly less aggressive in young adults, as compared to patients over age 40.[151] Young patients tend to have small primary lesions and extensive adenopathy, but even with local invasion survival is good. When it occurs in persons over the age of 45, it may show, on microscopic examination, areas of undifferentiation, and pursue a highly malignant clinical course. The lesions tend to be larger and more infiltrative, and to have fewer local metastases.[152] It is possible that persons dying in older age actually have had their disease since youth; it has simply evolved into a more malignant phase.[155,156]

Papillary carcinoma tends to metastasize locally to lymph nodes, and occasionally produces cystic structures near the thyroid that are difficult to diagnose because of the paucity of malignant tissue. The presence of nodal metastasis correlates with recurrence[155–157] but has little effect on mortality in patients under age 45. In some studies, cervical adenopathy even seems to confer a protective effect on young people.[156] In patients over 45, the presence of nodes is associated with greater recurrence rates and more deaths[158,159] (Fig. 18-13). The tumors often metastasize elsewhere, especially to lung or bones.

Papillary tumors may metastasize to the lungs and produce a few nodules, or the lung fields may have a snowflake appearance throughout. These tumors are amazingly well tolerated and may allow relatively

TABLE 18-4. TNM Clinical Classification of Thyroid Cancer

T - primary tumor
  T_0 - no palpable tumor
  T_1 - single tumor confined to the gland; no deformity
  T_1 - multiple tumors confined to the gland; no deformity
  T_2 - multiple tumors or a single tumor producing deformity of the gland
  T_3 - tumor extending beyond the gland
N - regional lymph nodes
  N_0 - no palpable nodes
  N_1 - movable homolateral nodes
  N_2 - movable contralateral or bilateral nodes
  N_3 - fixed nodes
M - distant metastases
  M_0 - no evidence of distant metastases
  M_1 - distant metastases present

normal physical activity for 10 to 30 years. At times the pulmonary metastases are active in forming thyroid hormone, and may even function as the sole source of hormone supply after thyroidectomy. The metastases may progress gradually to obstructive and restrictive pulmonary disease. They also may develop arteriovenous shunts, with hypoxia or cyanosis. Such shunts become more prominent during pregnancy, perhaps as an effect of the increased supply of estrogens.

The usual net extra mortality in papillary cancer is not great when compared to that of a control population—perhaps 10 to 20 percent over 20 to 30 years.[156,157,159] Mortality is rare in patients diagnosed before age 40, and is much greater in the patients found to be in clinical stages III and IV (Tables 18-4 and 18-5) at initial diagnosis (Fig. 18-14). About one-half of patients ultimately dying from this lesion do so because of local invasion. Frazell and Duffy[160] have noted that papillary carcinoma is not always so benign; they reported 35 patients with "invasive papillary carcinoma," which had a very malignant course.

We found that risk of death from cancer was increased by extrathyroidal invasion (6-fold) or metastasis (47-fold), age over 45 years (32-fold) and size over 3 cm (6-fold). Thyroiditis, multifocality and the presence of neck nodes had no effect on disease-induced mortality.

Long-Term Survival with Papillary Cancer
  P.P., a 51-year-old man, was first seen at age 41. At age 14, while living in Yugoslavia, he had developed a

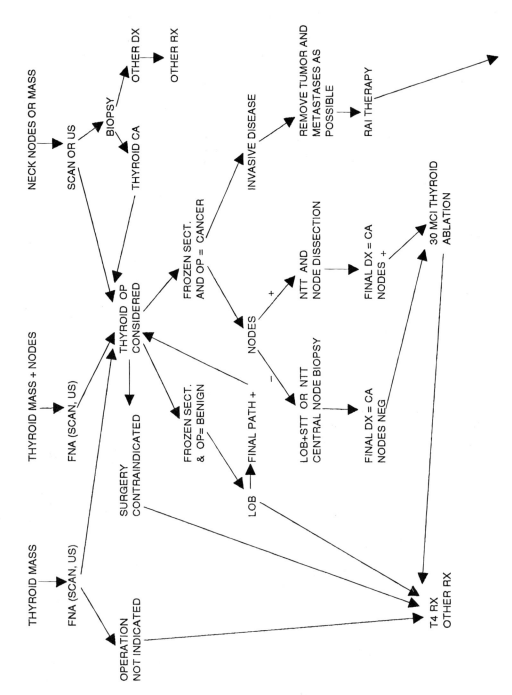

Fig. 18-14. Scheme for diagnosis and operative and radioactive iodide management of patients with various classes of thyroid disease presenting as a thyroid mass, with or without nodes.

TABLE 18-5. Comparison of Two Clinical Staging Systems

Clinical Stage	Comparable TNM Classification
I: Intrathyroidal	T_0, T_1, T_2, N_0, M_0
II: Cervical adenopathy	T_0—T_2, N_0—N_2, M_0
III: Locally invasive disease	T_3, N_3, M_0
IV: Distant metastases	M_1

mass in his neck. Tracheostomy was required because of dyspnea, and a biopsy of the mass was performed. A diagnosis of papillary thyroid carcinoma was made, and he was treated with radiotherapy to the neck. Because of an abnormal chest radiograph, presumed to be due to tuberculosis, he was given streptomycin and isoniazid for 2 months, but this therapy was discontinued when no improvement occurred. Extracts of calf thymus were injected. He was evaluated for hemoptysis at age 18, and chest radiographs again showed the infiltrates without evidence of change. The patient was not given thyroid hormone replacement therapy at any time. At age 39 he developed fatigue, substernal chest pain, occasional cough without production of sputum, and occasional hemoptysis. A thyroid scintiscan at another hospital revealed poor visualization of the thyroid and uptake of 4 percent, and ^{131}I uptake in the mediastinum.

Physical examination disclosed hyperpigmentation of the skin in the area of radiotherapy in the neck and supraclavicular areas. There was no evidence of a mass or lymphadenopathy. The tracheostomy site was well healed. The lungs were clear, BP was 100/70, pulse 68, and respiration 16/min, and there was no cyanosis. Routine complete blood count, urinalysis, and blood chemistry test results were normal. Chest radiographs showed multiple nodular densities throughout both lungs and a prominent left hilum. The results of a radiographic skeletal survey and a technetium pyrophosphate bone scan were normal. The FTI was 8.4 and TSH was 4.1 μU/ml. A whole body ^{131}I scan showed multiple areas of abnormal uptake in the area of the thyroid, and satellite areas of focal uptake around the thyroid bed. There was also focal activity in the mediastinum, in both hila, and in the lung fields. A 72-hour chest uptake was 8.9 percent. The serum TG level was 81 ng/ml.

The patient was treated multiple times with RAI and remained well while taking replacement T_4 for ten years. At age 51, the tumor grew more rapidly, failed to accumulate ^{131}I, and caused the patient's death.

This patient developed thyroid carcinoma at age 14 and probably had lymph node and lung metastases at that time. He lived a normal life during the ensuing 27 years, without suppressive thyroxine treatment, and

with only intermittent episodes of hemoptysis. The tumor responded at first to ^{131}I but later was uncontrolled. The common benign course of metastatic papillary thyroid carcinoma over many years is clearly shown, as is the equally typical later exacerbation and death.

Follicular Carcinoma

Follicular carcinoma has a peak incidence in the fifth decade of life in the United States and accounts for about one-quarter of all thyroid carcinomas.[151,153,156] Follicular carcinomas comprise up to 50 percent of thyroid malignancies in Europe, and sarcomas are also frequent. Whether this incidence is related to iodine deficiency or other factors is unknown. It is a slowly growing tumor and frequently is recognized as a nodule in the thyroid gland before metastases appear. Variation in the cellular pattern ranges from an almost normal-appearing structure to anaplastic tissue that forms no follicles or colloid. The tumor is three times as common in women as in men. At operation one-half to two-thirds of these tumors are resectable. Tumors that are small and well circumscribed (not surprisingly) tend to be less lethal than those actively infiltrating local structures at the initial operation. Local adenopathy does not appear to carry a greater risk, but extensive invasion of the tumor capsule and thyroid tissue increases mortality.[161] Local direct invasion of strap muscles and trachea is characteristic of the more aggressive tumors.[162] Resectability depends on this feature, and death may be caused by local invasion and airway obstruction.

Follicular carcinomas tend to invade locally and metastasize distantly, rather than to local nodes, and are especially prone to metastasize to bone or lung. In the Massachusetts General Hospital series,[152] one-half had metastasized at the time the diagnosis was originally established. Bony metastases are usually osteolytic, rarely osteoblastic, and the alkaline phosphatase level is rarely elevated. The tumor and metastases often retain an ability to accumulate and hold iodide, and are therefore sometimes susceptible to treatment with RAI. Indeed, some metastatic tumors synthesize thyroid hormone in normal or even excessive amounts. RAI therapy, as discussed below, improves survival in these patients.[161]

Occasionally the primary lesion of a follicular tumor appears to be entirely benign, but distant metastases are found. Invasion of vessels or the capsule, apart from the metastasis, is the only reliable criterion of malignancy. This variant has been called the benign metastasizing struma or malignant adenoma. It has a more prolonged course than do other varieties of follicular tumor, and is the type that has offered the best opportunity for the therapeutic use of [131]I.

The net extra mortality attributable to follicular cancer in the 10 to 15 years after diagnosis is 30 to 50 percent.[152,156,161] Of the patients dying from the lesion, three-fourths do so from the effect of distant metastases and the remainder from locally invasive disease.

Hürthle cell carcinomas are histologically distinct from other follicular tumors, but they pursue a similar course. They tend to invade and metastasize locally and have a strong propensity to recur after surgery. The course tends to be prolonged. These carcinomas often do not accumulate [131]I. In a large survey, however, Caplan et al[163] found that 4.4 percent of Hürthle cell neoplasms were hot on scan and 8.9 percent were warm. Serum TG levels may be normal or elevated.

A subset of thyroid carcinomas which give a histologic picture of islands of cells—thus "insular"—has been identified.[163] These tumors often look like anaplastic cancers, but are able to concentrate ^{131}I and thus are amenable to this excellent treatment. Whether these are properly considered a variety of follicular cancer is uncertain. The important message is that the histology in this instance does not reliably predict the utility of ^{131}I treatment, suggesting that all patients with thyroid cancer should at some point be studied to determine whether ^{131}I treatment is possible.

Medullary Carcinoma

Hazard et al.[134] first described a unique tumor in the thyroid characterized by sheets of cells with large nuclei, amyloid deposits, fibrosis, multicentricity,

and an unexpectedly benign course in view of the solid tumor appearance. Over 50 percent may have local or distant metastases at diagnosis. The tumors may metastasize locally, or to bones and soft tissues. The thyroid primary tumor and the metastases may show dense calcification on radiographs. The course tends to be progressive, and 10-year survivorship varies from 50 to 70 percent. These tumors, which constitute 2 to 8 percent of all thyroid cancers, are derived from the "light," or "C," or "parafollicular" cells. These are calcitonin (CT)-secreting cells, distinct from thyroid acinar cells, and are of ultimobranchial origin. The tumors may occur sporadically (about 70 percent of the total), in families, or as part of the MEN-II syndromes, which constitute about 10 to 20 percent of the cases, and are transmitted in families as dominant traits. In contrast with thyroid epithelial cell tumors, the female to male ratio is near unity. MEN-II includes patients with medullary thyroid cancers, pheochromocytomas, and parathyroid hyperplasia or adenomas. MEN-III (or, as sometimes designated, MEN-IIB) includes medullary thyroid carcinoma, mucosal neuromas, pheochromocytomas, which are usually bilateral and often malignant, occasionally cafe-au-lait spots, and possibly Gardner syndrome (mucocutaneous pigmented nevi and small intestinal polyps).[26–28,77,164–167] An occasional variant of medullary thyroid cancer appears to contain both CT and TG, suggesting the cells, surprisingly, have features of both medullary thyroid cancer and follicular cancer.[168] The origin of these tumors through mutation of specific oncogenes is described above.[168,169] Gastrointestinal symptoms including diarrhea, constipation, and megacolon are common in these patients and may occur long before the thyroid tumor is detected. Hyperplasia of C cells often precedes the development of familial cancers.[170] Medullary tumors derived from the C cells not only secrete CT, which may cause diarrhea,[171] but in addition may produce serotonin (with a carcinoid syndrome), prostaglandins, corticotropin releasing factor, and adrenocorticotropic hormone (causing Cushing syndrome), histaminase, and somatostatin. Interestingly, expression of somatostatin appears to correlate with improved prognosis.[172] Alcohol ingestion is reported to induce attacks of flushing and diarrhea, and to stimulate CT secretion by the tumors.[173] The CT secreted by these tumors rarely causes hypocalcemia,[174] but may possibly induce parathyroid hyperplasia. Most evidence suggests that the parathyroid hyperplasia is actually a separate part of a pleomorphic genetic syndrome.

The calcitonin assay provides a convenient screening procedure in families with this genetic trait.[175] Every member of one of these families with either a thyroid mass or elevated calcitonin levels should have a thyroidectomy. In MEN-II, the tumors follow a rather benign course somewhat akin to that of follicular cancer, and usually can be controlled by surgery. MEN-III tumors are much more aggressive and often cause death in the second or third decade. One patient has been reported with a medullary cancer that was suppressed by thyroid hormone.[176] Usually this treatment is not efficacious. Secretion of calcitonin by medullary cancer is remarkably increased by calcium or pentagastrin infusion.[177] This procedure can be helpful in establishing a diagnosis. At present the infusion of pentagastrin (0.5 μg/kg over 5 seconds), with determination of calcitonin levels at 0, 1, 2, 5, 10, and 15 minutes, appears to be the best test. Basal CT values are normally under (depending on the laboratory) 30 pg/ml.[177] Values of 30 to 100 after pentagastrin indicate hyperplasia, and values over 100 typically indicate the presence of cancer. Calcitonin should drop to levels of less than 30 pg/ml if the tumor is completely removed surgically. It should be noted that excess production of CT is not unique for medullary cancer, but can occur with granulomatous diseases and other cancers. Patients with the syndrome should also be studied with parathyroid hormone and catecholamine assays in order to determine the presence of other components of the syndrome.

The C cells also produce carcinoembryonic antigen (CEA) in large amounts. Serum CEA levels are elevated in medullary cancer with the same frequency as are CT levels.[178] Although CEA determination provides another parameter to follow, it does not offer any obvious advantage, and lacks the specificity of CT determinations. Tumor dedifferentiation is associated with a fall of CT and increasing CEA. This is an ominous sign.

Several specialized scanning procedures have been used in MTC. Total body imaging with T1-201 chloride and Tc-99m(V)DMSA have been successful in localizing metastases. [131]I MIBG and ^{131}I anti-CEA have been used both for localization and in attempts at therapy.[179] Most recently, radiolabelled somatostatin has been used as a whole body scanning agent.

Patients with MEN-IIA and IIB, and familial MTC, probably all have a germline mutation of the ret oncogene near the centromene of chromosome 10, and many patients with sporadic MTC have somatic mutations which allowed development of cDNA probes for the region which can be used to detect gene linkage in members of at-risk families.[177] PCR amplification of exons 10, 11, and 16, followed by single strand conformational electrophoretic analysis, allows recognition of most mutations.[180] This information is crucial in defining potential risk in young children and identifying need[169] for operation or frequent pentagastrin testing, and presumably will also screen out members of families who will not need to be repetitively screened by pentagastrin stimulation tests.

For readers with an interest in a somewhat broader view of oncogenesis, it may be noted that a syndrome entirely analogous to metastatic medullary thyroid carcinoma appears frequently in aged bulls.[181] Histologically similar adenomas are also frequently found. The lesion may be due to excessive dietary calcium; whether a similar stimulus could operate in human disease is unknown.

Undifferentiated Tumors

Undifferentiated tumors occur predominantly in persons over 50 years of age and constitute an increasing proportion of lesions in each subsequent age decade. Of great interest is the pathologic evidence that such tumors arise, in perhaps half of the cases, in a long-standing benign lesion or in differentiated carcinoma.[182] Although ^{131}I therapy for differentiated cancers has been blamed for this dedifferentiation, current evidence is against this hypothesis. Small-cell, spindle cell, and most giant-cell carcinomas of the thyroid grow rapidly and are very invasive. Local invasion may cause difficulty in breathing or swallowing, and tracheotomy is frequently required. These tumors metastasize to lymph nodes both locally and widely, but not characteristically to bone. Pulmonary metastases are frequent. Some patients present with a tender mass suggesting thyroiditis, and occasionally thyroid destruction induces hyperthyroidism.[183] The outlook for patients with this particular group of tumors is poor. By the time the diagnosis is made, the disease has spread in most patients beyond the area that can be attacked surgically, and they die within 6 months to 1 year. A few of these tumors, perhaps 10 percent, are entirely resectable when first discovered. There is nothing characteristic about the growth pattern of these tumors; their behavior is similar to that of any highly malignant tumor elsewhere in the body. The course of the epidermoid carcinoma and sarcoma of the thyroid is essentially the same. Small-cell anaplastic carcinomas are also found, but probably most tumors so classified in the past are actually lymphomas or lymphosarcomas.

Malignant Lymphomas

Lymphomas of the thyroid gland represent less than 5 percent of primary thyroid neoplasms.[184–187] Unlike most other thyroid neoplasms, lymphomas usually appear as rapidly enlarging masses; local symptoms are common. Many patients note hoarseness, dysphagia, and dyspnea or stridor. Hoarseness is often present in the absence of vocal cord paralysis. Rarely, patients may have the superior vena cava syndrome. The mean age at occurrence is 62 years. Primary lymphomas of the thyroid are two to three times more common in women than in men.

The incidence of hypothyroidism at the time of appearance is variable, ranging from 0 to 60 percent.[188,189] The co-occurrence of pathologic lymphocytic thyroiditis has ranged from 30 to 87 percent. These figures may underestimate the true incidence, as some patients have only had a biopsy examination and in others the entire gland has been replaced by the lymphoma. The frequent presence of thyroiditis has naturally led to the suggestion that the lymphoma might derive from preexisting thyroiditis.

The co-occurrence of thyroiditis may create difficulties in the proper interpretation of fine needle aspiration cytology. The clinical appearance must be carefully considered in accepting a diagnosis by fine needle aspiration of thyroiditis only or thyroiditis with lymphoma. An excisional or large needle biopsy may be necessary to make the correct diagnosis.

The majority of thyroid lymphomas are diffuse, large-cell lymphomas (formerly classified as diffuse, histiocytic or reticulum cell lymphomas), diffuse, mixed small and large cell lymphomas (formerly called diffuse, mixed lymphocytic-histiocytic), or diffuse, small cleaved-cell lymphomas (formerly classified as diffuse, poorly differentiated lymphocytic).

Although older series include reports of Burkitt's lymphoma, none were reported in larger, more recent series. Areas of diffuse large-cell lymphomas may have features similar to those characteristic of Burkitt's lymphoma or the Reed-Sternberg cells of Hodgkin's lymphoma.

Metastatic Carcinomas

Melanomas, breast tumors, pulmonary tumors, gastric, pancreatic, and intestinal carcinomas, renal carcinomas, lymphomas, carcinomas of the cervix, and tumors of the head and neck may metastasize to the thyroid. Sometimes the first indication of one of these tumors may be the appearance of a lump in the neck. Unless there is evidence for a primary site elsewhere, these tumors are easily mistaken for expanding tumors that have their origin in the thyroid gland. Usually by the time metastases appear in the thyroid, other metastases have occurred and the primary lesion may be discerned.

Cancer in Aberrant Thyroid Tissue

Thyroid tumors occasionally arise in lingual thyroids, along the thyroglossal duct, in substernal goiters, and even in struma ovarii.

Biochemical Studies

Interesting abnormalities in iodide metabolism have been found in thyroid adenomas (described above) and in thyroid carcinomas. In general, the tumors tend to lose the ability to accumulate iodide from the plasma, to bind iodide to TG, or to synthesize thyroid hormone.[19] The pattern is one of dedifferentiation, the loss of those functions peculiar to the thyroid gland. Most commonly there is a complete loss of selective uptake of iodide; this condition may be disclosed by the scintiscan, which shows an absence of ^{131}I accumulation over the mass in question. Follicular carcinomas tend to retain iodide metabolism more completely than other tumors, and therefore may be susceptible to treatment with RAI. Localization of ^{131}I in tumors, if present at all, is spotty rather than homogeneous.

Occasionally follicular tumors or their metastases produce significant amounts of thyroid hormone. In many instances the thyroid gland has been completely removed or destroyed, but the metastases have been sufficiently active to maintain the patient in a thyrotoxic state. More frequently, the metastases produce enough hormone to maintain the patient in a euthyroid condition, but not enough to produce thyrotoxicosis. This action indicates that the tumor may be responsive to thyrotrophic hormone, like the observation that thyrotropic hormone can induce growth of the tumors.

Robbins et al.[190] discovered that many of these tumors secrete an iodinated protein that has many of the physical properties of albumin. This iodinated protein moves electrophoretically with albumin and has a sedimentation constant of 4S. It contains iodotyrosines and possibly T_4. Evidently it is formed and iodinated in the thyroid. Since the original observation of Robbins et al., a similar protein has been found in the serum of patients with thyrotoxicosis and Hashimoto's disease. Much evidence suggests that a small amount of this "thyroalbumin" is a normal product of the gland, caused by iodination of serum albumin entering the thyroid. TG with an abnormal primary structure is also produced by most tumors; it retains immunologic relatedness to the normal protein.[191] Tumors unable to bind ^{131}I usually contain little or no mature TG, and instead contain poorly or noniodinated soluble proteins, possibly albumin, or fragments of the TG molecule. This dedifferentiation in proteins may relate to the loss of normal thyroid antigenicity that occurs in cancers.[133] In keeping with all goiters, carcinomas usually are associated with elevated serum TG levels. Growing differentiated tumors may cause levels of TG greater than 2000 mg/ml. In Hürthle cell tumors and anaplastic cancers, TG levels are usually minimally elevated.

Differentiated thyroid cancers retain a normal affinity and capacity for binding of TSH to their membrane receptors,[192] and TSH stimulates cAMP production normally in tumor tissue. Perhaps in keeping with the clinically recognized unresponsiveness to TSH, undifferentiated tumors lack high-affinity TSH receptors.[193] In autonomous thyroid nodules, TSH stimulates cAMP accumulation normally; hypersensitivity to the hormone has sometimes been found.[23,24]

Immunologic Studies

Differentiated thyroid cancers contain TG and microsomal (TPO) antigens cross-reacting with antibody to normal thyroid antigens; this fact can be very useful in identifying metastatic deposits.[194] (Fig. 18-15). Some tumors tend to lose the microsomal (TPO) antigen.[133,195] There is strong evidence that the immune system mounts a defense against the tumors, although an imperfect one. Tumors commonly are infiltrated by lymphocytes, and there is less tendency for nodal metastasis and a better prognosis with tumors so involved.[135] Antibodies to TG and microsomal antigen are more common in cancer patients than in control subjects.[196] We have shown, using in vitro assays, that 50 percent of patients develop immunity to TG, and some react to apparently specific thyroid tumor antigens.[197] The tumor antigen is recognized in both autologous and heterologous tumors, and is not present in Graves' disease tissue. Immunization with tumor preparation has been performed, and in a few cases has led to higher in vivo and in vitro reactivity and apparent partial tumor regression.[198] Nonspecific immune complexes are found in 10 percent of patients with differentiated cancers, and specific TG containing complexes are present at low levels in 30 percent of patients.[199] With progress of thyroid cancer, the immune system gradually loses responsivity, as with other tumors.[195,198,199]

The fibrosis and amyloid deposits in medullary cancers might suggest a host antitumor response, and indeed antitumor immune reactivity is detectable in vitro in most of these patients.[200]

Sometimes autoimmunity may play an adverse role. Graves' disease co-occurs with 4 to 8 percent of thyroid cancers, but whether this is by chance or through a true association is uncertain. The occurrence of TSH-like thyroid-stimulating antibodies in such patients could be related to the development or progress of tumors that have receptors recognizing these antibodies. In some reported cases, the thyroid-stimulatory autoantibodies seem clearly to stimulate the growth of the cancer, but overall, it is not clear that the co-occurrence of Graves' disease causes thyroid tumors to behave more aggressively.

Diagnosis

The question of thyroid carcinoma arises whenever a discrete solitary nodule is found in the thyroid gland by accident or because it has produced local symptoms. It also arises when an unusually hard or dominant nodule is found in multinodular goiter, when enlarged cervical lymph nodes are detected,

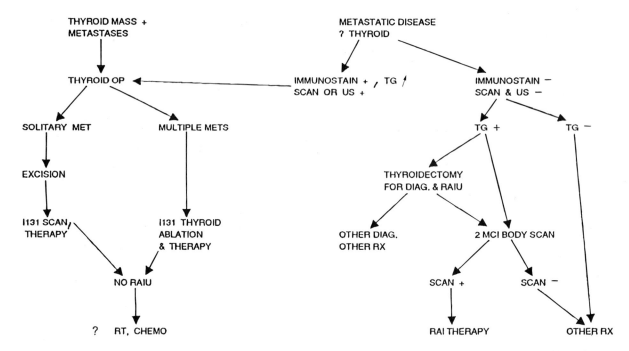

Fig. 18-15. Scheme for decisions in the management and therapy of metastatic tumor thought possibly to be thyroid cancer.

or when unidentified metastatic lesions are found elsewhere in the body. It must be strongly considered whenever an expanding lesion is present in the thyroid gland, especially when it is painful. Usually cancers present as discrete lumps, but occasionally papillary cancer may present as a diffuse goiter or as a "multinodular" goiter.[201] Anaplastic cancers and lymphomas commonly present as a smooth goiter. Stony hardness, fixation to the trachea, and damage to recurrent laryngeal or cervical sympathetic nerves are other important clinical signs. The problems of differentiating carcinoma from other lesions of the thyroid have been reviewed in the preceding discussion of thyroid nodules. A few additional comments are given here.

Scintiscanning is of some value in that it may demonstrate failure of the involved area to concentrate RAI. This reaction is typical of the malignant lesion. It in no way proves the presence of cancer, nor does its absence rule out this possibility. Whole body scintiscanning is useful to determine whether lesions in lung or bone are thyroid tumor metastases. Significant accumulation of RAI by the metastasis definitely proves thyroid origin. Occasionally uptake of RAI or the presence of stable iodine (by fluorescent scan-

ning) can be demonstrated in metastases in the neck before surgery. This finding is almost certain evidence for cancer, although rarely benign functioning bits of thyroid outside of but adjacent to the gland appear on scans. Usually normal thyroid tissue must be destroyed before a metastasis will accumulate ^{131}I. ^{131}I whole body scanning in management of previously diagnosed thyroid cancer is discussed later in this chapter.

Some tumors accumulate iodide but do not organify it. They are delineated by radiotechnetium scans done during the early "iodide phase" of isotope distribution, but not by scans using ^{131}I or ^{125}I done at 24 to 72 hours, when the storage of organified isotope is primarily recorded. Conversely, some metastases accumulate small amounts of ^{131}I but are not shown on short-term technetium scans.[202] Radiolabelled antithyroglobulin has shown potential in scanning for thyroid cancer metastasis, and in some studies has proven more sensitive than ^{131}Iodide.[203]

[^{32}P]-Phosphate and ^{75}Se-Selenium scanning did not prove useful.[75,204] Thallium[201] chloride is concentrated by most thyroid cancers and may be useful for identifying metastatic tumor.[205]

Ultrasonic scanning, angiography, thermography, iodopaque "thyrography," and fluorescent scanning have all been applied to the diagnosis of thyroid carcinoma. The techniques are discussed above. Of these approaches, only ultrasonic scanning has greatly improved diagnostic accuracy. Demonstration of the cystic nature of a thyroid lesion indicates, on a statistical basis, that it is probably benign. Since some papillary lesions are cystic, absolute reliance cannot be placed on this test. Currently, as described previously in the section on diagnosis of thyroid nodules, most reliance is placed on needle aspiration cytology. Scans, ultrasound studies, TG assay, and other tests are usually done, but tend to have a minor role in final therapeutic planning. Although TG assay has been suggested as an important marker for thyroid cancer,[206] practice shows that elevated TG levels can be caused by adenoma, multinodular goiter, and other diseases; thus the determination is of little absolute value before operation. In lesions which extend outside the thyroid, or have metastasis, ultrasound, CAT scanning, and MRI can provide useful information prior to surgery or when following disease progress.

Treatment

In past years the treatment of thyroid carcinoma has customarily been discussed in relation to the histopathologic condition, for example, papillary cancer, follicular cancer, etc. In discussing differentiated cancers, we have to some extent abandoned this approach, since contemporary medical and surgical practice depends much more on the clinical stage of the disease than on the exact histologic status. The anatomic stage can be defined precisely by the TNM system (see Table 18-4)[207,208] using information from the clinical and pathologic examinations. The classification can also be conveniently reduced to four categories that have some prognostic significance (Tables 18-4 and 18-5) and clear therapeutic relevance. It makes only a small difference in the initial surgical therapy whether a small focus of cancer in the gland is papillary or follicular. Even with ^{131}I therapy it makes little difference, because the therapeutic regimen depends on the function of the metastasis, not the structure of the primary lesion. Although follicular tumors are typically functional, metastases do not always follow the histologic or behavioral pattern of the primary tumor, and one

explores the possibility of ^{131}I therapy in most patients, regardless of the pathologic classification.

After the physical examination, radiographic examination of the chest, ^{131}I thyroid scintiscan, and aspiration cytology, thyroid tumors can be separated tentatively into four categories (which are further defined at operation): intrathyroid mass only (Clinical Stage I); intrathyroid mass plus enlarged, movable cervical lymph nodes (Clinical Stage II); fixed thyroid mass or fixed metastases in the neck (Clinical Stage III); and metastatic malignancy outside the neck (Clinical Stage IV).

Which operative procedure is indicated? The possible approaches range from a simple removal of the nodule to total thyroidectomy with bilateral radical neck dissection. If frozen section and operative examinations disclose no evidence of malignancy, only lobectomy is necessary for the benign lesion. On-the-spot examination should be followed by a careful study of multiple areas on permanent sections, since in a small percentage of nodules the diagnosis of malignancy can be made only from paraffin sections. Among patients with histologic or gross evidence of cancer within the gland, some will have cervical lymph node involvement and others will have no obvious spread. The surgeon has the option of removing the thyroid totally or in part, and performing a local or more radical excision of the cervical nodes. Prophylactic neck dissection is not done. Some patients will be found with cancer in the thyroid gland or in nodes only after examination of permanent histologic sections. One must then decide if a second surgical procedure is to be, performed or an attempt made to treat the tumor with [131]I.

Management of Clinical Stage I Differentiated Tumors (Intrathyroidal Disease Only)

Clinical Stage I differentiated cancers over 1 cm in size comprise half of total cases, occur in younger individuals, and have an excellent prognosis. After surgery (and often ^{131}I ablation), the survival was in our experience 95 to 98 percent at 15 years and about 95 percent at 30 years. Because of this excellent prognosis for treated patients, a controversy has continued during four decades over the appropriate extent of surgery, and necessity and value of postoperative ^{131}I ablation.[205–220]

At one extreme may be cited the position of Crile[218,219] and Cady,[156] who suggest that papillary carcinoma should be treated by excision of only the primary tumor (and grossly involved nodes), and afterward by administration of thyroid hormone. Cady doubts that thyroxine is needed and does not advise ^{131}I use. Among 307 patients with papillary cancer treated by Cady, 95 percent survived for 5 years or more. Only two patients died of their cancers.

Buckwalter and Thomas[209] and others suggested that lobectomy combined with dissection of nodes in the tracheosophageal groove is an adequate procedure for a Stage I differentiated cancer without evidence of multicentric involvement. In a series of 322 patients, total lobectomy (or total thyroidectomy) was a more effective procedure than subtotal lobectomy for Stage I well-differentiated cancer.[209] Interestingly, there were no cases of multicentricity in Stage I cancer in Buckwalter's series. Shands and Gatling,[221] in contrast, found an 11 percent contralateral recurrence rate after lobectomy, and one-half of these patients died. Tollefsen et al.[210] found a 4.6 percent recurrence rate after lobectomy for papillary cancer, and 7 of 17 patients with recurrence in the remaining lobe died of the disease.

A more aggressive approach for Stage I cancer is an ipsilateral total lobectomy and a contralateral intracapsular subtotal lobectomy with resection of nodes in the homolateral tracheoesophageal groove.[211] This operation minimizes damage to the parathyroids and to the recurrent laryngeal nerve on the contralateral side. Black et al.[212] found an 84 to 90 percent 10-year survival for Stage I papillary carcinoma and preferred this procedure to unilateral lobectomy because of the incidence of tumor involvement of the contralateral lobe. Rickey and Howard[211] and Buckwalter and Thomas[209] made no distinction between Stage I papillary and follicular cancers, but others treat Stage I follicular carcinoma more radically with total thyroidectomy[212,213] (see below). Prophylactic neck dissection is not recommended.

"Near-total" or total thyroidectomy is advocated by those who are impressed by the incidence of multicentricity of Stage I cancer, the fact that 2–5 percent of these young patients ultimately die of their disease, and the value of ^{131}I treatment. "Near-total" thyroidectomy refers to a procedure which may intentionally leave small portions of thyroid tissue near parathyroid glands or at the entry of the recurrent nerve into the larynx, but is associated with a marked reduction in possibility of hypoparathyroidism. It is frequently used with intended ^{131}I ablation of residual thyroid tissue. Multicentric involvement is reported to range from 25 to 90 percent. The wide variation of multicentricity (or intraglandular dissemination) can be explained in part by the finding that the incidence of multicentricity is doubled if one does whole gland histologic sections. There is little or no relationship between the size of a solitary nodule and the incidence of intraglandular dissemination, but an increasing degree of histologic malignancy is associated with the frequency of dissemination. Surprisingly, the incidence of pathologically detectable multicentricity always greatly exceeds that of clinical recurrence of tumor if the opposite lobe is left intact.[210] Whether this difference in incidence is a matter of time or of natural biologic defenses against tumor growth, is uncertain. It is clear, however, that multicentricity is not the only factor associated with an improved prognosis after more extensive surgery (and ^{131}I ablation), since in numerous studies multicentricity per se has been shown to have no clear effect on deaths or recurrences.

Mazzaferri et al., in their review of 576 cases of papillary carcinoma, found that total thyroidectomy statistically reduces the incidence of recurrences, and recurrences will presumably be correlated with deaths from disease.[150] Samaan et al[216] also support this procedure. Hay et al. prefer a slightly less extensive procedure, lobectomy plus contralateral subtotal lobectomy.

Total thyroidectomy carries an increased risk of hypoparathyroidism, recurrent nerve damage, and the necessity for tracheostomy.[214] Accidental unilateral nerve damage may reach 5 percent, but fortunately bilateral injury is rare.[215] All surgeons attempt to preserve those parathyroid glands that can be observed and spared, and an attempt is often made to transplant resected glands into the sternocleidomastoid muscles. Reports range from a 1 to a 25 percent incidence of hypoparathyroidism after total thyroidectomy.[159,210]

An alternative procedure for those who wish to have total thyroid removal, but who fear total thyroidectomy, is ipsilateral lobectomy and contralateral subtotal lobectomy followed by a dose of RAI to destroy the remaining remnant. The occurrence of hypoparathyroidism is close to zero after this procedure.

The most radical position advised in past years for the treatment of Stage I differentiated cancer was total thyroidectomy combined with homolateral prophylactic radical neck dissection.[217,220,222] Meissner and co-workers[223] found that when radical neck explorations were done, 65 percent of the patients without clinically apparent metastases were found by the pathologists to have lymph node involvement. Among 282 patients seen at Memorial Hospital in New York City, 46 percent with presumed Stage I disease were found in fact to have lymph node involvement in specimens obtained from homolateral radical neck dissection. Of 194 patients undergoing homolateral neck dissections, 177 had malignant nodes, as did 20 of 22 patients with contralateral neck dissection. Of 63 patients who did not have radical neck dissection, 21 percent later had further evidence of cancer, with a 33 percent mortality. It is not easy to reconcile such a high incidence of inapparent metastases with the low mortality among patients who did not have neck dissections, unless one assumes that the metastatic tumor in most instances failed to become clinically evident over a period of 10 to 20 years. Opinion has swung strongly away from prophylactic dissections. It is obviously impossible to predict which patients will derive benefit from this procedure. Nearly all surgeons now avoid enbloc dissections since such a resection is not required for long-term survival in thyroid carcinoma, and the procedure, which is mutilating, is especially undesirable in the young women who most frequently have such tumors.

Several groups have recently established criteria for low risk patients, including age under 45, lack of invasion or metastasis, tumor size under approximately 3 cm, and (in some analyses) low tumor grade on histologic criteria. These criteria categorize low and high risk patients very effectively.[224] Problems with such risk stratification is that the criteria are not available at the moment of surgery, and they fail to predict the few "low risk" patients (2.5 to 5 percent) who may behave as do "high-risk" patients, and might benefit from more extensive surgery.

Analysis of data on 269 papillary cancer patients followed at the University of Chicago for on average 12 years indicated that near-total thyroidectomy, or lobectomy plus contralateral thyroidectomy, compared to less extensive procedures, was associated with a statistically significant reduction in both recurrences and deaths in patients with Stage I and II cancers over 1 cm in size.

The current approach to surgery at the University of Chicago is outlined in Table 18-6. In unifocal papillary or follicular tumors under 1 cm detected at surgery, lobectomy plus contralateral subtotal thyroidectomy is done. This must be a sufficient procedure (some would say too aggressive) for these patients, who have a death rate (after therapy) not significantly different from that of normal persons over 10 to 20 years. Probably this procedure can be done regardless of age. This operation is also acceptable in a previously irradiated gland if the residual thyroid tissue appears to be entirely normal. If such minimal tumors are not recognized at surgery, but are found incidentally at pathologic examination of the tissue (e.g., after operation for Graves' disease), reoperation is not required.

In papillary or follicular tumors more than 1 cm, with multicentricity or with a history of neck irradiation associated with multiple abnormalities in the gland, we prefer a near-total thyroidectomy done by a surgeon with expertise in the field. This operation is an extracapsular thyroidectomy, but with the intention of and willingness to leave small amounts of tissue around the parathyroids and recurrent nerves, as necessary, to assure their viability.

In every procedure the tissue in the tracheoesophageal groove and the supraclavicular fossae should be palpated to the extent possible, and nodes in the homolateral groove should be biopsied. If nodes in this area are malignant, the supraclavicular area should be further explored; if the nodes are malignant, a modified neck dissection should be performed.[224–226] We do not favor enbloc dissection. The dissection should include all lymph node-bearing areas in the anterior neck as determined by inspection at surgery. Dissection of the upper mediastinum should be performed if malignant nodes are found, but rarely is a sternum-splitting operation justified. A more formal "block dissection" of involved nodes may be desirable in follicular cancer, since this tumor is more locally invasive.

It may also be possible and profitable to remove distant solitary metastases. The authors have, for example, removed a solitary metastasis in the skull of a woman who for 11 years after operation was entirely free of evidence of disease.

Most physicians who have considerable experience with the problem advise an ipsilateral "modi-

TABLE 18-6. Suggested Surgical Procedures in Thyroid Cancer

Type	Class	Operation
Papillary, follicular	I: <1 cm	Lobectomy + contralateral STT* (if a <1 cm tumor is detected in a resected specimen, do not reoperate)
Papillary, follicular	I: >1 cm, or multicentric or postradiation	NTT** or lobectomy + contralateral subtotal
Papillary, follicular	II	NTT + MND***
Papillary, follicular	III	Resection without mutilation
Papillary, follicular	IV	Resection without mutilation
Medullary	Any	NTT; MND
Anaplastic	Any	NTT or tumor resection, if possible

* STT = Subtotal thyroidectomy
** NTT = Near-total thyroidectomy
*** MND = Modified neck dissection

fied" dissection of node-bearing tissue, retaining the accessory nerve, jugular vein, and sternocleidomastoid muscle. Although some surgeons advised in the past a radical neck dissection,[227,228] it is obviously a much more mutilating procedure and there is no evidence that it offers a better prognosis. Those who favor a modified neck dissection cite the fact that the disease can usually be clinically cured by this procedure, and that, since the disease usually remains localized to the nodes for a long period of time, recurrent nodes may be removed at a second operation later on if necessary. Rickey and Howard found a 100 percent 10-year survival of papillary and follicular cancer patients after modified neck dissection,[211] and Buckwalter found that with radical neck dissection the survival in Stage II was the same as in Stage I.[206]

Stage III Disease

There is less controversy about the extent of required surgery in more advanced tumors. Patients with invasive papillary or follicular tumors should have as extensive a dissection as possible without mutilation. It appears that residual tumor can be left along one recurrent nerve, for example, to be ablated by ^{131}I therapy, without compromising the patient's life expectancy. Thus, in 97 patients with an incomplete procedure that left tumor in the neck, 83 percent had a 10-year survival.[229] It thus becomes obvious that survival cannot be directly correlated with the extent of surgery, and a certain degree of conservatism is warranted. In patients over age 45, since the papillary or follicular tumors are clearly more aggressive, more extensive resection including portions of the trachea may be required, and the

sternocleidomastoid muscle, jugular vein, and accessory nerve should be removed if this procedure allows apparently complete tumor resection.

Management of Stage IV Disease

Finally, one must consider the group of patients with metastases outside the confines of the neck. Those with a thyroid mass and solitary lung or bone metastases should undergo thyroidectomy and excision of the metastases if the latter are accessible. Prolonged survival may be observed. If there are multiple metastases, RAI ablation is attempted in addition to thyroidectomy. Unfortunately, the prognosis in Stage IV disease must be guarded. Patients with ^{131}I uptake in the lungs but no detectable nodules on radiographs or CAT scan tend to do well with ^{131}I therapy. Patients with other soft tissue or bone lesions, especially if multiple, however, have up to 75 percent mortality in ten years.[230]

A problem arises in patients with widely metastatic disease from an unknown primary site that is histologically and clinically compatible with thyroid cancer. If the diagnosis of thyroid cancer can be established, palliation or cure becomes occasionally possible, and accordingly one should take further steps to establish a definitive diagnosis. These steps include immunostaining of the tumor tissue, measurement of serum TG, sometimes ultrasound or CAT scans of the thyroid, a ^{131}I scan of the thyroid and metastases, and possibly thyroidectomy. If the scan is abnormal, it can be assumed that the diagnosis is probably thyroid cancer. A thyroidectomy is then done to establish a histologic diagnosis. With the thyroid removed, thyroid metastases are more likely to show uptake on scan, and if RAI treatment is contemplated, tumor uptake of the isotope is enhanced. If upon thyroidectomy the diagnosis of thyroid cancer is made, and if there is reasonable uptake of ^{131}I by the metastases, then the patient can be treated as outlined below. If the scan is negative, TSH stimulation of ^{131}I uptake should be attempted.

All medullary and anaplastic cancers are treated by near-total or total thyroidectomy, a more radical neck dissection, and if necessary, tumor resection if possible, as described below. When anaplastic cancers have infiltrated widely outside of the thyroid, only biopsy may be indicated, or a de-bulking procedure, or tracheostomy, as determined by operative findings.

After operation all patients are maintained indefinitely on thyroid hormone except when undergoing tests. Individuals with current active cancer (other than medullary or lymphoma) should have TSH suppressed to near zero. Patients who had cancer previously, but are currently believed free of disease, should have their replacement lowered to provide a TSH of 0.1 to 0.4 μU/ml, and ultimately as safety is assured, to the normal range. With the exception of persons under age 21 with no history of irradiation and unifocal papillary or follicular tumors less than 1 cm in size, all patients at the University of Chicago Clinics undergo postoperative ^{131}I ablation and ^{131}I therapy, if appropriate, as described below.

Patients with Stage III papillary or follicular tumors over age 55 also receive external irradiation therapy, as do patients of any age with Stage III medullary cancer. All patients with undifferentiated neoplasms or lymphomas, or with nonresectable neck recurrence of papillary or follicular cancer, also receive irradiation, or chemotherapy, as described below.

Radiation-Associated Cancers

Radiation-associated cancers have a high degree of multicentricity (54 percent in our series, more than double that in a control group of nonirradiated patients), are usually papillary or follicular tumors, tend to be the same size as cancers in nonirradiated persons, are often associated with other irradiation-induced lesions such as adenomas and fibrosis, and have at least as bad a prognosis as radiation-unassociated cancers. We accept lobectomy and contralateral subtotal thyroidectomy if there is only one lesion under 1 cm in size and the rest of the gland is nor-

mal. If there is multicentricity, a tumor more than 1 cm, adenopathy, or multiple abnormalities in the gland (the usual case), near-total thyroidectomy is performed.

Childhood Thyroid Cancer

Some special features of thyroid cancer occurring in children deserve comment. It is, of course, an uncommon disease. The tumors are usually papillary or mixed histologically, and tend to grow slowly, with a high frequency (50 to 80 percent) of neck metastases, but with a relatively favorable prognosis. The association with x-ray exposure has already been discussed. As in adults, the incidence in girls is double that in boys. Multicentricity of tumors is found in 30 to 80 percent. Metastases to lungs are common (perhaps 20 percent), but tumor is rarely found in the bones. Lung metastases usually accumulate ^{131}I and can often be eradicated with this isotope.

As with adult tumors there is no universally accepted surgical approach, but it is certain that sentiment has swung away from prophylactic and radical neck dissections to a more conservative position.[228,229,231] The operations employed are as described above. Thyroid remnants are destroyed with ^{131}I in patients with multicentric lesions and in all Clinical Stage II, III, and IV lesions. Detection of metastases is attempted, as described elsewhere in this chapter. Most childhood metastatic thyroid cancers are found to accumulate sufficient ^{131}I to allow useful and sometimes curative therapy. Although the 10-year survival is from 90 to 95 percent, long term follow-up demonstrates an eightfold greater than normal mortality[155] and emphasizes the need for comprehensive therapy and long term follow-up.

RA^{131}I Therapy

Many patients who have had a "total" thyroidectomy, and all patients who have had a subtotal resection, will have some functioning thyroid tissue remaining in the normal position after surgery, and will thus be candidates for ^{131}I ablation. There is no unanimity regarding the use of postoperative ^{131}I ablation in Stage I tumors, since absolutely convincing evidence of its value is lacking,[156,159] but for all patients with papillary and follicular cancers as a group, ^{131}I ablation correlates with improved survival.[157,159] Our data demonstrate that postoperative ^{131}I ablation correlated with decreased recurrences for all patients with papillary cancers over 1 cm in size. Samaan et al,[216] in a review of 1,599 patients, observed that ^{131}I treatment was the most powerful indicator for disease-free survival. Ablation can be accomplished in most instances by one dose of 30 mCi ^{131}I, giving the patients about 10 whole body rads.[232] We do not routinely use ablation in patients under age 21 with tumors under 1 cm. Patients with tumors above this size, older patients, or those with multicentricity or a history of neck irradiation are advised to take [131]I. This practice is not uniformly followed at other clinics. In patients with Stage II to IV disease, we proceed to destroy any residual thyroid and to treat demonstrable metastases if they can be induced to take up enough [131]I. Use of ^{131}I therapy is investigated in these patients, regardless of the histologic characteristics of the resected lesion, although significant uptake rarely is found in Hürthle tumors[163,233] or in patients with anaplastic lesions.

The patients are usually given full thyroid hormone replacement therapy for about 6 weeks after operation, so that any malignant cells disseminated at the time of thyroidectomy will not be stimulated by TSH. The value of this measure is admittedly unknown. Patients then receive 25 μg L-T$_3$ bid for 3 weeks, and therapy is then stopped for at least 2 weeks to allow endogenous TSH (which will reach 20 to 60 μU/ml) to stimulate uptake of the ^{131}I by the remaining fragments of thyroid tissue or metastatic lesions in the neck or elsewhere before proceeding with ^{131}I therapy. Some physicians proceed directly with ^{131}I therapy 2 to 4 weeks after surgery. We cannot prove any advantage to our approach. If possible, whole body scans are obtained about 5 to 7 days after the ablative dose of [131]I (or after therapeutic doses), since occasionally unsuspected metastasis may be visualized on scans at this time. Recently we have found that it is convenient to prepare patients for ^{131}I scanning simply by reducing replacement thyroxine to half the usual dose for 5 weeks. Patients feel more or less normal during this interval, and TSH is >25 μU/ml in most individuals. A longer period can be used as needed to elevate TSH.

After initial ablation, we replace hormone therapy at 24 hours and continue this therapy for 3 to 6 months. At this time, patients are switched to 50 μg L-T$_3$/day for 3 weeks. This medication is then stopped, and after 2 to 3 weeks imaging is again performed.

It has been the practice at the University of Chicago Clinics to perform whole body imaging with the gamma scintillation camera at 48 and 72 hours after administration of 2 to 5 mCi [131]I. The 48-hour study is done so that metastases showing a relatively active turnover of iodine will not be missed, to shorten the study if possible, and to allow early ordering of isotope. The 72-hour imaging is technically superior, since the background iodide is almost entirely excreted by this time. In whole body scanning there is a definite advantage to the use of the gamma camera with multiaperture parallel holes, over a diverging collimator. By comparing the counting rate over a metastasis with a known standard, the percentage uptake of the dose can be computed. The gamma camera is essential for this procedure since, with the multiaperture parallel collimation described, the counting rate is essentially distance independent, as compared to the usual broad-field thyroid uptake collimator in which distance is critical. Using this technique, it is possible to measure easily the exact percentage of dose retention at 24 to 72 hours. The method is much simpler and more accurate than measuring isotope retention by collecting urinary [131]I. The amount of ^{131}I used for scanning varies from 2 to 10 mCi, or even larger amounts. Clearly the larger doses detect more lesions, but this rarely alters treatment plans. More importantly, doses of 5 to 10 mCi have been shown to decrease tumor uptake of the subsequent treatment dose—to "stun" the tumor.[234] The exact importance of this phenomena is uncertain, but at this time, use of a 2 mCi dose seems to be a reasonable compromise. Patients who have significant uptake of ^{131}I in metastases (usually above 0.5 percent of the tracer) are given 150 to 250 mCi [131]I. This dose can be tolerated without acute radiation sickness, and is below the level that would promote pulmonary fibrosis if diffuse pulmonary metastases are present, unless uptake in the lungs exceeds 50 percent (see below).

In perhaps four-fifths of patients accumulating ^{131}I, it is possible to administer a dose of RAI that should be useful in destroying tumor. For normal thyroid tissue 10,000 to 15,000 rads is destructive, and a dose of 20,000 rads or more is probably needed for therapy of cancer. Assuming, for example, a standard 150 mCi ^{131}I dose, and delivery to tumor of about 100 rads per mCi retained per gram, a 1 percent tumor uptake distributed through 10 g of metastatic tissue could provide an effective treatment. The treatment dose can be estimated by the following formula:

Rads delivered = 74
  $\times$ energy of beta ray (.2 mev)
  $\times \dfrac{\mu\text{Ci given}}{\text{ml distribution volume}}$
  $\times$ fractional uptake
  $\times$ effective half-life in days

Obviously the distribution volume in tumor is difficult to ascertain, and great variation in tissue distribution and sensitivity may occur. Some groups have attempted to measure tumor volume by use of quantitative PET scanning.[235] The effective half-life can be determined from serial counts of the tracer over the metastasis. If 10 g of tumor in the neck accumulated 1 percent of a 150-mCi dose, and isotope turnover in the tumor was extremely slow, the radiation dose might be as follows:

$$\text{Rads} = 74 \times 0.19 \times \frac{150,000}{10} \times 0.01 \times 6$$
$$= 12,654$$

The question of whether a subcancericidal dose should be delivered in patients with low levels of tumor isotope accumulation needs further investigation, since radiobiologic studies suggest that radiation could preferentially spare the more radioresistant cells, ultimately leaving a more lethal tumor. It may be possible to give conventional x-ray therapy after ^{131}I in those instances in which ^{131}I uptake is present but the total dose delivered to the metastasis is less than adequate. This procedure may provide another therapeutic approach to the thyroid cancer patient, but it has not yet been given adequate trial. Maxon et al.[236] report that radiation doses of at least 30,000 rads for thyroid ablation, and 8,000 for therapy to metastasis, improve the rate of response.

In some patients tracer studies fail to show uptake, and serum TG is elevated. Some investigators recommend treating these individuals with large doses of [131]I (100 to 150 mCi) and report that tumor uptake can be visualized after treatment, and that serum TG may fall.[237] The clinical efficacy of this approach is not known. In some cases reported by Schlumberger et al,[238] TG became undetectable, clearly a striking and hopeful result. This approach is currently followed by many thyroidologists, but proof of efficacy (increased survival) is lacking (Fig. 18-23).

It is useful to do a scintiscan on patients who have received therapeutic doses of ^{131}I at 5 to 7 days following the treatment, thus using the treatment dose as a more powerful scanning dose. While often offering no new information, this may reveal unsuspected metastasis, especially in younger patients who have previously had ^{131}I treatment.[233]

After initial treatment, the patients are again given L-T_4 for 24 weeks, and then T_3 for 3 weeks, in order to accelerate the onset of hypothyroidism when hormone therapy is stopped. After 24 to 52 weeks the cycle is repeated, as long as there is no evidence of systemic radiation damage, and as long as the metastases continue to accumulate iodide (Fig. 18-16). The total ^{131}I dosage over several years may vary from 150 to (rarely) 2,000 mCi. It may be possible to induce further uptake of iodide and thus deliver additional radiation therapy after administration of TSH. We usually rely on endogenous TSH to stimulate uptake, since repeated administration of bovine TSH may lead to the development of neutralizing antibodies. Also, patients frequently develop an allergy to bTSH, with severe hives, fever, or serum sickness, after two or three courses of the drug. Occasionally TSH is given when prolonged hypothyroidism must be avoided. We believe that biosynthetic human TSH will become available for routine use in the near future, and allow ^{131}I therapy without induction of hypothyroidism.[239]

Another (although almost never employed) means of stimulating ^{131}I uptake in these patients is by administration of antithyroid drugs. Iodide depletion by dietary control and diuresis including furosemide or mannitol administration can also double the fractional uptake of ^{131}I in metastases.[240,241] Finally, when the scan shows no ^{131}I uptake, even with TSH, the potential benefits from this mode of therapy have been exhausted and permanent thyroid hormone replacement is prescribed.

The advent of TRH brought with it the hope of stimulating pituitary TSH secretion in the management of thyroid cancer. Unfortunately, intravenous TRH is probably of little value. Given intravenously, TRH is ineffective in releasing TSH until 3 to 10 days after hormone replacement therapy has been withdrawn. Until the patient has been without hormone for 2 to 3 weeks, it causes at best a minor and transient elevation of the TSH level, which is small in comparison to that induced by spontaneous hypothyroidism.

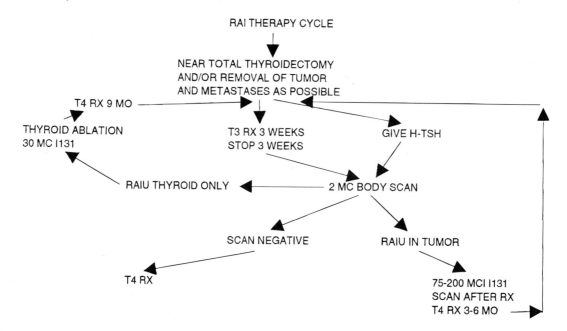

Fig. 18-16. Management of radioactive iodide for thyroid ablation and cancer treatment.

The therapeutic protocol used at Memorial Hospital in New York, by Maxon,[236] and as well at the other center, has for years been designed to give maximal-tolerable radiation doses to cancer patients.[242] The dose is calculated on the basis of prior isotope tracer kinetics. The aim is to give a blood dose of under 200 rads, or less than 120 mCi retained at 48 hours, or 80 mCi retained at 48 hours if diffuse lung metastases are present. This method has theoretical advantages since it potentially provides the most cancericidal dose, but in general the difficulties of calculating the dose and the occasional adverse reactions seem to outweigh the benefits.

Before radiation therapy, female patients should be carefully screened for pregnancy and lactation. Confirmed or possible pregnancy constitutes a firm contraindication to therapy because of the risk of damage to the fetus.

A patient who has ingested many milliCuries of ^{131}I can cause serious radiation contamination, and appropriate precautions must be followed. If less than 30 mCi ^{131}I is given, it is permissible to have the patient dispose of urine and feces into general sewage. If amounts of ^{131}I greater than 30 mCi are given, the patient should be kept in a private room in the hospital until less than 30 mCi is retained in the body. Urine should be collected by the patient and stored in bottles behind protective lead shield-

ing. After physical decay, usually after about 6 weeks, it may be discarded in the sewage. Contaminated bedding and utensils should be stored for 10 half-lives (80 days), thoroughly washed, and monitored for residual contamination before being used again. Alternatively, disposable bedding and utensils may be used.

Personnel caring for a patient who has received ^{131}I therapy are often concerned about exposure to excessive radiation. This is very rarely a real problem. Monitoring by means of a portable ionization chamber is important in making certain that no person receives more than an allowable radiation dose. Table 18-7 gives a rough estimate of the amount of radiation received while performing ordinary hospital tasks at various distances from a patient who has received [131]I. In general, all ordinary patient care can be performed without hazard. Even so, it is best to avoid close contact between personnel and patient during the first 48 hours after therapy because of undue apprehension that may be induced.

Definition of the amount of tracer ^{131}I collected by a tumor is difficult and inaccurate, and there is no firm basis for estimating the dose that must be localized in the tumor in order to produce a worthwhile effect. For these reasons, opinions vary on the practical value of ^{131}I therapy. Our operational rule is that if (1) a focal area of isotope concentration on

TABLE 18-7. Radiation Exposure to Personnel During Care of a Patient Who Has Received 100 mCi [131]I*

Distance From Source—e.g., The Patient	Reason for Exposure	Dose Rate (mrad/hr)	Duration of Exposure Permitted on Basis of Allowable 0.1 Rad/Week
½ in.	Direct handling of therapy dose or urine after therapy	136,000	None
1 ft.	Giving personal hygiene to treated patient	240	0.5 hr/week
3 ft.	Making the bed, mopping the floor	27	5.0 hr/week
9 ft.	In chair across the room	3	40.0 hr/week; allowable exposure cannot be reached

* Assuming 100% retention of the dose during the period of exposure.

scan is visible or (2) an area of tumor can be shown to collect over 0.5 percent of the ^{131}I tracer on scintiscan, then ^{131}I therapy is worth trying. Maxon[236] finds that a dose of 30,000 rads is needed to achieve thyroid ablation, at least 8,000 rads are needed to treat metastatic foci, and ideally 14,000 rads to treat nodes.

The use of RAI in large doses is not without hazard. The radiation dose delivered to the whole body, the gonads, or bone marrow is usually assumed to be the same as that of the blood. The blood dose depends on the amount of isotope administered; its distribution space and turnover; the degree of heterogeneity of distribution in the tumor; the uptake, synthesis, and secretion of labeled compound by the tumor; and perhaps other variables. The radiation is usually largely due to inorganic iodide, since little protein bound ^{131}I ordinarily appears in the blood. Sometimes tumor destruction is such that much PB[131]I appears in the blood and can yield a major fraction of the total whole body radiation dose. As a rough estimate, the blood, gonadal, or bone marrow radiation may be assumed to be 0.3 to 1.5 rad/mCi ^{131}I administered,[243] or 45 to 150 rads per treatment. The genetic risks are discussed in Chapter 11 and are not reviewed here. Ordinarily, when ^{131}I therapy is needed for carcinoma, the necessity of treating the patient outweighs the risks of genetic damage.

Various unwanted effects of radiation may occur in patients receiving large doses of [131]I. Mild radiation sickness is seen. Metastatic deposits or surrounding tissues may become painful over 2 to 4 weeks from radiation-induced inflammation. Damage to the salivary glands can cause sialadenitis, and xerostomia, and can lead to loss of teeth. Ovarian function is often temporarily suppressed,[244] and if there are

pelvic metastases that collect ^{131}I, the gonads may receive a sterilizing dose. Sperm count may be reduced for months. Leukemia occurs with increased frequency in patients who have received large doses of ^{131}I for cancer.[245] Transient hypoparathyroidism has been reported.[246] Transient or permanent alterations in liver function and lymphoma of the parotid gland have been reported as possible sequelae.[247] Pulmonary fibrosis has occurred in patients with functioning lung metastases who have received unusually large doses or who have very active metastases.[248,249] Leukopenia, thrombocytopenia, and anemia are encountered with accumulating doses. A mild effect on the bone marrow is seen with each therapeutic dose, and after several hundred mCi aplastic anemia may develop.[250] The hemoglobin level, white cell count, differential count, and platelets should be monitored periodically in order to judge recovery of the marrow between treatments and to prevent excess total radiation damage to the marrow. Large radiation doses may cause transient swelling of metastasis in the brain or spinal canal.

Two special complications need be noted. Occasionally withdrawal of hormone suppression, in preparation for isotope therapy, leads to rapid growth of the tumor, and reinstitution may not seem to return the patient to the prior condition. Special care should be taken if metastases are present in areas such as brain or spinal column, where growth could cause serious sequelae.

RAI was introduced into the treatment of thyroid carcinoma with the hope that it would be a panacea for this disease. Unfortunately, the results have not been universally beneficial. Most tumors in children appear to be treatable, and among adults 80 to 90 percent of metastatic carcinomas accumulate sufficient ^{131}I to warrant a serious therapeutic trial. Patients who harbor this form of the disease are fortunate, since ^{131}I may totally eradicate the metastases. Even multiple pulmonary metastases occasionally disappear after ^{131}I therapy (Fig. 18-7). The final value of ^{131}I therapy has been difficult to define, largely because of a lack of controlled series and because of other treatment (especially thyroid hormone) given at the same time.[250–253] Mazzaferri found that ^{131}I ablation and therapy significantly improved the prognosis in papillary cancer by decreasing recurrences.[159] Varma et al.[252] found that RAI treatment had no effect on the survival of persons under age 40 but did lower the death rate of patients over age 40. Leeper[253] concluded that ^{131}I treatment appears clearly to benefit patients under 40 years of age with papillary cancer, but the course of this cancer in older patients is rarely affected; follicular cancers in older patients are treatable, and survival is prolonged even if the disease is not eradicated. Soft tissue lesions, especially of the lung and mediastinum, respond best to [131]I. Osseous lesions are often highly functional but are infrequently totally destroyed by [131]I.[254] Lesions detected on whole body scans, with negative bone radiographs, are most likely to be cured. In another report, 59 of 400 patients were considered candidates for ^{131}I therapy after using antithyroid drugs or TSH to stimulate uptake. Of these, 61 percent with metastatic disease were benefited.[235] The follicular, papillary, and mixed cancers responded equally well. Numerous reports indicate that ablation of metastasis with ^{131}I is associated with a better prognosis than failure to ablate, but obviously this outcome may relate to the histologic nature and function of the lesion rather than to the therapy per se.

Disseminated pulmonary metastasis can sometimes be eradicated by ^{131}I, but radiation pneumonitis or fibrosis may be produced and may be fatal.[248,249] On first observation of pulmonary metastases, this therapy should be considered, but no more than 75 mCi should ever be deposited in the lungs in one treatment. Progress of the lesion and pulmonary function should be carefully evaluated before and between treatments.[250–255]

Follicular Carcinoma and [131]I Therapy

L.F., a 43-year-old woman, developed a thyroid mass, and a right lobectomy was done for follicular carcinoma. A recurrence was found 3 years later, and a left lobectomy and cervical lymph node dissection were carried out. The patient subsequently developed hypo-

parathyroidism. Cobalt therapy was given. Eight years after diagnosis, lytic lesions developed in the right humerus and right ileum, and she was given a course of x-ray therapy to the humerus. She was first seen in our clinic at this time. Her health was apparently good despite the known thyroid carcinoma, and she had no complaints. She was receiving replacement therapy of 120 mg desiccated thyroid daily. BP was 140/70 and pulse was 90. She was sweaty and tremulous. There were multiple small supraclavicular lymph nodes, a lobulated mass in the right hilar area, and osteolytic lesions in the right humerus, both femurs, and the right ileum. Ten days after thyroid therapy had been discontinued, the TT_4 level was 9.1 μg/dl and the FTI was 12.7, indicating that the metastases were sufficiently active to produce mild hyperthyroidism. Forty-seven percent of an RAI tracer was accumulated in the chest metastases after the patient was given 5 units of TSH daily for 3 days (Fig. 18-18). She was given 60 mCi ^{131}I at this time, and again 3 months later. Two months later, the patient received 100 mCi ^{131}I after a 17 percent RAIU was demonstrated in the pulmonary metastases. Four months later, there was clear evidence of reduction the size of the pulmonary and mediastinal metastases, and the RAIU was only 2 percent 3 weeks after withdrawal of thyroid medication. Metastases were visible in the lower lung fields, and in the pelvis, the right humerus, both femurs, and in the left first rib. Because of pain in the left shoulder area and the osteolytic metastasis, she was treated with 4,000 rads x-ray to the apex and given 100 mCi ^{131}I after 4 days of 5 units of TSH daily.

In 4 months the mediastinal and pulmonary lesions were largely gone, but there was obvious extension of metastatic deposits in the vertebrae D-2 and D-3. The patient developed spinal cord compression that required installation of a Wilson plate to stabilize the vertebrae. The next month, a scan, done 3 weeks after discontinuation of replacement therapy when the FTI was less than 1 and the TSH level was elevated to 60 μU/ml, indicated small amounts of uptake of isotope in the metastases in the vertebrae D-2 and D-3, the right humerus, the mediastinum, both lung fields, the right iliac crest, and both femurs. Total uptake was approximately 2 percent. She received 100 mCi [131]I.

Three months later, total isotope accumulation after a tracer was less than 0.5 percent of the dose in all the areas of the body containing visible metastases, and further ^{131}I uptake could not be stimulated by TSH (Fig. 18-18). Maximal tolerable radiation had been given to the metastatic lesions in the humerus and vertebrae. The leukocyte count hovered between 2,000 and 3,000. The patient received a course of bleomycin over 14 days without producing objective benefit. Later the same year she was immunized with homogenates of her own tumor and pertussis vaccine, and again there was no evidence of objective benefit. Progressive paraplegia and weakness occurred, and she died of the illness in August of the next year.

In this all too frequent story, initial lobectomy was followed by recurrence and dissemination. Functional pulmonary metastasis produced mild hyperthyroidism. These deposits were readily ablated with RAI therapy, but osseous metastasis progressed at the same time. The course, from first diagnosis to death, was 11 years.

Follow-up of Cancer Patients: The Serum TG Assay

In previous sections we have described diagnosis, surgery, and ^{131}I ablation. When these stages have been passed, patients should be followed in a regular manner at increasing intervals indefinitely in order to monitor replacement therapy and recognize recurrence or extension of disease. The serum TG assay is important in managing these patients.

All patients will receive thyroid hormone in a dose adequate to restore euthyroidism and to maintain TSH suppression. Doses above normal replacement levels,[256] should be used in patients with currently active disease (Fig. 18-17). If the patient can tolerate it, TSH should be suppressed close to zero in a sensitive assay, but this program must be related to the patient's symptoms, cardiac function, and potential for osteoporosis. Hyperphysiologic doses of T_4 clearly lead to osteoporosis.[257] Patients who recently were treated for cancer but have no known residual disease are probably best maintained with a just-depressed level of sTSH—0.1 to 0.4 μU/ml. Patients who have been followed for some time (1 to 2 years),

who had no evidence of metastasis at presentation, and who have no evidence of recurrent disease, should be managed by standard replacement dosage of the hormone.[54,258] Patients on suppressive doses of LT_4 for thyroid cancer can benefit from β-adrenergic blockage which provides improved sense of well being and reduces left ventricle overactivity.

Patients in category I are followed by physical examination, chest radiograph, serum FTI, and TG assay at least yearly (Table 18-8). Whole body ^{131}I scans are usually repeated in the third and fifth to sixth years after ^{131}I ablation. Measurement of serum TG, when the patient is on replacement, is of limited value, since serum TG may be suppressed. Elevated serum TG levels in the absence of medication is not a valid indicator of residual cancer or of recurrence if a thyroid remnant exists, but progressive elevation while receiving replacement hormone is an ominous sign, and elevation above 5 ng/ml, when off replacement therapy (after ablation) is also suggestive of recurrence (Fig. 18-18).

Most patients fall into category II (Table 18-8). Repeat whole body ^{131}I scan is usually done 6 to 9 months after the ablating dose of ^{131}I is given and, if negative, is repeated at 1 to 2 years and at 4 to 5 years if negative (Fig. 18-19, Fig. 18-20). Serum TG levels should be below 2 ng/ml when the patient is receiving replacement therapy if there is no thyroid remnant,[259] but the assay is more reliable and sensitive when the patient is not taking medication, since TG production by many tumors is suppressed by hormone therapy. A serum TG level after thyroid ablation that is above 5 ng/ml, on or off hormone therapy, suggests recurrence.[260–262] To be truly in-

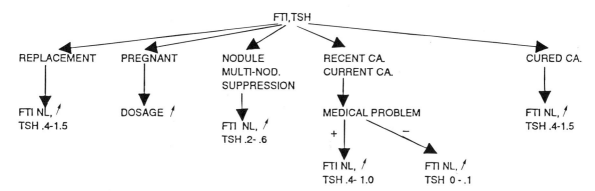

Fig. 18-17. Decisions in deciding the correct dosage of thyroxine in patients who are receiving this medication for various indications, including prior but presumed cured cancer, or who have had recent cancer, or currently have active thyroid malignancy.

TABLE 18-8. Medical Management After Surgery

Patient Category	Physical Examination, Chest Radiograph, Serum FTI and TSH	Repeat ^{131}I Body Scan	TG (Desired Level)
I. Tumor removed, residual thyroid in situ	Annually	—	Below 10 ng/ml while receiving therapy
II. Tumor ± nodes removed, thyroid ablated by surgery or ^{131}I	At least annually	At 6–9 months after ablation, then at 1, 3, and 6 years	Below 5 ng/ml when not taking hormone, preferably 0–1 ng
III. Tumor removed, thyroid ablated, metastatic disease treated	At 3–6 months, then at least annually	At 3–6 months after therapy, and annually for 3–5 years	Below 5 ng/ml when not taking hormone, preferably 0–1 ng

dicative of residual tumor, the assay must be done when the patient is not taking thyroid hormone. In most clinics, TG assay results are usually not available for 7 to 14 days, and the decision to treat with ^{131}I or not is based only on demonstration (or lack) of ^{131}I accumulation on whole body scan. It is possible that the serum TG assay will replace reliance on the ^{131}I whole body scan. At present we, and others,[263] believe that serum TG complements but does not substitute for scanning in this category of patients. After ^{131}I ablation, however, a TG less than 2 ng/ml, when the patient is off replacement, is indicative of absence of cancer. Although the serum TG assay will detect nonfunctioning metastases, such lesions are usually known from the prior history of the patient and from the physical or radiographic examination. In some patients serum TG levels of 5 to 10 mg/ml appear to gradually become lower over years of follow-up on thyroxine replacement, as if tiny metastatic tumor deposits were being destroyed by fibrosis or possibly an immune response (Fig. 18-18). Reexamination at yearly intervals also includes a chest radiograph, a serum FTI, and TSH determinations (Figs. 18-21, 18-22). Serial bone scans and bone radiographs are of little additional value in periodic follow-up examinations. The concept of treat-

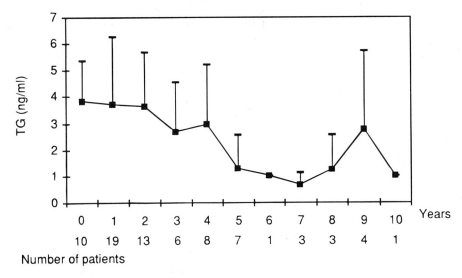

Fig. 18-18. Mean serum thyroglobulin values in patients with thyroid cancer given near-total or total thyroidectomy and radioactive iodide ablation and followed up to ten years. Without further treatment, there is a tendency for the serum thyroglobulin values to decline, suggesting the gradual death of residual normal or cancerous thyroid cells.

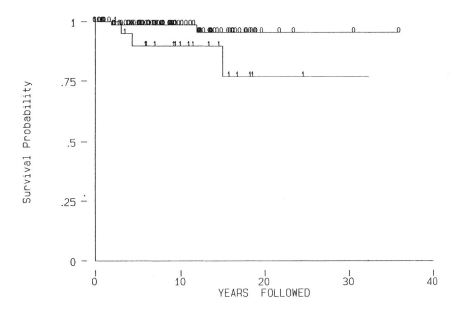

Fig. 18-19. Comparison of recurrence-free survival in patients with a "good prognosis" who had a limited (1) versus extensive (0) resection. Group 0 > Group 1, p = 0.05. Patients who had a good prognosis were less than 45 years old at diagnosis, in Class I or II with intrathyroidal disease or positive neck nodes, and had tumors less than 2.5 cm in diameter.

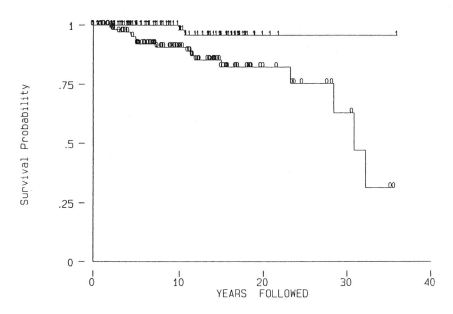

Fig. 18-20. The probability of survival without serious recurrence in Group (1) managed with surgery by an experienced surgeon, with at least lobectomy plus contralateral subtotal thyroidectomy, postoperative radioactive iodide ablation, and thyroid hormone replacement, versus probability without recurrence in Group (0), managed by surgeons outside the University of Chicago, with variable extent of operation and variable radioactive iodide ablation. All patients are in Clinical Classes I, II, and III, with intrathyroidal disease, cervical metastases, or invasive disease outside the thyroid capsule, but no distant metastases. The probability of Group 1 > Group 0, p = 0.01.

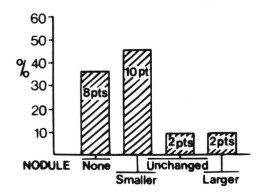

Fig. 18-21. The evolution of toxic thyroid nodules treated with ablative doses of radioactive ^{131}I, indicating that more than half the patients had a residual nodule after treatment during an extended follow-up. (From Goldstein and Hart,[59] with permission.)

ing patients who have negative 2 m li ^{131}I whole body scans, but elevated TG, with 100 m li doses of ^{131}I, is discussed above. We note that this practice is currently common, but is not without some danger, and the actual efficacy in terms of survival is not known (Fig. 18-23).

Patients in category III (Table 18-8) are given a complete physical and laboratory examination 3 to 6 months after ^{131}I therapy and, if the scan is negative, are reexamined at yearly intervals for 3 to 5 years and then with less frequency. Elevated TG levels while receiving therapy indicates persistent disease, even if ^{131}I whole body scans are negative during induced hypothyroidism or after TSH administration.

Patients may develop isolated metastases that can be approached surgically. Osseous metastases, especially from follicular cancer, may require radiother-

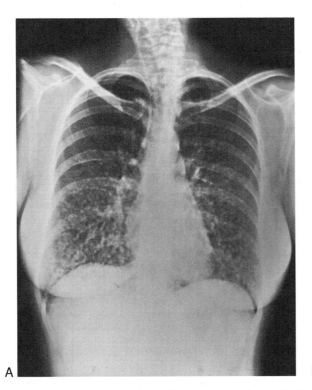
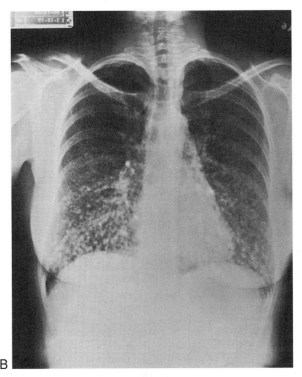

Fig. 18-22. X-rays of chest taken at ten year intervals (A, B) in a patient with extensive papillary thyroid cancer metastases treated with radioactive iodide. There was only modest evolution of the disease during this extended period of observation.

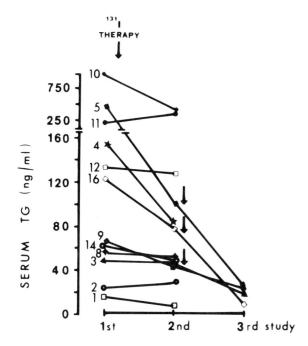

Fig. 18-23. Changes in serum TG after therapeutic doses of radioiodine in patients with negative basal whole body scans. The arrows indicate the administration of therapeutic doses of [131]I. The numbers represent individual patients. In most patients, thyroglobulin decreased, although only a few to an appropriately low level suggesting the absence of residual disease. (From Pacini et al,[237] with permission.)

apy or operative procedures for stabilization. Progressive growth of soft tissue or osseous metastases that are not amenable to thyroid hormone, ^{131}I therapy, or radiotherapy should lead to consideration of chemotherapy.

Medullary Thyroid Cancer (MTC)

MTC is unique since it can be detected in MEN-II or MEN-III families by screening tests measuring pentagastrin-stimulated CT secretion before the disease reaches clinical detectability. Repeatedly observed elevations to well above the normal range (e.g., peak values of 30 to 100 pg/ml) constitute a basis for operation. In these patients focal tumors or C-cell hyperplasia may be found after near-total or total thyroidectomy is performed. Since C-cell hyperplasia precedes the development of malignancy, it is currently believed logical to operate even at this stage of the disease.[264]

Patients with clinical tumor of any size, sporadic or familial, are also treated by near-total or total thyroidectomy. Invasive disease is resected if possible. Since cervical nodal metastasis occur in up to 90 percent of patients with palpable tumors, a careful modified radical neck dissection is performed with removal of nodes in the central and ipsilateral compartment. The exploration for nodes should include the upper mediastinum. Bilateral neck dissection may be appropriate in patients with hereditary tumors.

After these stages are reached, unanimity in approach is lost, and the authors present the University of Chicago approach. After operation, patients should be scanned and probably residual functioning thyroid ablated with ^{131}I, as in papillary or follicular tumors, since this procedure may ablate tiny foci of residual cancer.[265,266] The value of this procedure is not proven, and many groups do not routinely use [131]I. At a minimum, this treatment removes the often confusing issue of questionable small amounts of tissue in the thyroid bed, which may be normal thyroid or residual MTC. In patients with invasive disease, who are above age 45 to 50, radiotherapy (5,500 to 6,000 rads) should be given (see below). In all other patients, baseline CT levels should be followed. Pentagastrin stimulation may be done if the baseline CT level is normal. Occasionally CT levels fall gradually over a year. It is also possible to follow the serum level of CEA as a tumor marker, or CT-related peptide.[267] A discordant elevation of CEA in relation to CT may be an indicator of an aggressive tumor. In general, however, CT is the most informative marker.

What to do about the frequently-found elevated CT level without an obvious tumor source is less certain. A thorough workup including cervical ultrasound, bone scan, liver-spleen scan, and neck MRI and chest CAT scan, is in order. Thallium[201] chloride, [99]mTc DMSA, or somatostatin scanning may be informative. Neck dissection, if not done previously with a unilateral tumor, should be considered. Catheterization of the superior vena cava and internal jugulars, with an attempt to localize the tumor by means of multiple venous sampling for CT[268] during pentagastrin stimulation, is possible. The technical success of this approach has been demonstrated, but often the CT level is not reduced to normal, even if operation is subsequently performed on the identified area.[269] Residual or recurrent resectable disease should be approached surgically. In the best of hands, extensive microdissection of the neck may eliminate the source of CT in 30 percent of patients.[270] Radiotherapy may be given to identified nonresectable lesions. In many cases, no source for the CT is found. Mantle irradiation observation and chemotherapy have been recommended. We prefer to give mantle irradiation, especially if there is progressive elevation of the value. As shown by Simpson,[271] medullary tumors are radiosensitive, although a full response may not be seen for many months. Other investigators question the value of x-ray therapy, contending that patients with MEN-II have multicentric foci from the start, and that radiotherapy may actually worsen prognosis.[272] Chemotherapy is reserved for patients with proven symptomatic metastases, and the program is described below. New and semi-experimental therapies include treatment with [131I]-MIBG or [131I]-anti-CEA antibodies.[273]

MTC is associated in MEN-II with parathyroid adenomas and hyperplasia, and in both MEN-II and MEN-III with pheochromocytomas that are often bilateral and malignant. Parathyroid hormone, VMA, and catecholamine assays should be done to evaluate these problems, and pheochromocytoma, if present, should be treated before the thyroid cancer. Occasionally neuromas cause problems requiring surgery of the intestine or other organs, including the larynx.

Lymphomas

Once diagnosed, patients should be staged by chest radiograph, chest and abdominal CAT scans, bone marrow biopsy, and gallium scan. In 20 to 30 percent of patients, the lymphoma will be confined within the thyroid gland. Lymph nodes are involved in approximately 60 percent of the patients, and perithyroidal invasion is present in about half. When patients have undergone appropriate staging procedures, 20 to 30 percent will have Stage IIIE (lymphoma present in nodes below the diaphragm) or Stage IVE (distant extranodal metastases) disease.

The selection of appropriate therapy requires prior staging of the patient. As these tumors are radiosensitive, external radiation therapy is a satisfactory treatment for Stage I-E (local disease only, no nodal involvement) and has been used for Stage II-E (nodal involvement above the diaphragm only) disease. The dose to the neck is usually 4,000 rads

(40 Gy) over 4 to 5 weeks.[185] The radiation port should include the mediastinum even in the absence of clinical involvement. When evaluating the long-term survival of patients with Stage I and Stage II disease, Souhami et al. found that of seven patients treated with radiation to the neck only, five died within 5 years, whereas in five patients receiving radiation to the neck and mediastinum, there were no deaths.[186] Patients with unfavorable prognostic factors such as ages greater than 60 yr, large mass or tumor necrosis, may be given chemotherapy after radiotherapy. In radiation-treated patients with local extension or with malignant nodes, the survival after surgery is unaffected by the extent of surgery even when surgery was limited to a biopsy. With obvious extension or nodal involvement, surgery should be limited to obtaining an adequate diagnostic specimen since an attempt at complete excision may damage surrounding structures without improving survival. There is a suggestion that total thyroidectomy may improve the prognosis in patients with intrathyroidal disease only.[188] There is a growing tendency to use combination chemotherapy as the initial definitive treatment for Stage IE and IIE thyroid lymphoma. Programs may combine cyclophosphamide, adriamycin, vincristine, and prednisolone ("CHOP"). This approach may increase cure above the 30 to 50 percent found with radiotherapy alone.[184] Currently most patients with Stage II-E, and patients with Stage III-E or Stage IV-E disease, as well as those who relapse after radiation therapy, are treated with chemotherapy.

Although previous series report overall 5-year survivals of about 50 percent, certain subgroups have a more favorable prognosis. With appropriate staging to exclude Stage III-E and Stage IV-E patients, the Stanford group has reported a 3-year survival of 83 percent and at 3 years 75 percent of their Stage I-E and Stage II-E patients had no evidence of disease.[274] Matsuzuka et al[275] used both radiation therapy and six courses of "CHOP" chemotherapy, and report 100 percent survival for 8 years in a group of patients who received this treatment.

Undifferentiated Carcinomas

Undifferentiated carcinomas, if operable, may be treated by thyroidectomy and resection of all involved tissue in the neck. 5 to 10 percent can apparently be completely resected, and the patient can have a long survival. Prophylactic x-radiation (5,000 rads) should be given postoperatively in all cases. These tumors rarely concentrate ^{131}I, but it is probably useful to study their ability to accumulate the isotope spontaneously or after stimulation with TSH or with antithyroid drugs, at least on one occasion. If the lesion is obviously inoperable, x-ray therapy should be the initial treatment. In some instances, the rapidly growing tumors melt almost completely for a time after x-ray therapy, giving the patient a gratifying respite from the disease. Some tumors appear to be suppressed by thyroid hormone, and this therapy should be given a trial.[276]

Some anaplastic tumors have been treated with alkylating agents, and rarely, a rapidly proliferating and highly undifferentiated tumor has responded with a temporary regression. Chemotherapy is discussed below.

Kim and Leeper[277] have reported encouraging results combining low dose adriamycin (10 mg/m^2) and hyperfractionated radiotherapy (160 rads twice daily) to 5760 rads. Time of survival was prolonged and local recurrences largely prevented. There has been no confirmation of this study, unfortunately.

Radiation Therapy

The general indications for radiation therapy are given in Table 18-9. Other sources should be reviewed for details of the port, dose, and methods of irradiation.

Studies by Tubiana et al,[278] Simpson,[271] and Riccabona[279] have clearly established the efficacy of radiotherapy in all types of thyroid cancer. Although its therapeutic use is now well accepted, its prophylactic use (e.g., in papillary or follicular lesions with possible residual disease, or in papillary or follicular Stage III lesions after RAI ablation) is controversial. Currently, we would first treat all papillary or follicular invasive or possibly metastatic tumors with RAI. In patients under age 55, it is not clear that x-ray therapy should be added. Over age 55, ^{131}I therapy should be followed by x-ray treatment of Stage III or potentially Stage III lesions, and any recurrence or metastasis not responding to ^{131}I may also be treated,[280] since the prognosis is poor in this group of patients.

The indications for MTC have been described above. All Stage I-E lymphomas and anaplastic lesions are currently given radiotherapy after operation. It is possible that chemotherapy should be used instead of or in addition to radiotherapy in these lesions, but studies are needed to establish this point.

The exact dose must be individually determined, but usually the maximal dose is 5,000 to 6,000 rads, using ortho- or megavoltage, and a fractionated technique over several weeks. Dosage must be planned to assure that the spinal cord receives less than 3500 rads in order to avoid myelopathy.

Chemotherapy

Sporadic experience indicates that bleomycin,[281,282] adriamycin,[283] vinblastine,[284] methotrexate,[283] cisplatinum and other agents,[285] may have

TABLE 18-9. General Indications for Radiation Therapy

Tumor	Stage	Treatment (15–20 MV Electrons or ^{60}Co)
Papillary or Follicular	Invasive, under 55	Treat if invasive disease is thought not to be destroyed or if neck recurrence after [131]I. Dose is 4,500–5,000 rads
	Invasive, or possible residual, over 55	5,000 rads* to thyroid bed after RAI
	Recurrent, any age	5,000 rads* to thyroid bed if RAI treatment is thought not to be definitive
	Isolated lesion in bone	5,000–6,000 rads, as required for symptoms after RAI treatment
Medullary	Stage III	4,000–5,000 rads** to thyroid bed
	Abnormal or increasing TCT	5,000 rads** to mantle
	Recurrent tumor	5,000–6,000 rads* to thyroid bed
	Isolated metastasis	5,000–6,000 rads for symptoms
Lymphoma	Stage I-E, possibly II-E	5,000 rads** to thyroid and mantle
Anaplastic	All	4,500–5,500 rads** to thyroid and mantle

Note: Spinal cord dose not to exceed *3,000 rads or **3,500 rads.

TABLE 18-10. Chemotherapy for Thyroid Carcinoma

Primary tumor
    Progressive differentiated thyroid cancer, symptomatic medullary cancer, anaplastic cancer; two programs have been proposed
        Adriamycin + cis-diamine-dichloroplatinum + Vp-16
        Adriamycin + cis-diamine-dichloroplatinum
Secondary therapy for failure of primary treatment
    Differentiated cancer—bleomycin + cyclophosphamide
    Medullary cancer—5-fluorouracil + streptozotocin
    Anaplastic cancer—bleomycin + hydroxyurea

value in treating disseminated thyroid tumors. Metastatic papillary or follicular tumors grow slowly and may respond completely (often temporarily) to ^{131}I. Thus, chemotherapy is not indicated until the full value of ^{131}I has been exploited, and then only when the tumor is clearly growing progressively despite hormone suppression. Treatment of MTC is generally reserved for definite symptomatic disease. Currently, lymphomas and undifferentiated lesions are given routine postoperative radiotherapy, and chemotherapy for recurrence or known spread. Prophylactic chemotherapy may soon be developed for these lesions.

We offer for use the protocols developed by the Thyroid Cancer Treatment Cooperative Study Group (Table 18-10).

De Besi et al.[286] found combined bleomycin, adriamycin, and platinum therapy in advanced cancer "probably" increased survival.

SUMMARY

Thyroid adenomas occur in this country in approximately 2 percent of the population, and are far more frequent in women than men, by a ratio of 6:1. Histologic types include embryonal, fetal, and follicular adenomas, and the colloid nodule, which may be a variant of the follicular adenoma. Adenomas are neoplasms and probably arise from the same types of stimuli that cause carcinomas. Adenomas grow slowly and, if nonfunctioning, produce symptoms because of distortion of local anatomy. Hyperfunctioning adenomas may suppress the remainder of the gland or induce thyrotoxicosis. Occasionally bleeding into an adenoma causes sudden painful enlargement, and possibly destruction of the lesion. Very rarely, adenomas appear to change into carcinomas.

Thyroid nodules are evaluated by a review of features that may suggest malignancy, such as an increase in size, pain, undue firmness or fixation, and the presence of local adenopathy. Isotope scintiscans are of some value since the information they provide may suggest an alternative diagnosis, such as multinodular goiter or Hashimoto's thyroiditis, or may show hyperfunction of the adenoma, suggesting that it is a benign lesion. Currently, emphasis is placed upon fine needle aspiration cytology for evaluation of the possibility of malignancy. This diagnostic procedure appears to be 90 to 95 percent accurate in experienced hands.

Nodules that on fine needle aspiration cytology are benign may be treated conservatively by administration of thyroid hormone replacement therapy to suppress TSH and (possibly) prevent further growth. lesions that have suspicious clinical or physical signs, from which it is impossible to obtain adequate cytologic findings, or that have an abnormal cytology should be resected. Hyperfunctioning solitary thyroid nodules can be destroyed by administration of large doses of RAI or resected.

Thyroid carcinomas occur with an incidence of 30 to 60 new cases per million population per year and a mortality of approximately 4.5 per million population per year. Thyroid neoplasia can be caused by prior irradiation to the thyroid. Even small doses such as 7 to 20 rads have some adverse effect. Doses of several hundred rads may increase the incidence of malignancy over 100-fold. Chronic stimulation by TSH can also produce malignant change in the human thyroid. Occult cancers that are generally less than 0.5 cm in their greatest diameter occur in up to 6 percent of adult thyroids, but rarely appear to change into clinically significant thyroid tumors.

Papillary thyroid carcinomas grow very slowly, metastasizing primarily to cervical nodes and later to the lungs. Many persons survive for two to four decades with extensive metastatic disease. Follicular carcinomas invade more aggressively and are prone to metastasize to soft tissues and bones. Their mortality is 30 to 50 percent over 10 to 20 years. Medullary thyroid carcinomas develop from thyroid C cells and may occur sporadically or as part of familial syndromes associated with multiple endocrine tumors. These tumors secrete calcitonin, which aids in their detection and management. Undifferentiated thyroid carcinomas are extremely malignant. The vast majority cause death within 4 months to 1 year.

The basic therapy for thyroid carcinoma is surgical resection. The minimum desirable operation is a lobectomy on one side complemented by subtotal thyroidectomy on the opposite side. Many surgeons prefer a near-total thyroidectomy for any tumor larger than 1 cm in size. Modified neck dissection is done if local adenopathy is present. In most instances, residual thyroid tissue is destroyed by administration of [131]I. Metastatic thyroid disease that can be shown to accumulate isotope is treated by administration of large doses of ^{131}I on one or more occasions.

Radiotherapy is probably advisable in differentiated thyroid carcinoma that is invasive into the tissue of the neck, in patients over age 45, and is useful in recurrences resistant to ^{131}I therapy and in therapy for metastatic lesions elsewhere in the body. Radiotherapy to the thyroid bed is probably advisable in all anaplastic thyroid cancers.

Chemotherapy, depending primarily upon adriamycin, is occasionally valuable in some progressive differentiated, medullary, and anaplastic thyroid carcinomas.

REFERENCES

1. DeSmet MP: Pathological anatomy of endemic goiter. p. 315. In: Endemic Goiter. World Health Organization, Geneva, 1960
2. Vander JB, Gaston EA, Dawber TR: Significance of solitary non-toxic thyroid nodules. N Engl J Med 251:970, 1954
3. Vander JB, Gaston EA, Dawber TR: The significance of nontoxic thyroid nodules. Final report of a 15-year study of the incidence of thyroid malignancy. Ann Intern Med 69:537, 1968
4. Tunbridge WMG, Evered DC, Hall R et al: The spectrum of thyroid disease in an English community: the Wickham survey. Clin Endocrinol 7:481, 1977
5. Liechty RD, Stoffel PT, Zimmerman DE, Silverberg SG: Solitary thyroid nodules. Arch Surg 112:59, 1977
6. Wilems J-S, Lowhagen T: Fine needle aspiration cytology in thyroid disease. Clin Endocrinol Metab 2:247, 1981
7. Brown CL: Pathology of the cold nodule. Clin Endocrinol Metab 10:235, 1981
8. Mortensen JD, Woolner LB, Bennett WA: Gross and microscopic findings in clinically normal thyroid glands. J Clin Endocrinol Metab 15:1270, 1955
9. Silverberg SG, Vidone RA: Carcinoma of the thyroid in surgical and postmortem material. Ann Surg 164:291, 1966
10. Bisi H, Fernandes VSO, Asato de Camargo RY et al: The prevalence of unsuspected thyroid pathology in 300 sequential autopsies, with special reference to the incidental carcinoma. Cancer 64:1888, 1989
11. Werk EE, Vernon BM, Gonzalez JJ et al: Cancer in thyroid nodules: a community hospital survey. Arch Intern Med 144:474, 1984
12. Hedinger C, Dillwyn Williams E, Sobin LH: The WHO histological classification of thyroid tumors: a commentary on the second edition. Cancer 63:908, 1989
13. Namba H, Matsuo K, Fagin JA: Clonal composition of benign and malignant human thyroid tumors. J Clin Invest 86:120, 1990
14. Coclet J, Foureau F, Ketelbant P et al: Cell population kinetics in dog and human adult thyroid. Clinical Endocrinol 31:655, 1989
15. Hamburger JI: Evolution of toxicity in solitary nontoxic autonomously functioning thyroid nodules. J Clin Endocrinol Metab 50:1089, 1980
16. Silverstein GE, Burke G, Cogan R: The natural history of the autonomous hyperfunctioning thyroid nodule. Ann Intern Med 67:539, 1967
17. Evered DC, Clark F, Peterson VB: Thyroid function in euthyroid subjects with autonomous thyroid nodules. Clin Endocrinol 3:149, 1974
18. Horst W, Rosler H, Schneider C, Labhart A: 306 cases of toxic adenoma: clinical aspects, findings in radioiodine diagnostics, radiochromatography and histology; results of ^{131}I and surgical treatment. J Nucl Med 8:515, 1967
19. DeGroot LJ: Lack of iodide trapping in "cold" thyroid nodules. Acta Endocrinol Panam 1:27, 1970
20. Field JB, Larsen PR, Yamashita K et al: Demonstration of iodide transport defect but normal iodide organification in nonfunctioning nodules of human thyroid glands. J Clin Invest 52:2404, 1973
21. Fragu P, Nataf BM: Human thyroid peroxidase activity in benign and malign thyroid disorders. J Clin Endocrinol Metab 45:1089, 1977
22. Demeester-Mirkine N, Van Sande J, Corvilain H, Dumont JE: Benign thyroid nodule with normal iodide trap and defective organification. J Clin Endocrinol Metab 41:1169, 1975
23. Burke G, Szabo M: Dissociation of in vivo and in vitro "autonomy" in hyperfunctioning thyroid nodules. J Clin Endocrinol Metab 35:199, 1972
24. Sande Van J, Mockel J, Boeynaems JM et al: Regulation of cyclic nucleotide and prostaglandin forma-

tion in normal human thyroid tissue and in autonomous nodules. J Clin Endocrinol Metab 50:776, 1980

25. Thomas CG Jr, Buckwalter JA, Staab EV, Kerr CY: Evaluation of dominant thyroid masses. Ann Surg 183:464, 1976

26. Sipple JH: Association of pheochromocytoma with carcinoma of thyroid gland. Am J Med 31:163, 1961

27. Schimke RN, Hartmann WH, Prout TE, Rimoin DL: Syndrome of bilateral pheochromocytoma, medullary thyroid carcinoma, and multiple neuromas. N Engl J Med 279:1, 1968

28. Sapira JD, Altman M, Vandyk K, Shapiro AP: Bilateral adrenal pheochromocytoma and medullary thyroid carcinoma. N Engl J Med 273:140, 1965

29. Duffy BJ Jr, Fitzgerald PJ: Cancer of the thyroid in children: a report of twenty-eight cases. J Clin Endocrinol 10:1296, 1950

30. Clark DE: Association of irradiation with cancer of the thyroid in children and adolescents. JAMA 159:1007, 1955

31. Modan B, Ron E, Werner A: Thyroid cancer following scalp irradiation. Therap Radiol 123:741, 1977

32. DeGroot LJ, Frohman LA, Kaplan EL, Refetoff S (eds): Radiation-Associated Thyroid Carcinoma. Grune & Stratton, Orlando, 1977

33. Refetoff S, Harrison J, Karanfilski BT et al: Continuing occurrence of thyroid carcinoma after irradiation to the neck in infancy and childhood. N Engl J Med 292:171, 1975

34. DeGroot LJ, Paloyan E: Thyroid carcinoma and radiation: a Chicago endemic. JAMA 225:487, 1973

35. Sokal JE: The problem of malignancy in nodular goiter: recapitulation and a challenge. JAMA 170:61, 1959

36. Veith FJ, Brooks JR, Grigsby WP, Selenkow HA: The nodular thyroid gland and cancer. N Engl J Med 270:431, 1964

37. Hoffman GL, Thompson NW, Heffron C: The solitary thyroid nodule. Arch Surg 105:379, 1972

38. Kendall LW, Condon RE: Prediction of malignancy in solitary thyroid nodules. Lancet 1:1071, 1969

39. Miller JM, Hamburger JI: The thyroid scintigram. I. The hot nodule. Radiology 84:66, 1965

40. Attie JN: The use of radioactive iodine in the evaluation of thyroid nodules. Surgery 47:611, 1960

41. Dische S: The radioisotope scan applied to the detection of carcinoma in thyroid swellings. Cancer 17:473, 1964

42. Fujimoto Y, Oka A, Nagataki S: Occurrence of papillary carcinoma in hyperfunctioning thyroid nodule. Report of a case. Endocrinol Jpn 19:371, 1972

43. Scott MD, Crawford JD: Solitary thyroid nodules in childhood: is the incidence of thyroid carcinoma declining? Pediatrics 58:521, 1976

44. Messaris G, Evangelou GN, Tountas C: Incidence of carcinoma in cold nodules of the thyroid gland. Surgery 74:447, 1973

45. Thomas CG, Pepper FD, Owen J: Differentiation of malignant from benign lesions of the thyroid gland using complementary scanning with selenomethionine and radioiodide. Ann Surg 170:396, 1969

46. Hoffer PB, Gottschalk A, Refetoff S: Thyroid scanning techniques: the old and the new. Curr Probl Radiol 2:5, 1972

47. Clark OH, Okerlund MD, Cavalieri RR, Greenspan FS: Diagnosis and treatment of thyroid, parathyroid, and thyroglossal duct cysts. J Clin Endocrinol Metab 48:983, 1979

48. Hamlin E, Vickery AL: Needle biopsy of the thyroid gland. N Engl J Med 254:742, 1956

49. Walfish PG, Hazani E, Strawbridge HTG et al: Combined ultrasound and needle aspiration cytology in the assessment and management of hypofunctioning thyroid nodule. Ann Intern Med 87:270, 1977

50. Gershengorn MC, McClung MR, Chu WE et al: Fine-needle aspiration cytology in the preoperative diagnosis of thyroid nodules. Ann Intern Med 87:265, 1977

51. Gharib H, Goellner JR, Johnson DA: Fine needle aspiration cytology of the thyroid: A 12-year experience with 11,000 biopsies. Clin Lab Med 13:699, 1993

52. Miller JM, Hamburger JI, Kini S: Diagnosis of thyroid nodules: use of fine needle aspiration and needle biopsy. JAMA 241:481, 1979

53. McCowen KD, Reed JW, Fariss BL: The role of thyroid therapy in patients with thyroid cysts. Amer J Med 68:853, 1980

54. Papini E, Bacci V, Panunzi C et al: A prospective randomized trial of levothyroxine suppressive therapy for solitary thyroid nodules. Clin Endocrinol 38:507, 1993

55. Morita T, Tamai H, Ohshima A et al: Changes in serum thyroid hormone, thyrotropin and thyroglobulin concentrations during thyroxine therapy in patients with solitary thyroid nodules. J Clin Endocrinol Metab 69:227, 1989

56. Hakama M: Different world thyroid cancer rates. p. XII:66. In Hedinger CE (ed): Thyroid Cancer: International Union Against Cancer Monograph Series. Vol. 12. Springer-Verlag, Berlin, 1969

57. Young JL Jr, Percy CL, Asire AJ (eds): Surveillance, Epidemiology, and End Results: Incidence and Mortality Data, 1973–77. National Cancer Institute Publication NIH 81-2330, Washington, DC, 1981

58. Rafla S: Anaplastic tumors of the thyroid. Cancer 23:668, 1969

59. Goldstein R, Hart IR: Follow-up of solitary autono-

mous thyroid nodules treated with [131]I. New Engl J Med 309:1473, 1983

60. Gorman CA, Robertson JS: Radiation dose in the selection of ^{131}I or surgical treatment for toxic thyroid adenoma. Ann Intern Med 89:85, 1978

61. Paracchi A, Ferrari C, Livraghi T et al: Percutaneous intranodular ethanol injection: a new treatment for autonomous thyroid adenoma. J Endocrinol Invest 15:353, 1992

62. Treece GL, Georgitis WJ, Hofeldt FD: Resolution of recurrent thyroid cysts with tetracycline instillation. Arch Int Med 143:2285, 1983

63. Monzani F, Lippi F, Goletti O et al: Percutaneous aspiration and ethanol sclerotherapy for thyroid cysts. J Clin Endocrinol Metab 78:800, 1994

64. Woolner LB, Beahrs OH, Black BM et al: Long term survival rates. p. XII:326. In Hedinger CE (ed): Thyroid Cancer: International Union Against Cancer Monograph Series. Vol. 12. Springer-Verlag, Berlin, 1969

65. Fogelfeld L, Wiviott MBT, Shore-Freedman E et al: Recurrence of thyroid nodules after surgical removal in patients irradiated in childhood for benign conditions. N Engl J Med 320:835, 1989

66. Verby JE, Woolner LB, Nobrega FT et al: Thyroid cancer in Olmsted County, 1935–1965. J Natl Cancer Inst 43:813, 1969

67. Wahner HW, Cuello C, Correa P et al: Thyroid carcinoma in an endemic goiter area: Cali, Colombia. Am J Med 40:58, 1966

68. Curran PG, DeGroot LJ: The effect of hepatic enzyme-inducing drugs on thyroid hormones and the thyroid gland. Endocrine Rev 12:135, 1991

69. Farid NR, Shi Y, Zou M: Molecular basis of thyroid cancer. Endocrine Rev 15:202, 1994

70. Namba H, Gutman RA, Matsuo K et al: H-Ras protooncogene mutations in human thyroid neoplasms. J Clin Endocrinol Metab 71:223, 1990

71. Namba H, Rubin SA, Fagin JA: Point mutations of Ras oncogenes are an early event in thyroid tumorigenesis. Molecul Endocrinol 4:1474, 1990

72. Karga H, Lee J-K, Vickery AL et al: Ras oncogene mutations in benign and malignant thyroid neoplasms. J Clin Endocrinol Metab 73:832, 1991

73. Santoro M, Carlomagno F, Hay ID et al: Ret oncogene activation in human thyroid neoplasms is restricted to the papillary cancer subtype. J Clin Invest 89:1517, 1992

74. Larsson C, Skogseid B, Oberg K et al: Multiple endocrine neoplasia type I gene maps to chromosome 11 and is lost in insulinoma. Nature 332:85, 1988

75. Quadro L, Panariello L, Salvatore D et al: Frequent RET proto-oncogene mutations in multiple endocrine neoplasia type 2A. J Clin Endocrinol Metab 79: 590, 1994

76. Parma J, Duprez L, Van Sande J et al: Somatic mutations in the thyrotropin receptor gene cause hyperfunctioning thyroid adenomas. Nature 365:649, 1993

77. Suarez HG, du Villard JA, Caillou B et al: Gsp mutations in human thyroid tumors. Oncogene 6:677, 1991

78. Matsuo K, Friedman E, Gejman PV, Fagin JA: The thyrotropin receptor (TSH-R) is not an oncogene for thyroid tumors: structural studies of the TSH-R and the α-subunit of GS in human thyroid neoplasms. J Clin Endocrinol Metab 76:1446, 1993

79. Shi Y, Zou M, Farid NR: Expression of thyrotrophin receptor gene in thyroid carcinoma is associated with a good prognosis. Clin Endocrinol 39:269, 1993

80. Fagin JA, Matsuo K, Karmakar A et al: High prevalence of mutations of the p53 gene in poorly differentiated human thyroid carcinomas. J Clin Invest 91: 179, 1993

81. Lloyd KM, Dennis M: Cowden's disease: a possible new symptom complex with multiple system involvement. Annals Int Med 58:136, 1963

82. Harach HA, Williams GT, Williams ED: Familial adenomatous polyposis associated thyroid carinoma. Histopathology 25:549, 1994

83. Parkin JL: Familial multiple glomus tumors and pheochromocytomas. Ann Otol 90:60, 1981

84. Camiel MR, Mule JE, Alexander LL, Benninghoff DL: Association of thyroid carcinoma with Gardner's syndrome in siblings. N Engl J Med 278:1056, 1968

85. Wollman SH: Production and properties of transplantable tumors of the thyroid gland in the Fischer rat. Recent Prog Horm Res 19:579, 1963

86. Jacobs BB, Huseby RA: Neoplasms occurring in aged Fischer rats, with special reference to testicular, uterine, and thyroid tumors. J Natl Cancer Inst 39:303, 1967

87. Frantz VK, Kligerman MM, Harland WA et al: A comparison of the carcinogenic effect of internal and external irradiation on the thyroid gland of the male Long-Evans rat. Endocrinology 61:574, 1957

88. Doniach I: The effect of radioactive iodine alone and in combination with nethylthiouracil upon tumor production in the rat's thyroid gland. Br J Cancer 7:181, 1953

89. Maloof F, Dobyns BM, Vickery AL: The effects of various doses of radioactive iodine on the function and structure of the thyroid of the rat. Endocrinology 50:612, 1952

90. Dobyns BM, Didtschenko I: Nuclear changes in thyroidal epithelium following radiation from radioiodine. J Clin Endocrinol Metab 21:699, 1961

91. Pifer JW, Hempelmann LH, Dodge HJ, Hodges FJ: Neoplasms in the Ann Arbor Series of thymus-irradi-

ated children: a second survey. Am J Roent Rad Ther Nucl Med 103:13, 1968

92. Saenger EL, Silverman FN, Sterling TD, Turner ME: Neoplasia following therapeutic irradiation for benign conditions in childhood. Radiology 74:889, 1960

93. Beach SA, Dolphin GW: A study of the relationship between X-ray dose delivered to the thyroids of children and the subsequent development of malignant tumors. Phys Med Biol 6:583, 1962

94. Winship T, Rosvoll RV: Thyroid carcinoma in childhood. Cancer 14:734, 1961

95. Maxon H, Thomas SR, Saenger EL et al: Ionizing irradiation and the induction of clinically significant disease in the human thyroid gland. Am J Med 63: 967, 1977

96. Perkel VS, Gail MH, Lubin J et al: Radiation-induced thyroid neoplasms: evidence for familial susceptibility factors. J Clin Endocrinol Metab 66:1316, 1988

97. Hanford JM, Quinby EH, Frantz VK: Cancer arising many years after radiation therapy. JAMA 181:404, 1962

98. DeLawter DS, Winship T: Follow-up study of adults treated with Roentgen rays for thyroid disease. Cancer 16:1028, 1963

99. Parker LN, Belsky JL, Yamamoto T et al: Thyroid carcinoma after exposure to atomic radiation. Ann Intern Med 80:600, 1974

100. Conard RA: A twenty-year review of medical findings in a Marshallese population accidentally exposed to radioactive fallout. Brookhaven National Laboratory (BNL No. 50424), Upton, New York, 1975

101. Weiss ES, Rallison ML, London WT, Thompson GDC: Thyroid nodularity in southwestern Utah school children exposed to fallout radiation. Am J Public Health 61:241, 1971

102. Hancock SL, Cox RS, McDougall IR: Thyroid diseases after treatment of Hodgkin's disease. N Engl J Med 325:599, 1991

103. Favus JM, Schneider AB, Stachura ME et al: Thyroid cancer occurring as a late consequence of head-and-neck irradiation. N Engl J Med 294:1019, 1976

104. Royce PC, McKay BR, DiSabella PM: Value of postir-radiation screening for thyroid nodules. JAMA 242: 2675, 1979

105. Spitalnik PF, Straus FH: Patterns of human thyroid parenchymal reaction following low-dose childhood irradiation. Cancer 41:1098, 1978

106. Roudebush CP, Asteris GT, DeGroot LJ: Natural history of radiation-associated thyroid cancer. Arch Intern Med 138:1631, 1978

107. Rao DS, Frame B, Miller MJ et al: Hyperparathyroidism following head and neck irradiation. Arch Intern Med 140:205, 1980

108. Vickery AL: Thyroid alterations due to irradiation. p. 183. In: The Thyroid: International Academy of Pathology Monograph No. 5. Williams & Wilkins, Baltimore, 1964

109. Cantolino SJ, Schmickel RD, Ball M, Cisar CF: Persistent chromosomal aberrations following radioiodine therapy for thyrotoxicosis. N Engl J Med 275: 739, 1966

110. Sheline GE, Lindsay S, McCormack KR, Galante M: Thyroid nodules occurring late after treatment of thyrotoxicosis with radioiodine. J Clin Endocrinol Metab 22:8, 1962

111. Dobyns BM, Sheline GE, Workman JB et al: Malignant and benign neoplasms of the thyroid in patients treated for hyperthyroidism: a report of the cooperative thyrotoxicosis therapy follow-up study. J Clin Endocrinol Metab 38:976, 1974

112. Holm L-E, Eklund G, Lundell G: Incidence of malignant thyroid tumors in humans after exposure to diagnostic doses of iodine-131. II: Estimation of thyroid gland size, thyroid radiation, and predicted versus observed number of malignant thyroid tumors. J Natl Cancer Inst 65:1221, 1980

113. Holm L-E, Dahlqvist I, Israelsson A, Lundell G: Malignant thyroid tumors after iodine 131-therapy. N Engl J Med 303:188, 1980

114. Stanbury JB: Familial goiter. p. 273. In Stanbury JB, Wyngaarden JB, Fredrickson DS (eds): The Metabolic Basis of Inherited Disease. McGraw-Hill New York, 1960

115. McGirr EM, Clement WE, Currie AR, Kennedy JS: Impaired dehalogenase activity as a cause of goiter with malignant changes. Scott Med J 4:232, 1959

116. Elman DS: Familial association of nerve deafness with nodular goiter and thyroid carcinoma. N Engl J Med 259:219, 1958

117. Medeiros-Neto GA, Oliveira NRC: Follicular adenocarcinoma of thyroid associated with congenital hyperplastic goiter. Acta Endocrinol Panam 1:73, 1970

118. Cooper DS, Axelrod L, DeGroot LJ et al: Congenital goiter and the development of metastatic follicular carcinoma with evidence for a leak of nonhormonal iodide: clinical, pathological, kinetic, and biochemical studies and a review of the literature. J Clin Endocrinol Metab 52:294, 1981

119. Sloan LW: Of the origin, characteristics and behaviour of thyroid cancer. J Clin Endocrinol Metab 14: 1309, 1954

120. Ellenbert AH, Goldman L, Gordan GS, Lindsay S: Thyroid carcinoma in patients with hyperparathyroidism. Surgery 51:708, 1962

121. LiVolsi VA, Feind CR: Parathyroid adenoma and nonmedullary thyroid carcinoma. Cancer 38:1391, 1976

122. Shapiro SJ, Friedman NB, Perzik SL, Catz B: Incidence of thyroid carcinoma in Graves' disease. Cancer 26:1261, 1970

123. Belfiore A, Garofalo MR, Giuffrida D et al: Increased aggressiveness of thyroid cancer in patients with Graves' disease. J Clin Endocrinol Metab 70:830, 1990

124. Valenta L, Lemarchand-Beraud T, Nemec J et al: Metastatic thyroid carcinoma provoking hyperthyroidism,, with elevated circulating thyrostimulators. Am J Med 48:72, 1970

125. Greenspan FS, Lowenstein JM, West MN, Okerlund MD: Immunoreactive material to bovine TSH in plasma from patients with thyroid cancer. J Clin Endocrinol Metab 35:795, 1972

126. Greenspan FS, Lew W, Okerlund MD, Lowenstein JM: Falsely positive bovine TSH radioimmunoassay responses in sera from patients with thyroid cancer. J Clin Endocrinol Metab 38:1121, 1974

127. Mazzaferri EL: Thyroid cancer and Graves' disease. J Clin Endocrinol Metab 70:826, 1990

128. Panza N, Del Vecchio L, Maio M et al: Strong association between an HLA-DR antigen and thyroid carcinoma. Tissue Antigens 20:155, 1982

129. Sridama V, Hara Y, Fauchet R, DeGroot LJ: Association of differentiated thyroid carcinoma with HLA-DR7. Cancer 56:1086, 1985

130. Weissel M, Kains H, Hoefer R, Mayr WR: HLA-DR and differentiated thyroid cancer: Lack of association with the nonmedullary types and possible association with the medullary type. Cancer 62:2486, 1988

131. Sampson RJ, Woolner LB, Bahn RC, Kurland LT: Occult thyroid carcinoma in Olmsted County, Minnesota: prevalence at autopsy compared with that in Hiroshima and Nagasaki, Japan. Cancer 34:2072, 1974

132. Fukunaga FH, Yatani R: Geographic pathology of occult thyroid carcinomas. Cancer 36:1095, 1975

133. Goudie RB, McCallum HM: Loss of tissue-specific autoantigens in thyroid tumors. Lancet 1:348, 1963

134. Hazard JB, Hawk WA, Crile G Jr: Medullary (solid) carcinoma of the thyroid: a clinicopathologic entity. J Clin Endocrinol Metab 19:152, 1959

135. Meier DW, Woolner LB, Beahrs OH, McConahey WM: Parenchymal findings in thyroid carcinoma: pathologic study of 256 cases. J Clin Endocrinol Metab 19:162, 1959

136. Lindsay S, Dailey ME: Malignant lymphoma of the thyroid gland and its relation to Hashimoto's disease: A clinical and pathologic study of 8 patients. J Clin Endocrinol Metab 15:1332, 1955

137. Rayfield EJ, Nishiyama RH, Sisson JC: Small cell tumors of the thyroid: a clinicopathologic study. Cancer 28:1023, 1971

138. Black BM, Kirk TA Jr, Woolner LB: Multicentricity of papillary adenocarcinoma of the thyroid: influence on treatment. J Clin Endocrinol Metab 20:130, 1960

139. Iida F, Yonekura M, Miyakawa M: Study of intraglandular dissemination of thyroid cancer. Cancer 24:764, 1969

140. Hazard JB: Small papillary carcinoma of the thyroid. Lab Invest 9:86, 1960

141. Reed RJ, Russin DJ, Krementz ET: Latent metastases from occult sclerosing carcinoma of the thyroid. JAMA 196:233, 1966

142. Silverberg SG, Vidone RA: Metastatic tumors in the thyroid. Pac Med Surg 74:175, 1966

143. Studer H, Veraguth P, Wyss F: Thyrotoxicosis due to a solitary hepatic metastasis of thyroid carcinoma. J Clin Endocrinol Metab 21:1334, 1961

144. Hunt WB, Crispell KR, McKee J: Functioning metastatic carcinoma of the thyroid producing clinical hyperthyroidism. Am J Med 28:995, 1960

145. Pochin EE: Thyroid adenocarcinoma. A functioning tumor. Lancet 1:94, 1969

146. Wyse EP, Hill CS, Ibanez ML, Clark RL: Other malignant neoplasms associated with carcinoma of the thyroid: thyroid carcinoma multiplex. Cancer 24:701, 1969

147. Shimaoka K, Takeuchi S, Pickren JW: Carcinoma of thyroid associated with other primary malignant tumors. Cancer 20:1000, 1967

148. Halnan KE: Influence of age and sex on incidence and prognosis of thyroid cancer. Cancer 19:1534, 1966

149. Russel MA, Gilbert EF, Jaeschke WF: Prognostic features of thyroid cancer: a long term follow-up of 68 cases. Cancer 36:553, 1975

150. Rosvoll RV, Winship T: Thyroid carcinoma and pregnancy. Surg Gynecol Obstet 121:1039, 1965

151. Franssila KO: Prognosis in thyroid carcinoma. Cancer 36:1138, 1975

152. McDermott WV Jr, Morgan WS, Hamlin E Jr, Cope O: Cancer of the thyroid. J Clin Endocrinol Metab 14:1336, 1954

153. Woolner LB, Lemmon ML, Beahrs OH et al: Occult papillary carcinoma of the thyroid: study of 140 cases observed in a 30-year period. J Clin Endocrinol Metab 20:89, 1960

154. McConahey WM, Taylor WF, Gorman CA, Woolner LB: Retrospective study of 820 patients treated for papillary carcinoma of the thyroid at the Mayo Clinic between 1946 and 1971. p. 245. In Andreoli M, Monaco F, Robbins J (eds): Advances in Thyroid Neoplasia. Field Educational Italia, Rome, 1981

155. Schlumberger M, De Vathaire F, Travagli JP et al: Differentiated thyroid carcinoma in childhood: long

term follow-up of 72 patients. J Clin Endocrinol Metab 65:1088, 1987

156. Cady B, Sedgwick CE, Meissner WA et al: Changing clinical, pathologic, therapeutic, and survival patterns of differentiated thyroid carcinoma. Ann Surg 184:541, 1976

157. Mazzaferri EL, Young RL: Papillary thyroid carcinoma: a ten year follow-up report of the impact of therapy in 576 patients. Am J Med 70:511, 1981

158. Harwood J, Clark OH, Dunphy JE: Significance of lymph node metastasis in differentiated thyroid cancer. Am J Surg 136:107, 1978

159. Mazzaferri EL, Young RL, Oertel JE et al: Papillary thyroid carcinoma: the impact of therapy in 576 patients. Medicine 56:171, 1977

160. Frazell EL, Duffy BJ: Invasive papillary cancer of the thyroid. J Clin Endocrinol Metab 14:1362, 1954

161. Young RL, Mazzaferri EL, Rahe AJ, Dorfman SG: Pure follicular thyroid carcinoma: impact of therapy in 214 patients. J Nucl Med 21:733, 1980

162. Justin EP, Seabold JE, Robinson RA et al: Insular carcinoma: a distinct thyroid carcinoma with associated Iodine-131 localization. J Nucl Med 32:1358, 1991

163. Caplan RH, Abellera RM, Kisken WA: Hurthle cell neoplasms of the thyroid gland: reassessment of functional capacity. Thyroid 4:243, 1994

164. Manning PC, Molnar GD, Black M et al: Pheochromocytoma, hyperparathyroidism, and thyroid carcinoma occurring coincidentally. N Engl J Med 268:68, 1963

165. Gorlin RJ, Sedano HO, Vickers RA, Cervenka J: Multiple mucosal neuromas, pheochromocytoma, and medullary carcinoma of the thyroid—a syndrome. Cancer 22:293, 1968

166. Gagel RF, Robinson MF, Donovan DT, Alford BR: Medullary thyroid carcinoma: recent progress. J Clin Endocrinol Metab 76:809, 1993

167. Carney JA, Go VLW, Sizemore GW, Hayles AG: Alimentary-tract ganglioneuromatosis. N Engl J Med 295:1287, 1976

168. Noel M, Delehaye M-C, Segond N et al: Study of calcitonin and thyroglobulin gene expression in human mixed follicular and medullary thyroid carcinoma. Thyroid 1:249, 1991

169. Sobol H, Narod SA, Nakamura Y et al: Screening for multiple endocrine neoplasia type 2a with DNA-polymorphism analysis. N Engl J Med 321:996, 1989

170. Wolfe HJ, Melvin KEW, Cervi-Skinner SJ et al: C-cell hyperplasia preceding medullary thyroid carcinoma. N Engl J Med 289:437, 1973

171. Cox TM, Fagan EA, Hillyard CJ et al: Role of calcitonin in diarrhea associated with medullary carcinoma of the thyroid. Gut 20:629, 1979

172. Pacini F, Basolo F, Elisel R et al: Amer J Clin Pathol 95:300, 1991

173. Cohen SL, Graham-Smith D, MacIntyre I, Walker JG: Alcohol-stimulated calcitonin release in medullary carcinoma of the thyroid. Lancet 2:1172, 1973

174. Melvin KEW, Tashjian AH: The syndrome of excessive thyrocalcitonin produced by medullary carcinoma of the thyroid. Proc Natl Acad Sci USA 59:1216, 1968

175. Melvin KEW, Miller HH, Tashjian AH: Early diagnosis of medullary carcinoma of the thyroid gland by means of calcitonin assay. N Engl J Med 285:1115, 1971

176. Wahner HW, Cuello C, Aljure F: Hormone-induced regression of medullary (solid) thyroid carcinoma. Am J Med 45:789, 1968

177. Barbot N, Calmettes C, Schuffenecker I et al: Pentagastrin stimulation test and early diagnosis of medullary thyroid carcinoma using an immunoradiometric assay of calcitonin: comparison with genetic screening in hereditary medullary thyroid carcinoma. J Clin Endocrinol Metab 78:114, 1994

178. Calmettes C, Moukhtar MS, Milhaud G: Correlation between calcitonin and carcinoembryonic antigen levels in medullary carcinoma of the thyroid. Biomedicine 27:52, 1977

179. Hoefnagel CA, Delprat CC, Zanin D, Van der Schoot JB: New radionuclide tracers for the diagnosis and therapy of medullary thyroid carcinoma. Clin Nuclear Med 13:159, 1988

180. Pacini F, Ceccherini I, Martino E et al: Screening for ret gene mutations in multiple endocrine neoplasia (MEN) type 2 and in sporadic medullary thyroid carcinoma (MTC): clinical applications, abstracted. Report of the Sixty-eighth Annual Meeting of the American Thyroid Association, Chicago, IL, September 28–October 1, 1994

181. Black HE, Capen CC, Young DM: Ultimobranchial thyroid neoplasms in bulls. Cancer 32:865, 1973

182. Harada T, Ito K, Shimaoka K et al: Fatal thyroid carcinoma: anaplastic transformation of adenocarcinoma. Cancer 39:2588, 1977

183. Oppenheim A, Miller M, Anderson GH Jr, Davis B, Slagle T et al: Anaplastic thyroid cancer presenting with hyperthyroidism. Amer J Med 75:702, 1983

184. Leedman PJ, Sheridan WP, Downey WF et al: Combination chemotherapy as single modality therapy for state IE and IIE thyroid lymphoma. Med J Australia 152:40, 1990

185. Butler JS, Brady LW, Amendola BE: Lymphoma of the thyroid: Report of five cases and review. Amer J Clin Oncol (CCT) 13:64, 1990

186. Souhami L, Simpson WJ, Carrothers JS: Malignant lymphoma of the thyroid gland. Int J Radiat Oncol Biol Phys 6:1143, 1980

187. Kini SR, Miller JM, Hamburger JI: Problems in the cytologic diagnosis of the "cold" thyroid nodule in patients with lymphocytic thyroiditis. Acta Cytol 25: 506, 1981

188. Grimley RP, Oates GD: The natural history of malignant thyroid lymphomas. Br J Surg 67:475, 1980

189. Siroto DK, Segal RL: Primary lymphomas of the thyroid. JAMA 242:1743, 1979

190. Robbins J, Rall JE, Rawson RW: A new serum iodine component in patients with functional carcinoma of the thyroid. J Clin Endocrinol Metab 15:1315, 1955

191. Dunn JT, Ray SC: Changes in iodine metabolism and thyroglobulin structure in metastatic follicular carcinoma of the thyroid with hyperthyroidism. J Clin Endocrinol Metab 36:1088, 1973

192. Abe Y, Ichikawa Y, Muraki T et al: Thyrotropin (TSH) receptor and adenylate cyclase activity in human thyroid tumors: absence of high affinity receptor and loss of TSH responsiveness in undifferentiated thyroid carcinoma. J Clin Endocrinol Metab 52:23, 1981

193. Carayon P, Thomas-Morvan C, Castanas E, Tubiana M: Human thyroid cancer: membrane thyrotropin binding and adenylate cyclase activity. J Clin Endocrinol Metab 51:915, 1980

194. Franklin WA, Mariotti S, Kaplan D, DeGroot LJ: Immunofluorescence localization of thyroglobulin in metastatic thyroid cancer. Cancer 50:939, 1982

195. Pontius KI, Hawk WA: Loss of microsomal antigen in follicular and papillary carcinoma of the thyroid: an immunofluorescence and electron-microscope study. Am J Pathol 74:620, 1980

196. DeGroot L, Hoye K, Refetoff S et al: Serum antigens and antibodies in the diagnosis of thyroid cancer. J Clin Endocrinol Metab 45:1220, 1977

197. Aoki N, DeGroot LJ: Lymphocyte blastogenic response to human thyroglobulin in Graves' disease, Hashimoto's thyroiditis, and metastatic thyroid cancer. Clin Exp Immunol 38:523, 1979

198. Amino N, Pysher T, Cohen EP, DeGroot LJ: Immunologic aspects of human thyroid cancer. Cancer 36: 963, 1975

199. Mariotti S, DeGroot LJ, Scarborough D, Medof ME: Study of circulating immune complexes in thyroid diseases: comparison of Raji cell radioimmunoassay and specific thyroglobulin-antithyroglobulin radioassay. J Clin Endocrinol Metab 49:679, 1979

200. Rocklin ER, Gagel R, Feldman Z, Tashijan AH Jr: Cellular immune responses in familial medullary thyroid carcinoma. N Engl J Med 296:835, 1977

201. Wu PS-C, Leslie PJ, McLaren KM, Toft AD: Diffuse sclerosing papillary carcinoma of thyroid: a wolf in sheep's clothing. Clin Endocrinol 31:535, 1989

202. Meighan JW, Dworkin HJ: Failure to detect ^{131}I positive thyroid metastases with [99m]Tc. J Nucl Med 11: 173, 1969

203. Fairweather DS, Bradwell AR, Watson-James SF et al: Detection of thyroid tumors using radio-labelled thyroglobulin. Clin Endocrinol 18:563, 1983

204. Thomas CG, Pepper FD, Owen J: Differentiation of malignant from benign lesions of the thyroid gland using complementary scanning with [75]Selenomethionine and radioiodide. Ann Surg 170:396, 1969

205. Yano K, Morita S, Furukawa Y et al: Diagnosis of malignant neoplasms with [201]Ti chloride. Jpn J Nucl Med 15:989, 1978

206. Van Herle AJ, Uller RP: Elevated serum thyroglobulin: a marker of metastases in differentiated thyroid carcinomas. J Clin Invest 56:272, 1975

207. Harmer MH: Application of TNM classification rules to malignant tumors of the thyroid gland. p. XII: 64. In Hedinger CE (ed): Thyroid Cancer: UICC Monograph Series. Vol. 12. Springer-Verlag, Berlin, 1969

208. Staging of Cancer of Head and Neck Sites and of Melanoma. American Joint Committee on Cancer, Chicago, 1980

209. Buckwalter JA, Thomas CG: Selection of surgical treatment for well differentiated thyroid carcinomas. Ann Surg 176:565, 1972

210. Tollefsen HR, Shah JP, Huvos AG: Papillary carcinoma of the thyroid: Recurrence in the thyroid gland after initial surgical treatment. Am J Surg 124:468, 1972

211. Rickey O, Howard R: Cancer of the thyroid. Am J Surg 112:637, 1967

212. Black B, Yadeau R, Woolner L: Surgical treatment of thyroidal carcinomas. Arch Surg 88:610, 1964

213. Clark R, Ibanez M, White E: What constitutes an adequate operation for carcinoma of the thyroid? Arch Surg 92:23, 1966

214. Rustad WH, Lindsay S, Dailey ME: Comparison of the incidence of complications following total and subtotal thyroidectomy for thyroid carcinoma. Surg Gynecol Obstet 116:109, 1963

215. Thompson NW, Harness JK: Complications of total thyroidectomy for carcinoma. Surg Gynecol Obstet 131:861, 1970

216. Samaan NA, Schultz PN, Hickey RC et al: The results of various modalities of treatment of well differentiated thyroid carcinoma: a retrospective review of 1599 patients. J Clin Endocrinol Metab 75:714, 1992

217. Tollefson H, DeCosse J: Papillary carcinoma of the thyroid: the case for radical neck dissection. Am J Surg 108:547, 1964

218. Crile G Jr, Suhrer JG Jr, Hazard JB: Results of con-

servative operations for malignant tumors of the thyroid. J Clin Endocrinol Metab 15:1422, 1955

219. Crile G Jr: Changing end results in patients with papillary carcinoma of the thyroid. Surg Gynecol Obstet 132:460, 1971

220. Glass HG, Waldron GW, Allen HC Jr, Brown WG: A rational approach to the thyroid malignancy problem. Am Surg 26:81, 1960

221. Shands WC, Gatling RR: Cancer of the thyroid: review of 109 cases. Ann Surg 171:735, 1970

222. Hirabayashi RN, Lindsay S: Carcinoma of the thyroid gland: a statistical study of 390 patients. J Clin Endocrinol Metab 21:1596, 1961

223. Meissner WA, Colcock BP, Achenback H: The pathologic evaluation of radical neck dissection for carcinoma of the thyroid gland. J Clin Endocrinol Metab 15:1432, 1955

224. Hay ID, Bergstralh EJ, Goellner JR et al: Predicting outcome in papillary thyroid carcinoma: development of a reliable prognostic scoring system in a cohort of 1779 patients surgically treated at one institution during 1940 through 1989. Surgery 114:1050, 1993

225. Block GE, Wilson SM: A modified neck dissection for carcinoma of the thyroid. Surg Clin North Am 51:139, 1971

226. Mustard RA: Treatment of papillary carcinoma of the thyroid with emphasis on conservative neck dissection. Am J Surg 120:697, 1970

227. McGovern J, Mannex H Jr: Thirty year experience with thyroid cancer. NY State J Med 67:2207, 1967

228. Exelby P, Frazell E: Carcinoma of the thyroid in children. Surg Clin North Am 49:249, 1969

229. Klapp C, Rosvoli R, Winship T: Is destructive surgery ever necessary for treatment of thyroid cancer in children? Ann Surg 165:745, 1967

230. Ruegemer JJ, Hay ID, Bergstralh EJ et al: Distant metastases in differentiated thyroid carcinoma. A multivariate analysis of prognostic variables. J Clin Endocrinol Metab 67:501, 1988

231. Liechty RD, Safaie-Shirazi S, Soper RT: Carcinoma of the thyroid in children. Surg Gynecol Obstet 134:595, 1972

232. DeGroot LJ, Reilly M: Comparison of 30- and 50-mCi doses of iodine-131 for thyroid ablation. Ann Intern Med 96:51, 1982

233. Carcangiu ML, Bianchi S, Savino D et al: Follicular Hurthle cell tumors of the thyroid gland. Cancer 68:1944, 1991

234. Park H-M, Perkins OW, Edmondson JW et al: Influence of diagnostic radioiodines on the uptake of ablative dose of Iodine-131. Thyroid 4:49, 1994

235. O'Connell ME, Flower MA, Hinton PJ et al: Radiation dose assessment in radioiodine therapy. Dose-response relationships in differentiated thyroid carcinoma using quantitative scanning and PET. Radiotherapy-Oncology 28:16, 1993

236. Maxon HR, Thomas SR, Hertzberg VS et al: Relation between effective radiation dose and outcome of radioiodine therapy for thyroid cancer. N Engl J Med 309:937, 1983

237. Pacini F, Lippi F, Formica N et al: Therapeutic doses of iodine-131 reveal undiagnosed metastases in thyroid cancer patients with detectable serum thyroglobulin levels. J Nucl Med 28:1888, 1987

238. Schlumberger M, Arcangioli O, Piekarski JD et al: Detection and treatment of lung metastases of differentiated thyroid carcinoma in patients with normal chest x-rays. J Nucl Med 29:1790, 1988

239. Meier CA, Braverman LE, Ebner SA et al: Diagnostic use of recombinant human thyrotropin in patients with thyroid carcinoma (Phase I/II study). J Clin Endocrinol Metab 78:188, 1994

240. Hamburger JI: Diuretic augmentation of ^{131}I uptake in inoperable thyroid cancer. N Engl J Med 280:1091, 1969

241. Hamburger JI, Desai P: Mannitol augmentation of I^{131} uptake in the treatment of thyroid carcinoma. Metabolism 15:1055, 1966

242. Benua R, Cicale N, Sonenberg M, Rawson R: The relation of radioiodine dosimetry to results and complications in the treatment of metastatic thyroid cancer. Am J Roentgenol Rad Ther Nucl Med 87:171, 1962

243. Seidlin SM, Yalow RA, Siegel E: Blood radioiodine concentration and blood radiation dosage during I^{131} therapy for metastatic thyroid carcinoma. J Clin Endocrinol Metab 12:1197, 1952

244. Raymond JP, Izembart M, Marliac V et al: Temporary ovarian failure in thyroid cancer patients after thyroid remnant ablation with radioactive iodine. J Clin Endocrinol Metab 69:186, 1989

245. Pochin EE: Leukemia following radioiodine treatment of thyrotoxicosis. Br Med J 2:1545, 1960

246. Burch WM, Posillico JT: Hypoparathyroidism after I-131 therapy with subsequent return of parathyroid function. J Clin Endocrinol Metab 57:398, 1983

247. Wiseman JC, Hales IB, Joasoo A: Two cases of lymphoma of the parotid gland following ablative radioiodine therapy for thyroid carcinoma. Clin Endocrinol 17:85, 1982

248. Rall JE, Alpers JB, Lewallen CG et al: Radiation pneumonitis and fibrosis. A complication of I^{131} treatment of pulmonary metastases from cancer of the thyroid. J Clin Endocrinol Metab 17:1263, 1957

249. Exelby PE, Frazell EL: Carcinoma of the thyroid in children. Surg Clin North Am 49:249, 1969

250. Trunnell JB, Marinelli LD, Duffy BJ Jr et al: The

treatment of metastatic thyroid cancer with radioactive iodine: credits and debits. J Clin Endocrinol Metab 19:1138, 1949

251. Saenger EL, Barrett CM, Passino JW et al: Experiences with I[131] in the management of carcinoma of the thyroid. Radiology 83:892, 1964

252. Varma VM, Beierwaltes WH, Nofal MM et al: Treatment of thyroid cancer: death rates after surgery and after surgery followed by sodium iodide I.[131] JAMA 214:1437, 1970

253. Leeper RD: The effect of ^{131}I therapy on survival of patients with metastatic papillary or follicular thyroid carcinoma. J Clin Endocrinol Metab 36:1143, 1973

254. Marcocci C, Pacini F, Elisei R et al: Clinical and biologic behavior of bone metastases from differentiated thyroid carcinoma. Surgery 106:960, 1989

255. Harness JK, Thompson NW, Sisson JC, Beierwaltes WH: Differentiated thyroid carcinomas: treatment of distant metastases. Arch Surg 108:410, 1974

256. Lambert B-A, Rantanen M, Saarinen P et al: Suppression of the TSH response to TRH by thyroxine therapy in differentiated thyroid carcinoma patients. Acta Endocrinol 91:248, 1979

257. Diamond T, Nery L, Hales I: A therapeutic dilemma: suppressive doses of thyroxine significantly reduce bone mineral measurements in both premenopausal and postmenopausal women with thyroid carcinoma. J Clin Endocrinol Metab 72:1184, 1990

258. Gam AN, Jensen GF, Hasselstrom K et al: Effect of thyroxine therapy on bone metabolism in substituted hypothyroid patients with normal or suppressed levels of TSH. J Endocrinol Invest 14:451, 1991

259. Charles MA, Dodson LE, Waldeck N et al: Serum thyroglobulin levels predict total body iodine scan findings in patients with treated well-differentiated thyroid carcinoma. Am J Med 69:401, 1980

260. Pacini F, Pinchera A, Giani C et al: Serum thyroglobulin concentrations and 131-I whole body scans in the diagnosis of metastases from differentiated thyroid carcinoma (after thyroidectomy). Clin Endocrinol 13:107, 1980

261. Barsano CP, Skosey C, DeGroot LJ, Refetoff S: Serum thyroglobulin in the management of patients with thyroid cancer. Arch Intern Med 142:763, 1982

262. Pacini F, Pinchera A, Giani C et al: Serum thyroglobulin in thyroid carcinoma and other thyroid disorders. J Endocrinol Invest 3:283, 1980

263. Johansen K, Woodhouse NJ: Comparison of thyroglobulin and radioiodine scintigraphy during follow-up of patients with differentiated thyroid carcinoma. Eur J Med 1:403, 1992

264. Graze K, Spiler IJ, Tashijan AH Jr et al: Natural history of familial medullary thyroid carcinoma. N Engl J Med 299:980, 1978

265. Deftos LT, Stein MF: Radioiodine as an adjunct to the surgical treatment of medullary thyroid carcinoma. J Clin Endocrinol Metab 50:967, 1980

266. Hellman DE, Kartchner M, Van Antwerp JD et al: Radioiodine in the treatment of medullary carcinoma of the thyroid. J Clin Endocrinol Metab 48:451, 1979

267. Kim S, Morimoto S, Kawai Y et al: Circulating levels of calcitonin gene-related peptide in patients with medullary thyroid carcinoma. J Clin Chem Clin Biochem 27:423, 1989

268. Norton JA, Doppman JL, Brennan MF: Localization and resection of clinically inapparent medullary carcinoma of the thyroid. Surgery 87:616, 1980

269. Frank-Raue K, Raue F, Buhr HJ et al: Localization of occult persisting medullary thyroid carcinoma before microsurgical reoperation: high sensitivity of selective venous catheterization. Thyroid 2:113, 1992

270. Moley JF, Wells SA, Dilley WG, Tisell LE: Reoperation for recurrent or persistent medullary thyroid cancer. Surgery 114:1090, 1993

271. Simpson WJK: Radiotherapy in thyroid cancer. Can Med Assoc J 113:115, 1975

272. Samaan NA, Schultz PN, Hickey RC: Medullary thyroid carcinoma: prognosis of familial versus nonfamilial disease and the role of radiotherapy. Horm Metab Res 21:21, 1989

273. Hoefnagel CA, Delprat CC, Zanin D, Van Der Schoot JB: New radionuclide tracers for the diagnosis and therapy of medullary thyroid carcinoma. Clin Nucl Med 13:159, 1988

274. Chak LY, Hoppe RT, Burke JS, Kaplan HS: Non-Hodgkin's lymphoma presenting as thyroid enlargement. Cancer 48:2712, 1981

275. Matsuzuka F, Miyauchi A, Katayama S et al: Clinical aspects of primary thyroid lymphoma: diagnosis and treatment based on our experience of 119 cases. Thyroid 3:93, 1993

276. MacGregor CA, Ham DP: Hormonal dependent anaplastic thyroid carcinoma: a case report. Surgery 71:56, 1972

277. Kim JH, Leeper RD: Treatment of anaplastic and spindle cell carcinoma of the thyroid gland with combination adriamycin and radiation therapy. Cancer 52:954, 1983

278. Tubiana M, Lacour J, Monnier JP et al: External radiotherapy and radioiodine in the treatment of 359 thyroid cancers. Br J Radiol 48:894, 1975

279. Riccabona G: Radiotherapy and nuclear medicine in malignant tumors of the thyroid gland. Therapiewoche 29:3448, 1979

280. Tubiana M: External radiotherapy and radioiodine in the treatment of thyroid cancer. World J Surg 5: 75, 1981

281. Harada T, Nishikawa Y, Suzuki T et al: Bleomycin treatment for cancer of the thyroid. Am J Surg 122: 53, 1971

282. Gottlieb JA, Hill CS, Ibanez ML, Clark RL: Chemotherapy of thyroid cancer: an evaluation of experience with 37 patients. Cancer 30:848, 1972

283. Jereb B, Stjernsward J, Lowhagen T: Anaplastic giant-cell carcinoma of the thyroid. Cancer 35:1293, 1975

284. Shimaoka K, Reyes J: Chemotherapy of thyroid carcinoma. p. 434. In Robbins J, Braverman L (eds): Thyroid Research. Elsevier Biomedical, New York, 1975

285. Riccabona G, Zechmann W, Fill H: Cytostatic drug therapy of thyroid cancer. p. 432. In Robbins J, Braverman L (eds): Thyroid Research. Elsevier Biomedical, New York, 1975

286. De Besi P, Busnardo B, Toso S et al: Combined chemotherapy with bleomycin, adriamycin, and platinum in advanced thyroid cancer. J Endocrinol Invest 14:475, 1991

Acute and Subacute Thyroiditis

19

CLASSIFICATION

The diagnostic term *thyroiditis* comprises a group of inflammatory or inflammatory-like conditions. The terminology that has been employed is confusing, yet no classification is ideal. We prefer the following nomenclature, which takes into account the cause when known.

1. *Infectious thyroiditis*, also referred to as either acute or chronic (and which in fact may be either), along with the qualifying term suppurative, nonsuppurative, or septic thyroiditis. It includes all forms of infection, other than viral, and is caused by invasion of the thyroid by bacteria, mycobacteria, fungi, protozoa, or flatworms. The disorder is rare.

2. *DeQuervain's thyroiditis*, commonly known as subacute thyroiditis but also termed subacute nonsuppurative thyroiditis, granulomatous, pseudo-tuberculous, pseudo-giant cell or giant cell thyroiditis, migratory or creeping thyroiditis, and struma granulomatosa. This condition, probably of viral origin, lasts for a week to a few months and tends to recur. The eponym reflects its uncertain cause.

3. *Autoimmune thyroiditis*, commonly referred to as chronic, Hashimoto's, or lymphocytic thyroiditis and also known as lymphadenoid goiter and struma lymphomatosa. This indolent disease usually persists for years and is the principal cause of noniatrogenic primary hypothyroidism in the Western hemisphere. Nonspecific focal thyroiditis, characterized by local lymphoid cell infiltration without parenchymal changes, may be a variant of the autoimmune disease. The condition is covered in detail in Chapter 8.

Another form of thyroiditis, also believed to be of autoimmune cause, has been variably referred to as painless, silent, occult, subacute, subacute nonsuppurative, and atypical (silent) subacute thyroiditis, as well as hyperthyroiditis, transient thyrotoxicosis with low thyroidal RAIU, and lymphocytic thyroiditis with spontaneously resolving hyperthyroidism. There is no agreement on an inclusive name. The features of this disease overlap deQuervain's thyroiditis and Hashimoto's thyroiditis. The clinical course, with the

697

exception of a very high erythrocyte sedimentation rate, are indistinguishable from de Quervain's thyroiditis. Yet, histologically, the condition cannot be differentiated from a milder form of Hashimoto's disease. This condition often occurs in the postpartum period and is termed postpartum thyroiditis. All forms of autoimmune thyroiditis are considered in Chapter 8.

4. *Riedel's thyroiditis* is another disorder of unknown etiology. Synonyms include Riedel's struma, ligneous thyroiditis, and invasive fibrous or chronic sclerosing thyroiditis. This condition is characterized by overgrowth of connective tissue which often extends into neighboring structures.

5. Miscellaneous varieties of thyroid inflammation or infiltration including local manifestations of a generalized disease processes constitute a fifth category. Among these are sarcoid and amyloid involvement of the thyroid. Radiation and direct trauma to the thyroid gland may also cause thyroiditis.

ACUTE (INFECTIOUS) THYROIDITIS

The thyroid gland is remarkably resistant to infection. This has been attributed to its high vascularity, the presence of large amounts of iodine in the tissue, the fact that hydrogen peroxide is generated within the gland as a requirement for the synthesis of thyroid hormone, and its normal encapsulated position away from external structures. In certain situations, however, particularly in children, a persistent fistula from the pyriform sinus may make the left lobe of the thyroid particularly susceptible to abscess formation.[1-3] In the immunocompromised host, fungal infection may occur.[4-6] Rarely, infection will occur in a cystic or degenerated nodule. The principal differential diagnosis is generally between acute, meaning infectious, and subacute, meaning post-viral (non-infectious) inflammation of the gland (see below).

Etiology

Virtually any bacterium can infect the thyroid. *Streptococcus, Staphylococcus, Pneumococcus, Salmonella,*[7] *Bacteroides, T. pallidum* and *M. tuberculosis*[8,9] have all been described. The subject has been extensively reviewed.[5,10-12] In addition, certain fungi, including *Coccidioides immitis, aspergillus,* and *Candida albicans* have also been associated with thyroiditis.[4,13]

In the latter cases, the hosts have often been immunocompromised, either due to malignancy or to AIDS.

Most commonly, however—especially in children—infection of the thyroid gland is a result of direct extension from an internal fistula from the pyriform sinus.[1-3,12,14] This tract is thought to represent the course of migration of the ultimo branchial body from the site of its embryonic origin in the fifth pharyngeal pouch. Careful histopathologic studies of these fistulae have demonstrated that they are lined by squamous columnar or ciliated epithelium and occasionally form branches in the thyroid lobe.[1,3] In addition, occasional cells positive for calcitonin have been found in the fistulae and increased numbers of C cells were noted in the thyroid lobe at the point of termination of the tract. The predominance of acute thyroiditis in the left lobe of the thyroid gland, particularly in infants and children, is explained by the fact that the right ultimo branchial body is often atrophic and does not develop in the human (as well as in other species, such as reptiles). The reason for this phenomenon is not known. Acute thyroiditis may involve a normal gland, or arise in a multinodular goiter. At times, no source of infection can be demonstrated. The possibility of a persistent thyroglossal duct should be considered for patients with midline infections.

Pathology

Pathologic examination reveals characteristic changes of acute inflammation. With bacterial infections, heavy polymorphonuclear and lymphocytic cellular infiltrate is found in the initial phase, often with necrosis and abscess formation. Fibrosis is prominent as healing occurs. In material obtained by fine needle aspiration, the infectious agent may be seen on a gram, acid fast, or appropriate fungal stains. Fungal thyroiditis was clearly demonstrated in a patient with *Candida albicans*.[4]

Incidence

Acute thyroiditis is quite rare with no more than one to two patients per year observed in a large tertiary care hospital. It may be somewhat more common in the pediatric age group, although still quite unusual. The proper treatment of an acute thyroiditis in children generally requires the surgical removal of the fistula.[1-3] This almost always leads to a permanent cure.

Clinical Manifestations

The dominant clinical symptom is pain in the region of the thyroid gland which may subsequently enlarge and become hot and tender. The patient is unable to extend the neck and often sits with the neck flexed in order to avoid pressure on the thyroid gland. Swallowing is painful. There are usually signs of infection in structures adjacent to the thyroid, local lymphadenopathy, as well as temperature elevation and, if bacteremia occurs, chills. Symptoms are generally more obvious in children than in adults. Adults may present with a vague, slightly painful mass in the thyroid region without fever, which may raise the possibility of a malignancy. It may occur more commonly in the fall and winter following upper respiratory tract infections.

In general, there are no signs or symptoms of hyper- or hypothyroidism. Exceptions to both have been reported, however, particularly when the thyroiditis is generalized, as occurs with fungal processes. At times, even in patients with bacterial thyroiditis, destruction of the thyroid gland is sufficient to release thyroid hormone in amounts sufficient to cause symptomatic hyperthyroidism.[8] The adult thyroid gland contains approximately 600 μg of T$_4$/g.[15] Given a typical 15 to 20 g gland, sufficient hormone can be released to cause transient thyrotoxicosis.

Diagnosis

Pain in the anterior neck will usually lead to a consideration of the possibility of thyroiditis. Since the major differential diagnosis will lie between acute suppurative thyroiditis and subacute thyroiditis, it is critical to compare the history, physical, and particularly laboratory data in these two conditions (see Table 19-1). In general, the patient with acute thyroiditis appears septic, has greater and more localized pain in the thyroid gland, may have an associated upper respiratory infection, has lymphadenopathy, and may be immunocompromised. Localization of the tenderness to the left lobe should suggest the possibility of an infection, as should any erythema or apparent abscess formation. The presence of an elevated white blood count with a shift to the left would argue for infection; however, elevations in sedimentation rate are common in both acute and

subacute thyroiditis. As mentioned, patients with bacterial thyroiditis are not hyperthyroid, but exceptions do occur. This is more common but by no means universal in patients with subacute thyroiditis.

Depending on the age and clinical circumstances, one may wish to proceed with invasive or noninvasive studies. The most discriminating tests for recognizing a difference between the two conditions are either an iodine uptake or scan showing a very low value in subacute thyroiditis with a normal value found in the patient with localized bacterial thyroiditis.[12] If a thyroid ultrasound shows a localized process, a needle aspiration can be performed. This will be definitive. A CT scan may be useful in identifying the location of the abscess, but this is required only in unusual situations.[16] Gallium scans are sometimes performed in the course of an evaluation for a fever of unknown origin. Localization of gallium to the thyroid gland is a very useful finding confirming thyroid inflammation as the source of the problem.[13] If an infectious process is identified, particularly of the left lobe of a younger individual, then a barium swallow should be performed with attention to the possibility of a fistulous tract located on the left side between the pyriform sinus and the thyroid gland. In general, bacterial infections tend to be localized whereas the post-viral subacute thyroiditis is more often generalized, although intermediate conditions can certainly exist.

Occasionally, pain from an infectious process elsewhere in the neck will present as anterior neck tenderness. One of the authors has seen a very striking patient with retropharyngeal abscess presenting with typical symptoms of acute thyroiditis. The thyroid gland, however, had normal uptake, was normal on scan, and it was only on CT scan that the retropharyngeal abscess was recognized. The tendency for the pain of thyroid inflammation to be referred to the throat or ears should be kept in mind, although recognition of the anatomic source of the problem is usually not a difficult issue in patients with acute thyroiditis.

Treatment

The diagnosis and choice of antibiotic therapy are often aided by microscopic examination and appropriate staining of a fine needle aspirate. The procedure is best done under ultrasound guidance so that the source of the specimen is identified. It may also

TABLE 19-1. Features Useful in Differentiating Acute Suppurative Thyroiditis and Subacute Thyroiditis

	Characteristic	Acute Thyroiditis	Subacute Thyroiditis
History	Preceding upper respiratory infection	88%	17%
	Fever	100%	54%
	Symptoms of thyrotoxicosis	Uncommon	47%
	Sore throat	90%	36%
Physical examination of the thyroid	Painful thyroid swelling	100%	77%
	Left side affected	85%	Not specific
	Migrating thyroid tenderness	Possible	27%
	Erythema of overlying skin	83%	Not usually
Laboratory	Elevated white blood cell count	57%	25–50%
	Elevated erythrocyte sedimentation rate (>30 mm/hr)	100%	85%
	Abnormal thyroid hormone levels (elevated or depressed)	5–10%	60%
	Alkaline phosphatase, transaminases increased	Rare	Common
Needle aspiration	Purulent, bacteria or fungi present	~100%	0
	Lymphocytes, macrophages, some polyps, giant cells	0	~100%
	^{123}I uptake low	Uncommon	~100%
Radiologic	Abnormal thyroid scan	92%	—
	Thyroid scan or ultrasound helpful in diagnosis	75%	—
	Gallium scan positive	~100%	~100%
	Barium swallow showing fistula CT scan useful	Common	0
	CT scan useful	Rarely	Not indicated
Clinical course	Clinical response to glucocorticoid treatment	Transient	100%
	Incision and drainage required	85%	No
	Recurrence following operative drainage	16%	No
	Pyriform sinus fistula discovered	96%	No

(Modified from Szabo and Allen,[12] with permission.)

serve as a mechanism for drainage of an abscess and can be repeated to facilitate healing. Some abscesses will require surgical exploration and drainage. The choice of therapy will also depend on the immune status of the patient. Systemic antibiotics are required for severe infections. Candida albicans thyroiditis can be treated with amphotericin B and 5 fluconazol 100 mg/d. While patients with tuberculosis or parasitic infections tend to have a more indolent course, these infections can present with acute symptoms and this possibility should be considered if the epidemiology is consistent. For example, thyroidal echinococcosis occurs in countries in which this parasite is endemic.[17] Trypanosomiasis of the thyroid has also been reported.[12]

Prognosis

In some patients with thyroiditis, the destruction may be sufficiently severe that hypothyroidism eventuates. Thus, patients with a particularly diffuse thyroiditis should have follow-up thyroid function studies performed to determine that this has not occurred. Surgical removal of a fistula is required to prevent recurrence when this is present.

SUBACUTE (GRANULOMATOUS) THYROIDITIS

Subacute thyroiditis, sometimes referred to as granulomatous or DeQuervain's thyroiditis, is a spontaneously remitting inflammatory condition of the thyroid gland that may last for weeks to several months.[10,12,18] It has a tendency to recur. The gland is typically involved as a whole, and thyroidal RAIU is much depressed. Transient hyperthyroxemia, elevation of the serum TG concentration and the erythrocyte sedimentation rate, and sometimes the WBC during the early acute phase, are characteristic if not pathognomic.

Etiology

A cause can rarely be established. A tendency for the disease to follow upper respiratory tract infections or sore throats has suggested a viral infection. Earlier suggestions that the disease may represent a bacterial infection have been disproven. An autoimmune reaction is also unlikely. The development during the illness of cell-mediated immunity against various thyroid cell particulate fractions or crude antigens appears to be related to the release of these materials during tissue destruction.[19,20]

Although the search for a viral cause has usually been unrewarding, a few cases seem to be due to the virus that causes mumps.[18,21] The disease has occurred in epidemic form. High titers of mumps antibodies have been found in some patients with subacute thyroiditis, and occasionally parotitis or orchitis is associated with thyroiditis. The mumps virus has been cultured directly from thyroid tissue involved by subacute thyroiditis. Although the mumps virus seems to be one discrete etiologic factor, the disease has been reported in association with other viral conditions including measles, influenza, adenovirus infection, infectious mononucleosis, myocarditis, cat scratch fever, and coxsackie virus (Fig. 19-1).[22]

Numerous attempts to culture viruses from cases not associated with mumps have failed. Virus-like particles have been demonstrated in the follicular epithelium of a single patient suffering form subacute thyroiditis.[22] Viral antibody titers to common respiratory tract viruses are, however, often elevated in these patients. Since the titers fall promptly, and multiple viral antibodies may appear in the same patient, the elevation probably is an anamnestic response to the inflammatory condition[23] (Fig. 19-1). Histocompatibility studies show that 72 percent of patients with subacute thyroiditis manifest HLA-Bw35.[18,24] Thus, the susceptibility to subacute thyroiditis is genetically influenced.

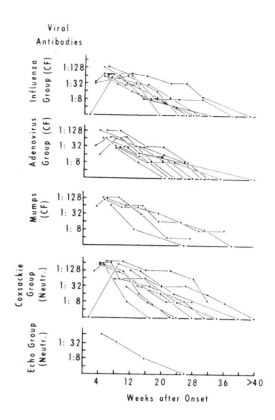

Fig. 19-1. Viral antibody titers in subacute thyroiditis. The graph shows serial viral antibody titers in 32 patients who had 4-fold changes in the dilution of these antibodies. Only the single viral antibody showing the greatest change in dilution during the period of observation is depicted for each patient. The antibody titers are characteristically high at the onset of the illness and gradually diminish. (From Volpé et al,[23] with permission.)

New treatments, particularly those in which there is manipulation of the immune system, have led to the development of a subacute thyroiditis. Infusion of interleukin 2 caused hyperthyroxinemia with a low radioiodine uptake in six patients who received this in combination with TNF α or α interferon.[25] The patients proceeded to pass through the pattern of hyperthyroidism and transient hypothyroidism, with a re-establishment of normal thyroid function typical of the patient with autoimmune painless thyroiditis. None of the patients, however, had detectable antithyroid antibodies. This condition is thus intermediate between subacute lymphocytic (painless) thyroiditis (Ch. 13) and subacute thyroiditis, which is typically painful.

Pathology

The thyroid gland may be adherent to its capsule or to the strap muscles but it can usually be dissected free, a feature distinguishing subacute thyroiditis from Riedel's thyroiditis. The involved tissue appears yellowish or white and is more firm than normal. The gland is enlarged, and the enlargement is usually bilateral and uniform, but it may be asymmetrical, with predominant involvement of one lobe. Although the lesion may extend to the capsular surface, it can also be confined to the thyroid parenchyma and merely be palpable as a suspiciously hard area.

The macroscopic pathologic picture of subacute thyroiditis frequently bears a striking resemblance to cancer. The lesion is firm to dense in consistency, pale white in color, and has poorly defined margins that encroach irregularly on the adjacent normal thyroid. Microscopically, one sees a mixture of subacute, chronic, and granulomatous inflammatory changes associated with zones of parenchymal destruction and scar tissue. Early infiltration with polymorphonuclear leukocytes is replaced by lymphocytes and macrophages. The normal follicles may be largely replaced by an inflammatory reaction, but a few small follicles containing colloid remain (Fig. 19-2). The most distinctive feature is the granuloma, consisting of giant cells clustered about foci of degenerating thyroid follicles (Fig. 19-2). The early literature contains accounts of *tuberculous thyroiditis,* a diagnosis largely based on the granulomatous tissue reaction, from which the descriptive but unfortunate term *pseudotuberculous thyroiditis* arose.[26]

Incidence

Subacute thyroiditis is encountered infrequently, but each year a handful of cases will be identified in a busy thyroid clinic. Woolner et al.[26] collected 162 cases diagnosed on clinical grounds at the Mayo Clinic over a 5-year period; during the same time, 1,250 patients with Graves' disease were seen. Thus, the disease had approximately one-eighth the incidence of Graves' disease in this clinic population. Although the disease has been described at all ages, it is rare in children. Female patients outnumbered male patients in a ratio of 3-6:1, and there is a preponderance of cases in the third to fifth decades.[10,11,26]

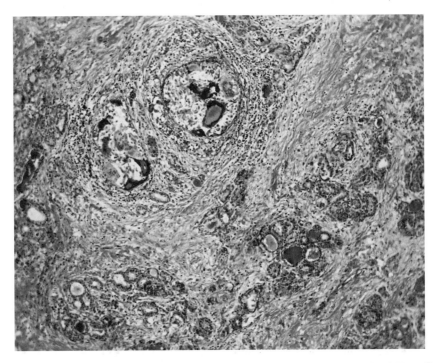

Fig. 19-2. Subacute thyroiditis. Note the discrete granulomas, with giant cells, and the diffuse fibrosis (85×).

Clinical Manifestations

Characteristically, the patient has severe pain and extreme tenderness in the thyroid region. When the symptom is difficulty in swallowing, the disorder may be initially mistaken for pharyngitis. At times, the pain begins in one pole and then spreads rapidly to involve the rest of the gland ("creeping thyroiditis"). It may radiate to the jaw or the ears. Malaise, fatigue, myalgia and arthralgia are common. A mild to moderate fever is expected, and at times a high, swinging fever causes temperatures to rise daily above 104°F (40.0°C). The disease may reach its peak within 3 to 4 days and subside and disappear within a week, but more typically, a gradual onset extends over 1 to 2 weeks and continues with a fluctuating intensity for 3 to 6 weeks. Several recurrences of diminishing intensity extending over many months may be the unhappy fate of the patient.

The thyroid gland is typically enlarged two or three times the normal size or larger and is tender to palpation, sometimes exquisitely so. It is smooth and firm.

Approximately one-half of the patients present during the first weeks of the illness, with symptoms of thyrotoxicosis, including nervousness, heat intolerance, palpitations, tremulousness, and increased sweating. These symptoms are caused by excessive release of thyroid hormone from the thyroid gland during the acute phase of the inflammatory process. As the disease process subsides, transient hypothyroidism occurs in about one-quarter of the patients. Ultimately, thyroid function returns to normal and permanent hypothyroidism occurs in less than 10 percent of the cases.[10–12]

Diagnosis

Table 19-1 provides a comparison between the clinical and laboratory findings of patients with subacute and acute thyroiditis.[12,27–39] Laboratory examination may disclose a moderate leukocytosis. A curious and striking elevation of the erythrocyte sedimentation rate, at times above 100 mm/hr, is a useful diagnostic clue. Short of tissue diagnosis, most helpful is the characteristic combination of elevated erythrocyte sedimentation rate, high serum T_4, T_3, and TG concentrations in the presence of low thyroidal RAIU, and an absent or low titer of circulating TG antibodies. Mild anemia and hyperglobulinemia may be present.

Subacute Thyroiditis

A.S., a 46-year-old woman, noted the onset of a tender, slowly enlarging swelling in the low anterior neck in December. There was no antecedent infection or virus-like syndrome. She was aware of associated increased nervousness, mild tremor, increased sweating, and anorexia, without alteration in weight. In January, increasing pain that radiated to the back of her head and orbits necessitated medical consultation. A family history of thyroid disease was not elicited.

On physical examination she appeared to be in pain. BP was 155/80, and pulse 112/min and regular. Clinically, she appeared to be euthyroid. The thyroid gland was estimated to be 40 g in weight and was tender, firm, and slightly irregular. The remainder of the examination was non-contributory.

Laboratory data included an erythrocyte sedimentation rate of 58 mm/min, FT_4I of 16.1 $\mu g/dl$ (normal, 3.6 to 9.3 $\mu g/dl$), TT_4 level of 14.9 $\mu g/dl$ (normal 4.2 to 9.4), and a Tg antibody titer of 1/40.

Figure 19-3 shows a sequence of ^{125}I and ^{241}Am scans obtained throughout the course of her illness. On presentation, there was no ^{125}I uptake seen on thyroid scintiscan, with an RAIU of 1 percent. At the same time, the ^{241}Am scan showed virtually no stable iodine in the thyroid. A ^{241}Am scan repeated in March showed continuing low ^{127}I levels in the thyroid, at which time the serum TT_4 level was 1.7 $\mu g/dl$ and the FT_4I was 0.8 $\mu g/dl$. The ^{241}Am scans on these two dates demonstrate mainly background radiation scatter. With the resolution of her clinical syndrome over the next few months, the results of the thyroid scans were seen to return to normal. The result of the ^{125}I scintiscan in June was completely normal, with an RAIU of 20 percent, at which time her TT_4 level and FT_4I had returned to the normal range. The ^{241}Am scan 3 months later showed some reaccumulation of ^{127}I, but the stable iodine store was still reduced. The last ^{241}Am scan 14 months after onset demonstrated total repletion of her thyroidal ^{127}I stores. At this time, the gland was normal in size (weight 20 g) and consistency.

If subacute thyroiditis affects only one part of the thyroid gland, the serum T_4 concentration and thyroidal RAIU may be entirely normal. A thyroid scan will demonstrate failure of the involved areas of the gland to concentrate iodide. When the thyroid is diffusely involved, which is more typical, a dramatic disturbance in iodine metabolism is observed.[27,28]

During the initial phase of the disease, the RAIU is depressed or entirely absent and the concentrations of serum T_4 and T_3 are often elevated. Due to the concomitant release of nonhydrolyzed iodoproteins from the inflamed tissue, the serum TG level is also high.[29,30] During this phase the serum TSH

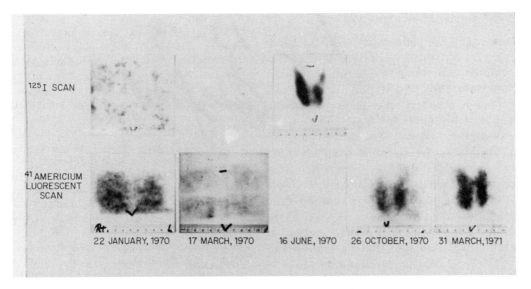

Fig. 19-3. Serial ^{125}I scintiscans and ^{241}Am fluorescent scans in a patient during the course of subacute thyroiditis. The first two fluorescent scans, done at a high sensitivity setting without background subtraction, have much neck "background" but demonstrate virtually no ^{127}I in the thyroid. (From Rapoport et al,[34] with permission.)

level is low, and the TSH response to TRH is suppressed[31] due to the high levels of circulating thyroid hormone. Iodide that is collected and metabolized by the gland is rapidly secreted because of the decreased ability to store colloid.[18] At this time, the involved tissue shows decreased but not necessarily depleted stores of iodine, as determined by x-ray fluorescence.[28,34] Administration of TSH usually fails to produce a normal increase in RAIU. Evidently, thyroid cell damage reduces the ability of the gland to respond to TSH. As the process subsides, the serum T_4, T_3, and TG levels decline, but the serum TSH level remains suppressed.

Later, during the recovery phase, the RAIU becomes elevated with the resumption of the ability of the thyroid gland to concentrate iodide. The serum T_4 concentration may fall below normal; the TSH level may become elevated. Usually after several weeks or months, all the parameters of thyroid function return to normal (Fig. 19-4). Restoration of iodine stores appears to be much slower and may take more than a year after the complete clinical remission.[28,34]

Differential Diagnosis

Diagnosis is usually not difficult. With an acutely enlarged, tender thyroid, an RAIU near zero, and elevated serum T_4 and Tg concentrations and ESR

the diagnosis is almost certain. Circulating thyroid autoantibodies are absent or the titer is low. Among the diagnostic alternatives, infectious thyroiditis must be considered and the possibility of invading bacteria excluded (see Table 19-1). The thyroid in Hashimoto's thyroiditis may be slightly tender and painful, but this event is rare, and the typical disturbances in iodine metabolism and erythrocyte sedimentation rate are not found. Hemorrhage into a cyst in a nodular thyroid gland may be confused with subacute thyroiditis. Hemorrhage is usually more sudden and transient, a fluctuant mass may be found in the involved region, and the erythrocyte sedimentation rate is normal. Occasionally, subacute thyroiditis mimics hyperthyroidism in a patient whose RAIU is suppressed by iodine. This event occurs particularly in transient thyrotoxicosis induced by iodine.[35] The sudden onset of subacute thyroiditis, the presence of toxic symptoms without the typical signs of long-term hyperthyroidism, the tender gland, the constitutional symptoms, and the high erythrocyte sedimentation rate are helpful in making the differentiation. In some instances, measurement of antibodies and thyroid-stimulating immunoglobulins, and observation of the course of the illness may be required to confirm the diagnosis.

The single disease entity that is probably most difficult to differentiate from subacute thyroiditis is sub-

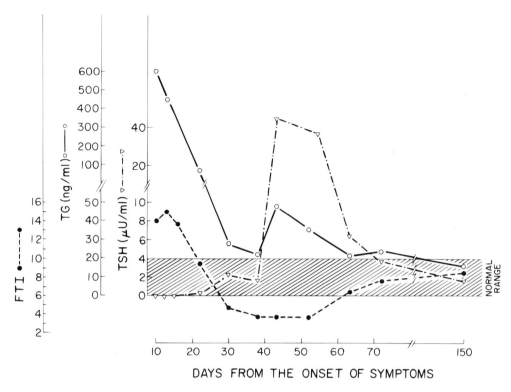

Fig. 19-4. Thyroid function in a patient during the course of deQuervain's (subacute) thyroiditis. During the thyrotoxic phase (days 10 to 20), the serum TG concentration was greatly elevated, the FTI was high, and TSH was suppressed; the erythrocyte sedimentation rate was 86 mm/hr, and the thyroidal RAIU was 2 percent. The TG level and FTI declined in parallel. During the phase of hypothyroidism (days 30 to 63), when the FTI was below normal, a modest transient increase in the serum TG level occurred in parallel with the increase in serum TSH. All parameters of thyroid function were normal by day 150, 5 months after the onset of symptoms.

acute lymphocytic thyroiditis.[37–39] This condition is unrelated to iodine ingestion and most likely is a variant of autoimmune thyroiditis. The patient presents with goiter, mild thyrotoxicosis, and a low RAIU. The course of the disease is indistinguishable from that of subacute thyroiditis and proceeds from a thyrotoxic phase through a hypothyroid phase to spontaneous remission with normalization of thyroid function. The goiter is painless, and there are no associated systemic symptoms. This condition has been formerly confused with subacute (deQuervain's) thyroiditis, whence come the misleading terms silent, painless, or atypical subacute thyroiditis. The most helpful distinguishing features, short of histologic examination of biopsy material, are the absence of pain and a normal erythrocyte sedimentation rate. (see also Ch. 13.) Localized subacute thyroiditis, with induration, mild tenderness, and de-

pressed iodine binding visualized on scan, can be very suggestive of thyroid cancer. Usually the degree of pain and tenderness, elevated erythrocyte sedimentation rate and leukocytosis, and remission or spread to other parts of the gland make clinical differentiation possible. Rarely, a fine needle aspiration is required for a definitive differentiation between these two processes.

Treatment

In some patients, no treatment is required. For many, however, some form of analgesic therapy is required to treat the symptoms of the disease until it resolves. At times, this relief of symptoms can be achieved with nonsteroidal anti-inflammatory agents or aspirin. If this fails, however, as it often does when the symptoms are severe, prednisone administration should be employed.[11,18] Large doses promptly relieve the symptoms through nonspecific anti-inflammatory effects. Treatment is generally begun with a single daily dose of 40 mg prednisone. After one week of this treatment, the dosage is tapered over a period of 6 weeks or so. The relief of the tenderness in the neck is so dramatic as to be virtually diagnostic of the problem as being due to subacute thyroiditis. As the dose is tapered, most patients have no recrudescence of symptoms, but occasionally this does occur and the dose must be increased again. Levothyroxine administration may be useful in situations where the patient is not already hyperthyroid due to the release of thyroidal contents into the circulation. It is thought that TSH suppression will reduce the thyroid stimulation which might otherwise prolong the inflammatory process.

It is also necessary to administer thyroid hormones, at least transiently, if the patient enters a phase of hypothyroidism subsequent to the acute inflammation. TSH-suppressive doses of levothyroxine should only be administered when there is evidence that exacerbation of the condition occurs when TSH is present. Otherwise, the return of thyroid function to normal, which presumably is facilitated by TSH, can be prevented or delayed. During the recovery process, there may be a marked but transient increase in the 24 hour radioactive iodine uptake, which can reach levels typical of Graves' Disease. This occurs prior to re-establishment of normal thyroid function and should not be confused with hyperthyroidism due to Graves' disease.

Prognosis

In 90 percent or more of patients, there is a complete and spontaneous recovery and a return to normal thyroid function. The thyroid glands of patients with subacute thyroiditis, however, may exhibit irregular scarring between islands of residual functioning parenchyma, although the patient has no symptoms. Up to 10 percent of the patients may become hypothyroid and require permanent replacement with levothyroxine. Elevated levels of serum TG may persist well over a year after the initial diagnosis, indicating that disordered follicular architecture and/or low grade inflammation can persist for a relatively long period.[30,40]

RIEDEL'S THYROIDITIS

In 1896 Riedel described a chronic sclerosing thyroiditis, occurring especially in women, that tends to progress inexorably to complete destruction of the thyroid gland and frequently causes pressure symptoms in the neck.[41-43] It is exceedingly rare. In the Mayo Clinic series it occurred approximately on-fiftieth as frequently as Hashimoto's thyroiditis. It is approximately twice as frequent in men as in women and is found most often in the 30- to 60-year age group. The thyroid gland is normal in size or enlarged, usually symmetrically involved, and extremely hard. Occasionally involvement may be unilateral. On pathologic examination the gland is replaced by dense fibrosis in which are scattered solitary follicular cells and occasional acini with small amounts of colloid. The fibrosis binds the thyroid firmly to the trachea and the strap muscles, from which it can be separated only with the greatest difficulty (*ligneous thyroiditis*).[44] The fibrosis may compress the trachea or esophagus. The disease may remain stable over many years, or it may progress slowly and produce hypothyroidism.

Dyspnea, dysphagia, hoarseness, and aphonia are caused by the local pressure, and if there is enough pressure on both recurrent laryngeal nerves, there may be stridor. Sometimes the disease is asymptomatic and discovered only incidentally. The pathologic process may advance to complete replacement of the gland, and then symptoms and signs of hypothyroidism appear. Involvement of the parathyroid glands by the fibrotic process may result in hypoparathyroidism.[45-47] Rarely, Riedel's thyroiditis may be associated with similar fibrosclerotic processes in other areas, including the lacrimal glands, orbits, parotid glands, mediastinum, lung, myocardium, retroperitoneal tissues, and bile ducts in varying combinations in the syndrome of multifocal fibrosclerosis.

The results of laboratory tests of thyroid function are usually normal, but about one-third are hypothyroid. The erythrocyte sedimentation rate is not elevated, as in subacute thyroiditis, and there is no leukocytosis. Antithyroid antibodies are present in 67 percent of reported cases[43] and a mixed population of B- and T cells is present in the thyroid, suggesting an autoimmune etiology or association.

The disease is rarely recognized on clinical grounds, and may be impossible to differentiate clinically from involvement of the thyroid with cancer. Unlike extensively invasive undifferentiated cancer, Riedel's thyroiditis is a slowly progressive, destructive process involving the thyroid and the perithyroidal structures. Carcinoma of a kind that would be confused with Riedel's struma would most probably rapidly increase the size of the goiter.

Surgery offers the only useful treatment. It may be necessary in order to establish a diagnosis or to relieve pressure on the trachea or esophagus. Resection of the isthmus may permit the two lobes to fall laterally, thereby relieving an obstruction.

When at surgery a diagnosis of Riedel's struma is suspected, a biopsy (specimen) of the involved area should be examined by a pathologist for confirmation and to rule out carcinoma. After this examination there is no good reason to attempt a thyroidectomy, and only relief of constriction should be sought. The denseness of the proliferated fibrotic process, with obliteration of landmarks and tissue planes, makes surgical exploration exceedingly difficult and, indeed, dangerous. Thyroid hormone should be administered postoperatively if there are signs or symptoms of hypothyroidism.

Hashimoto's disease may occasionally be associated with considerable fibrosis, but it is more frequently of the replacement type than the dense proliferative type of scar tissue of Riedel's thyroiditis. Involvement of perithyroidal structures does not occur. From a study of 16 patients with Hashimoto's thyroiditis who had repeated thyroid gland biopsies at an average interval of 5 years, there was little evidence to support the theory that progressive fibrosis is a regular feature of Hashimoto's disease. However, some reports strongly indicate that the progression of lymphocytic thyroiditis to Riedel's thyroiditis is at least one cause of the disease, a view that we share.[42,43] Occasionally, medullary carcinoma may be accompanied by massive fibrosis.

Riedel's Thyroiditis

A goiter known to be present for more than 20 years in M.R., a 45-year-old woman, had increased during the last 2 years. There was no difficulty in swallowing or breathing, or signs of abnormal metabolism. The patient had received iodine treatment on two occasions 10 years previously. Her medical history included rheumatic heart disease at age 16.

The thyroid was twice the normal size, and there was a nodule in each lobe. The left lobe was especially firm.

Because of a concern about possible carcinoma, thyroid exploration was advised.

At operation the left lobe and a portion of the right lobe were found to be completely replaced by a white, hard, fibrous mass that was sharply delineated from normally thyroid tissue. Each lobe also contained a nodule. Cutting of the tissue produced very little bleeding. Most of the right lobe and the isthmus and the involved tissue on the left were resected. Pathologic examination showed a 40-g mass with a multinodular goiter, Riedel's struma, and ectopic bone formation in the resected portion of the left lobe.

Seventeen years later, she was seen again because of hoarseness, a sensation of choking, and difficulty in breathing. There was a firm nodule in the left side of the neck measuring 3 × 4 cm in diameter. BP was 170/100, and she had atrial fibrillation. Radiographs of the trachea showed no abnormality. Serum T_4 was normal. Fluorescent scan showed normal iodine content on the left and some iodine in the small remnants of the right lobe. The result of the radioisotope scan was similar. The RAIU was 11 percent. The TSH level was 5 μU/ml, and the LATS test result was negative. Other findings included left ventricular hypertrophy on electrocardiogram and mild hyperglycemia. Administration of thyroid hormone moderately improved the sensation of choking but did not significantly alter the size of the left lobe.

In contrast to the usual experience, Riedel's thyroiditis did not produce overt hypothyroidism during the 17 years after surgical resection of much of the gland involved in this process.

RARE INFLAMMATORY OR INFILTRATIVE DISEASES

In addition to the varieties of thyroiditis already mentioned, which are diseases specifically of the thyroid gland, generalized or systemic diseases may also involve the thyroid gland.[11] The lesions of sarcoid may appear in the thyroid gland of patients with systemic sarcoidosis, and huge deposits of amyloid occasionally cause goiter in amyloidosis. Radiation during ^{131}I therapy produces thyroiditis, which is occasionally symptomatic. This situation is discussed in Chapters 11 and 18. Irradiation to the thyroid during therapy for breast cancer or lymphoma can also induce hypothyroidism. Therapy should be directed toward the primary disease rather than the thyroid, but administration of thyroid hormone may be necessary if destruction of thyroid tissue is sufficient to produce hypothyroidism.

SUMMARY

The thyroid, like any other structure, may be the seat of an acute or chronic suppurative or nonsuppurative inflammation. Various systemic infiltrative disorders may leave their mark on the thyroid gland as well as elsewhere. Infectious thyroiditis is a rare condition, usually the result of bacterial invasion of the gland. Its signs are the classic ones of inflammation: heat, pain, redness, and swelling, and special ones conditioned by local relationships, such as dysphagia and a desire to keep the head flexed on the chest in order to relax the peritracheal muscles. The treatment is that for any febrile disease, including specific antibiotic drugs if the invading organism has been identified and its sensitivity to the drug established. Otherwise, a broad-spectrum antibiotic may be used. Surgical drainage may be necessary and a search for a pyriform sinus fistula should be made, particularly in children with thyroiditis involving the left lobe.

Subacute (granulomatous) thyroiditis is a more common and protracted disease that usually involves the thyroid symmetrically. The gland is swollen and tender, and the systemic reaction may be severe, with fever and an elevated erythrocyte sedimentation rate. During the acute phase of the disorder, tests of thyroid function disclose a diminished thyroidal RAIU and increased serum concentrations of T_4, T_3, and TG. The cause of this disease has been established in only a few instances in which a viral infection has been the initiating factor. There may be repeated recurrences of diminishing severity. Usually, but not always, the function of the thyroid is normal after the disease has subsided. Subacute thyroiditis may be treated with rest, nonsteroidal anti-inflammatory drugs or aspirin, and thyroid hormone. If the disease is severe and protracted, it is usually necessary to resort to administration of glucocorticoids, but recurrence may follow their withdrawal.

Riedel's thyroiditis is a chronic sclerosing replacement of the gland that is exceedingly rare. The process involves the immediately adjacent structures, making any surgical attack very difficult. The cause is unknown, and no treatment is available beyond resecting the isthmus of the thyroid gland to relieve the symptoms of tracheal or esophageal compression. Sarcoid may involve the thyroid, and amyloid may be deposited in the gland in quantities sufficient to cause goiter. In all of these diseases it may be necessary to give the patient levothyroxine replacement therapy if the function of the gland has been impaired.

REFERENCES

1. Hatabu H, Kasagi K, Yamamoto K et al: Acute suppurative thyroiditis associated with piriform sinus fistula: sonographic findings. Am J Med 155:845, 1990
2. Lucaya J, Berdon WE, Enriquez G et al: Congenital pyriform sinus fustula: a cause of acute left-sided suppurative thyroiditis and neck abscess in children. Pediatr Radiol 21:27, 1990
3. Miyauchi A, Matsuzuka F, Kuma K, Takai S: Piriform sinus fistula: an underlying abnormality common in patients with acute suppurative thyroiditis. World J Surg 14:400, 1990
4. Gandhi RT, Tollin SR, Seely EW: Diagnosis of *Candida* thyroiditis by fine needle aspiration. J Infect 28:77, 1994
5. Berger SA, Zonszein J, Villamena P, Mittman N: Infectious diseases of the thyroid gland. Rev Inf Dis 5:108, 1983
6. Fernandez JF, Anaissie EJ, Vassilopoulou-Sellin R, Samaan NA: Acute fungal thyroiditis in a patient with acute myelogenous leukemia. J Intern Med 230:539, 1991
7. Chiovato L, Canale G, Maccherini D et al: Salmonella brandenburg: a novel cause of acute suppurative thyroiditis. Acta Endocrinol 128:439, 1993
8. Nieuwland Y, Tan KY, Elte JW: Miliary tuberculosis presenting with thyrotoxicosis. Postgrad Med J 68: 677, 1992
9. Das DK, Pant CS, Chachra KL, Gupta AK: Fine needle aspiration cytology diagnosis of tuberculous thyroiditis. A report of eight cases. Acta Cytol 36:517, 1992
10. Hamburger JI: The various presentations of thyroiditis. Ann Intern Med 104:219, 1986
11. Singer PA: Thyroiditis. Acute, subacute, and chronic. Med Clin North Am 75:61, 1991
12. Szabo SM, Allen DB: Thyroiditis—differentiation of acute, suppurative and subacute. Case report and review of the literature. Clin Pediatr 28:171, 1989
13. Bach MC, Blattner S: Occult candida thyroid abscess diagnosed by gallium-67 scanning. Clin Nucl Med 15: 395, 1990
14. Hopwood NJ, Kelch RP: Thyroid masses: approach to diagnosis and management in childhood and adolescence. Pediatr Rev 14:481, 1993
15. Larsen PR: Thyroidal triiodothyronine and thyroxine in Graves' disease: correlation with presurgical treatment, thyroid status and iodine content. J Clin Endocrinol Metab 41:1098, 1975

16. Bernard PJ, Som PM, Urken ML et al: The CT findings of acute thyroiditis and acute suppurative thyroiditis. Otolaryngol Head Neck Surg 99:489, 1988

17. Georgiades N, Papadimas B: Echinococcus cyst of the thyroid. Helliniki Chir 5:575, 1962

18. Volpé R: The management of subacute (DeQuervain's) thyroiditis. Thyroid 5:253, 1993

19. Galluzzo A, Giordano C, Andronico F et al: Leucocyte migration test in subacute thyroiditis: hypothetical role in cell-mediated immunity. J Clin Endocrinol Metab 50:1038, 1980

20. Tamai H, Nozaki T, Mikuta T et al: The incidence of thyroid stimulation blocking antibodies during the hypothyroid phase in patients with subacute thyroiditis. J Clin Endocrinol Metab 73:245, 1991

21. Eylan E, Zmucky R, Sheba CH: Mumps virus and subacute thyroiditis. Lancet 1:1062, 1957

22. Satoh M: Virus-like particles in the follicular epithelium of the thyroid from a patient with subacute thyroiditis (deQuervain). Acta Pathol Jpn 25:499, 1975

23. Volpé R, Row VV, Ezrin C: Circulating viral and thyroid antibodies in subacute thyroiditis. J Clin Endocrinol Metab 27:1275, 1967

24. Bech K, Nerup J, Thomsen M et al: Subacute thyroiditis deQuervain: a disease associated with a HLA-B antigen. Acta Endocrinol 86:504, 1977

25. Vassilopoulou-Sellin R, Sella A, Dexeus FH et al: Acute thyroid dysfunction (thyroiditis) after therapy with interleukin-2 Horm Metab Res 24:434, 1992

26. Woolner LB, McConahey WM, Beahrs OH: Granulomatous thyroiditis (deQuervain's thyroiditis). J Clin Endocrinol Metab 17:1202, 1957

27. Czernick P, Harrell-Steinberg A: The chronology of events in the development of subacute thyroiditis, studied by radioactive iodine. J Clin Endocrinol Metab 17:1448, 1957

28. Fragu P, Rougier P, Schlumberger M, Tubiana M: Evolution of thyroid [127]I stores measured by X-ray fluorescence in subacute thyroiditis. J Clin Endocrinol Metab 54:162, 1982

29. Van Herle AJ, Uller RP, Matthews NL, Brown J: Radioimmunoassay for measurement of thyroglobulin in human serum. J Clin Invest 52:1320, 1973

30. Glinoer D, Puttemans N, Van Herle AJ et al: Sequential study of the impairment of thyroid function in the early stage of subacute thyroiditis. Acta Endocrinol 77:26, 1974

31. Gordin A, Lamberg BA: Serum thyrotrophin response to thyrotrophin releasing hormone and the concentration of free thyroxine in subacute thyroiditis. Acta Endocrinol 74:111, 1973

32. Intenzo CM, Park CH, Kim SM et al: Clinical, laboratory, and scintigraphic manifestations of subacute and chronic thyroiditis. Clin Nucl Med 18:302, 1993

33. Ingbar SH, Freinkel N: Thyroid function and the metabolism of iodine in patients with subacute thyroiditis. Arch Intern Med 101:339, 1958

34. Rapoport B, Block MB, Hoffer PB, DeGroot LJ: Depletion of thyroid iodine during subacute thyroiditis. J Clin Endocrinol Metab 36:610, 1973

35. Savoie JC, Massin JP, Thomopoulos P, Leger F: Iodine-induced thyrotoxicosis in apparently normal thyroid glands. J Clin Endocrinol Metab 41:685, 1975

36. Larsen PR: Serum triiodothyronine, thyroxine, and thyrotropin during hyperthyroid, hypothyroid, and recovery phases of subacute thyroiditis. Metabolism 23:467, 1974

37. Gluck FB, Nusynowitz ML, Plymate S: Chronic lymphocytic thyroiditis, thyrotoxicosis, and low radioactive iodine uptake: report of four cases. N Engl J Med 293:624, 1975

38. Gorman CA, Duick DS, Woolner LB, Wahner HW: Transient hyperthyroidism in patients with lymphocyte thyroiditis. Mayo Clin Proc 53:359, 1978

39. Woolf PD: Transient painless thyroiditis with hyperthyroidism: a variant of lymphocytic thyroiditis? Endocr Rev 1:411, 1980

40. Izumi M, Larsen PR: Correlation of sequential changes in serum thyroglobulin, triiodothyronine, and thyroxine in patients with Graves' disease and subacute thyroiditis. Metabolism 27:449, 1978

41. Riedel BMCL: Die chronische, zur bildung eisenhaster tumoren fuhrende entzudung der schilddrus. Verh Dtsch Ges Chir 25:101, 1896

42. de Lange WE, Freling NJ, Molenaar WM, Doorenbos H: Invasive fibrous thyroiditis (Riedel's struma): a manifestation of multifocal fibrosclerosis? A case report with review of the literature. Quart J Med 72:709, 1989

43. Zimmermann-Belsing T, Feldt-Rasmussen U: Riedel's thyroiditis: an autoimmune or primary fibrotic disease? J Intern Med 235:271, 1994

44. Schwaegerle SM, Bauer TW, Esselstyn CB Jr.: Reidel's thyroiditis. Am J Clin Pathol 90:715, 1988

45. Chopra D, Wool MS, Crosson A, Sawin CT: Riedel's struma associated with subacute thyroiditis, hypothyroidism, and hypoparathyroidism. J Clin Endocrinol Metab 46:869, 1978

46. Marin F, Araujo R, Paramo C et al: Riedel's thyroiditis associated with hypothyroidism and hypoparathyroidism. Postgrad Med J 65:381, 1989

47. Best TB, Munro RE, Burwell S, Volpe R: Riedel's thyroiditis associated with Hashimoto's thyroiditis, hypoparathyroidism, and retroperitoneal fibrosis. J Endocrinol Invest 14:767, 1991

The Iodine Deficiency Disorders

20

With the Collaboration of Basil Hetzel, M.D., North Adelaide, Australia

The term "iodine deficiency disorders" (IDD) is now used to denote all the effects of iodine deficiency on growth and development, particularly that of the brain, that can be prevented by correction of iodine deficiency.[1] In previous editions of this book the term "endemic goiter" has been used to describe the effects of iodine deficiency. The term iodine deficiency disorders (IDD) has now been generally adopted in the field of international nutrition and health. This reconceptualization has been one factor in drawing much more attention to the problem of iodine deficiency in the last 10 years.

This chapter describes the effects of iodine deficiency on growth and development. These can be considered at the various stages of life; the fetus, the neonate, the child, the adolescent, and the adult. Special reference is made to the relation of the thyroid to the brain, which has now become a major focus of research and the area of particular concern for prevention of brain disfunction and public health programs.

Iodine deficiency is now recognized as a global problem, with large populations living in environments where the soil has been deprived of iodine at risk. This depletion arose from the distant past through glaciation, compounded by the leaching effects of snow, water, and heavy rainfall, which removes iodine from the soil. The mountainous regions of Europe, the northern Indian subcontinent, the extensive mountain ranges of China, the Andean region in South America, and the lesser ranges of Africa are all iodine deficient. But in addition we now know that the soil of flooded river valleys is also deprived of iodine—as with the Ganges Valley in India, the Irawaddy Valley in Burma, and the Songkala Valley in northern China—which indicates that

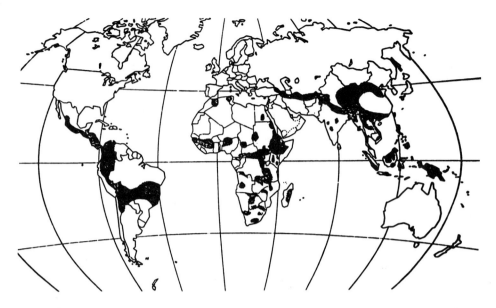

Fig. 20-1. Map showing worldwide distribution of IDD in developing countries. (from Hetzel,[5] with permission.)

the problem of iodine deficiency is more widespread than suspected. The deficiency in the soil leads to iodine deficiency in all forms of plant life and cereal grown in the soil. Populations living in systems of subsistence agriculture are, therefore, "locked into" iodine deficiency.[2]

The large populations at risk of IDD are in developing countries, particularly in Asia, Africa, and Latin America (Fig. 20-1). There is consensus that, in the developing world, a total population of at least 1 billion is at risk of IDD, (including 400 million in China) in excess of 200 million suffering from goiter and 5.7 million suffering from overt cretinism (Table 20-1).[3] In addition, there are three to five times the

number of individuals suffering from lesser degrees of brain damage. The estimate is in excess of 20 million suffering from varying degrees of brain damage in the developing world, due mainly to the effects of iodine deficiency in pregnancy. Significant populations in southern and eastern Europe, however, are still at risk to the effects of iodine deficiency. A more recent calculation including Europe estimates the total at-risk population to be in excess of 1.5 billion.[4] The elimination of IDD is recognized as feasible with available knowledge but its implementation remains a major challenge in international public health and nutrition.[2,3]

TABLE 20-1. Prevalence of IDD in Developing Countries and Numbers of Persons at Risk (In Millions)

	At Risk	Goiter	Overt Cretinism
Africa	227	39	0.5
Latin America	60	30	0.3
Southeast Asia	280	100	4.0
Asia (including China)	400	30	0.9
Eastern Mediterranean	33	12	—
Total	1,000	211	5.7

(From the World Health Organization,[3] with permission.)

THE IODINE DEFICIENCY DISORDERS IN THE LIFE CYCLE

The spectrum of the Iodine Deficiency Disorders (IDD) is shown in Table 20-2. All these effects are entirely preventable by correction of iodine deficiency.[1,2,5] This section contains a general description of these effects at the different stages of life. Reference will also be made to animal models. In the next section, specific attention is given to the most important types of IDD: endemic goiter, iodine induced hyperthyroidism, thyroid carcinoma, and endemic cretinism.

TABLE 20-2. The Spectrum of IDD

Fetus	Abortions
	Stillbirths
	Congenital anomalies
	Increased perinatal mortality
	Increased infant mortality
	Neurological cretinism (mental deficiency, deaf mutism, spastic diplegia, squint)
	Myxedematous cretinism (dwarfism, mental deficiency)
	Psychomotor defects
	Increased susceptibility of the thyroid gland to nuclear radiation (after 12 weeks)
Neonate	Neonatal goiter
	Neonatal hypothyroidism
	Increased susceptibility of the thyroid gland to nuclear radiation
Child and adolescent	Goiter
	Juvenile hypothyroidism
	Impaired mental function
	Retarded physical development
	Increased susceptibility of the thyroid gland to nuclear radiation
Adult	Goiter with its complications
	Hypothyroidism
	Impaired mental function
	Iodine induced hyperthyroidism
	Increased susceptibility of the thyroid gland to nuclear radiation

Iodine Deficiency in the Fetus

Iodine deficiency in the fetus is the result of iodine deficiency in the mother (Fig. 20-2). The condition is associated with a greater incidence of stillbirths, abortions, and congenital abnormalities, which can be reduced by provision of iodine. Many of the effects are similar to those observed with maternal hypothyroidism, and can be reduced by thyroid hormone replacement therapy[6], which of course provides both hormone and iodine to mother and fetus.

Another major effect of fetal iodine deficiency is endemic cretinism. This condition, which occurs when iodine intake is below 25 μg/d (compared to a normal intake of 100 to 150 μg/d) is still widely prevalent, affecting up to 10 percent of the populations living in severely iodine deficient areas in India, Indonesia, and China.[7] In its most common form, it is characterized by mental deficiency, deaf mutism, and spastic diplegia, which is referred to as

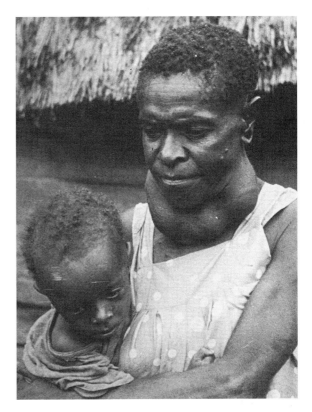

Fig. 20-2. A severely iodine deficient mother and child from a New Guinea village. The mother has a large goiter but the greater effect is on the child. The bigger the goiter, the more likely it is that she will have a cretin child. This can be prevented by correction of the iodine deficiency before pregnancy.

the "nervous" or neurologic type cretin in contrast to the less common "myxedematous" type characterized by hypothyroidism with dwarfism. (See *Specific Iodine Deficiency Disorders*, below.)

Cretinism also occurs in Africa and in South America in the Andean region (Ecuador, Peru, and Bolivia). In all these locations, with the exception of Zaire, neurologic features are predominant. In Zaire the myxedematous form is more common, probably due to the high intake of cassava (manioc or tapioka).[8] There is considerable variation, however, in the clinical manifestations of neurologic cretinism, which include isolated deaf mutism and mental defects of varying degrees.

The common neurologic form of endemic cretinism is not usually associated with severe clinical hypothyroidism, as is the case with myxedematous cretinism, although mixed forms with both the neurologic and myxedematous features do occur. Furthermore, the neurologic features are not reversed by the administration of thyroid hormones.[9]

Although isolated instances of cretinism can still be found, the apparent spontaneous disappearance of classic endemic cretinism in most of southern Europe raised considerable doubts as to the relation of iodine deficiency to the condition.[2] For this reason it was decided in 1966 to set up a controlled trial in the western highlands of Papua New Guinea to see whether endemic cretinism could be prevented by correction of iodine deficiency with the then recently available injection of iodized oil.[10] The study revealed that the injection of iodized oil given before pregnancy would prevent the occurrence of the neurologic syndrome of endemic cretinism in the infant (Fig. 20-3). The occurrence of the syndrome in those who were pregnant at the time of oil injection indicated that the damage probably occurred during the first half of pregnancy.[11] The controlled trial with iodized oil also revealed a significant reduction in recorded fetal and neonatal deaths in the treated group which is consistent with other evidence indicating the effect of iodine deficiency on fetal survival.[11] In a recent study from China, it was shown that in iodine deficiency, administration of iodine to pregnant women up to the end of the second trimester protects the fetal brain from the effects of iodine deficiency. Treatment later in pregnancy or after delivery may improve brain growth and developmental achievement slightly, but does not improve neurologic status.[12]

Further data from Papua New Guinea, indicates a relationship between the level of maternal thyroxine with the outcome of current and recent past pregnancies, including mortality and the occurrence of cretinism. There were proportionally more perinatal (i.e., stillbirths and neonatal) deaths and cretins among the offspring of women who showed the lowest levels of serum thyroxine.[13]

These data, indicating the importance of maternal thyroid function to fetal survival and development, are complemented by more recent studies. Study of experimental animal models,[14] and more recently in man,[15] indicate that there is a transfer of maternal thyroxine to the fetus early in pregnancy. It would seem likely, therefore, that the effects of iodine deficiency on the fetus are mediated by reduced transfer of maternal thyroxine before the onset of fetal thyroid function, and are not due solely to fetal defi-

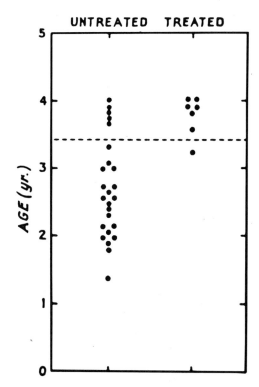

Fig. 20-3. The results of a controlled trial of iodized oil injection in the Jimi River District of the Highlands of Papua New Guinea. Alternate mothers were given an injection of iodized oil and saline in September 1966. All newborn children were followed for the next five years. Each dot represents a cretin child. The figure shows that mothers given iodized oil injections did not subsequently have cretin children, apart from those already pregnant at the time of injection. By contrast, cretinism persisted in the untreated group. (From Pharoah et al,[11] with permission.)

ciency of elemental iodine as originally suggested, because of the lack of evidence of transfer of T_4 at that time.[11]

Iodine Deficiency in the Neonate

An increased perinatal mortality due to iodine deficiency has been shown in Zaire from the results of a controlled trial of iodized oil injections alternating with a control injection given in the latter half of pregnancy.[16] There was a substantial fall in infant mortality with improved birth weight following the iodized oil injection. Low birth weight of any cause is generally associated with a higher rate of congenital anomalies and higher risk through childhood. This has been demonstrated in the longer term follow up of the controlled trial in Papua New Guinea in children up to the age of 12 years.[17]

Apart from mortality, the importance of the state of thyroid function in the neonate relates to the fact that the brain of the human infant at birth has only reached about one third of its full size and continues to grow rapidly until the end of the second year.[18] The thyroid hormone, dependent on an adequate supply of iodine, is essential for normal brain development as has been confirmed by the animal studies already cited. Recent data on iodine nutrition and neonatal thyroid function in Europe confirm the continuing presence of severe iodine deficiency which affecting neonatal thyroid function and, hence, poses a threat to early brain development.[19] A series of 1,076 urine samples were collected and analyzed from 16 centers from 10 different countries in Europe along with an additional series from Toronto, Canada.[19] The results of these determinations are shown in Table 20-3. The distribution was skewed so that arithmetic means were not used, but the results were expressed in percentiles. Some very high values were seen which could be attributed to the use of iodinated contrast media for radiologic investigation of the mother during pregnancy. There was a marked difference in the results from the various cities. The high levels in Rotterdam, Helsinki, and Stockholm differed from the low levels in Gottingen, Heidelberg, Freiburg, and Jena by a factor of more than 10. Intermediate levels were seen in Catania, Zurich, and Lille.

Data on neonatal thyroid function was analyzed for four cities where enough newborns (30,000 to 102,000) had been tested. The incidence of permanent congenital hypothyroidism was very similar in the four cities but the rate of transient hypothyroidism was much greater in Freiburg, associated with the lowest level of urine iodine excretion, than in Stockholm, with intermediate findings from Rome and Brussels. These data confirm the significance of iodine intake for neonatal thyroid function.

In developing countries with more severe iodine deficiency, observations have now been made using blood taken from the umbilical vein just after birth. Neonatal chemical hypothyroidism was defined by a T_4 level lesser than 3 μg/dl and TSH greater than 50 μU/ml.[20] In the most severely iodine deficient environments in northern India, where more than 50 percent of the population has urinary iodine levels below 25 μg per gram creatinine, the incidence of neonatal hypothyroidism was 75 to 115 per thousand births.[20] By contrast in Delhi, where only mild iodine deficiency is present with low prevalence of goiter and no cretinism, the incidence drops to 6

TABLE 20-3. Frequency Distributions of Urinary Iodine Concentrations in Healthy Full-Term Infants in 14 Cities in Europe and in Toronto, Canada

| City | Number of Infants | Urinary Iodine Concentration | | | Frequency (%) of Values Below 5 μg/dl |
		10th Percentile	50th Percentile	90th Percentile	
Toronto	81	4.3	14.8	37.5	11.9
Rotterdam	64	4.5	16.2	33.2	15.3
Helsinki	39	4.8	11.2	31.8	12.8
Stockholm	52	5.1	11.0	25.3	5.9
Catania	14	2.2	7.1	11.0	38.4
Zurich	62	2.6	6.2	12.9	34.4
Lille	82	2.0	5.8	15.2	37.2
Brussels	196	1.7	4.8	16.7	53.2
Rome	114	1.5	4.7	13.8	53.5
Toulouse	37	1.2	2.9	9.4	69.4
Berlin	87	1.3	2.8	13.6	69.7
Gottingen	81	0.9	1.5	4.7	91.3
Heidelberg	39	1.1	1.3	4.0	89.8
Freiburg	41	1.1	1.1	2.3	100.0
Jena	54	0.4	0.8	2.2	100.0

The European cities are listed according to decreasing values (50th percentile).
(From Delange et al.,[19] with permission.)

per thousand. In control areas without goiter the level was only one per thousand.

There is similar evidence from neonatal observations in neonates in Zaire in Africa where a rate of 10 percent of chemical hypothyroidism has been found.[21] This hypothyroidism persists into infancy and childhood if the deficiency is not corrected, with resultant retardation of physical and mental development.[22] These observations indicate a much greater risk of mental defect in severely iodine deficient populations than is indicated by the presence of cretinism. They provide strong evidence for the need to correct the iodine deficiency in Europe as well as in developing countries.

Another important aspect of iodine deficiency in the neonate and child is an increased susceptibility of the thyroid gland to radioactive fall-out. Delange[23] has shown that the thyroidal uptake of radioiodine reached its maximum value in the earliest years of life and then declined progressively into adult life. The apparent thyroidal iodine turnover rate was much higher in young infants than in adults and decreased progressively with age. In order to provide the normal rate of T_4 secretion, Delange has estimated that the turnover rate for intrathyroidal iodine must be twenty-five to thirty times higher in young infants than in adolescents and adults. In iodine deficiency a further increase in turnover rate is required to maintain normal thyroid hormone levels. This is the reason for the greatly increased susceptibility of the neonate and fetus to iodine deficiency. Iodine deficiency also causes an increased uptake of radioiodide, resulting from exposure to nuclear radiation. Protection against this increased uptake can only be provided by correction of iodine deficiency, which constitutes a further urgent indicator for the correction of iodine deficiency in Europe as well as in developing countries.

Iodine Deficiency in Childhood

Studies from a number of countries of schoolchildren living in iodine deficient areas indicate impaired school performance and IQs in comparison with matched groups from noniodine-deficient areas.[2]

More recently a meta-analysis of 100 studies, in which a comparison was made between the iodine deficient and the iodine sufficient groups, revealed that the mean scores were 13.5 IQ points apart.[24]

The differences in psychomotor development became apparent after the age of two and half years. In studies in China, lower intelligence quotient scores showed a relationship with nerve deafness, and the presence of abnormal neurologic signs similar to the pattern observed in overt neurologic cretins. It was concluded that iodine deficiency results in a shift of distribution of cognitive skills to a lower level for the entire population.[25]

The next question is whether these differences can be affected by correction of the iodine deficiency. In a pioneering study initiated in Ecuador in 1966, Feirro-Benitez et al.[26] studied the long-term effects of iodized oil injections by comparing observation in two highland villages: Tocachi was treated while La Esperanza served as a control. Particular attention was paid to 128 children aged 8 to 15 whose mothers had received iodized oil prior to the second trimester of pregnancy and a matched control group of 293 children of similar age. All children were periodically examined from birth at key stages in their development. The results indicated the significant role of iodine deficiency, but other factors were also considered to be important in the school performance of these Ecuadorean children, such as social deprivation and other nutritional factors. A controlled trial carried out with oral iodized oil in a small highland village (Tiquipaya) in Bolivia[27] showed improvement in IQ in those children who had significant reduction of goiter. This was particularly evident in girls. It was concluded that correction of iodine deficiency may improve the mental performance of school age children. These studies are now being followed up in a number of countries.

The major source of brain and pituitary T_3 is serum T_4. This contrasts with the liver, kidney, and muscle which derive a larger proportion of T_3 from the circulation[28] (see Ch. 3). Low levels of brain T_3 have been demonstrated in the iodine deficient rat in association with reduced levels of serum T_4 and these have been restored to normal with correction of iodine deficiency.[29] These animal studies are explanatory for suboptimal brain function in subjects with endemic goiter and lowered serum T_4 levels, and its improvement following correction of iodine deficiency. Thus, the relative increase in the secretion of T_3 from the thyroid glands of individuals exposed to low iodine does not adequately protect the brain.

Iodine Deficiency in the Adult

In Northern India, a high degree of apathy has been noted in populations living in iodine deficient areas. This may extend even to domestic animals, such as dogs. It is apparent that reduced mental function due to cerebral hypothyroidism is widely prevalent in iodine deficient communities which effects their residents' capacity for initiative and decision-making.[2] Clearly, iodine deficiency can be a major block to the human and social development of communities living in an iodine-deficient environment. An instructive example of the beneficial effect of iodine is provided by observations of the effect of an iodized salt program dating only from 1978 in the northern Chinese village of Jixian in northern Heilongjiang Province.[30] This village was locally regarded as "the village of the idiots." Between 1978 and 1983, productivity as measured by per capita income increased by a factor of 5; students' performance improved; recruits, for the first time, were provided for the People's Liberation Army—and girls from neighbouring villages were prepared to marry Jixian's men! True, this was also a time of significant economic development in China, but clearly the ability to benefit from such development required normal mental capacity.

Experimental Studies in Animals

Experimental studies on the effects of iodine deficiency in animals have confirmed the morphologic and biochemical modifications seen in the hyperplastic goiter of man (see below). More recently the effects of iodine deficiency on development, particularly those relating to the fetus, have been investigated. These studies on the rat, marmoset (*Callithrix jacchus jacchus*), and sheep have been particularly concerned with fetal brain development because of its relevance to the human problem of endemic cretinism and brain damage resulting from fetal iodine deficiency.

Iodine Deficiency in the Rat

Studies in rats using diets consumed in two endemic areas in China have been reported[31,32] following earlier work with artificial low iodine diets.[33,34] Extensive studies have been carried out using the diet consumed by the people of Jixian village by Li et al.[31]

This village was severely iodine deficient with 11 percent endemic cretinism. The diet included available main crops (maize, wheat), vegetables, and water from the area with an iodine content of 4.5 μg/kg. After the dam had received the diet for 4 months, there was obvious neonatal goiter, fetal serum T_4 was 3.6 μg percent compared to controls of 10.4 μg percent and they had higher ^{125}I uptake and reduced brain weight. The density of brain cells was increased in the cerebral hemispheres. The cerebellum showed delayed disappearance of the external granular layer with reduced incorporation of ^3H leucine in comparison to the control group.

Other more detailed studies have been carried out on the number and distribution of dendritic spines along the apical shaft of the pyramidal cells of the cerebral cortex of the rat.[35] These dendritic spines can be accurately measured and have been studied in relation to both iodine deficiency and hypothyroidism. Their appearance and development reflects the formation of synaptic contacts with afferents from other neurons. In normal rats there is a progressive increase in the number of spines from 10 to 80 days of age.

The studies have demonstrated a significant effect of an iodine deficient (Remington) diet on the number and distribution of the spines on the pyramidal cells of the visual cortex.[36] This effect is similar to that of thyroidectomy. More detailed studies following thyroidectomy indicated the importance of the timing of the procedure. If carried out before the tenth day of life, recovery is unlikely unless there is immediate replacement with L-T_4. At 40 or 70 days, replacement can restore a normal distribution of spines even if there is a 30 day delay in its initiation.[35] These differences confirm the need for early treatment of congenital hypothyroidism and prevention of iodine deficiency in the newborn infant. These effects at the neuronal level provide a firm basis for further studies of the effects of iodine deficiency at the subcellular and molecular level are now in progress.[37]

Iodine Deficiency in the Marmoset

Severe iodine deficiency has been produced in the marmoset (*Callithrix Jacchus Jacchus*) with a mixed diet of maize (60 percent), peas (15 percent), torula yeast (10 percent), and dried iodine deficient mutton

(10 percent) derived from the iodine-deficient sheep (described in the next section). The newborn iodine-deficient marmosets showed some sparsity of hair growth.[38] The thyroid gland was enlarged with gross reduction in plasma T_4 in both mothers and newborns, greater in the second pregnancy than in the first, suggesting a greater severity of iodine deficiency. There was a significant reduction in brain weight in the newborns from the second pregnancy but not from the first. The findings were more striking in the cerebellum with reduction in weight and cell number evident and histologic changes indicating, as in the rat and the sheep, impaired cell acquisition.[39] These findings demonstrate the significant effects of iodine deficiency on the primate brain.

Iodine Deficiency in the Sheep

Severe iodine deficiency has been produced in sheep[40] with a low-iodine diet of crushed maize and pelleted pea pollard (8 to 15 μg iodine/kg) which provided 5 to 8 μg iodine per day for sheep weighing 40 to 50 kg. The iodine deficient fetuses at 140 days were grossly different in physical appearance in comparison to the control fetuses. There was reduced weight, absence of wool growth, goiter, varying degrees of subluxation of the foot joints, and deformation of the skull (Fig. 20-4). There was also delayed bone maturation as indicated by delayed appearance of epiphyses in the limbs.[40,41] Goiter was evident from 70 days in the iodine-deficient fetuses and thyroid histology revealed hyperplasia from 56 days gestation, associated with a reduction in fetal thyroid iodine content and reduced plasma T_4 values. There was a lowered brain weight and DNA content as early as 70 days, indicating a reduction in cell number probably due to delayed neuroblast multiplication which normally occurs from 40 to 80 days in the sheep. Findings in the cerebellum were similar to those already described in rats.

A single intramuscular injection of iodized oil (1 ml = 480 mg iodine) given to the iodine deficient mother at 100 days gestation[41] was followed by partial restoration of the lambs brain weight and body weight with restoration of maternal and fetal plasma T_4 values to normal. The effects in the cerebellum and cerebral hemispheres are shown in Figure 20-5.

The effects of severe iodine deficiency on fetal brain development in the sheep were more severe

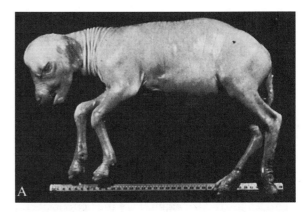
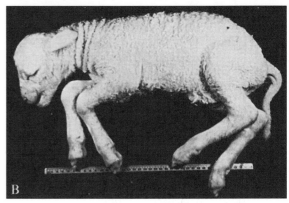

Fig. 20-4. Effect of severe iodine deficiency during pregnancy on lamb development. A 140-day-old lamb fetus (normal gestation period 150 days) was subjected to severe iodine deficiency (6A) through feeding the mother an iodine deficient diet (5 to 8 μg per day) for 6 months prior to and during pregnancy, compared to a control lamb given an iodine supplement (6B). The iodine deficient lamb shows absence of wool coat, subluxation of the leg joints, and a dome-like appearance of the head due to skeletal retardation. Compared to the control, the brain was smaller and contained a reduced number of cells. (From Hetzel and Potter,[41] with permission.)

but similar to those of fetal thyroidectomy carried out at 50 to 60 days.[41] Maternal thyroidectomy carried out about 6 weeks before pregnancy had a significant effect on fetal brain development in midgestation.[42] These data are in agreement with early observations of Man et al.[43] on human pregnancy, which demonstrated impaired intellectual performance in children born to hypothyroid mothers. They indicate the importance of maternal thyroid function for brain development consistent with pla-

CEREBELLUM   CEREBRAL HEMISPHERES

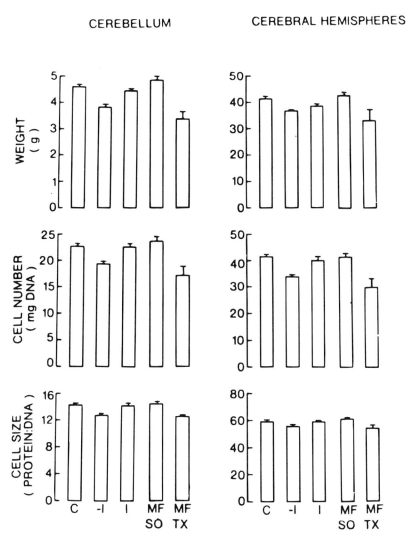

Fig. 20-5. Comparison of the brains of sheep fetuses at 140 days' gestation. The figure shows the effect of iodine deficiency, its reversal by iodized oil injection to the mother, and its reproduction by the effect of maternal and fetal thyroidectomy. C = control: −I = iodine deficient; I = iodine for 100 days; MFSO = mother + fetus sham operated; MFTX = mother + fetus thyroidectomised. (From Hetzel,[1] with permission.)

cental transfer of thyroid hormones. The combination of maternal thyroidectomy and fetal thyroidectomy at 98 days produces more severe effects than that of iodine deficiency and is associated with a greater reduction in both maternal and fetal thyroid hormone levels (Fig. 20-5). Thus, both maternal and fetal thyroid function are important for normal brain development. They confirm an early effect of iodine deficiency on neuroblast multiplication which could be significant in the pathogenesis of the neurologic form of endemic cretinism.[41,44]

SPECIFIC IODINE DEFICIENCY DISORDERS

Endemic Goiter

Epidemiology

The term endemic goiter is a descriptive diagnosis and reserved for a disorder characterized by enlargement of the thyroid gland in a significantly large fraction of a population group, and is generally considered to be due to insufficient iodine in the daily diet. Since nontoxic goiter also exists when there is abundant iodine in the diet, the distinction between endemic and nonendemic goiter is necessarily arbitrary. Endemic goiter may be said to exist in a population when more than 5 percent of the preadolescent (at 6 to 12) school-age children have enlarged thyroid glands, as assessed by the clinical criterium of the thyroid lobes being each larger than the distal phalanx of the subject's thumb. Detailed criteria are discussed further below.

Most of the significantly mountainous districts in the world are endemic goiter regions. The disease may be seen throughout the Andes, in the whole sweep of the Himalayas, in the Alps where iodide prophylaxis has not yet reached the entire population, in Greece and the Middle Eastern countries, in many foci in the People's Republic of China,[45] and in the highlands of New Guinea. There are also important endemias in nonmountainous regions, as for example, the belt extending from the Cameroon grasslands across northern Zaire and the Central African Republic to the borders of Uganda and Rwanda. An endemia existed in the Great Lakes region two generations ago. Measurements have indicated that these regions have in common a low concentration of environmental iodine. The iodine content of the drinking water is low, as is the quantity of iodide excreted each day by residents of these districts.

Goiter maps of various countries have been repeatedly drawn, requiring modification as successful prophylactic measures have been introduced. Although goiter was an important problem in many regions of the United States in the past,[46,47] more recent surveys have shown it in no more than 4 to 11 percent of schoolchildren, and with no evidence of iodine deficiency.[48] This finding is a testimony to the effectiveness of iodine prophylaxis in preventing endemic goiter.

The great arc of the Himalayas from west Pakistan across India and Nepal,[49,50] into northern Thailand[51] and Vietnam[52] and into Indonesia,[18] is one of the most highly endemic regions of the world. McCarrison made extensive studies of the Himalayan endemia in the early years of this century.[53] His epidemiologic findings have been confirmed in India by Ramalingaswami[49,54] and in Thailand by Suwanik[55] and their respective colleagues. The disease is a problem throughout the Andes.[56–58] Hercus and Roberts[59] have drawn a goiter map of New Zealand and have shown the incidence of goiter to be inversely proportional to the soil and food iodine. Such a map has also been drawn for Finland by Lamberg and his colleagues.[60] Goiter occurs in both domestic animals[61] and wild rodents[62] in conjunction with the disease in humans. The world distribution of goiter was exhaustively reviewed by Kelly and Snedden in 1960[62] and subsequently by others in 1980[63] and 1989.[2]

These surveys reveal striking differences in the rate of goiter in different endemic regions and even in adjacent districts. The geographic unevenness of an endemia undoubtedly has much to do with the habits of the population and their economic resources for the importation of foods. In attempting to account for the variability in the expression of endemic goiter from one locality to the next, the availability of iodine should be investigated before searching for some other subtle dietary or genetic factor. The key to the problem almost always lies in the availability of iodine. One must also consider the possibility that an observed goiter rate may not reflect current conditions, but rather may be a legacy of pre-existing iodine deficiency that has not yet been entirely resolved by an improvement in the supply of iodine.

The assessment of goiter in a population is discussed later in this chapter.

Causes

Iodine Deficiency

The arguments supporting iodine deficiency as the cause of endemic goiter are three: (1) the close association between a low iodine content in food and water and the appearance of the disease in the population; (2) the sharp reduction in incidence when iodine is added to the diet; and (3) the demonstration that the metabolism of iodine by patients with endemic goiter fits the pattern that would be expected from iodine deficiency and is reversed by iodine repletion. Further evidence lies in the observation that despite an assiduous search, no other seriously-considered cause has been identified. Finally, iodine deficiency causes changes in the thyroid glands of animals that are similar to those seen in humans. Almost invariably, careful assessment of the iodine intake of a goitrous population reveals levels considerably below the average in regions where the disease does not exist. Most reports place the mean between 15 and 40 μg/d urinary iodine excretion or 1.0 to 3 μg/dl. Severe iodine deficiency is still encountered up to the present. Thus, a mean iodine excretion as low as 24 and 31 μg per day in schoolchildren was reported from endemic goitrous regions in Sicily.[64] From two endemic goiter areas of Zimbabwe, mean iodine urinary excretion from adults was reported to vary between 1.0 and 2.1 μg/d.[65] In Senegal a mean iodine excretion of 17 μg/g creatinine (roughly equivalent to 24h) was also reported recently.[66] In the eastern part of Germany, a 24h iodine excretion of 16 μg has been recently reported.[67] This is only a small sample of many reports indicating that iodine deficiency, even in its severe form, is still present in many parts of the world.

From a pathophysiologic point of view, endemic goiter results from an excessive secretion of thyrotropic hormone. Whether this increased secretion is necessitated by an absolute dietary lack of iodine, or whether it is the aftermath of reduced thyroid function from some other cause such as ingestion of goitrogens, the end result is the same—namely, a stimulated and consequently enlarged thyroid gland. The TSH in the serum of patients with endemic goiter has been measured in many studies.[68-70] In some the values are moderately elevated, and on average they are higher than in control groups. A decrease in both the TSH concentration and the prevalence of goiter has been observed after correction of iodine deficiency.[71] A small but definite increase in the TSH level has also been reported in areas of mild or moderate deficiency.[72,73] Since iodine deficiency has been shown to increase the sensitivity of the thyroid to TSH, it is also possible that goitrogenesis can occur at serum TSH levels within the normal range.

Pathogenic Factors Other Than Absolute Iodine Deficiency

Although the relation of iodine deficiency to endemic goiter is well established, other factors may be involved. There are reasons to suspect that genetic factors and dietary goitrogens may also participate in the development of this condition.[74] A whole variety of naturally occurring agents have been identified that might be goitrogenic in man. Most of these have been tested in animals, have been shown to possess antithyroid effects in vitro, or both. These compounds belong to the following chemical groups.[75,76]: sulfurated organics (like thiocyanate, isothiocyanate, goitrin, and disulphides), flavonoids (polyphenols), polyhydroxyphenols and phenolderivatives, pyridines, phtalate esters and metabolites, polychlorinated (PCB) and polybrominated (PBB) biphenyls, other organochlorines (like DDT), polycyclic aromatic hydrocarbons (PAH), inorganic iodine (in excess), and lithium. Gaitan[76] divides goitrogens into agents acting directly on the thyroid gland and those causing goiter by indirect action. The former group is subdivided into those inhibiting transport of iodide into the thyroid (such as thiocyanate and isothiocyanate), those acting on the intrathyroidal oxidation and organic binding process of iodide and/or the coupling reaction (such as phenolic compounds), some phalate derivatives (disulfides and goitrin), and those interfering with proteolysis, dehalogenation, and hormone release (such as iodide and lithium).

Indirect goitrogens (such as 2,4-dinitrophenol, PCBs and PBBs) increase the rate of thyroid hormone metabolism. Soyabean, an important protein source in many third world countries, interrupts the enterohepatic cycle of thyroid hormone[77] and may cause goiter when iodine intake is limited. It should be recognized that goitrogens are usually active only if iodine supply is limited and/or goitrogen intake is of long duration.

Some of these goitrogens are synthetic and are used medicinally. Others occur in certain widely used food plants such as cabbage[78] and are discussed in Chapter 5. The initial recognition of dietary goitrogenesis is attributed to Chesney et al.[79] who in 1928 found that rabbits fed largely on cabbage developed goiters. In 1936, Barker[80] found that thiocyanate used in large doses to treat hypertension resulted in goiter. In 1936, Hercus and Purves,[81] reported their studies on the production of goiter in rats by feeding the seeds of several species of *Brassica* (rape, choumoellier, turnip, etc.). In 1943, both Mackenzie and MacKenzie[82] and Astwood[83] found that certain drugs such as thiourea and related compounds caused hyperplasia of the thyroid when administered to rats. Their investigations quickly led to the introduction of the thionamide series of antithyroid drugs, now so familiar in clinical therapeutics.

Thiocyanate and precursors of thiocyanate, such as the cyanogenic glycosides, form another group of widely distributed natural antithyroid substances. They have been found particularly in the widely used tuber cassava (manioc),[84] and in cabbage and other forms of brassica. Cassava causes goiter when fed to rats.[85] Certain sulfur-containing onion volatiles are also goitrogenic.[86] All of these substances interfere with the accumulation of thyroidal iodide, an effect that usually can be overcome by an increasing iodine intake.

Thilly and his co-workers[87] observed a striking difference in incidence of goiter in two regions of an isolated island in Kivu Lake in eastern Zaire. Although the iodine intake of both groups of ethnically identical people was approximately the same, there was a major difference in use of cassava. Delange, Ermans, and their colleagues have developed a strong case for cassava as the cause of endemic goiter, both in Zaire and in Sicily.[88–90] In a study of several communities in the Ubangi region of Zaire, they found an interesting relationship between goiter, on the one hand, and thiocyanate and iodide excretion, on the other. The thiocyanate was derived from intestinal breakdown of the cyanogenic glycoside, linamarin, from cassava and its conversion to thiocyanate by the liver. The results indicated a reciprocal relationship between iodide and thiocyanate, in that increasing amounts of iodide protected increasingly against the thiocyanate derived from the cassava. While it now seems well established that cassava may contribute to the severity of endemic goiter and probably the incidence of endemic cretinism, there are many severe endemics where cassava is not eaten. In these regions, it is possible that other goitrogens in the local food may contribute to the effects of a prevailing iodine deficiency. Cigarette smoking may cause goiter, possibly by inhaling thiocyanate.[91] Thiocyanate may cross the human placenta[92] and affect the thyroid of the fetus.

Excessive intake of iodine may itself cause goiter (see Ch. 5). A localized endemia has been reported on the coast of Hokkaido in northern Japan.[93,94] In this district the diet contained a huge amount of seaweed, and excretion of ^{127}I in the urine exceeded 20 mg/d. The uptake of RAI by the thyroid was low, and some of it could be discharged by administration of thiocyanate indicating impairment of organification. Similar findings have been reported from China.[45]

From Gaitain's review[95] it appears that firm evidence for goitrogenic action in humans has only

been shown for a few compounds: thiocyanate, goitrin, resorcinol, dinitrophenol, PBBs and their oxides, excess iodine, and high doses of lithium. Final proof for a definite role in endemic goiter has only been provided for sulfurated organics, although substantial and circumstantial evidence favors the view that natural goitrogens, acting in concert with iodine deficiency, may determine the pattern and severity of the condition.

Quite recently it has been shown that selenium deficiency may have profound effects on thyroid hormone metabolism and possibly also on the thyroid gland itself. In this situation the function of type I deiodinase (a selenoprotein) is impaired. Type I deiodinase plays a major role in T_4 deiodination in peripheral tissues (see Ch. 3). It has been shown[96,97] that when, in an area of combined iodine and selenium deficiency, only selenium is supplemented, serum T_4 decreases. This effect is explained by restoration of type I deiodinase activity leading to normalization of T_4 deiodination while T_4 synthesis remains impaired because of continued iodine deficiency.

Selenium deficiency also leads to a reduction of the selenium-containing enzyme, glutathione peroxidase. Glutathione peroxidase detoxifies H_2O_2, which is abundantly present in the thyroid gland as a substrate for the thyroperoxidase that catalyzes iodide oxidation and binding to thyroglobulin, and the oxidative coupling of iodotyrosines into iodothyronines (see Ch. 2). Reduced detoxification of H_2O_2 may lead to thyroid cell death.[98–101] Elevated H_2O_2 levels in thyrocytes may be more toxic under situations of increased TSH stimulation such as is present in areas with severe iodine deficiency. Last, but not least, decreased availability of glutathione peroxidase impairs thyroid hormone synthesis in the thyroid gland, a fact that could also contribute to decreased T_4 synthesis.

The Pathology of Endemic Goiter

There are no gross or microscopic features that distinguish the thyroid of endemic goiter from changes that may appear in simple and sporadic goiter. The changes evolve through stages. In the very young, or in older patients who have lived under constant iodide deprivation, the finding is extreme hyperplasia. In some instances only a cellular organ is found, with little or no colloid (Fig. 20-6). The evolution of pathologic findings in humans have been detailed

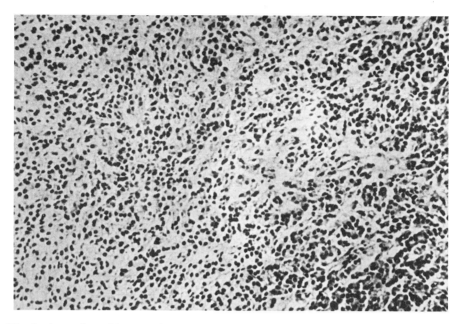

Fig. 20-6. Histologic section of large goiter removed because of pressure symptoms in Papua New Guinea, showing intense hyperplasia with no colloid. (From Buttfield and Hetzel,[10] with permission.)

and well illustrated by Correa[102] and Studer and Ramelli[103,104] and follow the pattern of events first described by Marine[105] and known as the *Marine cycle*. In this formulation, repeated episodes of hyperplasia induced by iodine deficiency are followed by involution and atrophy, the result being a gland containing a mixed bag of nodules, zones of hyperplasia, and involuting, degenerative, and repair elements. A laboratory model of endemic goiter has been produced in the hamster by exposing the animals intermittently to iodide deficiency.[106]

Diagnosis of Endemic Goiter

A diagnosis of endemic goiter implies that the cause is known, or at least strongly suspected. Usually water and food are found to have very low iodine content. The thyroid glands are often diffusely enlarged in childhood, but are almost always nodular in adults. The typical laboratory findings are elevated RAIU, normal or low T_4 and FT_4 levels, normal or elevated T_3 levels, normal or elevated TSH levels, and diminished urinary ^{127}I excretion. RAIU is typically suppressible when thyroid hormone is given, but not always. Scanning with radiodide or TcO_4^- shows a mottled distribution of the isotope. Serum thyroglobulin or thyroperoxidase antibodies

are usually absent. In an area of endemic goiter, the diagnosis can be presumed if the goiter is a community problem, but one must always be wary of missing individual patients with thyroiditis, thyrotoxicosis, or thyroid carcinoma.

Pathophysiology

The thyroid gland of a subject with endemic goiter has a high avidity for iodine.[107] A theoretic formulation of the relationship between dietary intake and thyroid avidity for iodine appears in Chapter 4, and this relationship has been confirmed many times. RAIU correlates inversely with the quantity of iodine excreted in the urine of patients in an endemic area. This result is illustrated by studies from Mendoza, Argentina.[107] There, patients with the smallest amount of stable iodine in the urine had the highest RAIU.

Compensation or adjustment to iodine deficiency is surprisingly good, providing the deficiency is not too severe. As recently reviewed,[107a] the ideal adaptation (i.e., more efficient hormone synthesis to ensure euthyroidism) is seen especially when no or only moderate goiter formation occurs. When large goiters ensue, however, adaptation is affected and *maladaptation* becomes the ultimate effect of iodine deficiency. The concentration of both T_4 and T_3 in the blood of patients from mildly endemic regions is often normal.[72] Nevertheless, in both rats and humans the initial response to a significant iodine deficiency is a fall in plasma T_4 levels. The pituitary is sensitive to plasma T_4, which is deiodinated to T_3 within the pituitary thyrotoph. The fall in plasma T_4 levels initiates an increased secretion of TSH, which in turn stimulates the thyroid to secrete an increased ratio of T_3 to T_4.[52,71,108–110] This action results in a normal or elevated concentration of T_3 in blood. Furthermore, normal serum T_3 levels in iodine deficiency may be maintained by increased T_3 production from T_4 in peripheral tissues[111] containing type II 5'deiodinase like the brain, as the activity of this enzyme is increased when serum T_4 falls (see Ch. 3). If the iodine deficiency is severe, the serum T_3 concentration may also fall. The iodine-deficient subject may appear to be euthyroid when the plasma T_3 is normal or elevated and the T_4 low, but this may not necessarily indicate euthyroid state. The iodine-deficient rat with normal serum T_3 concentrations may have reduced growth hormone, liver α glycerophosphate, and malic enzyme activity,[112–114] and may be sensitive to cold stress.[115] These results suggest the presence of at least mild hypothyroidism in some tissues. Supporting this view, it was recently reported that in iodine-deficient rats, tissue T_3 may be low despite normal levels of circulating T_3.[116] This was especially true for the brain, since this organ is dependent on T_3 generated from intracerebral T_4, a reaction catalyzed by type II deiodinase.[117] Although activity of this enzyme is increased in hypothyroxinemia, presumably as a compensatory mechanism to protect the brain from T_3 deficiency, intracerebral T_3 concentrations fall below normal if T_4 supply decreases substantially, as is the case in severe iodine deficiency.[118,119] Thus, while compensatory changes in TSH, the thyroid, and type II deiodinase can defend the organism against mild or moderate iodine deficiency, there is a limit to this capacity. The effects of iodine deficiency on brain development was the subject of a recent international meeting.[120]

In humans, T_4 values well below normal have been found in intensely endemic areas such as Zaire,[121] New Guinea,[122] the Himalayan region of North India, Nepal,[123] and North Algeria.[124] Vagenakis et al.[125] found that serum concentrations of T_4 were within the limits of normal in subjects with endemic goiter in Greece, but were lower than the average for a nonendemic region. T_3 concentrations in the goitrous individuals were significantly increased and TSH values were normal. In New Guinea, Patel et al.[126] found low T_4, and T_3 values ranging from low to elevated in goitrous persons. Serum TSH values correlated inversely with the serum T_4 concentrations, and those with goiter tended to have higher plasma levels of T_3. All had elevated levels of TSH[122] which returned to normal after administration of iodized oil.[127,128] Although a low T_4 level may reflect the severity of iodine deficiency, a relative increase in serum T_3 level, and possibly accelerated T_3 turnover, may maintain clinical euthyroidism. Several investigators have found normal or elevated plasma concentrations of T_3 but low T_4 levels in patients with severe endemic goiter.[21,72,126,129–131a] Since T_3 is the more potent hormone, these patients may appear to be metabolically normal, but the T_4 that is present probably makes a significant contribution to the final hormonal effect, as Chopra et al.[132] have shown.

Few clearly defined biochemical abnormalities have been detected in the thyroid glands of patients with endemic goiter. The most characteristic abnormality is a marked reduction of iodine concentration per gram of tissue, although total ^{127}I levels may be near normal or even high. There is no reservoir of unused inorganic iodide in these glands and no block in hormonogenesis, as is shown by the high iodine uptake and the failure of SCN^- or ClO_4^- to discharge previously accumulated RAI from the gland. Although low in iodine content, the proteins of the gland appear to be normal[133] except that an excess of a dense, insoluble iodoprotein different from TG or iodoalbumin has been found in some glands.[134] Recent reports suggest autoimmune phenomena playing a role in development of goiter in iodine deficiency. Iodine deficiency induces thyroid autoimmune reactivity in Wistar rats[135] and in histologic specimens of endemic goiters increased activity of antigen presenting cells was found,[136] and the presence of circulating thyroid growth stimulating immunoglobulins (TGI) in patients with endemic goiter has been reported,[137] but not found by others.[138] Doubts about a major role of TGI, if any, in the development of endemic goiter have been raised.[139–140b] A high incidence of thyroglobulin antibodies was found by some researchers. In goats in the Himalayan endemic region, more 27 S than 19

S TG becomes iodinated.[141] The same result occurs with the two components from normal thyroids, but 19 S TG is irreversibly converted to 27 S TG upon removal of sialic acid and galactose residues by glycosidase activity in the gland if the iodine content of the 19 S TG is high, but not if it is low. This activity would tend to increase the gland content of relatively high-iodine 27 S TG in the iodine-deficient gland[142] because the TG molecules of lower iodine content tend to escape the irreversible conversion to the 27 S fraction.[143]

No abnormal iodinated amino acid or other iodinated substance has been detected in the blood of patients with endemic goiter. In common with other situations in which there is hyperplasia, the monoiodotyrosine/diiodotyrosine (MIT/DIT) ratio in the thyroid may be high, and the quantity of iodothyronines may be quite low.[142] The increased MIT/DIT ratio presumably represents the effect of poor iodination of TG, as does the low iodothyronine/iodotyrosine ratio. The ratio of T_3 to T_4 in TG may be increased as a result of increased coupling of the available MIT to DIT residues. Some patients from endemic goiter zones exhibit marked heterogeneity in turnover of thyroid iodine—a small, rapidly turning-over pool providing most of the circulating hormone and a larger pool remaining relatively inert in the gland.[144,145] The response to TSH is normal,[130] but the response to TRH is increased suggesting compensated hypothyroidism.[146,147]

A search among euthyroid goitrous adults for inherited metabolic blocks in hormone biosynthesis or release has met with no success, except for the suggestive finding by Koutras et al. of an organification defect in certain individuals with endemic goiter in Greece.[148] Transport of iodide into the thyroid, organification of iodide, synthesis of TG, iodination and coupling of tyrosyl residues, and secretion of thyroid hormone all proceed qualitatively normally. Nor is there evidence of a deiodinase defect.[149] The extraordinarily wide range of total iodine content of these glands, which varies from a few micrograms in the whole gland to supranormal levels, is hard to understand. Nevertheless, the concentration of iodine per gram of gland is almost always lower than normal. Ermans et al.[150] have examined the intrathyroidal metabolism of iodine in patients with nontoxic goiter in Belgium. Their findings presumably also hold true for goiters from endemic regions, but their techniques have not yet been applied to such

glands. They found that, as the weight of the thyroid gland increases, there is a sharp reduction in the concentration of iodine, a fall in the DIT/MIT ratio, and a decreasing relative concentration of iodothyronine. Below a concentration of 0.1 percent iodine in TG, iodothyronine synthesis falls rapidly. Ermans et al.[150] considered that the increased size of the gland and the decreased concentration of iodine constituted, in effect, a positive feedback loop in the sense that as the iodine concentration decreased and the concentration of iodine in TG decreased, T_4 and T_3 synthesis become impaired and TSH release further accentuated the growth of the thyroid.

Iodine Induced Hyperthyroidism

An increase in the incidence of thyrotoxicosis has now been described following iodized salt programs in Europe and South America and use of iodized bread in Holland and Tasmania.[151–153] A few cases have been noted following iodized oil administration in South America. None have yet been described in New Guinea, or India. This is probably due to the scatter of the population into small villages with limited opportunities for observation,[154] and natural remission. The condition is largely confined to those over 40 years of age—a smaller proportion of the population in developing countries than in developed countries.

Detailed observations are available from the island of Tasmania.[152,155] Careful scrutiny of records in northern Tasmania revealed a rise in the incidence of thyrotoxicosis as early as 1964 associated with the rise in food imports and the introduction during 1963 of iodophors to the dairy industry.[152] There was a much larger rise in incidence from 1966 following the iodization of bread. It was clear that the increase was mainly seen in patients with toxic autonomous goiter and not Graves' disease.[155,156] A cohort effect was demonstrated because the peak was mainly composed of those over the age of 40 with life-long iodine deficiency and goiter with autonomous thyroid nodules which continued the rapid turnover of iodine after the increase in iodine intake. The findings were consistent with the original concept of Plummer and support the classical view of two types of hyperthyroidism—Graves' disease and Plummer's disease.[156]

Similar observations were subsequently made in Europe[156a] where the incidence of hyperthyroidism due to autonomy of the thyroid is much higher than in the United States. In Germany, 75 percent of hyperthyroidism is attributed to autonomous nodules with only 25 percent due to autoimmune disease.[157] This high rate reflects pre-existing, longstanding iodine deficiency which is now known to be highly prevalent in southern Europe. This form of hyperthyroidism should be regarded as predominantly an iodine deficiency disorder (IDD) since it is largely preventable. Its high prevalence in Europe provides a further indication for the correction of iodine deficiency. The costs of the diagnosis and treatment of thyroid disorders in the former Federal Republic of Germany have been estimated at DM 308 million for 1989.[157] This indicates that correction of iodine deficiency would be highly cost effective in Germany by preventing a major category of thyroid disorders. The same would apply to other countries.

Treatment of iodine induced thyrotoxicosis is effective with antithyroid drugs or, alternately, radioiodine is effective, provided that thyroidal uptake of ^{131}I is still high enough. Cardiac complications may occur because the condition is more common over the age of 40. The possibility of this condition in older age groups has been regarded as a contraindication to the correction of iodine deficiency in those over 40.[158] Use of iodized salt by older goitrous subjects may not be appropriate, although increased intake may still occur from increased iodine in milk and other sources in industrialized countries.

In Japan, where the intake of iodine from seaweed may be up to 5 mg/d, there is no evidence of an increased incidence of hyperthyroidism or of Hashimoto's disease.[159] These data provide strong reassurance that a higher intake of iodine can be tolerated, once the transition from a low intake to normal intake has been achieved and the cohort having hyperthyroidism due to autonomous nodules has been treated.

Thyroid Cancer in Relation to Iodine Deficiency

For many years thyroid cancer has been reported to be more frequent in autopsies from areas of endemic goiter than where iodine intake is adequate. Wegelin[160] found thyroid cancer in 1.04 percent of autopsies in Berlin in 1928, when goiter was endemic, but only 0.09 percent of autopsies in Berlin where endemic goiter was absent. Cuello et al.[161]

showed the incidence of anaplastic and follicular thyroid carcinoma in Colombia was greater than in the United States (Connecticut) but the incidence of papillary cancer appeared to be independent of iodine intake.[162]

Other studies show that follicular thyroid cancer is more common and papillary thyroid cancer is less common in iodine-deficient areas. Williams[163] has summarized these data which show that the ratio of follicular/papillary types exceeds 0.7 in iodine deficient areas, whereas in iodine sufficient areas, the ratio is 0.26 or below. Bubenhofer and Hedinger[164] reexamined all their cases of thyroid cancers from Zurich (1924–1974) and they found a relative reduction of anaplastic thyroid cancer after iodine prophylaxis. Different pathologists do not always agree on cancer classifications but slides of tissues from Argentina[165] before and after iodine prophylaxis were classified by the same two pathologists. Data from Argentina through the iodine transition period (1958–1967) and full prophylaxis (1967–1976) showed a relative reduction in anaplastic carcinoma and a decrease in the ratio of follicular/papillary carcinoma (Fig. 20-7).

TSH has an oncogene-like action,[166,167] and in cell cultures TSH has been shown to enhance expression of proto-oncogenes. Whether follicular cancer formation results from continuous and intense TSH action directly or synergistically through growth factors (as discussed in Ch. 17, the section: Other Thyroid-Stimulating Factors) is not known. As Van Middlesworth[168] points out, it is reasonable to consider that iodine deficiency may increase the invasiveness of thyroid cancer through TSH stimulation.

Endemic Cretinism

Epidemiology

This condition has been recognized for many centuries in the Alpine villages of Europe.[169] A survey carried out at Napoleon's order (1810) in what is now the Swiss canton of Valais, revealed 4,000 cretins among 70,000 inhabitants. This was followed by a series of surveys in virtually all cantons in the first half of the 19th century.[170] Deaf-mutism was well correlated with the prevalence of goiter and served as a marker for cretinism, which was variable in its manifestations and therefore hard to define. At the 1870 census in Switzerland, 24.5 per 10,000 inhabit-

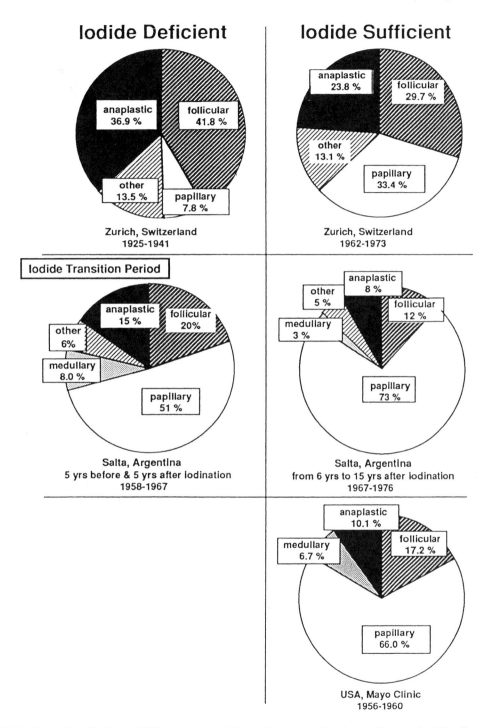

Fig. 20-7. Relative distribution of different types of thyroid cancer related to iodine intake. The figure shows the changing pattern of thyroid cancer after correction of iodine deficiency in Switzerland and Argentina. Data from an iodine sufficient area in the USA is shown for comparison (see text for further details). (From Middlesworth,[168] with permission.)

ants were deaf-mute, about three times more prevalent than in other European countries where cretinism was less common.[170]

When Sir Robert McCarrison described cretinism in northwestern India during the first decade of this century,[171] he delineated a *neurologic form*, with predominantly neuromotor defects, including strabismus, deaf-mutism, spastic diplegia, and other disorders of gait and coordination. The other form, which he called the *myxedematous form*, showed evidence of severe hypothyroidism, short stature, and markedly delayed bone and sexual maturation. The patient usually had a thyroid normal in size and position, and was seldom deaf.

The conditions result from two distinct pathologic processes that may coincide in the same individual. Usually the neurologic cretin is not hypothyroid. The condition is thought to result from maternal hypothyroidism affecting the fetus in the mid trimester of pregnancy. Myxedematous cretinism is the result of fetal hypothyroidism in late pregnancy and/or postnatal hypothyroidism.[22] The hypothyroid cretin resembles closely the sporadic cretin which occurs in all parts of the world due to an anatomic or biochemical anomaly of the thyroid. In contrast, the hypothyroid cretin occurs in the setting of severe iodine deficiency affecting a whole community with the full spectrum of IDD.

Neurological Cretinism

The three characteristic features of endemic cretinism in its fully developed form are mental deficiency, deaf-mutism, and motor spasticity with disorders of the arms and legs of a characteristic nature (Fig. 20-8). As would be expected with a deficiency disease, there is a wide range in the severity of the clinical features in the population affected. Recent studies by DeLong et al.[172] and by Halpern et al.[173] have provided new observations and insights.

Mental deficiency is characterized by a marked impairment of the capacity for abstract thought but vision is unaffected. Autonomic, vegetative, personal, social functions, and memory appear to be relatively well preserved except in the most severe cases.

Deafness is the striking feature. This may be complete in as many as 50 percent cretins. It has been confirmed by auditory brain stem evoked potential studies which showed no cochlear or brain stem responses even at the highest sound frequencies.

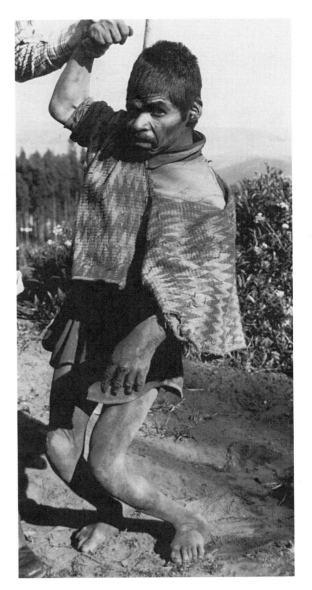

Fig. 20-8. Ecuadoran man about 40 years old, deaf-mute, unable to stand or walk. Use of the hands was strikingly spared, despite proximal upper-extremity spasticity. (From DeLong et al,[172] with permission.)

These findings suggest a cochlear lesion. In subjects with reduced hearing a high tone defect is apparent. Deafness is sometimes absent in subjects with other signs of cretinism. All totally deaf cretins were mute and many with some hearing had no intelligible speech.

The motor disorder shows a characteristic proximal rigidity of both lower and upper extremities and the trunk. There is a corresponding proximal spasticity with markedly exaggerated deep tendon reflexes at the knees, adductors, and biceps. Spastic involvement of the feet and hands is unusual or, if present, is much milder than that of the proximal limbs. Function of the hands and feet is characteristically preserved so that most cretins can walk. This observation is useful in differentiating cretinism from other forms of cerebral palsy commonly encountered in endemic areas, such as cerebral palsy from birth injury or meningitis.

In addition to frank cretinism, a larger proportion of the population (estimated to be three to five times as great) suffers from some degree of mental retardation and coordination defect. Comparative population based neuropsychological assessments of children in areas of iodine deficiency compared with areas with adequate iodine intake confirm a shift of the intelligence curve to the left in the iodine deficient areas. Careful examination of affected individuals in such areas reveals a pattern of neurologic involvement similar to that seen in frank cretins, although of milder degree.[25,173] In assessing these less severe defects, nonverbal tests are most helpful and school progress is a good indicator. After the age of 3 years drawings are very useful, indicating a defect in visual motor integration.

On the basis of his clinical observations, DeLong[45] suggests that the neuropathologic basis of the clinical picture includes underdevelopment of the cochlea for deafness; maldevelopment of the cerebral neocortex for mental retardation; and maldevelopment of the corpus striatum (especially putamen and globus pallidus) for the motor disorder. The cerebellum, hypothalamus, visual system, and hippocampus are relatively spared. Studies of human cretin brains by modern techniques are badly needed.

Pathophysiology

Developmental neuropathology and available epidemiologic data suggest that the period from about 12 to 14 weeks until 20 to 30 weeks of gestation may be the critical period during which damage occurs. Cortical and striatal neuron proliferation, migration, and early formation of neuropil occur between 12 and 18 weeks. Cochlear development occurs at the same time. These data correlate well with the data from the Papua New Guinea trial which indicated that iodine repletion must occur by three months of pregnancy to prevent cretinism.[11]

Studies already cited above on the effect of iodine deficiency on brain cell development in the newborn rat, sheep, and marmoset suggest that iodine deficiency has an early effect on neuroblast multiplication. Brain weight is reduced with a reduced number of cells as indicated by lowered DNA, a greater density of cells in the cerebral cortex, and reduced cell acquisition in the cerebellum.[14,174] In the light of the recent evidence that maternal thyroxine crosses the placenta,[15] it is now thought that neurologic cretinism is predominantly caused by maternal hypothyroidism due to iodine deficiency and hypothyroid cretinism by impaired fetal thyroid function. Recently it was found that an autosomal recessive predisposition, besides maternal iodine deficiency, may play an etiologic role in neurologic cretinism.[175]

Administration of PTU to pregnant mice also causes abnormalities in their pups in the tectorial membrane of the organ of Corti and results in deafness.[176] These experiments strongly suggest that it is the hypothyroidism per se that somehow damages the developing auditory system, causing deafness and other neurologic defects that are found characteristically in the endemic cretin. Patients with Pendred syndrome (see Ch. 16) also have goiter and deaf-mutism. Characteristically, when given SCN^- or ClO_4^-, a store of trapped but not yet oxidized iodide is discharged. There is no evidence that the Pendred syndrome can account for the deafness associated with endemic goiter.

Myxedematous Cretinism

The typical myxedematous cretin (Fig. 20-9) has severe mental and growth retardation, incomplete maturation of the features, myxedematous, thickened skin, and much delayed sexual maturation.[177] Movements are torpid, and the reflex relaxation is much prolonged. Radiographic studies disclose marked skeletal immaturity, with epiphyseal and metaphyseal dysgenesis. Electrocardiographic findings are consistent with myxedema. The thyroid is often atrophied and usually not much enlarged. Concentrations of T_4 in serum are low, and TSH levels are markedly elevated. Values for serum T_3 may be low in these patients.[21] RAIU is somewhat reduced below that of normal persons in the community. The scan shows a thyroid that is normal in size and position, but severely hypothyroid cretins show thyroid atrophy on ultrasound.[178]

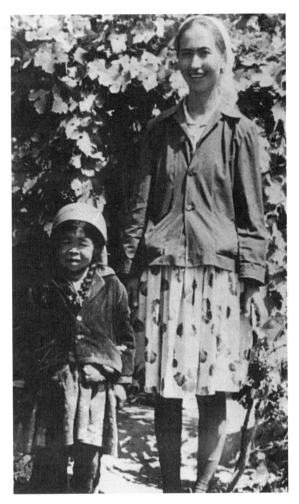

Fig. 20-9. Severe IDD: a dwarfed cretin woman with a "barefoot doctor" of the same age (35 years) from the Hetian district, Xinjiang, China. (Courtesy of Dr. Ma.)

Myxedematous cretinism is particularly common in Zaire where its higher incidence is attributed to cassava intake.[22] Two different mechanisms that may explain the myxedematous form have been advanced recently: autoimmunity based on the finding of growth-blocking immunoglobulins present in this type of cretin[179,180,181] and the coexisting selenium deficiency in areas of iodine deficiency.[98] Selenium deficiency results, among other things, in decreased thyroidal levels of glutathione peroxidase that detoxifies H_2O_2. Increased levels of H_2O_2 are damaging to the thyroid gland.[100,101] This combined deficiency is present in northern Zaire, an area known for its predominance of the myxedematous form of

cretinism.[98] Doubts about the role of thyroid autoimmunity in the pathogenesis of myxedematous cretinism have very recently been raised.[181a]

ASSESSMENT OF THE IDD STATUS OF A POPULATION

The assessment of the IDD status of a population is the basis for the development of a national IDD control program. Once an IDD control program has been initiated, monitoring and evaluation are required. The latter provide the basis for a program improvement.[2,182]

There are three major components of the data collection required for assessment and monitoring an iodine-deficient population. They are (1) the determination of thyroid size and estimation of the prevalence of goiter; (2) the determination of the urine iodine excretion; (3) the determination of the level of T_4 and TSH in the blood.

Apart from the techniques involved in these procedures, selection and sampling of the population has to be carried out using accepted criteria to provide valid indicators of the status of the population being studied. In general, observations have often been made on school children as one of the most vulnerable groups. A total sample of 200 children in the age range 10 to 14 years will suffice. Randomization is required to cover the variable distribution of goiter, which is related to hilly or mountainous terrain. This and other epidemiologic aspects are discussed more fully elsewhere.[182,183] Apart from these biologic aspects there is a need for assessment of the production and distribution of salt.

The Determination of Thyroid Size

The current definition of goiter[183] and the accepted criteria for estimation of thyroid size are summarized in Table 20-4. Earlier recommendations[184] have now been simplified. The problem of reproducibility of assessment by palpation, however, especially with the size estimation of smaller glands, particularly in children, has led to the use of more objective methods. The method of choice is now ultrasonography[185] which is reproducible with a maximum deviation of +10 percent.[186] Ultrasonography can be used repeatedly for assessing thyroid size and morphology. No untoward effects have been re-

TABLE 20-4. Proposed Classification of Goiter

Classification	Description
Grade 0	No palpable or visible goiter.
Grade 1	Mass in the neck that is consistent with an enlarged thyroid that is palpable but not visible when the neck is in the normal position. Moves upward in the neck as the patient swallows. Nodular alteration(s) can occur even when the thyroid is not enlarged.
Grade 2	Swelling in the neck that is visible when the neck is in a normal position and is consistent with an enlarged thyroid when the neck is palpated.

(From WHO/UNICEF/ICCIDD,[183] with permission.)

ported. Ultrasonography becomes inaccurate in large nodular goiters, since the formula applied for calculation is based on an ellipsoid model. Retrosternally located goiters, although detectable, cannot be precisely quantified by ultrasonography. For epidemiologic or clinical purposes, however, these limitations are negligible. In epidemiologic studies sonography can be performed on sitting subjects. Up to 200 individuals can be checked per day.

For surveys, a small portable apparatus weighing less than 10 kg is convenient. Transducers of 5 to 7.5 MHz are required to obtain a satisfactory resolution. Further details of the methodology are available elsewhere in references dealing with the public health aspect of such surveys.[183,186]

Urine Iodine Determination

The measurement of urine iodine excretion provides the best single measurement of the iodine intake of the population.[2,182] It can be used for both initial and follow up assessments.

Various methods are available using different procedures for the removal of chromogens and other substances such as thiocyanate which interfere with the sensitive colorimetry of the Sandell-Koltoff reaction.

Available methods have been reviewed by Bourdoux[187] and by Dunn et al.[188] The most practical and simple method involved mild acid digestion and colorimetric procedures timed with a stopwatch. Using this procedure some 150 samples can be processed in one day. The more traditional method of dry ashing is much more time consuming.

For epidemiologic studies a population distribu-

tion is required rather than individual levels. This means that less precision is needed, provided 40 different casual samples are taken from a particular group.[189] There is no need for the more difficult 24-hour urine collections. Casual samples from schoolchildren can be collected at the same time as the goiter is assessed.

In the past, levels have often been expressed per gram of creatinine excretion. More recent studies[182,187] have indicated that the creatinine level is variable depending on the general nutritional status of the population. This contributes an independent source of variation which invalidates the ratio. Urinary creatinine also decomposes after three days without refrigeration, whereas urine iodine remains stable for months. The values can be most conveniently expressed as a range with a median or by the proportions at a series of cut off points: less than 2 μg per dl, less than 5 μg per dl, and less than 10 μg per dl.[187]

Measurement of Thyroid Hormones

The serum thyroid hormone levels are a further index of the effects of iodine deficiency. Difficulties in obtaining venous blood samples, however, have often been encountered in populations due to apprehension about blood collection. By contrast, the use of whole blood from finger pricks, spotted on filter paper cards as for congenital neonatal hypothyroid screening, is well established in western countries. T_4 and T_3 in dried blood spots exposed to the natural environment are less stable, lasting only a few days.[189] One major advantage of TSH monitoring is that these specimens are stable and may be shipped long distances over periods of a month or more.[190] The use of this technology has now been applied to field conditions in countries such as India,[20] Zaire,[21] China, Indonesia, and Thailand. Rapid developments in technology for the measurement of T_4, T_3, and TSH by immunoassay have occurred with improved sensitivity, improved precision, greater convenience, and reduced costs. Developments in automation make the processing of large sample numbers feasible. The adaptation of the sensitive TSH assays to blood spots shows considerable promise in epidemiologic studies of iodine deficient populations.[154] This means TSH can be measured across the whole range from the low normal physiologic levels to the high levels of obvious

TABLE 20-5. Summary of IDD Prevalence Indicators and Criteria for a Public Health Problem

Indicator	Target Population	Severity of Public Health Problem (Prevalence) (%)		
		Mild	Moderate	Severe
Goitre Grade > 0	SAC*	5.0–19.9	20.0–29.9	≥30.0
Thyroid volume > 97th percentile by ultrasound	SAC	5.0–19.9	20.9–29.9	≥30.0
Median urinary iodine level (ug/dl)	SAC	5.0–9.9	2.0–4.9	<2.0
TSH > 5 mU/l whole blood	newborns	3.0–19.9	20.0–39.9	≥40.0

* SAC, school-aged children.
(From WHO/UNICEF/ICCIDD,[183] with permission.)

hypothyroidism. Such an approach uses all the TSH values in the population being monitored and does not rely solely on the levels observed in overt hypothyroidism to define the iodine status of the population.

At present it is believed that targeting the neonatal group gives the best hormonal indicator on the severity and risk of iodine deficiency disorders in the population. Women in the reproductive age group may also be a valuable target group but more information needs to be generated to enable a full assessment to be made. Using these three major criteria the severity of an endemic of iodine deficiency can be assessed. Three categories are now recognized: mild, moderate, and severe IDD.[183,191] (Table 20-5). Special and urgent attention needs to be given to areas of severe IDD in view of the need to prevent brain damage in fetuses and young children.

IODINE TECHNOLOGY

Iodized Salt

There are two forms of iodine which can be used to iodize salt: "iodide" and "iodate" usually as the potassium salt. Iodate is less soluble and more stable than iodide and is therefore preferred for tropical, moist conditions. Both are generally referred to as "iodized" salt.

The advantage of supplementing salt is that it is used by all sections of a community irrespective of social and economic status. It is consumed as a condiment at roughly the same level throughout the year. Its production is often confined to a few centers which means that processing can occur on a larger scale and with better controlled conditions. This is often not the case, however, in developing countries.

The minimum daily requirement of iodine is only 100 to 150 μg per person. The level of iodination of salt has to be sufficient to cover this requirement together with losses from the point of production to the point of consumption including the expected shelf life. It also has to take into account the per capita salt consumption in an area. Previously, generally accepted levels of salt consumption in the range 10 to 15 g per day are now regarded as excessive because of the increased liability to hypertension. For this reason, levels in the range of 3 to 5 g per day are being recommended in western countries. Iodinated salt will also be needed as a feed supplement for cattle and other livestock in iodine-deficient areas. Allowing for these factors, the level of iodine as iodate being used at present to provide 150 μg of iodine by day is in the range of 20 to 60 mg per kg.

The packaging of the iodized salt is very important. Jute bags have been used extensively but in humid conditions, the salt absorbs moisture. The iodate dissolves and will drip out of the bag if it is porous, with a heavy loss. This has been found to reach 75 percent over a period of nine months. To avoid this, waterproofing is required, achieved by either a polythene lining inside the jute bag or the use of a plastic bag. The additional cost of a plastic bag (50 to 80 percent more) would be justified by reduced losses and their resale value.[192]

Present Status of Iodized Salt Programs

Iodized salt was first introduced in Switzerland and in the United States in the 1920s when it was shown to be a successful measure.[170] New Zealand followed in 1941 but only very low levels were used in the first 20 years. Then in the 1950s and the 1960s a number of European countries followed with the expected benefits.

In general, iodination of salt was a simple procedure in these countries because the salt industries were large operations with automated refining plants. The addition of iodine was possible at little extra cost and production could be readily achieved.

It was with confidence from this experience that salt iodination programs were initiated in several Central and South American countries. In Guatemala, Colombia, Argentina, and Chile considerable progress was made with the control of IDD. There is recent evidence, however, of recurrence of the IDD problem in Guatemala and Colombia associated with social and political unrest. The initiation and successful maintenance of a public health program clearly is dependent on political stability. More recent studies in Europe have indicated serious defects in iodine nutrition in many countries. A review by a specially appointed committee of the European Thyroid Association[182] revealed that there is evidence of serious iodine deficiency of national significance in the Federal Republic of Germany (FRG), the former German Democratic Republic (GDR), Italy, Spain, Portugal, Rumania, Greece, and Turkey. None of these countries has a national iodinated salt program. There is evidence of a moderate to severe grade of IDD in all these countries. In Austria, Hungary, Poland, and Yugoslavia there are substantial areas with high goiter prevalence despite an iodinated salt program. This is due to inadequate Kl content (10 mg/kg) as the dietary iodine remains low. Increase to 20 mg Kl/kg was recommended in the report. These countries compare unfavorably with the complete control of IDD that has been achieved by Switzerland[170] and the Scandinavian countries.[193]

The report concluded that there is clearly a need for more effective national IDD control programs in all these countries. These programs are the responsibility of national governments. They will not succeed without the full political support of the Department of Health with appropriate cooperation from other relevant departments (Education, Media, Industry). An educational component is most important in view of the sensitivity of the social issue of food additives. This is despite the fact that iodine is an essential element and therefore an essential dietary ingredient at a level of 100 to 200 μg per day to maintain a normal output of thyroid hormones. The maintenance of an adequate level of iodination of salt requires continuous monitoring at the site of production, distribution, and consumption.

The report also pointed out that there was a need for continuous monitoring of iodine nutrition and the prevalence of IDD in schoolchildren at national and regional level in those countries with a continuing IDD problem. Suitable laboratories are required for the determination of urine iodine. Switzerland has achieved complete control of severe IDD with a well monitored iodized salt program.[170] This is a fine example to other countries. In 1993 an international meeting was held in Brussels[194] under the title "Iodine Deficiency in Europe: A Continuing Concern." This meeting was supported by many international bodies including UNICEF, WHO, NATO, the International Council for Control of Iodine Deficiency Disorders (ICCIDD, see below), the European Thyroid Association, and others. It was concluded that iodine deficiency was presently under control in Austria, Finland, Norway, Sweden, and Switzerland. Marginal or focal iodine deficiency was present in Belgium, former Czechoslovakia, Denmark, France, Hungary, Ireland, Portugal, and the United Kingdom. Iodine deficiency has recurred in Croatia, the Netherlands, and possibly other European countries. Moderate to severe iodine deficiency still persists in all other European countries: Bulgaria, the Common Wealth of Independent States, Germany, Greece, Italy, Poland, Romania, Spain, and Turkey. In other words, in most European countries iodine deficiency has recurred or still persists.

Special recommendations were made in order to eliminate iodine deficiency by the end of the century. Both the governments and the European community were called upon to initiate adequate legislation and other necessary measures to ensure the availability and use of iodized salt, which was considered to be generally the most appropriate measure for iodine supplementation. It was especially recommended that in pregnant and lactating women daily iodine intake should be at least 200 μg/day and 90 to 120 μg/day in young infants. To reach these objectives the mother's diet should be systematically supplemented with iodine whenever necessary, by vitamins/mineral tablets as prescribed by physicians. Since breast milk is the best source of iodine for the infant, exclusive breast feeding for 4 to 6 months should be encouraged. When infants require formula, the iodine content of the formula milk should be increased to 10 μg/dl for full term and 20 μg/dl for premature babies.

Use in Developing Countries

In Asian countries, salt iodization has not been successful, even after promising pilot programs in the Kangra Valley in India carried out by Sooch and Ramalingaswami and their colleagues between 1956 and 1972.[195] There have been great difficulties in the transfer of these successful results from populations of thousands to population of millions. A review of the IDD control situation by the Nutrition Foundation of India in 1983 revealed a major shortfall in production.[196] In fact only 15 percent of the total requirement for iodated salt was being produced. Obstacles identified then and since include gross ignorance both at a professional and consumer level of the effects of iodine deficiency on brain development, thousands of traditional small producers of salt, poor quality of salt leading to loss of iodine, poor packaging, and inadequate monitoring of salt at the retail and consumer level.

These problems are now being seriously addressed. In India there has been a remarkable improvement with the production of 2.5 million tons of iodized salt in 1991–92, an increase by a factor of 10 from 1983. Problems of transportation from the salt fields of Gujarat, Rajasthan, and Tamil Nadu to the subHimalayan belt have been largely overcome by better packaging and consignment of the salt as a priority in the railroad system.

The major requirement is for the iodized salt pro-

gram to be the responsibility of a multisectoral agency with political authority from the government. Such an agency must include adequate representation from the salt industry. Public education, planning, implementation, monitoring, and evaluation of the program must all be addressed.

Iodized Oil

Iodized oil ("lipiodol") was first used for the correction of iodine deficiency in Papua New Guinea as the result of a suggestion by a chest physician, Dr. Douglas Jamieson, in the late 1950s, to the then Director of Public Health, Dr. John Gunther.[2] The well known delay in excretion of the oil following its use for radiologic investigation suggested to Jamieson that this could be useful for the correction of iodine deficiency as a depot injection. Gunther requested Dr. Terry McCullagh carry out a controlled trial. After a preliminary study in a few subjects in Melbourne indicated the effects on thyroid function persisted over 2 years, it was decided to set up a controlled trial in the Boana area of the Huon Peninsula of New Guinea.[2] After a three year period, McCullagh carried out a double blind follow-up which revealed successful prevention of goiter.[197] In subsequent laboratory studies on the same population, Buttfield and Hetzel[10] demonstrated both severe iodine deficiency and the effectiveness of the single iodized oil injection (4 ml) in correcting iodine deficiency for a period of up to 4.5 years (Table 20-6).

A further advantage has been the subsidence of established goiter within one to three months of the

TABLE 20-6. The Effect of Iodized Oil on Thyroid Function in New Guinea Subjects[a]

Group	Urinary Iodine (μg/24 h)	[131]I Uptake (% at 24 h)	Serum PBI (μg/100 ml)
Untreated	11.5–12.4 (91)[b]	70–19 (181)	4.1–2.1 (204)
Treated 18 months before	119–114 (18)	31–20 (51)	8.2–2.6 (27)
Treated 3 years before	35–25 (29)	37–19 (43)	7.8–1.6 (52)
Treated 4 years before	23–21 (11)	44–18 (67)	6.4–2.4 (43)
Australian normal range	70–140	16–40	3.6–7.2

[a] Statistical analysis showed highly significant differences between the treated and untreated groups in urinary iodine. [131]I uptake and serum PBI (P < 0.001).
[b] Number of subjects.
(From Buttfield and Hetzel,[10] with permission.)

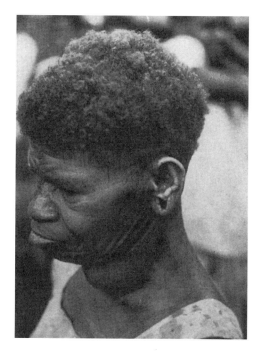
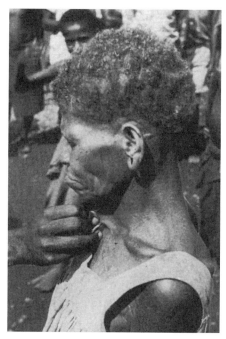

Fig. 20-10. Nodular goiter in a New Guinean (A) before and (B) three months after injection of iodized oil. The photos demonstrate the subsidence of goiter following the injection of iodized oil. (From Buttfield and Hetzel,[10] with permission.)

injection (Fig. 20-10). This is much appreciated by the goitrous subjects. When coupled with increased energy and well being consequent on the correction of hypothyroidism, there has been continued demand for the measure, originally in Papua New Guinea, and in many other countries since.

As the populations covered have increased, the injection dosage has been reduced to lower levels. Recent recommendations are 0.5 ml (240 mg) for children in the first year of life and 1 ml (480 mg) for all older subjects. Even a dose as low as 200 mg has been suggested to be sufficient for prophylaxis for one year in adults.[197a] Several studies from Latin America and Africa have shown that 1 ml will correct iodine deficiency for a minimum of 3 years. A dose of 3 ml will give coverage for 3 to 4 years. A larger dose will be indicated if the iodine deficient community lives in a more remote area in view of the transport costs of the injection team.

In excess of 20 million injections of iodized oil have been given since 1974 with very little in the way of side effects apart from a rare abscess at the site of injection. Refrigeration is not required, which is

a great advantage. Iodized oil is certainly an effective means for the correction of iodine deficiency and has opened up the possibility of elimination of IDD as a public health problem in the next decade. The necessity for an injection has been questioned, however, in view of the costs of the syringe and needles and the necessity to have specially trained staff give the injections. If the staff are readily available through the primary health care system, then the costs are comparable to those of iodated salt: 5 to 10 U.S. cents per person per year. On the other hand, if the oil can be given orally it would be possible to use village health volunteers to supervise the administration of the oil. This would make it much more readily available to village communities with severe IDD problems. Another advantage of the oral preparation is the freedom from the risk of AIDS or hepatitis B infection from contaminated syringes, although this should be eliminated by the proper sterilization of needles or use of disposable syringes. Recent experience has confirmed the convenience of the oral administration of iodized oil at yearly intervals through the primary health care system at a village level.[5] In general the effect of oral administration lasts half the time of the same dose given by injection.

Target Groups

An iodized oil supplementation program is necessary when other methods have been found ineffective or can be considered to be inapplicable. Iodized oil can be regarded as an emergency measure for the control of severe IDD until an effective iodinated salt program can be introduced. The spectacular and rapid effects of iodized oil in reducing goiter can be important in demonstrating the benefits of iodization, which can lead to community demand for iodized salt. In general iodized oil administration should be avoided over the age of 45 because of the possibility of precipitating hyperthyroidism (Jod Basedow) in subjects with longstanding goiter (see above). Pregnancy is not regarded as a contraindication. There is a considerable variation in the costs in various parts of the world as might be expected. One important factor is the availability of primary health care staff for the administration of the oil whether by mouth or by injection. The important feature of iodized oil administration is that it can be carried out without the legislation required for iodized salt.

The possibility of linking up an iodized oil program with other preventative programs including the Child Immunization Program, is now under active consideration.[198] Great progress has been made with child immunization programs in Africa and Asia. A series of injections are given covering diphtheria, tetanus toxoid, and whooping cough (3 injections), polio (usually double oral administration), and measles (single injection). The target group is young children (0 to 2 years). Tetanus toxoid is recommended for pregnant women as a preventive measure against tetanus in the neonate.

To this series of measures, iodized oil administration (by injection or by mouth) could readily be added to cover young children over the first 2 to 5 years of life, the second most important target group. Women of reproductive age would require separate coverage through the primary health care system, especially the family planning health care system or in antenatal services at the same time as with tetanus toxoid. These measures have now been recommended by the World Health Organization.[198]

Other Methods

Iodized bread was used in Tasmania in preference to both iodized salt and iodide tablets distributed through the schools, and shown to be effective.[199] Its use was discontinued because of the availability of other sources of iodine, notably from milk consequent to the use of iodophors in the dairy industry. It is for this reason that milk has become a major adventitious source of iodine in many western countries such as the United States and the United Kingdom, and in Northern Europe. A change in dairy practice would reverse the situation and increase the likelihood of iodine deficiency in the population.

Iodized water has been used in several countries. Reduction in goiter rate from 61 percent to 30 percent with 79 percent of goiters showing visible reduction has been demonstrated following iodation of the water supply in Sarawak. Significant rises in serum T_4 and falls in TSH were also shown. Measurement of urinary iodine excretion indicated iodine repletion.[200]

Similar results have been obtained from studies in Thailand by Dr Romsai Suwanik and his group at the Siriraj Hospital, Bangkok[201] and Squatrito et al[202] in Sicily. Most recently in Mali, West Africa, silicone cylinders have been introduced especially designed to provide a depot source in village wells for a period of 12 months.[203,203a] This method is appropriate at village level if a specific source of drinking water can be identified, otherwise there is a heavy cost as less than 1 percent of a general water supply is used for drinking purposes. More extensive trials are required to determine costs and feasibility.

NATIONAL IDD CONTROL PROGRAMS

In spite of the availability of effective technology, IDD control programs have until recently been conspicuous for their failure. It is now recognized that there is a social process involved which requires political will, community education, and training, as well as funding.[2,5] Resources have now become available to meet these challenges so that there is now better understanding, with an increasing number of effective national programs being established. Effective national IDD control program requires technical help. Assistance with surveys and laboratories, with the appropriate quality control, is now available to national governments through the World Health Organization, UNICEF, and a newly established expert network, the International Council for Control of Iodine Deficiency Disorders. The ICCIDD was established in 1986 to bridge the gap between existing knowledge of iodine deficiency by application of this knowledge in national programs in developing countries.[2,5,204] The ICCIDD consists of a global multidisciplinary network of 350 scientists, public health professionals, and technologists from 70 countries committed to the elimination of IDD by the year 2000. There is a board of 40 members, with a majority from developing countries and international agencies. The major objective of the ICCIDD is to cooperate with the major international agencies, particularly WHO and UNICEF, and key bilateral aid giving agencies, in the development of national IDD control programs in countries with significant IDD problems. These programs are the responsibility of national governments in developing countries yet there has been, until recently, no general awareness of the significance of IDD for national development.

One major function of the ICCIDD is, therefore, the communication of this IDD message to decision makers or national governments, international agencies, and a wide variety of health professionals and planners. To date the ICCIDD has received its funding support from UNICEF, WHO, and the international development programs of Australia, Canada, and Holland. To achieve the objective of assisting national governments the ICCIDD has established, in collaboration with WHO and UNICEF, Regional IDD Working Groups in all parts of the world, including Africa, Southeast Asia, the Middle East, Latin America, Indonesia, and China, to assist national governments in all aspects of the establishment of national IDD control programs. These Regional IDD Working Groups include representatives from WHO, UNICEF, and the International Council for Control of Iodine Deficiency Disorders (ICCIDD), interested bilateral agencies and representatives of national governments. Substantial progress has been made in Asia, Africa, and Latin America since the foundation of the ICCIDD in 1986. This has led to acceptance of the target of elimination of IDD as a public health problem by the year 2000 by the World Health Assembly (1990), and the World Summit for Children (1990).

THE ELIMINATION OF IDD AS A PUBLIC HEALTH PROBLEM BY THE YEAR 2000

The World Summit for Children was held at the United Nations, New York. It was attended by 71 heads of state and 80 other senior government representatives who signed a Plan of Action calling for the elimination of IDD by the year 2000, along with a number of other measures for the improvement of health and education of children throughout the world. Since the World Summit for Children, UNICEF, WHO, and ICCIDD have agreed on a series of targets to be met over the next 10 years in order to achieve the objective of elimination of IDD as a public health problem by the year 2000. For 1995, realization of the objective requires that all countries should have National Intersectoral Commissions operating national programs with access to laboratory assessment of salt iodine content and monitoring of the extent of iodine deficiency in the population by measurement of urine iodine levels and blood spot TSH determinations. Measurement of salt iodine requires only a simple chemical procedure, which can be made readily available. Bigger countries with large iodine deficient populations will need their own specialized laboratories, and expertise is already available in a number of them. For smaller countries access to regional specialized laboratories is now being organized.

There is therefore a steady tide of advance in the elimination of IDD. Europe and North America has nearly achieved it, with Latin America to follow next, and then Asia, where a number of national programs are making good progress. Finally, African countries have made excellent progress since 1987. Further details are available elsewhere.[2,5,204] Continued effort is required both in the initial achievement and the maintenance of that achievement in which thyroidologists are playing a significant part. A global partnership has coalesced involving the people and governments of affected countries, international agencies (WHO, UNICEF), the ICCIDD, the bilateral (country) agencies, the salt industry, and Kiwanis, a world service club based in the United States that has adopted a fund raising goal of $70 million for the elimination of IDD by the year 2000.[204] This concerted effort increases the authors' confidence that the elimination of an ancient scourge of mankind may be achieved by the year 2000.

REFERENCES

1. Hetzel BS: Iodine deficiency disorders (IDD) and their eradication. Lancet 2:1126, 1983
2. Hetzel BS: The Story of Iodine Deficiency: An International Challenge in Nutrition. Oxford University Press, Oxford, 1989
3. World Health Organization. Prevention Control Iodine Deficiency Disorders: Progress Report to 43rd World Health Assembly. Geneva, 1990
4. World Health Organization. Global prevalence of iodine deficiency disorders. Micronutrient Deficiency Information System (MDIS) Working Paper No. 1. Geneva, 1993
5. Hetzel BS: An overview of the prevention and control of iodine deficiency disorders. p. 7. In Hetzel BS, Dunn JT, Stanbury JB (eds): The Prevention and Control of Iodine Deficiency Disorders. Elsevier, Amsterdam, 1987
6. McMichael AJ, Potter JD, Hetzel BS: Iodine deficiency, thyroid function, and reproductive failure. p. 445. In Stanbury JB, Hetzel BS (eds): Endemic Goiter and Endemic Cretinism. John Wiley & Sons, New York, 1980
7. Pharoah POD, Delange F, Fierro-Benitez R, Stanbury JB: Endemic cretinism. p. 395. In Stanbury JB, Hetzel BS (eds): Endemic Goiter and Endemic Cretinism. John Wiley & Sons, New York, 1980
8. Delange F, Iteke FB, Ermans AM: Nutritional Factors Involved in the Goitrogenic Action of Cassava. IDRC, Ottawa, 1982
9. Fierro-Benitez R, Stanbury JB, Querido A et al: Endemic cretinism in the Andean region of Ecuador. J Clin Endocrinol Metab 30:228, 1970
10. Buttfield IH, Hetzel BS: Endemic goitre in Eastern New Guinea with special reference to the use of iodised oil in prophylaxis and treatment. Bull WHO 36:243, 1967
11. Pharoah POD, Buttfield IH, Hetzel BS: Neurological damage to the fetus resulting from severe iodine deficiency during pregnancy. Lancet 1:308, 1971
12. Cao X-Y, Jiang X-M, Dou Z-H et al: Timing of vulnerability of the brain to iodine deficiency in endemic cretinism. N Engl J Med 331:1739, 1994
13. Pharoah POD, Ellis SM, Ekins RP, Williams ES: Maternal thyroid function, iodine deficiency and fetal development. Clin Endocrinol 5:159, 1976
14. Hetzel BS, Mano MT: A review of experimental studies of iodine deficiency during fetal development. J Nutr 119:145, 1989
15. Vulsma T, Gons MT, De Vijlder JJM: Maternal-fetal transfer of thyroxine in congenital hypothyroidism due to a total organification defect on thyroid agenesis. N Engl J Med 321:13, 1989
16. Thilly CH: Goitre et cretinisme endemiques: role etiologique de la consommation de manioc et strategie d'eradication. Bull Acad Med Bel 136:389, 1981
17. Pharoah POD, Connolly KC: A controlled trial of iodinated oil for the prevention of endemic cretinism: a long term follow up. Int J Epid 16:68, 1987
18. Dobbing J: The later development of the brain and its vulnerability. p. 565. In Davis K, Dobbing J (eds): Scientific Foundations of Paediatrics. Heinemann Medical, London, 1974
19. Delange F, Heidemann P, Bourdoux P et al: Regional variations of iodine nutrition and thyroid function during the neonatal period in Europe. Biol Neonate 49:322, 1986
20. Kochupillai N, Pandav CS: Neonatal chemical hypothyroidism in iodine deficient environments. p. 85. In Hetzel BS, Dunn JT, Stanbury JB (eds): The Prevention and Control of Iodine Deficiency Disorders. Elsevier, Amsterdam, 1987
21. Ermans AM, Bourdoux P, Lagasse R et al: Congenital hypothyroidism in developing countries. p. 61. In Burrow GN (ed): Neonatal Thyroid Screening. Raven Press, New York, 1980
22. Vanderpas J, Rivera MT, Bourdoux P et al: Reversibility of severe hypothyroidism with supplementary iodine in patients with endemic cretinism. N Engl J Med 315:791, 1986
23. Delange F: Iodine nutrition and risk of thyroid irradiation from nuclear accidents. p. 45. In Rubery E, Smales E (eds): Iodine Prophylaxis Following Nuclear Accidents. Pergamon Press, Oxford, 1990
24. Bleichrodt N, Born MP: A metaanalysis of research in iodine and its relationship to cognitive development in iodine-deficient and noniodine-deficient populations. p. 195. In JB Stanbury (ed). The Damaged Brain of Iodine Deficiency. Cognizant Communication Corporation, New York, 1994.
25. Boyages SC, Collins JK, Maberly GF, Jupp JJ: Iodine deficiency impairs intellectual and neuromotor development in apparently-normal persons. Med J of Aust 150:676, 1989
26. Fierro-Benitez R, Cazar R, Stanbury JB et al: Long-term effect of correction of iodine deficiency on psychomotor and intellectual development. p. 182. In Dunn JT, Pretell E, Daza C, Viteri F (eds): Towards the Eradication of Endemic Goiter, Cretinism, and Iodine Deficiency. Pan American Health Organization, Washington, DC, 1986
27. Bautista A, Barker PA, Dunn JT et al: The effects of oral iodized oil on intelligence, thyroid status, and somatic growth in school-age children from an area of endemic goiter. Amer J Clin Nutr 35:127, 1982
28. Crantz FR, Larsen PR: Rapid thyroxine to 3,5,3′-

triiodothyronine conversion binding in rat cerebral cortex and cerebellum. J Clin Investigation 64:935, 1980

29. Obregon MJ, Santisteban P, Rodriguez-Pena A et al: Cerebral hypothyroidism in rats with adult-onset iodine deficiency. Endocrinol 115:614, 1984

30. Li J-Q, Wang X: Jixian: a success story in IDD control. IDD Newsletter 3:4, 1987

31. Li J-Q, Wang X, Yan Y et al: The effects of a severely iodine deficient diet derived from an endemic area on fetal brain development in the rat—observations in the first generation. Neuropathol Appl Neurobiol 12:261, 1985

32. Zhong F-G, Cao X-M, Liu J-L: Experimental study on influence of iodine deficiency on fetal brain in rats. Chinese J Pathol 12:205, 1983

33. Hetzel BS, Hay ID: Thyroid function, iodine nutrition and fetal brain development. Clin Endocrinol 11:445, 1979

34. McIntosh GH, Jones GH, Howard DA et al: Low iodine diet for producing iodine deficiency in rats. Aust J Biol Sci 33:205, 1980

35. Ruiz-Marcos A, Sanchez-Toscano F, Escobar Del Rey F, Morreale de Escobar G: Severe hypothyroidism and the maturation of the rat cerebral cortex. Brain Res 162:315, 1979

36. Obregon MJ, Mallol J, Pastor R et al: L-thyroxine and 3,5,3′ triodo-thyronine in rat embryos before onset of fetal thyroid function. Endocrinol 114:305, 1984

37. DeLong GR, Robbins J, Condliffe PG: Iodine and the Brain. Plenum Press, New York, 1989

38. Mano MT, Potter BJ, Belling GB, Hetzel BS: Low-iodine diet for the production of severe I deficiency in marmosets (*Callithrix jacchus jacchus*). Brit J Nutr 54:367, 1985

39. Mano MT, Potter BJ, Belling et al: Fetal brain development in response to iodine deficiency in marmosets (*Lallithrix, Jacchis, Jacchis*) J Neurolog Sc 179:287, 1987

40. Potter BJ, Mano MT, Belling GB et al: Retarded fetal brain development resulting from severe dietary iodine deficiency in sheep. Neuropath Appl Neurobiol 8:303, 1982

41. Hetzel BS, Potter BJ: Iodine deficiency and the role of thyroid hormones in brain development. p. 83. In Dreosti IE, Smith RM (eds): Neurobiology of the Trace Elements. Humana Press, Clifton, New Jersey, 1983

42. Potter BJ, McIntosh GH, Mano MT et al: The effect of maternal thyroidectomy prior to conception on fetal brain development in sheep. Acta Endocrinol 112:93, 1986

43. Man EB, Sally A, Seunian BA: Thyroid function in human pregnancy, IX: development of retardation of 7 year old progeny of hypothyroxinemic women. Am J Obstetr Gynecol 125:949, 1976

44. DeLong GR: Neurological involvement in iodine deficiency disorders. p. 49. In Hetzel BS, Dunn JT, Stanbury JB (eds): Elsevier, Amsterdam, 1987

45. Ma T, Lu T, Tan Y et al: The present status of endemic goitre and endemic cretinism in China. Food Nutr Bull 4:13, 1982

46. McClendon JF, Williams A: Simple goiter as a result of iodine deficiency. JAMA 80:600, 1923

47. Clesen R: Distribution of endemic goiter in the United States as shown by thyroid surveys. US Public Health Rep 44:1463, 1929

48. Hollingsworth DR, Butcher LK, White SD: Kentucky Appalachian goiter without iodine deficiency: evidence for evanescent thyroiditis. Am J Dis Child 131:866, 1977

49. Karmarkar MG, Deo MG, Kochupillai N, Ramalingaswami V: Pathophysiology of Himalayan endemic goiter. Am J Clin Nutr 27:96, 1974

50. Ramalingaswami V: Endemic goiter in Southeast Asia. New clothes on an old body. Ann Intern Med 78:277, 1973

51. Ibbertson HK, Gluckman PD, Croxson MS, Strang LJW: Goiter and cretinism in the Himalayas: a reassessment. p. 129. In Dunn JT, Medeiros-Neto G (eds): Endemic Goiter and Cretinism: Continuing Threats to World Health. Washington, DC, Pan American Health Organization, Sci Publ 292, 1974

52. Hershman JM, Due DT, Sharp B et al: Endemic goiter in Vietnam. J Clin Endocrinol Metab 57:243, 1983

53. Sinclair HM: The Work of Sir Robert McCarrison. Faber and Faber, London, 1953

54. Pandav CS, Kochupillai N: Endemic goitre in India: prevalence, etiology, attendant disability and control measures. Indian J Pediatr 50:259, 1982

55. Suwanik R, Nondasuta A: Field studies on iodine metabolism in an endemic goiter village. Prae, Thailand. J Natl Res Council Thailand 2(1):000, 1962

56. Ramirez I, Cruz M: Cretinismo endemico Andino: acotactiones socio-biologicas nuevos metodos de estudio. Politecnica 8:7, 1983

57. Gaitan E, Merino H, Rodriguez G et al: Epidemiology of endemic goiter in western Colombia. WHO Bull 56:43, 1978

58. Greene LS: Hyperendemic goiter, cretinism, and social organization in Highland Ecuador. p. 55. In Greene LS (ed): Malnutrition, Behavior and Social Organization. Academic Press, San Diego, 1977

59. Hercus CE, Roberts KC: Iodine content of foods, manures and animal products in relation to the prophylaxis of endemic goiter in New Zealand. J Hyg 27:49, 1927

60. Lamberg BA, Honkapohja H, Haikonen M et al: Iodine metabolism in endemic goitre in the east of Finland with a survey of recent data on iodine metabolism in Finland. Acta Med Scand 172:237, 1962

61. Orts S, Dustin P, Delange F: Goitrous enzootic in the wild rat with a geographic distribution similar to endemic human goiter. Acta Endocrinol 66:193, 1971

62. Kelly FC, Snedden WW: Prevalence and geographical distribution of endemic goiter. p. 27. In Clements FW, et al (eds): Endemic Goitre. World Health Organization, Geneva, 1960

63. Stanbury JB, Hetzel BS: Endemic Goiter and Endemic Cretinism. John Wiley & Sons, New York, 1980

64. Vermiglio F, Sidoti M, Finocchiaro MD: Defective neuromotor and cognitive ability in iodine-deficient schoolchildren of an endemic goiter region in Sicily. J Clin Endocrinol Metab 70:379, 1990

65. Todd CH, Bourdeux PP: Severe iodine deficiency in two endemic goitre areas of Zimbabwe. Centr Afr J Med 37:2237, 1991

66. Lazarus JH, Parkes AB, John R et al: Endemic goitre in Senegal—thyroid function, etiological factors and treatment with oral iodised oil. Acta Endocrinol (Copehn) 126:149, 1992

67. Delange F, Bürgi H: Iodine deficiency disorders in Europe. Bull World Health Org 67:317, 1989

68. Tonglet R, Bourdoux P, Minga T, Ermans AM: Efficacy of low oral doses of iodized oil in the control of iodine deficiency in Zaire. New Engl J Med 326:236, 1992

69. Todd CH, Sanders D: A high prevalence of hypothyroidism in association with endemic goitre in Zimbabwean schoolchildren. J Trop Pediatr 37:199, 1991

70. Biassoni P, Ceccarelli C, Marcia E et al: Ouham-Pende: a new endemic goiter area in Centro-African Republic (C.A.R.). Preliminary observations on schoolchildren. Thyroidal Clin Exp 2:35, 1990

71. Goslings BM, Djokomoeljanto R, Docter R et al: Hypothyroidism in an area of endemic goiter and cretinism in Central Java, Indonesia. J Clin Endocrinol Metab 44:481, 1977

72. Fenzi GF et al: Reciprocal changes of serum thyroglobulin and TSH in residence of a moderate endemic goiter area. Clin Endocrinol 23:115, 1985

73. Hershman JM et al: Endemic goiter in Vietnam. J Clin Endocrinol Metab 57:243, 1983

74. Elte JWF: Causes of non-toxic goitre other than mere iodine deficiency. Neth J Med 24:79, 1981

75. Gaitan E: Goitrogens. Clin Endocrinol Metab 2:683, 1988

76. Gaitan E: Goitrogens in food and water. Ann Rev Nutr 10:21, 1990

77. Van Wijk JJ, Arnold MB, Wynne J, Pepper F: The effects of a soybean product on thyroid function in humans. Pediatrics 24:752, 1959

78. Van Etten CH: Goitrogens p. 103. In Liener IE (ed). Toxic Constituents of Plant Foodstuffs. Academic Press, San Diego, 1969

79. Chesney AM, Clawson TA, Webster B: Endemic goiter in rabbits. Bull Johns Hopkins Hosp 43:261, 1928

80. Barker MH: The blood cyanates in the treatment of hypertension. JAMA 106:762, 1936

81. Hercus CB, Purves HD: Studies on endemic and experimental goitre. J Hyg 36:182, 1936

82. Mackenzie CG, MacKenzie JB: Effect of sulfonamides and thioureas on the thyroid gland and basal metabolism. Endocrinology 32:185, 1943

83. Astwood EB: Mechanisms of action of various antithyroid compounds. Ann NY Acad Sci 50:419, 1949

84. Bourdoux P, Delange F, Gerard M et al: Evidence that cassava ingestion increases thiocyanate formation: a possible etiologic factor in endemic goiter. J Clin Endocrinol Metab 46:613, 1978

85. Ekpechi OL: Pathogenesis of endemic goiter in eastern Nigeria. Br J Nutr 21:537, 1967

86. Cowan JW, Baghir AR, Salji JR: Antithyroid activity of onion volatiles. Aust J Biol Sci 20:683, 1967

87. Thilly CH, Delange F, Ermans AM: Further investigations of iodine deficiency in the etiology of endemic goiter. Am J Clin Nutr 24: 30, 1972

88. Delange F, Vigneri F, Trimarchi F et al: Etiological factors of endemic goiter in northeastern Sicily. J Endocrinol Invest 2:137, 1978

89. Ermans AM, Mbulamoko NM, Delange F, Ahluwalia R: Role of Cassava in the Etiology of Endemic Goitre and Cretinism. International Development Research Center, Ottawa, 1980

90. Delange F, Ahluwalia R: Cassava Toxicity and Thyroid Research and Public Health Issues. International Development Research Center, Ottawa, 1983

91. Hegedus L, Katrup S, Veiergang D et al: High frequency of goitre in cigarette smokers. Clin Endocrinol 22:287, 1985

92. Roti E, Grundi A, Braverman LE: The placental transport, synthesis and metabolism of hormones and drugs which affect thyroid function. Endocr Rev 4:131, 1983

93. Suzuki N, Higuchi T, Gawa M et al: Endemic coast goitre in Hokkaido, Japan. Acta Endocrinol 50:161, 1965

94. Suzuki N: Etiology of endemic goiter and iodide excess. p. 237. In Stanbury JB, Hetzel BS (eds): Endemic Goiter and Endemic Cretinism. John Wiley & Sons, New York, 1980

95. Gaitan E: Antithyroid activities of organic water pollutants in iodine sufficient endemic goiter areas. p.

25. In Haak A, Goslings BM, van der Heide D, Roelfsema F (eds): Schildklierziekten University Press, Leiden, The Netherlands, 1987

96. Berry M, Banu L, Larsen PR: Type I iodothyronine deiodinase is a selenocystein-containing enzyme. Nature 349:438, 1991

97. Contempré B, Duale L, Dumont JE et al: Effect of selenium supplementation on thyroid hormone metabolism in an iodine and selenium deficient population. Clin Endocrinol 36:576, 1992

98. Goyens P, Golstein J, Nsombola B et al: Selenium deficiency as a possible factor in the pathogenesis of myxedematous endemic cretinism. Acta Endocrinol (Copenh) 114:497, 1987

99. Contempré B, Vanderpas J, Dumont JE: Cretinism, thyroid hormones and selenium. Molec Cell Endocrinol 81:193, 1991

100. Contempré B, Denef J-F, Dumont JE, Many M-C: Selenium deficiency aggravates the necrotizing effects of a high iodide dose in iodine deficient rats. Endocrinology 132:1866, 1993

101. Contempré B, Dumont JE, Ngo B et al: Effect of selenium supplementation in hypothyroid subjects of an iodine and selenium deficient area: the possible danger of indiscriminate supplementation of iodine-deficient subjects with selenium. J Clin Endocrinol Metab 73:213, 1991

102. Correa P: Pathology of endemic goiter. p. 303. In Stanbury JB, Hetzel BS (eds): Endemic Goiter and Endemic Cretinism. John Wiley & Sons, New York, 1980

103. Studer H, Ramelli F: Simple goiter and its variants: euthyroid and hyperthyroid multinodular goiters. Endocrine Rev 3:40, 1982

104. Studer H, Gerber H, Peter H: Multinodular goiter. p. I:772. In DeGroot L (ed): Endocrinology. Vol. 1. WB Saunders, Philadelphia, 1989

105. Marine D: The pathogenesis and prevention of simple or endemic goiter. JAMA 104:2334, 1935

106. Follis R: Experimental colloid goitre produced by thiouracil. Nature 183:1817, 1959

107. Stanbury JB, Brownell GL, Riggs DS et al: Endemic Goiter: The Adaptation of Man to Iodide Deficiency. Harvard University Press, Cambridge, 1954

107a. Dumont JE, Ermans AM, Maenhaut C, Copée, Stanbury JB: Large goiter as a maladaptation to iodine deficiency. Clin Endocrinol 43:1, 1995

108. Larsen PR: Thyroid-pituitary interaction. N Engl J Med 306:23, 1982

109. Silva JE, Larsen PR: Contributions of plasma triiodothyronine to nuclear triiodothyronine receptor saturation in pituitary, liver, and kidney of hypothyroid rats. J Clin Invest 61:1247, 1978

110. Pazos-Moura CC, Moura EG, Dorris ML et al: Effect of iodine deficiency and cold exposure on thyroxine 5′-deiodinase activity in various rat tissues. Am J Physiol 260:E175, 1991

111. Lum SMC, Nicoloff JT, Spencer LA, Kaptein EM: Peripheral tissue mechanism for maintenance of serum triiodothyronine values in a thyroxine deficient state in man. J Clin Invest 73:570, 1984

112. Pharoah POD, Lawton NF, Elles SM et al: The role of triiodothyronine (T₃) in the maintenance of euthyroidism in endemic goitre. Clin Endocrinol 2:193, 1973

113. Okamura K, Taurog A, Krulich L: Hypothyroidism in severely iodine-deficient rats. Endocrinology 109:464, 1981

114. Santisteban P, Obregon MJ, Rodriguez-Pena A et al: Are iodine-deficient rats euthyroid? Endocrinology 110:1780, 1982

115. Nakashima T, Taurog A, Krulich L: Serum thyroxine, triiodothyronine, and TSH levels in iodine-deficient and iodine-sufficient rats before and after exposure to cold. Proc Soc Exp Biol Med 167:45, 1981

116. Escobar del Rey F, Ruiz de Ona, Bernal J et al: Generalized deficiency of 3,5,3′-triiodo-L-thyronine (T₃) in tissues from rats on a low iodine intake, despite normal circulating T₃ levels. Acta Endocrinol 120:490, 1989

117. Calfo R, Obregon MJ, Ruiz de Ona C et al: Congenital hypothyroidism as studied in rats. Crucial role of maternal thyroxine but not of 3,5,3′-triiodothyronine in the protection of the fetal brain. J Clin Invest 86:889, 1990

118. Obregon MJ, Ruiz de Oña C, Calvo R et al: Outer ring iodothyronine deiodinases and thyroid hormone economy: responses to iodide deficiency in the rat fetus and neonate. Endocrinology 129:2663, 1991

119. Morreale de Escobar G, Obregon MJ, Calvo R, Escobar del Rey F: Effects of iodine deficiency on thyroid hormone metabolism and the brain in fetal rats: the role of maternal transfer of thyroxine. Am J Clin Nutr, suppl. 57:280S, 1993

120. Stanbury JB: The Damaged Brain of Iodine Deficiency. Cognizant Communication Corporation, New York, 1994

121. Vanderpas JB, Rivera-Vanderhas MT, Bourdoux P et al: Reversibility of severe hypothyroidism with supplementary iodine in patients with endemic cretinism. N Engl J Med 315:791, 1986

122. Choufoer JC, Van Rhijn M, Kassenaar AH, Querido A: Endemic goiter in Western New Guinea: iodine metabolism in goitrous and non-goitrous and non-goitrous subjects. J Clin Endocrinol Metab 23:1203, 1963

123. Ibbertson HK, Pearl H, McKinnon J et al: Endemic

cretinism in Nepal. p. 71. In Hetzel BS, Pharoah POD (eds): Endemic Cretinism. Surrey Beatty & Sons, Chipping Norton, New South Wales, Australia, 1971

124. Bachtarzi H, Benmiloud M: TSH-regulation and goitrogenesis in severe iodine deficiency. Acta Endocrinol (Copenh) 103:21, 1983

125. Vagenakis AG, Koutras DA, Burger A et al: Studies of serum triiodothyronine, thyroxine, and thyrotropin concentrations in endemic goiter in Greece. J Clin Endocrinol Metab 37:485, 1973

126. Patel YC, Pharoah POD, Hornabrook RW, Hetzel BS: Serum triiodothyronine, thyroxine and thyroid-stimulating hormone in endemic goiter: a comparison of goitrous and nongoitrous subjects in New Guinea. J Clin Endocrinol Metab 37:783, 1973

127. Buttfield IH, Black ML, Hoffman MJ et al: Studies of the control of thyroid function in endemic goitre in Eastern New Guinea. J Clin Endocrinol Metab 26:1201, 1966

128. Buttfield IH, Hetzel BS, Odell WB: Effect of iodized oil on serum TSH determined by immunoassay in endemic goiter subjects. J Clin Endocrinol Metab 28:1664, 1968

129. Chopra IJ, Hershman JM, Hornabrook RW: Serum thyroid hormone and thyrotropin levels in subjects from endemic goiter regions of New Guinea. J Clin Endocrinol Metab 40:326, 1975

130. Kochupillai N, Karmarkar MG, Weightman D et al: Pituitary-thyroid axis in Himalayan endemic goiter. Lancet 1:1021, 1973

131. Squartito S, Delange F, Trimarchi F et al: Endemic cretinism in Sicily. J Endocrinol Invest 4:295, 1981

131a. Konde M, Ingenbleek Y, Daffe M et al: Goitrous endemic in Guinea. Lancet 344:1675, 1994

132. Chopra IJ, Solomon DH, Chuatteco GM: Thyroxine: just a prohormone or a hormone too? J Clin Endocrinol Metab 36:1050, 1973

133. Beckers C, DeVisscher M: Thyroid proteins in endemic goiter. Metabolism 10:695, 1961

134. Medeiros-Neto GA, Nicolau W, Ulhoa-Centra AB: Studies in the concentration of particulate iodoprotein, RNA, and DNA in normal and endemic goiter glands. p. 183. In Stanbury JB (ed): Endemic Goiter. Pan American Health Organization, Washington DC, 1969

135. Mooij P, de Wit HJ, Bloot AM et al: Iodine deficiency induces thyroid autoimmune reactivity in Wistar rats. J Clin Endocrinol Metab 133:1197, 1993

136. Wilders-Truschnig MM, Kabel PJ, Drexhage HA et al: Intrathyroidal dendretic cells, epitheloid cells, and giant cells in iodine deficient goiter. Am J Pathol 135:219, 1989

137. Wilders-Truschnig MM, Drexhage HA, Leb G et al: Clin Endocrinol Metab 70:444, 1990

138. Vitti P, Chiavato L, Tonacchera M et al: Failure to detect thyroid growth-promoting activity in immunoglobulin G of patients with endemic goiter. J Clin Endocrinol Metab 78:1020, 1994

139. Zakarya M, McKenzie JM: Do thyroid growth-promoting immunoglobulins exist? Editorial. J Clin Endocrinol Metab 70:308, 1990

140. Weetman AP: Is endemic goiter an autoimmune disease? Editorial. J Clin Endocrinol Metab 78:1017, 1994

140a. Brown R: Editorial: Immunoglobulins affecting thyroid growth: a continuing controversey. Endocrinology 80:1506, 1995

140b. Davies R, Lawry J, Bhatia V, Weetman AP: Growth stimulating antibodies in endemic goitre: a reappraisal. Clin Endocrinol 43:189, 1995

141. Karmarkar MG, Kochupillai N, Deo MG, Ramalingaswami V: Adaptation of the thyroid gland to iodine deficiency. Life Sci 8:1135, 1969

142. Ermans AM, Bastenie PA, Galperin H et al: Endemic goiter in the Uele region, II. Synthesis and secretion of thyroid hormones. J Clin Endocrinol Metab 21:996, 1961

143. Shifrin S, Consiglio E, Laccetti P et al: Bovine thyroglobulin: 27S iodoprotein interactions with thyroid membranes and formation of a 27S iodoprotein in vitro. J Biol Chem 257:9539, 1982

144. Ermans AM: Intrathyroid iodine metabolism in goiter. p. 1. In Stanbury JB (ed): Endemic Goiter. Pan American Health Organization, Washington DC, 1969

145. Platzer S, Groebner P, Hansen A et al: Schilddrusenproteine in endemischen Strumen und ihre Beziehung zur intrathyreoidalen Schilddrusenhormonkonzentration. Wien Klin Wochenschr, suppl. 92:88, 1980

146. Medeiros-Neto GA, Shenkman L, Penna M et al: The effects of synthetic TRH in patients with endemic goiter before and after iodized oil injection. p. 361. In Hypothalamic Hypophysiotropic Hormones: Proceedings of the Conference Held at Acapulco, June 1972. Excerpta Medica Foundation, Amsterdam, 1973

147. Medeiros-Neto GA: TSH secretion and regulation in endemic goiter and endemic cretinism. p. 119. In Soto R, Sartorio G, Forteza I (eds): Concepts in Thyroid Diseases. Alan R Liss, New York, 1983

148. Koutras DA, Souvatzoglou A, Pantos PG et al: Iodide organification defect in iodine deficiency endemic goiter. J Clin Endocrinol 47:610, 1978

149. Wellby ML, Powell K, Carman M, Hetzel BS: Comparative studies of diiodotyrosine deiodinase activities in endemic goiter and congenital goiter. J Clin Endocrinol Metab 35:762, 1972

150. Ermans AM, Kinthaert J, Camus M: Defective intrathyroidal iodine metabolism in nontoxic goiter: inadequate iodination of thyroglobulin. J Clin Endocrinol Metab 28:1307, 1968

151. Connolly RJ, Vidor GI, Stewart JC: Increase in thyrotoxicosis in endemic goiter area after iodination of bread. Lancet 1:500, 1970

152. Stewart JC, Vidor GI, Buttfield IH, Hetzel BS: Epidemic thyrotoxicosis in Northern Tasmania: studies of clinical features and iodine nutrition. Aust NZ J Med 1:203, 1971

153. Stewart JC, Vidor GI: Thyrotoxicosis induced by iodine contamination of food—a common unrecognized condition? Brit Med J 1:372, 1976

154. Larsen PR, Silva JE, Hetzel BS, McMichael AJ: Monitoring prophylactic programmes: general considerations. p. 551. In Stanbury JB, Hetzel BS (eds): Endemic Goiter and Endemic Cretinism. John Wiley & Sons, New York, 1980

155. Vidor GI, Stewart JC, Wall JR et al: Pathogenesis of iodine-induced thyrotoxicosis: studies in northern Tasmania. J Clin Endocrinol Metab 37:901, 1973

156. Hetzel BS, Hales IB: New Zealand, Australia, Papua, New Guinea. p. 123. In Stanbury JB, Hetzel BS (eds): Endemic Goiter and Endemic Cretinism. John Wiley & Sons, New York, 1980

156a.Baltisberger BL, Minder CE, Bürgi H: Decrease of incidence of toxic nodular goitre in a region of Switzerland after full correction of mild iodine deficiency. Europ J Endocrinol 132:546, 1995

157. Gutekunst G: The significance of increased iodine intake in Europe. Russian Problemy Endocrinologii 38:10, 1992

158. Stanbury JB, Ermans AM, Hetzel BS et al: Endemic goitre and cretinism: public health significance and prevention. WHO Chron 28:220, 1974

159. Nagataki S: Effects of iodide supplement in thyroid diseases. p. 31. In Vichayanrat A, Nitiyanant W, Eastman C, Nagataki S (eds): Recent Progress in Thyroidology. Crystal House Press, Bangkok, 1987

160. Wegelin C: Malignant disease of the thyroid gland and its relations to goitre in man and animals. Cancer Rev 3:297, 1928

161. Cuello C, Correa P, Eisenberg H: Geographic pathology of thyroid carcinoma. Cancer 23:230, 1969

162. Gaitan E, Nelson NC, Poole GV: Endemic goiter and endemic thyroid disorders. World J Surg 15:205, 1991

163. Williams ED: Dietary iodide and thyroid cancer. p. XXII:201. In Hall R, Kobberling J (eds): Thyroid Disorders Associated with Iodine Deficiency and Excess. Vol. 22. Raven Press, New York, 1985

164. Bubenhofer R, Hedinger C: Schilddrusenmalignome vor und nach Einfuhrung der Jodsalzprophylaxe. Schweiz Med Wschr 107:733, 1977

165. Harach HR, Escalante DA, Onativia A et al: Thyroid carcinoma and thyroiditis in an endemic goitre region before and after iodine prophylaxis. Acta Endocrinol 108:55, 1985

166. Frauman AG, Moses AC: Oncogenes and growth factors in thyroid carcinogenesis. p. 111:479. In Kaplan MM (ed): Endocrinology and Metabolism Clinics of North America. Vol. 3. WB Saunders, Philadelphia, 1990

167. Melmed S: Oncogenes and the thyroid. Thyroid Today 11:000, 1988

168. Van Middlesworth L: Relations between iodine deficiency disorders (IDD) and thyroid cancer. Russian Problemy Endocrinologii 38:56, 1992

169. Merke F: The History and Iconography of Endemic Goitre and Cretinism. MTP Press, Lancaster, 1984

170. Burgi H, Supersaxo Z, Selz B: Iodine deficiency diseases in Switzerland one hundred years after Theodor Kocher's survey: a historical review with some new goitre prevalence data. Acta Endocrinol 123:577, 1990

171. McCarrison R: Observations on endemic cretinism in Chitral and Gilgit valleys. Lancet 2:1275, 1908

172. DeLong R, Stanbury JB, Fierro-Benitez R: Neurological signs in congenital iodine deficiency disorders (endemic cretinism). Dev Med Childr Neurol 27:317, 1985

173. Halpern J-P, Boyages SC, Maberly GF et al: The neurology of endemic cretinism. Brain 114:825, 1991

174. Hetzel BS, Chavadej J, Potter J: The brain and iodine deficiency. Neuropathol appl neurobiol 14:93, 1988

175. Held KR, Cruz ME, Moncayo F: Clinical pattern and the genetics of the fetal iodine deficiency disorders (endemic cretinism): results of a field study in Highland Ecuador. Am J Med Gen 35:85, 1990

176. Deol M: An experimental approach to the understanding and treatment of hereditary syndromes with congenital deafness and hypothyroidism. J Med Genet 10:235, 1973

177. Delange F, Ermans A, Vis H, Stanbury JB: Endemic cretinism in Idjwi Island (Kivu Lake, Republic of the Congo). Clin Endocrinol 6:34, 1972

178. Boyages SC, Halpern J-P, Maberly GF et al: A comparative study of neurological and myxedematous endemic cretinism in Western China. J Clin Endocrinol Metab 67:1262, 1988

179. Tsuboi K, Lima N, Ingbar SH, Medeiros-Neto G: Thyroid atrophy in myxedematous endemic cretinism: possible role for growth-blocking immunoglobulins. Autoimmunity 9:201, 1991

180. Boyages SC, Halpern JP, Maberly GF et al: Endemic cretinism: possible role for thyroid autoimmunity. Lancet I:529, 1989

181. Medeiros-Neto GA, Tsuboik, Lima N: Thyroid auto-immunity and endemic cretinism. Lancet 335:111, 1990

181a. Chiovatol L, Vitti P, Bendinelli G et al. Humoral thyroid autoimmunity is not involved in the pathogenesis of myxedematous endemic cretinism. J Cain Endocrinol Metab 80:1509, 1995

182. Hetzel BS, Dunn JT, Stanbury JB (eds): The Prevention and Control of Iodine Deficiency Disorders. Elsevier, Amsterdam, 1987

183. Indicators for Assessing Iodine Deficiency Disorders and Their Control Programs Through Salt Iodination. WHO/UNICEF/ICCIDD Joint Report, Geneva. World Health Organization, 1994

184. Dunn JT, Pretell EA, Daza CH, Viteri FE: Towards the Eradication of Endemic Goiter, Cretinism, and Iodine Deficiency. p. 373. Pan American Health Organization, Washington DC, 1986

185. Vitti P, Martino E, Aghini-Lombardi F et al: Thyroid volume measurement by ultrasound in children as a tool for the assessment of mild iodine deficiency. J Clin Endocrinol Metab 79:600, 1994

186. Gutekunst R, Delange F: Assessment techniques and the epidemiology of iodine deficiency disorders in Europe. Euro J Internal Med 3, suppl. 1:71, 1992

187. Bourdoux PP: Measurement of iodine in the assessment of iodine deficiency. IDD Newsletter 4:8, 1988

188. Dunn JT, Crutchfield HE, Gutekunst R, Dunn AD: Methods for Measuring Iodine in Urine. ICCIDD/UNICEF/WHO, Wageningen, Netherlands, 1993

189. Follis RH: Patterns of urinary iodine excretion in goitrous and nongoitrous areas. Am J Clin Nut 114:253, 1964

190. Waite KV, Maberly GF, Eastman CJ: Storage conditions and stability of thyrotropin and thyroid hormones on filter paper. Clin Chem 33:853, 1987

191. Clugston GA, Hetzel BS: Iodine. p. 252. In Shils M, Shike R, Olson J (eds): Modern Nutrition in Health and Disease. 8th Ed. Lea & Febiger, Malvern, 1992

192. Mannar MGV: Control of iodine deficiency disorders by iodination of salt: strategy for developing countries. p. 111. In Hetzel BS, Dunn JT, Stanbury JB (eds): The Prevention and Control of Iodine Deficiency Disorders. Elsevier, Amsterdam, 1987

193. Scriba PC et al: Goitre and iodine deficiency in Europe. Lancet 1:1289, 1985

194. Delange F, Dunn JT, Glinoer D. Plenum Press, New York, 1993

195. Sooch SS, Deo MG, Karmarkar MG et al: Prevention of endemic goitre with iodised salt. Bull WHO 49:307, 1973

196. The National Goitre Control Programme: A Blueprint for Its Intensification. Nutrition Foundation of India, Scientific Report No. 1, 1983

197. McCullagh SF: The Huon Peninsula endemic: the effectiveness of an intramuscular depot of iodised oil in the control of endemic goiter. Med J Aust 1:769, 1963

197a. Elnagar B, Elton M, Karlssow FA et al: The effect of different doses of oral iodized oil on goiter size, urinary iodine, and thyroid-related hormones. J Clin Endocrinol Metab 80:891, 1995

198. Potential contribution of the expanded programme on immunization to the control of vitamin A deficiency and iodine deficiency disorders. EPI Report to EPI Global Advisory Group Meeting, Washington DC, November 9-13, 1987

199. Clements FW, Gibson HB, Coy JF: Goiter prophylaxis by addition of potassium iodate to bread. Lancet 1:489, 1970

200. Maberly GF, Eastman CJ, Corcoran JM: Effect of iodination of a village water-supply on goiter size and thyroid function. Lancet 2:1270, 1981

201. Pattanachak S, Tojinda N, Ingbar S, Suwanik R: An iodinator. p. 431. Vichayanrat A, Nitiyanant W, Eastman C, Nagataki S (eds): Recent Progress in Thyroidology. Crystal House Press, Bangkok, 1987

202. Squatrito S, Vigneri R, Runello F et al: Prevention and treatment of endemic iodine deficiency goitre by iodination of a municipal water supply. J Clin Endocrinol Metab 63:368, 1986

203. Fisch A, Pichard E, Prazuck T et al: A new approach to iodine deficiency: controlled release of iodine in water by a silicone elastomer. Am J Public Health 83:540, 1993

203a. Yasipio D, Ngoindiro LF, Barrière-Constantin L et al: Efficacitéd'mm système d'iodation de l'eau dans la luttle contre les troubles dus à la carence iodée en Afrique centrale. Cahiers Santé (Editions John Libbey Eurotert, Monterouge, France) 5:9, 1995

204. Hetzel BS, Pandav CS: SOS for a Billion: The Conquest of Iodine Deficiency Disorders. Oxford University Press, New Delhi, 1994

Surgery of the Thyroid Gland

21

Edwin L. Kaplan, M.D.
Reiko Tanaka, M.D.
Nidal Younes, M.D.

The extirpation of the thyroid gland . . . typifies, perhaps better than any operation, the supreme triumph of the surgeon's art. . . . A feat which today can be accomplished by any competent operator without danger of mishap and which was conceived more than one thousand years ago. . . . There are operations today more delicate and perhaps more difficult. . . . But is there any operative problem propounded so long ago and attacked by so many . . . which has yielded results as bountiful and so adequate?

Dr. William S. Halsted, 1920[1]

In the 75 years since these words were written, many additional improvements have made thyroidectomy even safer and more effective than it was in Halsted's time. In fact, in the best of hands, thyroid surgery can be performed today with a mortality that varies little from the risk of general anesthesia alone, and with a low morbidity as well. In order to obtain such enviable results, however, the surgeon must have a thorough understanding of the pathophysiology of thyroid disorders, be versed in the pre- and postoperative care of patients, have a clear knowledge of the anatomy of the neck region, and, finally, use an unhurried, careful, meticulous operative technique.

SURGICAL ANATOMY

Foremost in achieving surgical expertise is a working knowledge of the normal anatomy of the neck region (Fig. 21-1). The normal thyroid gland varies in

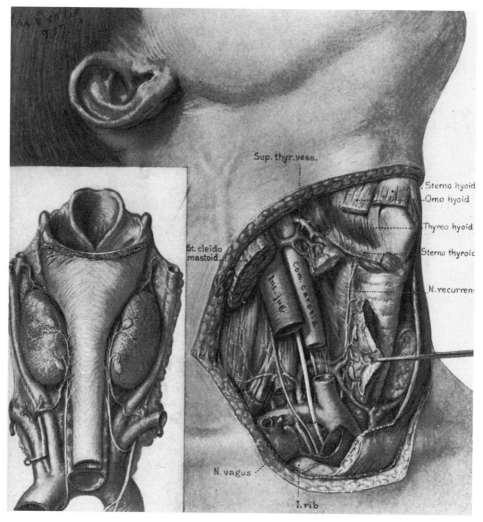

Fig. 21-1. The normal anatomy of the neck in the region of the thyroid gland. (From Halsted,[1] with permission.)

size in different parts of the world, depending in large part upon the iodine content of the diet; in the United States it is about 15 g (Fig. 21-2). It is convex anteriorly and concave posteriorly as a result of its relation to the anterolateral portions of the trachea and larynx, to which it is firmly fixed by fibrous tissue. The lateral lobes extend along the sides of the larynx, reaching the level of the middle of the thyroid cartilage. Each lobe resides in a bed between the trachea and larynx medially and the carotid sheath and sternocleidomastoid muscles laterally. The thyroid gland is enveloped by a thickened fibrous capsule. The deep cervical fascia divides into an anterior and a posterior sheath, creating a loosely applied false capsule for the thyroid. Anterior to the

thyroid lobes are the strap muscles. Situated on the posterior surface of the lateral lobes of the gland are the parathyroid glands and the recurrent laryngeal nerves; the latter usually lie in a cleft between the trachea and the esophagus. The lateral lobes are joined by the isthmus that crosses the trachea. A pyramidal lobe is often present. This is a long, narrow projection of thyroid tissue extending upward from the isthmus lying on the surface of the thyroid cartilage. It represents a vestige of the embryonic thyroglossal duct.

Vascular Supply

The thyroid has an abundant blood supply. Its four major arteries are the paired *superior thyroid ar-*

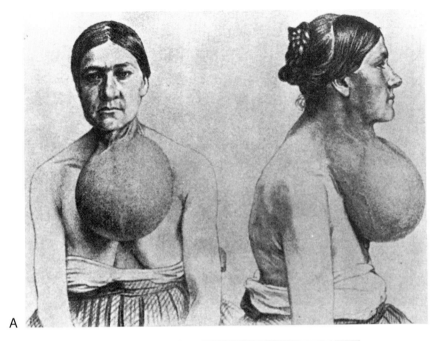

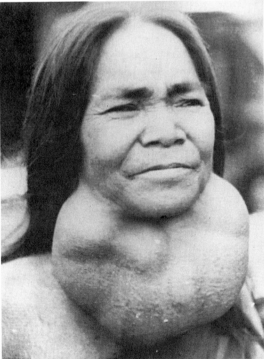

Fig. 21-2. Large goiters are prevalent in areas of iodine deficiency. (A). A woman from Switzerland operated upon by Dr. Theodor Kocher (From Kocher.[37]) (B). One hundred years later, large goiters still occur in many parts of the world, as demonstrated in this woman from a mountainous region of Viet Nam, 1970.

teries, which arise from the external carotid arteries and descend several centimeters in the neck to reach the upper poles of each thyroid lobe, where they branch, and the paired *inferior thyroid arteries,* each of which arises from the thyrocervical trunk of the subclavian artery and enters the lower or midpart of the thyroid lobe from behind. A fifth artery, the *thyroidea ima,* is sometimes present; it arises from the arch of the aorta and enters the thyroid in the midline.

A venous plexus forms under the thyroid capsule. Each lobe is drained by the *superior thyroid vein* at the upper pole and the *middle thyroid vein* at the middle part of the lobe, both of which enter the internal jugular vein. Arising from each lower pole are the *inferior thyroid veins,* which drain directly into the innominate vein.

Nerves

The thyroid gland receives its innervation from sympathetic and parasympathetic divisions of the autonomic nervous system. The sympathetic fibers arise from the cervical ganglia and enter with blood vessels, whereas the parasympathetic fibers are derived from the vagus and reach the gland via branches of the laryngeal nerves.

The thyroid gland's relation to the *recurrent laryngeal nerves* and to the *external branch of the superior laryngeal nerves* is of major surgical significance, since damage to these nerves leads to a disability of phonation. In a study by Hunt et al.,[2] it was shown that in 100 cases the right recurrent laryngeal nerve resided in the tracheoesophageal groove in 64 percent, whereas the left nerve was similarly located on the left side in 77 percent. The nerve was lateral to the trachea in 33 percent of cases on the right side and 22 percent on the left side. In six cases on the right side and four on the left, the nerve was anterolateral to the trachea and therefore was in greater danger of division during a thyroidectomy. On one occasion, a direct "recurrent" laryngeal nerve was given off in the neck without looping around the subclavian artery—that is, it was nonrecurrent.

A nonrecurrent, recurrent laryngeal nerve occurs more commonly on the right side than on the left.[6] On each side, this occurs because of a vascular anomaly—an aberrant take off of the right subclavian, artery from the descending aorta results in a right nonrecurrent, recurrent laryngeal nerve while, less commonly, a right-sided aortic arch is associated with a left-sided nonrecurrent nerve. Such an anomaly on either side puts the recurrent laryngeal nerve at greater risk of damage at the time of operation (Fig. 21-3).

The recurrent laryngeal nerve passed anterior to the inferior thyroid artery in 37 percent of cases on the right side and 24 percent on the left. In 50 percent of cases, the nerve was embedded in the ligament of Berry, which is of importance because traction on the gland would put the nerve on stretch and make it more prone to accidental division during lobectomy (Fig. 21-4).[3] Damage to the recurrent laryngeal nerve produces paresis or paralysis of the intrinsic musculature of the larynx on that side and usually results in a huskiness or hoarseness of the voice.

Bilateral recurrent laryngeal injury is a very serious complication which usually results in tracheostomy.

On each side, the *external branch of the superior laryngeal nerve* innervates the cricothyroid muscle[4] In 85 percent of cases, these nerves lie close to the vascular pedicles of the superior poles of the thyroid glands requiring that the vessels be ligated with care to avoid their injury (Fig. 21-5). In 21 percent these nerves are intimately associated with the superior thyroid vessels. In only 15 percent of cases is the superior laryngeal nerve sufficiently distant from the superior pole vessels to be protected from manipulation by the surgeon.

Parathyroid Glands

The parathyroids are small glands that secrete parathyroid hormone, the major hormone that controls serum calcium homeostasis in humans. Usually four glands are present, but three to six glands have been found.[5] Each gland normally weighs 30 to 40 mg but may be larger if more fat is present. Because of their small size, their delicate blood supply, and their usual anatomic position adjacent to the thyroid gland, these structures are at risk of being accidentally removed, traumatized, or devascularized during thyroidectomy.

The upper parathyroid glands arise embryologically from the fourth pharyngeal pouch[7] (Fig. 21-6C). They descend only slightly during embryologic development, and their position in adult life remains quite constant. This gland is usually found adjacent to the posterior surface of the middle part of the

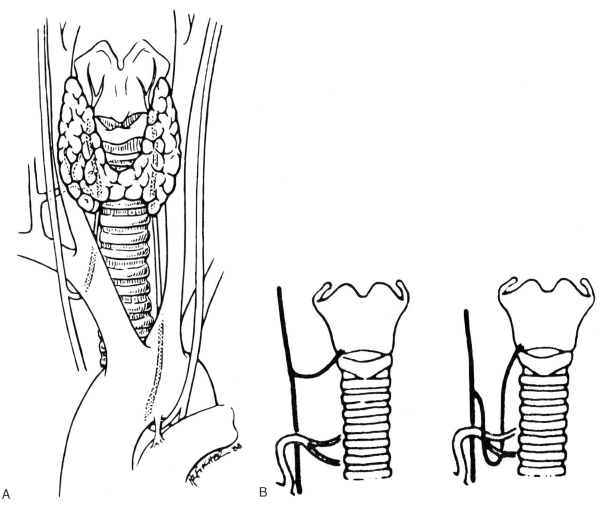

Fig. 21-3. A. Normal anatomy of the recurrent laryngeal nerve. Note that on the right side the recurrent laryngeal nerve hooks around behind the subclavian artery, while on the left side this nerve passes around behind the aortic arch before ascending in the neck. **B.** When there is a vascular anomaly of the right subclavian artery, the recurrent laryngeal nerve no longer "recurs" around this artery but proceeds from the vagus nerve in a more transverse direction to the larynx. In such a situation, the nerve is much more likely to be damaged during operation unless care is taken to visualize its course in the neck. (From Skandalakis et al,[3] with permission.)

thyroid lobe, often just anterior to the recurrent laryngeal nerve as it enters the larynx.

The lower parathyroid glands arise from the third pharyngeal pouch along with the thymus. Hence, they often descend with the thymus. Because they travel so far in embryologic life, they have a wide range of distribution in the adult, from just beneath the mandible to the anterior mediastinum. Usually, however, these glands are found on the lateral or posterior surfaces of the lower part of the thyroid gland or within several centimeters of the lower thyroid pole within the thymic tongue.

Parathyroid glands can be recognized by their tan appearance, their small vascular pedicle, the fact that they bleed freely when biopsy is performed, as opposed to fatty tissues, and their darkening color of hematoma formation when they are traumatized. With experience, one becomes much more adept in recognizing these important structures and in differentiating them from either lymph nodes or fat. Fro-

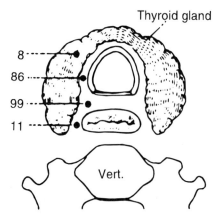

Fig. 21-4. The location of 204 recurrent laryngeal nerves in dissection of 102 cadavers. Note that the recurrent laryngeal nerve was found *anterior* to the tracheoesophageal groove in 42 percent of cases and *within* the thyroid gland in 3.9 percent of cases. In both of these locations, the nerve is more prone to be damaged if its course is not carefully visualized by the surgeon. (From: Skandalakis et al[3] with permission.)

zen section examination during operation can be helpful, at times, for their identification.

Lymphatics

A practical description of the lymphatic drainage of the thyroid gland for the thyroid surgeon has been proposed by Taylor.[8] The results of his studies, which are clinically relevant to the lymphatic spread of thyroid carcinoma, are summarized as follows:

1. The most constant site to which dye goes when injected into the thyroid is the trachea, where there is a rich network of lymphatics in the wall. This fact probably accounts for the frequency with which the trachea is involved by thyroid carcinoma, especially when it is anaplastic. This involvement is sometimes the limiting factor in surgical excision.
2. A chain of lymph nodes lies in the groove between the trachea and the esophagus.
3. Lymph can always be shown to drain toward the

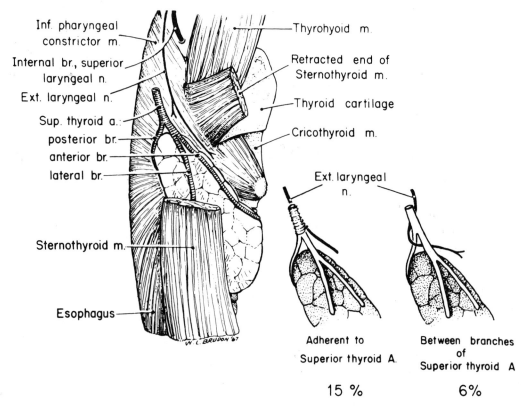

Fig. 21-5. Proximity of the external branch of the superior laryngeal nerve to the superior thyroid vessels is clearly shown. (From Moosman and DeWeese,[4] with permission.)

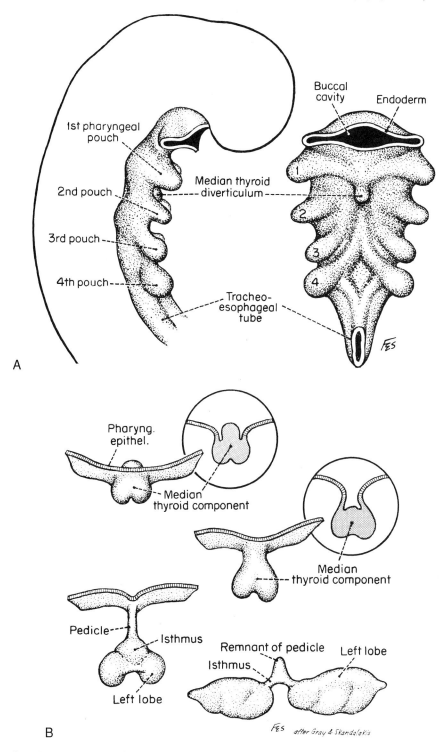

Fig. 21-6. Embryologic development of the thyroid and parathyroid glands. (**A**). Early embryologic development of the pharyngeal anlage. (**B**). Schematic representation of early thyroid gland development from the midline floor of the pharyngeal anlage with later downward growth and division into lobes connected by an isthmus. (*Figure continues.*)

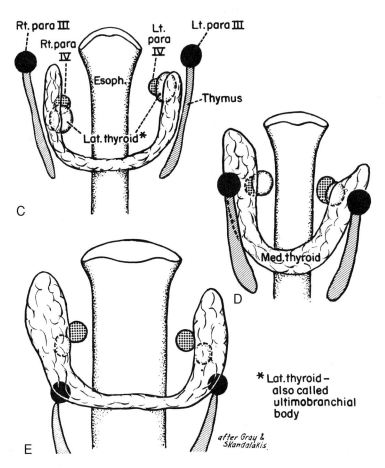

Fig. 21-6. *(Continued)* **(C–E)** Schematic view of the shifts in location of the parathyroid glands, thymus, and lateral thyroid lobes. Approximate adult location. Note that although the upper parathyroid glands (para. IV) remain relatively constant in location, the lower glands (para. III) descend with the thymus gland. The lateral thyroid lobes (ultimobranchial bodies) contain the C cells (calcitonin containing cells), which are incorporated into the thyroid tissue. (From Sedgwick and Cady,[7] with permission.)

mediastinum and to the nodes intimately associated with the thymus.

4. A group of nodes lying above the isthmus and therefore in front of the larynx is sometimes involved. These have been called the *Delphian nodes* (named for the Oracle of Delphi) because it has been said that, if palpable, they were diagnostic of carcinoma. This clinical sign, however, is often misleading.

5. There is a constant group of nodes lying along the jugular vein on each side of the neck. The lymph glands that are found in the supraclavicular fossae may also be involved in the more distant spread of malignant disease from the thyroid gland.

6. Finally, it should not be forgotten that the thoracic duct on the left side of the neck is a lymph vessel of considerable size, arching up out of the mediastinum and passing forward and laterally to drain into the left subclavian vein, usually just lateral to its junction with the internal jugular vein. If the thoracic duct is damaged, the wound is likely to fill with lymph; in this case, the duct should always be sought and tied. A wound that discharges lymph postoperatively should always raise the suspicion of damage to the thoracic duct or a major tributary.

The space from carotid artery to carotid artery and down into the mediastinum is called the central space while lateral to the carotid is referred to as

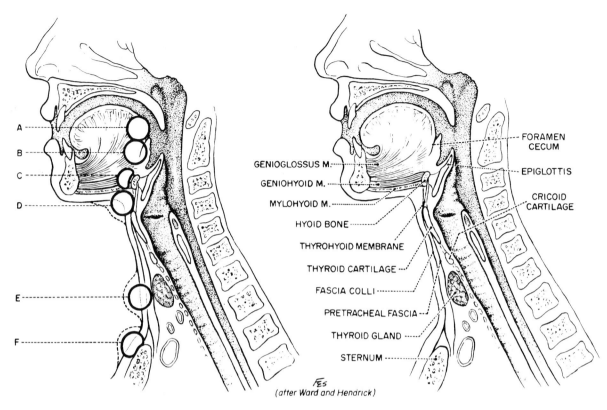

GENIOGLOSSUS M.
GENIOHYOID M.
MYLOHYOID M.
HYOID BONE
THYROHYOID MEMBRANE
THYROID CARTILAGE
FASCIA COLLI
PRETRACHEAL FASCIA
THYROID GLAND
STERNUM

FORAMEN CECUM
EPIGLOTTIS
CRICOID CARTILAGE

FES
(after Ward and Hendrick)

Fig. 21-7. Developmental abnormalities of the thyroid gland in humans. Location of thyroglossal cysts. (**A**). In front of the foramen cecum. (**B**). At the foramen cecum. (**C**). Suprahyoid. (**D**). Infrahyoid. (**E**). Area of the thyroid gland. (**F**). Suprasternal. (From Sedgwick and Cady,[7] with permission.)

the lateral compartment. A careful, extensive central lymph node dissection is particularly important in medullary cancer, for example. A modified radical neck dissection differs from a radical neck dissection in that the sternocleidomastoid muscle and internal jugular vein are not removed and the spinal accessory nerve is left intact.

THYROID ANOMALIES

The thyroid is embryologically an offshoot of the primitive alimentary tract, from which it later becomes separated (Figs. 21-6A and 21-6B). A median anlage arises from the pharyngeal floor in the region of the foramen cecum of the tongue. The main body of the thyroid descends into the neck from this origin and is joined by a pair of lateral components originating from the ultimobranchial bodies of the fourth and fifth branchial pouches (Fig. 21-6C). It is from

these lateral components that the C cells enter the thyroid lobes. C cells contain and secrete calcitonin and are the cells that give rise to a medullary carcinoma of the thyroid gland.

The median thyroid anlage may rarely fail to develop, causing athyreosis, that is, absence of the thyroid gland, or it may differentiate in locations other than the isthmus and lateral lobes. The most common of these is as the pyramidal lobe, which has been reported in as many as 80 percent of patients in whom the gland was surgically exposed. Usually the pyramidal lobe is small; however, in Graves' disease or lymphocytic thyroiditis it is often enlarged and is frequently clinically palpable. Other variations involving the median thyroid anlage represent an arrest in the usual descent of part or all of the thyroid-forming material. These variations include the development of a lingual thyroid, suprahyoid and infrahyoid thyroid tissue, and persistence of the thyroglossal duct as a sinus tract or cyst (Fig. 21-7).

A thyroglossal duct cyst is the most common of the clinically important anomalies of thyroid development.

Before removal of what appears to be a thyroglossal duct cyst, the surgeon must be certain that a normal thyroid gland is present. Instead of a cyst, this mass might rarely be undescended thyroid tissue, and resection of it might remove the infant's only thyroid tissue.

Lingual Thyroid

Lingual thyroid is relatively rare, estimated to occur in 1 in 3,000 cases of thyroid disease. It does, however, represent the most common location for functioning ectopic thyroid tissue. Lingual thyroids are associated with an absence of the normal cervical thyroid in 70 percent of cases and occur much more commonly in women than in men.

The diagnosis is usually made by the discovery of an incidental mass in the back of the tongue in an asymptomatic patient (Fig. 21-8). The mass may en-

large and cause dysphagia, dysphonia, dyspnea, or a sensation of choking. As with other undescended thyroid tissue, hypothyroididm. Hypothyroidism is frequently present, but hyperthyroidism is very unusual. The incidence of malignancy is extremely low. The diagnosis of lingual thyroid should be suspected when a mass is detected in the region of the foramen cecum of the tongue, and is established by radioisotope scanning.

The usual treatment is replacement with thyroid hormone to suppress the lingual thyroid and reduce its size. Only rarely is surgical excision necessary.

Thyroglossal Duct Cysts

Both cysts and sinus tracts can develop along the course of the thyroglossal duct (Fig. 21-7). Normally the thyroglossal duct becomes obliterated early in embryonic life, but occasionally it may persist as a cyst or a draining sinus tract. The lesions usually appear in the midline or just off the midline between the isthmus of the thyroid and the hyoid bone. Cysts

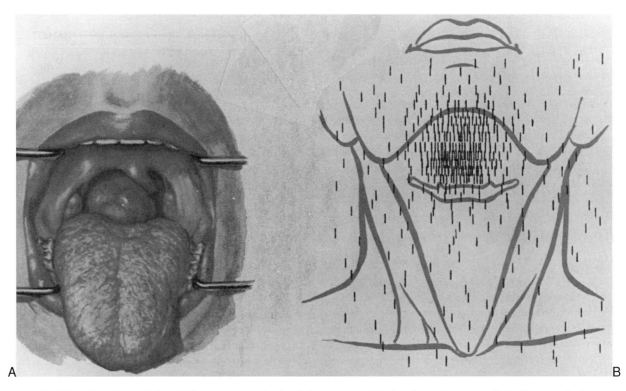

A   B

Fig. 21-8. (A). Lingual thyroid is seen in the back of the tongue. (B). On thyroid scan, radioiodine uptake is present only in the lingual thyroid, demonstrating that no thyroid tissue is present in its normal cervical location.

often become infected and may rupture spontaneously. Removal of the cyst or sinus usually requires excision of the central part of the hyoid bone and dissection of the tract to the base of the tongue (the Sistrunk operation), if recurrence is to be minimized. Thyroid carcinoma can develop from thyroid cells in the thyroglossal duct, especially if the individual has received low-dose irradiation to the head and neck.

Lateral Aberrant Thyroid Rests

True lateral aberrant thyroid tissue is rare since the lateral anlages are normally incorporated into the expanding lateral lobes of the median thyroid anlage. It is now recognized that a mass of thyroid in the lateral neck previously called lateral aberrant thyroid, almost always represents well-differentiated, metastatic thyroid cancer within cervical lymph nodes rather than an embryonic rest and should be treated as such.

INDICATIONS FOR THYROIDECTOMY

Thyroidectomy is usually performed (1) as therapy for some persons with thyrotoxicosis, (2) to remove benign and malignant tumors, (3) to alleviate pressure symptoms or respiratory obstruction attributable to the thyroid, and (4) occasionally, to remove an unsightly goiter. Finally some thyroid masses are still removed in order to establish their pathologic diagnosis. This is much less commonly done, however, because of the effectiveness of fine needle aspiration with cytologic analysis as a diagnostic tool.

A detailed discussion of the selection of patients for operation with thyrotoxicosis is presented in Chapter 11. In general, most young adults with thyrotoxicosis due to Graves' disease are treated first by antithyroid drug therapy, whereas older patients are most often treated with RAI therapy. When antithyroid medication is used, it is usually stopped after control is achieved for 6 months or longer. If a recurrence of disease occurs after all medication is stopped, a *definitive* form of therapy is necessary. Often, in young persons, subtotal thyroidectomy is chosen. Older persons with Graves' disease who do not want to receive RAI therapy are also treated with thyroidectomy. Other indications for surgery include selected pregnant women, children who cannot be controlled with drugs, patients who suffer drug reactions, and others who have thyroid nodules with Graves' disease.

Advantages of this technique include an avoidance of the potential harmful effects of irradiation therapy and a lower incidence of hypothyroidism than occurs after RAI treatment. Perhaps of greatest value is the rapidity with which such patients are returned to a euthyroid state and to a productive life after thyroidectomy. We have been impressed by the absence of operative mortality and by the low operative morbidity in such patients who have been operated on at the University of Chicago Medical Center.[9] Thyroidectomy is of benefit in the treatment of selected persons with toxic adenomas and toxic nodular goiters as well.

Thyroid Nodules

It has been estimated that 4 percent of all adults living in the United States have a clinically nodular thyroid gland. The incidence of thyroid cancer, on the other hand, is about 40 to 50 persons per million population per year. Thus, it is apparent that most persons with thyroid nodules do not have cancer. Care should be exercised to choose those patients for operation who are at greatest risk of having cancer.

Clinically of greatest concern are thyroid masses that are solitary, hard, recent in origin, found in young persons or men of any age, cold on isotope scan, and solid on ultrasound. Our current algorithm makes far less use of isotope or sonographic scanning, however, (Fig. 21-9) but relies much more heavily on fine needle aspiration biopsy with cytologic examination for selection of operative cases (Fig. 21-10); we have been impressed by its diagnostic value. Using this method, patients with thyroid cancers or follicular neoplasms are operated upon while those diagnosed as having colloid nodules are not operated upon unless pressure symptoms or obstructive symptoms are present or unless the patient wishes the nodule to be removed electively. Such a diagnostic regimen has reduced the number of colloid nodules that are operated upon and increases the yield of carcinomas in the surgical cases.

A history of *low-dose external irradiation* to the head or neck is probably the most important historic fact that can be obtained, for it indicates that a cancer of the thyroid is more likely even if the gland is multi-

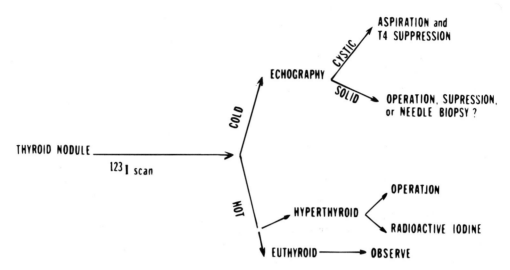

Fig. 21-9. Former algorithm for diagnosing solitary thyroid nodules. This algorithm used mainly the results of isotope scanning and ultrasonographic studies.

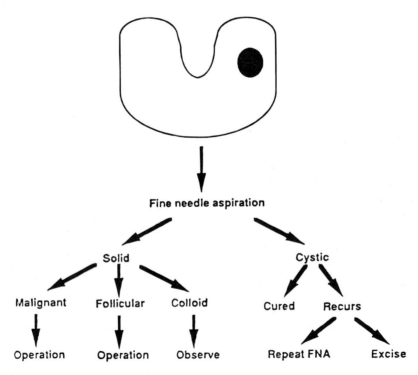

Fig. 21-10. Our current algorithm for the diagnosis of a thyroid nodule utilizes fine needle aspiration (FNA) with cytologic analysis. (Courtesy of Dr. Jon Van Heerdon.)

nodular. This fact is clearly apparent when the results of our operative series are examined.[10] Before the use of aspiration needle biopsy with cytologic evaluation, 15 percent of our nonirradiated but carefully selected patients with solitary nodules were found to have carcinoma. In the irradiated group, on the other hand, less stringent criteria were used for selection, and most single and multiple nodules were operated upon. Nevertheless, close to 40 percent of patients with single or multiple nodules were found to harbor carcinoma within their thyroid gland. Prior low-dose external irradiation has also been associated with later skin cancers, benign and malignant brain and salivary gland tumors, parathyroid adenomas, and even breast cancer.

Recently, we and others have documented the fact that *high-dose external irradiation therapy*, that is, more than 2,000 rads, does not confer safety from thyroid carcinoma, as was previously thought.[11] Rather, an increased prevalence of thyroid carcinoma has been found, particularly in patients with Hodgkin's disease and other lymphomas who received mantle irradiation, which included the thyroid bed. Both benign and malignant thyroid nodules are beginning to be recognized, now that these persons survive for longer periods of time. If a thyroid mass appears in such a patient, it should be treated aggressively. These patients should also be observed carefully for the development of hypothyroidism.

PREOPERATIVE PREPARATION

Most patients with a mass of the thyroid are euthyroid and require no specific preoperative preparation other than the usual examinations to determine their risk for a general anesthetic. Indirect laryngoscopy to determine preoperative vocal cord function is especially important if the person has already had a thyroid or parathyroid operation or if hoarseness or other changes of the voice are present.

Hypothyroidism

If a person is hypothyroid, it is appropriate to use T_4 treatment preoperatively if time permits. Although mild hypothyroidism probably has little deleterious effect, severe hypothyroidism increases both the anesthetic and surgical risks. Although surgery with general anesthesia can be performed safely in an emergency if close attention is paid to all associ-

ated problems in the profoundly hypothyroid patient, it is preferable to defer operation until the patient has been made euthyroid in nonemergent cases. The treatment program for severe myxedema is the administration of small doses of T_4 at the outset, and the gradual increase of this hormone to the normal maintenance dose after a period of time.

Hyperthyroidism

Persons with Graves' disease or other thyrotoxic states should be treated preoperatively in order to restore a euthyroid state and to prevent *thyroid storm*, a severe accentuation of the symptoms and signs of hyperthyroidism that can occur during or after operation. Thyroid storm results in tachycardia, or cardiac arrhythmias, fever, disorientation, coma, and even death. In the early days of thyroid surgery, operations on the toxic gland were among the most dangerous surgical procedures because of the frequent occurrence of severe bleeding and of all the complications described above. Now, with proper preoperative preparation, operations on the Graves' gland can be performed with the same degree of safety as with other thyroid conditions.

In mild cases of thyrotoxicosis, iodine therapy alone can be used for preoperative preparation, although we do not usually recommend this approach. Lugol's solution or a saturated solution of potassium iodide (SSKI) is given for several weeks. Although only several drops per day are needed to block the release of T_4 by the toxic thyroid gland, it is our practice to administer 3 drops, two or three times daily. This medication is taken in milk or orange juice to make it palatable.

Most of our patients with Graves' disease are treated initially with the antithyroid drugs, PTU or methimazole (Tapazole), until they approach a euthyroid state.

Then iodine is added to the regimen for 10 days to 2 weeks before operation. The iodine decreases the vascularity and increases the firmness of the gland. Sometimes T_4 is added to this regimen to prevent hypothyroidism and to decrease the size of the gland.

The β-adrenergic blocker propranolol (Inderal) has increased the safety of thyroidectomy for Graves' disease. We use it frequently with antithyroid drugs to block β-adrenergic receptors and ameliorate the major signs of Graves' disease by decreasing the patient's pulse rate and eliminating tremor. Some surgeons recommend the use of propranolol alone or in combination with iodine for 1 to 2 weeks as the total preoperative management.[12] These regimens, they feel, shorten the preparation time of patients with Graves' disease for operation and make the operation easier since the thyroid gland is smaller and less friable than it would otherwise be. We do not favor these regimens as our routine preparation, for they do not appear to offer the same degree of safety as do those preoperative programs that restore a euthyroid state before operation.

Several instances of fever and tachycardia have been reported in persons with Graves' disease who were taking only propranolol.[13] Yet we have used propranolol therapy alone or with iodine without difficulty in some patients who were allergic to antithyroid medications. In such patients it is essential to continue the propranolol for 1 to 2 weeks postoperatively; they are still thyrotoxic immediately after operation, although the peripheral manifestations of their disease have been blocked.

SURGICAL APPROACH TO THYROID NODULES AND CANCER

Benign Lumps and Differentiated Thyroid Cancer

In nonirradiated patients, our approach is to excise the mass completely and widely, which means performing a lobectomy on the side of the lesion. We then await the frozen section diagnosis while the patient is anesthetized. If the lesion is interpreted as a colloid nodule and the other side is normal, no further resection of the thyroid is usually performed. Because of the difficulties of both fine needle aspiration biopsy and frozen section analysis in differentiating a follicular adenoma from a follicular cancer, if a follicular neoplasm is diagnosed at the time of operation, an ipsilateral lobectomy with a subtotal resection of the contralateral lobe is also usually performed. This prevents the need for a second operation if a follicular cancer is later diagnosed on permanent section analysis, for the remaining thyroid tissue can be ablated by radioiodine treatment. It is our practice to prescribe thyroxine therapy following lobectomy for a benign or malignant lesion in any event.

When papillary or follicular cancer is diagnosed, a near-total or total thyroidectomy is performed in

most cases.[14,15] But for small sclerotic cancers, less than 1 cm diameter and without lymph node involvement or known distant spread, a lobectomy may be satisfactory therapy, especially in a young individual. In addition, any abnormal lymph nodes that are present in the central compartment of the neck, along the tracheoesophageal groove or in the superior mediastinal areas, are removed. Abnormal-feeling lymph nodes from the lateral neck are biopsied. A lymph node biopsy specimen is also routinely taken from along the jugular chain for staging purposes, even if abnormal lymph nodes are not palpable.

A modified radical neck dissection is performed only if enlarged lateral lymph nodes are found to be involved with tumor. This procedure is done by extending the collar incision laterally, retracting the sternocleidomastoid muscle, and removing the nodes from the clavicle to the carotid bifurcation. Occasionally, in a large man, the dissection requires dividing the sternocleidomastoid muscle, but it later can be reinserted. One should always try to preserve the spinal accessory nerve; the internal jugular vein is also saved if nodes are not adherent to it. Furthermore, the phrenic nerve, the brachial plexus, and the sympathetic nervous chain should all be carefully preserved. This operative procedure is quite satisfactory for differentiated thyroid cancer and creates a more favorable cosmetic result than does a classic radical neck dissection since the hollowness that follows removal of the sternocleidomastoid muscle is avoided as are all vertical neck incisions. So-called "cherry-picking" operations, in which individual enlarged lymph nodes are removed, should be avoided. A prophylactic lateral node dissection (i.e., performed when lateral nodes are normal) should not be done.

In *irradiated* patients our overall operative approach is somewhat different. Here, because of the high incidence of small cancers away from the dominant nodule that are often found only on permanent section, a lobectomy on the ipsilateral side and a subtotal lobectomy on the other is usually performed even if the frozen section diagnosis of the mass is benign. In many cases, bilateral thyroid masses are present in this patient population and in such cases most of the thyroid is removed, as well. If a malignancy is diagnosed intraoperatively, a near-total or total thyroidectomy is performed. A modified neck dissection is performed when indicated, as described for the nonirradiated patient. The parathyroid glands can usually be left in place even if a total thyroidectomy is performed. A parathyroid gland is transplanted only if it appears to be clearly devitalized and after histologic confirmation of its identity.

We base these operative approaches for patients with papillary or follicular cancer first and foremost on the fact that such operations have been performed in our hands with no mortality and with very low morbidity.[10] Papillary carcinoma has such an excellent prognosis in most young persons that unless one can perform a near-total or total thyroidectomy with a very low morbidity, these procedures should not be used and a less extensive operation should be performed or the patient should be sent to a center which specializes in thyroid cancer. It is far better, we feel, to leave a small amount of normal thyroid tissue away from the tumor to protect the viability of the parathyroid glands or the integrity of the recurrent laryngeal nerve than to suffer a high incidence of complications when dealing with differentiated thyroid cancers in the young patient. We have also tried to preserve the recurrent laryngeal nerve in such patients even if it means shaving tumor from around it. When a small amount of normal thyroid tissue is left, it can be ablated with postoperative ^{131}I treatment. If tumor is shaved from the recurrent laryngeal nerve, a combination of RAI and external irradiation is usually used.

Removal of most or all of the thyroid gland for significant thyroid carcinomas offers the following advantages for differentiated thyroid cancer:[16]

1. Multicentricity of microscopic papillary tumor is present in up to 80 percent of cases, especially those with a history of radiation exposure. In approximately 7 to 18 percent of patients with an initial lesser procedure, clinical cancer develops in the remaining lobe. Often this event portends widespread dissemination.
2. One-fourth to one-half of all patients who die of thyroid cancer do so because of central neck disease.
3. Follow-up scanning and treatment programs for metastatic papillary or follicular cancer by RAI are facilitated if most or all of the thyroid gland has been removed.
4. The use of serum TG levels as a tumor marker is facilitated, for after total thyroidectomy and ^{131}I ablation of residual tissue, the presence of measurable levels of TG indicates that metastatic disease is present.

After thyroidectomy, all persons with papillary or follicular carcinoma should be given suppressive doses of thyroid hormone for life, whether or not the entire thyroid has been removed. Other ancillary modes of treatment such as RAI, external irradiation, and chemotherapy are used when they are deemed appropriate.

Usually, one to two months after near-total or total thyroidectomy for papillary or follicular carcinoma, thyroxine therapy is stopped and T_3 (Cytomel) therapy is begun for several weeks to a month. Then T_3 is also stopped for several weeks in order to induce hypothyroidism and an elevation of the serum TSH levels. Then RAI is administered and a total body scan is performed. It is our practice to ablate any small thyroid remnant that is present in the neck after thyroidectomy and to treat metastases with RAI when they are demonstrated to take up the isotope.[17] In general, RAI, 30 mCi is given for ablation of normal tissue while 100mCi or more is used for therapeutic regimen. External radiation therapy is used in these types of carcinoma if proved metastases are nonfunctional or when local invasion of the trachea or esophagus is present in the neck and resection is not feasible. Chemotherapy is reserved for progressive disease that cannot be treated by other modalities.[18] Adriamycin appears to be the single best drug for palliation of these thyroid cancers; however, combination chemotherapy regimens are being tried.

When patients are referred to us after thyroid surgery for carcinoma performed elsewhere, we frequently find it advantageous to reoperate if a large amount of normal thyroid tissue, such as an entire thyroid lobe, or if metastatic disease is present in the neck. Occasionally we have found it helpful to administer a small dose of RAI preoperatively. In such cases, a hand-held Geiger counter has been used intraoperatively to locate all of the sites of metastatic disease.

Anaplastic Carcinoma

Anaplastic carcinoma is still one of the most virulent of all human cancers. Without question, if it is possible, a total thyroidectomy and a radical lymph node dissection should be done if the tumor is resectable, and no distant metastases are present. These lesions, however, are almost always nonresectable for cure.

Not uncommonly, the surgeon is called upon in such cases to make the diagnosis, to relieve pressure on the trachea, or to perform a tracheostomy. Most patients are then usually treated with hyperfraction-ation schedules of external irradiation with chemo-therapeutic regimens, since this tumor does not con-centrate RAI. Currently protocols using adriamycin, bleomycin, cis-platinum, Taxol and other agents are being evaluated. The prognosis is dismal except in the rare case in which a small anaplastic carcinoma is accidently found very early and is resected for cure.

Medullary Carcinoma

Medullary carcinoma of the thyroid is an "apu-doma" derived from the C cells of the thyroid. It frequently occurs in a sporadic fashion but in 25 to 30 percent of cases it is part of the multiple endo-crine neoplasia (MEN)-IIA syndrome, a familial dis-order that includes pheochromocytomas that are often bilateral, hyperparathyroidism that is usually due to parathyroid hyperplasia, and bilateral medul-lary carcinoma of the thyroid.[19] Sometimes C-cell hyperplasia and adrenal medullary hyperplasia are present instead of frank tumors.

Another syndrome, (MEN)-IIB, also occurs in a sporadic or familial pattern. Such patients have bilat-eral medullary carcinoma (or C-cell hyperplasia) and pheochromocytomas (or adrenal medullary hyper-plasia) but do not have hyperparathyroidism. In ad-dition, they have a characteristic facial appearance, with thick lips and neuromas of the tongue, conjunc-tiva and buccal mucosa, a Marfan-like body habitus, and ganglioneruromas of the bowel (Fig. 21-11). Their medullary carcinoma is generally an aggres-sive tumor, and few people have lived to adulthood with this disease. Finally, another rarely found group has familial medullary cancer without manifestations of the MEN syndrome.

The MEN-IIA and IIB syndromes are transmitted as an autosomal dominant trait, so that 50 percent of the offspring would be expected to have these tumors. Thus, it is essential that the family members of every patient who is found to have a medullary cancer be screened for this disease. In the past screening was best done by measurement of serum calcitonin values following injections of calcium, pentagastrin, or both of these agents on a yearly basis. Now it has been shown that the MEN-IIA and IIB syndromes are due to mutations of the *ret* onco-gene in the central region of chromosome 10. Hence, now family members can be best tested by analyzing for mutations of the *ret* oncogene. If no

abnormality is detected, the child will *not* develop the MEN-II syndrome. If, on the other hand, a muta-tion of *ret* is present, such a patient is at great risk of developing the MEN syndrome.[20-22] On the basis of this abnormal genetic testing, Wells recommends prophylactic total thyroidectomy with careful follow-up and testing for other manifestations of the syn-drome.[23] All patients with medullary carcinoma and all of their family members should also be evaluated for other manifestation of the MEN syndromes—hy-perparathyroidism and pheochromocytoma. This can be accomplished by regular screening of the blood pressure, serum calcium, and parathyroid hormone determinations and urinary studies for epi-nephrine, norepinephrine, metanephrine, normeta-nephrine, and vanyl mandelic acid (VMA).

Medullary carcinoma, whether sporadic or famil-ial, can also secrete adrenocorticotropic hormone (ACTH) ectopically, which results in adrenal cortical hyperplasia and Cushing syndrome. In such cases a bilateral adrenalectomy is sometimes necessary. Re-moval of all the thyroid cancer in such a case would also be curative but this is rarely possible since usu-ally widely metastatic disease is present when the ec-topic ACTH syndrome occurs. Finally, some persons develop diarrhea. This condition is usually associ-ated with bulky deposits of metastatic disease and may be the result of serotonin, prostaglandin, or cal-citonin secretion.

If a patient with medullary carcinoma is also rec-ognized to have a pheochromocytoma, the adrenal tumor should be operated on first because of the dangers inherent in this tumor during daily life and especially under anesthesia. Preoperative treatment with α-adrenergic blockade using phenoxybenza-mine (Dibensyline) is routine. β-Adrenergic receptor blockade is used selectively for tachycardia or ar-rhythmias. It is an absolute maxim that proper moni-toring, careful anesthetic management, skillful phar-macologic manipulations to prevent hypertension and hypotension, and a gentle, "nontraumatic" op-erative approach are necessary to achieve excellent results. Frequently a bilateral total adrenalectomy is necessary to remove all tumor or to ablate the adre-nal medullary hyperplasia completely.

A total thyroidectomy is always indicated for med-ullary carcinoma of the thyroid.[24] In addition, a very extensive central node dissection should be per-formed. Single or bilateral lateral node dissections should be performed if the lymph nodes in these

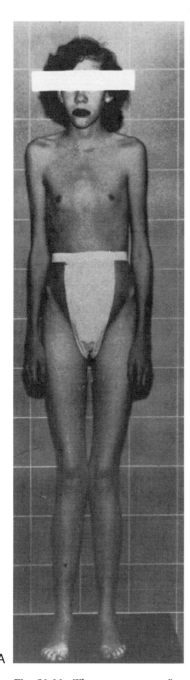

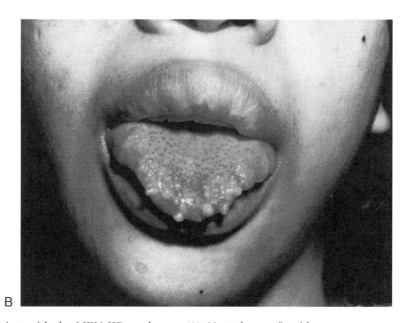

A   B

Fig. 21-11. The appearance of a patient with the MEN-IIB syndrome. (**A**). Note the marfanoid appearance, with kyphosis and long extremities. (Courtesy of Dr. Glen Sizemore.) (**B**). Neuromas of the tongue and the typical thick lips are present

areas are involved with tumor.[25] Few would disagree with this aggressive operative regimen because medullary carcinoma, a C-cell tumor, does not concentrate RAI and is not responsive to T_4 therapy. Radiotherapy is used for invasive or nonresectable residual tumor; however, the tumor is sometimes not very radiosensitive. Occasional metastatic tumors have responded favorably to adriamycin and other agents, but chemotherapeutic regimens have not been generally effective. Treatment with multiple agents is being evaluated. Tisell[26] has performed very extensive reoperations in the neck when calcitonin levels remain elevated postoperatively and no distant metastases are present. He and others[27] have been able to restore about one quarter to one-third of such patients normocalcitoninemic postoperatively.

Hyperparathyroidism associated with medullary cancers is generally not severe, although renal stones and other complications may occur. Enlarged parathyroid glands should be removed at the time of total thyroidectomy, but care should be taken not to produce permanent hypoparathyroidism. Finally, as with most endocrine neoplasms, tumor growth is often relatively slow and patients may suffer from symptoms related to their humoral secretions. Thus in some cases, palliative removal of the bulk of tumor should be performed even if a curative resection is not feasible, since this procedure often improves symptoms such as diarrhea, for example. The use of octreotide therapy, however, may benefit the diarrhea and flushing of patients with medullary carcinomas as it does patients with the carcinoid syndrome, and should be tried before operation.

OPERATIVE TECHNIQUES

Surgeons who take unnecessary risks and operate by the clock are exciting from the onlooker's standpoint, but they are not necessarily those in whose hands you would by preference choose to place yourself.
    Theodor Kocher (1841–1917)[28]

Today, thyroidectomy is almost always performed under general endotracheal anesthesia, although there was a time when local anesthesia was popular in some clinics. The patient's neck is extended by inflating a pillow or inserting a thyroid roll beneath the shoulders. A symmetrical, low, collar incision is made in the line of a natural skin crease approximately 1 to 2 cm above the clavicle (Fig. 21-12). The incision is carried through the skin, subcutaneous tissue, and platysma muscle down to the dense cervical fascia that overlies the strap muscles and anterior jugular veins. The upper flap is raised to the level of the notch of the thyroid cartilage. Despite care, it is difficult to avoid cutting some sensory nerves, which usually results in some temporary loss of sensation above the incision postoperatively. A small lower flap is also elevated to the level of the manu-

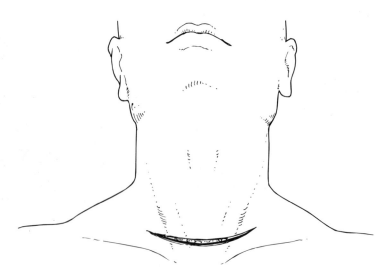

Fig. 21-12. Operative technique of thyroid lobectomy. The neck is extended and a symmetrical, gently curved incision is made 1 to 2 cm above the clavicle.

brial notch. If dissection of the flaps is performed in the plane between the platysma muscle and the fascia overlying the strap muscles, bleeding is minimal. The cervical fascia is then incised vertically in the midline from the upper margin of the thyroid cartilage to the sternal notch (Fig. 21-13).

Exposure of the superior and lateral aspects of the thyroid gland is achieved by retracting the sternohyoid and sternothyroid muscles laterally or occasionally by dividing these muscles. Division of these muscles is associated with little or no disability, but is not necessary unless the gland is markedly enlarged. High transection is preferable, since the ansa cervicalis nerve innervates the muscles from below. This procedure diminishes the amount of muscle that is paralyzed.

Digital or blunt dissection frees the thyroid from the surrounding fascia. We then prefer to rotate one lobe medially and continue the dissection bluntly (Fig. 21-14). The middle thyroid veins are first encountered and are ligated and divided. This maneuver facilitates exposure of the superior and inferior poles of the thyroid lobe. The suspensory ligaments

are transected craniad to the isthmus, and the pyramidal lobe and Delphian nodes are mobilized. The cricothyroid space is opened in order to separate the superior pole from the surrounding tissue. During dissection of the superior lobe, care is taken to avoid injury to the superior laryngeal nerve (Fig. 21-5). The internal branch of the nerve, which provides sensory fibers to the epiglottis and larynx, is rarely in the operative field. It is the external branch, which supplies motor innervation to the inferior pharyngeal constrictor and the cricothyroid muscles, that must be protected. This purpose is achieved by dissecting the nerve away from the superior pole vessels if it can be identified, or by separately ligating and dividing the individual branches of the superior thyroid vessels at the level of the upper pole of the thyroid lobe rather than cephalad to it[29] (Fig. 21-15).

The lobe is then retracted mediad to permit identification of the inferior thyroid artery and the recurrent laryngeal nerve (Fig. 21-16). It is essential that meticulous hemostasis be achieved during this part of the dissection. The inferior thyroid artery is isolated, but I rarely, if ever, ligate it laterally. Rather,

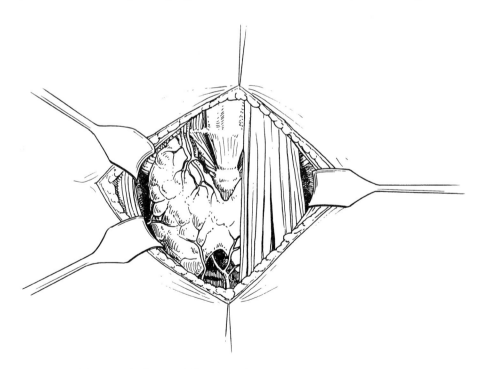

Fig. 21-13. Upper and lower subplatysmal flaps are developed. The deep cervical fascia is divided in the midline and the strap muscles are retracted laterally, exposing the anterior surface of the thyroid lobe. Occasionally, in cases of large goiters, better exposure can be obtained by dividing the strap muscles transversely.

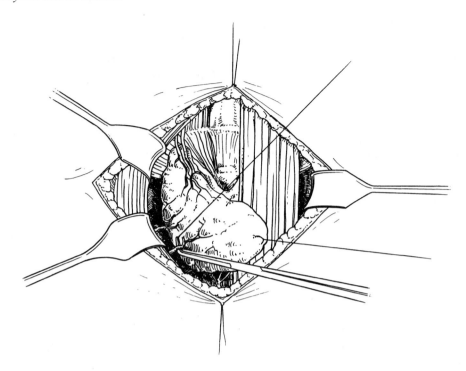

Fig. 21-14. The thyroid lobe is retracted medially and is bluntly dissected from the surrounding fascia. The middle thyroid vein is encountered and is ligated close to the thyroid.

when performing a lobectomy, it is preferable to ligate and divide each small arterial branch near the thyroid capsule at a point after branches to the parathyroid glands have been given off. This technique lessens the incidence of devascularization of the parathyroid gland and plays a role in reducing permanent hypoparathyroidism. The recurrent laryngeal nerve is then identified along its course by blunt dissection. The nerve is treated with care, for excessive trauma or its division will result in an ipsilateral vocal cord paralysis. At the junction of the trachea and larynx, the recurrent laryngeal nerve is immediately adjacent to the thyroid lobe and is most easily damaged. The lobe may be totally removed as indicated for tumor, or a small remnant of posterior thyroid tissue on each side should be left in those patients in whom the operation is being performed for the diffuse goiter of Graves' disease.

During exposure of the posterior surface of the thyroid gland, the parathyroid glands should be identified and preserved, along with their vascular pedicles (Fig. 21-16). Care should be taken to ensure that the parathyroid glands are not excised or devascularized. Once the recurrent laryngeal nerve and

the parathyroid glands have been preserved, the thyroid lobe is then dissected from the lateral aspect of the trachea, and the dissection is continued along the pretracheal fascia in order to separate the isthmus from the anterior trachea. If a pyramidal lobe is present, it is also removed at this time. When performing a lobectomy, it is important that the isthmus also be removed so that a mass due to hypertrophy of the thyroid in this region is not later felt. When a lobectomy is performed of the remaining thyroid lobe is oversewn by a continuous suture technique. When a total thyroidectomy is performed, the remaining thyroid lobe is removed in a similar manner.

The entire wound is then inspected, and careful hemostasis is obtained before closure. It is mandatory that the operative field show no evidence of bleeding. In most instances, we use a suction catheter to drain the bed of the thyroid lobes, employing a small, soft plastic drain that is brought out through a stab wound inferior to the incision (Fig. 21-17). Others feel that little is accomplished by this maneuver. Although I concede that rapid bleeding leading to respiratory distress cannot be adequately evacu-

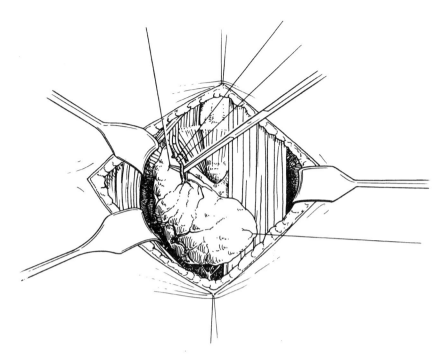

Fig. 21-15. The superior thyroid vessels are then individually ligated and divided at the level of the superior pole, rather than cephalad to it, in order to protect the external branch of the superior laryngeal nerve from damage. This nerve can be seen in many patients.

ated by this small drain, the postoperative wound appearance with this technique is far superior to that obtained when either no drainage or a Penrose drain is employed. If the sternothyroid and sternohyoid muscles have been transected, they are reapproximated. The midline vertical fascial incision is only loosely approximated by one interrupted suture, and the drain is positioned superficial to the strap muscles. I rarely suture the platysma muscle and use a technique of approximating the dermis with interrupted 5-0 Vicryl subcuticular sutures. Finally, the epithelial surfaces are approximated with sterile skin tapes.

A tracheostomy set is left at the patient's bedside for 24 hours so that the wound can be opened rapidly if there is a need. The drain is usually removed on the first postoperative morning or soon thereafter. The patient is almost always discharged on the first or second postoperative days. When a neck dissection has also been performed, the drains are usually left in place for several days. The skin tapes are removed at the time of the first outpatient visit, about 8 to 10 days postoperatively.

Intrathoracic Goiter

In a small percentage of patients undergoing thyroidectomy, a significant part of the thyroid tissue is intrathoracic. Intrathoracic goiter usually represents a benign process in which there is an extension of cervical thyroid tissue into the chest rather than aberrant glandular tissue (Fig. 21-18). Since the lesion usually retains its connection to the cervical thyroid and receives its blood supply from the inferior thyroid artery, it can generally be removed through the conventional collar incision described above. In the case of a very large mass, however, it is sometimes very difficult to elevate the thoracic portion of the goiter through the thoracic inlet. In such instances, the semiliquid colloid and degenerated portions can sometimes be evacuated to permit delivery of the remaining mass with its capsule into the neck. The indications for transsternal or transpleural thyroidectomy are few, but might include (1) an inability to remove the tumor totally through a cervical approach, (2) a large mass with an extensive blood supply within the mediastinum, (3) evidence of superior vena caval obstruction, (4) the possibility that the

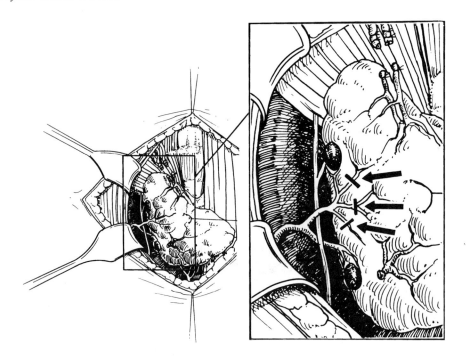

Fig. 21-16. The thyroid lobe is retracted medially again and, by careful blunt dissection, the recurrent laryngeal nerve, the inferior thyroid artery, and the parathyroid glands are identified. The inferior thyroid artery is not ligated laterally as a single trunk. Rather, each small branch is ligated and divided at a point distal to the parathyroid glands (see *arrows* in insert) in order to preserve their blood supply. The thyroid lobe can then be removed from its tracheal attachments if a lobectomy is to be performed.

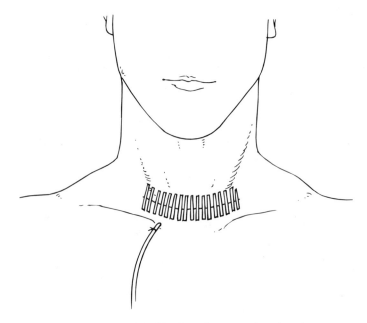

Fig. 21-17. Closure of the wound is accomplished by loosely approximating the strap muscles in the midline. A small suction catheter is usually inserted through a stab wound. The dermis of the flaps is approximated with interrupted 5-0 sutures, and the epithelium is apposed by sterile skin tapes.

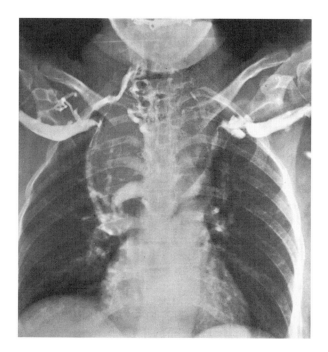

Fig. 21-18. Massive substernal goiter causing partial obstruction to the innominate veins. Dye has been injected into both arm viens.

large mass is a thyroid carcinoma, and (5) an undiagnosed superior mediastinal lesion of nonthyroid origin.

Transsternal thyroidectomy can be performed by using a partial or complete sternum-splitting incision. In the partial sternotomy, the sternum is transected horizontally at the level of the third interspace and vertically from the suprasternal notch down to the level of the horizontal transection. This procedure permits extrapleural resection of the gland and provides excellent visualization of the recurrent laryngeal nerves and the vascular supply. Sometimes a full sternotomy is preferable, however.

COMPLICATIONS OF THYROIDECTOMY

The mortality accompanying thyroidectomy is very low. Gould et al.[30] reviewed 1,000 patients operated on consecutively by a large group of surgeons over a 5-year period and reported no deaths. The mortality reported by Colcock and King[31] was 0.12 percent with no deaths between 1954 and 1962. Their morbidity was about 13 percent when all complications, including the most minor types, were considered. Pulmonary problems and wound infections are relatively uncommon. Four major complications classically have been associated with thyroidectomy: (1) thyroid storm, which is related to the patient's thyrotoxicosis. (2) wound hemorrhage with hematoma formation. (3) recurrent laryngeal nerve injury, and (4) hypoparathyroidism. The latter three are regarded as complications of technique.

Thyroid Storm

Thyroid storm occurs in patients with preexisting thyrotoxicosis who either have not been treated at all or have been treated incompletely. It is usually seen in patients with Graves' disease but may occur with toxic adenomas or multinodular goiter as well. In the past, before adequate preparation with antithyroid drugs, surgical treatment was the most common precipitating factor. Presently thyroid storm is a rare complication of surgical treatment and is more frequently precipitated by trauma, infection, diabetic acidosis, toxemia of pregnancy or non-thyroid operations.

When thyroid storm is related to surgical treatment, the manifestations usually develop during the operative procedure or in the recovery room. The patient becomes markedly hyperthermic, with profuse sweating and tachycardia. Nausea, vomiting, and abdominal pain are common. Initial tremor and restlessness may progress to delirium with eventual coma.

Treatment is directed toward inhibiting the production of thyroid hormone and antagonizing the effects of thyroid hormone (Table 21-1).[32] Sodium or potassium iodide or ipodate should be administered intravenously *after* an antithyroid drug, PTU (preferably) or methimazole has been started. Oxygen should be given, and glucose may be administered intravenously as therapy for the hypermetabolic state. Fluid and electrolytes must be maintained in view of the losses. A hypothermia blanket may be applied to reduce the temperature. Propranolol is given to antagonize β-adrenergic effects. Large doses of propranolol may be needed in toxic patients to control tachycardia, for thyroid storm has been reported to occur postoperatively in patients receiving 40 mg propranolol every 6 hours preoperatively. In severe cases, cortisol is administered to eliminate the possibility of a relative adrenal cortical insuffi-

TABLE 21-1. Treatment of Thyroid Storm

Treatment	Dose or Description
Propranolol	60–80 mg q6h PO, or 1–3 mg IV, slowly, q4h
Hydrocortisone	100–500 mg IV q12h
Sodium iodide *or*	1 g in 1 L of saline q12h
SSKI[a] *or*	5 drops tid PO
Lugol's solution *or*	5 drops tid PO
Ipodate	0.5 g PO daily or 3.0 g PO every 2–3 days
Supportive measures	Mild sedation, fluid replacement, oxygen, vitamins, cooling, and antibiotics, as needed
Propylthiouracil *or*	100–200 mg q4h PO
Methimazole	10–20 mg q4h PO

Abbreviation:[a] SSKI, saturated solution of potassium iodide.
(From Burman,[32] with permission.)

ciency state and to suppress T_4 to T_3 conversion. If this customary therapy is effective peritoneal dialysis, resin or charcoal hemoperfusion or plasma pheresis can be attempted if the patient is seriously ill.

Wound Hemorrhage

Wound hemorrhage is a problem of the early postoperative period, usually within the first 12 hours. It has been reported in 0.3 to 1.0 percent of consecutive thyroidectomies. Hemorrhage in the neck is a significant problem since a small amount of blood that forms a hematoma deep to the strap muscles might be sufficient to obstruct the airway and result in respiratory death. This complication is usually caused by bleeding from branches of the inferior or superior thyroid artery, and the rate of bleeding is such that the commonly employed drains do not afford protection.

The patients are rarely in shock. The initial manifestations are swelling of the neck and bulging of the wound; these conditions demand immediate attention. If they remain untreated, respiratory obstruction due to compression of the trachea eventually ensues. Treatment consists of opening the incision, evacuating the clot, and securing the bleeding vessel. This constitutes an emergency procedure; if it is

thought to be necessary, the wound should be opened, the clot evacuated at the bedside and the bleeding point compressed. Later, the patient can be brought to the operating room. Tracheostomy is not required if the clot is removed early. Prolonged endotracheal intubation is occasionally necessary. Usually, however, the crisis is totally relieved as soon as the hematoma is evacuated.

Recurrent Laryngeal Nerve Injury

Damage to the recurrent laryngeal nerve can be unilateral or bilateral and temporary or permanent. Injury occurs more commonly when thyroidectomy is being performed for malignant disease. In one series of 1,011 thyroidectomies, there were 28 examples of vocal cord paralysis, three of which proved to be permanent. Gould et al.[30] reported the incidence of recurrent nerve injury of 1,000 patients to be 0.2 percent. Colcock and King,[31] evaluating 1,246 thyroid operations, noted 1 bilateral recurrent laryngeal nerve paralysis. Thompson and Harness[33] reported an incidence of accidental unilateral nerve injury of 4.8 percent when total thyroidectomy was employed for carcinoma. Clark[16] reported that after total thyroidectomy was employed for carcinoma, 2 of 82 patients suffered transient bilateral recurrent laryngeal nerve injuries, but no permanent nerve injury occurred. Total thyroidectomy results in a greater incidence of recurrent laryngeal nerve injuries than does a lesser procedure. Undoubtedly, this complication occurs more frequently when thyroidectomy is performed by less experienced neck surgeons.

Loss of function of the recurrent laryngeal nerve can result from excessive trauma to the nerve during its dissection, inclusion of the nerve in a ligature, or inadvertent sectioning of the nerve. Other uncommon causes are damage to the vagus nerve in the neck and damage due to pressure from the cuff of the endotracheal tube. A unilateral recurrent laryngeal nerve injury produces a loss of abduction of the ipsilateral vocal cord, which assumes a median or paramedian position. This injury is usually suggested by a huskiness of the speaking voice and can be confirmed by postoperative laryngoscopy. The involved cord is initially flaccid, but with the passage of time the flaccidity is often replaced by spasticity. If the injury is related to trauma but the nerve is not divided, function should return usually within 3 to 6 months and invariably within 9 months.

Bilateral recurrent nerve injury is much more serious than unilateral injury. Many patients require immediate tracheostomy. If this is not done initially, patients often suffer progressive difficulties with respiratory toilet and obstruction to the airway. In some patients the voice gets better within several months, but breathing becomes worse. This occurs as the cords move progressively toward the midline and the glottic aperture narrows. A tracheostomy may become necessary at that time.

The incidence of recurrent nerve injury can be markedly reduced by identifying the nerves routinely during thyroidectomy. The recurrent laryngeal nerve is in greatest jeopardy at the level of the two upper tracheal rings, where the middle third of the thyroid lobe is in closest contact with it. The lobe is attached by a strong process of pretracheal fascia, called the *suspensory ligament of Berry,* to the cricoid cartilage and trachea. This fascia must be divided before a total lobectomy can be performed. Although the recurrent laryngeal nerve usually runs posteriorly to this connective tissue zone, in 25 percent of patients it courses through the ligament of Berry and thus is in greater danger of injury during thyroidectomy.

At the time of operation, removal of any ligatures on the nerve or direct repair of the transected recurrent laryngeal nerve should be performed if either complication is recognized. Using magnification and microsurgical technique for reapproximation, the chance for successful reinnervation is good.

Asymptomatic paralysis of a vocal cord does not require correction. In other cases, if the airway is adequate, no attempts to perform corrective procedures upon the paralyzed cord or cords are undertaken until 6 to 12 months have elapsed from the time of injury in order to permit spontaneous return of cord function. Attempts at reinnervation of the abductor muscles of the vocal cords, by implanting an innervated omohyoid muscle into the posterior cricoarytenoid muscle, have resulted in occasional clinical successes. In unilateral cord injuries, injection of Teflon or collagen into the paralyzed cord will bring it to the midline and result in an improvement in the voice. Finally, if the glottic aperture is not adequate, as might occur in bilateral cord paralysis, it can be widened by moving one vocal cord laterally, by arytenoidectomy or by laser excision of a vocal cord. These procedures provide a more adequate airway but cause further deterioration of the voice.

Injury to the external branch of the superior laryngeal nerve is not as serious as a recurrent laryngeal nerve injury. However, it should be avoided because it results in a limitation of the force of projection of one's voice and impairs a singer's high tones. Not infrequently these disabilities improve during the first 3 months after thyroidectomy.

Hypoparathyroidism

Overt manifestations of hypocalcemia occur in a minority of patients after thyroidectomy. This syndrome is usually *temporary* and is related to dissection in the region of the parathyroid glands. To prevent permanent hypoparathyroidism, it is probably necessary to leave only one gland in situ with an adequate blood supply or to autotransplant one parathyroid gland successfully.

Permanent hypoparathyroidism is a serious complication that requires lifetime therapy and should thus be avoided whenever possible. Mazzaferri[34] showed that the incidence of this complication was related to the magnitude of the thyroid operation. It was greatest (20 percent) when a total thyroidectomy and a radical neck dissection were performed for thyroid cancer. In the same series, total thyroidectomy alone resulted in an incidence of 13.5 percent. Less than a total thyroidectomy with a radical neck dissection resulted in a 2.5 percent incidence of permanent hypoparathyroidism; in contrast, this complication occurred in only 0.9 percent of cases when less than a total thyroidectomy was performed alone. This study was performed by a large group of surgeons. With surgeons who are particularly experienced in thyroid surgery, the incidence of permanent hypoparathyroidism is considerably lower. In our series,[14] for example, permanent hypoparathyroidism is an uncommon event following near-total or total thyroidectomy. Postthyroidectomy hypoparathyroidism may be due to the inadvertent removal of all of the parathyroid glands, but more frequently is caused by damage to their blood supply. The parathyroid end arteries probably have to be damaged in order to infarct the glands. We make it a practice not to ligate the inferior thyroid artery laterally, however, because of the danger that this procedure will decrease blood flow to the parathyroid glands when a lobectomy is performed.

Despite the care used by the surgeon in attempting to preserve the integrity and blood supply to the parathyroid glands, a parathyroid gland sometimes appears to be severely damaged or devascularized at the end of the lobectomy. In such cases, the parathyroid gland can be minced into 1 to 2 mm cubes. After it has been identified by frozen section analysis, it is autotransplanted into small pockets in the sternocleidomastoid or the forearm musculature using the technique described by Wells et al.[35] Some surgeons routinely autotransplant one parathyroid gland in this manner whenever they perform a total parathyroidectomy, and feel that it reduces the incidence of permanent hypoparathyroidism. We prefer to individualize patients and use this technique only in the rare instance in which parathyroid function is deemed to be in jeopardy by the thyroidectomy.

The clinical manifestations of hypoparathyroidism usually occur within the first few days after operation and almost invariably within the first week. The initial symptoms are circumoral numbness, tingling, and intense anxiety. The Chvostek sign appears early, followed by Trousseau's sign and carpopedal spasm. As the disease progresses, muscle cramps and frank tetany develop. The greatest danger is from convulsions and respiratory stridor, which can occur with severe hypocalcemia and have occasionally resulted in hypoxia and even death, especially in children. Prolonged hypoparathyroidism may cause cataracts, convulsive episodes, and psychoses.

The diagnostic findings consist of reduced serum calcium and increased serum phosphorus levels, a decrease or absence of calcium in the urine, and a lowered urinary phosphorus concentration. Serum concentrations of parathyroid hormone are low or absent. Postoperative hypoparathyroidism must be differentiated from tetany caused by alkalosis associated with anxiety and hyperventilation. This condition causes a reduction of ionized calcium levels, but the manifestations can be promptly reversed by inhalation of carbon dioxide or by breathing through an increased dead space. Another cause is "bone hunger." In severely thyrotoxic patients, for example, bone turnover is increased. After thyroidectomy calcium ions and phosphorus may return to bone, resulting in hypocalcemia and a low serum phosphorus level. Since patients are made euthyroid before operation, this event does not often occur.

Treatment of Postoperative Hypocalcemia[36]

When postoperative hypocalcemia is mild, no treatment is needed but careful, watchful waiting should be employed. Serum calcium levels should be determined every 12 hours for the first few days and then daily thereafter. If the patient becomes symptomatic, 1 g calcium gluconate can be slowly given intravenously; then 2 g of this preparation should be added to the intravenous bottle and dripped continuously every 8 hours. This therapy will alleviate most symptoms although more calcium may be needed. Usually, within several days all calcium therapy can be stopped. This condition is called *transient hypoparathyroidism*.

Because of pressures to discharge patients soon after operation, or because of more persistent hypocalcemia, oral calcium is also used in a dose of 1.5 to 2.0 g calcium ion per day. It is important to note that in order to provide 1.0 g elemental calcium, one must administer 4.0 g calcium acetate, 5.5 g hydrated calcium chloride, 8.0 g calcium lactate, or 11.0 g calcium gluconate. Calcium gluconate or calcium carbonate is generally used. If the serum calcium level returns to normal on this regimen, the patient can be sent home while taking oral calcium therapy; this medication can usually be discontinued after several weeks. Ideally, it is preferable not to add vitamin D to this early regimen unless one strongly suspects that permanent hypoparathyroidism has occurred. From a practical point of view, however, the fastest way to attain a normal serum calcium value postoperatively is to add a vitamin D analogue to the oral calcium regimen and this is frequently done.

If *permanent hypoparathyroidism* has occurred, in addition to the oral calcium therapy the patient must be given vitamin D. Vitamin D_3, 50,000 to 100,000 units/day (1.25 to 2.5 mg/day) can be used but acts slowly. Others prefer to use dihydrotachysterol, 0.125 to 1.0 mg/day. Larger initial doses of these compounds are often used to achieve a more rapid response. I prefer to use Rocaltrol, $(1,25(OH)_2D_3)$, the active metabolite of vitamin D. Its use is advantageous since it is faster acting and more readily reversed if an overdose is given. Initially it is given in a divided oral dose of 1 to 2 μg daily. The maintenance dose is usually 0.5 μg or less per day. Regardless of the preparation used, the serum calcium concentration must be checked frequently, since some patients are insensitive and need larger doses, whereas others develop vitamin D intoxication with severe hypercalcemia while taking relatively small doses.

Serum intact parathyroid hormone concentrations should be checked at intervals in patients being treated for permanent postoperative hypoparathyroidism. Several patients whom we have seen have been treated unnecessarily with vitamin D for many years because postoperative tetany had occurred. When serum parathyroid hormone is detectable, vitamin D therapy should be slowly tapered and finally stopped, if possible.

Other factors may influence the treatment of hypocalcemia. A diet high in phosphate or oxalate should be avoided, since it may impair calcium absorption. Concomitant ingestion of anticonvulsants and tranquilizers may lower intestinal absorption of calcium both directly and by interfering with vitamin D metabolism. Estrogen and oral contraceptive therapy lower serum calcium levels by suppressing bone resorption. Diuretics such as furosemide result in increased calcium excretion in the urine. Hypomagnesemia should be avoided since it leads to resistance to vitamin D therapy. Finally, the role of emotional stress in vitamin D resistance and hypocalcemia may be important.

Tracheomalacia

Tracheomalacia, a softening of the tracheal rings due to pressure necrosis of the cartilaginous tracheal rings from a large goiter, is a frequently discussed but rarely encountered complication. If it is present, dangerous consequences can result after removal of the thyroid, for collapse or narrowing of the trachea would occur with inspiration, resulting in respiratory embarrassment. Although tracheal resection may be performed in some cases, the treatment of choice for this complication is endotracheal intubation. Usually this procedure leads to fixation of the trachea, and with time the endotracheal tube can be removed. In severe cases a tracheostomy is necessary.

ACKNOWLEDGEMENT

The work was supported in part by a grant from the Nathan and Frances Goldblatt Society for Cancer Research

REFERENCES

1. Halsted WS: The operative story of goiter. Johns Hopkins Hosp Rep 19:71, 1920
2. Hunt PS, Poole M, Reeve TS: A reappraisal of the surgical anatomy of the thyroid and parathyroid glands. Br J Surg 55:63, 1968
3. Skandalakis JE, Droulias C, Harlaftis N et al: The recurrent laryngeal nerve. Am Surg 42:629, 1976
4. Moosman DA, DeWeese MS: The external laryngeal nerve as related to thyroidectomy. Surg Gynecol Obstet 127:1011, 1968
5. Gilmour JR: The embryology of the parathyroid glands, the thymus and certain associated rudiments. J Pathol 45:507, 1937
6. Henry JF, Audiffret J, Denizot A, Plan M: The nonrecurrent inferior laryngeal nerve: review of 33 cases, including two on the left side. Surgery 104:997, 1988
7. Sedgwick CE, Cady B: Embryology and developmental abnormalities. p. 6. In Sedgwick CE, Cady B (eds): Surgery of the Thyroid and Parathyroid Glands. WB Saunders, Philadelphia, 1980
8. Taylor S: Surgery of the thyroid gland. p. 776. In DeGroot LJ Stanbury JB (eds): The Thyroid and Its Diseases. 4th Ed. New York, John Wiley & Sons 1975
9. Sridama V, McCormick M, Kaplan EL et al: Long-term follow-up study of compensated low-dose ^{131}I therapy for Graves' disease. N Engl J Med 311:426, 1984
10. Kaplan EL: An operative approach to the irradiated thyroid gland with possible carcinoma: criteria, technique and results. p. 371. In DeGroot LJ, Frohman LA, Kaplan EL, Refetoff S (eds): Radiation Associated Carcinoma of the Thyroid. Grune & Stratton, Orlando, 1977
11. Naunheim KS, Kaplan EL, Straus FH II et al: High-dose external radiation to the neck and subsequent thyroid carcinoma. p. IV:51. In Kaplan EL (ed): Surgery of the Thyroid and Parathyroid Glands. In: Clinical Surgery International. Vol. 4. Churchill Livingstone, Edinburgh 1983
12. Michie W, Hamer-Hodges DW, Pegg CAS et al: Beta-blockade and partial thyroidectomy for thyrotoxicosis. Lancet 1:1009, 1974
13. Eriksson M, Rubenfeld S, Garber AJ et al: Propranolol does not prevent thyroid storm. N Engl J Med 296:263, 1977
14. DeGroot LJ, Kaplan EL, McCormick M, Straus FH: Natural history, treatment, and course of papillary thyroid carcinoma. J Clin Endocrinol Metab 71:414, 1990
15. DeGroot LJ, Kaplan EL, Straus FH II, Shukla MS: Does the management of papillary thyroid carcinoma

make a difference in outcome? World J Surg, 18:123, 1994

16. Clark OH: Total thyroidectomy: the treatment of choice for patients with differentiated thyroid cancer. Ann Surg 196:361, 1982

17. Beierwaltes WH: Treatment of metastatic thyroid cancer with radioiodine and external radiation therapy. p. IV:103. In Kaplan EL (ed): Surgery of the Thyroid and Parathyroid Glands. In Clinical Surgery International. Vol. 4. Churchill Livingstone, Edinburgh, 1983

18. Hill JR, Stratton C: Chemotherapy of thyroid cancer. p. IV:120. In Kaplan EL (ed): Surgery of the Thyroid and Parathyroid Glands. Vol. 4. In: Clinical Surgery International. Churchill Livingstone, London, 1983

19. Sizemore GW, van Heerden JA, Carney JA: Medullary carcinoma of the thyroid gland and the multiple endocrine neoplasia type 2 syndrome. p. IV:75. In Kaplan EL (ed): Surgery of the Thyroid and Parathyroid Glands. Vol. 4. In: Clinical Surgery International. Churchill Livingstone, Edinburgh 1983

20. Chi DD, Toshima K, Donis-Keller H, Wells SA Jr: Predictive testing for multiple endocrine neoplasia type 2A (MEN2A) based on the detection of mutations in the ret protooncogene. Surgery 116:124, 1994

21. Ledger GA, Khosla S, Lindor NM et al: Genetic testing in the diagnosis and management of multiple endocrine neoplasia type II: a review. Ann Int Med 122: 118, 1995

22. Lips CH, Landsvater RM, Hoppener JW et al: Clinical screening as compared with DNA analysis in families with multiple endocrine neoplasia type 2A. N Engl J Med 331:828, 1994

23. Wells SA Jr, Chi DD, Toshima K et al: Predictive DNA testing and prophylactic thyroidectomy in patients at risk for multiple endocrine neoplasia type 2A. Ann Surg 220:237, 1994

24. van Heerden JA, Grant CS, Gharib H et al: Long term course of patients with persistent hypercalcitoninemia after apparent curative primary surgery for medullary thyroid carcinoma. Ann Surg 212:395, 1990

25. Dralle H, Damm I, Scheumann GFW et al: Compartment-oriented microdissection of regional lymph nodes in medullary thyroid carcinoma. Jpn J Surg 24: 112, 1994

26. Tisell LE, Hansson G, Jansson S, Salander H: Reoperation in the treatment of asymptomatic metastasizing medullary thyroid carcinoma. Surgery 99:60, 1986

27. Moley JF, Wells SA, Dilley WG, Tisell LE: Reoperation for recurrent or persistent medullary thyroid cancer. Surgery, 114:1090, 1993

28. Theodor Kocher quoted by Harvey Cushing in Fulton JF: "Arnold Klebs and Harvey Cushing at the 1st International Neurological Congress at Berne in 1931." Bull Hist Med 8:345, 1940

29. Thompson NW, Olsen WR, Hoffman GL: The continuing development of the technique of thyroidectomy. Surgery 73:913, 1973

30. Gould EA, Hursh E, Brecher I: Complications arising in the course of thyroidectomy. Arch Surg 90:81, 1965

31. Colcock BP, King ML: The mortality and morbidity of thyroid surgery. Surg Gynecol Obstet 114:131, 1962

32. Burman KD: Hyperthyroidism. p. 345. In Becker KL (ed): Principles and Practice of Endocrinology and Metabolism. JB Lippincott, Philadelphia, 1990

33. Thompson NW, Harness JK: Complications of total thyroidectomy for carcinoma. Surg Gynecol Obstet 131:861, 1970

34. Mazzaferri EL: Papillary and follicular cancer: a selective approach to diagnosis and treatment. Annu Rev Med 32:73, 1981

35. Wells SA, Farndon JR, Dale JK et al: Long-term evaluation of patients with primary parathyroid hyperplasia managed by total parathyroidectomy and heterotopic autotransplantation. Ann Surg 192:451, 1980

36. Kaplan EL, Sugimoto J, Yang H, Fredland A: Postoperative hypoparathyroidism: diagnosis and management. p. IV: 262. In Kaplan EL (ed): Surgery of the Thyroid and Parathyroid Glands. In: Clinical Surgery International. Vol. 4. Churchill Livingstone, Edinburgh 1983

37. Kocher T: Zur pathologie und therapie deKropfes (parts 1 and 2). Dtsch Z Chir 4, 1874

Index

Page numbers followed by f *indicate figures, those followed by* t *indicate tables.*